ORTHOTIC INTERVENTION

for the Hand and Upper Extremity: Splinting Principles and Process

THIRD EDITION

ORTHOTIC INTERVENTION
for the Hand and Upper Extremity

SPLINTING PRINCIPLES AND PROCESS

THIRD EDITION

MaryLynn A. Jacobs, MBA, MS, OTR/L, CHT
Senior Director, National Hand Therapy Services
ATI Physical Therapy
Bolingbrook, Illinois

Noelle M. Austin, MS, PT, CHT
Owner/Educator
CJ Education & Consulting, LLC
Nashville, Tennessee

Hand Therapist
STAR Physical Therapy
Nashville, Tennessee

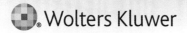 Wolters Kluwer

Philadelphia • Baltimore • New York • London
Buenos Aires • Hong Kong • Sydney • Tokyo

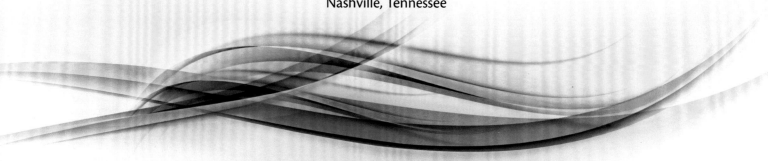

Acquisitions Editor: Matt Hauber
Senior Development Editor: Amy Millholen
Editorial Coordinator: Vinoth Ezhumalai
Production Project Manager: Barton Dudlick
Design Coordinator: Steve Druding
Manufacturing Coordinator: Margie Orzech
Prepress Vendor: TNQ Technologies

Third edition

Copyright © 2022 Wolters Kluwer.

9 8 7 6 5 4 3 2 1

Printed in China

Library of Congress Cataloging-in-Publication Data

ISBN-13: 978-1-975140-95-3

Cataloging in Publication data available on request from publisher.

shop.lww.com

Dedication

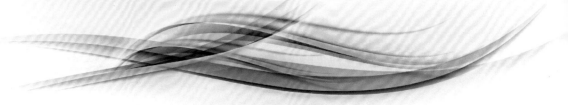

To our families and all the patients we have treated throughout the years,
and to

Judy C. Colditz, OT/L, CHT, FAOTA

A master clinician, a skilled teacher, a committed leader, a mentor to many, and an expert orthotic fabricator.

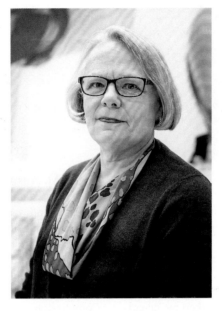

"When You Learn It, Teach It"

This is Judy's motto and if you have had the unique opportunity to attend one of her in-person courses, hear her present at professional meetings, read any of her articles/chapters from an extensive list of her publications, viewed her educational videos, or had the occasion to learn from her at hand conferences, you are able to fully appreciate this motto. She teaches with passion, intrigue, depth of knowledge, and relentless energy.

Judy has had an enormous and lasting impact on the field of Hand Therapy through her various professional contributions. To name a few, she has taught us the value of the intrinsics, the intricacies of the dorsal apparatus, a casting technique to mobilize stiffness (CMMS), and further enhanced our knowledge of the thumb CMC joint.

Judy's commitment to hand therapy has extended beyond her clinical work and into leadership roles. She has been president of both the International Federation of Societies of Hand Therapists (IFSHT) and the American Society of Hand Therapists (ASHT), helping to advance and shape Hand Therapy policy.

We are enormously grateful for Judy's ongoing support and guidance throughout our careers and encouraging our passion for teaching and writing—she kindly wrote the foreword to our second edition. In this latest edition, we are especially thankful for her generous sharing of her various Clinical Pearls that are scattered throughout this textbook and the fabrication manual derived from her world-known Clinical Pearl series from her company HandLab.

Through her 40+ years of hand therapy work, she has pushed us all to be better, think deeper, think "what else," be innovative, and always stay intellectually challenged. We are hopeful that future generations will continue to be inspired by her work and live by her motto of "when you learn it, then teach it".

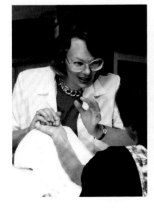
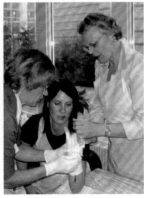
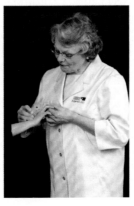
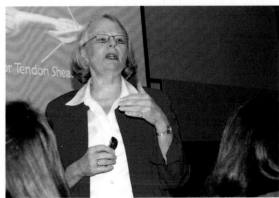

About the Authors

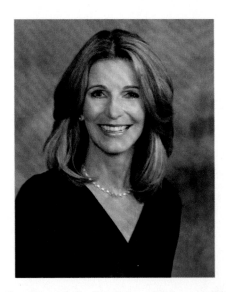

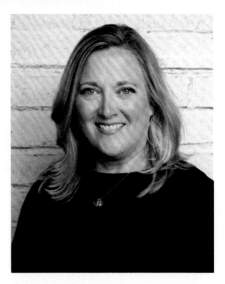

MaryLynn Jacobs earned a Bachelor of Science in Rehabilitation Medicine from Springfield College, Springfield, MA; a Master of Science in Occupational Therapy from Boston University, Boston, MA; and a Master in Business Administration in Entrepreneurial Thinking and Innovative Practices from Bay Path University, Longmeadow, MA. She has been a certified hand therapist (CHT) for most of her professional career.

Her academic, clinical, and business expertise spans well over three decades. She has developed several hand therapy departments, consulted to physician practices, industry, hospitals, home health care agencies, and software development companies. She has been teaching hand therapy and upper extremity orthosis/splinting courses across the country for over 35 years.

MaryLynn coedited and coauthored *Orthotic Intervention of the Hand and Upper Extremity, Splinting Principles and Process* published by Lippincott Williams and Wilkins, 2003/2013/2021. MaryLynn has contributed to the hand therapy literature with several journals, newspaper articles and coauthored *Orthotics in the Management of Hand Dysfunction in Orthotics and Prosthetics in Rehabilitation*, second edition, Saunders/Elsevier, 2005.

MaryLynn cofounded Attain Therapy + Fitness, a private practice, Physical and Occupational Therapy Company with a large footprint in Western MA. In 2015, Attain Therapy + Fitness merged with ATI Physical Therapy. Presently she is the Senior Director of National Hand Therapy services, overseeing the growth and development of hand therapy throughout ATI Physical Therapy nationwide. She is a member of the American Society of Hand Therapists (ASHT), past ASHT chair of the Legislation and Reimbursement Committee, and past chair of ASHT's Practice Management Committee. She is on several advisory boards as a board member of the Springfield College Board of Trustees, Springfield, Massachusetts.

Noelle M. Austin, MS, PT, CHT, is a graduate of Quinnipiac University, Hamden, CT with a Bachelor of Science in Physical Therapy and later obtained her Master of Science from the University of Connecticut, Storrs, CT with a special focus on Allied Health Education. She owns CJ Education and Consulting, LLC, offering private clinical education events on orthotic fabrication, as well as consulting services related to orthotic product development. Noelle was initially certified by the Hand Therapy Certification Commission as a Certified Hand Therapist (CHT) in 1996, and most recently recertified in 2021. She is an active member of the American Society of Hand Therapists. Noelle has been teaching the art and science of orthotic fabrication for over 25 years. In addition to conducting conferences both nationally and internationally, she has presented multiple sessions at Annual ASHT meetings, various State Chapter meetings, and for Hand Therapy Special Interest Groups on the topic of orthotic fabrication.

Noelle has been practicing in Hand Therapy for 30 years and most recently accepted a position with STAR Physical Therapy in the Nashville TN area. She was previously employed at OrthoVirginia in Lynchburg, VA and ProPT in Hamden, CT. She has also been adjunct faculty/guest lecturer in the Physical Therapy Programs at Lynchburg College in Virginia and Sacred Heart University in Connecticut, presenting lectures/labs on the topics of hand anatomy/kinesiology, examination/intervention, and orthotic fabrication. Noelle also consults with Kinetec USA as a Senior Clinical Specialist, assisting in product development and education with their Manosplint thermoplastics.

Noelle is coauthor and coeditor of the book: *Orthotic Intervention for the Hand and Upper Extremity: Splinting Principles and Process* published by Lippincott Williams and Wilkins, 2003/2013/2021. In addition, she authored the chapter "Wrist and Hand Complex" in the fourth/fifth/sixth edition of *Joint Structure and Function: A Comprehensive Analysis* (Levangie and Norkin) published by FA Davis in 2005/2011/2019. Noelle also authored "Orthotics in the Management of Hand Dysfunction" in the second and third edition of *Orthotics and Prosthetics in Rehabilitation* (Lusardi and Nielsen) published by Elsevier 2007/2012.

Foreword

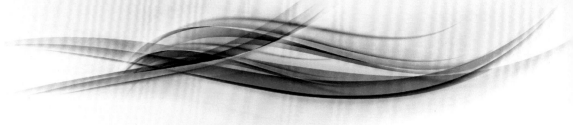

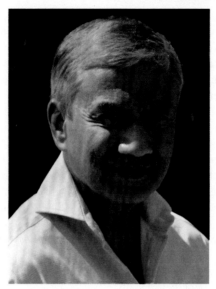

It is with the utmost respect and best wishes that I am honored to write this Foreword for the Third Edition of *Orthotic Intervention for the Hand and Upper Extremity: Splinting Principles and Process.*

In 2021, I will be entering into the fifth decade of my clinical practice and synchronously, this latest edition will be available to healthcare practitioners such as physical therapists, occupational therapists, hand therapists, physicians, surgeons, and clinical nurse specialists. This is the second time I have had the opportunity to write a chapter in this textbook on orthotics for arthritic conditions. Over the years, I have admired MaryLynn Jacobs and Noelle Austin for working tirelessly in compiling the previous two editions, and again with this third edition. Having compared the previous two editions, I found the third editions (main text and the *Fabrication Process Manual*) both to have new improved, simplified, and innovative orthotic prescription, fabrication, and application techniques.

As a clinician, educator, administrator, and researcher, and having practiced for five decades, I have witnessed the understanding of orthotic applications and how they have evolved significantly over time. Historically, after World War I, orthoses were primarily used for fracture fixation, providing rest to the healing tissues and/or correction of deformities. Over the years, with greater understanding of anatomy, healing processes, tissue engineering, and biomechanics, the orthotic fabrication and its clinical application has made a world of difference in restoring motion of human joints.

This third edition offers substantial clinical reasoning considering all avenues that are necessary to regain and restore extremity function. I find this textbook extremely valuable to clinicians and healthcare practitioners who are either prescribing or fabricating orthotics for their patients or clients. The extensive descriptions presented in the main textbook and the *Fabrication Process Manual* enable the clinician to have an edge on problem identification and evidence-based clinical reasoning for achieving specific orthotic goals. The step-by-step illustrations and instructions for the various mobilization orthoses empowers the practitioner to custom tailor the orthotic fabrication, and make necessary alterations for the best clinical outcome. Moreover, the chapters included in these books assist the healthcare provider in making the correct judgement of orthotics prescription and applications.

The Third Edition of *Orthotic Intervention for the Hand and Upper Extremity: Splinting Principles and Process* presents descriptions of a wide variety of diagnoses. This textbook and its companion manual undoubtedly are a valuable resource for healthcare practitioners. In addition, these books offer highlights of anatomical and mechanical principles, and biomechanics of normal and altered pathomechanics; discusses associated indications and precautions; and promotes clinical reasoning skills by presenting a wide variety of expert pearls and patient case studies. This wide-ranged approach allows practitioners to confidently present their clinical reasoning to referring physicians and surgeons and utilize techniques in their clinical practice to promote and advance the hand therapy profession for greater recognition.

This publication has many new and well-thought-out added features, including new chapters on Relative Motion Orthoses and Prosthetics, a separate *Fabrication Process Manual* for every orthotic design, full-color images with a larger format, Expert Pearls shared by the international experts, surgeons' comments, addressing Frequently Asked Questions by the practitioners for specific clinical diagnoses, instructional videos, and the printable patterns for orthotic fabrication. These additions to the textbook make the third edition a most desirable resource material for the practitioner of all levels. Reading this book, as well as exploring the extensive references, will undoubtedly bring the professionals a long way in improving their knowledge and skills that are necessary in an evidence-based clinical practice environment.

I know that the compilation of material presented in this third edition by MaryLynn Jacobs and Noelle Austin will help improve clinical practice for this generation and many generations to come.

With due respect and best wishes.

Shrikant J. Chinchalkar, MThO, BScOT, OTR, CHT, OTReg(ON)
Roth-McFarlane Hand & Upper Limb Centre
St. Joseph's Health Care London
London, Ontario,
Canada

Foreword (from Second Edition)

As a therapist who has written about and taught hand splinting (now accurately called orthotic fabrication) for many years, I commend MaryLynn A. Jacobs and Noelle Austin on giving you, the reader, this second edition of *Splinting the Hand and Upper Extremity: Principles and Process*, which now has the updated title of *Orthotic Intervention for the Hand and Upper Extremity: Splinting Principles and Process*.

This book is your doorway into the complex, skill-based, real world of orthotic intervention for the upper extremity. Therapists who want to specialize in treating upper extremity patients must have a wide range of knowledge and ability in orthotic intervention by developing an understanding of the underlying anatomical principles, how tissue heals and matures, how to apply mechanical principles to orthotic design, how to skillfully handle orthotic tools and materials, and how to evaluate and determine the need for and the appropriate design of an orthosis. Then they must be able to design, fabricate, fit, adjust, and describe for billing, as well as reevaluate the effectiveness of the orthotic intervention. This book delivers all of this information and more to the reader.

WHY SHOULD YOU READ THIS BOOK?

I have observed therapists in the clinic wanting a book, which will give them a pattern for an orthosis and how to construct it but nothing more. But an orthosis is only part of the treatment approach and cannot be separated from a comprehensive understanding of the pathology and how a therapist can influence the outcome. This book combines the "how to" with the "why" and directs you to resources, which can further your understanding. To appreciate the entire therapy process and not just the construction, an orthosis should be every therapist's goal.

A number of features of this book set it apart from others on this subject. Not all orthoses need to be made of low-temperature thermoplastics, and the authors' discussion of casting, taping, use of neoprene, and prefabricated orthoses completes your armamentarium to address the wide range of specific patient needs. The real-life "Clinical Pearls" included throughout the book give you insight from experienced clinicians who have learned on-the-job tips and tricks to increase efficiency and patient comfort.

For therapists who are looking for a starting point, the section on "Orthotic Fabrication" gives a step-by-step design and construction process, while concurrently the section on "Orthotic Intervention for Specific Diagnoses and Populations" provides deeper insight to the appropriate orthotic intervention for specific diagnostic problems. The case study accompanying each chapter in this latter section illustrates direct application to a specific situation.

Reading this book as well as some of the recommended references will take you a long way toward gaining orthotic skills. In our current busy clinic climate, time to practice and learn orthotic skills is scarce, and we must find innovative methods and resources to build and maintain this skill set.

WHY WAS I WILLING TO WRITE THIS FOREWORD?

I wrote this because it matters that we, as therapists, develop and maintain a high level of orthotic intervention skills for our patients as part of our treatment spectrum. No one else can integrate the use of an orthosis into the treatment but us. My recommendation is to keep this book at your bedside as well as next to your treatment area. Read a few pearls each day and incorporate them into your clinical practice or make an unfamiliar orthosis on a coworker as self-training. You will build your skill and knowledge arsenal each day.

Who knows… perhaps you will contribute to the text on orthotic intervention for the next generation.

Judy C. Colditz, OTR/L, CHT, FAOTA
HandLab
Raleigh, North Carolina
June 1, 2013

Preface

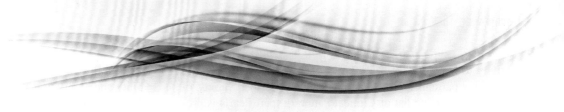

Orthotic Intervention for the Hand and Upper Extremity: Splinting Principles and Process, Third Edition, along with the complementary *Fabrication Process Manual*, was inspired by clinicians and students who, in our teaching experience, were requesting one resource that would clarify all appropriate traditional orthosis fabrication/splinting, casting, and taping managements for upper extremity diagnoses. Although an upper extremity therapist tends to fabricate thermoplastic orthoses most of the time, there are many situations when casting, taping, neoprene, or even a prefabricated orthosis is a more appropriate choice. These books are unique in that they provide orthosis patterns for most upper extremity diagnoses as well as in-depth discussions and instructions for choosing and fabricating with these other options. This feature truly distinguishes these books from all others currently on the market. We do not delve into the specifics of rehabilitation techniques and surgical interventions; instead, we provide contemporary overviews of the various diagnoses described to clarify a particular rationale specific to an orthosis design or evidence-based protocol. New authors have contributed to the following chapters: **Concepts of Orthotic Fundamentals, Tissue Healing, Prefabricated Orthoses, Taping Techniques, Stiffness, Arthritis, Flexor Tendon Injuries, Peripheral Nerve Injuries, Burns, The Musician,** and **Hand and Upper Extremity Transplantation.** New chapters include: **Relative Motion Orthoses, Upper Extremity Prosthetics, Orficast® and Orficast More®, Delta-Cast®** and **Tendon and Nerve Transfers.**

ORGANIZATION HIGHLIGHTS AND FEATURES

The main text is divided into three sections. **Section I** focuses on the **Fundamentals of Orthotic Fabrication.** Much of the mystery surrounding orthotic fabrication can be eliminated if the therapist has a good working knowledge of appropriate nomenclature (to interpret referrals), upper extremity anatomy, tissue healing guidelines, and a concrete understanding of mechanical principles. This section provides the foundation necessary to plan and create an orthosis. **Chapter 1** presents a modified version of the American Society of Hand Therapists (ASHT) orthosis nomenclature, various types of orthoses, and objectives for orthosis intervention which is used consistently throughout the book. **Chapter 2** systematically reviews the bony and neuromuscular anatomy, specifically as it relates to the application of orthoses. **Chapter 3** describes the stages of healing, factors that influence healing, and the relationship of specific stages of healing to orthosis selection and application. **Chapter 4** defines the fundamental mechanical terms and concepts pertinent to orthosis design and fabrication and discusses the clinical relevance and application of these basic principles using specific examples. **Chapter 5** surveys the proper equipment crucial to effective orthosis fabrication. **Chapter 6** outlines the entire process of creating an accurate orthosis design, from obtaining an appropriate referral to properly dispensing the device. It also introduces the PROCESS concept used in the *Fabrication Process Manual*.

Section II entitled **Optional Methods** describes alternative interventions for immobilization, mobilization, or restriction of a body part. Because of time constraints, monetary issues, or perhaps lack of product availability, it is not always practical or appropriate to make an orthosis from thermoplastic materials. The chapters included in this section provide information on alternative means of orthotic fabrication. **Chapter 7** presents how to integrate relative motion orthoses into everyday practice, **Chapter 8** provides an overview of upper extremity prosthetics. **Chapter 9** outlines the considerations and options related to the use of prefabricated orthoses, including information on how to become an educated consumer on the availability, application, and modification of these devices. **Chapters 10-12** describe casting as a treatment technique that has the ability to provide outcomes that no other orthotic intervention approach can offer—including traditional casting, Orficast® and Delta-Cast® techniques. This new content familiarizes the clinician with the characteristics of casting products and outlines the ideal material to be chosen that best meets the patient's needs. **Chapter 13** provides information on the most common taping methods: traditional athletic taping, McConnell taping, and elastic therapeutic taping. Each technique is described with specific instructions and multiple clinical examples. **Chapter 14** is a noteworthy chapter because neoprene is becoming increasingly popular. This unique content reviews the basic information regarding the benefits of neoprene, qualities of neoprene materials, and a variety of thought-provoking options and alternatives for orthotic management.

Each chapter in **Section III** on **Orthotic Intervention for Specific Diagnoses and Populations** goes into depth regarding the following: stiffness, fractures, arthritis, extensor and flexor tendon injuries, peripheral nerve injuries, tendon and nerve transfers, the athlete, adult neurologic dysfunction, the pediatric patient, burns, the musician, and upper extremity transplantation.

After an overview of the specific topic, these chapters include common orthotic interventions and specific considerations. Many chapters include tables that clarify information and decrease redundancy within the text. **Case Studies** and **Chapter Review Questions** accompany each chapter and are meant to stimulate clinical reasoning and synthesize information reviewed in the text. **Expert Pearls** are a new feature in these chapters which provide unique ideas regarding intervention for that population. The addition of **MD notes** and **Field Notes** in Section III allows for alternative perspectives from the world of hand surgery/therapy.

The *Fabrication Process Manual* is a hands-on working manual and organized into four chapters that cover immobilization (**Chapter 1**), mobilization (**Chapter 2**), restriction (**Chapter 3**), and nonarticular (**Chapter 4**) orthoses.

Each chapter includes pattern illustrations and accompanying photography of the orthosis described. Most of the pattern descriptions include **Clinical Pearls**, **Pattern Pearls,** and newly added **Expert Pearls** that apply to that particular orthosis. The Clinical and Pattern Pearls relate to our personal experience and the Expert Pearls were contributed by our colleagues working in the field of Hand Therapy. They include fabrication and orthosis modification tips as well as insight for improving cost containment and maximizing time efficiency. Most orthosis patterns have alternative design options in the event that the therapist cannot fabricate a custom orthosis. Common diagnoses and general positioning are recommended. However, one must appreciate that the diagnoses appropriate for an orthosis and the recommended positioning can be varied and depend on many factors. The pattern designs illustrated are suggestions of the ones we have found simple to visualize and use. The Pattern Pearls give alternative pattern designs that we have used in our clinical practice. The therapist is encouraged to modify the pattern according to specific patient needs. The manual is meant as a guideline for orthosis construction—use your creativity to individualize each device. The pearls are not always unique to a particular orthosis, and many apply to a variety of orthoses. A complete list of Clinical/Pattern/Expert Pearls is provided at the front of the book to help the student locate specific points of interest.

Appendix A is a list of orthotic vendors/resources that offer equipment, materials, and prefabricated orthoses. **Appendices B** and **C** provide examples of forms used in a clinical setting. The **Index** allows the reader to access information about orthoses by their common names as well as by the ASHT terminology.

FEATURES

- **Chapter Objectives:** At the beginning of each chapter, these guide both students and instructors to the material in the chapter and help prepare for the information provided.
- **Key Terms:** Appearing at the beginning of each chapter, these are defined in the glossary to emphasize basic terminology associated with orthotic fabrication.
- **FAQs:** List common questions that therapists have related to orthotic fabrication and other intervention strategies for a specific patient population.
- **MD Note:** Respected surgeons contributed their thoughts highlighting the important collaborative relationship between a surgeon and hand therapist.
- **Field Notes:** Written by chosen clinical experts highlighting a unique perspective on that chapter's content.
- **Case Studies:** Located in the chapters and online, these foster critical thinking to apply concepts to clinical practice.
- **Expert Pearls:** New feature added in both main text and manual, generously shared by dozens of hand therapy experts from around the world including unique orthotic ideas, tips, and material usage. This unique feature includes select pearls authored by Judy C. Colditz, OT/L, CHT, FAOTA.
- **Clinical Pearls:** Appearing in main text and manual, these illustrate tips on ways to modify the design or alter the fabrication process to improve efficiency or maximize patient specificity.
- **Pattern Pearls:** Presented in manual, these provide alternative pattern designs or other orthotic options.
- **ASHT Orthotics Nomenclature:** Nomenclature is described in detail for better understanding.
- **Chapter Review Questions:** Located at the end of each chapter in the main textbook, these help students review and retain the information they have encountered in each chapter.
- **Discussion Points:** At the end of *Fabrication Process Manual* chapters, these questions challenge students to use critical thinking to recall concepts and theories learned in these chapters.

- **Printable Patterns:** Available online to allow for easy accessibility and ability to resize for lab/clinic use. Orthotic fabrication for a spectrum of diagnoses and special populations (available with *Fabrication Process Manual* only).
- **Full Color/Large Format:** This updated presentation of images provides a more intimate view of the orthoses presented.
- **Glossary:** This provides a list of terms and definitions.

This book reviews numerous pattern designs and other options for orthotic management for the upper extremity. Although this endeavor documents a spectrum of orthotic management, the possibilities for different options extend far beyond a single text. New challenges face the clinician daily; and it is with each patient that we learn something new, building on our previous knowledge. This book is meant to stimulate clinical skills and clinician creativity, encouraging the integration of principles and process from which a clinician can create new orthoses.

ADDITIONAL RESOURCES

Orthotic Intervention for the Hand and Upper Extremity: Splinting Principles and Process includes additional resources for both instructors and students that are available on the book's companion website at http://thePoint.lww.com.

Instructor Resources

Approved adopting instructors will be given access to the following additional resources:

- Image Bank
- PowerPoint Presentation as "Clinic in the Classroom"
- Sample Syllabi
- Lab Exercises
- Answers to Chapter Review Questions
- Answers to Discussion Points

Student Resources

Students who have purchased *Orthotic Intervention for the Hand and Upper Extremity: Splinting Principles and Process* and *Fabrication Process Manual* have access to the following additional resources:

- Videos detailing the Fabrication process and common orthoses
- Interactive Quiz Bank
- Online Case Studies
- Checklist
- Anatomy Reference Tables
- Appendix A: Distributors of Orthotic Fabrication Products
- Appendix B: Occupational/Physical Therapy Examination
- Appendix C: Care and Use of Your Custom Orthosis
- References

Contributors

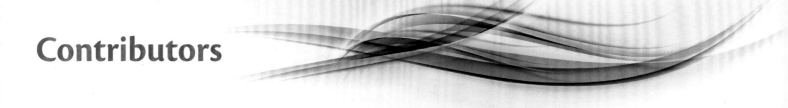

Gary P. Austin, PT, PhD, OCS, FAAOMPT, FAFS
Chair and Professor
School of Physical Therapy
Belmont University
Nashville, Tennessee

Noelle M. Austin, MS, PT, CHT
Owner/Educator
CJ Education & Consulting, LLC
Nashville, Tennessee

Hand Therapist
STAR Physical Therapy
Nashville, Tennessee

Nancy Beaman, MBA, OTR/L, CHT
Senior Hand Therapist
Coordinator of Clinical Excellence – Hand Therapy
ATI Physical Therapy
Westfield, Massachusetts

Richard A. Bernstein, MD, FAAOS
Hand Surgeon
CT Orthopaedics
Hamden, Connecticut

Assistant Clinical Professor, Orthopaedic Surgery
Yale University School of Medicine
New Haven, Connecticut

Salvador Bondoc, OTD, OTR/L, BCPR, CHT, FAOTA
Chair and Professor of Occupational Therapy
Quinnipiac University
Hamden, Connecticut

Occupational Therapist
Griffin Hospital
Derby, Connecticut

Sabrina Cassella, MEd, OTR/L, CHT
Senior Hand Therapist
ATI Physical Therapy
Wilbraham, Massachusetts

Nancy Chee, OTD, OTR/L, CHT
Hand Therapist IV
CA Pacific Medical Center
San Francisco, California

Adjunct Assistant Professor
Samuel Merritt University
Oakland, California

Shrikant Chinchalkar, M.Th.O, BSc.OT, OTR, CHT
Hand Therapist
Hand Therapy Division
Roth-McFarlane Hand & Upper Limb Center
St. Joseph's Health Care London
London, Ontario, Canada

President
Advanced Clinical Education Inc.
Mississauga, Ontario, Canada

Jennifer Stephens Chisar, PT, MS, CHT
Supervisor of Outpatient Rehabilitation Services
John Muir Health
Pleasant Hill, California

Guest Lecturer
Samuel Merritt University
Oakland, California

University of CA
San Francisco, California

San Francisco State University
San Francisco, California

Courtney Condon, MEd, OTR/L
Occupational Therapist
Advanced Clinician
Shriners Hospitals for Children
Boston, Massachusetts

Kimberly Gross, MEd, OTR/L, CHT, CKTP, CDTI
Senior Hand Therapist
ATI Physical Therapy
Springfield, Massachusetts

Adjunct Faculty
Western New England University
Springfield, Massachusetts

Melissa Hirth, B (OT), MSc (OT - Hand & Upper Limb Rehab)
Senior Occupational Therapist, Hand Therapy Stream Leader
Austin Health
Heidelberg, Victoria, Australia
Senior Occupational Therapist & Co-Director
Malvern Hand Therapy
Malvern, Victoria, Australia

PhD Candidate
Monash University, Peninsula Campus
Frankston, Victoria, Australia

Julianne Wright Howell, PT, MS, CHT
Self-employed
Saint Joseph, Michigan

MaryLynn A. Jacobs, MBA, MS, OTR/L, CHT
Senior Director, National Hand Therapy Services
ATI Physical Therapy
Bolingbrook, Illinois

Lorna Canavan Kahn, PT, CHT
Advance Practice Clinician
Milliken Hand Rehabilitation Center
Washington University School of Medicine
Program in Occupational Therapy
St. Louis, Missouri

Debra Ann Latour, OTD, MEd, OTR/L
Assistant Professor of Occupational Therapy
Division of Occupational Therapy
Western New England University
Springfield, Massachusetts

Owner
Single-Handed Solutions, LLC
Springfield, Massachusetts

Marsha Lawrence, PT, DPT, CHT
Senior Hand Therapist
University of Iowa Hospitals & Clinics
Iowa City, Iowa

Kristen MacDonald, MScOT, CHT, OT Reg. (Ont)
Hand Therapist
Hand Therapy Division
Roth-McFarlane Hand & Upper Limb Center
St. Joseph's Health Care London
London, Ontario, Canada

Alexandra MacKenzie, OTR/L, CHT
Clinical Supervisor of Hand Therapy
Hospital for Special Surgery
New York, New York

Jamie McMillan, OTR, CHT
Director of Upper Extremity Products
Hely & Weber
Santa Paula, California

Anna VanVoorhis Miller, MS, OTR/L, CHT
Clinical Specialist
Milliken Hand Rehabilitation Center
Washington University School of Medicine
Program in Occupational Therapy
St. Louis, Missouri

Jill Peck-Murray, MOTR/L, CHT
Continuing Education Instructor
Rehab Education
Del Mar, California

Rebecca Neiduski, PhD, OTR/L, CHT
Dean of the School of Health Sciences
Professor of Health Sciences
Elon University
Elon, North Carolina

Katherine Hartigan Norris, MS, OTR/L
Occupational Therapist
Advanced Clinician
Clinical Education Coordinator
Shriners Hospitals for Children
Boston, Massachusetts

Joey Pipicelli, MScOT, CHT, OT Reg. (Ont)
Sessional Instructor
School of Occupational Therapy
Western University
London, Ontario, Canada

Hand Therapist
Hand Therapy Division
Roth-McFarlane Hand & Upper Limb Center
St. Joseph's Health Care London
London, Ontario, Canada

Deborah A. Schwartz, OTD, OTR/L, CHT
Product and Educational Specialist, Physical Rehabilitation
Orfit Industries America
Leonia, New Jersey

Adjunct Professor
Touro College
Department of Occupational Therapy
New York, New York

Gayle Severance, MS, OT/L, CHT
Hand Therapy Team Leader
Good Shepherd Penn Partners
Philadelphia, Pennsylvania

Gary Solomon, MS, OTR/L, CHT
Director
Chicago Metro Hand Therapy, LLC
Arlington Heights, Illinois
Past President
American Society of Hand Therapists
Board of Directors
　　American Association for Hand Surgery
　　American Hand Therapy Foundation
　　Chicago Metro Hand Study Group

Kimberly Goldie Staines, OTR, CHT
Senior Hand Therapist
Department of Physical Medicine and Rehabilitation
Michael E. DeBakey Veterans Affairs Medical Center
Houston, Texas

Adjunct Faculty
Department of Rheumatology
Baylor College of Medicine
Houston, Texas

Visiting Scientist
Houston Methodist Hospital
Center for Performing Arts Medicine
Department of Orthopedics
Houston, Texas

Visiting Faculty
University of Texas, Medical Branch
Department of Occupational Therapy
Galveston, Texas

Macy Miller Stonner, OTD, OTR/L
Occupational Therapist
Milliken Hand Rehabilitation Center
Washington University School of Medicine
Program in Occupational Therapy
St. Louis, Missouri

Janine Thomas, OTR/L, CHT, COMT
Hand Therapist, Assistant Director of Therapy
OrthoVirginia
Lynchburg, Virginia

Amy Vissing, MHS, OTR/L, CHT
Hand Therapist
Good Shepherd Penn Partners
Philadelphia, Pennsylvania

Aviva Wolff, EdD, OT/L, CHT
Clinician Scientist
Leon Root, MD Motion Analysis Laboratory
Hospital for Special Surgery
New York, New York

Assistant Professor of Clinical Rehabilitation
Weill Cornell Medical College
New York, New York

Hand Therapist Consultant
The Juilliard School
New York, New York

Owner
Music Hands Therapy
New York, New York
Paramus, New Jersey

Danielle Wojtkiewicz, MSOT, OTR/L, CHT
Hand Therapist – Director of Bellevue Hand Therapy
Washington Hand Therapy – RET Physical Therapy
Bellevue, Washington

Field Note Contributors

Jeanine Beasley, EdD, OTR, CHT, FAOTA
Grand Valley State University
Michigan

Carolyn Brown, OTR/L, CLT, OTD candidate
Hospital for Special Care
Quinnipiac University
Connecticut

Aimee Chiasson, PT, DPT
Shriners Hospital for Children
Massachusetts

Michelle Coil, MOT, OTR, CHT, PYT, CEAS
Virtual Hand Care
Texas

Debbie Fisher, MS, OTR, CHT
Baylor Scott and White Institute of Rehab
Texas

Ginny Gibson, OTD, OTR/L, CHT
Samuel Merritt University
California

Mojca (Mo) Herman, MA,OTR/L, CHT
Advanced Therapy Center: Hand and Upper Extremity Specialists
California

Amanda Higgins, BScOT, OT Reg (NB)
Saint John Regional Hospital
Canada

Julianne Wright Howell, PT, MS, CHT
Self-employed
Michigan

Melissa Jayne Hirth, B (OT), MSc (OT-Hand & Upper Limb Rehab)
Malvern Hand Therapy
Australia

MaryLynn A. Jacobs, MBA, MS, OTR/L, CHT
ATI Physical Therapy
Illinois

Robin Janson, OTD, MS, OTR, CHT
Indiana University
Indiana

Mary Matthews-Brownell OTR/L, MHA, CHT, PTA, CLT
Veterans Health Administration
Washington

Wyndell H. Merritt, MD, FACS
Private Practice
Virginia

Robyn Midgley, BSc (Hons) OT, AHT (BAHT), ECHT (EFSHT)
Hand Therapy Consulting
South Africa

Maria Josette S. Mullins, PT, DPT
Memorial Hospital Miramar
Florida

Virginia H. O'Brien, OTD, OR/L, CHT
University of Minnesota Health-Hand Center
Minnesota

Marie Pace, OTR/L, CHT
University of Pittsburgh Medical Center
Pennsylvania

Rita M. Patterson, PhD
Texas College of Medicine
Texas

Ben Salatin, MS
VA Healthcare System
New Mexico

Sandra P. Salinas, OTR, CHT
Memorial Hospital Miramar
Florida

Alison Taylor, OTR/L, CHT, CKTP, CKTI
Baylor Scott & White Health
Texas

Aviva Wolff, EdD, OT/L, CHT
Hospital for Special Surgery
Weill Cornell Medical College
The Juilliard School
Music Hands Therapy
New York

Kimberly Zeske-Maquire, MS, OTR/L, CHT
University of Pittsburgh Medical Center
Pennsylvania

Expert Pearl Contributors

Natalie Alfaro, OT, CHT
Macquarie Hand Therapy
Australia

Baptiste Arrate, OT
Institut Sud Aquitain de la Main et du Membre Supérieur
France

Michele Auch, OTR/L, CHT
ATI Physical Therapy
Illinois

Larissa Póvoa Alves Barradas, OT
Hamato Rehabilitation
Brazil

Nancy Beaman, MBA, OTR/L, CHT
ATI Physical Therapy
Massachusetts

Jeanine Beasley, EdD, OTR, CHT, FAOTA
Grand Valley State University
Michigan

Theresa Bell-Nagle, OTR/L, CHT
2 Thumbs Up Hand Therapy
Massachusetts

Carolyn Brown, OTR/L, CLT, OTD candidate
Hospital for Special Care
Quinnipiac University
Connecticut

Laura Carter, OT
Advanced Health and Hand Therapy
Australia

Sabrina Cassella, MEd, OTR/L, CHT
ATI Physical Therapy
Massachusetts

Melissa Cepeda, OTR/L
Peak Physical Therapy & Wellness
Colorado

Ana Candice Coelho, PT
Quiros Reabilitação Integrada
Brazil

Michelle Coil, MOT, OTR, CHT, PYT, CEAS
Virtual Hand Care
Texas

Diane Coker, PT, DPT, CHT
South County Orthopedic Specialists
California

Judy C. Colditz, OT/L, CHT, FAOTA
HandLab/BraceLab
North Carolina

Laura Conway, OTR, CHT, COMT UE
Select Medical
Florida

Bruce Curtis, OT
Performance Health
Illinois

Mary Anne Dykstra, OTR/L, CHT
ATI Physical Therapy
Illinois

Chantal Etcheverry, OT
Institut Sud Aquitain de la Main et du Membre Supérieur
France

Sheri B. Feldscher, OTR/L, CHT
Philadelphia Hand to Shoulder Center
Pennsylvania

Debbie Fisher, MS, OTR, CHT
Baylor Scott and White Institute of Rehab
Texas

Angela Frigerio, OT, CHT
Pacific Hand Therapy
Australia

Ginny Gibson, OTD, OTR/L, CHT
Samuel Merritt University
California

Trish Griffiths, OT
Christian Barnard Memorial Hospital
South Africa

Amanda Hall, PT, MPT, PCS, ATP
The HSC Pediatric Center
The Center
Washington, Dc

Emma Hirst, OT
The Hand Therapy Group
New Zealand

Clyde Johnson, PT, CHT
Bellevue Bone and Joint Orthopedics
Washington

Joanna Jourdan, OT
HLO Handtherapie and Ergotherapeutin
Germany

Saba Kamal, OTR, CHT
Hands-On-Care,
California

Magdalena Kolasińska, PT
Józef Piłsudski University of Physical Education
Poland

Hannah Leaman, OTR/L, OTD
University of Virginia Medical Center
Virginia

Julianne Lessard, OTR/L, CHT
ATI Physical Therapy
Massachusetts

Niamh Masterson, OT
UrbanRehab
Australia

Grégory Mesplié, PT
Institut Sud Aquitain de la Main et du Membre Supérieur
France

Andrea Moser, OT, Hand Therapist
Trauma Hospital Klagenfurt
Private practice – St. Veit/Glan
Austria

Alfred Ninja, OTR/L, CHT
Fortis Hand Therapy Clinic
Kenya

Anna Ovsyannikova, MD, Hand Therapy
University Clinic
Russia

Jill Peck-Murray, MOTR/L, CHT
Rehab Education
California

Kirsten C. Pedersen, OT
K.C. Pedersen / Ergoklinikken
Denmark

Beth Perko, OTR/L, CHT
OrthoVirginia
Virginia

Bob Phillips, OTR/L, CHT
Optim Orthopedics
Georgia

Ceri Pulham, OT, CHT
Norwest Hand Therapy
Australia

Lisa Ray, OTR/L, CHT
OrthoVirginia
Virginia

Kerry A. Raymond, MS, OTR, CHT, CFCE
Key Therapy Services
New Hampshire

Kathy Riley, PT, CHT
University of Virginia/Healthsouth
Virginia

Kim Rosinski, OTR/L, CSCS, CHT
NovaCare Rehabilitation
Pennsylvania

Veruschka Moreira Coêlho Savoldeli, OT
Hamato Rehabilitation
Brazil

Debby Schwartz, OTD, OTR/L, CHT
Orfit Industries America
New Jersey

Erfan Shafiee, OT, Hand Therapist
University of Western Ontario
Canada

Mary Sommer, OTR/L, CHT
ATI Physical Therapy
Washington

Kimberly Goldie Staines, OTR, CHT
Michael E. DeBakey Veterans Affairs Medical Center
Texas

Alison Taylor, OTR/L, CHT, CKTP, CKTI
Baylor Scott & White Health
Texas

Janine Thomas, OTR/L, CHT, COMT
OrthoVirginia
Virginia

Hoang Tran, OT/L, CHT
Hands on Therapy Services
CHT Secrets
Florida

Ngaire Turnbull, OT, Hand Therapist
Hand Spark
Australia

Kathy Villacres, OTR/L, CHT
Hand and Arm Therapy Specialists
Ohio

Anne Wajon, PT, CHT
Macquarie Hand Therapy
Australia

Karol Young, OTD, OTR/L, CHT
HandLab/BraceLab
North Carolina

MD Contributors

Ajay K. Balaram, MD
Hand to Shoulder Associates
Illinois

Gregory M. Buncke, MD
The Buncke Medical Clinic
California

Benjamin Chang, MD, FACS
Children's Hospital of Philadelphia
Pennsylvania

Alfred Gelhorn, MD
Weill Cornell Medicine
New York

Don Lalonde, MD
Dalhousie University
Canada

Steve K. Lee, MD
Lenox Hill Hospital
New York

L. Scott Levin, MD, FACS
Children's Hospital of Philadelphia
Pennsylvania

Susan E. Mackinnon, MD
Washington University School of Medicine
Missouri

Wyndell H. Merritt, MD, FACS
Private Practice
Virginia

David T. Netscher, MD
Houston Methodist
Texas

Mitchell A. Pet, MD
Washington University Physicians
Missouri

Janet Pope, MD
St. Joseph's Health Centre
Canada

Robert L. Sheridan, MD
Shriners Hospitals for Children
Massachusetts

Alyse Sicklick, MD
Gaylord Specialty Healthcare
Connecticut

C. Douglas Wallace, MD
Rady Children's Hospital
California

Acknowledgments

The undertaking of this third edition would not be possible if it were not for the patience and guidance provided by our experienced team at Wolters Kluwer including: Matt Hauber, Acquisitions Editor; Amy Millholen, Development Editor; Cody Adams and Vinoth Ezhumalai, Editorial Coordinators; Barton Dudlick, Production Project Manager; Steve Druding, Design Coordinator; Margie Orzech, Manufacturing Coordinator. We truly value their time and experience with assisting us in updating the design of this new edition including dividing the original text into two separate books. We want to thank them for allowing us the space to expand our content including the overwhelming task of organizing the hundreds of additional color photographs and contributions from dozens of therapists. We truly appreciate the hard work provided by Oviya Balamurugan, Project Manager at TNQ Technologies during this revision; she successfully conquered the daunting task of creating a user-friendly format to present the images and information.

No book is solely the work of its authors. We would like to thank all the patients who were so generous in allowing us to photograph them and provide such a plethora of clinical examples for our book. We would like to express our gratitude to the many therapists and physicians we have worked with over the years who contributed to our knowledge base, professional growth, and clinical skills. So many of you have urged and supported us to always dig deeper and be as creative as possible! Your trust in our expertise and appreciation for what we do has fueled the underlying passion for the writing of this book. We also want to acknowledge the generosity of therapists from around the world who were eager to contribute their unique ideas that will provide the reader with so many options when it comes to orthosis selection.

We would like to especially thank Performance Health, especially Paul England, former Director of Marketing, Orthopedics for the generous support in supplying the majority of thermoplastic materials and components used in the Fabrication Manual for the professional photographs. We have thoroughly enjoyed working with TailorSplint which has stood the test of time since our first edition. Thanks so much!

Finally, we would like to express our sincere thanks to our families who have been so patient and understanding during the writing process—from our first edition nearly 20 years ago to this third edition. Without their love, support, and ongoing patience, we would not have been able to tackle such a huge, detail-oriented task successfully.

Contents

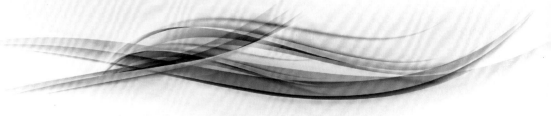

SECTION 1 Fundamentals of Orthotic Fabrication

1 **Concepts of Orthotic Fundamentals** 2
by MaryLynn A. Jacobs, MBA, MS, OTR/L, CHT and Marsha Lawrence, PT, DPT, CHT

2 **Anatomical Principles** 25
by Noelle M. Austin, MS, PT, CHT

3 **Tissue Healing** 63
by Richard A. Bernstein, MD, FAAOS and Nancy Beaman, MBA, OTR/L, CHT

4 **Mechanical Principles** 82
by Gary P. Austin, PT, PhD, OCS, FAAOMPT, FAFS and MaryLynn A. Jacobs, MBA, MS, OTR/L, CHT

5 **Equipment and Materials** 99
by Noelle M. Austin, MS, PT, CHT

6 **Fabrication Process** 120
by Noelle M. Austin, MS, PT, CHT*

SECTION 2 Optional Methods

7 **Relative Motion Orthoses** 138
by Julianne Wright Howell, PT, MS, CHT and Melissa Hirth, B (OT), MSc (OT -Hand & Upper Limb Rehab)

8 **Upper Extremity Prosthetics** 150
by Debra Ann Latour, OTD, MEd, OTR/L

9 **Prefabricated Orthoses** 177
by Jamie McMillan, OTR, CHT

10 **Casting** 196
by MaryLynn A. Jacobs, MBA, MS, OTR/L, CHT

11 **Orficast® and Orficast® More** 219
by Deborah A. Schwartz, OTD, OTR/L, CHT

SECTION 3   Orthotic Intervention for Specific Diagnoses and Populations

CLINICAL PEARLS

EXPERT PEARLS

Fundamentals of Orthotic Fabrication

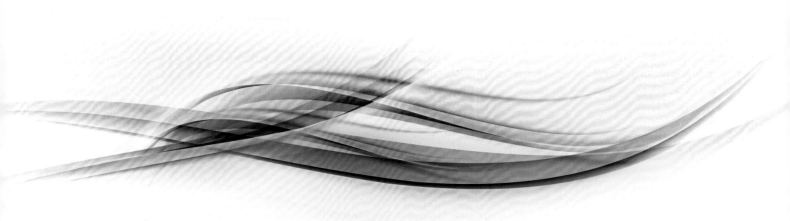

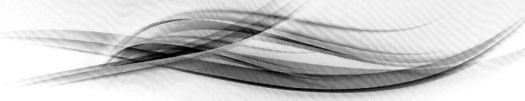

1

Concepts of Orthotic Fundamentals[a]

MaryLynn A. Jacobs, MBA, MS, OTR/L, CHT
Marsha Lawrence, PT, DPT, CHT

CHAPTER OBJECTIVES

After study of this chapter, the reader should be able to:
• Identify the proper nomenclature used to describe orthoses for communication to peers, payers, and referral sources.
• Understand the clinical reasoning process for selecting the most appropriate orthosis for a patient.
• Explain the specific differences and appropriate uses for the term's *static, dynamic, serial static,* and *static progressive orthoses.*
• List the objectives for immobilization, mobilization, and restrictive orthoses and describe an example of each.

KEY TERMS
American Society of Hand Therapists (ASHT)
Articular orthosis
Centers for Medicare & Medicaid Services (CMS)
Current Procedural Terminology (CPT)
Custom fabricated
Durable Medical Equipment, Prosthetics, Orthotics, and Supplies (DMEPOS)
Dynamic orthosis

Immobilization orthosis
L-Code
Medicare Administrative Contractors (MAC)
Mobilization orthosis
Modified Orthosis Classification System (MOCS)
Modifier
National Supplier Clearinghouse (NSC)
Nonarticular orthosis
Prefabricated orthosis

Provider Enrollment, Chain and Ownership System (PECOS)
Restriction orthosis
Serial static orthosis
Splint Classification System (SCS)
Static progressive orthosis
Static orthosis

FAQ

Will Medicare Pay for Replacement Orthoses?
The Medicare Supplier Manual has specific policies regarding replacement of DME for Medicare beneficiaries. The standard reasonable useful lifetime for DMEPOS is 5 years unless a specific policy indicates otherwise. There is no such exceptions policy in place for upper limb orthoses so by default, the expectation is a 5-year wear expectancy. A treating physician or practitioner's order is required in order to confirm medical necessity.

   If the replacement is due to loss, irreparable damage, or theft, the replacement orthosis is bill with a modifier and appropriate documentation must be submitted to confirm the loss such as an insurance claim or police report and a signed patient affidavit must be in the medical record.

Can I Bill for Replacement of Parts for an Orthosis?
Code L4210 can be used to bill for replacement orthosis components lacking specific codes: screws, elastic, rivets, etc. Must provide proof of component cost (i.e., original ordering invoice). The claim should include laterality modifiers: RT, LT, and RB (replacement of a part of DME furnished as a component of repair of the item).

   The narrative portion of the claim should describe the parts or if filing by paper claim, the description must be attached to the claim.

Will Medicare Cover Digit Ring Orthoses?
Medicare limits the number of ring orthoses billable on a single day of service to 3 but only one per finger. Medicare will cover two ring orthoses per digit (proximal interphalangeal [PIP] and distal interphalangeal [DIP]) but both cannot be billed on the same date of service. This applies regardless of the material that makes up the orthosis (thermoplastic versus precious metals) and the reimbursement fee is the same for either. Replacements are not billable within a calendar year, and this policy may vary depending on the DME MAC jurisdiction.

---

[a]**Disclaimer:** The information provided in this chapter reflects payment and coding policies active at the time of publication. Medicare regulations are updated annually, and private insurer's policies are also subject to change. New regulations and payment policies are typically initiated at the start of the calendar year. The reader is advised to consult with individual private payers and review payment updates from CMS in November of each year in order to anticipate policy changes.

Can I Bill an Orthosis for a Patient Receiving Home Health Services?

Services provided to individuals under the care of a certified home health plan of care are paid to the Home Health Agency under the Consolidated billing rules. DME, including orthoses billed using the Level II HCPCS codes (L-Codes), are NOT included in consolidated billing. They can be billed directly by the therapist to their DME Medicare Administrative Contractor.

Can I Bill for Bilateral Orthoses?

Yes. The code should appear with "2" as the quantity and the both the RT and LT modifiers on the same billing line.

Will Medicare Pay for Two Orthoses for the Same Extremity?

Yes, as long as they are not the same code on the same part, i.e., two ring orthoses for the same digit.

What is a Cast Material Versus a Thermoplastic Material?

Casting materials are considered materials such as plaster of Paris or fiberglass.

   Thermoplastic materials can also include thermoplastic tapes such as Orficast and QuickCast. The product name uses the word cast; however, its properties are consistent with those of thermoplastic materials.

What Codes to Use for Cast Materials and Thermoplastic Tapes?

Casting material—CPT 29000 series.

Thermoplastic material/tape—L-Codes.

What Should a Therapist Consider or do When Coding for Multiple Adjustments or "New" Cast/Orthoses?

- Cost of materials: Thermoplastic material versus plaster/fiberglass materials
- Code reimbursement: What does an L-Code versus CPT Code reimburse?
- Check with your local DME MAC for coverage of L-Codes versus CPT codes
- Check with individual payer/plan coverage
- Find out what the patient's financial responsibility is (coinsurance, copay, DME deductibles, etc.)
- Check employer specific directives and policies on how they recommend coding for these services
- For Medicare, always be compliant with the 8-minute rule for CPT codes (97760, 97763)

INTRODUCTION

Fabrication of upper extremity orthoses requires a unique combination of the therapist's creative abilities and a sound knowledge of anatomical, biomechanical, physiologic, and healing principles as they relate to injury, surgery, and disease. Orthotic design and fabrication can be one of the most challenging and enjoyable aspects of being a therapist. Before delving into the fabrication process, therapists must develop a solid understanding of the clinical reasoning process for selecting the most appropriate orthosis for the patient, learn the physical skills required to manipulate the materials and must also be familiar with the recognized standard orthosis descriptions for consistent communication among all stakeholders.

   Regional and historical differences in nomenclature previously led to confusion and emphasized the need for development of a standard language that clearly and uniformly described an orthosis to those who refer, fabricate, use and/or pay for the device. The **American Society of Hand Therapists (ASHT)** recognized the importance of uniform terminology and in 1992 developed the **Splint Classification System (SCS)** that grouped orthoses into progressively more refined categories (American Society of Hand Therapists [ASHT], 1992). This detailed system clearly described the design, purpose, and direction of any applied force on the extremity. Unfortunately, the system was not adopted by payers. In 2006, ASHT created an L-Code task force which worked closely with **Centers for Medicare & Medicaid Services (CMS)** to improve code descriptors for custom fabricated upper extremity devices and aligned the codes with designs actually being used in clinical practice. The term *splint* had been used in medical professions, in particular the therapy world for decades. For coding purposes, CMS defines a splint as a device used in physicians' offices following reductions of fractures or dislocations, similar to a cast.

Billing/coding for splints uses different codes. The term *orthotic devices* (orthoses) was adopted in the 2008 **Durable Medical Equipment, Prosthetics, Orthotics, and Supplies (DMEPOS) Quality Standards** manual as the reimbursable language (CMS, 2008) and has been retained in the most recent version of the DMEPOS manual to date (CMS, 2018).

NOMENCLATURE: ORTHOSIS VERSUS SPLINT

DEFINITION
Orthosis

Orthotic Devices: Rigid and semirigid devices used for the purpose of supporting a weak or deformed body member or restricting or eliminating motion in a diseased or injured part of the body.

(CMS, 2008; Coverdale, 2012)

   An orthosis can also be used for prevention or correction of a deformity, maintain or improve alignment, improve or restrict motion, and ultimately to increase function.

- **Orthosis** is a noun and should be used in place of the word *splint.*
- **Orthoses** is a plural noun and should be used to replace the term for more than one orthosis.
- **Fabricating an orthosis** or orthotic fabrication should be used in place of the verb *splinting.*
- **Orthotic** is an adjective and is used to describe a noun associated with the science of orthotics, such as orthotic device, orthotic treatment plan, orthotic intervention, orthotic fabrication, or orthotic coding.

(ASHT, 2009)

This terminology should be used in all documentation and communication with physicians, payers, patients, and colleagues.

Orthotic devices are described by CMS using L-Codes that are found in the **Healthcare Common Procedure Coding System (HCPCS) Level II** manual. Additional codes have been added in the past few years including codes for two categories of prefabricated orthoses. Following CMS' lead, this group of codes has been adopted by payers. Chapter 9 goes into more detail on prefabricated orthoses and information on how to code for these products. While therapists and payers are aligned, some referring providers continue to use traditional names when ordering orthoses (e.g., thumb spica, wrist cock-up, etc.), so the task falls to therapists and orthotists to continue educating referring providers in order to achieve consistency with the use of *orthosis* as proper nomenclature.

REGULATORY CHALLENGES OVER THE YEARS

In 2000, orthotic and prosthetic quality concerns led to attempts to define standards of excellence for custom fabricated orthoses. A series of modifications of the Social Security Act of 1935 (SSA), which governs Medicare services, was mandated in legislation and passed over the last 20 years (Federal Register). These mandates included requirements to define quality standards, create independent accrediting organizations, and identify which providers and facilities were eligible to fabricate, dispense, and be compensated for providing orthoses and prostheses for Medicare beneficiaries. A committee was formed to determine how to implement these new regulations, but consensus was never reached, and the committee was dissolved. In 2009, the Health and Human Services (HHS) Secretary was given the right to exempt eligible professionals, including occupational therapists (OTs), physical therapists (PTs), and "other persons" such as orthotists and prosthetists from the quality standards and accreditation requirements.

In January 2017, CMS published a Proposed Rule (CMS-6012-P) clarifying requirements to qualify for payment for custom fabricated orthoses and prostheses. This regulation included requirements for facilities and providers and mandated that eligible providers must be either licensed by their state in orthotics, pedorthics, or prosthetics or certified by one of two organizations as Orthotists and/or Prosthetists in order to be compensated by Medicare for the provision of these devices. This led to multiple professional organizations joining together to contest the regulation. This grassroots advocacy effort resulted in withdrawal of the regulation in October of 2017 (Federal Register). While therapists were relieved, it is important to remember that the certification requirements remain law and the ability of OTs and PTs to be exempted from these requirements remains at the discretion of the HHS Secretary.

OTs and PTs have the educational background, clinical exposure, and clinical assessment/reasoning skills to design, fabricate, fit, and educate a client safely and effectively with an orthotic device. This education includes, but is not limited to, orthosis training, knowledge of anatomy, biomechanics, kinesiology, disease/injury processes (including surgical procedures and wound healing physiology), and the psychosocial aspects of injury/disease. There are no uniform standards or certifications for orthosis fabrication and fitting. While all states mention orthotics in Occupational Therapy Practice Acts, the language for Physical Therapists' Practice Acts is not uniformly clear. Both OTs and PTs should remain vigilant going

forward to adhere to the standards established by CMS and follow legislation and regulation impacting the provision of orthotics and prosthetics.

The lead author of this chapter has taken the ASHT SCS and the current CMS **L-Codes** and developed a simplified orthosis classification system: the **Modified Orthosis Classification System (MOCS)** to help guide organization and decision-making in this text. A comprehensive and detailed description of the expanded ASHT SCS can be found in *Rehabilitation of the Hand*, Sixth Edition (Fess, 2011). The reason for combining these two systems follows. Clinicians are responsible for correct orthosis coding, including documentation consistent with the billed code descriptors. These coding descriptions are frequently not sufficiently detailed to specify the design or purpose of the orthosis. In order to guide the aspiring clinician in the decision-making process, more detail is needed (Table 1–1; Fig. 1–1).

OVERVIEW OF ORTHOSIS CLASSIFICATION

This section is dedicated to assisting in proper L-Code selection and to promote consistency across our profession.

CMS does not reimburse for all published L-codes, and private payers *selectively* reimburse for orthoses. CMS publishes reimbursement rates quarterly for each code, and these rates vary by location. Private payers are free to establish their own fee schedules for orthoses and can establish different reimbursement rates for different plans. Each clinic/organization must abide by the contract they have with the individual insurance carriers and accept the negotiated rates that are mutually agreed upon through the contract period. Patients should be directed, whenever possible, to contact the insurance provider in advance of services provided, in order to be clear on possible out of pocket responsibility.

CHOOSING THE CORRECT L-CODE

Clinicians should ask the following questions when determining the correct L-Code for a specific orthosis.

Is the Orthosis Custom Fabricated or Prefabricated?

A custom fabricated orthosis is one designed for a specific patient and involves measuring, molding, cutting, assembling, etc. Prefabricated or "off-the-shelf" orthoses are broken down into two categories: (1) prefabricated, requiring minimal adjustment, and (2) prefabricated, expert adjustment required. The prefabricated orthoses are reimbursed at different rates to reflect the *expertise required* to apply them to the individual (refer to Chapter 9 for more detail).

What Body Parts Are Included in the Orthosis?

Orthoses codes are based on the extremity on which they are applied and further broken down to the segments and or joints affected by the orthosis. Upper extremity orthoses are coded based on whether they include the shoulder (S), elbow (E), wrist (W), hand (H), or fingers (F). Each joint or segment is recognized with the first letter of that joint. For example, "SO" would represent shoulder orthosis; "EO," elbow orthosis; "WHO," wrist and hand orthosis; etc. The combination of each letter will determine the structures that the orthosis crosses (refer to Table 1–3).

TABLE 1–1	**Relevant Terminology Definitions**
CMS	Centers for Medicare & Medicaid Services is a federal agency within the US Department of Health and Human Services that administers the Medicare program and works in partnership with state governments to administer Medicaid and other Such programs.
CPT	Current Procedural Terminology
	This refers to a number/code assigned to the majority of tasks and services a medical practitioner may provide to a patient. It is then linked to a determined amount of reimbursement by the insurer. Level II of the HCPCS is a standardized coding system that is used primarily to identify products, supplies, and other services *not* included in these CPT codes (such as orthoses). CPT codes are developed and published by the American Medical Association (AMA, 2018) and revised yearly.
DME	Durable Medical Equipment
	This is a term used to describe any medical equipment used in the home to aid in an improved quality of life. Examples are walkers, wheelchairs, power scooters, hospital beds, and home oxygen equipment. Clinicians often refer to orthoses as DME equipment; however, the proper terminology is DMEPOS.
DMEPOS	Durable Medical Equipment, Prosthetics, Orthotics, and Supplies
	Durable medical equipment is often referred to as DMEPOS because Medicare also covers prosthetics, orthotics, and certain supplies (POS). Prosthetics are devices that can replace a missing body part, such as a hand or leg. Orthotics are devices that help to immobilize, mobilize, or restrict a body part.
HCPCS	Healthcare Common Procedure Coding System
	HCPCS is a comprehensive, standardized system that classifies similar products that are medical in nature into categories for the purpose of efficient claim processing and ensures uniformity. It is used primarily to identify products, supplies, and services *not* included in the CPT codes, such as durable medical equipment, prosthetics, orthotics, and supplies (DMEPOS) when used outside a physician's office. Because Medicare and other insurers cover a variety of services, supplies, and equipment that are *not* identified by CPT codes, the level II HCPCS codes were established for submitting claims for these items.
L-Code	L-Codes describe orthoses by identifying which body parts they are used for (**S**, shoulder; **E**, elbow; **W**, wrist; **H**, hand; and **F**, finger), followed by the letter **O** for orthosis. They are also described as static (without joint) or dynamic (nontorsion joint and elastic bands and turnbuckles) and specify whether an orthosis is custom or prefabricated. The L-Code is the number linked to the specific description of a custom or prefabricated orthosis for proper communication to the insurance carrier.
MAC	Medicare Administrative Contractors
	L-Codes are not billed to CMS directly but rather through regional/jurisdiction MAC. There are currently four jurisdictions based on which region of the United States you are billing from.
Modifiers	A code added to the end of a CPT code to clarify the services and increase accuracy regarding what is being billed. Modifiers offer a way in which the service can be altered without changing the procedure code.
NPI	National Provider Identification number
	This is a unique 10-digit identification number issued to healthcare providers in the United States by CMS. This number is a required identifier for Medicare services and is used by other payers, including commercial healthcare insurers. All healthcare providers and facilities must obtain an NPI number to use in all standard transactions. Therefore, a clinician and/or facility must have this number in order to bill for orthotic services.
NSC	National Supplier Clearinghouse
	This organization processes the enrollment applications submitted by DMEPOS suppliers for their NSC (DMEPOS) number. This process is done online via PECOS enrollment.
PECOS	Provider Enrollment Chain Ownership System
	Allows DME suppliers to initially enroll for an NSC (DMEPOS) number, make changes to an existing number, update information (such as adding a new provider), check on the status of an application or reenroll online. Anyone wishing to become a Medicare provider must apply through PECOS. In addition, as the supplier of the **DMEPOS**, you will be denied payment **if** your referral source is not enrolled in PECOS.

Which current procedural terminology descriptors should I choose? How do I differentiate between immobilization and mobilization orthoses?

The CPT manual describes the differences in orthoses using the following language. Orthoses intended to

1. Immobilize a body part and/or joint(s) are described as being *without joint(s) or rigid.*
2. Mobilization: If the orthosis allows or encourages joint motion, the description will contain words such as "dynamic, double uprights, adjustable position locking joint, dynamic hinge, nontorsion joints," indicating there is at least one joint whose movement is influenced by the orthosis.

3. Mobilization with force applied: If additional force is applied to the included joint(s), the description may include "elastic bands, springs, or turnbuckles."

How do I Identify the Extremity in Which I Am Applying the Orthosis?

In order to identify the treated extremity, a ***modifier*** is required on the billing form to designate laterality: RT for right upper extremity and LT for the left upper extremity, and RTLT for bilateral orthoses. Table 1–2 lists the modifiers used to designate specific digits.

The L-Code includes orthosis evaluation, cost of base materials, time required for fabrication, fitting, and minor adjustments to the orthosis on subsequent visits. An evaluation CPT code

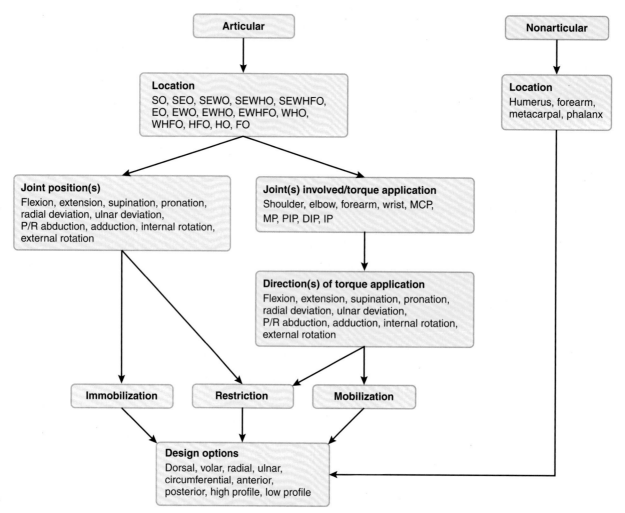

FIGURE 1–1 **The authors recommended Modified Orthosis Classification System (MOCS).** Note that the Centers for Medicare & Medicaid Services (CMS) does not recognize the thumb as a separate body part. The thumb is classified as F, the same distinction used for the index, middle, ring, and small digits.

(97165-97167 for OTs or 97161-97163 for PTs) should only be coded at the time of orthotic fabrication/dispensing if additional evaluation procedures are performed as part of an ongoing treatment plan.

Orthotics and prosthetics management and training codes are additional CPT codes that can be used to describe and receive reimbursement for additional services for adjustments, training, and fitting of an orthosis or prosthesis. The code 97760 may be used during the *initial* orthosis fabrication visit in addition to the L-Code *only* if training goes above and beyond what is considered customary or when assessment and fitting are otherwise not reported (CMS, 2018). This code can also be used for a therapist to assess and adjust the fit of an orthosis even if it was issued prior

by a physician or fabricated by another provider. Because this is the initial encounter for this provider, the 97760 code can be used. This CPT code should not be used for basic and routine training for use and care. It is imperative that documentation justifies why the additional training time was necessary and what that training entailed. The code 97761 can be used for the initial encounter for prosthetic training. On subsequent visits, 97763 can be used if additional orthosis or prosthesis training or modification(s) are needed. For example, if a patient returns for education, modifications and/or adjustments due to tissue changes the 97763 would be the appropriate code to use. The orthotic and prosthetic management and training codes (97760, 97761, 97763) are **timed** codes and reflect the time spent in providing the additional services. For

TABLE 1–2	**Digit Modifiers**			
LEFT HAND			**RIGHT HAND**	
Thumb	FA		Thumb	F5
Index	F1		Index	F6
Middle	F2		Middle	F7
Ring	F3		Ring	F8
Small	F4		Small	F9

TABLE 1–3	**Key to Anatomical Headings**
SEWHFO	Shoulder, elbow, wrist, hand, finger/thumb Orthosis
SEWHO	Shoulder, elbow, wrist, hand orthosis
SEO	Shoulder, elbow orthosis
EWO	Elbow, wrist orthosis
EWHFO	Elbow, wrist, hand, finger/thumb orthosis
EWHO	Elbow, wrist, hand orthosis
WHFO	Wrist, hand, finger/thumb orthosis
WHO	Wrist, hand orthosis
HFO	Hand, finger/thumb orthosis
SO	Shoulder orthosis
EO	Elbow orthosis
HO	Hand orthosis
FO	Finger/thumb orthosis

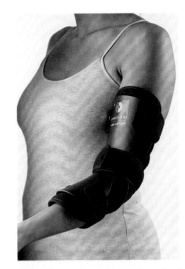

FIGURE 1–2 Immobilization prefabricated orthosis (EO). L3762 EO, rigid, without joints, includes soft interface material, prefabricated, and includes fitting and adjustment. The Ventral Cubital Tunnel Splint positions elbow in slightly flexed position to relieve stress on the cubital tunnel region. (Photo courtesy of Corflex Inc (Manchester, NH).)

these CPT codes, the treating clinician must document and support the services provided such as education, training, instruction, and modifications.

The following coding examples include the anatomical headings (Table 1–3) and the CMS descriptions of the corresponding L-Codes. In the coding examples (Figs. 1–2 to 1–5), the actual numerical number associated with that L-Code description (e.g., L3908) has been recommended.

When a therapist receives a referral for a patient who is covered by Medicare with the diagnosis of bilateral distal radius fractures and the prescription is for bilateral wrist orthoses, evaluation, and treatment, if all services are performed at the initial encounter with the patient, the clinician can code for an evaluation CPT code as well as treatment CPT codes, which are billed directly to CMS. The L-Code (L3906 in this example) is billed using modifiers RT and LT to denote that two orthoses that were fabricated, one for the right and one for the left upper extremities. The L-Codes are billed to the **National Supplier Clearinghouse (NSC)** via regional **Medicare Administrative Contractors (MACs)** instead of directly to CMS and require that the provider have a supplier number, also known as a DMEPOS number. Therapists apply for this DMEPOS number via the Internet through the **Provider Enrollment, Chain and Ownership System (PECOS)**. The therapist would also perform an evaluation and develop a treatment plan for the additional medically necessary services identified by the evaluation. If the referral was *only* for bilateral wrist orthoses, then the therapist would not perform the evaluation or bill the evaluation CPT code but only the WHO (L3906) code using the right and left modifiers.

CHALLENGES IN THE USE OF L-CODES

There are some challenges using the L-Code terminology. Because of the vast possibilities of designs, it is impossible to have a unique code description for every orthosis. If a code cannot be found to match up with the orthosis fabricated, then the code that *best* describes the orthosis should be chosen. Clear, proper, and meticulous documentation must justify this choice.

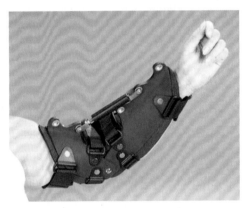

FIGURE 1–3 Mobilization prefabricated orthosis (EO). L3760 EO, with adjustable position locking joint(s), prefabricated, includes fitting and adjustments, any type; Turnbuckle elbow orthosis. (Photo courtesy of Tiburon Medical Enterprises, Inc (San Jacinto, CA).)

For example, there is no code that accounts for using an immobilization orthosis to function as a static progressive (mobilization) device that can be sequentially adjusted over several treatment sessions. The CPT code 97763 may be used when it is necessary to serially modify the immobilization orthosis in order to provide a mobilizing force. Remember that this code is considered a *timed code* based on 15-minute increments. Consistent with **all** timed codes billed to Medicare, the service performed must take a minimum of 8 minutes in order to be billing eligible.

An additional challenge is the limited options for codes describing nonarticular orthoses, with the exception of a hand orthosis (HO) that can be used for midshaft metacarpal fractures or a finger orthosis (FO) such as a pulley ring. Therefore, if a therapist fabricates a custom humeral orthosis to protect a midshaft humeral fracture, then the code chosen for billing would have to closely describe this orthosis. A choice could be a custom-fabricated immobilization orthosis or L3671 shoulder orthosis (SO); "shoulder joint design, without joints, may include soft interface, straps, custom fabricated, and includes fitting and adjustments" (HCPCS, 2019). Even though the description actually states it immobilizes the shoulder joint, it is the closest description offered. Details regarding the rationale for the specific code choice should be noted in the medical record (Fig. 1–6).

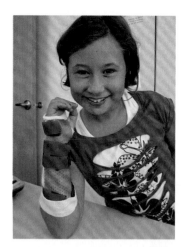

FIGURE 1–4 Immobilization custom-fabricated orthosis (WHO). L3906
WHO, without joints, may include soft interface, straps, custom fabricated, includes fitting and adjustment.

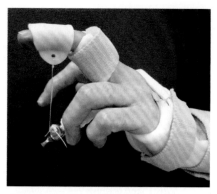

FIGURE 1–5 Mobilization custom-fabricated orthosis (WHFO). L3806
WHFO, includes one of more nontorsion joint(s), turnbuckles, elastic bands/ springs, may include soft interface material, straps, custom fabricated, includes fitting and adjustment. This is using the Merit™ component. WHFO, wrist, hand, finger orthosis.

Orthoses may be coded using the same L-Codes, but the goal for each may be quite different. If these goals are not clearly documented, the orthoses may be at risk for denial. An example would be a WHFO applied to protect a flexor tendon repair and a WHFO designed to progressively lengthen the repaired tendons once danger of rupture has passed. Both are coded as L3808 but have different placement, design, and goals. In general, duplicate codes for the same site during a single episode of care will be denied and the clinician should expect an appeal will be needed. As stated previously, documentation is crucial to distinguish the differences between the orthoses. The authors strongly recommend obtaining a signed photographic release and including photos of the completed orthosis in the patient record.

The third edition of this book has adopted the terminology put forth by CMS while addressing historical nomenclature in the orthosis pattern section of this book, under *common names*. The editors and contributors of this publication strongly believe that unified terminology is paramount when referring to orthoses in every aspect of our professions. Weaved throughout this chapter, the reader will find examples of CMS language (WHO, SO, etc.) and in Figures 1–2 to 1–5 corresponding L-Codes for the orthosis described. The reader must note that the L-Codes described in this chapter are only discussed in this chapter as examples and are reflective of the time of this publication. L-Codes can be changed or altered by CMS at any time. It is important to keep current with individual insurance carrier changes (including CMS) and the associated reimbursements. It is the authors' intent to continually reinforce the important relationship between documentation and billing.

SUMMARY OF THE MODIFIED ORTHOSIS CLASSIFICATION SYSTEM

ARTICULAR AND NONARTICULAR ORTHOSES

Orthoses are divided into two broad groups: **articular** and **nonarticular**. Articular orthoses are those that cross one or more joints. Nonarticular orthoses provide support and protection to a healing bone (e.g., humerus, metacarpal, or phalanx) or to a soft tissue structure (e.g., annular pulley or musculotendinous junction of the medial or lateral epicondyle). There are far fewer nonarticular orthoses than articular orthoses (Fig. 1–7).

When interpreting a referral, it is advantageous to distinguish between articular and nonarticular orthoses so that a joint is not unnecessarily immobilized. For example, if the word *nonarticular* does not precede the words *proximal forearm immobilization orthosis* on the referral, then the therapist may assume that the elbow and/or wrist needs to be included in the design. By adding the word *nonarticular*, the description becomes far more specific. In the pattern section of this book, the articular orthoses are separated from the nonarticular to aid in pattern location; the term *articular* does not need to appear in the description because the name of the orthosis (e.g., wrist immobilization orthosis or WHO) indicates whether a joint is included. However, the term *nonarticular* does need to appear in the descriptions (e.g., nonarticular humerus orthosis or SO L3671 and nonarticular metacarpal orthosis or HO L3919), so there is no ambiguity as in Figures 1–6 and 1–7. Note: for billing purposes, the CMS codes chosen here are the best choice (to this publication date) available to describe these devices for reimbursement.

LOCATION

Location, the next level in the MOCS, refers to the joint, set of joints, or body part on which the orthosis acts according to its main intent. Therefore, in order to simplify naming, if there are several joints

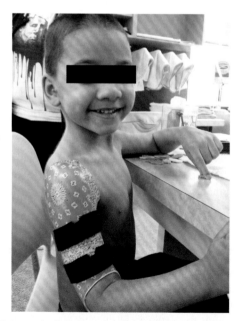

FIGURE 1–6 Nonarticular humerus orthosis (SO). A humeral fracture brace used to stabilize and protect a healing midshaft humerus fracture. Although labeled as nonarticular, the orthosis partially crosses the shoulder joint. The most appropriate L-Code is L3671.

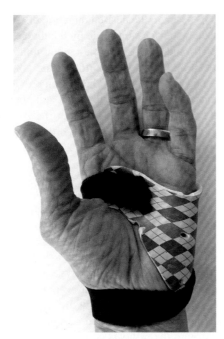

FIGURE 1−7 Nonarticular hand orthosis (HO). A hand immobilization orthosis for treatment of a midshaft fifth metacarpal fracture; the pressure applied through the volar-dorsal nature of this device during fabrication minimizes the tendency for the bone fragments to shift. The most appropriate L-Code is L3919. (Printed thermoplastic material courtesy of Kinetec® (Jackson, WI).)

involved, as commonly seen after a severe crushing injury to the hand, MOCS groups the joints together. For example, if a crush injury involves all the metacarpophalangeal (MCP), proximal interphalangeal (PIP), and distal interphalangeal (DIP) joints, the proper name would be a hand and digit immobilization orthosis or HFO. If the crush injury involves the three joints of only the middle finger (MF), then the orthosis is described as a digit immobilization orthosis or FO.

Nonarticular orthoses are described in much the same way. For example, an orthosis used to immobilize a fifth metacarpal fracture is described as a nonarticular fifth metacarpal orthosis or HO (Fig. 1–7). Similarly, an orthosis used to protect a recently reconstructed annular pulley is described as a nonarticular proximal phalanx orthosis or FO (Fig. 1–8).

JOINT(S) INVOLVED/TORQUE APPLICATION

A mobilization orthosis may require immobilization support of adjacent joints or, occasionally, mobilization in more than one direction *within* the same orthosis. When noting the anatomical locations

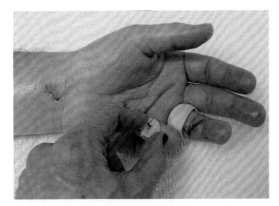

FIGURE 1−8 Nonarticular proximal phalanx orthosis (FO). This circumferential designed orthosis provides protection to a recently reconstructed A2 annular pulley.

that the orthosis crosses, it is imperative to note which joint(s) are immobilized and which joint(s) have torque applied to them. An example would be managing metacarpal phalangeal (MCP) joint extension contractures after a distal radius fracture. The wrist may require continued immobilization, whereas the MCPs would benefit from flexion mobilization, as shown in Figure 1–24. This orthosis would be noted for billing as a WHFO (L3806), and the written documentation would reflect a statement such as "wrist extension immobilization, MCP flexion mobilization orthosis." A mobilization orthosis may also require torque application to more than one joint and in different directions. An example would be managing a claw hand deformity from a long-standing ulnar nerve injury where the patient exhibits MCP extension and interphalangeal (IP) flexion contractures. The joint torque in this case would be applied to the MCPs in the direction of flexion and simultaneously to the IPs in the direction of extension. This orthosis would be noted for billing as an HFO (L3921) and for documentation as a small finger and ring finger (SF/RF) MCP flexion/IP extension mobilization orthosis.

DIRECTION

The **direction** descriptor, the next level in the MOCS, refers to the position of the primary joint in an immobilization orthosis, the joint boundary of a restrictive orthosis, and the direction of torque in a mobilization orthosis. The direction descriptor provides critical information necessary for accurately fabricating the orthosis. Prior to fabrication, the specific purpose of the orthosis must be known before the therapist can add the direction descriptor. Direction defines the position of the involved joints (immobilization orthosis), the desired direction of the mobilizing force (mobilization orthosis), or the direction in which motion is to be blocked (restriction orthosis). For example, by adding a direction term (e.g., RF PIP extension orthosis), the orthosis' intent is further clarified, in this case by indicating that the joint is to be extended. As noted in the next section—by then following "direction" by the use of the words *immobilization, mobilization,* or *restriction*—there will be even more clear information about what that direction really means: is it to gain PIP extension (mobilize), to rest (immobilize) the PIP in extension, or to block a portion of PIP extension (restriction)?

INTENT: IMMOBILIZATION, MOBILIZATION, AND RESTRICTION

Intent, the next level of the MOCS, refers to the overall function or primary purpose of the orthosis, which is generally **immobilization, mobilization,** or **restriction.** Adding the orthosis' purpose to the description provides the fabricator with a clearer understanding of what is being requested. For example, a prescription for an RF PIP extension mobilization orthosis tells the fabricator that an extension force needs to be exerted on the PIP joint of the RF. The purpose of an RF PIP extension immobilization orthosis, on the other hand, is to immobilize the PIP joint in extension. Finally, an RF PIP extension restriction orthosis restricts full extension of the PIP joint but allows active flexion (as often requested for management of a finger with a swan-neck deformity).

In the pattern section of this book, the orthoses are organized according to their most common purpose, although additional functions are also defined. For example, the RF PIP immobilization orthosis is discussed in Chapter 1 of the Fabrication Manual. However, because it is essentially the same pattern used for an RF PIP extension mobilization orthosis (serial static design), this use is referenced under the heading "Additional Functions." The cross-reference list provided in this book will also help in quick pattern location.

DESIGN DESCRIPTORS

The design descriptor improves understanding of the type of orthosis that is requested. In this text, the descriptors are used as an aid whenever necessary. Design descriptors include non-MOCS nomenclature that is still widely used by hand surgery and hand therapy specialists throughout the world; some examples are *gutter*, *spica*, *static*, *dynamic*, *static progressive*, and *serial static*. These terms are discussed separately later in this chapter.

In the MOCS, design descriptors, which are selectively included, appear in parentheses after the name of the orthosis. In this book, however, the descriptors are most often found at the beginning of the name to help readers with critical thinking and decision-making processes. The descriptive terms include the following:

- Digit-based: Originating from the digit, allowing MCP joint motion, and possibly extending to the distal phalanx
- Hand-based: Originating from the hand, allowing wrist motion, and possibly extending to the distal phalanx
- Thumb-based: Originating from the thenar eminence or thumb and incorporating one or more joints of the thumb
- Forearm-based: Originating from the forearm, allowing full elbow motion, and possibly extending to the distal phalanx
- Arm-based: Originating from the upper arm and possibly including the wrist, elbow, and/or shoulder joints
- Circumferential: Encompassing the entire perimeter of a body part
- Gutter: Including only the radial or ulnar portion of a body part
- Radial: Incorporating the radial aspect of a body part
- Ulnar: Incorporating the ulnar aspect of a body part
- Dorsal: Traversing the dorsal aspect of the hand or forearm
- Volar: Traversing the volar aspect of the hand or forearm
- Anterior: Traversing the anterior aspect of the elbow and upper arm
- Posterior: Traversing the posterior aspect of the elbow and upper arm

NON-MODIFIED ORTHOSIS CLASSIFICATION SYSTEM NOMENCLATURE

The widely used terms *static*, *serial static*, *dynamic*, and *static progressive* are not included in the MOCS. These terms designate choices of designs that a therapist can incorporate to achieve immobilization, mobilization, or restriction of the intended structure(s). These choices are noted under "Common Names" in the pattern section of this book and are listed in the book's index.

Static Orthoses

Static orthoses have a firm base and immobilize the joint(s) they cross. They can be used to facilitate dynamic functions, for example, by blocking one joint to encourage movement of another. In some cases, a static orthosis is considered to be nonarticular—having no direct influence on joint mobility—while providing stabilization, protection, and support to a body segment, such as the humerus or metacarpal. Static orthoses are the most common orthoses that therapists are called upon to make. They can be used as an alternative to mobilization devices when ease of application and compliance are potential issues (Riggs, Lyden, & Chung, 2011). An example of this would be using a simple wrist immobilization orthosis instead of a more complicated mobilization orthosis to support a radial nerve injury.

Serial Static Orthoses

Serial static orthoses or casts are applied with the tissue at its near maximum length; they are worn for long periods to accommodate elongation of soft tissue in the desired direction of correction. They are remolded or new devices are made by the therapist to maintain the joint(s), soft tissue, and/or muscle-tendon units they cross in a lengthened position. Serial static orthoses are constructed to be circumferential and nonremovable. This option provides for greater patient compliance and assures the therapist and physician that the tissue is being continually stressed without the risk of the tissue rebounding, which could happen if the orthoses were removed (Brand & Thompson, 1993; Colditz, 2011a; Schultz-Johnson, 2003a).

Dynamic Orthoses

Dynamic orthoses generate a mobilizing or supportive force on a targeted tissue that results in passive gains or passive-assisted range of motion (ROM) (Fess & Phillips, 1987; Glascow, Tooth, Fleming, & Peters, 2011). Dynamic orthoses have a static base that provides the foundation for some type of outrigger attachment. Controlled mobilizing forces are applied via a dynamic (elastic) assist, which may include but are not limited to rubber bands, springs, neoprene, or wrapped elastic cord. The dynamic force applied through the orthosis continues as long as the elastic component can contract, even when the shortened tissue reaches the end of its elastic limit (Schultz-Johnson, 1992, 2003b). As soon as appropriate, dynamic forces should be applied to the targeted tissue because this provides better opportunity for contracture resolution and/or tissue elongation. The less mature the scar tissue, the better the tissue will respond to the intermittent force application of a dynamic orthosis (Colditz, 2011b; Glascow et al., 2011). Mature, dense scar tends to respond more favorably to a prolonged static progressive force (Colditz, 2011b). A dynamic orthosis can also be used as an active-resistive exercise modality against its line of pull.

Static Progressive Orthoses

Static progressive orthoses achieve mobilization by applying unidirectional, low-load force to the tissue's maximum end ROM until the tissue accommodates. Construction is similar to dynamic orthoses, except these use nonelastic components to deliver the mobilizing force, including, but not limited to nylon cord, strapping materials, screws, hinges, turnbuckles, and nonelastic tape (Sueoka & DeTemple, 2011). Once the joint position and tension are set, the orthosis does not continue to stress the tissue beyond its elastic limit (Schultz-Johnson, 1992, 2003a, 2003b). The force can be modified only through progressive adjustments. Some patients may tolerate static progressive application better than dynamic application, perhaps because the joint position is constant while the tissue readily accommodates to the tension and is less subject to the influences of gravity and motion (Colditz, 2011b; Schultz-Johnson, 1992, 1996, 2002, 2003b).

FUNCTION OF ORTHOSES AND OBJECTIVES FOR INTERVENTION

This section reviews the objectives for orthotic intervention and provides appropriate clinical examples for immobilization, mobilization, and restriction. Remember that not all orthoses can be simply classified, and the primary objective may not always be clear-cut. There may be multiple objectives for orthotic intervention. For example, a wrist/hand immobilization orthosis (WHFO) for a patient with rheumatoid arthritis may be designed to immobilize inflamed arthritic joints while placing the MCP joints in near extension and a gentle radially deviated position to minimize ulnar drift and periarticular deformity.

The discussion that follows covers general and common examples to emphasize how critical thinking is necessary when fabricating orthoses. Experienced therapists recognize that managing complex injuries requires much overlap and problem-solving in order to determine the best approach.

IMMOBILIZATION ORTHOSES

Although the **immobilization orthosis** is the most common and simplest form of orthotic intervention, it can be used for the most complex of injuries. Static orthoses are considered immobilization orthoses because they do not allow motion of the joints to which they are applied. Immobilization orthoses can be considered either articular or nonarticular, immobilizing the joints they cross (articular), or stabilizing the structure to which they are applied (nonarticular), as in the case of a humerus orthosis (Fig. 1–6).

The common objectives for immobilization are as follows:

- Provide symptom relief after injury or overuse
- Protect and properly position edematous structure(s)
- Aid in maximizing functional use of the hand
- Maintain tissue length to prevent soft tissue contracture
- Protect healing structures and surgical procedures
- Maintain and protect reduction of a fracture
- Protect and improve joint alignment
- Block or transfer power of movement to enhance exercise
- Reduce tone and contracture of a spastic muscle

These objectives and examples of orthotic intervention are discussed in the following sections.

Provide Symptom Relief

An immobilization orthosis can provide significant pain relief when applied as soon as possible after injury or even after prolonged functional activity. The injured or fatigued structures should be placed in a resting, nonstressed position, minimizing movement that can influence pain (Callegari, Resende, & Filho, 2018). This orthosis is initially worn day and night and may be removed for only short periods of exercise and hygiene. After the initial symptoms have subsided, orthosis use is decreased; eventually, the orthosis may be used only for preventing the risk of reinjury. For example, a person who has sustained a wrist sprain may present with exquisite pain when wrist motion is attempted. The use of a wrist immobilization orthosis (WHO custom or prefabricated) is appropriate for approximately 1 month or until pain subsides. After the period of immobilization, the orthosis may be used for only sleeping and/or at-risk activities (Fig. 1–9).

EXAMPLE: WRIST/HAND IMMOBILIZATION ORTHOSIS (WHFO) (Fig. 1–9).

A wrist/thumb immobilization orthosis (WHFO) can assist in decreasing inflammation and pain within the first dorsal compartment (deQuervain's tenosynovitis) by preventing simultaneous wrist ulnar deviation and thumb flexion. The wrist is positioned in neutral to 20° extension with 0° to 5° of ulnar deviation. This position keeps the extensor pollicis brevis (EPB) and the abductor pollicis longus (APL) tendons in alignment with the radius as they exit the pulley about the radial styloid (Eaton, 1992). The thumb carpometacarpal (CMC) joint is positioned in slight abduction, and the MP joint is included in a slightly flexed, comfortable position (Fig. 1–10). The orthosis is generally worn full time for 3 to 4 weeks, and then use is gradually reduced to

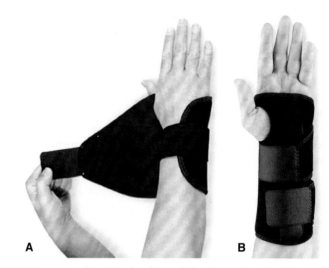

FIGURE 1–9 **A** and **B, Wrist/hand immobilization orthosis (WHO).** A simple prefabricated wrist orthosis can be used to stabilize a painful wrist when a custom design is not warranted or feasible. Shown here is the Modabber™ wrist orthosis which has an adjustable volar stay. (Photo courtesy of Hely & Weber (Dallas, TX).)

nights only once the day symptoms have resolved. The orthosis is discontinued when the patient is asymptomatic to provocative (painful) positioning.

EXAMPLE: WRIST/THUMB IMMOBILIZATION ORTHOSIS (WHFO) (Fig. 1–10).

Protect and Position Edematous Structures

Edema is often the first observable reaction to injury yet not always the first addressed. Its immediate reduction is critical to facilitate proper healing with minimal complications (such as tight joint capsules and ligaments, which could lead to joint and soft tissue contracture). An edematous hand may be a painful hand that has associated injuries that must be considered before orthosis application. For

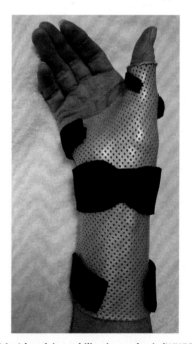

FIGURE 1–10 **Wrist/thumb immobilization orthosis (WHFO).** Immobilization of the thumb and wrist can provide relief for a patient with acute deQuervain's tenosynovitis.

example, consider fabricating an orthosis that places the digital joints in a safe position (MCP flexion, IP extension) and can be donned and doffed easily to allow access for wound or pin care. Attention to joint positioning in the orthosis, elevation, massage, compression wraps, and gentle active ROM of adjacent structures (if appropriate) all contribute to reducing edema and preventing deformity (e.g., MCP extension and PIP flexion contractures).

Compression bandages or gloves (e.g., Coban™ and Isotoner® gloves) can be worn under the orthosis for edema reduction and can complement the device's effectiveness. As noted in Figure 1–11C, a light compressive tubular stockinette is applied to a recent repair of the small finger FDS tendon. This stockinette also assists in keeping the gauze bandages against the incision site (Fig. 1–11B) and makes for a less bulky dressing.

Caution is necessary when donning and doffing these compression devices to avoid inadvertently moving the involved tissues to a harmful position or causing reinjury of the healing bones, tendons, and/or ligaments. The therapist must also consider the type and placement of the straps that will be used. A narrow strap placed across an edematous area may cause pooling of edema proximal and distal to the strap and may irritate superficial sensory nerves. Circumferentially wrapping or encompassing the orthosis, distal to proximal, with an elasticized wrap or compressive garment (e.g., Ace™ wrap, elasticized stockinette, or Coban™) may help distribute pressure evenly along the extremity and aid in minimizing edema.

In addition, patient education regarding the importance of the use of an orthosis, in conjunction with other edema management methods, facilitates early reduction of edema. Crush injuries are often complex and may involve one or more structures, including bone, ligament, tendon, and nerve. Patients often do well during the initial stages of healing with a simple wrist/hand/thumb immobilization orthosis to keep the involved structures positioned, supported, and protected. Therapists working with these patients should strive to achieve optimal joint positioning. One of the most important goals is to maintain the antideformity position of the hand (also referred to as the intrinsic plus or safe position): MCP flexion, IP extension, and thumb palmar abduction. If this is not accomplished early after injury, MCP joint collateral ligament shortening and PIP joint volar plate contracture may occur, which can result in MCP extension and PIP flexion contractures. Optimal joint positions may be difficult to achieve initially owing to stiffness, pain, and significant edema. Be persistent, fabricate the orthosis within a comfortable ROM, monitor, and serially adjust the orthosis as pain and healing allows (Fig. 1–11A).

EXAMPLE: WRIST/HAND/THUMB IMMOBILIZATION ORTHOSIS (WHFO) (Fig. 1–11).

Aid in Maximizing Functional Use

An orthosis can enhance function by correctly positioning and supporting structures that are injured or unstable. During the day, these supportive, lightweight, functional orthoses can often help patients use their hands to engage in vocational, academic, or recreational activities. Without support, function is diminished, and deforming forces may dominate. Figure 1–12A–D shows a patient with advanced scleroderma and how a small, light orthosis can allow the simple act of turning a key. These orthoses can be fabricated to position and support with minimal bulk. The bulkier the orthosis, the more likely it will interfere with functional use.

EXAMPLE: INDEX FINGER RADIAL DEVIATION ORTHOSIS (HFO) (Fig. 1–12).

A thumb CMC joint that presents subluxed and painful when a pinch is attempted may benefit from the use of a well-molded first

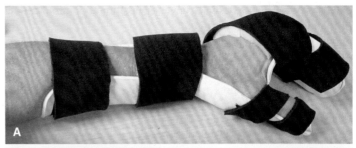
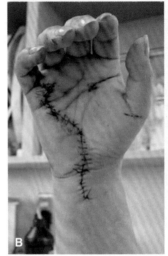
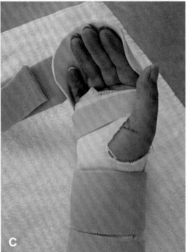

FIGURE 1–11 A–C, Wrist/hand/thumb immobilization orthosis (WHFO). A, Traditionally named a "resting hand splint," this simple device can provide the support, proper positioning (MCP flexion, IP extension, thumb palmar abduction), and healing environment that crush injuries require. **B,** Postoperative SF FDS and FDP repair. **C, Wrist/hand immobilization orthosis (WHFO)**—Dorsal design. The elasticized stockinette underneath this orthosis allows for gentle compression to the incision site and assists in securing the surgical dressing. The elastic nature of the stockinette allows for execution of the postoperative protocol, in this case PROM to the involved digits within the orthosis.

CMC immobilization orthosis (Colditz, 1995a; Sillem, Backman, Miller, & Li, 2011; Gil, Ebert, & Blanchard, 2019). Function and comfort are gained by careful attention to molding and pressure distribution about the base of the first metacarpal bone and the CMC joint. These types of orthoses (rigid or soft) offer a degree of stabilization to the thumb CMC joint and places the first metacarpal bone in a better anatomical position of abduction. Small devices can significantly relieve pain during active use of the thumb and enable the patient to grasp and pinch more effectively (Fig. 1–13A,B).

EXAMPLE: THUMB CMC IMMOBILIZATION ORTHOSIS (HFO) (Fig. 1–13).

Maintain Tissue Length

Orthoses can preserve tissue length when applied carefully and accurately, within the appropriate time frame. Contractures of soft tissue can occur from many sources. One such cause is nerve injury, resulting in muscle-tendon imbalances in the hand. Left untreated, these imbalances often result in tendon-ligament shortening, which in turn may create some degree of joint contracture.

During the initial stages of injury, the goal for orthotic intervention should be to place the joints in a position that inhibits tissue shortening and enables functional use. During the end stages of scar maturation (3-6 months or longer), the goal would be to keep the tissue at its achieved maximum length to prevent regression of tissue tightness (Genova, Lester, & Walsh, 2010; McFarlane, 1997). At this stage, the orthosis is not influencing the tissue length but is maintaining the desired and previously achieved ROM. Gains

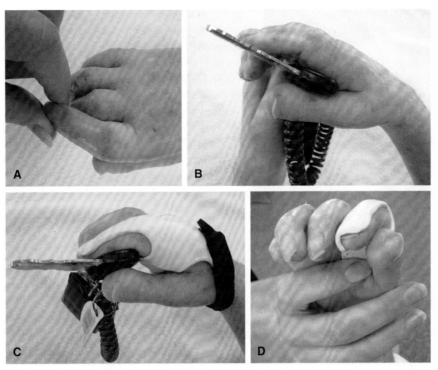

FIGURE 1-12 A-D, Digit immobilization orthosis (HFO). A, Severe MCP/PIP instability and ulnar deformity of the index finger makes it nearly impossible for this patient with scleroderma to turn a key **(B)**. **C,** A small orthosis holding the index finger in neutral deviation allows for a stable post for the thumb to hold the key against. **D,** Note how the material wraps along the ulnar border, keeping the volar-radial border free for tactile input.

attained in therapy sessions and at home can be maintained with a balanced program of proper immobilization and exercise.

Adduction contractures of the thumb can occur after injury to or repair of the median nerve. To prevent this, an orthosis should be applied as soon as possible after nerve repair. The orthosis can be forearm-based, with the wrist slightly flexed, intimately molded into the first web space, and extending distally to the thumb IP joint crease. Care should be taken to avoid undue stress on the ulnar collateral ligament of the thumb MP joint during fabrication. This orthosis position maintains the thumb in maximum abduction, preventing a possible adduction contracture while placing the nerve repair in a shortened position to allow for healing (Fig. 1–14A). As the nerve heals and greater extension of the wrist is allowed, a small hand-based device can be made to fit over a wrist immobilization orthosis. This can be worn at night to maintain tissue length of the first web space. Another option that can be considered when trying to prevent web space contracture is a small orthosis that maintains maximum

palmar abduction but allows for intermittent exercise of adjacent joints as healing progress. This may be an option as patients begin to attempt functional use of the hand (Fig. 1–14B). The goal of these orthoses is to prevent an adduction contracture of the first web space.

EXAMPLE: WRIST/THUMB CMC PALMAR ABDUCTION IMMOBILIZATION ORTHOSIS (WHFO) (Fig. 1–14).

Protect Healing Structures and Surgical Procedures

A therapist may be called on to fabricate an immobilization orthosis to rest and protect an extremity that has undergone an operative procedure (Fig. 1–15A–E). This may involve a simple orthosis or an intricate one that must immobilize several structures in specific positions because of a complex injury or surgical repair. For postoperative orthotic fabrication, close communication with the surgeon is critical to guide proper selection of orthosis. Consideration needs to be given to fabricating the orthosis around or over drains, wounds,

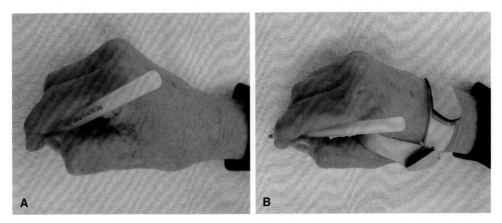

FIGURE 1-13 A and B, Thumb immobilization orthosis (HFO). A, Note the thumb posture before application of the orthosis. **B,** A thumb CMC immobilization orthosis is being used for stabilization of this joint while writing is attempted. This small device is only one of many design options available that can help prevent subluxation of the first CMC joint during functional use.

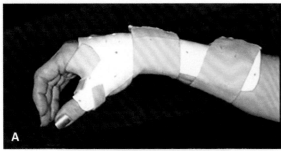

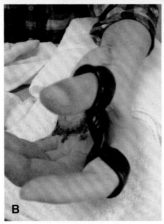

FIGURE 1–14 A and B, Wrist/thumb CMC palmar abduction immobilization orthosis (WHFO). A, This immobilization orthosis used to prevent adduction contractures of the first web space after median nerve injury or repair. It can be fabricated to incorporate the wrist and first web space as shown here. **B, Palmar abduction orthosis (FO).** This removable orthosis acts as a spacer to maintain palmar abduction while engaging in functional use or therapeutic exercise.

external pins, or skin grafts. These issues, as well as the pain level and psychological trauma of injury and surgery, make fabrication of the orthosis in the postoperative extremity quite a challenge.

Support, comfort, and protection of a patient's hand after a Dupuytren's contracture release can be achieved by using a hand immobilization orthosis. This orthosis is applied after the bulky dressing is removed, new hand and digit dressings are reapplied, and the orthosis is then fabricated over these dressings. The patient is able to take the device off and perform the exercise regime dictated by the therapist/surgeon (Fig. 1–15A–C). As shown in Figure 1–15D,E, an orthosis can be fabricated to protect external hardware from environment insults or harm. The patient is instructed in pin and wound care and, along with careful donning and doffing of the orthosis.

EXAMPLE: HAND/DIGIT IMMOBILIZATION ORTHOSIS (HFO) (Fig. 1–15).

Maintain and Protect Reduction of a Fracture

An orthosis can provide fracture stabilization and maintain reduction when applied by an experienced therapist and supervised by a physician. There are times when casting is not appropriate for a patient and an orthosis can be used as an alternative. The use of thermoplastic material can often provide an intimate fit around detailed areas, such as the metacarpal heads and phalanges, which may be harder to achieve with traditional casting materials. Some patients are more comfortable with the lighter thermoplastic material and better functional use of the hand that comes with orthotic intervention versus casting.

Stable fractures, such as some fifth metacarpal fractures, may be treated effectively with an RF-SF MCP immobilization orthosis (Fig. 1–16A,B). This type of orthosis, when molded intimately

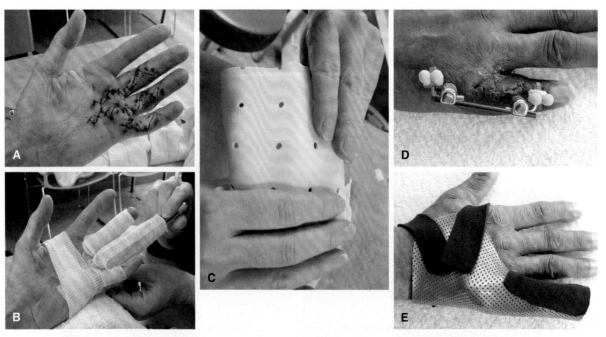

FIGURE 1–15 A–C, Hand/digit immobilization orthosis (HFO). An orthosis is applied after a Dupuytren's contracture release to support the MCP and IP joints of the involved digits in comfortable extension postoperatively. **A,** Following postoperative dressing removal. **B,** Dressings are applied. **C,** Thermoplastic material is applied over the dressings and molded at the patient's tolerable digit extension end range. **Hand/digit protection immobilization orthosis (HFO). D,** Postoperative external fixator for comminuted fifth proximal phalanx fracture. **E,** Orthosis molded directly over area to protect the vulnerable region.

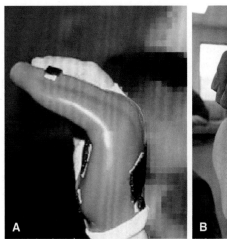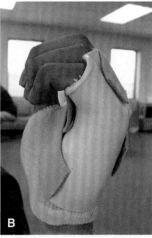

FIGURE 1–16 **A** and **B, RF-SF MCP flexion/IP extension immobilization orthosis (HFO). A,** An orthosis used for treatment of a fifth metacarpal head fracture with concomitant PIP joint sprain. The pressure applied through the volar-dorsal nature of this device during the molding process minimizes the tendency for the bone fragments to shift. **RF-SF MCP flexion immobilization orthosis (HFO). B,** A similar orthosis used to stabilize a nondisplaced fifth metacarpal head fracture (boxer's fracture), allowing unimpeded motion of the IP joints.

and carefully, provides continued alignment and protection for the healing fracture, maintains the RF-SF MCP collateral ligaments in a lengthened position, and can allow for active ROM of the wrist, and proximal and distal joints. In Figure 1–16A, the orthosis is designed to keep IPs extended due to the complexity of the injury. The position of the fourth and fifth MCP joints is generally 60° of flexion, with the wrist, PIP, and DIP joints often left free. Because the fourth and fifth metacarpals are mobile compared to the second and third metacarpals, the hand portion of the orthosis should encompass the second and third metacarpal bases to improve stability and provide adequate purchase of the orthosis on the hand (Colditz, 2011a).

EXAMPLE: RF-SF MCP FLEXION IP EXTENSION IMMOBILIZATION ORTHOSIS (HFO) (Fig. 1–16).

Protect and Improve Joint Alignment

An orthosis can be fabricated to align subluxed and/or deviated joints to an improved anatomical position. In certain conditions, such as rheumatoid arthritis, joint laxity and/or tendon ruptures may disrupt proper joint mechanics, resulting in significant functional loss. Immobilization orthoses may work well to provide support and protection; they also redirect and attempt to position ligaments properly during healing (Beasley, 2011; Dell & Dell, 1996; Philips, 1995).

Patients with arthritis can wear a comfortable and supportive wrist and hand immobilization orthosis at night; the orthosis aids in maintaining proper joint alignment, protects against deforming forces, and prevents or minimizes soft tissue contractures. Not only can the orthosis be molded to support the larger joints involved, but strategically directed soft straps can also aid in repositioning the small joints of the digits within the design. Without attention to corrective positioning, joint deformity and limitation of function may occur sooner rather than later. Figure 1–17A is the radiograph of a patient with subluxed and ulnarly deviated MCP joints prior to surgery. Figures B and C show postoperative positioning with attention to joint alignment. The person with arthritis often welcomes the rest and support that the immobilization orthosis provides (Fig. 1–17A–C).

EXAMPLE: WRIST/HAND/DIGIT IMMOBILIZATION ORTHOSIS (WHFO) (Fig. 1–17).

Block or Transfer the Power of Movement

Applying a cast or orthosis to an individual joint can be used to block or transfer the power of movement to another joint in the same plane of motion. By blocking movement at a particular joint, the power of that movement is then transferred either proximally or distally. This can be especially useful when the goal is to glide a tendon through scar tissue or facilitate movement of a stiff joint. These devices are often used in the field of hand rehabilitation as a home exercise tool.

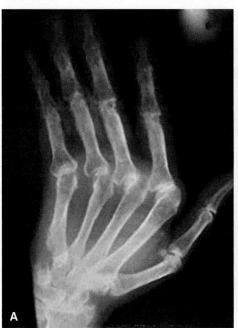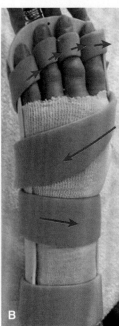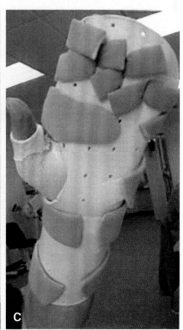

FIGURE 1–17 **A–C, Wrist/hand/digit immobilization orthosis (WHFO). A,** Radiograph of a patient with rheumatoid arthritis (presurgical). **B,** Immobilization orthosis with strategically positioned straps provides support to and maintains near optimal positioning of the involved joints post-surgery. **C,** Volar view—notice slits cut in thermoplastic material to allow for individual strapping to each digit.

A circumferential orthosis or cast to block PIP joint motion, leaving the DIP free, transfers the force of flexion to the DIP joint. The PIP orthosis acts as a mechanical block, eliminating flexor digitorum superficialis function and encouraging the flexor digitorum profundus tendon to work independently to move the distal phalanx (Fig. 1–18A). This same concept can be applied to the DIP joint. If the DIP joint is held in extension, the forces of flexion are then transferred to the PIP joint (Fig. 1–18B). If the other digits are held in extension, the orthosis will help block flexor digitorum profundus motion and isolate flexor digitorum superficialis glide. Another great example of an orthosis to block or transfer the power of movement is a relative motion orthosis (Hirth, Howell, & O'Brien, 2016). This relative motion flexion orthosis is utilized to address an active PIP extension lag at middle finger; by relatively flexing the middle finger MCP joint compared to the adjacent digits, the force of extension is directed to PIP joint (Fig. 1–18C,D). Refer to Chapter 7 for more detailed information.

EXAMPLE: PIP IMMOBILIZATION ORTHOSIS (FO) and RELATIVE MOTION FLEXION ORTHOSIS (FO) (Fig. 1–18).

Reduce Tone and Contracture of a Spastic Muscle

There is controversy in the literature regarding which design and therapeutic approaches are most effective for inhibiting tone in a spastic muscle. However, most therapists agree that early orthotic intervention is beneficial for decreasing muscle tone, preventing or reducing contractures, and preventing maceration of skin in the palm (Botte, Kivirahk, & Kinoshita, 2011; Mathiowetz, Bolding, & Trombley, 1983; McPherson, 1981; Neuhaus, Ascher, & Coullon, 1981; Rose & Shah, 1987).

The choice of design is influenced by the severity of the muscle tone, any existing contracture(s), and the ability to position the patient for the actual fabrication. Two people may be needed to fabricate these orthoses. Tone-reducing techniques performed before orthosis application often helps. See Chapter 23 for details regarding options for orthoses and patient positioning for ease of fabrication. There are many prefabricated or preformed orthoses available that provide support and alignment to the upper extremity and can be applied with greater ease for the patient. These may be better choices for patients that live alone or are dependent on others to don and doff the orthosis. These can be found and further described in Chapter 9.

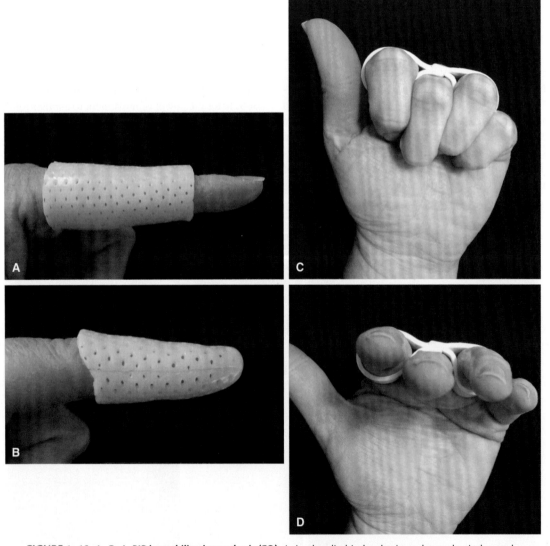

FIGURE 1–18 A–D, A, PIP immobilization orthosis (FO). A simple cylindrical orthosis can be used to isolate and promote flexor digitorum profundus glide. **B, DIP immobilization orthosis (FO).** A simple cylindrical orthosis can be used to isolate and promote flexor digitorum superficialis glide. **C and D, Middle finger relative motion extension orthosis (FO).** Notice that all joints have unimpeded motion with the MF MCP joint positioned in relative extension throughout the range of motion.

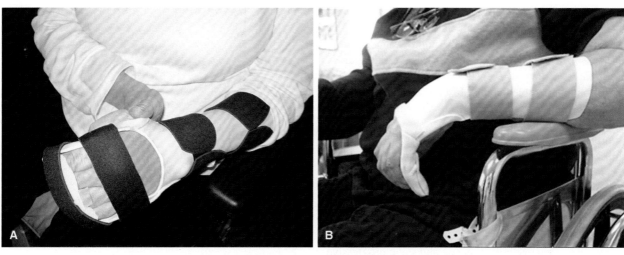

FIGURE 1–19 A and **B, Wrist/hand immobilization orthosis (WHFO).** A wrist/hand immobilization orthosis (volar-dorsal approach) is often a common choice for managing high tone in the wrist and hand and to prevent skin breakdown. This orthosis design can often be easier for the patient to apply. **A,** Dorsal view; **B,** side view.

Fabrication of orthoses to address contractures (or prevent the development of) due to an increase in tone can be challenging. The use of additional materials such as hard cones, finger spreaders, or neoprene straps (attached or incorporated into the orthosis) can sometimes aid in better positioning of the digits, thumb, and wrist while fabricating the device (Fig. 1–19).

EXAMPLE: WRIST/HAND/THUMB IMMOBILIZATION ORTHOSIS (WHFO) (Fig. 1–19).

MOBILIZATION ORTHOSIS

The rationale of fabricating **mobilization orthoses** is based on a physiologic theory that controlled tension applied over a long period of time alters cell proliferation. Brand and others have well described and documented the benefits of using different forms of mobilization techniques as a treatment modality (Bell-Krotoski, 1995; Bell-Krotoski & Breger-Stanton, 2011; Bell-Krotoski & Figarola, 1995; Brand & Thompson, 1993; Colditz, 1995b; Fess, 1995, 2011; Fess & McCollum, 1998; Flowers & LaStayo, 1994, 2012; Glascow et al., 2011; Gyovai & Wright Howell, 1992; Krotoski, 2011; Prosser, 1996; Rose & Shah, 1987; Tribuzi, 1995). The effectiveness of mobilization of tissue using an orthosis is not based on the concept of stretching tissue but relies on actual facilitation of cell growth. The target tissue lengthens when the living cells of the contracted tissues are stimulated to grow. The stimulation occurs when consistent external tension is applied through the orthosis over time (Brand & Thompson, 1993; Krotoski, 2011). The living cells recognize the tension placed on them, permitting the older cells of collagen to be actively absorbed and replaced with new collagen cells oriented in the direction of the applied tension.

This concept of tissue growth has been demonstrated in several African groups for whom it is deemed fashionable to stretch out certain body parts, such as earlobes, lips, and necks. For example, a small dowel is placed in the earlobes of a young child; the diameter of the dowel is serially increased as the tissue expands and accommodates to each new size (Fig. 1–20).

Mobilization orthoses can be challenging to plan and fabricate. The therapist has many options (dynamic, serial static, static progressive) when contemplating which type of mobilization orthosis is most appropriate to produce the desired result. The integration of

specific information gathered in the initial assessment—for example, age, motivation, psychological status, associated trauma or disease, avocational or vocational demands, quality of the joint's end ROM (soft, hard, elastic), length of time since injury or surgery, active versus passive ROM, and function—contributes to the decision-making process. For example, a patient with a dense, longstanding PIP joint flexion contracture may be better served with a serial static or static progressive orthosis than with a dynamic orthosis. Serial static or static progressive orthoses maintain the PIP joint in extension for a set period of time. A dynamic orthosis may not offer enough time within the orthosis (because it is removable) or enough force to overcome a dense contracture (Bell-Krotoski & Breger-Stanton, 2011; Colditz, 2011b; Flowers, 2002; Schultz-Johnson, 2002).

Dynamic and static progressive orthoses differ only in the way mobilizing forces are applied and delivered to the target tissue. Tension through both types of orthoses is initially set by the therapist and can be adjusted by the well-informed patient. The patient may be instructed to decrease the tension for night comfort and to increase the tension between treatment sessions. With dynamic orthoses, the effectiveness of the dynamic forces (especially rubber bands) may diminish over time because of the tendency of the elastic properties of the bands to fatigue under tension. Gravity may

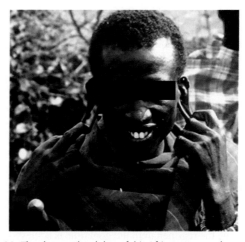

FIGURE 1–20 The elongated earlobes of this African man are the result of stretching owing to the lifelong use of graded ear dowels.

also adversely affect the elasticity of the dynamic force by progressively stretching out the bands.

The use of dynamic orthoses through the night is generally not encouraged. The nature of this orthosis is to deliver continuous tension to the target structure, even though the tissue may have reached its maximum tolerable length. Most patients cannot endure this persistent tension at night and end up removing the device (Schultz-Johnson, 1996, 2002, 2003b). Furthermore, sleeping with a dynamic orthosis may be awkward and cumbersome, and there is a possibility that the line of pull could get caught up in bedding or clothing. When applied properly, static progressive and serial static orthoses may be worn throughout the night; these devices hold the target structure at or close to maximum tolerable length but not beyond this position (Bell-Krotoski & Breger-Stanton, 2011; Schultz-Johnson, 1996).

Patients are able to remove both dynamic and static progressive orthoses for hygiene, completion of active exercise, and functional use. Serial static casts are generally fabricated to be nonremovable. They can be changed when the tissue has accommodated to the tension placed on them. Generally, this occurs between 3 and 6 days. Some serial static orthoses are made to be worn for a long period of time (e.g., throughout the night) but allow for periods of exercise and rest. For patients who require an uninterrupted stretch in one direction (as in a PIP flexion contracture secondary to a central tendon injury), an orthosis that is removable may **not** be the best choice. Once the orthosis has been removed, the tissue is able to rebound back to its original resting position, and the gains that were achieved may be at least partially lost. A nonremovable circumferential serial static cast should be considered in these situations.

Attempts should be made to measure and document all forces applied to the hand. Too much tension can cause discomfort, edema, and tissue reaction; too little tension may not be effective. Various force gauges can be used to document tension applied through a "dynamic" orthosis (see Chapter 4). The tension should be measured and adjusted on a consistent basis because the forces may lessen as the hand heals and tissues relax. Observation and clinical judgment are important means of assessing tension parameters; however, patient education is paramount. A patient wearing an MCP extension mobilization orthosis following an MCP joint arthroplasty will require significantly less tension than a patient whom the clinician is attempting to elongate contracted tissues (Fess, 2005; Jacobs & Austin, 2003, 2013). This information needs to be clearly communicated with the patient and/or family members. If not, harm can occur.

Orthosis wearers should be aware of the signs of too much tension (e.g., blanching skin, pain, numbness/tingling, and color changes) and what they should perceive (e.g., slight discomfort or a mild stretching sensation) (Fig. 1–21). If redness persists (does not fade) 30 minutes after removal of the orthosis, tension/position will need to be adjusted. Too much tension that has been generated over a short duration of time may create microtearing of soft tissue structures. This in turn will increase inflammatory and proliferative activity of cells resulting in increased scar tissue (Bell-Krotoski & Breger-Stanton, 2011; Brand & Thompson, 1993; Fess, 2005, 2011; Schultz-Johnson, 2002, 2003a, 2003b).

Initially, a general rule of thumb may be to attempt to wear the orthosis for 1 hour. If there is no discomfort or sign of tissue distress, gradually increase the wearing time by 1 hour per day. If none of the warning signs have been noted, yet the patient perceives a slight stretching sensation, continue the regimen until the goal time is achieved.

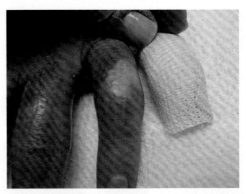

FIGURE 1–21 Note the blanching of the skin from too much localized force on the dorsum of the PIP joint of this serial static PIP extension mobilization cast. Once pressure areas have been resolved, wearing time can be gradually reintroduced.

The common objectives for mobilization orthoses are as follows:

- Remodel long-standing, dense, mature scar tissue
- Elongate soft tissue contractures, adhesions, and musculotendinous tightness
- Increase passive joint ROM
- Realign and/or maintain joint and ligament profile
- Substitute for weak or absent motion
- Maintain reduction of an intra-articular fracture with preservation of joint mobility
- Provide resistance for exercise

These objectives and examples of orthotic intervention are discussed in the following sections.

Remodel Long-standing, Dense, Mature Scar Tissue

A soft tissue contracture can often be addressed with some form of mobilization using an orthosis. The choice of orthosis types depends on many factors, including information obtained from the physician such as bony union or neurovascular status, maturity of the scar, end feel of the tissue, and the patient's anticipated compliance and motivation level. Mature scar tends to respond well to serial casting, and static progressive and serial static orthosis fabrication (Bell-Krotoski & Breger-Stanton, 2011; Schultz-Johnson, 1992, 2002, 2003a). Softer, less mature scar may respond better to gentle dynamic forces, which are applied with proper mechanical principles (Fess, 2011; Fess & Phillips, 1987; Flowers & LaStayo, 1994, 2012). Soft tissue contracture that is associated with Dupuytren's disease and contractures secondary to fibrotic tissue do not respond to mobilization with an orthotic device.

A cylindrical extension mobilization orthosis (cast) applied to a long-standing, dense PIP flexion contracture may be effective in elongating the contracture and maintaining the desired lengthened position (Colditz, 2011b). Therapeutic techniques (e.g., heat, ultrasound, joint mobilization, passive stretching, and massage) used before casting or fabrication of an orthosis may aid in preparing the tissue's responsiveness to stretch. As the tissue lengthens or the ROM increases, the serial static orthoses or casts are changed to support the joint in the new position. Each new device helps remodel the tissue to a further lengthened position (Fig. 1–22). The cast or orthosis is changed every 3 to 6 days, depending on individual protocols and the tissues response until the contracture is resolved (Flowers, 2002; Flowers & LaStayo, 1994, 2012; Glascow et al., 2011, 2012; Means, Saunders, & Graham, 2011). Many more examples and principles can be found in Chapters 10 and 15.

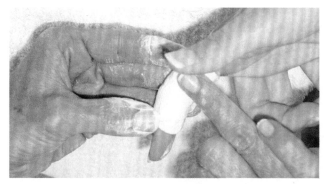

FIGURE 1–22 **Digit extension mobilization orthosis (FO).** Intimately molded cast (here fabricated with plaster of paris) can be applied and changed frequently to allow for tissue remodeling. Serial casting can be effective in resolving PIP joint contractures.

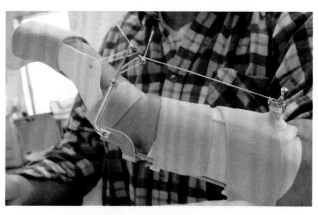

FIGURE 1–23 **Wrist/hand extension mobilization orthosis (WHO).** A static progressive wrist/hand extension mobilization orthosis using a Phoenix wrist hinge, MERiT™ Static Progressive component and simple soft strapping influences adherent volar forearm soft tissue.

EXAMPLE: PIP EXTENSION MOBILIZATION ORTHOSIS (FO) (Fig. 1–22).

Elongate Soft Tissue Contractures, Adhesions, and Musculotendinous Tightness

Several factors are thought to contribute to the outcome of contracture resolution and soft tissue elongation when using an orthotic device. Some of these include the amount and quality of pretreatment stiffness and intervention, diagnosis, time since injury, age, gender, insurance status, and family support (Glascow et al., 2011, 2012; Glascow, Wilton, & Tooth, 2003). Fabrication of an orthosis for mobilization can be effective in elongating contracted tissue and stretching adhesions and tight muscle-tendon units during the proliferative stage of scar formation. Judiciously and incrementally applied tension during this phase of wound healing can greatly enhance tissue accommodation (see Chapter 3, for details). Preparing the tissue, usually by heating and stretching before the orthotic application, maximizes the device's benefit.

Forearm, wrist, and digit motion can be significantly limited by soft tissue adherence after flexor tendon injury and repair. A wrist/hand extension mobilization orthosis is one treatment option for addressing flexor tendon adhesions and musculotendinous extrinsic tightness in the volar forearm (Fig. 1–23). The static progressive nature of the orthosis holds tension at the wrist and digit's maximum extension ROM, thereby longitudinally stressing the volar forearm's contracted soft tissue structures. Orthosis adjustments occur only when the tissue response allows. This type of orthosis can be taken off for hygiene purposes or to work on active and/or passive ROM. Refer to Chapters 10 and 15, and Chapter 2 in the Fabrication Manual for more information.

EXAMPLE: WRIST/HAND EXTENSION MOBILIZATION ORTHOSIS (WHO) (Fig. 1–23).

Increase Passive Joint Range of Motion

Orthotic fabrication is one of the most effective ways of increasing passive mobility of stiff joints. It has been shown that the amount of increase in passive ROM of a stiff joint is proportional to the amount of time the joint is held at its end ROM (Colditz, 2011b; Flowers, 2002; Flowers & LaStayo, 1994, 2012; Schultz-Johnson, 2002). Serial static and static progressive mobilization devices may accomplish this goal effectively (Schultz-Johnson, 1996). Both types of orthoses are applied after the joint has been prepared (warmed and stretched in therapy) at the tissue's near maximum end range and held there until the tissue response allows repositioning to accommodate a change in length (Glascow, Tooth, & Fleming, 2008). This should be a comfortable, tolerable position for the patient.

An MCP flexion mobilization orthosis can be effective in increasing the passive ROM of the MCP joints. This orthosis addresses MCP collateral ligament shortening that can occur after bony or soft tissue injury to the hand or cast immobilization that hinders full MCP motion. Before applying flexion forces to the MCP joint(s), check with the physician regarding possible issues such as bony union, neurovascular status, and/or tendon repair strength. This orthosis applies flexion forces to the tight MCP joints via two different static progressive approaches. The therapist should be certain that the distal volar border of the orthosis clears the distal palmar crease, allowing for unrestricted MCP flexion (Fig. 1–24).

EXAMPLE: FOREARM-BASED MCP FLEXION MOBILIZATION ORTHOSIS (WHFO) (Fig. 1–24).

Realign and/or Maintain Joint and Ligament Profile

When ligaments surrounding a joint become tight, stretched, or damaged from disease or injury, the joint may sublux or deviate. This process causes an alteration of joint mechanics. Patients may experience pain, note an inability to use the hand, and often develop harmful substitution patterns. Surgical intervention, such as an MCP arthroplasty or extensor tendon rebalancing, can be a treatment option for these patients. After surgery, a therapist may fabricate a mobilization orthosis for protective positioning. Correctly applied, a postsurgical orthosis can maintain joint-tendon alignment, thereby decreasing previous substitution patterns and

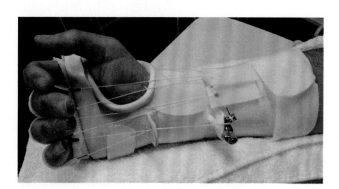

FIGURE 1–24 **Forearm-based MCP flexion mobilization orthosis (WHFO).** An MCP flexion mobilization orthosis using two different methods for a static progressive approach. A MERiT™ static progressive component is used for the small digit, because of the severity of the extension contracture and simple loop to hook with static line is used for the ring and middle digits. This orthosis is aimed at improving MCP joint flexion secondary to collateral ligament shortening.

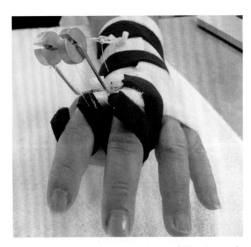

FIGURE 1–25 Forearm-based MCP extension mobilization orthosis (WHFO). This wrist and MCP extension mobilization orthosis is applied after an MCP joint arthroplasty of the IF and MF. Slings can be adjusted on the outrigger to guide alignment of the MCP joints into slight radial deviation and desired extension (Phoenix Outrigger system shown).

deforming forces while increasing the functional capabilities of the hand during the course of healing.

An MCP extension mobilization orthosis is often used in the postoperative care of a patient who has undergone MCP joint arthroplasty. The orthosis gives support to the wrist, provides a stable base for outriggers to assist the weakened digital extensors, and prevents undue stress on the reconstructed joints (Swanson, 1995). The orthosis should be fabricated only after the operative procedure, integrity of the joints/surrounding soft tissue, and ligament reconstruction have been discussed with the surgeon. The purpose of this device is to provide well-controlled guided motion to the MCP joints and to allow for remodeling of the new capsule with proper balance between stability and motion (Fig. 1–25).

The force applied to the MCP joints should be just enough to position them in passive extension with some degree of radial deviation yet allow for gentle active digital flexion. The force used here is much less than the amount used to elongate a soft tissue contracture. Reconstruction of the radial collateral ligament to the index

finger (IF) MCP joint is commonly seen in association with MCP arthroplasty. A radially placed outrigger (also known as a supinator attachment) can be added to the orthosis to correct any IF pronation deformity (Bell-Krotoski & Breger-Stanton, 2011; DeVore, Muhleman, & Sasarita, 1986; Philips, 1995). Refer to Chapter 17, for more information.

EXAMPLE: FOREARM-BASED IF-MF MCP EXTENSION MOBILIZATION ORTHOSIS (WHFO) (Fig. 1–25).

Substitute for Weak or Absent Motion

A mobilizing force through an orthosis may aid functional use of the hand by substituting for absent musculature or assisting in the motion of weak muscles. The dynamic force replaces or assists the motion performed by specific or absent musculature. However, a primary goal when using these orthoses is to preserve good passive motion (Fess, 2011; Fess & McCollum, 1998; Fess & Phillips, 1987). Orthoses that take advantage of the natural tenodesis action of the hand are commonly fabricated to assist functional use after nerve injury. Such substitution orthoses can greatly enhance function, prevent joint contracture, and minimize the overstretching of involved muscle-tendon units. Chapter 20 provides further information.

An orthosis that addresses the loss of radial nerve function was first fabricated at the Hand Rehabilitation Center (Chapel Hill, NC) and later described by Colditz (1987). The orthosis has a thermoplastic component that rests on the dorsum of the forearm but does not cross the wrist joint. By using a static line directed from the forearm base to the proximal phalanges, the MCP joints are suspended in extension. This orthosis re-creates the tenodesis action of the hand by allowing passive wrist extension through active finger flexion as well as passive finger extension via active wrist flexion. The device enables the digits to extend, span, and grasp/release light objects-critical motions for functional use (Fig. 1–26A–C).

EXAMPLE: RECIPROCAL WRIST EXTENSION, MCP FLEXION/WRIST FLEXION, MCP EXTENSION MOBILIZATION ORTHOSIS (WHFO) (Fig. 1–26).

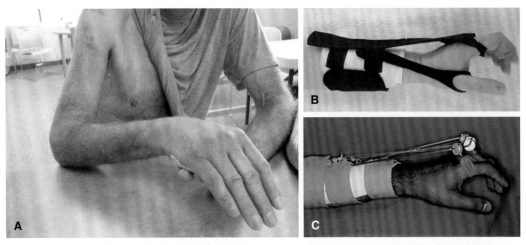

FIGURE 1–26 A–C, Wrist/MCP extension mobilization orthosis (WHFO). A, Patient with radial nerve injury— notice loss of active digit/thumb and wrist extension. **B,** Various types of orthoses can be used to manage loss of active extensors. Neoprene material imparts the extension force, and tension can be adjusted to allow for specific activity requirements. **C,** The Phoenix Radial Nerve Outrigger Kit is used as another option to generate passive wrist extension, allowing functional grasp.

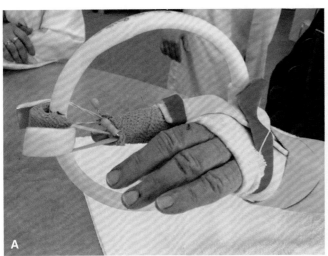
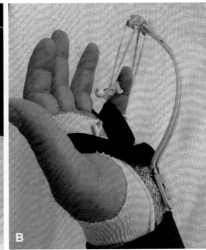
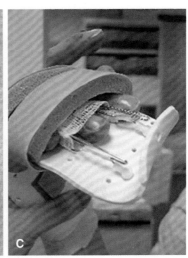

FIGURE 1–27 **A–C, Intra-articular PIP traction mobilization orthoses (WHFO). A,** Traditional Schenck design for managing complex intra-articular fractures. **B,** This modified version of the original Schenck-designed intra-articular orthosis maintains gentle traction and fracture alignment while allowing guarded, controlled passive motion of the PIP joint. **C,** An immobilization orthosis is used as the foundation for stabilization and alignment of the RF PIP intra-articular fracture.

Maintain Reduction of an Intra-articular Fracture

The application of a gentle traction force to a healing intra-articular fracture site during monitored, controlled ROM maintains fracture alignment, facilitates healing, and contributes to the preservation of joint mobility (Dennys, Hurst, & Cox, 1992; Schenck, 1986; Wong, 1995). Such orthoses are often fabricated in the operating room or shortly thereafter and are most often created by an experienced therapist who has close, ongoing communication with the surgeon.

Intra-articular PIP fractures can be selectively managed with external traction using an orthosis. Schenck (1986) originally developed and described one such traction orthosis. The surgeon places a wire horizontally through the middle phalanx leaving the ends of the wire protruding. The wire is bent to hold rubber bands or springs that are then attached to a hoop that extends from the orthosis base. The rubber band or spring attachment is commonly made with a bent aluminum device or thermoplastic material that can easily glide along the hoop. The traction from the PIP joint to the hoop can be cautiously moved through a specific degree of motion hourly or as prescribed by the physician. The completed orthosis should be checked by the surgeon to ensure proper fracture alignment and force application (Fig. 1–27A). This method may be applied to other joints, such as the MCP joint, and many variations (Fig. 1–27B, C) of this orthosis have been described since Dr. Schenck's original article (Dennys et al., 1992; Schenck, 1986; Wong, 1995). Refer to Chapter 16 for more information.

> *EXAMPLE: CIRCULAR TRACTION (SCHENCK DESIGN) PIP INTRA-ARTICULAR MOBILIZATION ORTHOSIS (WHFO) and DIGIT IMMOBILIZATION ORTHOSIS TO PROTECT HEALING FRACTURE WITH TRACTION APPARATUS IN PLACE (HFO)* (Fig. 1–27).

Provide Resistance for Exercise

Dynamic orthoses can be used as an exercise tool to apply resistance in the opposite direction of the patient's active force. This can be a useful way to facilitate tendon excursion through scar, gain tensile strength of specifically targeted muscles, and provide resistance to adherent tendons.

Providing resistance to an adherent tendon, such as a flexor digitorum superficialis or flexor pollicis longus, can facilitate tendon gliding through scar and contribute to increasing tensile strength once a strengthening program has begun. To facilitate flexor digitorum superficialis glide, the orthosis is fabricated to position the MCP joint in extension, and the DIP is held in extension via a cast or with thermoplastic material. A sling is then applied to the middle portion of this DIP cast (Fig. 1–28). Resistance to the line of pull is felt when PIP flexion is attempted.

> *EXAMPLE: PIP EXTENSION MOBILIZATION ORTHOSIS (HFO)* (Fig. 1–28).

RESTRICTION ORTHOSES

Restriction orthoses limit a specific aspect of joint mobility. These orthoses can be a challenge to fabricate, especially when made for patients who have multiple injuries with a combination of needs. Static orthoses and dynamic orthoses can also be considered types of restrictive orthoses because they can be made to restrict some portion of joint motion while allowing the rest of the joint to move freely. A therapist may be asked to fabricate a device that completely immobilizes a joint and creatively allows motion or partial motion of other joints. This scenario requires integration of problem-solving skills,

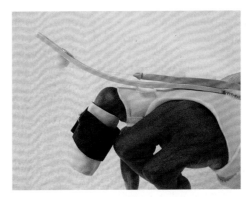

FIGURE 1–28 **PIP extension mobilization orthosis (HFO).** A PIP extension mobilization orthosis being used for controlled resistance to an adherent flexor digitorum superficialis tendon. The DIP is held in extension by a small circumferential orthosis to eliminate any motion at the DIP joint. Increasing flexor digitorum superficialis tendon glide and gentle strengthening are the goals of this orthosis. This orthosis is shown with the Digitec System.

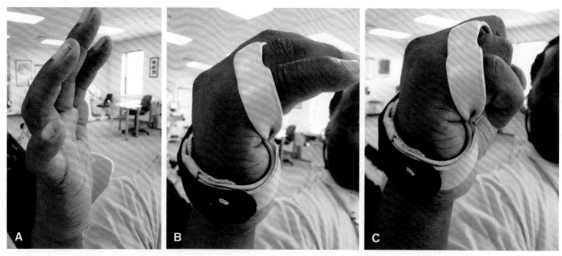

FIGURE 1–29 A–C, RF-SF MCP extension restriction orthosis (HFO). After low ulnar nerve injury, preventing hyperextension at the MCP joints facilitates extension at the IP joints. The fourth and fifth MCP joints are generally positioned between 45° and 70° of flexion to optimize function within the orthosis while awaiting nerve regeneration. **A,** Subtle claw deformity noted, **B,** IP extension, and **C,** near composite digit flexion.

clinical judgment, critical thinking, and understanding of how wound healing stages apply to specific tissues. Careful attention to the construction and fit of these orthoses is crucial because of the expected motion and use of the extremity within the orthosis.

The common objectives for restriction orthoses are as follows:

- Limit motion after nerve injury or repair.
- Limit motion after tendon injury or repair.
- Limit motion after bone-ligament injury or repair.
- Provide and improve joint stability and alignment.
- Assist in functional use of the hand.

These objectives and examples of orthotic intervention are discussed in the following sections.

Limit Motion After Nerve Injury or Repair

Restrictive orthoses can effectively block potentially deforming and abnormal forces to the hand secondary to nerve injury. They allow the healing nerve or reinnervated nerve to glide within a protected ROM, minimizing tension at the repair site, decreasing the risk of adherence to soft tissue structures, increasing blood flow, and improving the nutritional environment. Chapter 20 provides specific design details.

A restriction orthosis can prevent the common claw deformity of the ring and small digits that occurs after low ulnar nerve injuries (Fig. 1–29A–C). Such an orthosis restricts extension motion at the MCP joints by applying well-distributed pressure at the dorsum of the proximal phalanxes and allowing the transfer of force from the extrinsic extensors to the dorsal hood mechanism of the digits. By placing the MCP joints in some degree of flexion, extension of the IP (PIP and DIP) joints is made possible in the absence of the ulnar innervated intrinsic muscles by means of the radial nerve–innervated extrinsic extensors. This position provides the extensor tendons with a mechanical advantage that greatly enhances composite grasp and release, which is quite awkward and difficult without the orthosis.

EXAMPLE: RF-SF MCP EXTENSION RESTRICTION ORTHOSIS (HFO) (Fig. 1–29).

Limit Motion After Tendon Injury or Repair

After soft tissue injury or surgical repair, limited motion is often necessary to promote tissue healing, prevent joint contractures, maintain tissue length, and facilitate gliding of structures to minimize adhesion formation. There are numerous protocols that address orthotic intervention for these types of injuries, and only one technique is discussed here. Refer to Chapters 18 and 19 for a discussion of various tendon protocols.

Extensor tendon injuries in zones V to VII can be managed with a restrictive orthosis (Fig. 1–30). The wrist is held in static extension (35°-45°) while the involved MCP joint(s) are passively extended using rubber band traction. Active MCP flexion against the rubber bands can be performed to a set volar block or a block placed on the monofilament as it meets the Phoenix wheel. Initially, the block is restricted to approximately 30° of MCP joint motion or per MD protocol. Gradually, as healing progresses, the block is adjusted to allow greater MCP flexion. The adjustments are generally done each week as long as the tendon healing allows (Evans, 2011; Evans & Burkhalter, 1986; Thomas, Moutet, & Guinard, 1996). This type of orthosis promotes early protected motion and tendon excursion for optimal healing with less risk of adhesion formation and tendon rupture; however, there are numerous combinations of orthoses and motion protocols for the treatment of extensor tendons that should be explored by the reader (Wong et al., 2017). This includes immobilization, mobilization, and restriction orthoses. The decision of which approach to choose is dependent on many factors including but not limited to geographical practice patterns, experience level, patient commitment, and patient compliance.

EXAMPLE: WRIST EXTENSION IMMOBILIZATION, DIGIT EXTENSION MOBILIZATION ORTHOSIS (with flexion restriction) (WHFO) (Fig. 1–30).

Limit Motion After Bone-Ligament Injury or Repair

After fracture reduction or surgical fixation, an orthosis that allows a restricted ROM can be used to promote bone growth, healing of associated ligaments, joint mobility, and soft tissue/tendon gliding. The initial amount of joint restriction depends on the surgical procedure, the severity of the fracture dislocation, the extent of ligament involvement, and the physician protocol. The therapist and/or physician monitor the amount and degree of allowed extension or flexion exercise and gradually may increase the limits of motion as healing progresses. The permitted, restricted arc of motion promotes healing of the injury or repair and aids in minimizing tendon adherence (Blazer & Steinberg, 2000; Gallagher & Blackmore, 2011; Kadelbach, 2006; Schenck, 1986).

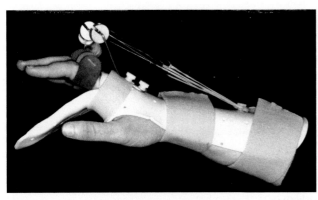

FIGURE 1–30 Wrist extension immobilization, MCP extension mobilization/ flexion restriction (WHFO). This restrictive orthosis (using a Phoenix Outrigger Kit) immobilizes the wrist in slight extension while providing dynamic MCP flexion to a predetermined range. The patient actively flexes the digits to the volar block, allowing passive excursion of the extensor tendons. Dynamic forces, via the rubber bands, return the digits to full extension.

Limiting full extension after a posterior elbow dislocation is the key to preventing reinjury. A static or dynamic orthosis can minimize lateral movement of the elbow, decrease motions of pronation and supination, and restrict elbow extension. The degree of elbow extension restriction is determined by the severity of the fracture dislocation and the position required, preventing subluxation. The position may be altered as the involved structures heal and the physician permits. Care is taken to minimize the risk of flexion contracture by carefully extending the motion allowed as healing progresses. By applying an elbow extension restriction orthosis, the distal forearm straps may be removed to allow unrestricted functional elbow flexion while limiting elbow extension to the confines of the device (Fig. 1–31A,B). A hinged extension restriction orthosis includes an elbow hinge applied to forearm and humerus circumferential "cuff." The hinge is locked to prevent a specific degree of extension while allowing unrestricted

elbow flexion (Fig. 1–31C). The degree of extension block is determined by the physician protocol. Refer to Chapter 3 in the Fabrication Manual for more examples and information.

EXAMPLE: ELBOW EXTENSION RESTRICTION ORTHOSIS (EWHO) (Fig. 1–31).

Provide and Improve Joint Stability and Alignment

A restrictive orthosis, such as an IF-SF MCP ulnar deviation orthosis, can help support and realign subluxed and/or deviated joints to an improved anatomical position while preserving some functional use of the extremity. Such restrictive devices can block or restrict harmful movement patterns that place undue stress on joints, ligaments, and tendons. Functional orthoses often allow patients to use their hands in a natural way while limiting pain and edema and without contributing to further joint or soft tissue breakdown.

A small dorsal thumb IP joint orthosis can limit lateral IP deviation deformities sometimes seen in the patient with rheumatoid arthritis (Fig. 1–32A,B). This orthosis realigns the proximal and distal phalanxes and places the IP joint in better alignment and preparation for function. This positioning greatly improves stability during pinch. An elastic wrap is recommended for securing the proximal portion of the orthosis about the proximal phalanx of the thumb if rotation or slippage becomes an issue (Terrono, Nalebuff, & Philips, 1995). Applied in this way, the orthosis allows functional IP pinch with minimal deforming forces. Therapy should also include gentle ROM exercises to avoid soft tissue contractures, intrinsic muscle tightness, and collateral ligament shortening. Refer to Chapter 17 for more information.

EXAMPLE: THUMB IP RADIAL DEVIATION RESTRICTION ORTHOSIS (FO) (Fig. 1–32A,B).

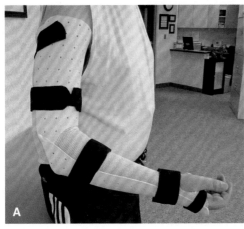
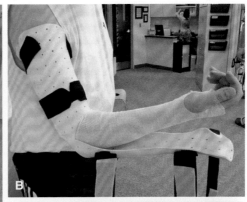
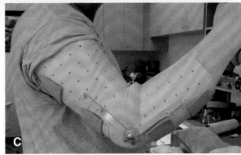

FIGURE 1–31 A–C, Elbow extension restriction orthoses. A, Immobilization (EWHO): When this elbow extension restriction orthosis' distal straps are removed, the patient is able to **(B)** slide the wrist out and flex the elbow within the orthosis' parameters. **C,** Mobilization (EO): This elbow extension restriction orthosis (with a Phoenix elbow hinge component that includes a mechanical block) limits the amount of elbow extension yet allows unimpeded flexion.

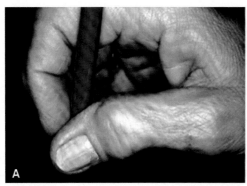
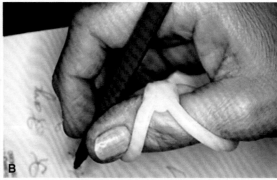

FIGURE 1–32 **A** and **B, Thumb IP radial deviation restriction orthosis (FO).** This thumb IP restriction orthosis provides stability and protection to an unstable IP joint. The orthosis prevents radial deviation and realigns the IP joint in order to do light activities that require pinching.

Assist in Functional Use of the Hand

Orthoses are an excellent way to assist and ready the hand for functional use (Deshaies, 2008; Sillem et al., 2011). Chronic, improper positioning as a result of a poorly fit orthosis can lead to contractures, functional lengthening or shortening of tendons, pain, and prolonged edema. Orthosis fabrication can be used advantageously to position joints and tendons while preventing the possible deforming consequences. The key to independence is maintaining function for as long as possible.

A small lightweight orthosis can be used to manage a supple swan-neck deformity (PIP hyperextension, DIP flexion). Such a device balances digital extension by applying three-point pressure about the PIP joint (Fig. 1–33A). Dorsal pressure applied proximal and distal to the PIP joint limits the joint's extension; volar pressure directly supports the joint. Hyperextension is not permitted; however, flexion of the digit is preserved (Fig. 1–33B). Intervention should also include a program of intrinsic stretching and ROM exercises for the wrist and uninvolved joints. Patients can manage quite well with these small devices, which allow them to have better stability during pinching and grasping activities. Refer to the clinical pearls and field notes throughout this book for further information and ideas.

EXAMPLE: PIP EXTENSION RESTRICTION ORTHOSIS (FO) (Fig. 1–33).

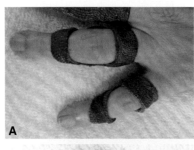
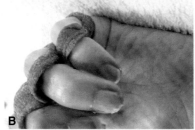

FIGURE 1–33 **A** and **B, PIP extension restriction orthosis (FO).** These are worn during functional use to manage long-standing swan-neck deformities. **A,** Digit extension. **B,** Digit flexion.

CONCLUSION

This chapter describes the blended nomenclature important to all therapists working with upper extremity patients. It also provides practical clinical examples of various orthoses, outlines common objectives for intervention, and offers insight in the use of L-Codes in billing for orthoses. The MOCS provides clarity and a mechanism to define orthoses through a sequence of analytic steps that combines historical nomenclature, the CMS coding language, and parts of the ASHT splint classification system. The editors and authors of this publication strongly believe that unified terminology is paramount when referring to orthotic devices in every aspect of our professions.

Fabricating orthoses for the injured extremity is only one part of a comprehensive rehabilitation program. For successful orthotic intervention, the clinician must help the patient (and/or caregiver) understand the importance of compliance and make certain they are aware of the orthosis function; why are they wearing it? The orthosis must be comfortable to wear and convenient to apply and should have an acceptable aesthetic appearance for the wearer. The orthosis needs to be accepted into the patient's lifestyle; otherwise, it may have a detrimental effect (Callinan, 2008; Deshaies, 2008; McKee & Rivard, 2004, 2011; Sandford, Barlow, & Lewis, 2008).

CHAPTER REVIEW QUESTIONS

1. Explain the terms:
   A. Orthotic
   B. Orthosis
   C. Orthoses
   D. Splint
2. What is an L-Code?
3. What is the difference between an immobilization, a mobilization, and a restrictive orthosis?
4. What is a nonarticular orthosis? Give an example.
5. What are the three basic mobilization approaches and how do they differ from each other?
6. What must a clinician take into consideration when choosing the most appropriate orthosis for a patient?
7. Why is it important to eliminate the word *Splint* and adapt the word *Orthosis* into our medical nomenclature?

2

Anatomical Principles

Noelle M. Austin, MS, PT, CHT

CHAPTER OBJECTIVES

After study of this chapter, the reader should be able to:

- Appreciate the normal architecture of the hand and upper extremity.
- Name the three arches that comprise the arch system in the hand and describe the importance of including these arches within a molded orthosis.
- Recognize the precautions related to orthosis application and how this relates to patient education.
- Give examples of the various bony prominences and superficial nerves that are at risk for irritation from orthosis application.

KEY TERMS

Acromioclavicular joint
Articular capsule
Articular cartilage
Axillary artery and nerve
Brachial artery
Brachial plexus
Carpometacarpal (CMC) joints
Collateral ligaments

Deep palmar arterial arch
Distal interphalangeal (DIP) joints
Distal palmar crease
Glenohumeral joint
Humeroradial and humeroulnar joint
Longitudinal arch
Median nerve
Metacarpophalangeal (MCP) joints
Palmar creases
Proximal interphalangeal (PIP) joints

Proximal palmar crease
Proximal and distal radioulnar joint
Proximal and distal transverse arch
Radial artery and nerve
Radiocarpal joint
Superficial arterial and venous arch
Thumb interphalangeal (IP) joint
Ulnar artery and nerve

INTRODUCTION

The anatomy of the upper extremity is composed of a complex arrangement of bones, joints, nerves, muscles, and vascular structures, which work together to permit a wide range of functional capabilities. To be effective as clinicians, therapists must have a comprehensive understanding of how these structures function conjointly under normal and abnormal conditions, such as injury and disease. This chapter focuses on the anatomical structures of the upper extremity and notes how they are specifically related to orthotic intervention.

THE BONES AND JOINTS OF THE UPPER EXTREMITY

The skeletal structure of the upper extremity is defined proximally by the shoulder girdle and distally by the finger joints (Fig. 2–1A–C). This complex configuration of bones allows each joint to move in specific ways, permitting mobility and function of the hand in space. Dysfunction of even one joint in the upper extremity can affect the ability of the other joints to function normally (Calliet, 1994).

Except for the scapulothoracic joint, the joints of the upper extremity are considered synovial joints, which have a joint cavity, articular cartilage lining the bony ends, and an **articular capsule** containing **synovial fluid** (Fig. 2–2) (Moore, 2017; Moore, Agur, & Dalley, 2019). Synovial joints are categorized by their bony configuration and the amount of motion they allow. Each type of synovial joint is represented in the upper extremity (Fig. 2–3A–F) (Moore, 2017; Moore et al., 2019). **Ligaments** are composed of thick connective tissue that emanates from the **joint capsule**; they provide stability to the joint. The ligaments of each joint are shown in the figures throughout this chapter.

Wherever the patient's problem lies—from the shoulder to the distal interphalangeal (DIP) joint—the therapist's goal is to appreciate normal joint mechanics; to preserve, as much as possible, the normal anatomical alignment; and to provide the opportunity for maximal functional use. Therapists must understand how the upper extremity structures interact under normal and abnormal conditions and must ultimately be aware of how therapy intervention can influence the final outcome.

THE SHOULDER

In the proximal upper extremity, the shoulder complex includes the **sternoclavicular**, **acromioclavicular**, **scapulothoracic**, and **glenohumeral joints**. The first three of these joints are discussed here because they link the upper extremity to the trunk and their status can affect the ultimate function of the limb. The sternoclavicular joint is a **saddle joint** consisting of the medial end of the

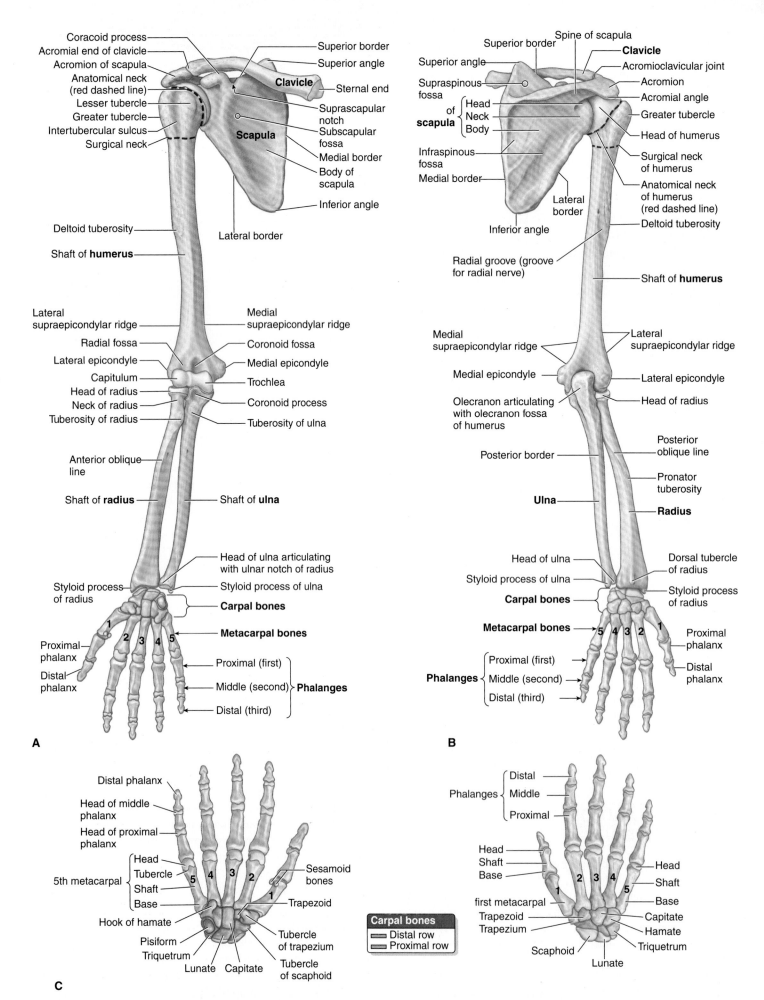

FIGURE 2–1   Bones of the upper limb. A, Anterior view. **B,** Posterior view. **C,** Anterior (palmar) and posterior (dorsal) views: bones of hand. (Reprinted with permission from Moore, K. L., Agur, A. M., & Dalley, A. F.II. (2019). *Moore's Essential clinical anatomy* (6th ed.). Philadelphia, PA: Wolters Kluwer.)

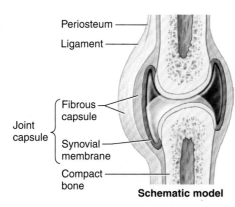

FIGURE 2–2 In a **synovial joint** (articulation), the two bones are separated by the characteristic joint cavity (containing synovial fluid) but are joined by an articular capsule (fibrous capsule lined with synovial membrane). The bearing surfaces of the bones are covered with articular cartilage. Synovial joints are functionally the most common and important type of joint. They provide free movement between the bones they join and are typical of nearly all joints of the limbs. (Reprinted with permission from Moore, K. L., Agur, A. M., & Dalley, A. F.II. (2019). *Moore's Essential clinical anatomy* (6th ed.). Philadelphia, PA: Wolters Kluwer.)

clavicle and the lateral aspect of the manubrium; it allows motion in several directions (Fig. 2–4) (Moore, 2017; Moore et al., 2019). The acromioclavicular joint is a **plane joint** formed by the lateral end of the clavicle and medial portion of the acromion; it permits rotation and anterior to posterior movement of the acromion on the clavicle (Fig. 2–5) (Moore, 2017; Moore et al., 2019). The articulation between the scapula and thorax is considered a **pseudo joint** (false joint); it allows the scapula to glide along the thoracic wall as the arm moves in space (Fig. 2–6) (Kapandji, 1982). The **ball-and-socket** arrangement of the glenohumeral joint is formed by an articulation between the glenoid fossa of the scapula and the head of the humerus. This loose configuration provides a highly mobile arrangement; however, mobility is achieved by sacrificing stability. The joint allows the arm to move freely in extension and flexion, abduction and adduction, and internal and external rotation (Fig. 2–7A–D) (Kapandji, 1982; Moore, 2017; Moore et al., 2019).

THE ELBOW

The **elbow joint** is composed of the **humeroulnar** and **humeroradial joints** (Moore, 2017; Moore et al., 2019). The humeroulnar joint consists of the trochlea of the distal humerus as it joins the trochlear notch of the proximal ulna. The humeroradial joint is made up of the capitulum of the distal humerus and the head of the radius. The elbow joint is generally considered a **hinge joint**, which allows extension and flexion (Fig. 2–8A–E). There is a normal valgus carrying angle of 5° in males and 10° to 15° in females (Hoppenfeld, 1976). When fabricating elbow orthoses with the forearm positioned in supination, the therapist must incorporate the valgus angle into the design to ensure an appropriate fit.

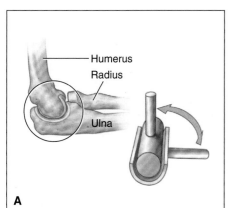

A

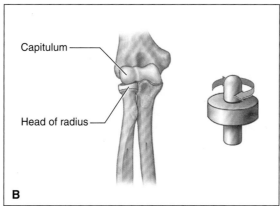

B

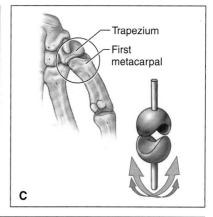

C

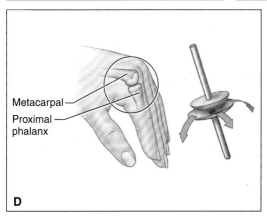

D

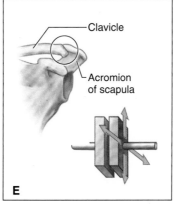

E

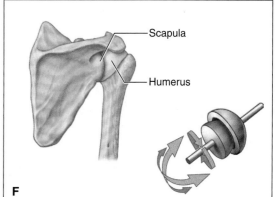

F

FIGURE 2–3 **Types of upper extremity synovial joints. A,** Uniaxial hinge joints, such as the humeroulnar joint, permit only flexion and extension. **B,** Uniaxial pivot joints, such as humeroradial joint, allow rotation. A round process on one bone fits into a ligamentous socket in the other bone. **C,** One bone of a biaxial saddle joint, such as the trapeziometacarpal joint, is concave and the other is convex at the point of articulation. **D,** Biaxial condyloid joints, such as the metacarpophalangeal joint, permit flexion and extension, abduction and adduction, and circumduction. **E,** Plane joints, such as the acromioclavicular joint, permit gliding or sliding movements. **F,** Multiaxial ball-and-socket joints, such as the glenohumeral joint, permit flexion and extension, abduction and adduction, medial and lateral rotation, and circumduction. The rounded head of one bone fits into a concavity in the other bone. (Adapted with permission from Moore, K. L., Agur, A. M., & Dalley, A. F.II. (2019). *Moore's Essential clinical anatomy* (6th ed.). Philadelphia, PA: Wolters Kluwer.)

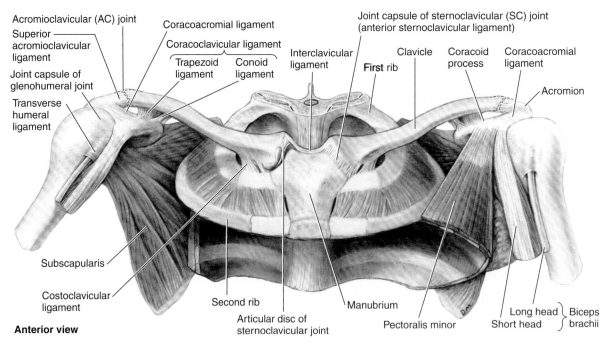

FIGURE 2–4 The sternoclavicular joint. Joints of pectoral girdle and associated tendons and ligaments. (Reprinted with permission from Moore, K. L., Agur, A. M., & Dalley, A. F.II. (2019). *Moore's Essential clinical anatomy* (6th ed.). Philadelphia, PA: Wolters Kluwer.)

THE FOREARM

The **proximal radioulnar joint** consists of the articulation of the radial head with the radial notch of the ulna. The **distal radioulnar joint** (DRUJ) is made up of the ulnar notch of the radius and the head of the ulna. These articulations are both considered **pivot joints**; they permit the radius to rotate about the ulna during supination and pronation (Fig. 2–9A–D) (Moore, 2017; Moore et al., 2019). Stability is provided proximally by the annular and quadrate ligaments and distally by the anterior and posterior radioulnar ligaments along with the triangular fibrocartilage complex (TFCC) (Levangie, Norkin, Lewek, & 2019; Tubiana, Thomine, & Mackin, 1996). The interosseous membrane helps bind the radius and ulna together by virtue of its fiber orientation from the radius to the ulna (Levangie et al., 2019). Therapists applying forearm-based orthoses must appreciate the variation in

muscle bulk during forearm rotation and compensate for this by rotating the forearm at the end of the molding process to ensure adequate fit.

THE WRIST

The wrist complex incorporates the radiocarpal and midcarpal joints. The **radiocarpal joint** is a **condyloid joint** created by the connection between the distal radius with the scaphoid and lunate. The midcarpal joint is a **plane joint** formed by the intimate union of the proximal (scaphoid, lunate, triquetrum, and pisiform) and distal (trapezium, trapezoid, capitate, and hamate) carpal rows (Moore, 2017; Moore et al., 2019). In combination, the radiocarpal and midcarpal joints allow extension and flexion, radial and ulnar deviation, and a small amount of circumduction (Fig. 2–10A–D; Table 2–1).

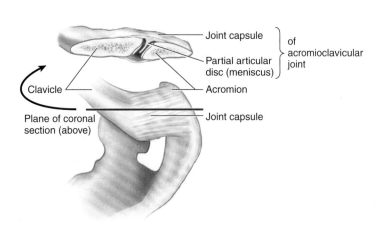

FIGURE 2–5 Acromioclavicular joint. Joint capsule and partial articular disc. (Reprinted with permission from Moore, K. L., Agur, A. M., & Dalley, A. F.II. (2019). *Moore's Essential clinical anatomy* (6th ed.). Philadelphia, PA: Wolters Kluwer.)

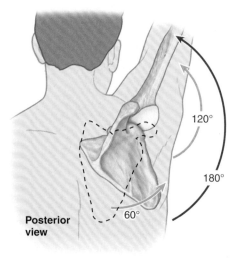

FIGURE 2–6 Scapulohumeral rhythm. The scapula and humerus move in a 1:2 ratio. When the arm is abducted 180°, 60° occurs by rotation of the scapula and 120° by rotation of the humerus at the shoulder joint. (Modified from Hamill, J., Knutzen, K. M., & Derrick, T. R. (2015). *Biomechanical basis of human movement* (4th ed.).)

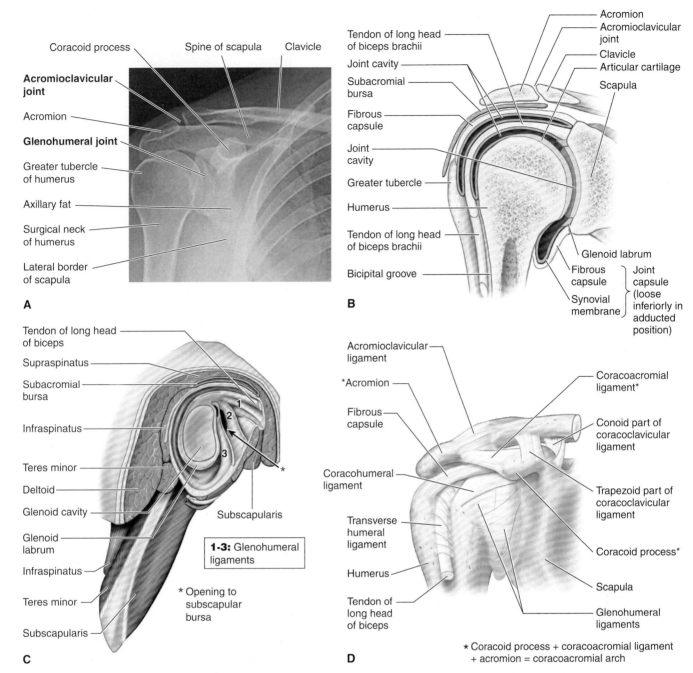

FIGURE 2–7 Glenohumeral joint and acromioclavicular joints. A, Anteroposterior radiograph. **B,** Coronal section of glenohumeral joint. **C,** Lateral view of glenoid cavity and related structures following disarticulation of humerus. **D,** Anterior view of ligaments. (A, Courtesy of Dr. E. Lansdown, University of Toronto, Ontario, Canada. B-D, Reprinted with permission from Moore, K. L., Agur, A. M., & Dalley, A. F.II. (2019). *Moore's Essential clinical anatomy* (6th ed.). Philadelphia, PA: Wolters Kluwer.)

THE HAND

The **carpometacarpal (CMC) joints** of the digits are considered plane joints; they provide minimal motion at the index and middle fingers and progressively more mobility in the ring to small fingers (Moore, 2017; Moore et al., 2019). This arrangement allows humans to grasp objects tightly (Fig. 2–10A–C). The CMC joint of the thumb, formed by the articulation of the trapezium with the base of the first metacarpal, is considered a saddle joint. It permits radial abduction and adduction, palmar abduction and adduction, and opposition (Fig. 2–10A–C) (Moore, 2017; Moore et al., 2019).

The digital **metacarpophalangeal (MCP) joints** are condyloid joints formed by the union of the metacarpal heads with the base of the proximal phalanges. They allow flexion and extension, abduction and adduction, and circumduction (Fig. 2–11A–C; Table 2–2)

(Moore, 2017) (Moore et al., 2019). The thumb MCP joint is unique in its ability to allow a few degrees of abduction and rotation, which improves precision pinch function (Fess & Philips, 1987).

Distally, the digital **proximal interphalangeal**, **distal interphalangeal (DIP)**, and **thumb interphalangeal (IP) joints** are considered simple hinge joints, allowing only extension and flexion (Fig. 2–11A–C) (Moore, 2017; Moore et al., 2019). Therapists must appreciate the tension placed on the ligamentous structures when applying orthoses to the digits. Depending on the specifics of the diagnosis, the goal is to utilize the antideformity position (MCP flexion/IP extension). The MCP joint **collateral ligaments** are taut in flexion and slack in extension, but the opposite is true for the palmar plate (taut in extension; slack in extension). Therefore, the MCP joints should be positioned in flexion to place these ligaments at maximal length, to prevent shortening and

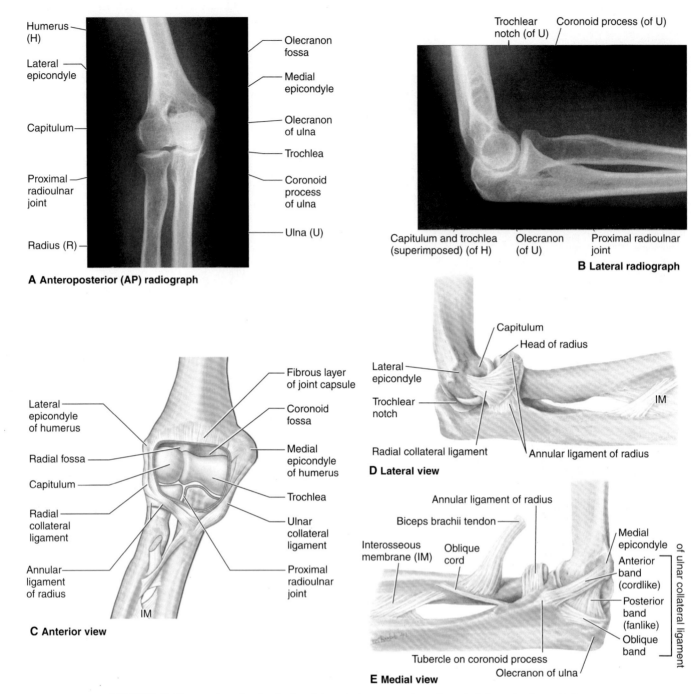

FIGURE 2–8 Elbow and proximal radioulnar joints. A, Anteroposterior radiograph. **B,** Lateral radiograph. **C,** Articulating surfaces. The thin anterior aspect of the joint capsule has been removed. **D,** Lateral ligaments. **E,** Medial ligaments. (A and B, Courtesy of Dr. E. Becker, University of Toronto, Ontario, Canada. C-E, Reprinted with permission from Moore, K. L., Agur, A. M., & Dalley, A. F.II. (2019). *Moore's Essential clinical anatomy* (6th ed.). Philadelphia, PA: Wolters Kluwer.)

MCP extension contractures (Fig. 2–11B,C) (Fess & Philips, 1987; Pratt, 2011a). Similarly, when addressing the IP joints, the therapist must remember that the volar plate is taut in extension and slack in flexion. Ideally, these joints are positioned in full PIP extension to prevent shortening and PIP flexion contractures (Fig. 2–12).

Arches of the Hand

The bony architecture, along with the muscles of the hand, contributes to the formation and maintenance of the arches in the hand (Fig. 2–13A,B) (Bowers & Tribuzi, 1992; Fess & Philips, 1987; Pratt, 2011a; Tubiana et al., 1996). The **proximal transverse arch** is a rigid arrangement at the level of the distal carpal bones and forms the base of the carpal tunnel. In comparison, the

distal transverse and **longitudinal arches** are mobile and add depth to the hand. The distal transverse arch is located at the level of the metacarpal heads and provides the ability of the hand to grasp objects of different sizes. The mobility afforded by the ring- and small-finger CMC joints allows for this mobile arch. The longitudinal arch courses from the carpal level through the four digital rays. This highly mobile arch adapts to meet the needs of specific grasping activities. When fabricating orthoses for metacarpal fractures, the therapist must appreciate the differences in mobility of the CMC joints. For example, small-finger metacarpal fractures require inclusion of the middle- and ring-finger metacarpals to gain adequate purchase, stability, and immobilization of the fracture.

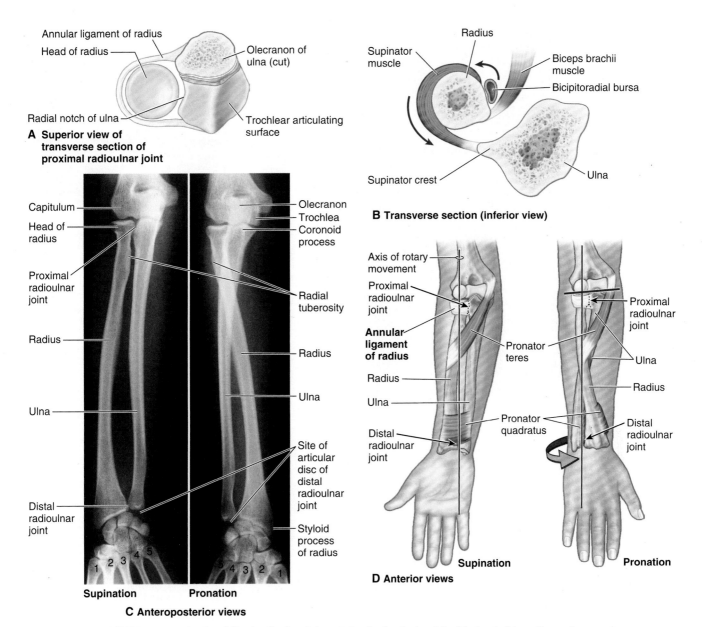

FIGURE 2–9 Proximal and distal radioulnar joints. A, Proximal radioulnar joint. The head of the radius rotates in the "socket" formed by the annular ligament. **B,** Actions of supinator and biceps brachii in producing supination are shown. **C,** Radiograph. **D,** Position of radius and ulnar in supination and pronation. (A, B, and D, Reprinted with permission from Moore, K. L., Agur, A. M., & Dalley, A. F.II. (2019). *Moore's Essential clinical anatomy* (6th ed.). Philadelphia, PA: Wolters Kluwer. C, Courtesy of Dr. J. Heslin, University of Toronto, Ontario, Canada.)

When the hand is injured, the arch system can be compromised, altering hand function. For example, ulnar nerve injury and the subsequent loss of intrinsic function (active MCP flexion/IP extension) disrupt the normal arch system, causing virtual collapse into a claw deformity (MCP hyperextension/IP flexion) (Fig. 2–14A–C). During the orthotic fabrication process, therapists must endeavor to create the mobility and stability the arches provide and should incorporate them into each orthosis to maximize the functional potential of the hand. In addition, a well-contoured orthosis that incorporates the arches minimizes migration of the orthosis on the body and better stabilizes a mobilization orthosis on the extremity when force is applied (Fig. 2–15A,B).

Creases of the Hand

Palmar creases are distributed throughout the hand in a relatively consistent pattern (Bowers & Tribuzi, 1992; Fess & Philips, 1987; Pratt, 2011b). These creases form in direct relation to the underlying structures and the functional demands placed on that region. To properly apply orthoses to the hand, the therapist must gain awareness of which specific joints underlie each crease (Fig. 2–16). The therapist can use the creases as boundaries when creating patterns and molding orthoses. To permit motion distally, the orthosis must clear the creases proximally (Fig. 2–17A–C). For example, wrist orthoses must clear the **proximal palmar crease** (PPC) and **distal palmar crease** (DPC) to allow unimpeded digital range of motion. (To maintain wrist position, the orthosis should extend distally as far as possible in the palm.) Differences in metacarpal length contribute to the obliquity of the PPC and DPC, requiring an oblique angle at the distal edge of a volar wrist orthosis (Fig. 2–18A,B). An additional consideration involves the importance of recognizing each patient's individual anatomical characteristics. For example, in one patient, clearing for the DPC on the radial side of the palm may be enough to allow full motion of the MCP joints, but in another patient, the orthosis must clear the PPC to allow full motion.

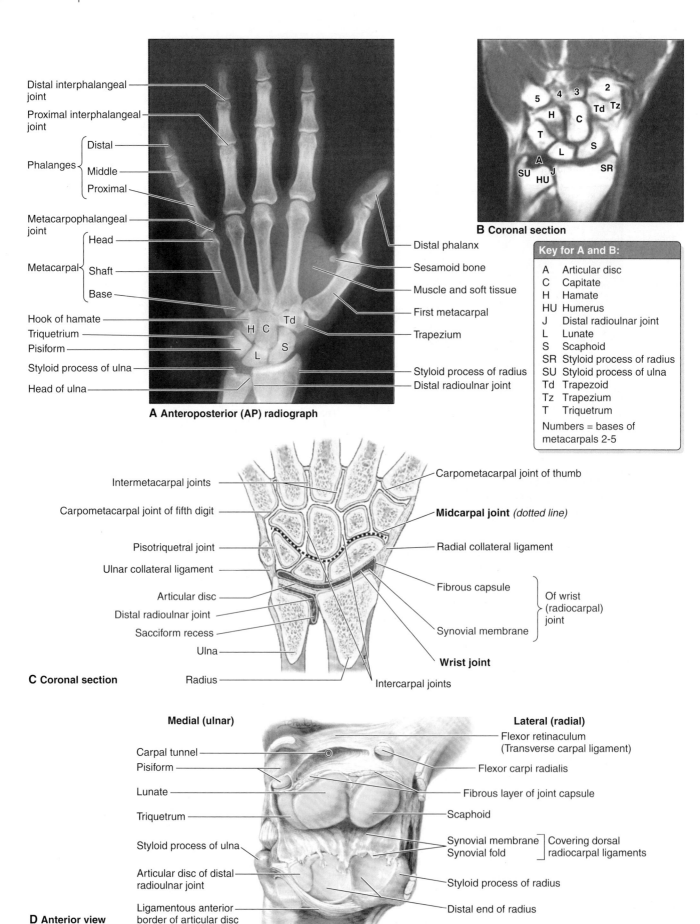

FIGURE 2–10 Wrist and hand joints. A, Radiograph. **B,** Coronal MRI of wrist. **C,** Coronal section of distal radioulnar, wrist, and carpal joints. **D,** Dissection. The wrist is opened anteriorly, with the dorsal radiocarpal ligaments acting as a hinge. (Reprinted with permission from Moore, K. L., Agur, A. M., & Dalley, A. F.II. (2019). *Moore's Essential clinical anatomy* (6th ed.). Philadelphia, PA: Wolters Kluwer.)

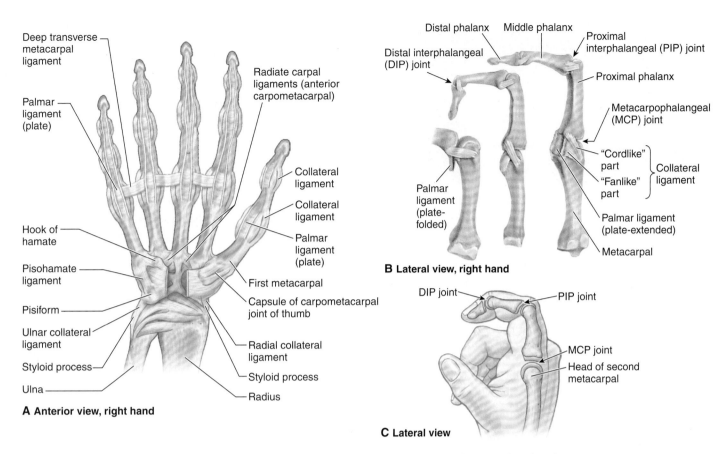

A Anterior view, right hand

B Lateral view, right hand

C Lateral view

FIGURE 2–11 Joints of hand. A, Palmar ligaments. **B,** MCP and interphalangeal IP joints. The palmar ligaments (plates) are modifications of the anterior aspect of the MCP and IP joint capsules. **C,** Joints of digit. (Reprinted with permission from Moore, K. L., Agur, A. M., & Dalley, A. F.II. (2019). *Moore's Essential clinical anatomy* (6th ed.). Philadelphia, PA: Wolters Kluwer.)

ORTHOTIC IMPLICATIONS

The bony prominences that exist throughout the upper extremity skeleton must be taken into consideration when molding an orthosis (Fess & Philips, 1987; Pratt, 2011b). These areas tend to be vulnerable to irritation because of minimal soft-tissue covering. Avoiding pressure over these areas by the orthotic material and/or strapping is of extreme importance, along with educating the patient about what to watch for in terms of warning signs. Signs of too much pressure include the following:

- Pain
- Redness
- Skin necrosis (breakdown from ischemia)

The primary prominences to consider include the following (Fig. 2–19A–D):

- Clavicle
- Spine of scapula
- Acromion
- Olecranon
- Medial and lateral epicondyles
- Radial and ulnar styloid processes
- Base of first metacarpal
- Dorsal thumb MP and IP joints
- Dorsal MCP, PIP, and DIP joints
- Pisiform

Clinical Example

A well-molded orthosis that disperses the area of pressure application can prevent the aforementioned complications by providing a custom fit with accommodations, such as padding or flaring of the orthosis' edges in the at-risk areas (Fig. 2–20A–G). For example, when molding the ulnar border of a volar wrist support, the therapist should flare the edge adjacent to the ulnar styloid process to help prevent the bone from abutting the hard orthotic material during forearm rotation motions.

NERVES AND MUSCLES OF THE UPPER EXTREMITY

The nerve supply to the upper extremity arises from the **brachial plexus** (Fig. 2–21; Table 2–3) (Moore, 2017; Moore et al., 2019). The plexus originates from the cervical level of the spinal cord via the brachial plexus, receiving contributions from the ventral rami of spinal nerves C5-T1. Variations may exist with some contribution from C4 and T2. These five nerve roots combine to form the **superior, middle,** and **inferior trunks.** Posterior to the clavicle, the three trunks in turn divide into the three anterior divisions and three posterior divisions. The divisions then give rise to the **posterior, lateral,** and **medial cords** of the plexus. The cords are named according to their relationship to the axillary artery. The cords provide the origin for the terminal nerve branches: **musculocutaneous, axillary, radial, median,** and **ulnar nerves.** Figure 2–21 and Table 2–3 outline the specific origins of the small branches throughout the plexus.

Each terminal nerve branch traverses through the upper extremity, passing through and innervating specific muscles along its path toward the hand (Fig. 2–22A–E; Table 2–4) (Rayan, 1992;

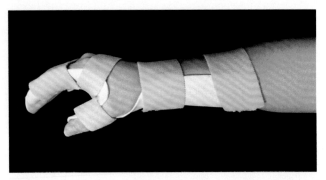

FIGURE 2–12 In the antideformity position, the MCP joints are flexed and the IP joints are extended with the thumb CMC joint midway between palmar and radial abduction.

Spinner, 1995; Wolfe, Pederson, Kozin, & Cohen, 2016). (Chapter 24 includes a detailed discussion of nerve anatomy, including pathways, innervations, and compression sites.) In general, the radial nerve innervates the dorsal extensor muscles of the elbow, forearm, wrist, and hand. The median and ulnar nerves provide innervation to the volar flexor muscles and the intrinsic muscles of the hand. Sensation of the upper extremity is provided by various cutaneous nerves as shown in Figure 2–22. Throughout each nerve's individual pathway, areas exist in which the nerves are vulnerable to compression by other anatomical structures, such as muscles and ligaments. These nerves are also vulnerable to external forces, such as those associated with wearing an orthosis—thermoplastic and strapping.

Therapists must have a working knowledge of peripheral neuroanatomy, along with full comprehension of the muscular and cutaneous innervations in the upper extremity. Table 2–5 lists the muscular attachments, innervations, and actions and serves as a handy reference when making decisions about orthotic fabrication and therapy intervention. The muscles of the anterior compartment of the forearm are divided into four layers (Fig. 2–23A–C). The extrinsic digital flexors pass through the carpal tunnel region as they enter the hand (Fig. 2–23D). The muscles of the posterior compartment are arranged in two layers (Fig. 2–24A,B). These extrinsic muscles traverse the dorsal wrist in separate compartments within the extensor retinaculum (Fig. 2–24C,D). Chapters 22 and 23 provide a detailed discussion of the muscular anatomy of the forearm and hand.

ORTHOTIC IMPLICATIONS

Therapists must avoid compression of the superficial nerves while molding the orthosis and again when applying straps or mobilization components (Fess & Philips, 1987). Similar to educating patients regarding bony prominences, the therapist must explain to the patient the symptoms of nerve compression and what to do if they occur. Symptoms of nerve irritation include the following:

- Numbness
- Paresthesias (tingling)
- Burning
- Motor control changes
- Pain

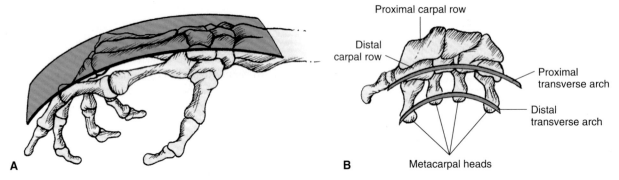

FIGURE 2–13 **A,** The longitudinal arch of the hand spans the length of the rays and carpus. **B,** The proximal and distal transverse arches of the hand.

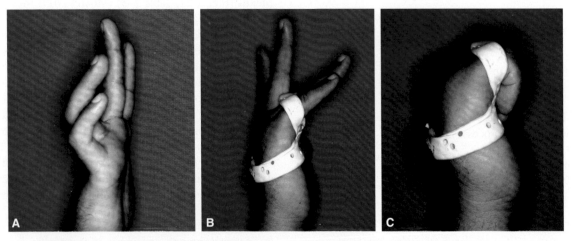

FIGURE 2–14 **A,** After ulnar nerve injury, there is a loss of the arch system. MCP extension-restriction orthosis during active digit extension **(B)** and active digit flexion **(C).**

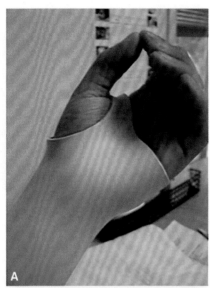

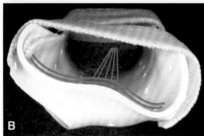

FIGURE 2–15 **A,** Gently opposed position helps to capture arches during the molding process. **B,** A wrist immobilization orthosis that includes the transverse and longitudinal arches to ensure a stable fit.

Timely orthotic modification or strap adjustment is necessary if the patient reports any of these signs. Patient education regarding this matter is the key to preventing long-term nerve damage and ensuring maximal compliance with orthosis wearing schedule. Patients are more inclined to wear a comfortable orthosis than one that is causing undue symptoms. Specific nerves that are vulnerable

to compression because of their superficial location include the following (Fig. 2–25A–C):

- Suprascapular nerve
- Axillary nerve
- Radial nerve at radial groove
- Ulnar nerve at cubital tunnel
- Superficial branch of ulnar nerve
- Superficial branch of radial nerve
- Median nerve at wrist
- Digital nerves

Clinical Example

When fabricating an orthosis, the therapist must be aware of the underlying anatomy and anticipate any potential nerve irritation to prevent the aforementioned complications. Accommodations include applying padding, flaring the orthosis edges, and using straps and slings of adequate width to disperse pressure about the at-risk areas (Fig. 2–26A–D). For example, when applying a dorsal wrist and hand immobilization orthosis to a patient who has sustained a flexor tendon injury, the therapist must recognize that the superficial branch of the radial nerve is highly susceptible to irritation at the radial wrist. The nerve may be irritated by both the wrist-flexed position along with the dorsally applied material. Furthermore, the orthosis must be worn on a full-time basis. The therapist must be sure there is no excess pressure along the dorsal and radial forearm over the path of this nerve. Any signs of skin redness or patient complaints of numbness or paresthesias in the dorsoradial hand indicate the need for timely intervention by the therapist. Modifications or adjustments to the orthosis include flaring the thermoplastic away from the nerve region, padding the area with soft foam or gel, and being sure to trim away any offending material (Fig. 2–27A–C).

VASCULAR SUPPLY OF THE UPPER EXTREMITY

The blood supply to the upper extremity arises proximally from larger vessels that bifurcate to form smaller vessels that provide circulation distally throughout the extremity (Fig. 2–28; Table 2–6) (Moore, 2017; Moore et al., 2019). In the shoulder area, the **axillary artery** originates from the **subclavian artery** at the border of the first rib. The axillary artery in turn continues as the brachial artery, passing the inferior border of the teres major. The **brachial artery** provides the main blood supply to the arm. In the inferior portion of the cubital fossa, at the level of the neck of the radius, the brachial artery divides to form the **radial artery** and the larger **ulnar artery**. These arteries descend through the forearm into the hand to unite and form the **superficial** and **deep palmar arterial arches**. The ulnar artery primarily forms the superficial arch, whereas the radial artery primarily forms the deep arch. The superficial and deep palmar arches provide circulation to the hand and give rise to the digital arteries.

Superficial and **deep venous arches** lie close in relation to the superficial and deep arterial arches. The dorsal digital veins drain into the dorsal metacarpal veins, forming the dorsal venous network. This network continues as the **cephalic** and basilic veins proximally (Fig. 2–29A,B). The therapist must be familiar with the circulation of the upper extremity when forming orthoses, especially for patients with injury to, surgical repair of, or compromise of these structures.

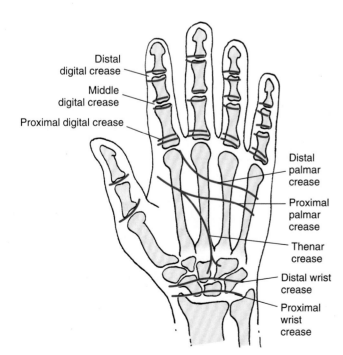

FIGURE 2–16 The relationship between the palmar creases and their underlying joints.

Distal digital crease

Middle digital crease

Proximal digital crease

Distal palmar crease

Proximal palmar crease

Thenar crease

Distal wrist crease

Proximal wrist crease

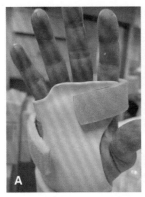
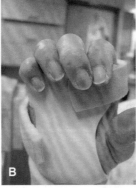
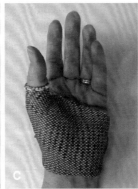
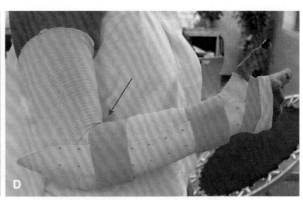

FIGURE 2–17 A and B, An MCP extension immobilization orthosis that clears the middle digital creases of all digits to allow unimpeded PIP flexion. This orthosis is being used to protect healing sagittal band repair. **C,** A thumb MP immobilization orthosis with full clearance at the IP joint; be mindful not to "over clear" which would decrease effectiveness of immobilizing the MP fully. This device was fabricated using X-Lite PLUS° material. **D,** An elbow extension-restriction orthosis with a proximal strap that extends too far proximally into the antecubital fossa, not allowing full flexion of the elbow joint.

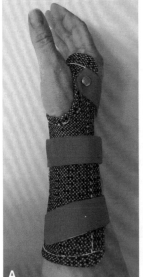
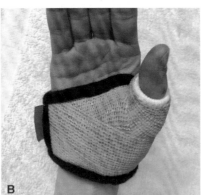

FIGURE 2–18 A, A wrist immobilization orthosis with inadequate clearance of the PPC, impeding full flexion at the index MCP joint. This device was fabricated using X-Lite PLUS°. **B,** A thumb MP immobilization orthosis that does clear the DPC and PPC to allow the digits full range of motion. This device was fabricated using Delta-Cast° Conformable material.

ORTHOTIC IMPLICATIONS

When orthoses, straps, casts, or edema wraps are applied too tightly, circulation to tissue may be compromised (Fess & Philips, 1987). Therapists must educate their patients on the signs of impaired blood flow:

- Color changes (deep red, blue, or blanched)
- Temperature changes (cool/cold or extreme warmth)
- Excessive throbbing sensation

Prompt alterations must be made to correct the problem. There may also be vascular problems related solely to the position of the body part in the orthosis. For example, in a patient who has undergone surgical arterial repair, the therapist must carefully position the joints above and below the repair to prevent undue tension at the surgical site.

Clinical Example

Careful application of circumferential orthoses, wraps, and straps is imperative to prevent disruption of blood flow to and from the body part (Fig. 2–30A–C). An edema response follows trauma from injury, surgery, or both. One of the therapist's primary goals is to decrease edema to prevent the problematic sequelae of stiffness and adhesion formation. Therapists commonly use elasticized

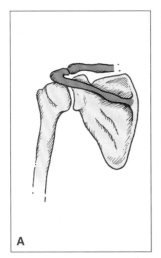
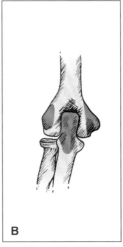
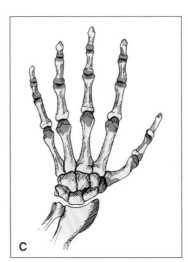
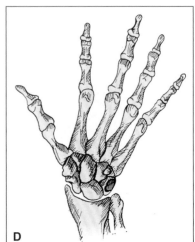

FIGURE 2–19 Bony prominences of the shoulder **(A)**, elbow **(B)**, dorsal wrist and hand **(C)**, and volar wrist and hand **(D)**.

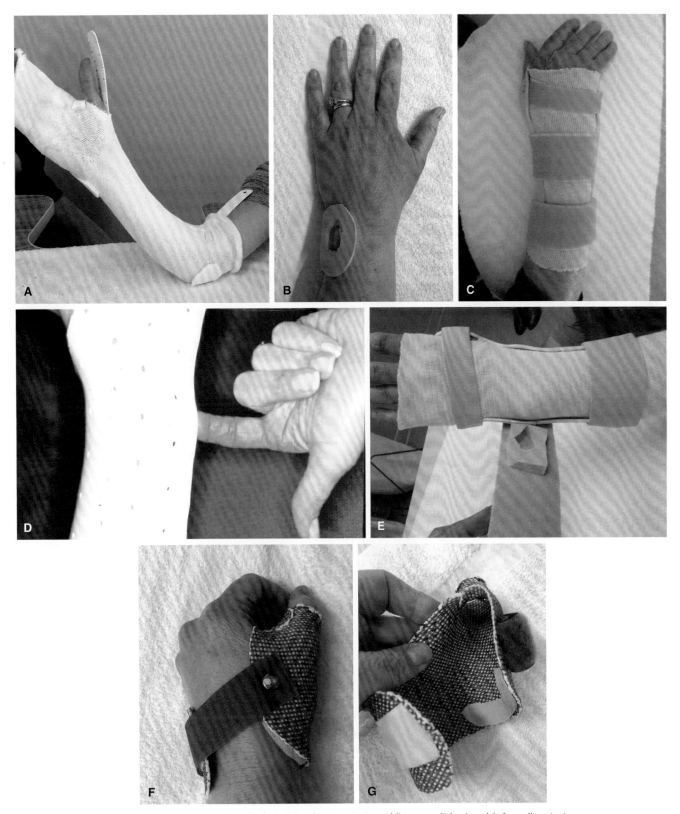

FIGURE 2–20 **Accommodations for bony prominences. A,** Prepadding at medial epicondyle for a elbow/wrist immobilization orthosis fabricated from Delta-Cast® Conformable material. **B,** Prepadding with a donut at the distal ulna. Thumb orthosis fabricated from X-Lite PLUS® material. **C,** Padding of the strap that traverses the index MCP joint. **D,** Flaring at the distal ulna on a wrist immobilization orthosis. **E,** Padding on wrist strap with donut for sensitive distal ulna. **F and G,** Foam padding adhered to base of CMC joint immobilization orthosis.

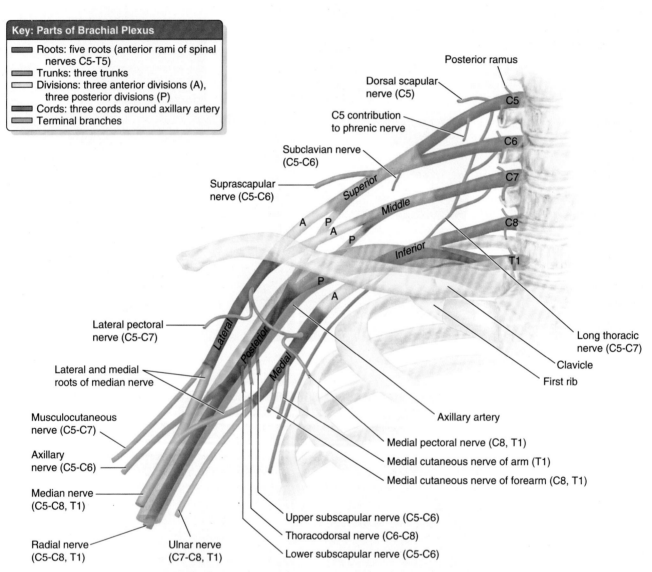

Key: Parts of Brachial Plexus

- Roots: five roots (anterior rami of spinal nerves C5-T5)
- Trunks: three trunks
- Divisions: three anterior divisions (A), three posterior divisions (P)
- Cords: three cords around axillary artery
- Terminal branches

FIGURE 2–21 Brachial plexus. (Reprinted with permission from Moore, K. L., Agur, A. M., & Dalley, A. F., II. (2019). *Moore's essential clinical anatomy* (6th ed.). Philadelphia, PA: Wolters Kluwer. Fig. 3.27.)

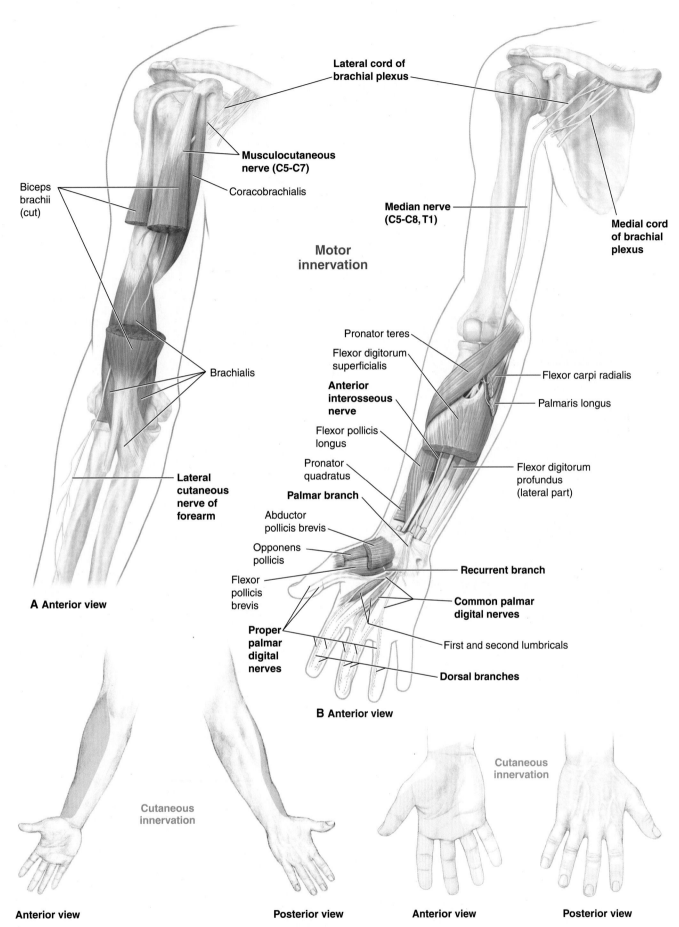

FIGURE 2–22 Overview of peripheral nerves of upper limb. A, Musculocutaneous nerve. **B,** Median nerve. **C,** Ulnar nerve. **D,** Radial nerve. (Reprinted with permission from Moore, K. L., Agur, A. M., & Dalley, A. F., II. (2019). *Moore's essential clinical anatomy* (6th ed.). Philadelphia, PA: Wolters Kluwer. Fig. 3.17.)

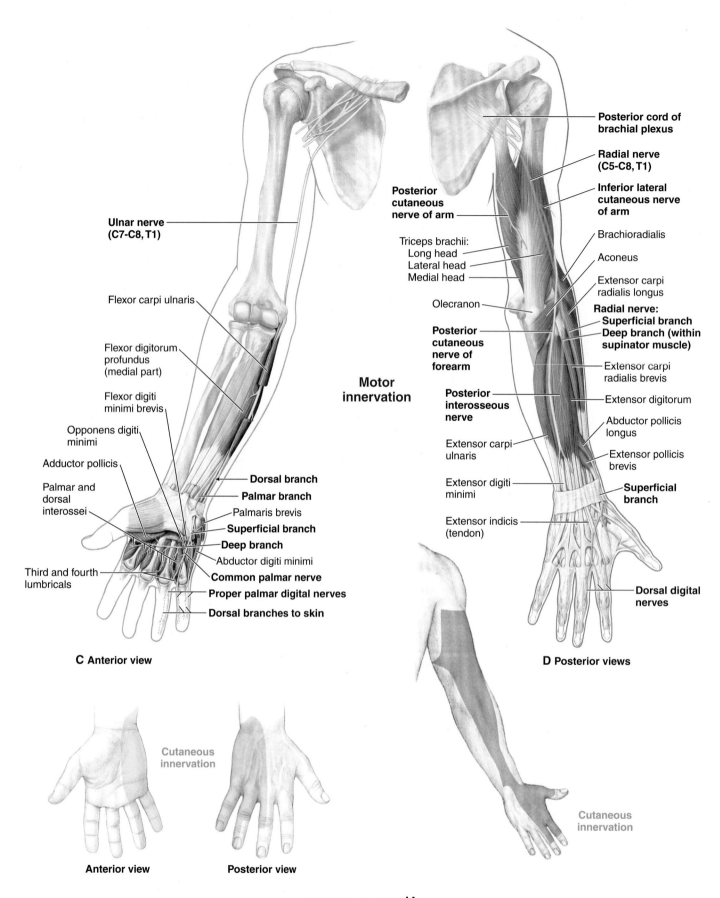

Ulnar nerve
(C7-C8, T1)

Flexor carpi ulnaris

Flexor digitorum
profundus
(medial part)

Flexor digiti
minimi brevis

Opponens digiti
minimi

Adductor pollicis

Palmar and
dorsal
interossei

Third and fourth
lumbricals

Dorsal branch

Palmar branch

Palmaris brevis

Superficial branch

Deep branch

Abductor digiti minimi

Common palmar nerve

Proper palmar digital nerves

Dorsal branches to skin

C Anterior view

**Motor
innervation**

Posterior
cutaneous
nerve of arm

Triceps brachii:
Long head
Lateral head
Medial head

Olecranon

**Posterior
cutaneous
nerve of
forearm**

**Posterior
interosseous
nerve**

Extensor carpi
ulnaris

Extensor digiti
minimi

Extensor indicis
(tendon)

**Posterior cord of
brachial plexus**

**Radial nerve
(C5-C8, T1)**

**Inferior lateral
cutaneous nerve
of arm**

Brachioradialis

Aconeus

Extensor carpi
radialis longus

**Radial nerve:
Superficial branch
Deep branch (within
supinator muscle)**

Extensor carpi
radialis brevis

Extensor digitorum

Abductor pollicis
longus

Extensor pollicis
brevis

**Superficial
branch**

**Dorsal digital
nerves**

D Posterior views

Cutaneous
innervation

Anterior view   **Posterior view**

Cutaneous
innervation

FIGURE 2-22 cont'd

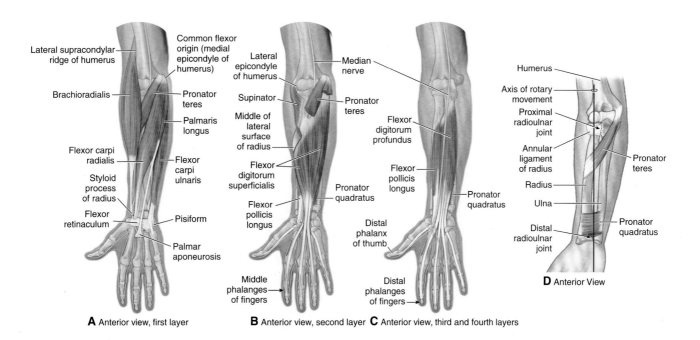

A Anterior view, first layer

Lateral supracondylar ridge of humerus
Brachioradialis
Flexor carpi radialis
Styloid process of radius
Flexor retinaculum
Common flexor origin (medial epicondyle of humerus)
Pronator teres
Palmaris longus
Flexor carpi ulnaris
Pisiform
Palmar aponeurosis

B Anterior view, second layer
Lateral epicondyle of humerus
Supinator
Middle of lateral surface of radius
Flexor digitorum superficialis
Flexor pollicis longus
Pronator quadratus
Middle phalanges of fingers

C Anterior view, third and fourth layers
Median nerve
Pronator teres
Flexor digitorum profundus
Flexor pollicis longus
Pronator quadratus
Distal phalanx of thumb
Distal phalanges of fingers

D Anterior View
Humerus
Axis of rotary movement
Proximal radioulnar joint
Annular ligament of radius
Radius
Ulna
Distal radioulnar joint
Pronator teres
Pronator quadratus

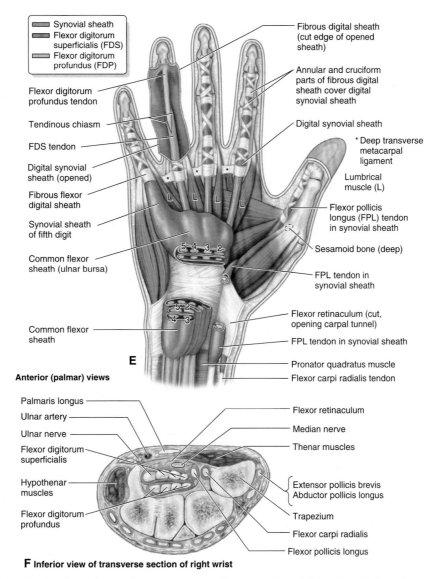

Synovial sheath
Flexor digitorum superficialis (FDS)
Flexor digitorum profundus (FDP)

Flexor digitorum profundus tendon
Tendinous chiasm
FDS tendon
Digital synovial sheath (opened)
Fibrous flexor digital sheath
Synovial sheath of fifth digit
Common flexor sheath (ulnar bursa)
Common flexor sheath

Fibrous digital sheath (cut edge of opened sheath)
Annular and cruciform parts of fibrous digital sheath cover digital synovial sheath
Digital synovial sheath
* Deep transverse metacarpal ligament
Lumbrical muscle (L)
Flexor pollicis longus (FPL) tendon in synovial sheath
Sesamoid bone (deep)
FPL tendon in synovial sheath
Flexor retinaculum (cut, opening carpal tunnel)
FPL tendon in synovial sheath
Pronator quadratus muscle
Flexor carpi radialis tendon

E

Anterior (palmar) views

Palmaris longus
Ulnar artery
Ulnar nerve
Flexor digitorum superficialis
Hypothenar muscles
Flexor digitorum profundus

Flexor retinaculum
Median nerve
Thenar muscles
Extensor pollicis brevis
Abductor pollicis longus
Trapezium
Flexor carpi radialis
Flexor pollicis longus

F Inferior view of transverse section of right wrist

FIGURE 2–23 **Muscles of the anterior compartment of forearm and hand. A,** First layer. **B,** Second layer. **C,** Third layer. **D,** Fourth layer. 1, Wrist joint; 2, carpometacarpal joint; 3, metacarpophalangeal joint; 4, proximal interphalangeal joint; 5, distal interphalangeal joint. **E,** Dissection of common flexor sheath and synovial sheaths of digits 1-5 (purple). **F,** Transverse section of wrist showing carpal tunnel and its contents. (Reprinted with permission from Moore, K. L., Agur, A. M., & Dalley, A. F.II. (2019). *Moore's Essential clinical anatomy* (6th ed.). Philadelphia, PA: Wolters Kluwer.)

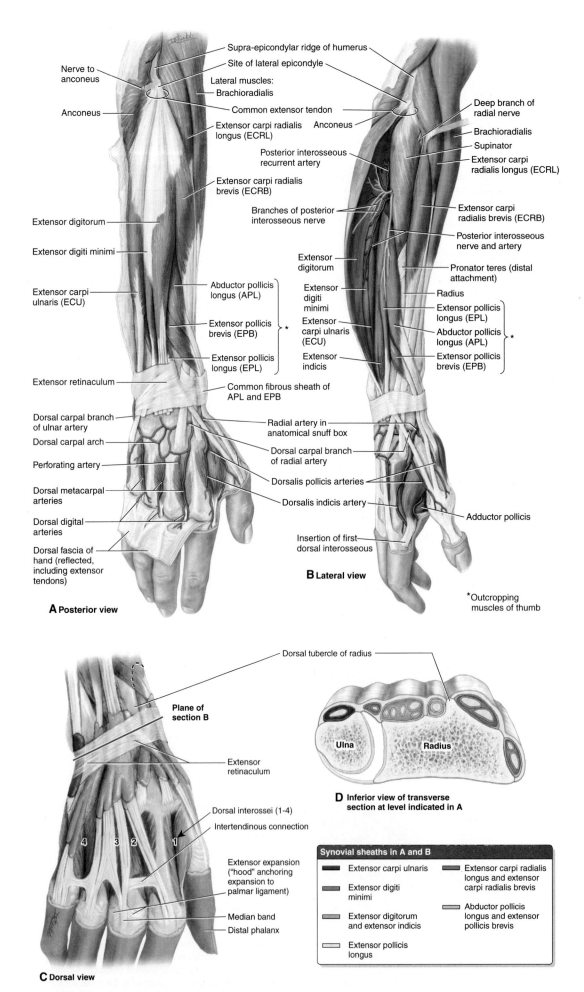

FIGURE 2-24 Muscles and neurovascular structures of the posterior compartment of forearm and hand.
A, Superficial dissection. **B,** Deep dissection. **C,** Synovial sheaths of extensor tendons on distal forearm and dorsum of hand. **D,** Transverse section through distal end of radius and ulna to show extensor tendons in their synovial sheaths. (Reprinted with permission from Moore, K. L., Agur, A. M., & Dalley, A. F.II. (2019). *Moore's Essential clinical anatomy* (6th ed.). Philadelphia, PA: Wolters Kluwer.)

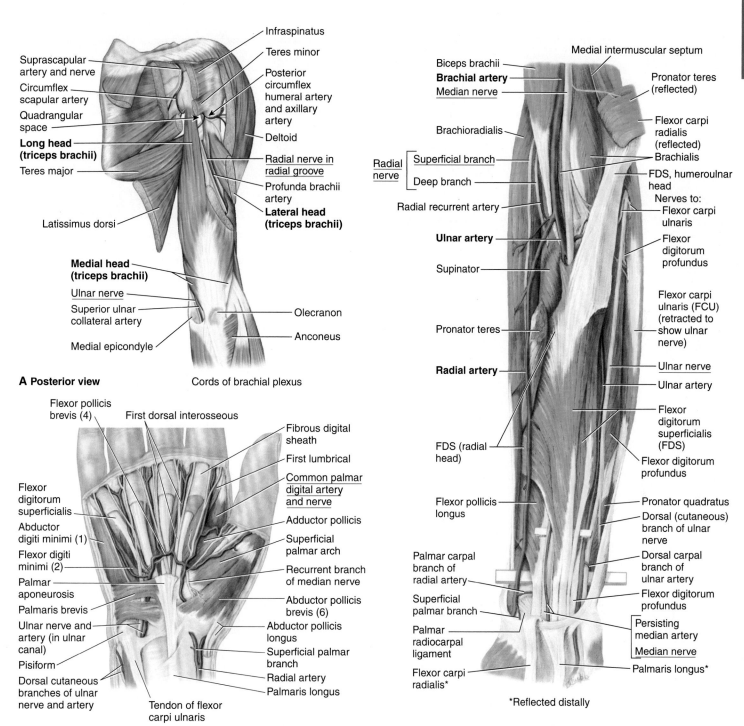

A Posterior view

- Suprascapular artery and nerve
- Circumflex scapular artery
- Quadrangular space
- **Long head (triceps brachii)**
- Teres major
- Latissimus dorsi
- Infraspinatus
- Teres minor
- Posterior circumflex humeral artery and axillary artery
- Deltoid
- Radial nerve in radial groove
- Profunda brachii artery
- **Lateral head (triceps brachii)**
- **Medial head (triceps brachii)**
- Ulnar nerve
- Superior ulnar collateral artery
- Medial epicondyle
- Olecranon
- Anconeus
- Cords of brachial plexus

B Anterior view

- Biceps brachii
- **Brachial artery**
- Median nerve
- Brachioradialis
- Radial nerve
  - Superficial branch
  - Deep branch
- Radial recurrent artery
- **Ulnar artery**
- Supinator
- Pronator teres
- **Radial artery**
- FDS (radial head)
- Flexor pollicis longus
- Palmar carpal branch of radial artery
- Superficial palmar branch
- Palmar radiocarpal ligament
- Flexor carpi radialis*
- Medial intermuscular septum
- Pronator teres (reflected)
- Flexor carpi radialis (reflected)
- Brachialis
- FDS, humeroulnar head
- Nerves to:
  - Flexor carpi ulnaris
  - Flexor digitorum profundus
- Flexor carpi ulnaris (FCU) (retracted to show ulnar nerve)
- Ulnar nerve
- Ulnar artery
- Flexor digitorum superficialis (FDS)
- Flexor digitorum profundus
- Pronator quadratus
- Dorsal (cutaneous) branch of ulnar nerve
- Dorsal carpal branch of ulnar artery
- Flexor digitorum profundus
- Persisting median artery
- Median nerve
- Palmaris longus*

*Reflected distally

C Anterior view

- Flexor pollicis brevis (4)
- First dorsal interosseous
- Flexor digitorum superficialis
- Abductor digiti minimi (1)
- Flexor digiti minimi (2)
- Palmar aponeurosis
- Palmaris brevis
- Ulnar nerve and artery (in ulnar canal)
- Pisiform
- Dorsal cutaneous branches of ulnar nerve and artery
- Tendon of flexor carpi ulnaris
- Fibrous digital sheath
- First lumbrical
- Common palmar digital artery and nerve
- Adductor pollicis
- Superficial palmar arch
- Recurrent branch of median nerve
- Abductor pollicis brevis (6)
- Abductor pollicis longus
- Superficial palmar branch
- Radial artery
- Palmaris longus

FIGURE 2–25 **Nerves of the upper limb** that are highly susceptible to compression. **A,** Upper arm. **B,** Elbow/forearm region. **C,** Hand. (Adapted with permission from Moore, K. L., Agur, A. M., & Dalley, A. F.II. (2019). *Moore's Essential clinical anatomy* (6th ed.). Philadelphia, PA: Wolters Kluwer.)

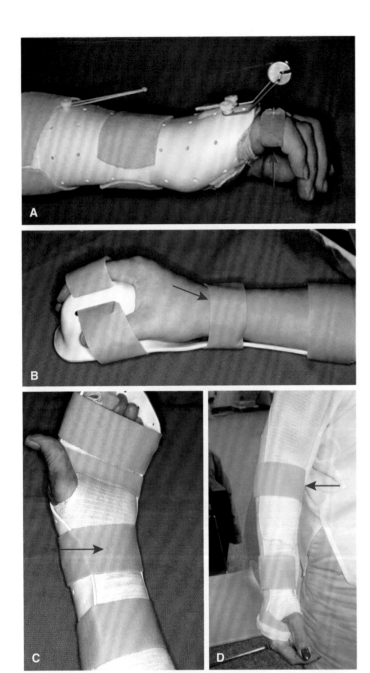

FIGURE 2–26 **A,** This MCP extension mobilization orthosis puts the digital nerves at risk for compression volarly as the weight of the fingers rests volarly the slings. **B,** The wrist strap on this antispasticity orthosis is neither wide nor made of soft flexible material; thus, the radial sensory nerve is at risk for irritation. **C,** The wrist strap on this wrist/hand immobilization orthosis, if placed too tightly, combined with the necessary wrist flexed positioning, can place undue pressure on the median nerve at the carpal tunnel level. **D,** If the proximal strap on this forearm rotation-restriction orthosis is applied to tightly, it can result in ulnar nerve irritation with distal paresthesias in the hand.

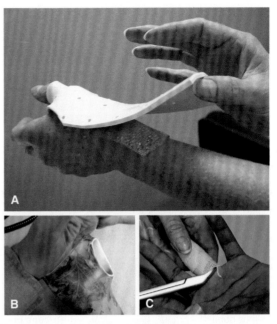

FIGURE 2–27 **A,** Gel padding underneath this radial-based thumb orthosis to protect a hypersensitive radial sensory nerve. **B,** The therapist's palm is being used to "flare and smooth" the distal edge of this orthosis. **C,** Trimming proximally on this PIP joint cast to prevent sharp edge from irritating digital nerves.

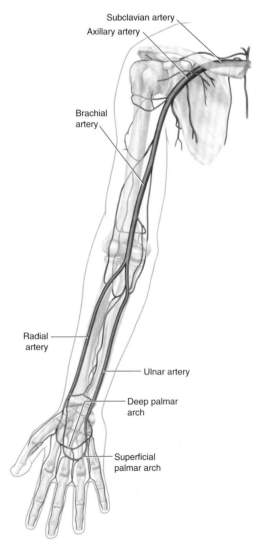

Anterior view

FIGURE 2–28 **Arterial supply of upper limb.** (Reprinted with permission from Moore, K. L., Agur, A. M., & Dalley, A. F., II. (2019). *Moore's essential clinical anatomy* (6th ed.). Philadelphia, PA: Wolters Kluwer. Fig. 3.13 (not images – just center drawing).)

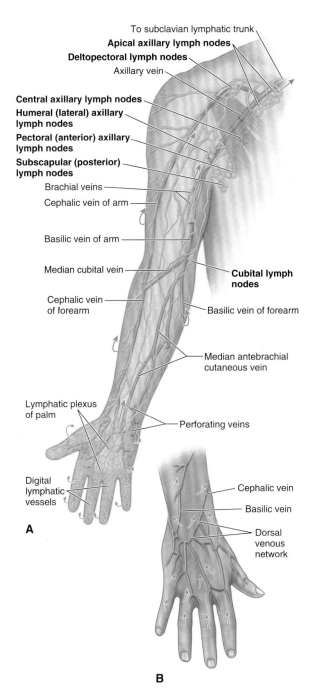

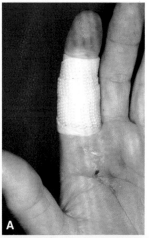

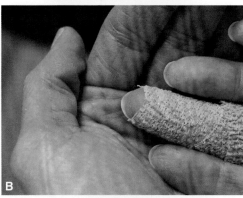

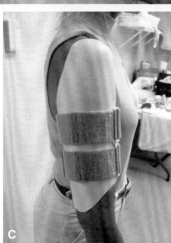

FIGURE 2–29 **Superficial venous and lymphatic drainage of upper limb.** **A,** Anterior (palmar) view of upper limb. **B,** Posterior view of distal forearm and hand. Green arrows, superficial lymphatic drainage to lymph nodes. (Reprinted with permission from Moore, K. L., Agur, A. M., & Dalley, A. F., II. (2019). *Moore's essential clinical anatomy* (6th ed.). Philadelphia, PA: Wolters Kluwer. Fig. 3.11.)

FIGURE 2–30 **A,** Note change in color of the fingertip with this circumferential cast indicating excess pressure on the digital blood supply. **B,** When any circumferential wrap is applied to a body part, the patients should remain in the clinic to monitor for any vascular changes so timely adjustments can be made prior to sending them home. **C,** Patients wearing circumferential orthotic designs, such as this humerus orthosis, should be educated regarding signs and symptoms of neurovascular compromise. Oftentimes, these designs can be modified into a bivalve or clamshell-type design with a strapping system as shown here to allow for easy adjustments of circumferential pressure.

compression products for management of edema; they must be applied judiciously, and the patient should be informed regarding any adverse signs. The problem may be resolved by simply adjusting the amount of tension on the wrap or by changing the wear schedule to intermittent use.

CONCLUSION

The anatomy of the hand and upper extremity is an intricate arrangement of bones, muscles, vessels, and other soft-tissue structures that interact to allow for functional use of the upper limb. To appropriately apply orthoses, the therapist must understand how these structures function together and how they interact with orthoses.

CHAPTER REVIEW QUESTIONS

1. What are the three arches in the hand?
2. How can the creases of the hand be used during the orthotic fabrication process?
3. Describe two techniques to accommodating for bony prominences.
4. What are the signs of nerve irritation?
5. What precautions must a therapist educate a patient to be aware of when dispensing these devices?

TABLE 2–1   Joints of the Wrist and Hand

Joint	Type	Articulation	Joint Capsule	Ligaments	Movements	Blood Supply	Nerve Supply
Wrist (radiocarpal)	Condyloid synovial joint	Distal end of radius and articular disc with proximal row of carpal bones (except pisiform)	Fibrous layer of joint capsule surrounds joint and attaches to distal ends of radius and ulna and proximal row of carpal bones; lined by synovial membrane	Anterior and posterior ligaments strengthen fibrous capsule; ulnar collateral ligament attaches to styloid process of ulna and triquetrum; radial collateral ligament attaches to styloid process of radius and scaphoid	Flexion-extension, abduction-adduction, circumduction	Dorsal and palmar carpal arches	
Carpal (intercarpal)	Plane synovial joint	Between carpal bones of proximal row; joints between carpal bones of distal row *Midcarpal joint:* synovial joint between proximal and distal rows of carpal bones *Pisiform joint:* synovial joint between pisiform and triquetrum	Fibrous layer of joint capsule surrounds joints; lined by synovial membrane; pisiform joint is separate from other carpal joints	Carpal bones united by anterior, posterior, and interosseous ligaments	Small amount of gliding movement possible; flexion and abduction of hand occur at midcarpal joint	Dorsal and palmar carpal arches	Anterior interosseous branch of median nerve, posterior interosseous branch of radial nerve, and dorsal and deep branches of ulnar nerve
Carpometacarpal (CMC) and intermetacarpal (IM)	Plane synovial joints, except for CMC joint of thumb (saddle-shaped synovial joint)	Carpals and metacarpals with each other; CMC joint of thumb between trapezium and base of first metacarpal	Fibrous layer of joint capsule surrounds joints; lined on internal surface by synovial membrane	Bones united by anterior, posterior, and interosseous ligaments	Flexion-extension and abduction-adduction of CMC joint of first digit; almost no movement at second and third digits; fourth digit slightly mobile; fifth digit very mobile	Dorsal and palmar metacarpal arteries and deep carpal and deep palmar arches	

Reprinted with permission from Moore, K. L., Agur, A. M., & Dalley, A. F.II. (2019). Moore's Essential clinical anatomy (6th ed.). Philadelphia, PA: Wolters Kluwer.

CHAPTER 2

TABLE 2–2   **Joints of the Digits**

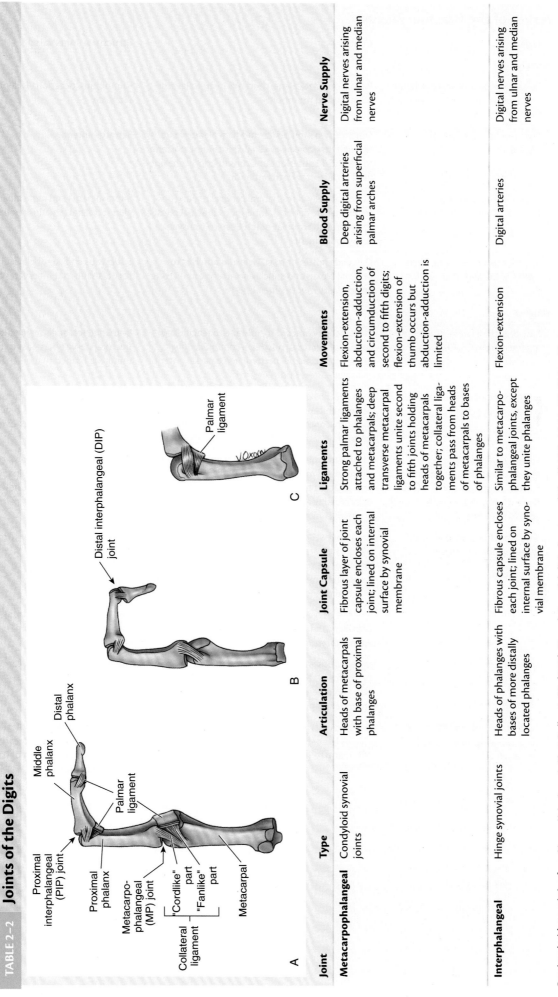

A

B

C

Joint	Type	Articulation	Joint Capsule	Ligaments	Movements	Blood Supply	Nerve Supply
Metacarpophalangeal	Condyloid synovial joints	Heads of metacarpals with base of proximal phalanges	Fibrous layer of joint capsule encloses each joint; lined on internal surface by synovial membrane	Strong palmar ligaments attached to phalanges and metacarpals; deep transverse metacarpal ligaments unite second to fifth joints holding heads of metacarpals together; collateral ligaments pass from heads of metacarpals to bases of phalanges	Flexion-extension, abduction-adduction, and circumduction of second to fifth digits; flexion-extension of thumb occurs but abduction-adduction is limited	Deep digital arteries arising from superficial palmar arches	Digital nerves arising from ulnar and median nerves
Interphalangeal	Hinge synovial joints	Heads of phalanges with bases of more distally located phalanges	Fibrous capsule encloses each joint; lined on internal surface by synovial membrane	Similar to metacarpophalangeal joints, except they unite phalanges	Flexion-extension	Digital arteries	Digital nerves arising from ulnar and median nerves

Reprinted with permission from Moore, K. L., Agur, A. M., & Dalley, A. F.II. (2019). Moore's Essential clinical anatomy (6th ed.). Philadelphia, PA: Wolters Kluwer.

TABLE 2–3   Nerves of the Brachial Plexus

Nerve	Origin[a]	Course	Structures Innervated
Supraclavicular Branches			
Dorsal scapular	Posterior aspect of anterior ramus of **C5** with a frequent contribution from C4	Pierces middle scalene; descends deep to levator scapulae and rhomboids	Rhomboids; occasionally supplies levator scapulae
Long thoracic	Posterior aspect of anterior rami of **C5, C6,** C7	Superior two rami pierce middle scalene; passes through cervicoaxillary canal, descending posterior to C8 and T1 anterior rami; runs inferiorly on superficial surface of serratus anterior	Serratus anterior
Suprascapular	Superior trunk, receiving fibers from **C5,** C6, and often C4	Passes laterally across lateral cervical region (posterior triangle of neck), superior to brachial plexus; then through scapular notch deep to transverse scapular ligament	Supraspinatus and infraspinatus muscles; glenohumeral (shoulder) joint
Subclavian nerve (nerve to subclavius)	Superior trunk, receiving fibers from C5, **C6,** and often C4	Descends posterior to clavicle and anterior to brachial plexus and subclavian artery; often giving an *accessory root to phrenic nerve*	Subclavius and sternoclavicular joint (accessory phrenic root innervates diaphragm)
Infraclavicular Branches			
Lateral pectoral	Side branch of lateral cord, receiving fibers from C5, **C6,** C7	Pierces costocoracoid membrane to reach deep surface of pectoral muscles; a *communicating branch to the medial pectoral nerve* passes anterior to axillary artery and vein	Primarily pectoralis major, but some lateral pectoral nerve fibers pass to pectoralis minor via branch to medial pectoral nerve
Musculocutaneous	Terminal branch of lateral cord, receiving fibers from C5-C7	Exits axilla by piercing coracobrachialis; descends between biceps brachii and brachialis, supplying both; continues as *lateral cutaneous nerve of forearm*	Muscles of anterior compartment of arm (coracobrachialis, biceps brachii, and brachialis); skin of lateral aspect of forearm
Median	*Lateral root of median nerve* is a terminal branch of lateral cord (C6, C7 fibers); *medial root of median nerve* is a terminal branch of medial cord (C8, T1 fibers)	Lateral and medial roots merge to form median nerve lateral to axillary artery; descends through arm adjacent to brachial artery, with nerve gradually crossing anterior to artery to lie medial to artery in cubital fossa	Muscles of anterior forearm compartment (except for flexor carpi ulnaris and ulnar half of flexor digitorum profundus), five intrinsic muscles in thenar half of palm and palmar skin
Medial pectoral	Side branches of medial cord, receiving fibers from C8, T1	Passes between axillary artery and vein; then pierces pectoralis minor and enters deep surface of pectoralis major; although it is called *medial* for its origin from medial cord, it lies lateral to lateral pectoral nerve	Pectoralis minor and sternocostal part of pectoralis major
Medial cutaneous nerve of arm		Smallest nerve of plexus; runs along medial side of axillary and brachial veins; communicates with *intercostobrachial nerve*	Skin of medial side of arm, as far distal as medial epicondyle of humerus and olecranon of ulna
Median cutaneous nerve of forearm		Initially runs with ulnar nerve (with which it may be confused) but pierces deep fascia with basilic vein and enters subcutaneous tissue, dividing into anterior and posterior branches	Skin of medial side of forearm, as far distal as wrist
Ulnar	Larger terminal branch of medial cord, receiving fibers from C8, T1, and often C7	Descends medial arm; passes posterior to medial epicondyle of humerus; then descends ulnar aspect of forearm to hand	Flexor carpi ulnaris and ulnar half of flexor digitorum profundus (forearm); most intrinsic muscles of hand; skin of hand medial to axial line of digit 4

TABLE 2–3 · Nerves of the Brachial Plexus (Continued)

Nerve	Origin[a]	Course	Structures Innervated

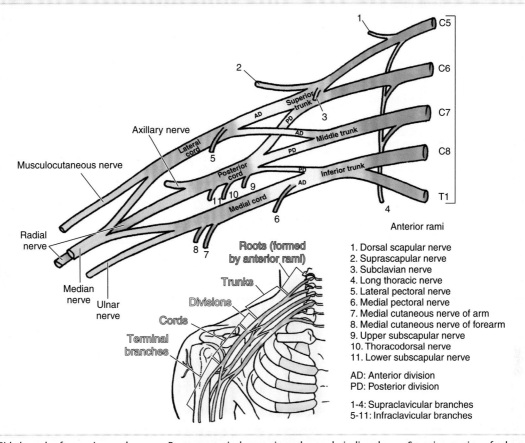

Anterior rami

Roots (formed by anterior rami)

Trunks
Divisions
Cords
Terminal branches

1. Dorsal scapular nerve
2. Suprascapular nerve
3. Subclavian nerve
4. Long thoracic nerve
5. Lateral pectoral nerve
6. Medial pectoral nerve
7. Medial cutaneous nerve of arm
8. Medial cutaneous nerve of forearm
9. Upper subscapular nerve
10. Thoracodorsal nerve
11. Lower subscapular nerve

AD: Anterior division
PD: Posterior division

1-4: Supraclavicular branches
5-11: Infraclavicular branches

Labels on figure: Axillary nerve, Musculocutaneous nerve, Lateral cord, Superior trunk, Middle trunk, Inferior trunk, Posterior cord, Medial cord, Radial nerve, Median nerve, Ulnar nerve, C5, C6, C7, C8, T1

Nerve	Origin[a]	Course	Structures Innervated
Upper subscapular	Side branch of posterior cord, receiving fibers from **C5**	Passes posteriorly, entering subscapularis directly	Superior portion of subscapularis
Lower subscapular	Side branch of posterior cord, receiving fibers from **C6**	Passes inferolaterally, deep to subscapular artery and vein	Inferior portion of subscapularis and teres major
Thoracodorsal	Side branch of posterior cord, receiving fibers from C6, **C7**, C8	Arises between upper and lower subscapular nerves and runs inferolaterally along posterior axillary wall to apical part of latissimus dorsi	Latissimus dorsi
Axillary	Terminal branch of posterior cord, receiving fibers from **C5**, C6	Exits axillary fossa posteriorly, passing through quadrangular space[b] with posterior circumflex humeral artery; gives rise to *superior lateral brachial cutaneous nerve*; then winds around surgical neck of humerus deep to deltoid	Glenohumeral (shoulder) joint; teres minor and deltoid muscles; skin of superolateral arm (over inferior part of deltoid)
Radial	Larger terminal branch of posterior cord (largest branch of plexus), receiving fibers from C5 to T1	Exits axillary fossa posterior to axillary artery; passes posterior to humerus in radial groove with profunda brachii artery between lateral and medial heads of triceps; perforates lateral intermuscular septum; enters cubital fossa, dividing into *superficial* (cutaneous) and *deep* (motor) *radial nerves*	All muscles of posterior compartments of arm and forearm; skin of posterior and inferolateral arm, posterior forearm, and dorsum of hand lateral to axial line of digit 4

Modified with permission from Moore, K. L., Agur, A. M., & Dalley, A. F.II. (2019). Moore's Essential clinical anatomy (6th ed.). Philadelphia, PA: Wolters Kluwer.
[a]*Boldface indicates primary component of the nerve.*
[b]*Bounded superiorly by the subscapularis, head of humerus, and teres minor; inferiorly by the teres major; medially by the long head of the triceps; and laterally by the coracobrachialis and surgical neck of the humerus.*

TABLE 2–4	**Nerves of the Upper Extremity**

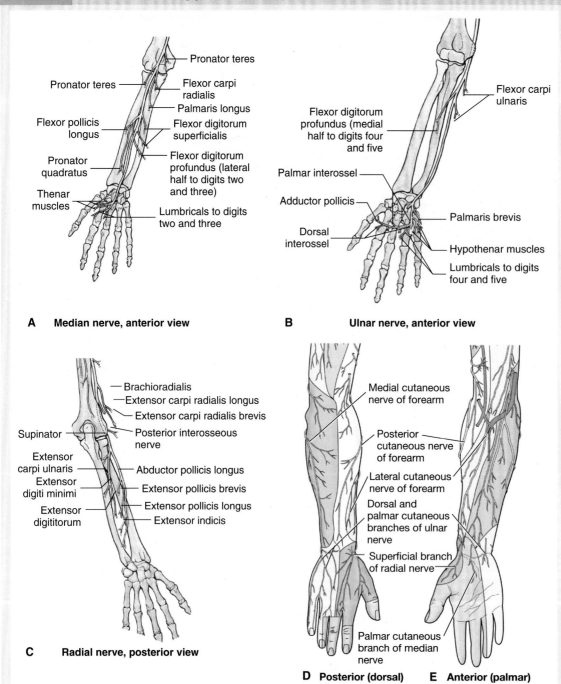

A Median nerve, anterior view

B Ulnar nerve, anterior view

C Radial nerve, posterior view

D Posterior (dorsal) view

E Anterior (palmar) view

Nerve	Origin	Course in Forearm
Median	By union of lateral root of median nerve (C6, C7, from lateral cord of brachial plexus) with medial root (C8, T1) from medial cord	Enters cubital fossa medial to brachial artery; exits by passing between heads of pronator teres; descends in fascial plane between flexors digitorum superficialis and profundus; runs deep to palmaris longus tendon as it approaches flexor retinaculum to traverse carpal tunnel
Anterior interosseous	Median nerve in distal part of cubital fossa	Descends on anterior aspect of interosseous membrane with artery of same name, between FDP and FPL, to pass deep to pronator quadratus

TABLE 2–4   **Nerves of the Upper Extremity   (Continued)**

Nerve	Origin	Course in Forearm
Palmar cutaneous branch of median nerve	Median nerve of middle to distal forearm, proximal to flexor retinaculum	Passes superficial to flexor retinaculum to reach skin of central palm
Ulnar	Larger terminal branch of medial cord of brachial plexus (C8, T1, often receives fibers from C7)	Enters forearm by passing between heads of flexor carpi ulnaris, after passing posterior to medial epicondyle of humerus; descends forearm between FCU and FDP; becomes superficial in distal forearm
Palmar cutaneous branch of ulnar nerve	Ulnar nerve near middle of forearm	Descends anterior to ulnar artery; perforates deep fascia in distal forearm; runs in subcutaneous tissue to palmar skin medial to axis of fourth digit
Dorsal cutaneous branch of ulnar nerve	Ulnar nerve in distal half of forearm	Passes posteroinferiorly between ulna and flexor carpi ulnaris; enters subcutaneous tissue to supply skin of dorsum medial to axis of fourth digit
Radial	Larger terminal branch of posterior cord of brachial plexus (C5-T1)	Enters cubital fossa between brachioradialis and brachialis; anterior to lateral epicondyle divides into terminal superficial and deep branches
Posterior cutaneous nerve of forearm	Radial nerve, as it traverses radial groove of posterior humerus	Perforates lateral head of triceps; descends along lateral side of arm and posterior aspect of forearm to wrist
Superficial branch of radial nerve	Sensory terminal branch of radial nerve, in cubital fossa	Descends between pronator teres and brachioradialis, emerging from latter to arborize over anatomical snuff box and supply skin of dorsum lateral to axis of fourth finger
Deep branch of radial/posterior interosseous nerve	Motor terminal branch of radial nerve, in cubital fossa	Deep branch exits cubital fossa winding around neck of radius, penetrating and supplying supinator; emerges in posterior compartment of forearm as posterior interosseous nerve; descends on membrane with artery of same name
Lateral cutaneous nerve of forearm	Continuation of musculocutaneous nerve distal to muscular branches	Emerges lateral to biceps brachii on brachialis, running initially with cephalic vein; descends along lateral border of forearm to wrist
Medial cutaneous nerve of forearm	Medial cord of brachial plexus, receiving C8 and T1 fibers	Perforates deep fascia of arm with basilic vein proximal to cubital fossa; descends medial aspect of forearm in subcutaneous tissue to wrist

Modified with permission from Moore, K. L., Agur, A. M., & Dalley, A. F.II. (2019). Moore's Essential clinical anatomy (6th ed.). Philadelphia, PA: Wolters Kluwer.
FCU, flexor carpi ulnaris; FDP, flexor digitorum profundus; FPL, flexor pollicis longus.

TABLE 2–5	Muscles of the Upper Extremity

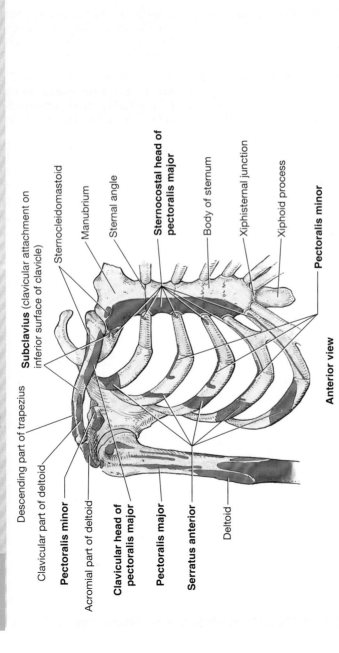

Descending part of trapezius

Subclavius (clavicular attachment on inferior surface of clavicle)

Clavicular part of deltoid

Sternocleidomastoid

Pectoralis minor

Manubrium

Acromial part of deltoid

Sternal angle

Clavicular head of pectoralis major

Sternocostal head of pectoralis major

Pectoralis major

Body of sternum

Serratus anterior

Xiphisternal junction

Xiphoid process

Deltoid

Pectoralis minor

Anterior view

Anterior Axioappendicular Muscles

Muscle	Medial Attachment	Lateral Attachment	Innervation[a-g]	Main Action(s)
Pectoralis major	*Clavicular head:* anterior surface of medial half of clavicle *Sternocostal head:* anterior surface of sternum, superior six costal cartilages, aponeurosis of external oblique muscle	Lateral lip of intertubercular sulcus (groove) of humerus	Lateral and medial pectoral nerves; clavicular head (C5, **C6**), sternocostal head (**C7**, **C8**, T1)	Adducts and medially rotates humerus; draws scapula anteriorly and inferiorly Acting alone, clavicular head flexes humerus and sternocostal head extends it from the flexed position
Pectoralis minor	Third to fifth ribs near their costal cartilages	Medial border and superior surface of coracoid process of scapula	Medial pectoral nerve (C8, T1)	Stabilizes scapula by drawing inferiorly and anteriorly against thoracic wall
Subclavius	Junction of first rib and its costal cartilage	Inferior surface of middle third of clavicle	Subclavian nerve (**C5**, C6)	Anchors and depresses clavicle
Serratus anterior	External surfaces of lateral parts of first to eighth ribs	Anterior surface of medial border of scapula	Long thoracic nerve (C5, **C6**, **C7**)	Protracts scapula and holds against thoracic wall; rotates scapula

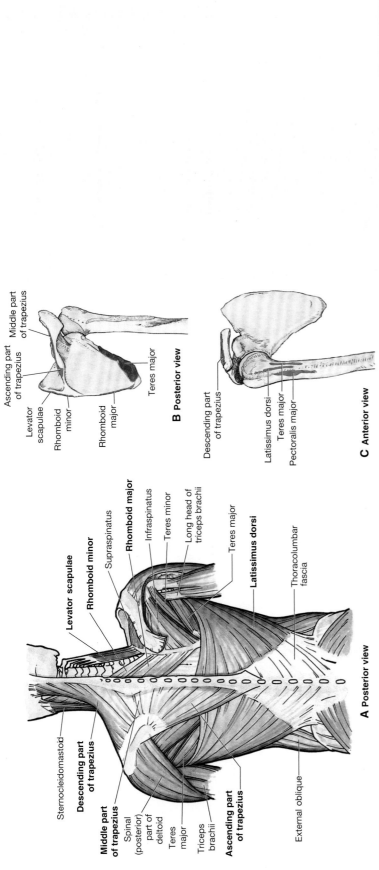

A Posterior view

Ascending part of trapezius — Middle part of trapezius

Levator scapulae
Rhomboid minor
Rhomboid major
Teres major

B Posterior view

Descending part of trapezius

Latissimus dorsi
Teres major
Pectoralis major

C Anterior view

Labels (A Posterior view): Sternocleidomastoid; Descending part of trapezius; Middle part of trapezius; Spinal (posterior) part of deltoid; Teres major; Triceps brachii; Ascending part of trapezius; External oblique; Levator scapulae; Rhomboid minor; Supraspinatus; Rhomboid major; Infraspinatus; Teres minor; Long head of triceps brachii; Teres major; Latissimus dorsi; Thoracolumbar fascia

Posterior Axioappendicular Muscles

Muscle	Medial Attachment	Lateral Attachment	Innervation[a-g]	Main Action(s)
Superficial posterior thoracoappendicular (extrinsic shoulder) muscles				
Trapezius	Medial third of superior nuchal line; external occipital protuberance; nuchal ligament; spinous processes of C7-T12 vertebrae	Lateral third of clavicle; acromion, and spine of scapula	Spinal accessory nerve (CN XI) (motor fibers) and C3, C4 (pain and proprioceptive fibers)	*Descending (superior) part* elevates; *ascending (inferior) part* depresses; and *middle part* (or all parts together) retracts scapula; descending and ascending parts act together to rotate glenoid cavity superiorly
Latissimus dorsi	Spinous processes of inferior six thoracic vertebrae, thoracolumbar fascia, iliac crest, and inferior three or four ribs	Floor of intertubercular sulcus (groove) of humerus	Thoracodorsal nerve (**C6, C7**, C8)	Extends, adducts, and medially rotates humerus; raises body toward arms during climbing
Deep posterior thoracoappendicular (extrinsic shoulder) muscles				
Levator scapulae	Posterior tubercles of transverse processes of C1-C4 vertebrae	Medial border of scapula superior to root of spine	Dorsal scapular (C5) and cervical (C3, C4) nerves	Elevates scapula and tilts its glenoid cavity inferiorly by rotating scapula
Rhomboid minor and major	*Minor:* nuchal ligament; spinous processes of C7 and T1 vertebrae *Major:* spinous processes of T2-T5 vertebrae	*Minor:* triangular area at medial end of scapular spine *Major:* medial border of scapula from level of spine to inferior angle	Dorsal scapular nerve (C4, **C5**)	Retract scapula and rotate it to depress glenoid cavity; fix scapula to thoracic wall

(Continued)

TABLE 2-5 Muscles of the Upper Extremity (Continued)

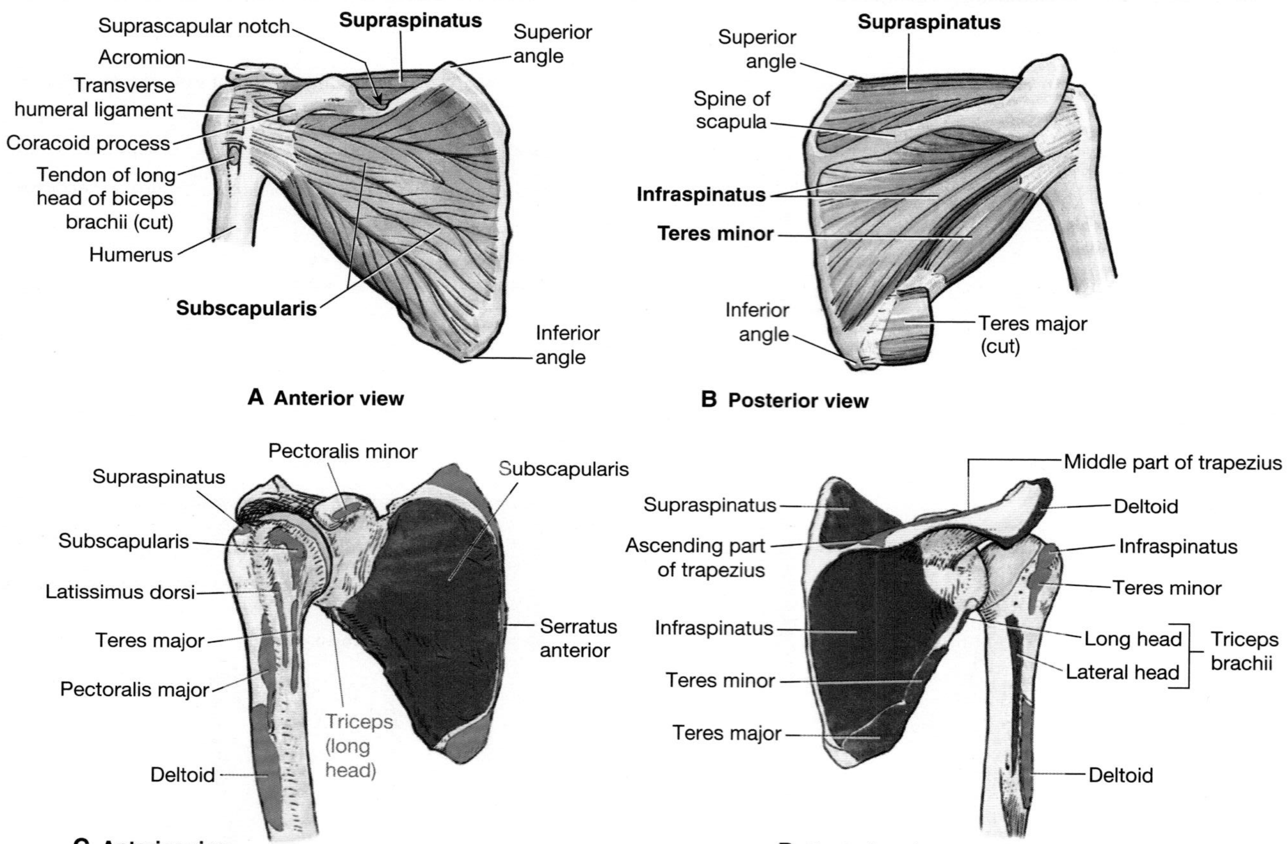

Supraspinatus
Superior angle
Spine of scapula
Infraspinatus
Teres minor
Inferior angle
Teres major (cut)

B Posterior view

Suprascapular notch
Acromion
Transverse humeral ligament
Coracoid process
Tendon of long head of biceps brachii (cut)
Humerus
Supraspinatus
Superior angle
Subscapularis
Inferior angle

A Anterior view

Pectoralis minor
Subscapularis
Supraspinatus
Subscapularis
Latissimus dorsi
Teres major
Pectoralis major
Triceps (long head)
Serratus anterior
Deltoid

C Anterior view

Middle part of trapezius
Deltoid
Infraspinatus
Teres minor
Long head / Lateral head — Triceps brachii
Deltoid
Supraspinatus
Ascending part of trapezius
Infraspinatus
Teres minor
Teres major

D Posterior view

Scapulohumeral (Intrinsic Shoulder) Muscles

Muscle	Medial Attachment	Lateral Attachment	Innervation[a–g]	Main Action(s)
Deltoid	Lateral third of clavicle; acromion, and spine of scapula	Deltoid tuberosity of humerus	Axillary nerve (**C5**, C6)	Clavicular (anterior) part flexes and medially rotates arm; acromial (middle) part abducts arm; spinal (posterior) part extends and laterally rotates arm
Supraspinatus[h]	Supraspinous fossa of scapula	Superior facet	Suprascapular nerve (C4, **C5**, C6)	Initiates and assists deltoid in abduction of arm and acts with other rotator cuff muscles[h]
Infraspinatus[h]	Infraspinous fossa of scapula	Middle facet — Of greater tubercle of humerus	Suprascapular nerve (**C5**, C6)	Laterally rotate arm; help hold humeral head in glenoid cavity of scapula
Teres minor[h]	Middle part of lateral border of scapula	Inferior facet	Axillary nerve (**C5**, C6)	

Muscle	Medial Attachment	Lateral Attachment	Innervation	Main Action(s)
Teres major	Posterior surface of inferior angle of scapula	Medial lip of intertubercular groove of humerus	Lower subscapular nerve (C5, **C6**)	Adducts and medially rotates arm
Subscapularis[h]	Subscapular fossa (most of anterior surface of scapula)	Lesser tubercle of humerus	Upper and lower subscapular nerves (C5, **C6**, C7)	Medially rotates and adducts arm; helps hold humeral head in glenoid cavity

A Anterior view

Labels: Pectoralis minor; Coracobrachialis; Brachialis; Biceps brachii (short head) and coracobrachialis; Biceps brachii; Brachialis

B Posterior view

Labels: Long head; Lateral head (Triceps brachii); Brachialis; Triceps brachii, medial head; Triceps brachii; Anconeus

Muscles of Arm

Muscle	Medial Attachment	Lateral Attachment	Innervation[a–g]	Main Action(s)
Biceps brachii	*Short head:* tip of coracoid process of scapula *Long head:* supraglenoid tubercle of scapula	Tuberosity of radius and fascia of forearm via bicipital aponeurosis	Musculocutaneous nerve[i] (C5, **C6**)	Supinates forearm and, when it is supinated, flexes forearm; flexes arm; short head resists dislocation of shoulder
Brachialis	Distal half of anterior surface of humerus	Coronoid process and tuberosity of ulna		Flexes forearm in all positions
Coracobrachialis	Tip of coracoid process of scapula	Middle third of medial surface of humerus	Musculocutaneous nerve (C5, **C6**, C7)	Helps flex and adduct arm; resists dislocation of shoulder
Triceps brachii	*Long head:* infraglenoid tubercle of scapula *Lateral head:* posterior surface of humerus, superior to radial groove *Medial head:* posterior surface of humerus, inferior to radial groove	Proximal end of olecranon of ulna and fascia of forearm	Radial nerve (C6, **C7**, **C8**)	Chief extensor of forearm; long head extends arm and resists dislocation of humerus (especially important during abduction)
Anconeus	Lateral epicondyle of humerus	Lateral surface of olecranon and superior part of posterior surface of ulna	Radial nerve (C7, **C8**, T1)	Assists triceps in extending forearm; stabilizes elbow joint; abducts ulna during pronation

(Continued)

| TABLE 2–5 | Muscles of the Upper Extremity | (Continued) |

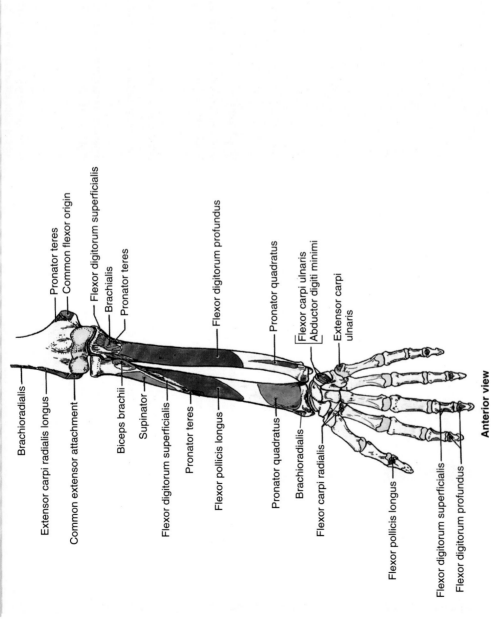

Anterior view

Muscles of Anterior Compartment of Forearm

Muscle	Medial Attachment	Lateral Attachment	Innervation[a–g]	Main Action(s)
Superficial (first) layer				
Pronator teres (PT)	*Ulnar head:* coronoid process of ulna	Middle of convexity of lateral surface of radius	Median nerve (C6, **C7**)	Pronates and flexes forearm (at elbow)
	Humeral head: Medial epicondyle of humerus			
Flexor carpi radialis (FCR)		Base of second (third) metacarpal		Flexes and abducts hand (at wrist)
Palmaris longus	Medial epicondyle of humerus	Distal half of flexor retinaculum, palmar aponeurosis	Median nerve (C7, C8)	Flexes hand (at wrist) and tenses palmar aponeurosis

Muscle	Proximal Attachment	Distal Attachment	Innervation	Main Action
Flexor carpi ulnaris (FCU): Humeral head, Ulnar head	Olecranon and posterior border (via aponeurosis)	Pisiform, hook of hamate, fifth metacarpal	Ulnar nerve (C7, **C8**)	Flexes and adducts hand (at wrist)
Intermediate (second) layer				
Flexor digitorum superficialis (FDS)	*Humeroulnar head:* medial epicondyle of humerus and coronoid process of ulna *Radial head:* oblique line of radius	Shafts (bodies) of middle phalanges of medial four digits	Median nerve (C7, C8, T1)	Flexes proximal interphalangeal joints of middle four digits; acting more strongly, it also flexes proximal phalanges at metacarpophalangeal joints
Deep (third) layer				
Flexor digitorum profundus (FDP)	Proximal three quarters of medial and anterior surfaces of ulna and interosseous membrane	Bases of distal phalanges of second, third, fourth, and fifth digits	*Lateral part (to digits 2 and 3):* median nerve (C8, **T1**) (anterior interosseous branch) *Medial part (to digits 4 and 5):* ulnar nerve (**C8**, T1)	Flexes distal interphalangeal joints of digits 2, 3, 4, and 5; assists with wrist flexion
Flexor pollicis longus (FPL)	Anterior surface of radius and adjacent interosseous membrane	Base of distal phalanx of thumb	Anterior interosseous nerve, from median nerve (**C8**, T1)	Flexes phalanges of first digit (thumb)
Pronator quadratus	Distal quarter of anterior surface of ulna	Distal quarter of anterior surface of radius		Pronates forearm; deep fibers bind radius and ulna together
Muscles of Posterior Compartment of Forearm				
Superficial layer				
Brachioradialis	Proximal two-thirds of lateral supraepicondylar ridge of humerus	Lateral surface of distal end of radius proximal to styloid process	Radial nerve (C5, **C6**, C7)	Relatively weak flexion of forearm, maximal when forearm is in midpronated position
Extensor carpi radialis longus	Lateral supraepicondylar ridge of humerus	Dorsal aspect of base of second metacarpal	Radial nerve (C6, C7)	Extend and abduct hand at the wrist joint; extensor carpi radialis brevis active during fist clenching
Extensor carpi radialis brevis	Lateral epicondyle of humerus (common extensor origin)	Dorsal aspect of base of third metacarpal	Deep branch of radial nerve (**C7**, C8)	
Extensor digitorum		Extensor expansions of medial four fingers	Posterior interosseous nerve (**C7**, C8), continuation of deep branch of radial nerve	Extends medial four fingers primarily at metacarpophalangeal joints, secondarily at interphalangeal joints
Extensor digiti minimi		Extensor expansion of fifth finger		Extends fifth finger primarily at metacarpophalangeal joint, secondarily at interphalangeal joint
Extensor carpi ulnaris	Lateral epicondyle of humerus; posterior border of ulna via a shared aponeurosis	Dorsal aspect of base of fifth metacarpal		Extends and adducts hand at wrist joint (also active during fist clenching)
Deep layer				
Supinator	Lateral epicondyle of humerus; radial collateral and annular ligaments; supinator fossa; crest of ulna	Lateral, posterior, and anterior surfaces of proximal third of radius	Deep branch of radial nerve (C7, **C8**)	Supinates forearm; rotates radius to turn palm anteriorly or superiorly (if elbow is flexed)

(Continued)

TABLE 2–5 **Muscles of the Upper Extremity** (Continued)

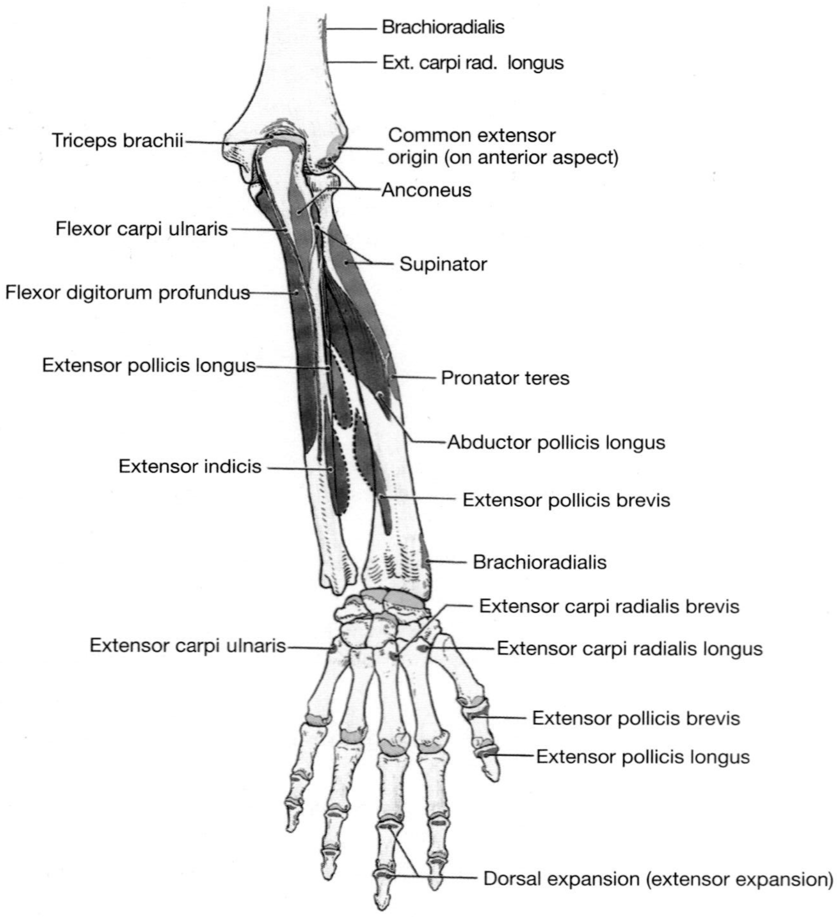

Triceps brachii
Brachioradialis
Ext. carpi rad. longus
Common extensor origin (on anterior aspect)
Anconeus
Flexor carpi ulnaris
Supinator
Flexor digitorum profundus
Pronator teres
Extensor pollicis longus
Abductor pollicis longus
Extensor indicis
Extensor pollicis brevis
Brachioradialis
Extensor carpi radialis brevis
Extensor carpi radialis longus
Extensor carpi ulnaris
Extensor pollicis brevis
Extensor pollicis longus
Dorsal expansion (extensor expansion)

Posterior view

"Outcropping" muscles of deep layer

Abductor pollicis longus	Posterior surface of proximal halves of ulna, radius, and interosseous membrane	Base of first metacarpal	Posterior interosseous nerve (C7, **C8**), continuation of deep branch of radial nerve	Abducts thumb and extends it at carpometacarpal joint
Extensor pollicis longus	Posterior surface of middle third of ulna and interosseous membrane	Dorsal aspect of base of distal phalanx of thumb		Extends distal phalanx of thumb at interphalangeal joint; extends metacarpophalangeal and carpometacarpal joints
Extensor pollicis brevis	Posterior surface of distal third of radius and interosseous membrane	Dorsal aspect of base of proximal phalanx of thumb		Extends proximal phalanx of thumb at metacarpophalangeal joint; extends carpometacarpal joint
Extensor indicis	Posterior surface of distal third of ulna and interosseous membrane	Extensor expansion of second finger		Extends second finger (enabling its independent extension); helps extend hand at wrist

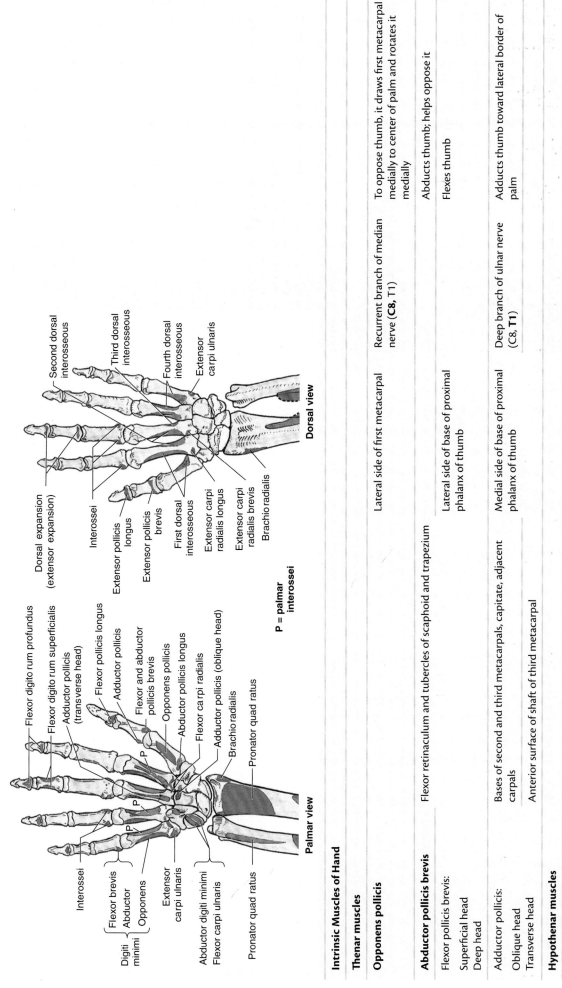

Palmar view

- Interossei
- Digiti minimi { Flexor brevis, Abductor, Opponens
- Extensor carpi ulnaris
- Abductor digiti minimi
- Flexor carpi ulnaris
- Pronator quad ratus

- Flexor digito rum profundus
- Flexor digito rum superficialis
- Adductor pollicis (transverse head)
- Flexor pollicis longus
- Adductor pollicis
- Flexor and abductor pollicis brevis
- Opponens pollicis
- Abductor pollicis longus
- Flexor carpi radialis
- Adductor pollicis (oblique head)
- Brachio radialis
- Pronator quad ratus

P = palmar interossei

- Second dorsal interosseous
- Third dorsal interosseous
- Fourth dorsal interosseous
- Extensor carpi ulnaris

- Dorsal expansion (extensor expansion)
- Interossei
- Extensor pollicis longus
- Extensor pollicis brevis
- First dorsal interosseous
- Extensor carpi radialis longus
- Extensor carpi radialis brevis
- Brachio radialis

Dorsal view

Intrinsic Muscles of Hand

Thenar muscles

Muscle	Origin	Insertion	Nerve	Action
Opponens pollicis	Flexor retinaculum and tubercles of scaphoid and trapezium	Lateral side of first metacarpal	Recurrent branch of median nerve (**C8**, T1)	To oppose thumb, it draws first metacarpal medially to center of palm and rotates it medially
Abductor pollicis brevis		Lateral side of base of proximal phalanx of thumb		Abducts thumb; helps oppose it
Flexor pollicis brevis:				Flexes thumb
Superficial head				
Deep head				
Adductor pollicis:	Bases of second and third metacarpals, capitate, adjacent carpals	Medial side of base of proximal phalanx of thumb	Deep branch of ulnar nerve (C8, **T1**)	Adducts thumb toward lateral border of palm
Oblique head				
Transverse head	Anterior surface of shaft of third metacarpal			

Hypothenar muscles

Muscle	Origin	Insertion	Nerve	Action
Abductor digiti minimi	Pisiform	Medial side of base of proximal phalanx of fifth finger	Deep branch of ulnar nerve (C8, **T1**)	Abducts fifth finger; assists in flexion of its proximal phalanx
Flexor digiti minimi brevis	Hook of hamate and flexor retinaculum			Flexes proximal phalanx of fifth finger
Opponens digiti minimi		Medial border of fifth metacarpal		Draws fifth metacarpal anterior and rotates it, bringing fifth finger into opposition with thumb

(Continued)

TABLE 2-5   Muscles of the Upper Extremity   (Continued)

	Proximal attachment	Distal attachment	Innervation	Main actions
Short muscles				
Lumbricals				
1 and 2	Lateral two tendons of flexor digitorum profundus (as unipennate muscles)	Lateral sides of extensor expansions of second to fifth fingers	Median nerve (C8, **T1**)	Flex metacarpophalangeal joints; extend interphalangeal joints of second to fifth fingers
3 and 4	Medial three tendons of flexor digitorum profundus (as bipennate muscles)			
Dorsal interossei, 1-4	Adjacent sides of two metacarpals (as bipennate muscles)	Bases of proximal phalanges; extensor expansions of second to fourth fingers	Deep branch of ulnar nerve (C8, **T1**)	Abduct second to fourth fingers from axial line; act with lumbricals in flexing metacarpophalangeal joints and extending interphalangeal joints
Palmar interossei, 1-3	Palmar surfaces of 2nd, 4th, and 5th metacarpals (as unipennate muscles)	Bases of proximal phalanges; extensor expansions of second, fourth, and fifth fingers		Adduct second, fourth, and fifth fingers toward axial line; assist lumbricals in flexing metacarpophalangeal joints and extending interphalangeal joints

Modified with permission from Moore, K. L., Agur, A. M., & Dalley, A. F.II. (2019). Moore's Essential clinical anatomy (6th ed.). Philadelphia, PA: Wolters Kluwer.

[a]The spinal cord segmental innervation is indicated (e.g., "C5, C6" means that the nerves supplying the subclavius are derived from the fifth and sixth cervical segments of the spinal cord). Numbers in boldface (C5) indicate the main segmental innervation. Damage to one or more of the listed spinal cord segments or to the motor nerve roots arising from them results in paralysis of the muscles concerned.

[b]The spinal cord segmental innervation is indicated (e.g., "C6, C7, C8" means that the nerves supplying the latissimus dorsi are derived from the sixth through eighth cervical segments of the spinal cord). Numbers in boldface (C6, C7) indicate the main segmental innervation. Damage to one or more of the listed spinal cord segments or to the motor nerve roots arising from them results in paralysis of the muscles concerned.

[c]The spinal cord segmental innervation is indicated (e.g., "C5, C6" means that the nerves supplying the deltoid are derived from the fifth and sixth cervical segments of the spinal cord). Numbers in boldface (C5) indicate the main segmental innervation. Damage to one or more of the listed spinal cord segments or to the motor nerve roots arising from them results in paralysis of the muscles concerned.

[d]The spinal cord segmental innervation is indicated (e.g., "C5, C6" means that the nerves supplying the biceps brachii are derived from the fifth and sixth cervical segments of the spinal cord). Numbers in boldface (C6) indicate the main segmental innervation. Damage to one or more of the listed spinal cord segments or to the motor nerve roots arising from them results in paralysis of the muscles concerned.

[e]The spinal cord segmental innervation is indicated (e.g., "C6, C7" means that the nerves supplying the pronator teres are derived from the sixth and seventh cervical segments of the spinal cord). Numbers in boldface (C7) indicate the main segmental innervation. Damage to one or more of the listed spinal cord segments or to the motor nerve roots arising from them results in paralysis of the muscles concerned.

[f]The spinal cord segmental innervation is indicated (e.g., "C7, C8" means that the nerves supplying the extensor carpi radialis brevis are derived from the seventh and eighth cervical segments of the spinal cord). Numbers in boldface (C7) indicate the main segmental innervation. Damage to one or more of the listed spinal cord segments or to the motor nerve roots arising from them results in paralysis of the muscles concerned.

[g]The spinal cord segmental innervation is indicated (e.g., "C8, T1" means that the nerves supplying the opponens pollicis are derived from the eighth cervical segment and first thoracic segment of the spinal cord). Numbers in boldface (C8) indicate the main segmental innervation. Damage to one or more of the listed spinal cord segments or to the motor nerve roots arising from them results in paralysis of the muscles concerned.

[h]Collectively, the supraspinatus, infraspinatus, teres minor, and subscapularis muscles are referred to as the rotator cuff, or SITS, muscles. Their primary function during all movements of the glenohumeral (shoulder) joint is to hold the humeral head in the glenoid cavity of the scapula.

[i]Some of the lateral part of the brachialis is innervated by a branch of the radial nerve.

TABLE 2–6   Blood Supply of the Upper Extremity

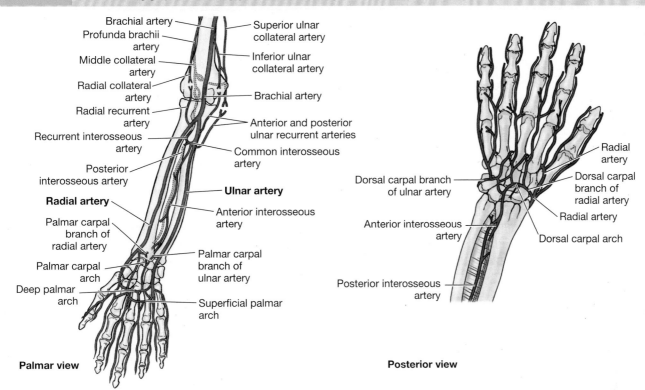

Palmar view

Posterior view

Arteries of Forearm and Wrist

Artery	Origin	Course
Ulnar	As larger terminal branch of brachial artery in cubital fossa	Descends inferomedially and then directly inferiorly deep to superficial pronator teres, palmaris longus, and flexor digitorum superficialis to reach medial side of forearm; passes superficial to flexor retinaculum at wrist in ulnar (Guyon) canal to enter hand
Anterior ulnar recurrent artery	Ulnar artery just distal to elbow joint	Passes superiorly between brachialis and pronator teres, supplying both; then anastomoses with inferior ulnar collateral artery anterior to medial epicondyle
Posterior ulnar recurrent artery	Ulnar artery distal to anterior ulnar recurrent artery	Passes superiorly, posterior to medial epicondyle and deep to tendon of flexor carpi ulnaris; then anastomoses with superior ulnar collateral artery
Common interosseous	Ulnar artery in cubital fossa, distal to bifurcation of brachial artery	Passes laterally and deeply, terminating by dividing into anterior and posterior interosseous arteries
Anterior interosseous	As terminal branches of common interosseous artery, between radius and ulna	Passes distally on anterior aspect of interosseous membrane to proximal border of pronator quadratus; pierces membrane and continues distally to join dorsal carpal arch on posterior aspect of interosseous membrane
Posterior interosseous		Passes to posterior aspect of interosseous membrane, giving rise to recurrent interosseous artery; runs distally between superficial and deep extensor muscles, supplying both
Recurrent interosseous	Posterior interosseous artery, between radius and ulna	Passes superiorly, posterior to proximal radioulnar joint, to anastomose with middle collateral artery (from deep artery of arm)
Palmar carpal branch	Ulnar artery in distal forearm	Runs across anterior aspect of wrist, deep to tendons of flexor digitorum profundus, to anastomose with the palmar carpal branch of the radial artery, forming **palmar carpal arch**

(Continued)

TABLE 2-6	Blood Supply of the Upper Extremity (Continued)	
Artery	**Origin**	**Course**
Dorsal carpal branch	Ulnar artery, proximal to pisiform	Passes across dorsal surface of wrist, deep to extensor tendons, to anastomose with dorsal carpal branch of radial artery, forming **dorsal carpal arch**
Radial	As smaller terminal branch of brachial artery in cubital fossa	Runs inferolaterally under cover of brachioradialis; lies lateral to flexor carpi radialis tendon in distal forearm; winds around lateral aspect of radius and crosses floor of anatomical snuff box to pierce first dorsal interosseous muscle
Radial recurrent	Lateral side of radial artery, just distal to brachial artery bifurcation	Ascends between brachioradialis and brachialis, supplying both (and elbow joint); then anastomoses with radial collateral artery (from profunda brachii artery)
Palmar carpal branch	Distal radial artery near distal border of pronator quadratus	Runs across anterior wrist deep to flexor tendons to anastomose with the palmar carpal branch of ulnar artery to form palmar carpal arch
Dorsal carpal branch	Distal radial artery in proximal part of snuff box	Runs medially across wrist deep to pollicis and extensor radialis tendons, anastomoses with ulnar dorsal carpal branch forming dorsal carpal arch
Arteries of Hand		
Superficial palmar arch	Direct continuation of ulnar artery; arch is completed on lateral side by superficial branch of radial artery or another of its branches	Curves laterally deep to palmar aponeurosis and superficial to long flexor tendons; curve of arch lies across palm at level of distal border of extended thumb

Anterior view

Lateral view (isolated third digit)

Posterior view

Deep palmar arch	Direct continuation of radial artery; arch is completed on medial side by deep branch of ulnar artery	Curves medially, deep to long flexor tendons; is in contact with bases of metacarpals
Common palmar digitals	Superficial palmar arch	Pass distally on lumbricals to webbing of fingers
Proper palmar digitals	Common palmar digital arteries	Run along sides of second to fifth digits
Princeps pollicis	Radial artery as it turns into palm	Descends on palmar aspect of first metacarpal; divides at base of proximal phalanx into two branches that run along sides of thumb
Radialis indicis	Radial artery; but may arise from princeps pollicis artery	Passes along lateral side of index finger to its distal end
Dorsal carpal arch	Radial and ulnar arteries	Arches within fascia on dorsum of hand
Palmar carpal arch	Radial and ulnar arteries	Arches on anterior aspect of wrist

Modified with permission from Moore, K. L., Agur, A. M., & Dalley, A. F.II. (2019). Moore's Essential clinical anatomy (6th ed.). Philadelphia, PA: Wolters Kluwer.

3

Tissue Healing[a]

Richard A. Bernstein, MD, FAAOS
Nancy Beaman, MBA, OTR/L, CHT

CHAPTER OBJECTIVES

After study of this chapter, the reader should be able to:

- Define the three stages of tissue healing.
- Understand which types of orthoses are appropriate to apply at each stage of wound healing.
- Explain how lifestyle factors can influence a patient's ability to heal.
- Give a minimum of one diagnosis and the most appropriate orthosis intervention for each of the following: immobilization, restriction, and mobilization of healing tissue.
- Recognize the impact preexisting medical conditions have on the healing process.
- Discuss the importance of patient education regarding precautions for orthosis wear.

KEY TERMS

Antideformity position
Collagen synthesis
Edema
Elastic behavior
Fibroblasts
Fibroplasia and proliferative stage

Granulation tissue
Infections
Inflammatory stage
Macrophages
Maturation and remodeling stage
Osteoblasts
Osteoclasts
Plastic behavior

Primary closure
Secondary intention
Stages of tissue healing
Tensile strength
Tissue oxygenation
Tissue remodeling
Viscoelastic properties

INTRODUCTION

The biology of soft-tissue healing is paramount to the treatment of hand and upper extremity disorders. Whether undergoing traumatic or elective surgery, understanding the biologic processes involved is important to predict patient outcomes. Both the surgeon and therapist need to understand, and to a large degree predict, how the tissue will respond to the injury. This understanding guides the patients' rehabilitation, use of orthoses, modalities, and progression of functional tasks. The **stages of tissue healing** influence the use and extent of orthotic intervention and therapy; the status and stage of a healing wound direct the specifics of orthotic selection, fabrication, and patient use.

STAGES OF WOUND HEALING

The stages of tissue healing are inflammation, fibroplasia (proliferative), and scar maturation (chronic stage or remodeling) (Figure 3–1). The response to injury is proportional to the nature and severity of the trauma, associated injuries, and tissue contamination. For instance, a sharp laceration with a "clean" knife through nerve and tendon will respond acutely and chronically different than a 50-lb dirty weight crushing a finger and transecting the nerve and tendon. Sharp injuries do better than crush, and clean better than contaminated. Inflammation sometimes has a negative connotation, but inflammation is a necessary biologic response to injury. Scavenger cells such as **macrophages** and **osteoclasts** migrate into

the area to biologically debride the injured tissue, and the inflammatory response also brings in healing cells including **fibroblasts** and **osteoblasts**.

Tissue oxygenation is essential for wound healing. Oxygen is carried in blood, dissolved in plasma, and bound to hemoglobin. Biologic function and tissue processes are dependent on adequate tissue oxygenation, which requires adequate vascularization (Stotts & Wipke-Tevis, 1997). Orthoses and edema management products need to help stabilize the tissue environment, allow adequate blood flow, and avoid impeding arterial inflow or venous outflow.

INFLAMMATORY STAGE

The first stage, the inflammatory stage lasts for less than 1 week and is characterized by an influx of white blood cells, especially macrophages, and an increase in local vascularity (Figure 3–1). These scavenger cells help cleanse the area of bacteria, necrotic debris, and foreign material. Edema occurs from the body's inflammatory response to injury, increased vascularity, and often some degree of venous congestion (Smith & Dean, 1998; Strickland, 1987, 2000). At this stage, rest is more important than exercise; immobilization orthoses are useful for protecting, supporting, and resting the injured part (Figure 3–2A–C). Because of the tendency for venous congestion, elevation can help improve the tissue congestion, and orthoses help decrease the stress or tension on a surgically repaired structure, such as bone, tendon, or nerve. The orthosis should maintain the injured part in a position that is best for subsequent restoration of function. Classically, this involves the position of function, **antideformity position**: slight wrist extension

---

[a]This chapter is based on the first edition chapter written by Steven Wenner, MD and Ellen Smithline, RN.

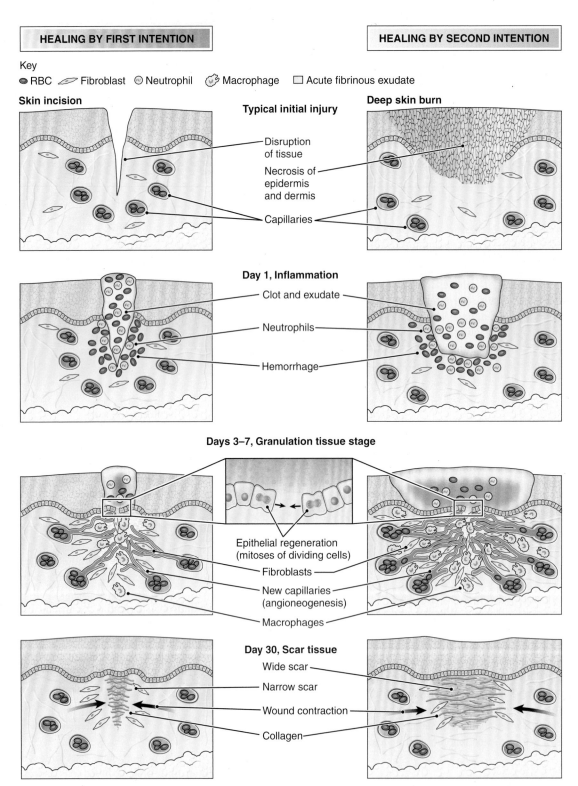

FIGURE 3–1 Healing by first and second intention. Small, narrow wounds heal by first intention (**left**), usually in less than a week, and leave a small scar. Large wounds heal by second intention (**right**), have more inflammatory tissue, take several weeks to heal, and leave a larger scar. (Borrowed with permission from McConnell, T. H. (2007). *The nature of disease: Pathology for the health professions.* Philadelphia, PA: Lippincott Williams & Wilkins.)

along with metacarpophalangeal (MCP) joint flexion and proximal interphalangeal (PIP) joint extension (Figure 3–3A and B). This posture places the collateral ligaments of the MCP joints and volar plates at the PIP joints at maximal tension to help counteract scarring and contracture that can subsequently impede motion (risk of MCP extension and PIP flexion contracture). By placing these soft-tissue structures at maximal tension, once therapy begins, one does not need to counteract tissue tightness. Simultaneously, adjacent structures should be positioned to prevent unwanted deformity and to facilitate prompt return to function (Smith & Dean, 1998).

FIBROPLASIA AND PROLIFERATIVE STAGE

The second stage of fibroplasia begins 4 or 5 days after the injury and lasts for 2 to 6 weeks (Figure 3–1). Fibroblasts enter the wound and begin synthesizing collagen, which ultimately becomes the scar tissue. Whereas bone is the only tissue to regenerate itself, collagen proliferation, although, on the positive side, augments healing, on the negative side, interferes with the normal tissue. **Granulation tissue** depends on adequate angiogenesis and tissue oxygenation. Early in the fibroblastic stage, immobilization allows neovascularization and protects the newly deposited immature collagen fibers,

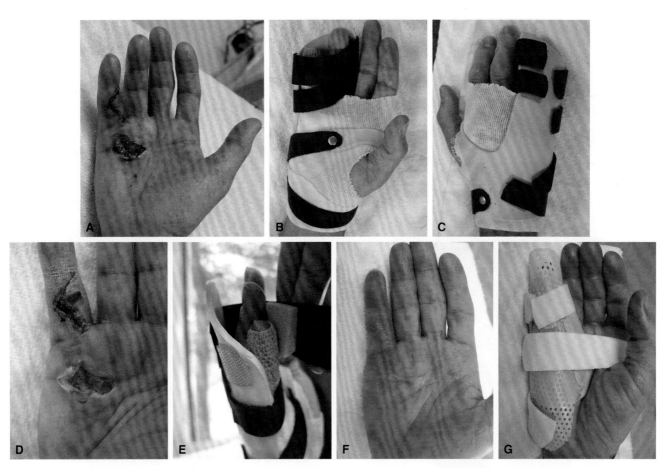

FIGURE 3-2 A, Inflammatory stage of healing characterized by fibrin depositing and forming the initial gel of the wound matrix. First day postoperative Dupuytren's release, notice skin closed in digit with sutures, while the palm was left open to heal by secondary intention. **B and C,** Hand-based ring and small finger immobilization orthosis used postoperatively to position digits in maximal extension. Note use of elasticized wrap to control edema. **D,** Proliferative stage of healing during which collagen is laid down, giving the wound strength. Shown is 10 days postoperative—sutures have been removed and open palm area is beginning to close. **E,** Orthosis modified by adding foam to provide gentle extension stretch to the PIP joint, counteracting tendency for flexion contracture. **F,** Scar maturation stage shown when collagen, responsible to structure and integrity of the wound, is formed in a generally random manner. Note complete wound closure at 6 weeks postoperative. **G,** Volar orthosis with Elastomer™ included for scar management; used at night for 6 additional months.

thereby facilitating an increase in tensile strength of the wound. Between weeks 3 and 6, cellularity diminishes, and the extracellular matrix, largely collagen, increases both in volume and in tensile strength (Smith & Dean, 1998; Strickland, 1987, 2000). During this stage, appropriately applied stress can facilitate tissue growth (Figure 3–2D and E). Mobilization orthoses, which take advantage of tissue's elasticity and responsiveness to external stress, are useful. A balance must be achieved between applying enough stress to encourage positive scar remodeling and avoiding excessive stress, which could cause further tissue damage (Figure 3–4A and B).

MATURATION AND REMODELING STAGE

During the stage of scar maturation (Figure 3–1), the collagen fibers become better organized and remodel along the lines of stress, thus enhancing the **tensile strength** of the healing wound. The load per cross-sectional area is referred to as tensile strength, which occurs at a rate equal to that of **collagen synthesis** (Fess & McCollum, 1998; Strickland, 1987, 2000). Therefore, understanding a tissue's tensile strength influences the decision process of orthotic intervention and therapy (Figure 3–2F and G). Bone, tendon, and nerve healing occur at varying rates and influence the therapy protocol.

Tensile strength is 30% at 3 weeks, 60% at 6 weeks, and 90% at 6 months (Figure 3–5). Therefore, orthotic use and the therapy regimen need to keep these tissue factors in mind during the

rehabilitative process (Kane, 1997). Although tensile strength of the flexor tendon is still diminished in the first 6 weeks postoperatively, with current surgical techniques, a supervised active protocol is typically begun during this period; early tendon gliding diminishes scarring within the flexor tendon sheath. (Refer to Chapter 23 for additional information.)

Although scars soften during the maturation and remodeling stage, they also contract and shorten. In certain circumstances, such as a partial fingertip amputation, wound contracture is a favorable process. Amputations without exposed bone measuring less than 1 cm² heal favorably by **secondary intention**. However, for instance, a laceration perpendicular to a flexor crease can lead to a permanent painful contracture. With shortening, the scar's elasticity decreases; thus, stretching and corrective orthoses are valuable for preventing unwanted contractures (Figure 3–6A and B). The length of the maturation phase depends on several factors, including age, comorbidities (such as diabetes or rheumatoid arthritis), genetic background, location of the wound, and length and intensity of the inflammatory phase. Scar maturation is a continual process, and remodeling can occur for up to a year (Smith & Dean, 1998; Strickland, 1987, 2000).

The stages of wound healing are a fluid process, not necessarily segmental as staging suggests (Figure 3–7). Just as the healing stages overlap, so do the time frames for using specific orthoses

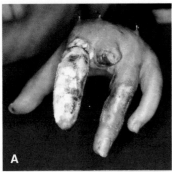

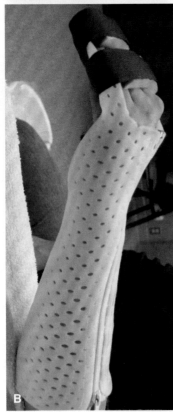

FIGURE 3–3 **A,** A press injury led to the amputation of the middle finger and replantation of the index and ring fingers. **B,** A simple immobilization orthosis promotes healing by providing a safe position for the joints: wrist extension, MCP joint flexion, IP joint extension, and thumb palmar abduction.

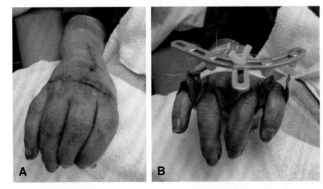

FIGURE 3–4 **A and B,** RA patient 10 days after MCP arthroplasty using mobilization orthosis during the encapsulation process to promote optimal collagen alignment. (Digitec Outrigger System, Performance Health, Warrenville, IL).

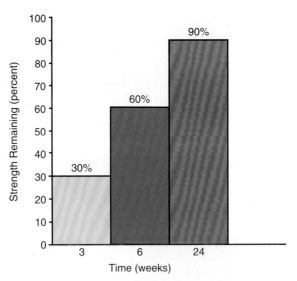

FIGURE 3–5 Tensile strength at 3 weeks, 6 weeks, and 6 months.

(Figure 3–8). For example, immobilization orthoses may be indicated throughout the healing process but typically more in the inflammatory phase. In subsequent phases, immobilization orthoses may have a role, especially during sleep, but mobilization orthoses are often used during the later stages (Colditz, 2011; Fess, Gettle, Phillips, & Janson, 2005).

EFFECT OF ORTHOSES ON TISSUE HEALING

During the inflammatory and early fibroblastic stages, certain tissues such as bone and nerve are best managed with immobilization orthoses; protection is more important than exercise (Figure 3–9A–D). Fractures need protection until callous begins to stabilize the bone; nerves repaired microsurgically need protection based on the intraoperative findings of the degree of tension at the repair site. When edema subsides, mobilization orthoses may be appropriate. Stress should be applied to the healing tissue to the degree that it favorably influences scar remodeling but not so much that it further damages tissues (Figure 3–10A–E). However, timing requires balance with biology; the degree of tissue trauma, persistent contamination or infection, or an immunocompromised host can prolong the inflammatory phase and retard healing.

Healthy healing tissue benefits from early therapy and responds favorably to continuously applied gentle stress. Edema and pain should diminish, and function should increase if the mobilizing orthosis is appropriately applied and working well. However, the overly aggressive use of mobilization orthoses (dynamic, static progressive, or serial static) during the fibroblastic stage or their premature use may reinjure healing tissues and retard recovery. For example, unstable fractures and torn collateral ligaments are injuries for which active range of motion (ROM) and accompanying mobilizing orthoses should be delayed until the likelihood of disruption of healing owing to a repeat injury is diminished (Fess & McCollum, 1998; Strickland, 1987, 2000).

For most tissues, the stress that can be safely applied and the degree and duration of the force increase at approximately 6 weeks after injury, when generally speaking tensile strength is 60% normal. At this point, the scar maturation or remodeling stage commences, and it is the sensible time to introduce serial static or static progressive orthoses (Figure 3–11).

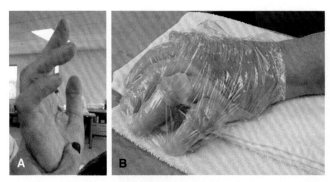

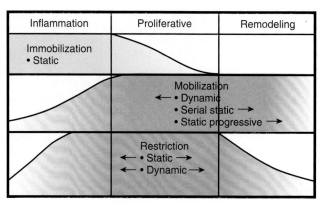

FIGURE 3–6 **A and B,** Patient with long-standing PIP joint flexion contractures caused by ulnar neuropathy using prefabricated PIP extension mobilization orthoses in conjunction with paraffin/heat application. This preconditioning of joints is helpful prior to manual therapy intervention.

FIGURE 3–8 Orthotic management for the patient should be based on the current stage of healing. The most common orthotic intervention is shown here; however, special conditions may require deviation from these guidelines.

TISSUE REMODELING

Soft tissue possesses **viscoelastic properties** that allow it to lengthen and shorten within a certain anatomical range. When soft tissue has shortened, perhaps as a consequence of scar contracture, orthotic and casting techniques are useful adjuncts for stretching the tight tissue.

Tissue remodeling may be favorably encouraged by gentle stretching over a period of time, allowing an alteration in cellular structure and alignment in response to the applied forces. Old cells are phagocytosed and new cells are created, orienting themselves in the direction of the tension. Through remodeling, the length of the previously contracted tissue increases—termed **elastic behavior**. On the other hand, tissue fibers that are stretched beyond their elastic limits will exhibit **plastic behavior** and tear or rupture. When plastic deformation occurs, enzymatic proteins are released from the cells and more scarring can occur (Brand & Thompson, 1993) (Figure 3–12).

CLINICAL CONSIDERATIONS

During the rehabilitation of injured tissue, the goal is gaining length of contracted tissue without causing further tissue damage, the latter can lead to inflammation, hemorrhage, and further scarring. This may occur with an overzealous stretching program or excessive force applied with an orthosis. Such tissues become reactive, stiff, and painful, possibly leading to problems such as a complex regional pain syndrome (CRPS), previously known as reflex sympathetic dystrophy (RSD) (Figure 3–13). Brand and Thompson (1993) noted that if tissue is held stretched to its tolerable limit for a longer time, it has a greater chance of undergoing permanent remodeling and lengthening. When applying mobilization orthoses, using a tolerable tension (lower stress) for a longer period of time is more beneficial than increasing the tension (high stress) for short periods of time (Brand & Thompson, 1993; Fess, Gettle, Phillips, & Janson, 2005).

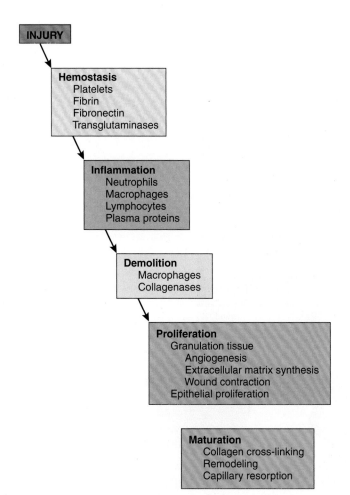

FIGURE 3–7 **The repair cascade.** Repair can be viewed as a chain of events, each stage completing the previous one and initiating the subsequent one. (Borrowed with permission from Rubin, E., & Farber, J. L. (1999). *Pathology* (3rd ed.). Philadelphia, PA: Lippincott Williams & Wilkins.)

CONDITIONS AND FACTORS THAT INFLUENCE TISSUE HEALING

Tissue healing and remodeling are influenced by several factors, including the magnitude of soft-tissue trauma, the extent of bony involvement, tissue contamination and infection, and vascular injury on both the venous and arterial sides. A stable skeletal platform is critical for healing; if one fails to achieve bony stability, soft-tissue healing can be compromised. Revascularization allows the influx of macrophages to remove debris, and increased tissue oxygenation aids cellular proliferation. Rigid internal fixation is the gold standard to treat unstable fractures; this not only provides the best biomechanical construct to allow bony healing but also helps diminish the stresses on the soft-tissue envelope. Plates or screws are most often utilized; Kirschner wires (K-wires) can also provide stability but not the same rigid mechanical construct. In the most extreme conditions, temporary or definitive treatment can be obtained through external fixation.

Some injuries include nerve damage that may lead to a loss of protective sensation. Once the orthosis is applied, the patient,

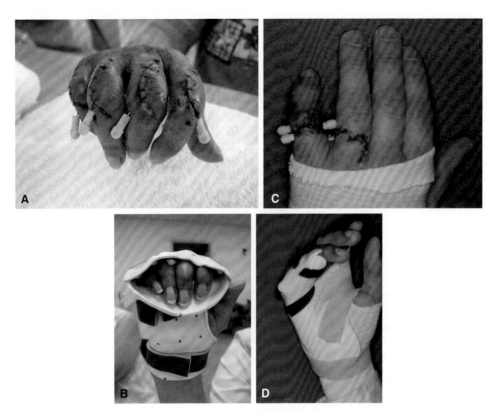

FIGURE 3–9 A and B, Patient with RA 2 days following PIP joint reconstruction to reverse swan-neck deformities; immobilization orthosis used to rest and protect reconstruction. Note position of MCP flexion to prevent collateral ligament shortening. **C and D,** Comminuted fractures of the small finger with percutaneous pinning and a hand-based protective orthosis to rest digit 5 days s/p surgery.

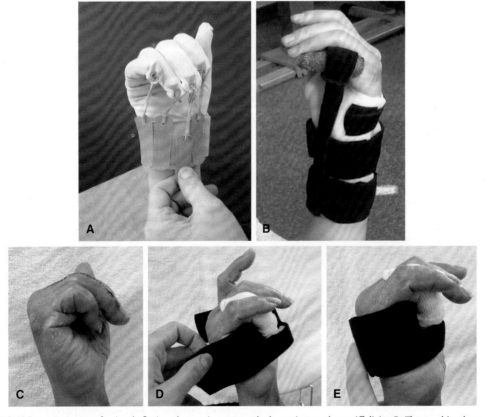

FIGURE 3–10 A, Use of a simple flexion glove to impart gentle dynamic stretch to stiff digits. **B,** The combined use of a wrist immobilization orthosis, digit cast using Orficast® and neoprene to mobilize a PIP flexion contracture into extension while imparting a gentle flexion force to a stiff MCP joint. **C–E,** A neoprene strap used to gently maintain flexion stress on a postsurgical extensor tenolysis of the ring finger.

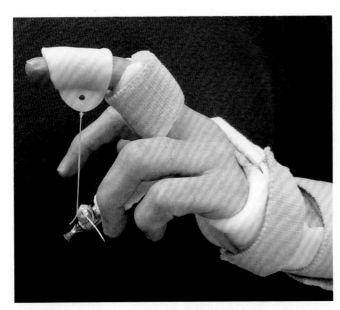

FIGURE 3–11 Middle finger PIP flexion mobilization orthosis used 8 weeks after a proximal phalanx fracture. A MERiT™ component provides the static progressive force. Note the extended outrigger on which the MERiT™ device rests. This allows for an accurate 90° angle of force application (Performance Health).

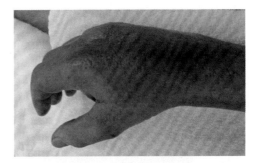

FIGURE 3–13 Right hand presents after carpal tunnel release (CTR) and trigger finger release (TFR) with excessive hypersensitivity, pain, and swelling—typical complex regional pain syndrome (CRPS).

family, medical staff, and therapist need to understand the importance of monitoring the extremity for possible skin irritation or breakdown caused by the orthosis (Figure 3–14A–F). Often, patients cannot fully appreciate the orthosis' contact with the skin, and pressure areas can develop. Any redness, erythema, or potential for skin breakdown needs to be immediately addressed to avoid frank ulceration. For patients at risk, the orthosis should be of lighter weight, incorporate protective padding, or be made with soft-lined materials to aid in protecting the at-risk tissue. Edges need to be smoothed and sharp or jagged borders avoided. Wide, soft, and strategically placed straps may aid in minimizing shear and compression stresses along the orthosis-skin interface and are of particular importance when applying an orthosis to an individual with vascular insufficiency.

AGE

Age strongly influences the healing process. The younger the patient, the more likely the tissue(s) involved will heal quickly and without complications. In general, younger patients need to wear orthoses and casts for shorter periods of time, since healing occurs sooner, and ROM is initiated earlier than for older patients. Stotts and Wipke-Tevis (1997) noted, "fetal wound healing is virtually

scarless." Comorbidities also increase with age. Diabetes, vascular insufficiency, steroid use, and associated peripheral neuropathies increase with age and are associated with a poorer prognosis.

LIFESTYLE FACTORS

Nutrition

Dietary factors have a profound effect on wound healing. On the most simplistic level, a diet with an appropriate balance of fat, proteins, and carbohydrates is essential. Caloric requirements are dramatically elevated after trauma; however, with massive trauma, often, a patient's ability to eat may be compromised. Parenteral nutrition can help if the gastrointestinal tract is poorly functioning. Measuring serum albumin levels can help guide a patient's nutritional status, while high-caloric supplements are often necessary. A deficient diet may contribute to weight loss, an increased risk of infection, and poor wound healing (Pinchocofsky-Devin, 1997). In thin patients or those with minimal subcutaneous fat, consider using soft prefabricated orthoses or orthotic materials made of neoprene; straps should be placed away from bony prominences, especially in cachectic or malnourished individuals.

Tobacco Use

Nicotine is a POTENT vasoconstrictor and restricts blood flow to the skin, thereby creating low oxygen levels and markedly diminishes the body's ability to heal. Nicotine, carbon monoxide, and hydrogen cyanide are inhaled with each puff and clearly cause delayed wound healing (Jenson, 1991; Silverstein, 1992; Smith & Feske, 1996). At the microvascular level, nicotine results in increased blood viscosity and platelet aggregation. At the bone marrow level, nicotine decreases the formation of red blood cells, fibroblasts, and macrophages (the cellular elements required to repair wounds). Carbon monoxide, the inhaled by-product of smoking, has 300 times the affinity for hemoglobin than does oxygen. When it binds with hemoglobin, oxygen transport is decreased and thus there is less oxygen within the tissues. This leads directly to slower wound healing; for many reasons notwithstanding the index injury, therapists should review with each patient the effects of continued nicotine use on healing rates (Figure 3–15).

Alcohol Use

Excessive alcohol intake can also impair the immune system, lead to malnourishment, and cause liver damage (Rund, 1997). Malnutrition is common in alcoholics: albumin and protein levels are diminished, and the bodies' reserves to heal are severely impaired. Delirium tremens, commonly known as "DTs," can occur with abrupt alcohol withdrawal. Orthoses need to be protective and carefully placed, especially if restraints are required in an inpatient setting. As with tobacco use, patient education is paramount.

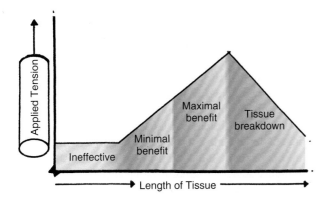

FIGURE 3–12 Length-tension curve depicting elastic and plastic behaviors of tissue.

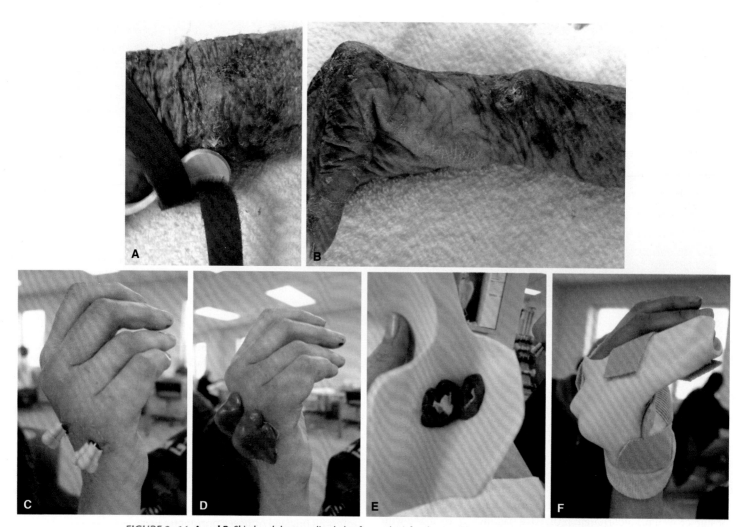

FIGURE 3–14 **A and B,** Skin breakdown at distal ulna from edge of orthosis rubbing against skin in this elderly patient. **C–F,** Relieving pressure over a pin site or an area of irritation can be simple by creating a space while molding the orthosis. In this case, a space was created by applying a temporary "dome" using Xeroform over the pins, followed by putty and then topped with another light layer of Xeroform. Thermoplastic material is then gently draped and molded over the putty and formed to the hand. Once it is set, the putty dome is removed **(E)** forming a space.

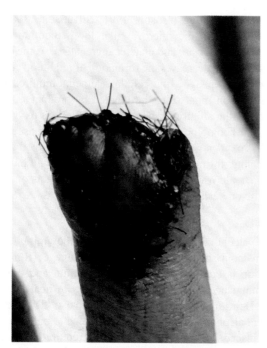

FIGURE 3–15 Necrotic flap noted in a patient who is a heavy smoker.

MEDICAL CONDITIONS

Connective tissue disorders and systemic diseases not only have a generalized effect on the body but also may be associated with impaired tissue oxygenation, which can delay local tissue healing (LeRoy, 1996). With any of the medical conditions mentioned in this chapter, orthotic intervention should be only one aspect of the medical and therapeutic intervention. When an orthosis is fabricated for a patient who has a medical condition that affects tissue healing, vascular compromise, or impaired sensation, both the therapist and the patient should inspect the skin frequently. The therapist should adjust the orthosis and modify the straps as soon as any signs of redness or irritation occur. Affected patients may not perceive the discomfort of the orthosis on the body part owing to nerve and/or vascular involvement.

Buerger's Disease

Buerger's disease, also known as thromboangiitis obliterans, is characterized by progressive inflammation and thrombosis of small and medium arteries and veins of the hands and feet associated with tobacco smoking. Affected individuals frequently have nonhealing ulcerations; arterial and venous occlusion may occur. Cessation of smoking is paramount, although many patients with Buerger's disease are highly addicted. Initially, nonhealing ulcers occur; subsequently, gangrene is unfortunately common. If vascular problems persist, these individuals may have to undergo amputation later in the course of the disease.

Raynaud's

Raynaud's is a condition caused by spasticity or occlusion of the digital arteries, with blanching and numbness in the digits (Figure 3–16) (LeRoy, 1996). Three different conditions exist, Raynaud's syndrome, Raynaud's disease, and Raynaud's phenomenon. Raynaud's syndrome is *secondary* to immune-mediated inflammatory arthritis or an autoimmune connective tissue disease. Raynaud's disease is the name given when the findings are not associated with either condition. Finally, the term Raynaud's phenomenon is used when the cause is unknown. Initially, patients report cold sensitivity, sometimes from simple exposure such as reaching for food in a freezer. In advanced stages, the skin may become firm, thickened, and leathery. Flexion contractures can develop because the skin becomes tightly bound to the underlying subcutaneous tissue. Cold temperatures and autoimmune diseases are among the many factors that precipitate the onset of symptoms. Orthotic materials that are soft, flexible, and contribute to retaining warmth (e.g., neoprene) may be a sensible option for these patients.

Systemic Lupus Erythematosus

Systemic lupus erythematosus (SLE) is an autoimmune disease that can affect any major organ and occurs more predominantly in women, with a variable course of symptomatology (LeRoy, 1996). As with other autoimmune diseases, the body's own immune system attacks the body's normal cells and tissue, resulting in inflammation and tissue damage. The course of the disease is unpredictable, but musculoskeletal manifestations are common, specifically affecting joints and skin. The disease can wax and wane with periodic "flares" of illness balanced with periods of remission. Not only is the disease itself pertinent to this discussion but also treatment. Corticosteroids, immunosuppressants, and medications commonly used in the treatment of cancer are often used in lupus patients. These medications significantly retard the function of the immune system and interfere with healing.

Diabetes

Patients with diabetes may be one of the most difficult groups of patients to treat and apply orthoses. Patients are typically subclassified as insulin-dependent diabetes mellitus (IDDM) and non–insulin-dependent diabetes mellitus (NIDDM). The former have a much more severe form of the disease and, consequently, greater difficulty with wound healing (Davidson, 1999). Peripheral neuropathy is also more common, leading to a loss of protective sensation. Retarded wound healing occurs based on tissue ischemia and neuropathy. Glucose control is critical; individuals with poor blood sugar control, commonly known as "brittle diabetics," are at greater risk of complications. Diabetic neuropathy demands attention to the details of orthotic fabrication. Patients may lack protective sensation; orthotic pressure may, therefore, cause unnoticed skin injury (Figure 3–17). It is important that the patient and therapist perform frequent, regular inspection of the area for early signs of pressure and redness.

Rheumatoid Arthritis

Rheumatoid arthritis (RA) is a systemic immunologic disorder primarily affecting synovial tissue, although most major organ systems can be directly or indirectly affected. Synovial tissue commonly surrounds joints and tendons and, in the normal situation, aids in tissue nutrition, oxygenation, and lubrication. In RA, the autoimmune response causes synovial proliferation producing excess fluid and the fibrous tissue hyperplasia can form "pannus." Destructive enzymes produced by the hypertrophic synovium can be destructive

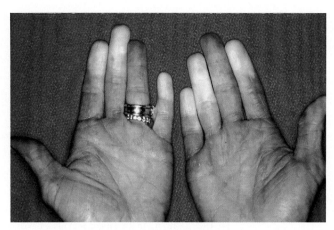

FIGURE 3–16 Note the blanching of the digits because of Raynaud's syndrome, a vasospastic disorder triggered by cold temperatures.

to the articular cartilage, ligaments, and joint. Because of the high incidence of small joint involvement, orthotic fabrication of the hands and wrists are common. Orthoses have an important role not only during a period of exacerbation to protect inflamed painful joints but also have, in the long term, to prevent further joint deformity (Figure 3–18A–C). Over the last few years, the use of disease-modifying agents (e.g., disease-modifying antirheumatic drugs [DMARDs]) has flourished. Use of these biologic agents has significantly altered the natural history of rheumatoid arthritis and many of the other autoimmune disorders. Awareness of the side effect profile, the increased risks of infection, and their possible effects on wound healing are all important considerations.

Pharmacologic treatment often involves medications that retard healing; corticosteroids, for instance, inhibit the normal development of tensile strength in a healing wound and should be taken into account when formulating a treatment plan. Corticosteroids also inhibit the natural inflammatory response, and patients are at higher risk of infection. When possible, thin, lightweight, soft, and flexible materials should be used to fabricate orthoses. Many patients have fragile skin and require additional protection at the orthosis-skin interface. Refer to Chapter 17 for further information.

Sickle Cell Disease

Sickle cell disease is a group of inherited blood diseases that can cause severe pain, damage to vital organs, and occasionally death

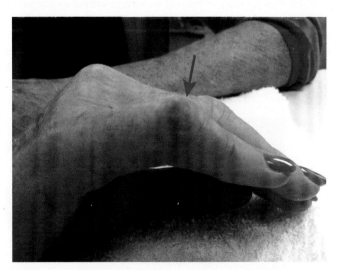

FIGURE 3–17 Reddened area (red arrow) over PIP joint caused by pressure from orthosis. The patient did not perceive this sore area because of diabetic neuropathy and did not inspect the skin as instructed. If the orthosis was not modified, this could have resulted in skin breakdown.

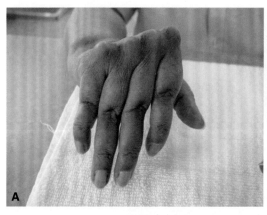
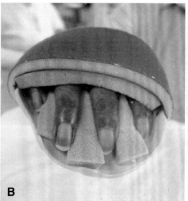
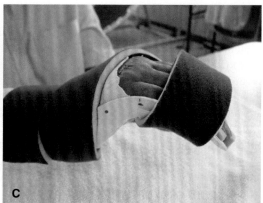

FIGURE 3–18 **A,** An RA patient with ulnar deviation and MCP subluxation deformity **B and C,** s/p MCP arthroplasty. A forearm-based ulnar deviation, MCP extension orthosis to support the MCP reconstruction in a neutral position.

in childhood or early adulthood (Sickle Cell Disease Research Foundation, 2001). The geometrically deformed red blood cells cannot pass easily through the blood vessels, creating a sludging effect and preventing oxygen from reaching the tissues. This results in severe pain and damage to the organs; wound healing is also inhibited. Orthoses fabricated for these patients should be made with caution; straps and other materials should not compress tissue, which could further impede vascular flow.

Peripheral Vascular Disease

Patients with peripheral vascular disease (PVD) are at risk for impaired wound healing because of tissue hypoxia (Figure 3–19A and B). Improvement in arterial circulation and/or venous drainage improves wound healing; therefore, any signs of orthotic compression should be addressed promptly. Orthosis straps should be applied firmly enough to secure the orthosis on the body part but not so tight that circulation is affected. Edema control especially in patients with venous stasis disease is critical. Venous congestion can not only contribute to significant changes in tissue oxygenation but also cause irritation or loosening of orthoses depending upon the status of the edema.

MEDICAL TREATMENT AND COMPLICATIONS

Radiation Therapy

Radiation therapy has a dramatic benefit in curing or controlling certain cancers but also can have damaging effect on previously healthy tissue. Vascular deterioration occurs, creating a hypoxic environment for the tissue; and the adverse consequence of radiation therapy may not become apparent until several years after

treatment. Management of these wounds is difficult because of circulatory compromise. Orthoses and straps should be applied cautiously to these areas for the reasons described previously.

Steroids

Corticosteroid use can impair all phases of wound healing. Because these drugs slow the healing process, they may increase the risk of infection, but the signs and symptoms may be masked by the suppressed inflammatory response (Stotts & Wipke-Tevis, 1997). Patients on chronic steroids often suffer from thinning of the skin, giving it a tissue paper–type appearance and are prone to skin tears and breakdown. Therapists need to evaluate potential areas of friction or pressure when applying orthoses to patients who are using steroid medications. Steroids, like tobacco and alcohol, slow the healing process and increase the risk of skin breakdown. Daily skin inspection and timely orthotic modification can accommodate the risks associated with steroid use.

Edema

Tissue **edema** is the physiologic response to injury often resulting from tissue congestion, diminished venous drainage, and decreased capillary blood flow (Figure 3–20A and B). The increase of interstitial fluid may decrease oxygen diffusion to the tissues. Edema can result from the overly aggressive manipulation of healing tissue by manual techniques or orthotic fabrication methods, and, if occurring, the therapy protocol should be modified. Caution should be taken when applying a mobilization orthosis to a severely edematous part (Fess et al., 2005). Rest, by use of an immobilization orthosis along with edema management techniques/products, may be a better plan until the edema has subsided enough to allow for more aggressive techniques.

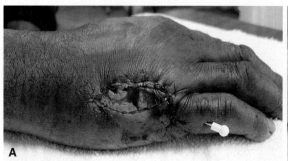
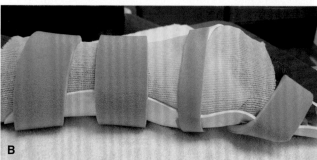

FIGURE 3–19 **A,** Tissue breakdown due to maceration and slow wound healing after open reduction internal fixation for metacarpal fracture in this patient with peripheral vascular disease (PVD). **B,** Wrist and ring/small finger immobilization orthosis with light gauze dressing covering the open area.

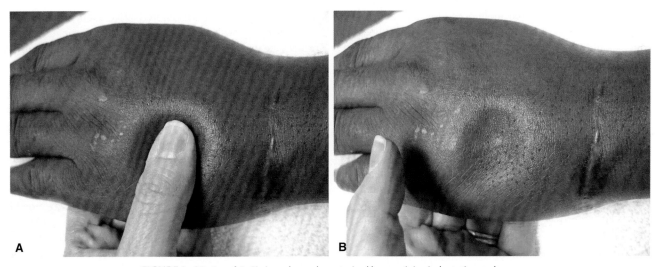

FIGURE 3–20 A and B, Pitting edema characterized by remaining indentation as shown.

Techniques to reduce edema before orthotic application include elevation, massage, compression garments (Isotoner® gloves), circumferential bandages (Ace™ or Coban™ wrapping), or therapeutic elasticized taping methods (Figure 3–21A–H). These can be worn under orthoses, and straps can be modified to prevent window edema (swelling between straps) (Villeco, 2012). Circumferential dressings should be rewrapped periodically during the day to avoid specific areas of increased pressure and to allow progressive control of edematous tissue. However, too much compression may decrease arterial blood flow, thereby creating vascular compromise

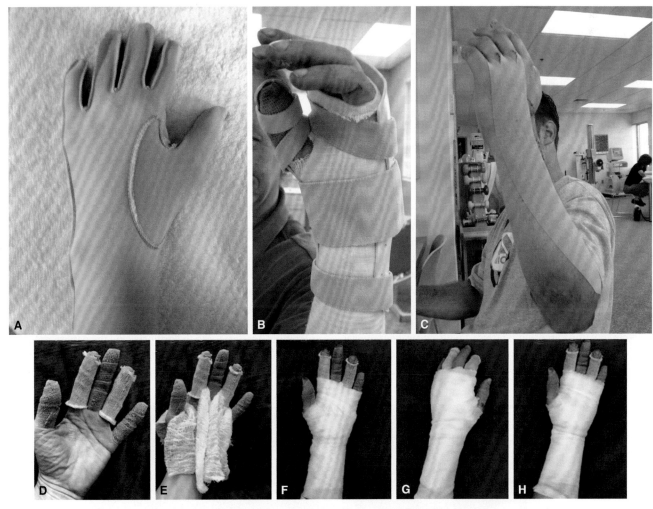

FIGURE 3–21 Edema management techniques including **(A)** compressive glove, **(B)** compression via circumferential wrapping with Coban™ for the thumb and elasticized stockinette, and **(C)** use of Kinesio® Tex Tape for edema control. A bulky Littler dressing with Coban™ wrap on the digits to reduce edema: **D,** Coban™ wraps lightly from distal to proximal. Tubegauz® keeps fingers from sticking together and allow movement. **E,** Kurlix™ strips between the digits. **F,** Kurlix™ or cast padding applied in a figure-of-8 configuration from distal to proximal. **G and H,** Stockinette is applied to keep dressing in place and as another layer of light dressing. Take care to apply lightly so as not to impede the lymph collectors.

to the limb. Circulation should be monitored after and during the application of compression garments and circumferential bandages, and patients should be informed about the signs and symptoms of diminished arterial blood flow (e.g., dusky or blue nail beds; numbness, tingling, or coolness of skin). As edema diminishes, the orthosis will need to be remolded to ensure an adequate fit.

Edema itself can cause significant restriction in the ROM of the joint. Reactive, stiff, painful, edematous tissue does not permit motion; the therapeutic program must be modified to restore tissue homeostasis (Brand & Thompson, 1993). More rest and less movement of the injured part are usually appropriate, and any stress applied to the healing tissue by the orthosis should be monitored closely.

Infection

Infections involve the invasion of tissue by microorganisms: viruses, bacteria, fungi, or atypical organisms (Thompson & Taddonio, 1997). Infection increases oxygen demand and decreases oxygen delivery to tissues secondary to edema and collagen breakdown. These changes prolong and accelerate the inflammatory phase of wound healing. Common signs of infection include warmth, erythema, purulence, and wound drainage but also may include wound discoloration, friable granulation tissue, pain or tenderness out of proportion, and delayed wound healing. Infected tissue interferes with the normal cascade of wound healing, and immobilization through orthotic application helps diminish motion that consequently aids in the body's natural ability to treat the infection. Orthoses should be carefully applied to allow access and free drainage of open areas as well as ease of application and removal to facilitate wound care. Consider using perforated thermoplastic materials to increase air exchange under orthoses that have dressings. One of the most severe infections is necrotizing fasciitis when beta-hemolytic streptococcus invade the tissue. If there is any sign of gas in the soft tissue, emergent evaluation is necessary.

Vacuum-Assisted Wound Closure

A great advance in the treatment of open wounds is commonly referred to as "wound vac treatment" (Von Der Heyde & Evans, 2011; Webb, 2002). Once surgically debrided, a specially designed sponge is contoured to cover the open area; sealed with an impervious cover; and finally, negative pressure is applied through a closed system. With suction applied, exudates, serous fluid, and edema are removed from the wound, facilitating wound granulation and reepithelialization. Wounds previously requiring rotational flaps, free flaps, and skin grafting can often be treated without further surgery as healing occurs through secondary intention. Appropriately placed orthoses help protect the injured area, facilitating drainage and allowing the growth of healthy granulation tissue. Orthoses should protect the extremity and avoid kinking of the suction apparatus.

Thermal Injuries to the Hand

The dorsal skin is thin and highly mobile, providing minimal protection to deeper structures but allowing for flexion and extension of digits. Due to this, the extensor tendon is quite superficial and highly susceptible to injury with the central slip insertion at the PIP joint most injured with dorsal hand burns. The coordination and balance of extrinsic tendons, intrinsic muscles, ligaments, and joints may also be affected with dorsal hand injury. Volarly, the hand has a thick layer to fatty tissue, which provides more protection to deeper structures (Wolfe, Hotchkiss, Pederson, & Kozin, 2011).

Burns may be due to heat, cold, or chemical. First-degree burns are superficial without blistering and heal quickly: usually within 2 to 3 days. Orthosis wear is not needed. Second-degree burns, both superficial and partial thickness, present with protein-rich fluid-filled blisters (Figure 3–22A and B). Deep partial-thickness second-degree burns do not present with blisters and may be either pale or erythemic in color. Third-degree burns involve damage to beyond the dermis, and the hand has a leathery pale or brown appearance. Fourth-degree represents significant damage to deeper structures such as tendon and bone. The latter classification of burns requires orthotic intervention (Skirven, Osterman, Fedorczyk, & Amadio, 2011; Wolfe et al., 2011).

Immediate edema management via elevation is paramount as is positioning of the hand in an orthosis to maintain soft-tissue length. Literature differs on exact degrees; however, the hand should be placed in an "intrinsic plus" or "antideformity" position of wrist extension, MCP joint flexion, IP joint extension, and thumb in abduction and extension (Beredjiklian & Bozentka, 2004; Skirven et al., 2011; Trumble, Rayan, Baratz, Budoff, & Slutsky, 2016; Weinzweig & Weinzweig, 2005; Wolfe et al., 2011). Refer to Chapter 25 for further information on orthosis intervention for this patient population.

ORTHOTIC APPLICATION FOR SPECIFIC TISSUES

For the therapist and surgeon to treat the condition and to correct it, they must understand the integrity of the anatomical structures: the articular surfaces, bones, ligaments, capsules, tendons, nerves, vessels, skin, and subcutaneous tissues. The type of orthotic application (static, serial static, static progressive, or dynamic), the technical considerations for designing the orthosis, and the pattern used depend on the specifics of the tissue pathology (Strickland, 1987, 2000).

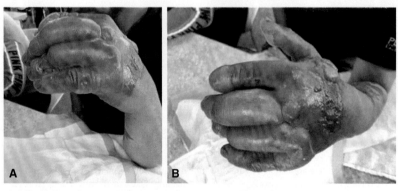

FIGURE 3–22 **A and B,** Partial-thickness second-degree burns on the dorsal hand.

SKIN

Wounds heal by either primary or secondary intention. With **primary closure**, wound healing occurs when wound edges are anatomically aligned and held by suture, "steri-strips," or skin glue (Figure 3–23A–E). With adequate approximation, collagen synthesis binds the edges together, accelerating the healing curve.

Healing by secondary intention refers to the process of a wound closing from the inside out (Figure 3–24A and B). The wound base fills with granulation tissue and then is covered with epithelial cells. As this occurs, the wound edges are gradually drawn centripetally until closure has been achieved. This method may be chosen if the wound is contaminated or infected and when there may be inadequate skin coverage. Wound healing by secondary intention is often advantageous as in partial, superficial fingertip amputations (Figure 3–25). Wounds less than 1 cm^2 can often be treated with this technique; it avoids the general risks associated with surgery as well as donor site morbidity from harvesting skin grafts. In the author's experience, it allows better reinnervation and return of sensation and, often, a better cosmetic appearance. Secondary wound healing was used by McCash (1964) in his so-called open palm technique of Dupuytren's fasciectomy and has seen resurgence in utilization (Figure 3–2). A transverse palmar incision is made to debride the pathologic palmar fascia and is then left open at the conclusion of surgery. This diminishes the risk of hematoma formation, seroma and obviates the need for skin grafting or undo tension on the surgical wound.

Skin grafts and flaps demand specific dressing and orthotic application measures to ensure their survival (Levin, 2011) (Figure 3–26A–E). A partial- or full-thickness skin graft obtains its nutrition initially by diffusion from the surrounding tissues. Vascularized granulation tissue enters the graft from its bed, and capillaries enter the sutured wound edges and allow its incorporation as living skin. The incorporation of grafts depends on the health of the granulation bed, the host's nutritional and metabolic status, comorbidities, and age and takes approximately 2 weeks during which time the graft must be held close to the underlying bed. Surgically placed stents, dressings, and orthoses should minimize motion at the graft site to facilitate incorporation. Generally speaking, the orthosis should only rigidly immobilize the grafted area; adjacent joints should be unencumbered and free to move to prevent adjacent joint stiffness and arthrofibrosis. For example, a skin graft used for a Dupuytren's fasciectomy should be immobilized to facilitate revascularization of the graft, but the adjacent joints released as part of the surgery should be free and mobilized to obtain the desired surgical and therapeutic result.

Skin and soft-tissue flaps require specific attention to their pedicles, the source of arterial inflow, and venous outflow. The pedicle must not be compromised, compressed, or kinked by the position of the operated site in the orthosis or by the straps.

TENDON

Tendon healing occurs because of intrinsic and extrinsic contributions (Gelberman, Khabie, & Cahill, 1991; Legrand, Kaufman, Long, & Fox, 2017; Lundborg & Rank, 1980; Lundborg, 1976; Lundborg, Holm, & Myrhage, 1980). Intrinsic healing, which depends on cells bridging the injury site directly, relies on vincular blood flow; blood flow from the proximal synovial fold in the palm and the bone insertion distally; and diffusion of synovial fluid (and the nutrients it contains) (Figure 3–27A–C). At one point in time, it was believed that flexor tendon healing occurred via extrinsic fibroblast ingrowth and thus required rigid immobilization. The

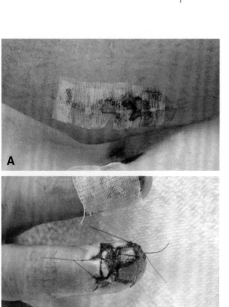
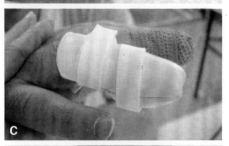
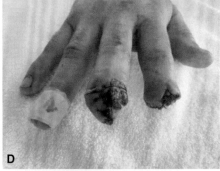
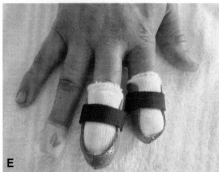

FIGURE 3–23 **A,** Skin closure using running suture and steri-strips post ulnar nerve release at the elbow. **B and C,** Sutured nail bed repair and protective orthosis. **D and E,** Partial amputation with revision and protective orthoses.

consequence was dense adhesions between the tendon and fibroosseous canal. Lundborg (1976) demonstrated that flexor tendon healing occurs intrinsically via the intratendinous vascular arcade. Although tenosynovial fluid undoubtedly provides an anatomically conducive milieu, fibroblastic ingrowth from the tendon sheath is counterproductive to the desired end result: a strong tendon junction free of external adhesions. Adhesions cause scar at the site of tendon injury; if the adhesions are too thick or inelastic, they

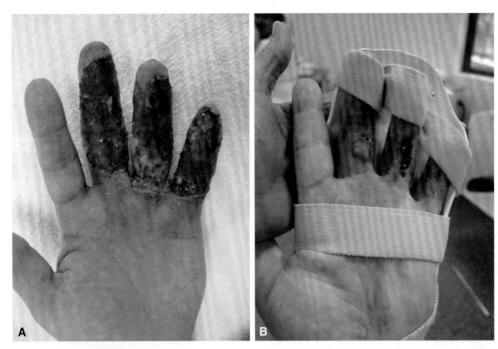

FIGURE 3–24 A and B, Burn injury healing by secondary intention, with orthosis keeping gentle extension positioning during collagen formation.

restrict tendon gliding and often require further surgeries such as a tenolysis (Wang, 1998). Refer to Chapters 18 and 19 for further information.

The stages of tendon healing are the same as for other wounds—inflammatory, fibroblastic, and remodeling—and the timing is also similar to that described previously. However, the critical need to restore tendon gliding, to regain active digital motion, and the nature of the healing present challenges to the surgeon and therapist. The surgeon must create a repair that has maximum strength, permits early motion, and minimizes bulk at the repair site to ease gliding. The therapist must then initiate an early ROM program to establish gliding of the tendon in its fibroosseous canal. The orthosis must facilitate exercise but limit stress on the repair (Wang, 1998) (Figure 3–28A–F). Tendons that are mobilized soon after repair heals with fewer and less restrictive adhesions, achieve greater tensile strength sooner, and establish better gliding than immobilized tendons. Multiple clinical studies reflect this favorable biology of healing and are beyond the context of this chapter.

The precise rehabilitation program depends on the surgeon's and therapist's experience, the nature of the injury, technical factors of the tendon repair (integrity of repair, suture strength), and presence

of associated injuries (Duran, Houser, Coleman, & Stover, 1978; Evans, 2012; Lister, Kleinert, Kutz, & Atasoy, 1977; Pettengill, 2005; Trumble et al., 2010). While trends once favored a modified Duran (early passive mobilization), Kleinert-type program with rubber band–type traction (early passive mobilization), current trends are moving toward an early active mobilization protocol including place hold exercises (Duran et al., 1978; Evans, 2012; Lister et al., 1977; Pettengill, 2005; Trumble et al., 2010) and true active movement (Chye et al., 2013; Gibson, Sobol, & Ahmed, 2017; Higgens & Lalonde, 2016; Neiduski & Powell, 2018; Starr, Snoddy, Hammond, & Seiler, 2013). In all situations, the custom-fabricated orthosis should protect the repair, MCP joint flexion, and wrist position according to the protocol of either slight flexion or extension. The Kleinert protocol can be more labor intensive to make and requires a very precise orthosis that adequately protects the repair with biomechanically appropriately placed bands and pulleys. Common to all protocols, though, is the focus on reestablishing early tendon gliding. Significant advances in tendon surgery have occurred in the last decade. Traditionally, a two-strand core suture was used; current trends and research uses four-strand with an epitendinous repair (Gibson et al., 2017; Starr et al., 2013). The greater number of strands across the repair site helps increase the initial strength of the repair to allow the therapists to institute active tendon protocols at an earlier stage. The dilemma is how many core strands is optimal. When one is striving for strength, a greater number of sutures of greater suture caliber are favored. However, the negative consequence is first, the more strands crossing the repair site diminishes the cross-sectional area of actual tendon available for healing. Second, theoretically, more foreign body can cause more peritendinous scar tissue, greater adhesions, and poorer gliding. Finally, advances have been made in the epitendinous sutures regarding suture technique—for example, locking. The epitendinous sutures have two significant purposes: first, it helps "tidy" the repaired tendon to minimize bulk and aid gliding, and second, despite the small caliber of suture used, it does provide significant increased strength to the repair. The pulley system is an important component when addressing a flexor tendon injury. Doyle and Blythe (1977) demonstrated the critical importance of the A2 and

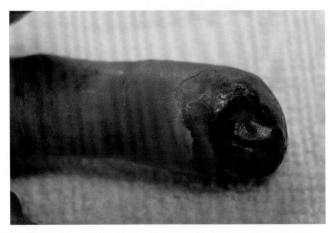

FIGURE 3–25 Partial fingertip amputation healing by secondary intention may result in less sensory deficits versus surgical repair.

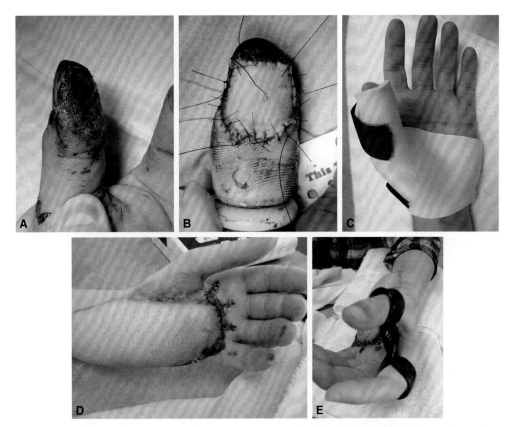

FIGURE 3–26 A and B, Split-thickness graft (upper arm donor site) to provide coverage for soft-tissue loss at the thumb. **C,** Protective thumb immobilization orthosis to protect graft from external forces. **D,** Flap coverage in distal forearm/palm following extensive burn injury. **E,** Thumb carpal metacarpal (CMC) immobilization orthosis to prevent first web space contracture: this unique design prevents need for any contact on healing flap.

A4 pulleys, but, when possible, all pulleys should be preserved and surgically induced trauma minimized. When possible, the pulleys should be left in situ; however, current surgical techniques emphasize pulley maintenance, venting, repair, or reconstruction when necessary. The author of this chapter refers the reader to Chapters 18 and 19 in this book or other external resources for further information.

PERIARTICULAR SOFT TISSUE

Joint stiffness results either from direct injury to the articular surfaces, capsule, and ligament apparatus; or secondarily from edema, scar formation, and contracture affecting the soft tissues around the joint and its associated muscle-tendon units. Anatomical restoration of joint congruity and soft-tissue support and the elimination

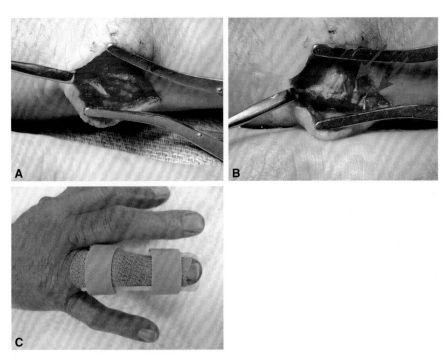

FIGURE 3–27 A and B, Repair of extensor mechanism at lateral PIP joint. **C,** Digit immobilization orthosis, initial weeks of rehabilitation.

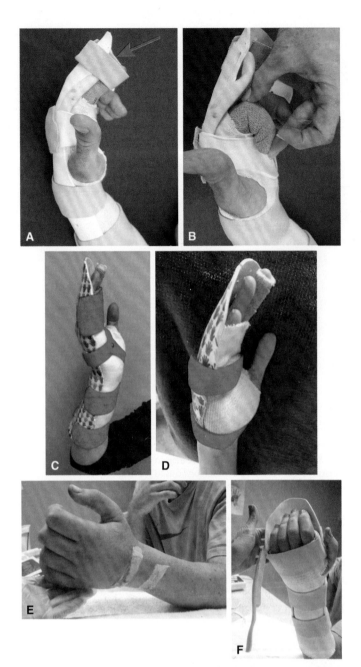

FIGURE 3-28 A and B, Index finger flexor tendon repair with wrist/hand immobilization orthosis in place. Note use of Coban™ for edema and thermoplastic palmar strap (verses a loop strap) to better maintain position of hand in orthosis. Additional piece of thermoplastic added dorsal and distal to MCP joint to allow digit strap to impart gentle extension stretch at the PIP joint, which was developing a flexion contracture. **C,** True active motion protocol positions the wrist in up to 45° extension with the MCPs in 30° of flexion. **D,** The Manchester short orthosis allows wrist motion with up to 45° of extension with the MCPs in 30° of flexion and continues the true active motion protocol. **E and F,** Extensor tendon repair at wrist level and wrist/hand immobilization orthosis with removable hand segment to allow IP joint motion for exercise.

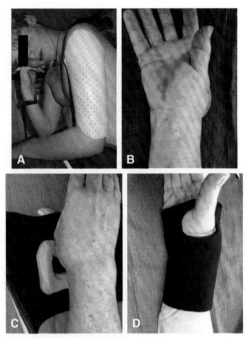

FIGURE 3-29 A, Patient s/p midshaft humeral fracture. An elastic-based material was chosen in order to allow for repeated remolding of the orthoses as edema lessens. **B,** Patient s/p carpal metacarpal (CMC) fascial arthroplasty with implant herniation and reactive synovitis. **C and D,** Neoprene and a donut-shaped piece of soft adhesive-backed foam creates a space for the inflamed soft tissue and at the same time provides lightweight, gentle support to the affected area.

operative treatment, was it done open or closed? With closed reduction techniques, additional soft-tissue damage is lessened. However, anatomical restoration is paramount; open treatment usually requires a surgical incision (and subsequent scar) around the tendon, ligaments, and joint capsule. Finally, was rigid internal fixation applied? Screw or plate fixation generally holds the reduction better; but not only the implants but also the soft-tissue dissection can lead to more scar formation. When open reduction internal fixation (ORIF) techniques are used, the goal is to obtain rigid stability to allow a more aggressive postoperative rehabilitation protocol. However, in some situations, fragment size or fracture pattern is not conducive, and K-wires or sutures may be used but do not have the same mechanical stability. How much damage occurred to the soft-tissue support of the joint, specifically ligaments, capsule, and for the PIP joint, the volar plate? If the trauma disrupted any or all of these structures, were they allowed to heal with closed treatment or, if operated, were they surgically released to treat the fracture and/or were they repairable at closure? What was the extent of the trauma and the extent of surgical treatment to the supporting musculotendinous units? The early response of the soft tissue will often predict the tissue's and patients' response to treatment. The patients' affect is also an important determining factor in how aggressive the team can be with therapy. Recurrent inflammation may demand a less aggressive approach, whereas a more rapid improvement in the clinical situation may necessitate a change in the precise configuration of the orthosis (Figure 3–29A–D). As edema changes, as motion improves, and as radiographs delineate progressive healing, orthoses might require frequent modifications to accommodate changes in status. In certain instances, a contracted ligament will lengthen just so much; further increases in joint motion may be the result of a hinge-open effect rather than to concentric articular gliding (Brand & Thompson, 1993; Strickland, 1987, 2000).

Commonly encountered contractures include elbow flexion, wrist flexion, MCP joint extension, PIP joint flexion, and thumb

of edema help prevent such joint stiffness. Several questions must be addressed to achieve successful treatment of a stiff joint. First, what was the extent of traumatic damage to the joint and how well was it restored? Simple articular fractures, especially in younger individuals, often involves a minimally or noncomminuted injury through the joint. In contrast, the elderly may have significant comminution with multiple small fragments often too small to reconstruct requiring removal. How was the fracture addressed? How well was the articular surface restored? Was a small amount of displacement accepted and treated nonoperatively? If it required adduction. Such contractures may be the result of direct joint trauma (e.g., intra-articular fractures), periarticular crushing, sprains, articular surface contusions (e.g., jammed finger), and other injuries. However, contractures may also occur secondarily from edema, improper positioning, and subsequent soft-tissue contracture that follow injury elsewhere in the upper extremity. These and other contractures may respond to a therapy program that includes edema control, exercise, and application of a mobilization orthosis (usually dynamic, static progressive, or serial static) (McKee, Hannah, & Prignac, 2012) (Figure 3–30A–E). Occasionally, in the multiple traumatized patient, the extremities are neglected while the major organ system damage is addressed. Education is important with other healthcare providers that early application of orthoses in a trauma patient can minimize contractures and aid in minimizing the need for future rehabilitation intervention. When a contracture is severe and unresponsive to therapy and orthotic application, surgical release is sometimes required, after which a resumption of therapy, with orthoses, is indicated (Slade & Chou, 1998). Refer to Chapter 15 on "Stiffness" for further information.

BONE AND CARTILAGE

Fracture healing follows the same sequence as the healing of other tissues (Figure 3–31). Inflammation, edema, and hemorrhage occur at the time of injury. The fibroblastic stage is characterized cellularly by migration of both scavenger osteoclasts and healing osteoprogenitor cells from their endosteal and periosteal origins adjacent to the fracture site. The initial inflammatory response is critical to the healing cascade; anti-inflammatories have been shown in spine fusion models to interfere with bony healing and fusion rates and consequently should be avoided. The collagen matrix deposited by osteoblasts eventually calcifies. The developing callus remodels during the scar maturation stage and responds to the controlled application of stress. As bone healing progresses, the requirements of external immobilization change. In nonsurgically treated fractures, casts, and subsequently, orthoses protect the bone to allow osseous consolidation (Figure 3–32A–D). As healing progresses, it is important to allow stress and/or joint mobility, so orthoses should be lessened during callous maturation and remodeling (Slade & Chou, 1998). Orthoses are usually less bulky and can be contoured more precisely than casts. Their use with fractures permits earlier and more complete mobilization of nearby joints. This can lessen fracture site, distal limb, and digit edema with its concomitant fibrosis, ligament and capsular contracture, and tendon adherence. Refer to Chapter 16 for further information.

NERVE

Nerve injury results in degeneration of the axon and the myelin sheath distal to the wound and for a short distance proximally (Wallerian degeneration) (Figure 3–33A–E). During the inflammatory stage of nerve healing, macrophages clear the cellular debris. Subsequently, axonal buds migrate proximally through the endoneural tube, and Schwann cells envelop the axon in a new myelin sheath as the stage of fibroplasia progresses.

During the fibroblastic stage, protection of the nerve repair against tensile forces is crucial. The surgeon must observe intraoperatively the effect of movement of nearby joints on tension at the site of the repair because this will guide the early postoperative rehabilitation program of the nearby joints. If only a nerve repair was performed, the area was immobilized 3 to 4 weeks; however, Chao et al. (2001) demonstrated that without undue tension on the repair site, nerves can be mobilized earlier in conjunction with tendon repair protocols.

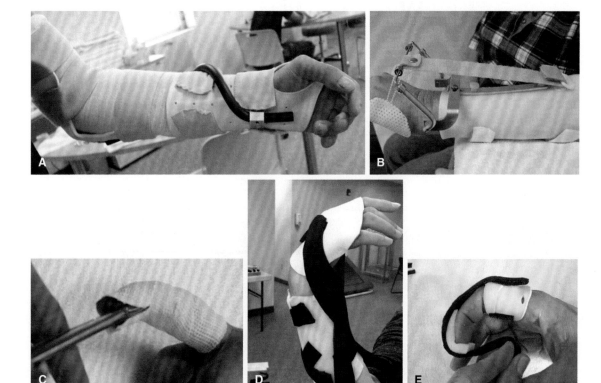

FIGURE 3–30 Types of mobilization orthoses: **A,** dynamic forearm supination (Rolyan® Dynamic Pronation/Supination Kit), **(B)** static progressive wrist extension (Phoenix Wrist Hinge), **(C)** serial static PIP extension (QuickCast 2) (most products available through Performance Health), **(D)** wrist flexion mobilization using neoprene strapping for the dynamic mobilization component, **(E)** IP flexion mobilization with neoprene for a gentle dynamic approach—digit based.

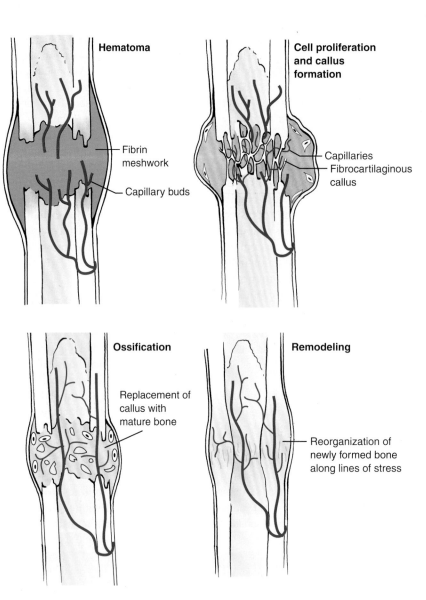

FIGURE 3–31 The stages of bone healing: The hematoma stage provides the fibrin meshwork and capillary buds needed for subsequent cellular invasion. Cellular proliferation and callus formation represent the stages during which osteoblasts enter the area and form the fibrocartilaginous callus that joins the bone fragments. The ossification stage involves the mineralization of the fibrocartilaginous callus, and the remodeling stage involves the reorganization of mineralized bone along the lines of mechanical stress. (Borrowed with permission from Porth, C. M. (2005). *Pathophysiology concepts of altered health states* (7th ed.). Philadelphia, PA: Lippincott Williams & Wilkins.)

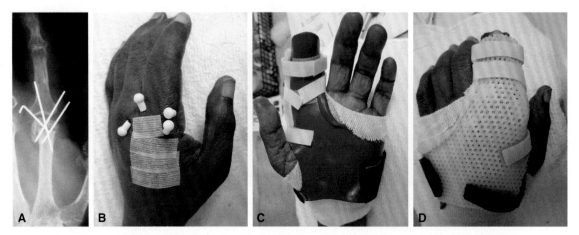

FIGURE 3–32 A and B, Metacarpal fracture with closed reduction and external pinning. **C and D,** Hand-based index finger immobilization orthosis with dorsal clamshell segment for protection of protruding pins. Perforated dorsal material chosen to allow air exchange.

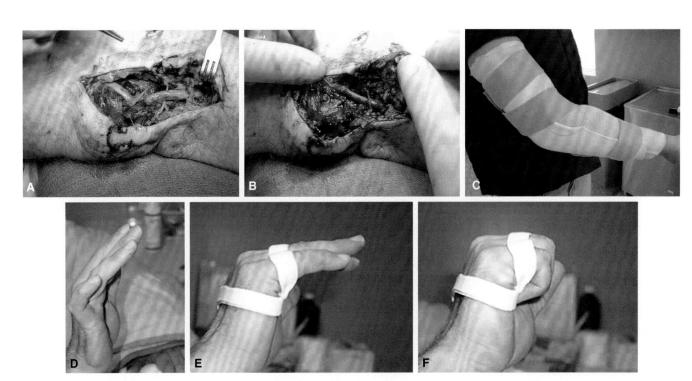

FIGURE 3–33 A and B, Ulnar nerve laceration and repair at level of the elbow. **C,** Postoperative positioning in an elbow immobilization orthosis. **D–F,** Hand-based orthosis used once claw deformity became evident, **(D)** allowing full functional flexion and extension via the long extensors (radial nerve innervated).

Advances in nerve grafting techniques have provided alternatives to a nerve repair under tension. Biocompatible collagen tubes are available in various lengths and diameters and are useful in cases of segmental nerve loss. The conduits provide a biologically conducive milieu for axonal regeneration. Occasionally, autogenous nerve grafts taken from the sural, posterior, interosseous, or antebrachial cutaneous nerve or nerve allografts are also available. A study by Evans, Bain, Mackinnon, Makino, and Hunter (1991) suggested that actually leaving a 5-mm gap between nerve ends can aid in the correct realignment of motor and sensory nerve fibers in mixed nerve repairs. Refer to Chapter 20 for further information.

CONCLUSION

Knowledge of the sequence of events of tissue healing is critical for understanding how and when to intervene—both surgically and conservatively. The selection of a particular treatment program by the surgeon and therapist, including the timely use of specific orthoses, is determined by the nature of the injury and its repair, the techniques used in treatment, the stage of tissue healing, factors that may influence the healing process, and the response of the tissues to previous therapeutic measures.

CHAPTER REVIEW QUESTIONS

1. What are the three stages of tissue healing?
2. Describe the importance of the antideformity position.
3. Should a patient be placed immediately into a digit mobilization orthosis 2 days after wrist fracture repair if he or she presents with swollen and stiff fingers? Why or why not?
4. What factors may negatively influence a patient's ability to heal?
5. What precautions should be stressed when dispensing an orthosis for a patient with diabetes and rheumatoid arthritis?

4

Mechanical Principles

Gary P. Austin, PT, PhD, OCS, FAAOMPT, FAFS
MaryLynn A. Jacobs, MBA, MS, OTR/L, CHT

CHAPTER OBJECTIVES

After study of this chapter, the reader should be able to:

- Understand the basic terminology of mechanics related to the application of an orthosis on the upper extremity.
- Appreciate the various types of force and stress that relate to orthotic fabrication.
- Describe the three lever systems and the term "mechanical advantage" as it relates to the design and fit of an orthosis.
- Identify the various modes in which a mobilization force can be delivered.
- Be able to determine which type of force delivery is best for a given outcome.
- Evaluate the proper fit and function of an immobilization and a mobilization orthosis.

KEY TERMS

Angle of application	Fulcrum	Resistance arm
Axis of rotation	High-profile designs	Rotational force
Bending	Hysteresis	Second-class lever
Compression	Levers	Shear stress
Creep	Linear force	Stress
Effort arm	Low-profile designs	Tensile stress
Elastic force	Magnitude	Third-class lever
First-class lever	Mechanical advantage	Torque
Friction force	Moment of force	Torsion
	Pressure	Translational force

INTRODUCTION

Orthotic intervention is the intentional application of external loads to specific anatomical structures to manipulate the internal reaction forces and thus enhance or restore function of the extremity. Mechanics is the science that addresses the effects of forces on structures. Ideally, the effective therapist integrates basic mechanical concepts into all facets of design and fabrication of an orthosis. A potential barrier to understanding and incorporating these concepts is the confusing mechanical terminology. Therefore, the purposes of this chapter are twofold: to define the fundamental mechanical terms and concepts pertinent to the design and fabrication of an orthosis and to discuss the clinical relevance and application of these basic principles using specific examples.

FORCE

As clinicians and students are interested in the therapeutic application of force, it is essential that the concept of force be clearly defined. Force is an action or influence that either arrests, produces, or changes the direction of motion (LeVeau, 1992). A force can be sufficiently described using the following parameters:

- Nature: the type or kind of force (e.g., push or pull)

- Magnitude: the amount or quantity of influence present
- Line or angle of application: the path or direction along which the force acts
- Point of application: the location on the structure at which the line of force acts

An unbalanced force with a point of application other than the center of the object results in the rotation of an object around a fixed axis. Such a force is referred to as a **moment of force** or **torque**. An example of torque is pulling down on a lever to open a door (Fig. 4–1A). A force with a point of application directly through the center of the object results in the translation of an object along a straight or curvilinear path. This is referred to as **linear force**. An example of linear force is the act of pushing a box along a floor (Fig. 4–1B). Although it may appear that **rotational force** should be the principal focus when discussing orthotic intervention, in fact, most motions incorporate both rotational and **translational** components.

As will become evident, an orthosis is fundamentally the sum of translational and rotational forces acting on anatomical structures for a specific therapeutic purpose. Thus, the different applications of force and force systems must be appreciated. Although it might seem that two forces equal in magnitude would have the same therapeutic effect, this is rarely the case. Furthermore, therapists must understand that the system with the greater force does not always yield the greatest benefit.

There are different forms or types of force. The most pertinent forces for the design and fabrication of orthoses are torque (moment of force), elastic force, and friction force.

TORQUE

The vast majority of articulations in the human body consist of segments or levers assembled around an **axis of rotation**, that is, the proximal and distal segments rotate around a joint axis. By virtue of this structure, the point of application of force is at a distance from the joint axis, producing joint motion that is rotational in nature. Rotational motion is produced, changed, or prevented by force applied in the form of torque. Torque, or the moment of force, is the potential for a force to produce the rotation of a lever around an axis.

The magnitude of torque is a function of two components: the magnitude of applied force and the perpendicular distance from the axis of rotation to the point of application of the force, otherwise known as the moment arm. More specifically,

$$T = F \times d$$

where T is torque, F is force, and d is the perpendicular distance from the axis of rotation to the point of application (Fig. 4–2A). It is important to note that the torque about an axis, or joint, can be modified by manipulating either the distance from the axis of rotation at which the force is applied (Fig. 4–2B) or the quantity of the applied force (Fig. 4–2C). Increases in the force and/or distance produce increases in torque; in other words, torque is directly proportional to both force and distance.

LEVER SYSTEMS AND MECHANICAL ADVANTAGE

For orthoses, torque is commonly applied to a joint via leverage. **Levers** are rigid structures through which a force can be applied to produce rotational motion about a fixed axis. A lever system is composed of a **fulcrum**, or fixed axis, and two arms: the **effort arm** (EA) and the **resistance arm** (RA). The effort arm, also referred to as the force arm, is the segment of the lever between the fulcrum and the effort force (EF) that is attempting to stabilize or mobilize a structure. With respect to orthotic fabrication, the fulcrum typically coincides with the anatomical axis of the target joint, the effort arm

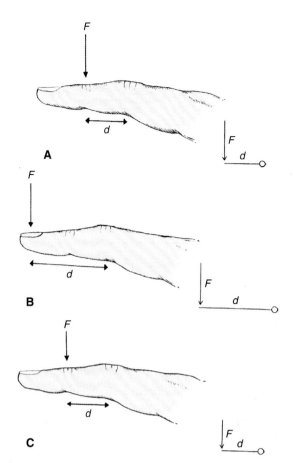

FIGURE 4–2 The torque (τ), or moment of force, can be affected by changes in either the distance (d) from the axis of rotation at which the force (F) is applied or the magnitude of the force applied. **A,** $F = 5$, $d = 5$, $\tau = 25$. **B,** $F = 5$, $d = 10$, $\tau = 50$. **C,** $F = 3$, $d = 5$, $\tau = 15$.

is the segment of the orthosis that applies the effort force, and the resistance arm is the segment of the limb that resists the effort force. The effort force and resistance force (RF), in acting about a fixed axis, create opposing torques about the fulcrum (Fig. 4–3).

The components of the lever system can be arranged to create different types, or classes, of levers, each with a characteristic **mechanical advantage** (MA) or efficiency. The mechanical advantage of a lever system is defined by the relation between the length of the effort arm and the length of the resistance arm:

$$MA = EA/RA$$

Thus, there are three possible relations and three classes of lever systems (Fig. 4–4A–C). Examples of a **first-class lever** system are a seesaw, a pair of scissors, pliers, and a crowbar. Because the fulcrum is between the effort and the resistance arms, the mechanical advantage can be greater than, less than, or equal to 1. Common **second-class lever** systems include the wheelbarrow and the nutcracker. In each of these, the mechanical advantage is greater than 1 because the resistance is between the effort force and the fulcrum. Examples of **third-class lever** systems are a spoon, a fork, tweezers, a shovel, and a fishing rod. In this case, the effort force is applied between the fulcrum and the resistance force; because the effort arm is shorter than the resistance arm, the mechanical advantage is less than 1. Note that the majority of orthoses are first-class lever systems.

Clinical Considerations

The goal when designing an orthosis (i.e., a lever system) is to deliver the intended therapeutic stress to the target structure in the

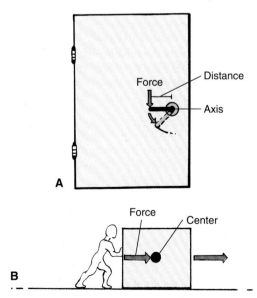

FIGURE 4–1 A, Force is applied at a distance from the axis, causing a rotation of the lever. **B,** Linear force is applied directly through the center of the box, causing a translation across the surface.

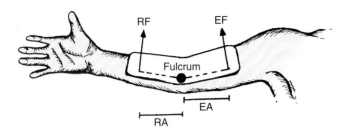

FIGURE 4–3 In this anterior elbow immobilization orthosis, the effort arm (EA) is the proximal segment of the orthosis, which applies the effort force (EF); the resistance arm (RA) is the distal segment of the limb, which applies the resistance force (RF). These forces, acting about the elbow joint axis, create opposing torques.

most efficient and effective manner. The length of the resistance arm greatly influences the mechanical advantage of the applied force. The effort arm of the orthosis can also affect the mechanical advantage by the manner in which it is molded to the body part. Both the effort and the resistance arms should conform to the structures they contact and should incorporate adequate surface area for proper pressure distribution. It is important to consider how pressure distribution within an orthosis can vary depending on joint position. This in turn will influence functional performance within the orthosis (Cha, 2018). The net effect of the forces acting on a joint or structure should result in an optimal therapeutic effect and minimal negative effects. If the opposing force (effort arm) is not properly distributed relative to the distal force (resistance arm), the orthosis may become uncomfortable and thus ineffective. Therapists can create mechanical advantages through meticulous orthosis fabrication techniques and the judicious application of basic mechanical principles.

- The longer the resistance arm, the less force required to generate sufficient torque (Fig. 4–5). And, conversely, the shorter the resistance arm, the more force required to produce sufficient torque.
- The effort arm is most comfortable when adequate length and depth are incorporated into the orthosis (Fig. 4-6A,B). A short, narrow, and shallow effort arm is likely to create excessive pressure and discomfort; a well-molded effort arm more effectively dissipates pressure.
- The greater the force generated through the resistance arm, the broader and longer the shape of the effort arm.

As a clinical example, consider fabricating an orthosis to mobilize a stiff proximal interphalangeal (PIP) joint in the direction of flexion. The effort arm (on the volar proximal phalanx) is fabricated in the direction of extension. If the surface contact area of the effort arm is not of adequate length, circumference, and/or contour, this may result in localized shear and compression stress and potential migration of the orthosis (shear and compression stress are discussed later in this chapter). When the proximal segment migrates or shifts, the resistance arm is not able to provide a perpendicular angle of pull to the PIP joint axis of rotation, causing the resistance arm to alter the sling's fit on the middle phalanx (Fig. 4–7A–C).

ANGLE OF APPLICATION

The angle of application of the moment of force or torque is critical to the proper design and fabrication of orthoses. Ideally, the force should be applied so that the angle of application is oriented 90° to the lever. This maximizes the therapeutic effect of the external force because the total force influencing the target segment acts

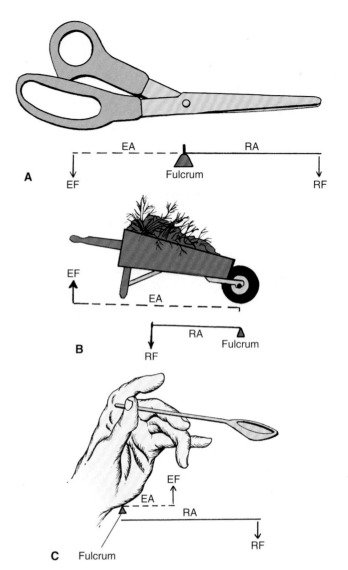

FIGURE 4–4 A, A first-class lever system. **B,** A second-class lever system. **C,** A third-class lever system. EA, effort arm; EF, effort force; RA, resistance arm; RF, resistance force.

in the intended direction. When the force is applied in a purely perpendicular orientation to the target segment, there are no forces in other directions (Fig. 4–8A–E). However, at an angle other than 90°, a portion of the force acting on the segment is applied in a direction other than the desired trajectory (either compression or tension), thereby effectively diminishing the perpendicular component and decreasing the therapeutic torque (Fig. 4–8F). Thus, when the angle of application is either greater or less than 90°, the beneficial effect of the application of torque cannot be optimized and potentially damaging compression and/or shear stress is applied. Nonrigid and forgiving materials such as neoprene can be used to impart a gentle mobilizing force. Neoprene and neoprene-like materials can be an option for light joint positioning (i.e., radial nerve palsy) or to gently impart a mobilizing force in a desired direction. The reader is directed to Chapter 14 for more information regarding the use of neoprene material.

Design Considerations

General

- To achieve a near-90° angle of application, use line guides and pulleys to aid in the orientation (Fig. 4–9A–E).
- To prevent undue torque or stress on the surrounding soft tissues, view the orthosis from all angles to ensure that the pull of the line

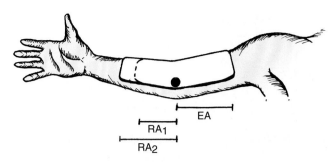

FIGURE 4–5 When the resistance arm (RA$_2$) is lengthened, less force is required to generate sufficient torque to prevent elbow joint movement. When the resistance arm (RA$_1$) is shortened, greater force is required to immobilize the elbow joint.

is directed centrally over the digit or limb and oriented properly in all planes (Fig. 4–9B–G).

- With a few exceptions, the general rule of thumb when using a mobilization orthosis to improve flexion of the digits, the anatomical configuration of the hand requires that the line of application converge toward the scaphoid. If this orientation is not incorporated into the orthosis design, excessive stress may be placed on the metacarpophalangeal (MCP) joints, potentially causing discomfort and/or harm.
- Fess (1989, 2004) describes the importance of differentiating single-finger versus multiple-finger flexion alignment while considering the construction of a mobilization orthosis. It is recommended that the reader further study this work (Fess, 1989, 2004, 2011).
- Isolated, *individual* finger flexion converges toward the center of the volar wrist (Fig. 4–9C).
- During *simultaneous* finger flexion, the merging of the digits points to the radial middle third of the forearm. The dorsal rotation of the fourth and fifth metacarpals changes the alignment of the longitudinal axis of the ulnar digits away from the direction of the scaphoid and to an ulnarly directed position.

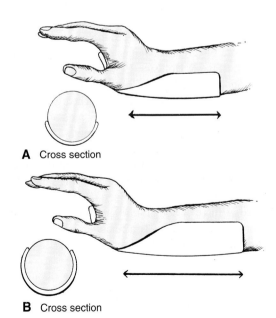

FIGURE 4–6 **A,** An orthosis with a short, narrow, and shallow effort arm is likely to cause discomfort from inadequate pressure distribution. **B,** An orthosis with a longer, broader, and deeper effort arm adequately distributes pressure and thus increases comfort. The depth of the orthosis should encompass two-thirds of the circumference of the body part, not only adding strength but also allowing for adequate placement of straps without the risk of compressing soft tissue.

- Occasionally, a force applied in either a radial or ulnar direction is indicated, for example, after MCP joint arthroplasties or sagittal band repairs (Fig. 4–10A–D). (Except for special circumstances such as these, the line of application should be centrally located over the longitudinal axis of the bone being mobilized.)
- All orthoses described in this chapter are removeable. Research has shown that removable orthoses are effective even with a mobilizing force applied. The ability to remove the orthosis to wash, inspect tissue, and generally move the immobilized parts, is imperative (McVeigh et al., 2019).

High-Profile Design

- **High-profile designs**—mobilization orthoses that have high vertical outriggers—are commonly thought to require fewer adjustments to maintain the optimal 90° angle of application than a low-profile orthosis. However, this conjecture has been called into question, and the actual deviations from 90° line of pull are approximately 1° for each degree of motion gained (Austin, Slamet, Cameron, & Austin, 2004). Adjustments must be made when large improvements are seen in joint motion; otherwise, the line of pull will no longer be at 90°. Deviation of the line of pull from 90° results in both a reduction in the therapeutic corrective force and an increase in the dangerous shear component of the applied force (Austin et al., 2004).
- Patient compliance is often a challenge because the orthosis is large. The dimensions of the high-profile design can make it cumbersome to engage in activities of daily living, such as putting the arm through a shirt sleeve.
- When using high-profile designs, the therapist should be careful to firmly attach the outrigger to the orthosis base because this attachment site has the potential of low stability.

Low-Profile Design

- With **low-profile designs**—mobilization orthoses that have low, close to the surface outriggers—the force required to mobilize a joint may be uncomfortable and difficult to tolerate for extended periods of time.
- Low-profile designs may be cosmetically appealing. However, when greater resistance is necessary, such as when mobilizing a dense 60° PIP flexion contracture, it may be more appropriate to incorporate a higher outrigger into the orthosis design. In such a situation, the force is applied at a greater distance from the joint axis to produce a greater amount of torque on the contracture.
- A low-profile design is an excellent choice for an orthosis that is used to substitute for weak or absent musculature, as seen when managing a radial nerve injury. Typically, less torque is needed to hold the distal segments (wrist and MCP joints in this case) in the proper position to substitute for the loss of muscle action than is needed to try to mobilize a stiff joint. For this purpose, only minimal adjustments are necessary, and the low-profile design tends to enhance function.
- Although dynamic orthoses require periodic adjustments to maintain an optimal 90° angle of pull, many make the unsubstantiated claim that high-profile dynamic orthoses require less frequent adjustment of the outrigger than do low-profile dynamic orthoses. However, it appears that it may be best to assume that the actual deviation from 90° line of pull is quite small for both low- and high-profile devices, and these likely require adjustments at the same frequency to maintain the optimal 90° line of pull on the target segment (Austin et al., 2004, Fig. 2).

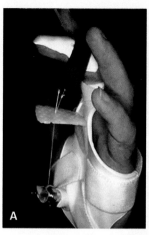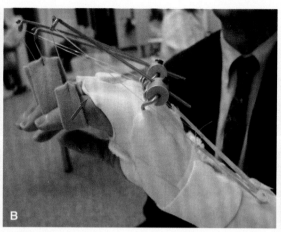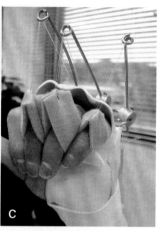

FIGURE 4–7 A, A dorsal thin thermoplastic "cuff" aids in pressure distribution due to its adequate length and circumference therefore the static progressive force into PIP flexion is best tolerated (MERiT™ component, Performance Health, Warrenville, IL). **B,** There is a potential for shear stress at the distal orthosis/dorsum of small-finger (SF) interface. **C,** However, when viewed during digital flexion, the distal portion of the orthosis is molded to accommodate for the convex/concave nature of the dorsum of the digits. This design distributes the shear stress adequately (Rolyan® Adjustable Outrigger Kit, Performance Health).

- Low-profile orthosis designs can be less cumbersome for performance of activities of daily living and often fit under loose clothing.
- Low-profile outriggers may undergo alternations in alignment more rapidly when applied for the purpose of correcting a contracture because of the short angle of application (Fess, 2011).

ELASTIC FORCE

Elastic force is the influence on the motion of an object or segment that is the result of the amount of applied stretch. Elastic force is directly proportional to both the stiffness of a structure and the amount of displacement present. Specifically,

$$F = -k\Delta l$$

where F is elastic force, k is stiffness, and Δl is the change in length or displacement. Elastic force can be increased by increasing the stiffness of the structure and/or increasing the amount of displacement or stretch. Stiffness is the relationship between the amount of force produced and the applied stretch:

$$-k = \frac{F}{\Delta l}$$

In other words, a stiffer structure produces a large amount of resistance to a small stretch, whereas a less stiff structure offers little resistance in response to the same stretch.

Clinically, when a therapist fabricates an orthosis to influence tissue response, he or she must consider the elastic nature of both the target tissues and the materials used to make the orthosis. The therapist should be familiar with the properties of the materials, including such factors as resistance to stretch, rigidity, and conformability (see Chapter 5 for more information).

Torque-Angle Measurement

The notion of elastic force and stiffness applies not only to the materials used to produce external loads (e.g., rubber bands, elastic cord, and spring coils) but also to the internal reaction forces of the limb. An example is the torque-angle measurement proposed by Brand and Hollister (1993), in which torque is measured at several joint angles. These measurements provide the clinician with information regarding the magnitude of resistance to motion at

particular joint angles throughout an arc of movement. A stiff hand, for example, offers more resistance at different angles than does a "normal" hand.

Clinical Considerations

When using elastic force to mobilize stiff structures, the therapist must take into account the clinical objectives. Is the goal to mobilize a mature, dense joint contracture or to stabilize the MCP joints in extension after MCP joint arthroplasty? Both situations may employ an elastic force; however, the amount of force and the materials used to achieve these goals may differ considerably.

To date, the ideal relationship between the amount of elastic force for mobilization of a specific structure remains unknown. However, the amount of force applied likely depends on such factors as individual tolerance, diagnosis, stage of tissue healing, chronicity of the problem, severity of the contracture, density of the contracture, age, lifestyle factors (smoking, alcohol use), and other health-related issues. A range of 100 to 300 g has been suggested for mobilization of the small joints of the hand, whereas higher parameters (350+ g) seem to be more effective for larger structures (Bell-Krotoski & Figarola, 1995; Brand & Hollister, 1993; Flowers & LaStayo, 1994, 2012; Giurintano, 1995; Glasgow, Tooth, Fleming, & Hockey, 2012; Glasgow, Tooth, Fleming, & Peters, 2011). The estimate of 300 g is based on what is tolerated per unit of surface area of the skin, not on the tolerance of the contracted tissue to tension. Therefore, in most cases, skin tolerance becomes the limiting factor in determining appropriate orthosis tension, not the specific targeted tissue. "While the optimum force has yet to be calculated, the amount of force applied to the tissues must be determined relative to the tissues that are contracted. A force of 800 grams may be on the high end of the spectrum for the PIP joint but is a relatively small amount when considering remodeling at the elbow or shoulder" (Bell-Krotoski & Figarola, 1995, p. 135).

The therapist will nearly always rely on the tissue's response to the tension in determining the effectiveness of the mobilizing forces. Indicators of excessive stress include edema, skin blanching, vascular changes, and pain. With tools such as a tension gauge (e.g., Haldex gauge), the therapist can obtain a general estimate of the amount of tension a dynamic orthosis is applying to the involved area (Fig. 4–11A). Occasionally, mobilizing forces can be delivered using a product such as neoprene or elastic-based loop

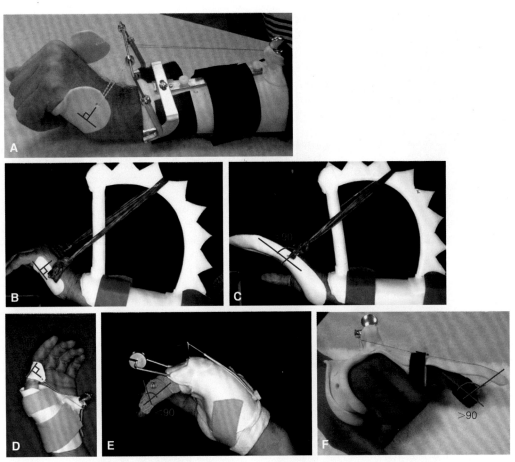

FIGURE 4–8   A, Demonstrating the optimal 90° angle of application with Phoenix Wrist Hinge (Performance Health). **B and C,** A homemade wrist extension mobilization orthosis, nicknamed the "Dinosaur orthosis" is shown here with a near 90° angle of application. For a true 90° angle, the TheraBand® would need to move one segment proximally (Performance Health). **C,** is modified to include the digits; note the pressure is distributed along the entire volar hand with the line of pull originating at the border of the MCP joints. **D,** A thumb IP flexion mobilization orthosis (Splint-Tuner™; North Coast Medical, Morgan Hill, CA). **E,** The angle of force application is very close to 90° in this hand-based PIP extension mobilization orthosis (Phoenix Single Finger Outrigger, Performance Health). **F,** The angle of force application is greater than 90° in this IP extension orthosis, leading to shear stress at the proximal volar edge of the sling with potential migration off the distal phalanx (MERiT™ component, Performance Health, Warrenville, IL).

materials. The tension applied to the tissue is difficult to monitor; therefore, clinician experience and patient monitoring are crucial (Fig. 4–11B,C). A few of the common devices a therapist can use to generate an elastic force for mobilizing the soft tissue are discussed in the next sections.

Rubber Bands

The length and thickness of a rubber band determine its effectiveness when used for fabrication of a mobilizing orthosis. Thinner (narrow) rubber bands tend to elongate more easily than do thicker ones (i.e., narrow bands are less stiff). A rubber band, made of latex and rubber, does not return to its exact original shape after being *stretched, relaxed, and then restretched*. This phenomenon is called **hysteresis**.

If a rubber band has been held in a *constant* stretched position for a long period of time, eventually, there will be a *permanent* change in length. The structure of the rubber band has been permanently altered; this is called **creep**. The clinician should appreciate that rubber bands do not behave exactly like a spring and will undergo some degree of hysteresis and creep as the orthosis is worn. Therefore, attention to the rubber band's effectiveness should be monitored and reassessed accordingly.

The therapist must consider the purpose of the orthosis when selecting the properties of the rubber band (i.e., thickness, length, width). For example, a narrow rubber band may not be stiff enough to aid in mobilizing a dense PIP flexion contracture but may generate adequate force to maintain a PIP joint in extension after an extensor tendon repair.

Wrapped Elastic Cord

Wrapped elastic cord is made of a light layer of cotton wrapped around an elastic cord and often provides a greater degree of resistance or stiffness when stretched. With wrapped elastic cord, less stretch is required to generate movement of a stiff joint than with a rubber band; therefore, caution should be used.

Spring Coils

Spring coils can produce an elastic force as well. They are available in various sizes (diameters and lengths) that offer different degrees of resistance. The composition, stiffness, and length of the coil aid the therapist in the appropriate selection for the tissue involved. Spring coils produce a consistent controlled force with little material breakdown, an advantage over rubber bands. However, they are more costly and less readily available than rubber bands.

Neoprene

Neoprene has grown in popularity over the years as an efficient and cost-effective means of imparting a mobilization force to tissue

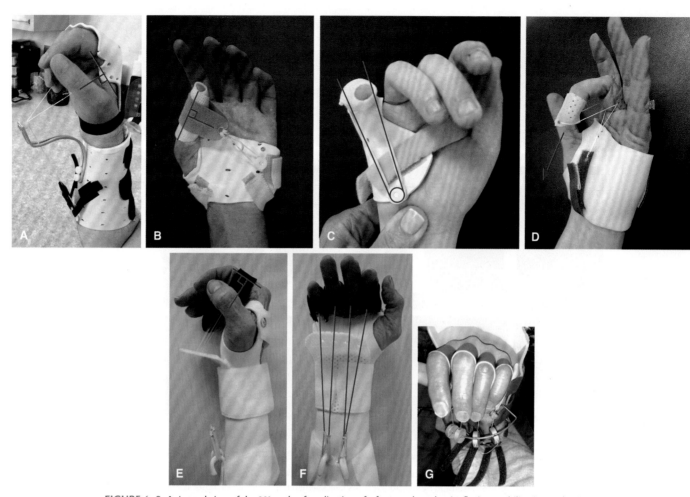

FIGURE 4–9 A, Lateral view of the 90° angle of application of a forearm-based wrist flexion mobilization orthosis. The modified outrigger and screw-on plastic line guide allows for simple orthosis adjustments as the wrist range of motion improves (Base 2™ Outrigger Kit North Coast Medical). The thermoplastic "cuff" creates a wide base for pressure distribution. **B,** The application of a circumferential orthosis to the thumb IP joint aids in dispersing pressure distal to the thumb MP (effective lever arm) and allows for an adequate surface area to apply stress (the sling) for focused MP flexion. **C,** Volar view highlighting the line of force application directed toward the center of the wrist. **D,** With this isolated middle-finger (MF) composite IP flexion mobilization orthosis, the convergence of the line of application is toward the base of the thumb/scaphoid. Note the line guide that was made by "lifting" a small segment of thermoplastic material from the base and creatively forming a line guide. **E and F,** The radial view **(E)** of this MCP flexion mobilization orthosis with a near 90° angle of force application. A piece of perforated thermoplastic material was applied and used as a line guide. The line of pull can then be readily adjusted as motion improves. **F,** This demonstrates the convergence of the lines of pull of each digit. It is important for the clinician to appreciate the natural flexion direction of the digits when fabricating an orthosis and incorporate this into the design. A distal view **(G)** of a similar orthosis appreciating the natural direction of digital flexion.

(Figure 4–11B,C). Although clinical evidence of its effectiveness is currently lacking, individual clinical experience suggests this may provide a reasonable and effective option for select patients. With escalating costs and decreasing reimbursements for many therapy services, it can be expensive for facilities to maintain proper stock of the components necessary (pulleys, outriggers) to fabricate mobilization orthoses. Based on the elastic properties of neoprene, the material can be used as a "dynamic" force in the fabrication of mobilization orthoses in lieu of traditional rubber bands or wrapped elastic cord. "Orthoses made of neoprene material have the advantage of being pliable and at the same time can be constructed as dynamic orthoses" (Punsola-Izard, Rouzaud, Thomas, Lluch, & Garcia-Elias, 2001). In some instances, neoprene may effectively replace traditional outriggers which can often be cumbersome (and costly). Additionally, custom neoprene mobilization may provide a cost-effective and easily adjustable option for lower profile orthoses. Utilization of neoprene requires the therapist use care to ensure safe and effective application of force. Interested readers are directed to Chapter 14 for more information.

FRICTION FORCE

Friction force is a type of **translational force**, sometimes referred to as either static friction or kinetic friction. Friction opposes movement between two surfaces and acts parallel to the surfaces. The force of friction (F_x) is proportional to the coefficient of friction (μ) and the contact force (F_c):

$$F_x = \mu F_c$$

The coefficient of friction is specific to each material. At rest, the opposing force of friction is categorized as static and depends on the coefficient of static friction (μ_s) and F_c. When motion occurs, friction is classified as kinetic, or moving, friction and depends on the coefficient of kinetic friction (μ_k) and F_c.

In situations of either motion or equilibrium, friction is directly proportional to (1) the coefficient of friction specific to the material(s) and (2) the amount of contact force. The therapist, therefore, can minimize friction by using materials with lower coefficients of friction, such as smooth, nonperforated

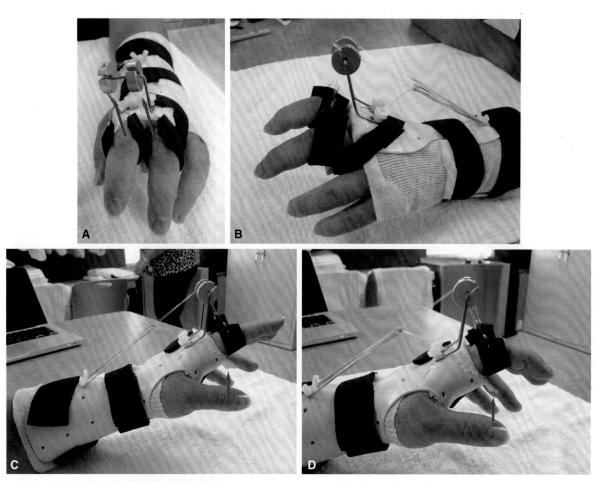

FIGURE 4−10 **A-D,** This MCP IF/middle-finger (MF) extension mobilization orthosis has a radially directed pull to protect the reconstruction of the radial collateral ligaments of the MCP joints and the silicone implant arthroplasties in this young patient with rheumatoid arthritis. **C and D,** Radial view of MCP digit extension and digit flexion to the thermoplastic block that is incorporated into the orthosis (Phoenix Single Finger Outrigger, Performance Health).

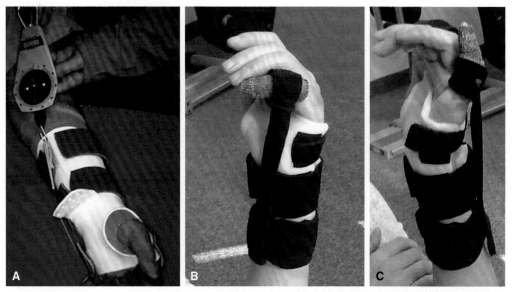

FIGURE 4−11 **A,** A tension gauge applied to a mobilization orthosis determines the approximate forces on the intended tissue. **B and C,** Neoprene is used to impart both flexion and extension forces on the fifth MCP joint. When using such a material, the tension applied is left to the discretion of the therapist, patient feedback, and tissue monitoring/response. The patient should be closely monitored.

thermoplastics (instead of gel or foam-lined thermoplastic materials). In addition, friction can be reduced by decreasing the contact force generated by rubber bands and straps. Often, friction must be minimized to prevent skin irritation or breakdown, such as chaffing or blistering. Sources of potential harmful friction include orthosis borders, poor-fitting straps, attachments that rub against the skin (e.g., the underside of rivets or rubber band posts), and edges that extend beyond joint creases.

Clinical Considerations

Friction may be desired to prevent the migration of an orthosis along the skin. In such cases, friction can be increased by applying straps to increase the contact force or by simply lining the orthosis with thin foam strips or a tape (e.g., Microfoam™ Tape, Performance Health) to increase the coefficient of friction.

At times, a small amount of orthosis migration is inevitable; for example, a wrist immobilization orthosis causes some degree of friction along the orthosis-skin interface as the patient moves the digits and elbow. An attempt must be made to decrease this friction force; it can be lessened by covering the involved area with materials such as cotton stockinette, TubiGrip™, or TubiPad® (Performance Health).

Friction, also referred to as drag, may be present in the pulley systems used for dynamic mobilization orthoses. As the monofilament line passes through the line guide or pulleys, the point of contact can be a source of friction, thereby increasing unwanted resistance through the orthosis. This can be the result of the coefficient of friction of the monofilament, the orthosis line, or the line guide itself (Fig. 4–12A–C). The amount of friction present is increased when the angle at which the monofilament line enters one of these devices is increased.

Most manufactures of orthosis fabrication components have attempted to address these issues. For example, the Phoenix outrigger has a tubular plastic insert in which the monofilament line passes, and the Rolyan® adjustable outrigger is completely rounded and smooth to reduce drag as the line traverses the outrigger (see Chapter 5 for additional information). Therapists should be aware of this problem when fabricating homemade line guides. Friction can be minimized by smoothing and rounding the edges and by carefully monitoring the angles of force application.

STRESS

When designing and fabricating orthoses, the therapist must understand the **stress** produced by external forces. By definition, stress is the response of, or resistance offered by, a surface to the deformation caused by an externally applied force or moment (Nordin & Frankel, 2001; Soderberg, 1986). Stress (σ), often simply referred to as pressure, is described according to the amount of force (F) per unit area (A), specifically:

$$\sigma = \frac{F}{A}$$

Stress, therefore, is directly proportional to F and inversely proportional to A. In other words, stress is increased when either the magnitude of the force applied to the surface area is increased or the amount of area over which the force is applied is decreased (Fig. 4–13A,B). Stress can occur in different forms, the most important of which are compression, shear, tensile, bending, and torsion.

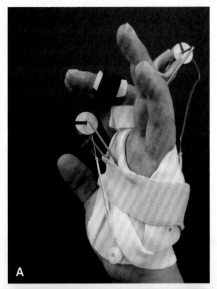

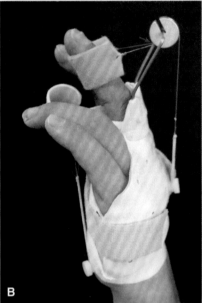

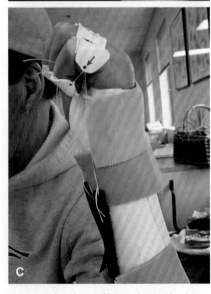

FIGURE 4–12 A-C, Examples of monofilament line guides that approach at different angles. Note the point of contact and potential sites of friction: **A and B,** Phoenix Outrigger Kit (Performance Health) used in a combination orthosis to address both PIP flexion and extension deficits; note the friction created with this less than 90° angle of pull where the monofilament meets the wheel. In both the PIP flexion and extension modes, the monofilament is not gliding through the wheel at a 90° angle therefore creating drag upon exit. **C,** Custom-made thermoplastic outrigger fabricated to guide this composite flexion orthosis.

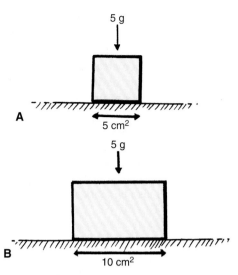

CHAPTER 4

FIGURE 4-13 Different magnitudes of stress (g/cm²) can result from the application of a 5-g force to different-sized areas. **A,** Small area (5 cm²): stress = 1 g/cm². **B,** Large area (10 cm²): stress = 0.5 g/cm².

COMPRESSION

Compression, often mistakenly referred to simply as **pressure,** is the special case of stress in which opposing loads push toward one another along the same line of application (Fig. 4–14). A compressive stress (σ) is distinguished by the perpendicular angle of application of the load. Usually, compression results in a squeezing type of force, causing a broadening and flattening of the object (Nordin & Frankel, 2001). Compressive stress is maximized by the perpendicular nature of the force application. Notably, pure compression lacks a force component parallel to the surface (defined as shear). Compression is proportional to the perpendicular force (F_{perp}) and inversely proportional to the surface area:

$$\sigma_c = \frac{F_{perp}}{A}$$

For a constant magnitude of force, compression can be minimized by increasing the surface area over which the force can be distributed. For a constant surface area, compression can be reduced by decreasing the perpendicular force.

Clinical Considerations

The therapist must be sure to fabricate the base of an orthosis with sufficient length, depth, and contour. In addition to offering greater mechanical advantage, a longer orthosis base provides greater surface area over which to distribute the contact force. A wider and deeper orthosis base is not only stronger but also minimizes shear stress and maximizes pressure distribution.

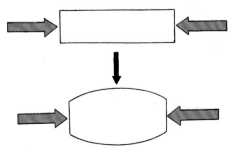

FIGURE 4-14 To maximize compressive stress, force should be applied in a perpendicular fashion.

Optimizing the conformity of materials to the shapes, contours, and curvatures of the body part being immobilized can minimize compressive stress. If care is not taken to meticulously pad vulnerable areas such as the ulnar or radial styloid and pin sites, increased compressive stress can result in discomfort, possible pin migration, and probable noncompliance.

Straps, although necessary to secure the orthosis firmly on the extremity, can be sources of compressive stress. A narrow strap width, especially in conjunction with shallow orthoses (less than two-thirds of the circumference), can produce high compressive stresses on the soft tissue it contacts. This can lead to uncomfortable, ill-fitting orthoses (Fig. 4–15A,B). Increasing the width and conformability of the straps can aid in distribution of the compressive forces over a greater surface area and help minimize orthosis migration (Fig. 4–15C).

Orthosis borders should be fabricated so that they lie flush with the skin surface that the strap traverses. The strap should not bridge the two borders of the orthosis; it should come in light contact with

CHAPTER 4

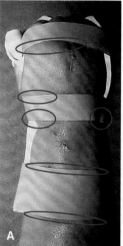

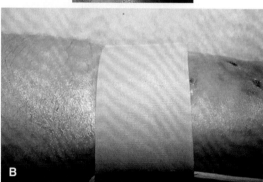

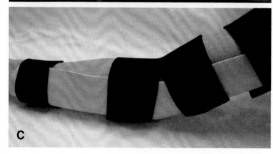

FIGURE 4-15 A, Improper selection and placement of straps can create high and uncomfortable compressive and shear forces. The borders of this orthosis are inadequate (too low) in order to support the bulk of the hand and forearm. The narrow straps are also a source of high compressive stress. **B,** Lateral view of sheer stress. **C,** Other options such as elasticized straps can distribute forces and add comfort to the patient. Shown is custom cut neoprene straps. The straps are simply cut to allow accommodation about the anterior elbow fossa.

the skin. For example, the lateral borders of a volar forearm orthosis base should be just at the level of the dorsal forearm. The strap(s) can then be applied to rest lightly on the dorsal forearm. As previously mentioned, if the lateral borders of the orthosis do not rise high enough to reach the dorsal skin surface, the straps cannot lie flush; they instead wrap around the dorsal skin and underlying soft-tissue structures, causing potential neurovascular compression, pinching of the skin against the orthosis border, and discomfort for the wearer.

Excessively high orthosis borders can cause a "bridging" of the straps where there is no contact with the skin surface beneath the strap. This type of closure will not adequately secure the orthosis onto the extremity. There will be too much room left between the orthosis strap and the skin, allowing unwanted movement of the immobilized part (Fig. 4–16A–F).

The therapist should remember that slings and loops can also be sources of compression stress. Several techniques help the orthosis fabricator avoid compression to the lateral, dorsal, or volar aspects of the digit (or body part in the sling or loop). One orthosis line can be attached to each side of a sling (two pieces of line) and then joined after they pass through the pulley. This prevents the circumferential compression created when one line is threaded through both ends of the loop, an important consideration when addressing a digit with edema or neurovascular issues (Fig. 4–17A). Alternatively, a well-contoured cuff fabricated from thermoplastic, plaster, or QuickCast may be placed under the sling as a support. The thermoplastic cuff with a soft sling disperses the compressive forces applied through the sling by lifting the borders away from the skin and increasing the area of force application (Fig. 4–17B). Circumferential cuffs can also be fabricated to maximize pressure distribution (Fig. 4–17C–E).

SHEAR

Shear stress results from force being applied parallel to the surface and produces a tendency for an object either to deform or to slide

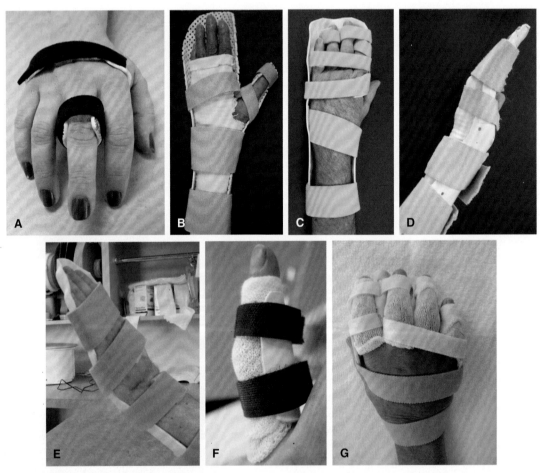

FIGURE 4–16 A, Note the floating straps on this hand-based middle-finger (MF) MCP immobilization orthosis. **B,** When the orthosis borders are too generous, the straps tend to "float" between the lateral borders and hardly braze the skin, leaving room for unintended motion. Although the strap widths in this figure are appropriate, the borders on this orthosis are too high in order to properly secure the wrist and forearm into the device. Note the use of adhesive foam between the strap and skin in order to "absorb" the extra room. **C,** When adjustment of the orthosis borders is not an option, originating the strap from a lower spot on the inside of the orthosis may offer better purchase and effectiveness of the strap as it traverses the tissue it is intended to hold in place. This technique is often used for the patient with rheumatoid arthritis (as shown here) because it can assist in managing the zigzag forearm and hand deformity often seen in these patients. **D,** This orthosis demonstrates appropriate border height and strap placements. **E,** Note how the straps have the potential to "push" the skin against the low border. The narrow width and "too" proximal placement of the wrist strap can contribute to discomfort during wear. **F,** This small PIP extension immobilization orthosis has been fabricated with low lateral borders that inadequately support the proximal and middle phalanges. The dorsal straps need to push the digit into the orthosis, leading to possible compression stress and edema pooling between straps ("window edema"). **G,** Strategically placed straps, accommodating to the oblique cascade of the digits, can make all the difference in a well-fitting orthosis. Note here that the thermoplastic material has been molded to provide "gulleys" for the digits to rest in. This aides in positioning and comfort.

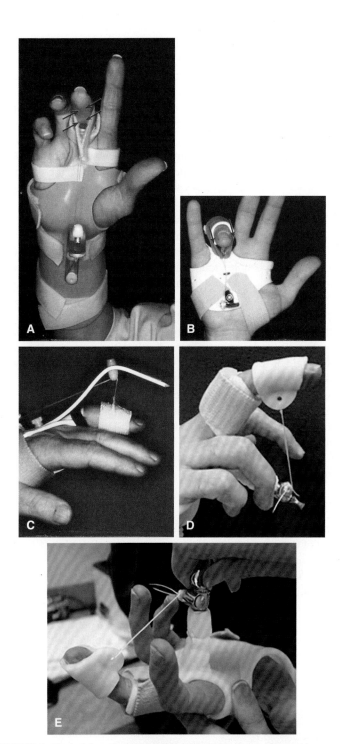

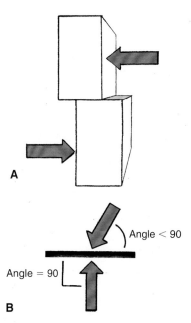

CHAPTER 4

FIGURE 4–18 Shear stress results from force being applied parallel to the surface and can occur when two parallel opposing forces are applied in the same plane (coplanar) but not along the same line (noncollinear) **(A)** and when two oblique opposing forces share the same point of application but are neither parallel nor perpendicular **(B)**.

high owing to the parallel force and compressive stress is negligible in the absence of perpendicular force. In the second case, in which the angle of application does not equal 90°, there exists both a parallel component (shear) and a perpendicular component (compression). Although difficult to measure, the amount of shear in the latter case can be inferred from the angle of application. Shear is inversely proportional to the angle of application, thus, as the angle approaches 0° (as in the former case), the shear dominates, and as it becomes more perpendicular, it decreases.

Shear is often accompanied by other stresses, for example, compression, tension, and torsion (as seen in orthoses that attempt to mobilize forearm rotation). In addition, static or kinetic friction may be present as a counterforce to the shear stress. If static friction is high, it may impart high shear stresses to the subcutaneous tissue interfaces. For example, ineffective strapping on a posterior elbow immobilization orthosis may quickly lead to noncompliance because of discomfort. If 1″ traditional loop straps (instead of conforming soft or elasticized straps) are applied in an oblique fashion to secure the anterior elbow into the orthosis, the loop strap edges are likely to rub along the skin. Rather than applying a direct compressive stress (i.e., perpendicular), the straps impart an oblique compressive stress and produce shear stress in the tissues over which they traverse (especially in the presence of high static friction) (Fig. 4–19A,B). In such cases, the therapist should consider using soft, conforming 2″ straps made from neoprene, soft foam such as Rolyan® SoftStrap® (Performance Health), or a circumferential wrap that is applied along the entire length of the orthosis for even compression.

Clinical Considerations

The therapist should use care to smooth out, roll, and/or flare uneven or sharp orthosis edges. This is especially important near joint creases where movement will occur (e.g., the volar distal portion of a wrist immobilization orthosis where the MCP joints are free to move).

When using circumferential bandages or wraps to assist in the molding of an orthosis (e.g., when a second set of hands is needed), the therapist should avoid applying them too tightly. During the

FIGURE 4–17 A, A forearm-based PIP flexion mobilization orthosis with one monofilament line converging at the volar aspect of the digit creating compressive stress along the dorsum and lateral aspect of the digit. **B,** A hand-based PIP flexion mobilization orthosis with a custom-molded thermoplastic cuff (under the sling) on the middle phalanx. This technique can be used to decrease compression of the lateral borders of the digit or thumb by lifting the sling borders off the segment being mobilized. **C,** Circumferential sling is constructed with QuickCast 2 (Performance Health), and the monofilament line is incorporated into the circumferential sling owing to better pressure distribution. **D and E,** A thermoplastic sling can also be used to maximize surface area while delivering a gentle flexion force to the PIP joint as shown here (Base 2™ Outrigger Kit and Splint-Tuner™; North Coast Medical). Note the extended homemade outrigger to accommodate for the correct angle of application.

along the surface. This can occur in two instances: when two parallel opposing forces are applied in the same plane (coplanar) but not along the same line (noncollinear) and when two oblique opposing forces share the same point of application but are neither parallel nor perpendicular (Fig. 4–18A,B). In the first case, shear stress is

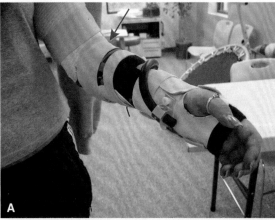

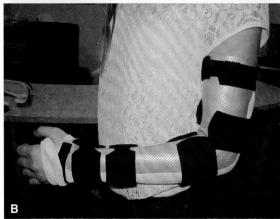

FIGURE 4–19 **A,** The 2″ straps, placed just proximal and distal to the elbow crease, assist in distributing shear and compression stress to the tissue beneath (Rolyan® Dynamic Supination Pronation Kit, Performance Health). **B,** Conforming, soft 2″ straps better distribute the force and improve patient comfort whether it is an anterior or posterior design.

wrapping process, orthosis borders may inevitably be pushed in toward the body part. This makes it difficult to smooth the borders away from the skin and may cause shear stress along the entire length of the orthosis-skin interface. Alternative options include very light stockinette (nonelastic) or prewraps/underwraps often used by athletic trainers beneath athletic taping (Fig. 4–20A–C).

When fabricating a mobilization orthosis, the therapist must consider both compression and shear stresses. Mobilizing forces, which are attached to the proximal orthosis base, usually traverse the length of the orthosis and terminate distally to the intended joint(s). If the proximal base of the orthosis is not adequately secured to the limb, motion at the distal joints will result in an undesirable migration or dragging and shearing of the proximal base over the skin. The amount of shear stress depends on the coefficient of friction of the materials used and the direction and amount of force necessary to make the change at the intended joint(s) (Fig. 4–21A–C).

The therapeutic effect of a mobilization orthosis is to increase the range of motion, thereby causing the angle of application to shift from 90° (Fig. 4–8F). Alterations in the angle of application through a sling can create an uneven pull, resulting in shear stress proximally on the orthosis base and distally on the sling. The patient may cease to use the orthosis because of discomfort. When tissue is changing rapidly owing to the use of a mobilization orthosis, the patient should visit the clinic frequently so the therapist can adequately monitor the orthosis line and adjust it as necessary to ensure a 90° angle of force application. Commercially available outriggers make adjustment simple.

Orthosis bases must be fabricated to the correct length and circumference. The proximal orthosis border of a short forearm-based orthosis is likely to pivot on the volar aspect of the forearm (because of attempted distal movement by the patient), causing shear stress at the proximal orthosis border and irritation of the superficial sensory nerves and skin (Fig. 4–22A–C).

TENSILE

Tensile stress is opposite in nature to compressive stress and is the result of opposing loads pulling away from a surface along the same line of application (Fig. 4–23). Tensile stress, also referred to as tension and distraction, results in stretching as evidenced by the lengthening and narrowing of an object to which it is applied. As is true with compression, tensile stress is the greatest when the force is applied perpendicular to the surface. Thus, to optimize the effect of tensile stress, the pulling force should be applied at a 90° orientation to the target surface.

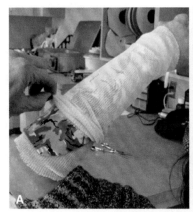

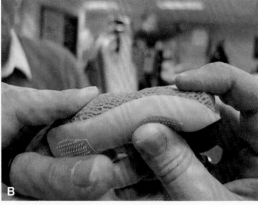

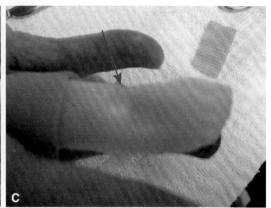

FIGURE 4–20 **A,** Use caution when applying a circumferential wrap to secure an orthosis while molding. The wrap can cause shear at the borders if not applied carefully; this can be avoided by leaving a small border of thermoplastic material outside the wrap so that this edge will not be pushed into the skin by the bandage. If the only option is an elasticized bandage, wrap the orthosis lightly and uniformly. An alternative is using a nonelastic stockinette to assist in securing the material to the body part. This will not cause undue stress at the borders of the material. **B and C,** Caution should also be taken with finger placements when molding an orthosis. The therapist creating the orthosis should use a *"light and moving"* touch when molding. As shown in this picture, the pressure created by prolong application can cause harm.

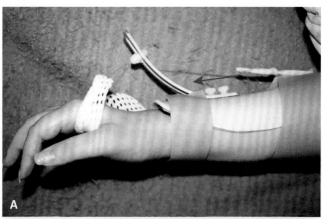

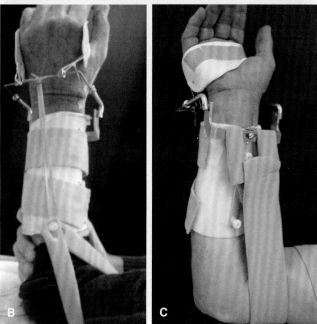

FIGURE 4-21 **A,** Wrist extension mobilization orthosis using components of the Digitec Outrigger System (Performance Health). This is a dynamic approach. Shear stress is increased proximally as the mobilizing force drags the orthosis base distally. Although there is some natural mobility of the skin (proximally and distally), this mobility is increased with the force generated through the orthosis **and** if the orthosis is not adequately contoured and secured. Therefore, the base has no choice but to migrate/translate distally. Note the distal volar portion of the strap causing potential shear stress. **B and C,** These are similar mobilization orthoses using an elastic (dynamic) force. Consider either of these proximal strap techniques; the straps are applied from the proximal base of the orthosis to above the elbow joint. These strategies can minimize the distal migration of the orthosis.

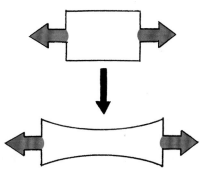

FIGURE 4-23 Tensile stress results from opposing forces pulling away from a surface along the same line of application. It is also referred to as tension, distraction, and stretching.

Clinical Considerations

When the goal of orthotic fabrication is to gain thumb abduction, the therapist may find it challenging to optimize tensile stress. Force applied to the proximal phalanx does not deliver tensile stress to the tight first dorsal interossei or to the adductor pollicis (thumb web); rather, it produces excessive stress at the ulnar collateral ligament of the thumb MP joint. The therapist should take care when fabricating an orthosis that delivers tensile stress directly to the distal aspect of the first metacarpal. The sling should conform around the head of the first metacarpal (which may cause discomfort in the web space if not molded well), and the angle of application should be directed 90° from the long axis of the first metacarpal (Fig. 4–24A–D).

Tensile stress can be used to maintain reduction of an intra-articular fracture while preserving joint mobility. The application of a gentle traction force to a healing intra-articular fracture site can help maintain bone alignment, facilitate healing, and preserve joint range of motion. An example is the circular traction PIP intra-articular mobilization orthosis designed by Schenck (1986). The surgeon places a wire horizontally through the bone proximal to the fracture site, leaving the ends of the wire protruding. The wire is bent to place rubber bands or springs, which are then attached to a hoop extending from the orthosis base. Tensile stress is then delivered from the wire to the hoop via the rubber band or spring. The hoop allows for segmental changes in range of motion while maintaining consistent stress throughout the range. These orthoses are often fabricated during the immediate postoperative period (Fig. 4–25A–D).

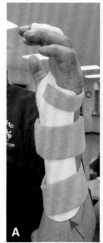
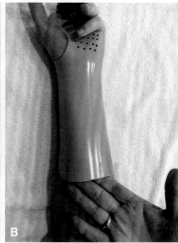
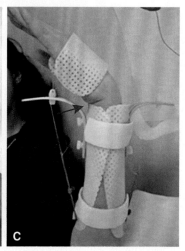

FIGURE 4-22 **A,** The proximal border of this short forearm-based orthosis is pivoting on the volar aspect of the forearm and digging into the skin. **B,** The proximal borders should be flared away from the skin as they are cooling during the fabrication process. **C,** The volar distal border of this wrist flexion mobilization orthosis is abutting the flexion angle causing discomfort and potential skin breakdown.

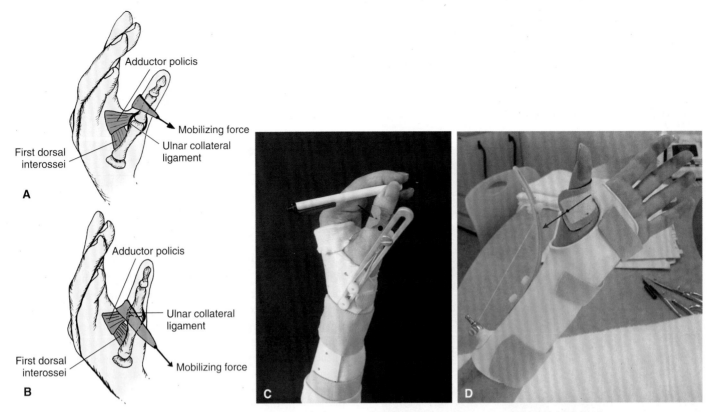

FIGURE 4–24 **A,** An incorrectly applied thumb sling stressed the ulnar collateral ligament at the thumb MP joint. **B,** A correctly applied thumb sling mobilizes the first dorsal interossei and the adductor pollicis muscles. **C,** The soft sling shown here will stress the UCL during writing with this patient. **D,** A combined soft strap and QuickCast 2 material (Performance Health) make a comfortable sling. This was molded to orient stress to the distal portion of the first metacarpal instead of the ulnar collateral ligament—making for a gentle stress applied to the first web space versus the UCL (Digitec Outrigger System, Performance Health).

BENDING AND TORSION

Compression, shear, and tensile stresses can be present in two particular combinations. **Bending** is the application of loads to a structure in such a manner that the object simultaneously undergoes tension, compression, and shear as it bends about a transverse axis (Fig. 4–26). Compression develops on the concave aspect of the structure, and tension forms across the convex aspect. In addition, shear stress develops as a result of the opposing parallel forces producing the bending (LeVeau, 1992). The bending stress is directly proportional to both the magnitude of the force and the distance from the transverse axis at which it is applied.

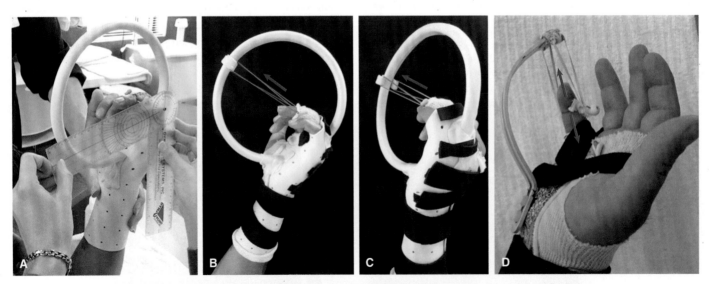

FIGURE 4–25 **A,** The clinician is shown here measuring the distance from the distal pin site on the middle phalanx to the traction point on the "hoop." **B,** Completed design using elastic "rubber band" traction. **C,** A dorsal to volar view to appreciate the role of the attachment device on the hoop. This small device plays a significant role in the ability to gently and segmentally change angles while keeping the tension uniform throughout the range. **D,** Variation of a PIP intra-articular orthosis. Note the perpendicular line of application of the rubber bands attached to a surgically placed horizontal wire through the middle phalanx. Gentle tension is applied to the PIP joint, maintaining ligament length and bone alignment while providing supervised periods of limited joint range of motion (Components of the Digitec Outrigger System used, Performance Health).

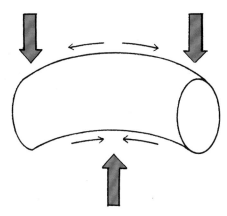

FIGURE 4–26 Bending is the application of force in such a manner that the object simultaneously undergoes tension, compression, and shear as it bends about a transverse axis.

Torsion is stress produced when a rotational force is applied to a rod or cylinder, causing a portion of the structure to turn around the longitudinal axis (Fig. 4–27) (Nordin & Frankel, 2001). Torsion, also referred to as twisting, is directly proportional to the distance from the longitudinal axis to the point of application of the force. To generate greater torsion, apply the force farther from the axis about which the intended twisting will occur. Torsion results in the simultaneous generation of compression, tension, and shear forces.

Clinical Considerations

Bending

A clinical example of the effects of bending stress is when a therapist attempts to elongate an elbow extension contracture by using an elbow flexion mobilization orthosis.

The therapist must appreciate the tensile stress present along the posterior aspect of the elbow, while compression stress is applied to the soft-tissue structures along the anterior aspect of the elbow (Fig. 4–28A–D). Shear stress simultaneously may occur at the skin-orthosis interface of both the humeral and forearm cuffs owing to orthosis migration. The force applied through the device attempts to mobilize the distal segment (forearm cuff) in the direction of elbow flexion. In doing so, the proximal segment tends to migrate distally, whereas the distal segment migrates proximally. This shifting of the orthosis can cause shear stress along the orthosis-skin interface.

Torsion

The concept of torsion stress is demonstrated by a supination-pronation mobilization orthosis used to gain forearm rotation (Shah, Lopez, Escalante, & Green, 2002).

To appreciate this concept, the therapist must first understand that forearm rotation is created by the simultaneous effort of both the proximal and the distal radioulnar joints. The nature of this design imparts a torsion stress along the entire length of the forearm, which

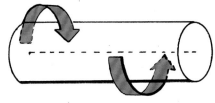

FIGURE 4–27 Torsion stress, or twisting, is produced when a rotational force is applied to a rod or cylinder, causing a portion of the structure to turn around the longitudinal axis.

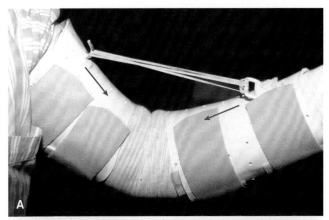
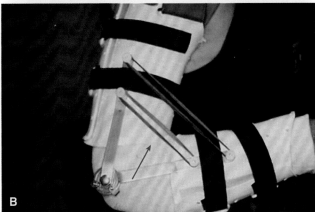
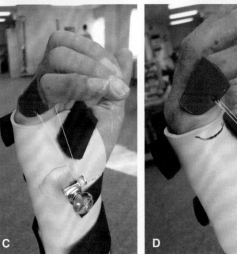
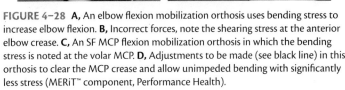

FIGURE 4–28 A, An elbow flexion mobilization orthosis uses bending stress to increase elbow flexion. **B,** Incorrect forces, note the shearing stress at the anterior elbow crease. **C,** An SF MCP flexion mobilization orthosis in which the bending stress is noted at the volar MCP. **D,** Adjustments to be made (see black line) in this orthosis to clear the MCP crease and allow unimpeded bending with significantly less stress (MERiT™ component, Performance Health).

is considered the axis of rotation. Therefore, the principles of adequate orthosis length, pressure distribution, and precise orthosis molding along the entire forearm are critical for the construction of these orthoses (Fig. 4–29A,B). The potential pressure points include the proximal and distal ends of the orthosis where the force originates and terminates (elbow and wrist joints). With this orthosis, compression and shear stresses and distal migration (the result of a linear force) are inevitably present at the orthosis-skin interface during force application. The effectiveness of this type of orthosis depends on proper fit, which requires careful monitoring by the therapist along with education of the patient.

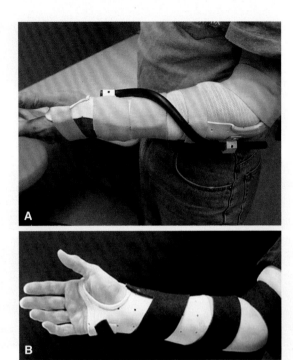

FIGURE 4-29 **A,** A forearm supination-pronation mobilization orthosis uses torsion stress to increase the supination of the forearm (Rolyan® Dynamic Supination Pronation Kit, Performance Health). **B,** Similar forearm supination force applied using gentle elastic force with neoprene strapping.

CONCLUSION

The application of an orthosis enhances or restores function of the extremity via the intentional application of external loads to manipulate the internal reaction forces of specific anatomical structures.

This chapter defined and clarified the fundamental mechanical terms and concepts pertaining to the design and fabrication of orthoses. In addition, the clinical relevance of these terms and concepts was discussed in light of specific clinical application. The effective therapist successfully integrates basic mechanical concepts into all facets of orthosis design and fabrication.

CHAPTER REVIEW QUESTIONS

1. What is the optimal angle of force application and how can a therapist ensure this is maintained in an orthosis?
2. Give an example of compressive stress and how it relates to orthotic application.
3. Why should orthoses be fabricated as long and wide as possible?
4. What is the difference between a high- and a low-profile design?
5. Name two potential areas of friction force in a typical wrist immobilization orthosis.
6. Give three different methods of how to impart a mobilization force on a body segment?

5

Equipment and Materials

Noelle M. Austin, MS, PT, CHT

CHAPTER OBJECTIVES

After study of this chapter, the reader should be able to:
- Name the various tools to have in the clinic for orthotic fabrication.
- Recognize the importance of different thermoplastic characteristics and how these influence optimal material selection.
- Appreciate the various types of strapping and lining/padding materials and understand how to choose appropriately.
- Understand the basic components of mobilization orthoses.

KEY TERMS

Bonding
Combination plastic and rubber-like materials
Conformability
Drape
Elastic materials
Finger loops
Finger slings
Fingertip attachment
Hand drills
Heat guns
Heating pans

Heating time
Hinges
Hook
Line connector
Line guide
Line stops
Lines
Lining material
Loop
Low-temperature thermoplastic orthotic materials
Memory
Mobilization force
Nonperforated materials

Outrigger systems
Perforated materials
Plastic materials
Proximal attachment device
Resistance to stretch
Rigidity
Rubber materials
Rubber-like materials
Working time

INTRODUCTION

This chapter presents the fundamentals of orthotic fabrication, including review of the equipment and materials needed to create orthoses effectively and efficiently. With today's rising healthcare costs, it has become increasingly important to be economical. Thus, therapists have been forced to change the way they buy and use rehabilitation products. They must educate themselves about what is available by researching online and conversing with their sales representatives as resources regarding new products. Such measures can help therapists make more fiscally prudent decisions. If therapists take the time to research a particular item, they will usually be able to find a lower cost or less-expensive substitute. Unfortunately, there may be restrictions in ordering practices in some settings due to that particular facility's contract with rehabilitation product distributors—this may limit purchasing options. Spending time with management to gain a better understanding will help ease this ordering process. The constant innovation in orthotic fabrication techniques and methods has spurred the need for consumers to be discriminating when purchasing products. Experimenting with new materials and providing feedback to vendors can promote positive changes in the available rehabilitation products.

Before fabricating an orthosis, the therapist must be sure to have the necessary equipment, tools, materials, and accessories readily accessible. These products can be purchased from rehabilitation vendors (see Appendix A for contact information). To provide patients with the best orthotic options, therapists must be aware of what is currently available. Therapists should be familiar with the major rehabilitation catalogs and their websites which often include links to videos or other resources demonstrating how best to use the product. There are also ways to connect with other therapists sharing ideas on social media including LinkedIn, Facebook, and Instagram as well as YouTube videos demonstrating techniques. Also spend some time browsing local hardware and hobby stores for creative ideas and products to incorporate into orthoses and/or rehabilitation. Discount dollar stores also offer inexpensive options for both handmade orthotic options as well as functional exercise tools. When attending continuing education courses, therapists should visit vendor booths and make an effort to obtain hands-on experience with new or unfamiliar products; these measures increase the therapist's comfort with using various products. Note that each vendor has its own version of common rehabilitation items and mobilization component kits. Vendors may offer the same products as their competitor, or something very similar, but they may call the item by a different name. Other invaluable resources are hand therapy journals featuring practical information on orthosis fabrication and unique ideas/hints from fellow therapists often presented in case study format.

ESSENTIAL EQUIPMENT

This section discusses the equipment needed to fabricate upper extremity orthoses efficiently and effectively. In Section 2, the Clinical, Pattern and Expert Pearls provide detailed information and helpful hints on how to use specific products and offer alternative and cost-saving strategies.

HEATING SOURCES

Thermoplastic materials need to be heated to a softened state before they can be molded to the body part. Heating pans and heat guns provide the most common means to warm the material for orthotic fabrication. Most recently the dry heat oven has been introduced which is a water-free means to fully heat and activate thermoplastic materials (Fig. 5–1A).

Orthotic Heating Pans

Ideally, dedicated **heating pans** are used to heat materials; however, if they are not available, electric frying pans will suffice. Drain water and dry pan thoroughly at the end of each clinic day to prevent any water contamination issues. This will also help preserve the bottom surface of the pan, preventing the breakdown of nonstick coating or the adherence of hard water deposits. Although hot pack heaters are readily available in most clinics, their use to soften thermoplastics includes the following disadvantages: inability to control water temperature, difficult to remove materials without overstretching (especially if attempted in a vertical manner), and possibility of contamination from dirty water.

Commercial heating pans are available in several sizes, ranging from a pan that is spacious enough to accommodate large pieces of orthotic material to a small household electric frying pan (Fig. 5–1B). Small pans may be easier to manage in the clinic because they are easy to clean (can be emptied daily), quick to heat, and do not require too much counter space. Each type of orthotic material must be heated to a specific temperature per the manufacturer's specifications to take advantage of that material's specific properties (check with each individual manufacturer for recommendations). The water temperature should be adjusted accordingly. Some of the newer pan designs have thermal regulators; a thermometer can also be used to check the temperature before heating the material. Be aware that owing to the location of the heating coils, materials may be heated unevenly when using a heating pan. This can be avoided by moving the material around the pan during the heating process.

There are several ways to prevent orthotic material from sticking to the bottom and sides of the pan, including keeping the material moving by use of a spatula and the addition of a drop of liquid hand soap, dish washing liquid, or lotion to the water. Another strategy is to employ the use of pan netting. Not only does this stop material from sticking to the pan, but it also protects hands from being burned, prevents the overstretching of softened materials, and eases the task of removing the heated material from the water. Remember that netting may leave an imprint on material that is very contouring. An alternative is to layer the bottom of the pan with paper towels. Spatulas help when removing heated material from the pan and prevent imprints in the material. Consider adding a liquid disinfectant when changing the water to prevent contamination. Utilizing distilled water may prevent mineral buildup on the inside metal surfaces.

Heat Guns

Heat guns provide a source of dry heat that can be used to spot warm specific areas of thermoplastic material. Care must be taken

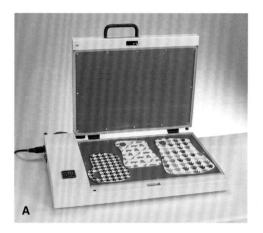

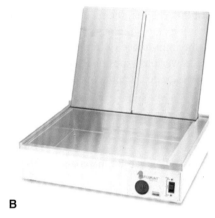

FIGURE 5–1 **A,** Large heat pan; **B,** dry heat oven offering hygienic water-free technology. [Photos courtesy of Kinetec USA. (Jackson, WI)].

when using this device to adjust an orthosis; inadvertent overheating of adjacent regions can cause irregular surfaces and the loss of contour or fit of the orthosis (especially problematic when using materials with memory that may shrink). Special nozzles are available to direct the heat to a small area; the Precision Point Heat Gun provides a concentrated source of heat (North Coast Medical, Morgan Hill, CA) (Fig. 5–2). Minor changes in contour and edge finishing can be accomplished with a heat gun as well.

The heat gun can be used to prepare the surface of the thermoplastic material for bonding, as when applying components such as outriggers. These devices are particularly useful when heating components before applying them to the orthosis, allowing them to be embedded into the thermoplastic. In addition, if experiencing difficulty with adherence of adhesive hook material onto the

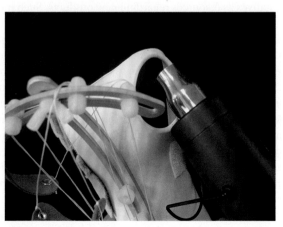

FIGURE 5–2 A Precision Point Heat Gun being used to adjust web space in metacarpophalangeal (MCP) flexion mobilization orthosis (Base 2™ Outrigger Kit, North Coast Medical).

thermoplastic (commonly an issue when using coated thermoplastics), heating the adhesive just to the point of getting tacky prior to application can ensure that it will be strongly attached.

ORTHOTIC TOOLS

The use of high-quality tools is extremely important when fabricating orthoses. Using tools that are not appropriate for the specific task can be frustrating and ineffective, making the fabrication process more difficult than otherwise. In the long run, an initial investment in quality products saves time and money. Well-maintained tools help avoid the need for replacement and guard the therapist against developing a repetitive stress injury.

In addition to cutting devices, other mandatory tools include pliers, hole punch, hand drill, wire cutters, and benders. Many other tools can assist in making the fabrication process easier. The therapist should browse through rehabilitation catalogs to learn about other tools and how they are used in the fabrication process. Be aware that less costly alternatives may be available through Amazon or local hardware stores.

Cutting Devices

Thermoplastic materials are most commonly sold in large sheets, which need to be cut into specific shapes or patterns for a particular design. Many types of cutting devices are found in hand therapy catalogs. When cutting unheated materials, use a utility knife or heavy-duty shears or snips. Some distributors offer time-saving precut thermoplastic materials (to be discussed in detail later in this chapter), eliminating the need to cut up large sheets; these precut forms are ready to be warmed in the water and molded onto the body part.

Using dull, improperly chosen scissors to cut out orthotic patterns from warmed material can be frustrating. Invest in a quality pair of scissors such as Gingher Super Shears (Performance Health

Warrenville, IL) that are comfortable to use (Fig. 5–3A). Designating a "thermoplastic-material only" pair of scissors can help prevent premature blade dullness and adhesive from sticking to the blades, which causes the warm material to stick to the scissors' blades later. Assign the use of other, less expensive scissors for cutting adhesive-backed products, such as hook, lining, and padding. Special Non-Stick Scissors are coated to minimize adhesives from sticking to the blades (Performance Health) (Fig. 5–3B). Adhesive can be removed from the scissors with solvent, Goo Gone®, rubbing alcohol, or nail polish remover. Sharpen the blades frequently to maintain sharp, smooth edges; inquire at a local fabric or craft store about sharpening services. Furthermore, sharp blades will help protect the therapist from developing overuse syndromes, which can result from making the repetitive, forceful strokes needed to operate dull scissors. Left-handed scissors are available online since utilizing those commonly found in clinics are not easy to operate for left handed users resulting in challenges with obtaining smooth trimming of thermoplastics.

When cutting with scissors, practice using *smooth, long strokes* rather than short snips, which cause multiple irregular sharp edges and can lead to an uncomfortable, unsightly orthosis. All borders and corners should be smooth and slightly rounded to maximize patient comfort, provide an aesthetically pleasing result, and add strength and rigidity to the orthosis.

Other scissors may be useful in the clinic. Bandage scissors, which remove surgical or wound dressings, have a protective blunt tip to prevent injury to the patient. Mini Serial Cast Cutter Scissors (North Coast Medical), designed to remove digit casts, are essential when using serial casting techniques for digit flexion contractures regardless of material used (Fig. 5–3C). They provide a safe way to remove a finger cast effectively and without risk of cutting the skin. Joyce Chen Scissors allow for precise trimming techniques (North Coast Medical).

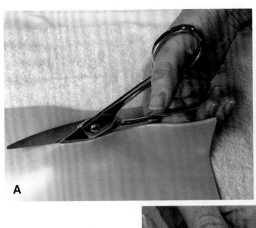

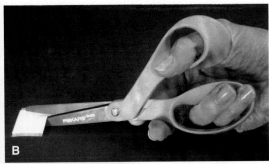

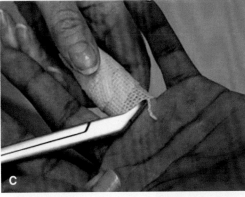

FIGURE 5–3 **A,** To obtain a smooth cut edge, the scissors should be sharp, and the material should be warm—Gingher Scissors (Performance Health). **B,** Special Non-Stick Scissors shown here trimming adhesive-backed foam product (Performance Health). **C,** A Serial Cast Cutter Scissors is used to trim a serial static finger cast (North Coast Medical).

Pliers

Pliers are important for various fabrication tasks, including cutting metal components, bending wire for outriggers, embedding small components such as eyelets into warm thermoplastic material, setting speedy rivets in place, and holding components or adhesive hook to warm over a heat gun (Fig. 5–4A,B). Various types of pliers are available in a range of styles and sizes, although the most common are blunt and needle-nose pliers. Having both types on hand in the clinic is essential to manipulate various components. Long handles are preferred to allow for less force to operate.

Hole Punches

A high-quality hole punch with a range of hole sizes is necessary for creating holes in thermoplastic materials for strapping or custom finger loops/slings and also for punching holes in hard thermoplastic materials for straps application, outriggers, rivets, and hinge components (Fig. 5–5). When the tubes on the tool grow dull, it becomes difficult to punch a hole; therefore, it is wise to buy a heavy-duty tool with replaceable tubes.

Hand Drills

Electric **hand drills**, such as the Dremel® (available with a cord or rechargeable battery pack), can be used to make holes in an orthosis in locations that the traditional hole punch cannot reach, such as applying an elbow hinge to a humeral and/or forearm cuff (Fig. 5–6A). This prevents the potentially dangerous task of heating a sharp device, such as an awl, over a heat gun to make the hole. The drill can be used to add custom perforations to specific regions of an orthosis, which help prevent skin maceration or rash caused by excess perspiration. Slits can also be drilled into thermoplastic materials to allow for custom strapping of individual digits (Fig. 5–6B,C).

Wire Cutters and Benders

Wire cutters and benders provide a way to customize an outrigger for specific anatomical requirements. When component kits are not available or appropriate for a patient, the therapist must fabricate the orthosis from scratch, using outrigger wire and ingenuity to create the desired effect. By bending the wire, the therapist can create a customized orthosis to accommodate a difficult anatomical configuration or situation, for example, fabricating over postsurgical dressings, wounds, casts, or external pins or fixators.

LOW-TEMPERATURE THERMOPLASTIC ORTHOTIC MATERIALS

Numerous types of **low-temperature thermoplastic orthotic materials** are available through various rehabilitation vendors (AliMed, Chesapeake Medical Products, DeRoyal Industries, Kinetec USA, North Coast Medical, Orfit Industries America, Performance Health); see Table 5–1 for contact information). Many therapists are justifiably confused about how to choose the right material for a specific orthosis. Unfortunately, there is no easy answer. Some therapists learned on one type of material, developed a comfort level with its use and utilize that material for all orthoses. Or perhaps the clinic is restricted in what they are allowed to purchase, one or two materials which can limit a therapists development of fabrication skills. Other therapists may have access to a multitude of materials and reap the benefit of having a choice during the fabrication process. Therapists must use their clinical knowledge and experience when making the choice of what material to order—not defaulting to previously ordered products. Often, sorting through the options is just a matter of learning more about the products and not being afraid to try different materials. During the planning stage, consider which types of materials have the best handling and physical features for that particular orthotic application. The key handling characteristics include resistance to stretch and memory. The important physical qualities consist of bondability, thickness, and perforations/colors. Assessing these factors in advance will improve the ability of the orthosis to meet that particular patient's needs.

A single type of material is not suitable for all orthoses or for all patients; there are many factors that must be taken into account when it comes to selecting the appropriate material. Therapists must recognize each material's unique characteristics (e.g., conformability and resistance to stretch) and understand the desired function of the orthosis in terms of the required rigidity and ventilation. In

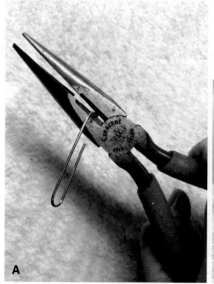
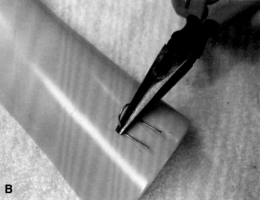

FIGURE 5–4 Blunt-nosed pliers help bend wires **(A)** to create homemade components and hold them to heat and imbed into thermoplastic **(B)**.

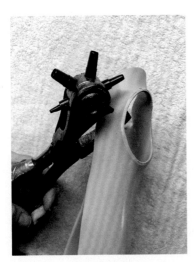

FIGURE 5–5 A hole punch is used to create hole to prepare for application of a rivet.

addition, they need to appreciate the particular nuances of each patient in terms of diagnosis, compliance, and age as well as recognize the limitation of their own fabrication skills and experience.

The novice therapist should develop a comfort level with a few types of materials before venturing on to others. The more experienced therapist who is comfortable using only a few types of materials, however, should broaden his or her selection choices by experimenting with other available materials. Expanding material options ultimately benefits the patients. Remember, however, that material selection may also be limited by other factors, including availability, budgetary constraints, and physician preferences.

To help the therapist begin to understand the multitude of orthotic material options, the following sections introduce the terms used to describe the materials' characteristics (i.e., drapability and resistance to stretch). Later sections discuss the general categories of orthotic materials (i.e., plastic and rubber-like). Specific brand name materials are not examined in depth because the availability of materials often changes; refer to manufacturers' catalogs and Websites for current availability. If the therapist understands the particular characteristics and general categories of orthotic materials, he or she should be able to select the correct one from almost any vendor.

Some distributors describe a material's conformability, whereas others label this same factor as drapability or moldability. This can be confusing for a therapist who is trying to decide which material to use. The two largest companies that offer thermoplastic materials, North Coast Medical and Performance Health, both describe their thermoplastic product line in relation to the resistance to stretch, allowing for some comparison between their products. It can be more challenging to relate the smaller company's products because there is variability with the descriptive terms used. The following

sections simplify the nomenclature as much as possible and present broad concepts and key points to aid the selection of a particular orthotic material.

HANDLING CHARACTERISTICS
Conformability and Resistance to Stretch

To meet the requirements of a specific patient, the therapist must choose a material with the optimal conformability and resistance to stretch for that particular orthosis. **Conformability** or **drape** is the degree to which a heated material is able to mold well and produce an intimate fit that encompasses the contours and irregularities of the body part (North Coast Medical, 2019; Performance Health, 2018-2020). **Resistance to stretch** is the degree to which a heated material is able to counteract being stretched or pulled, giving the therapist valuable information on how much handling the material can tolerate (North Coast Medical, 2019; Performance Health, 2018-2020). Resistance to stretch is generally inversely related to the degree of conformability (Breger Lee & Buford, 1992). Ranging from minimum to maximum, thermoplastics can be sorted on a continuum of resistance to stretch (Fig. 5–7A,B). To demonstrate this property, thoroughly heat a small piece of material in water and try to pull it apart. Resistance to stretch determines the degree of conformability. The more resistance to stretch, the less conformable the material will be when applied; less resistance to stretch results in more conformability and contouring during application. Refer to Table 5–2 for more information on how thermoplastic materials from various companies are organized on this continuum of resistance to stretch.

High Conformability/Low Resistance to Stretch

- Requires only light handling during the molding process to achieve a precisely formed orthosis (Fig. 5–8A).
- Best used when gravity can assist in the orthotic fabrication process (Fig. 5–8B).
- Often the material of choice for the skilled therapist because little handling is needed during the molding process.
- Recommended when the patient is best approached with minimal handling (i.e., the patient who is postsurgical, extremely painful, or arthritic).
- Recommended for smaller orthoses (i.e., finger and hand) because the therapist can achieve a precise fit, maximizing patient comfort and preventing orthosis migration.

Low Conformability/High Resistance to Stretch

- Requires firm handling during the molding process to obtain a well-conformed orthosis.
- Can be used when the orthosis cannot be formed with the assistance of gravity.

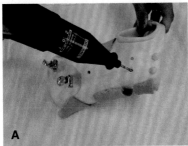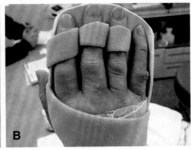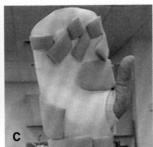

FIGURE 5–6 Dremel used to **(A)** create a hole in this mobilization orthosis and **(B and C)** cut slits in material to allow for customization of strapping system.

TABLE 5–1	**Distributors of Thermoplastic Materials**

AliMed
297 High Street, Dedham, MA 02026
800–225–2610
www.alimed.com

Chesapeake Medical Products
9629 Philadelphia Road, Suite 110, Baltimore, MD 21237
888–560–2674
www.chesapeakemedical.com

DeRoyal Industries
200 DeBusk Lane, Powell, TN 37849
800–251–9864
www.deroyal.com

Kinetec USA
W225N16708 Cedar Park Court, Jackson, WI 53037
262–677–1248
www.kinetecusa.com

North Coast Medical
18305 Sutter Blvd, Morgan Hill, CA 95037
800–821–9319
www.ncmedical.com

Orfit Industries America
810 Ford Drive, Norfolk, VA 23523
516–935–8500
www.orfit.com

Performance Health
28100 Torch Parkway, Suite 700, Warrenville, IL 60555
800–323–5547
www.performancehealth.com

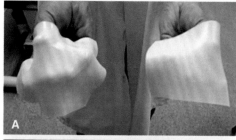

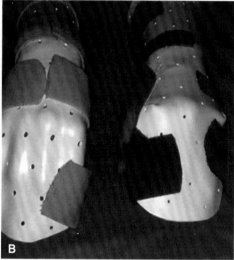

FIGURE 5–7 A and B, Demonstration of resistance to stretch: material on left with least resistance to stretch, and material on right with maximal resistance to stretch—notice difference in conformability.

- Comfortable for the novice therapist, who may feel more in control with a hands-on approach.
- Circumferential wraps may be used to aid in the molding process when fabricating without an assistant, molding against gravity, or applying material to a large area. Wrapping too tightly may cause the orthotic borders to dig and results in skin irritation (Fig. 5–9A).
- Recommended for larger orthoses (i.e., forearm, elbow, and shoulder) for which an intimate fit is not crucial, and a greater degree of control may be needed (Fig. 5–9B).

Memory

Memory is the degree to which a material is able to return to its original shape once molded and then reheated (North Coast Medical, 2019; Performance Health, 2018-2020). This quality ranges from 100% to 0% (no) memory (Fig. 5–10A,B).

High-Memory Material

- Recommended when fabricating an orthosis that will require frequent remolding (i.e., a serial static orthosis); once the material is reheated, it tends to return to the shape of the original pattern.
- Cost-efficient to remold an existing orthosis instead of making a new one to accommodate for any change in tissue status.
- Recommended for novice therapists; they can place the material back in the water and start over if a mistake is made during the molding process.
- Do not remove the molded orthosis from the body part until it is completely set, or it will return to its original shape. This may alter the final fit of the orthosis, which is especially consequential when the material is wrapped circumferentially, as in a thumb immobilization orthosis. If the material is removed too soon, shrinking can occur and the patient may not be able to don the orthosis after setting is complete.

- Be careful when using a heat gun for spot heating; ridges can form, which may adversely affect the comfort and fit of the orthosis.

Rigidity

Rigidity is the ultimate stiffness or strength of a material or the degree to which a molded orthosis is able to resist deformation when external forces are applied (North Coast Medical, 2019). This quality ranges from highly rigid to highly flexible (Fig. 5–11A).

- High-rigidity materials are recommended when the potential forces placed on the orthosis will be significant (i.e., a hand orthosis for a construction worker who applies excessive force to the hands).
- Thicker materials (1/8″) are more rigid than thinner materials (1/16″).
- Overstretching during the fabrication process creates weakened areas in the orthosis, which may decrease rigidity.
- Specific diagnoses (i.e., metacarpal fractures) require more rigid materials to support the healing structures.
- A circumferential design provides a more rigid support than a volar or dorsal approach even if the material is thin (Fig. 5–11B).

Bonding

Bonding is the ability of a material to adhere to itself once heated (North Coast Medical, 2019; Performance Health, 2018-2020). Bondability refers to the presence of coating, which acts as a barrier to prevent unwanted adherence. Some materials are available with or without this coating—be sure to read the specific description before placing an order. If there is "mystery material" in your clinic, consider experimenting with small pieces to determine whether a coating is present and label accordingly. When in doubt, assume there is no coating and be cautious with overlapping using

TABLE 5–2   Thermoplastic Materials

Company Name	Resistance to Stretch				
	Minimum	Minimum to Moderate	Moderate	Moderate to Maximal	Maximal
AliMed[a]	Multiform™		Multiform™ Clear Elastic		
Chesapeake[b]	Excel™	Infinity™	FiberForm™-Soft	Colours™	FiberForm™-Stiff
			Rebound™		Marque-Easy™
DeRoyal[c]	LMB Drape™		LMB Blend™		
Kinetec USA[d]		Manosplint® Arizona	Manosplint® Wisconsin	Manosplint® Ohio	Manosplint® Carolina
North Coast Medical[e]	Clinic®	Encore™	Vanilla™	Omega Max™	Omega™ Plus
		Preferred®	Spectrum™	Solaris™	Omega™ Black
			Prism™		
Orfit[f]	Orfit® Flex NS		Orfit® Classic Soft		Orfit® Classic Stiff
	Orfit™ Crystal NS		Orfit® NS Soft		Orfit® NS Stiff
			Orfit® Colors NS		Orfit® Eco
			Orfilight™		Orfibrace™ NS
			Orfit® Natural NS		
Performance Health[g]	Polyform™	Kay-Splint II™	Aquaplast™ ProDrape™-T	Aquaplast™ Original	Aquaplast™ Original Resilient™
		Polyflex II™	TailorSplint™	Aquaplast-T™	Aquaplast™-Resilient™T
		Orthoplast II™	Kay-Splint III™	Aquaplast T™ Watercolors™	Synergy™
		CuraDrape™		Ezeform™	San-Splint™

[a]www.alimed.com.
[b]2019 brochure/catalog and www.chesapeakemedical.com.
[c]www.deroyal.com.
[d]2019 brochure/catalog and www.kinetecusa.com.
[e]2019 brochure/catalog and www.ncmedical.com.
[f]2019 brochure/catalog and www.orfit.com.
[g]2019 brochure/catalog and www.performancehealth.com.

techniques described in the following text to prevent inadvertent sticking. Some manufacturers offer specific hints for best handling their materials, such as Orfit products. To decrease surface tackiness and improve handling ability, they recommend rubbing talcum powder on the surface of the thermoplastic prior to heating and adding liquid soap to the heating pan water.

- Coated thermoplastic does not bond to itself unless overheated, overstretched, scratched, or treated with solvent.
- Coated material does not bond to itself when heated. For example, this helps when fabricating thumb orthoses, allowing the therapist to create a trap door to ease removal (Fig. 5–12A).
- Coated material also allows for temporary bonding when two heated pieces are overlapped, which can assist with the fabrication process. Once the material has cooled completely, this area can easily pop apart as long as the material was not overstretched.
- Coated material has a reduced tendency to adhere to the patient's skin, hair, and wound dressings. It is generally easier to clean as well.
- Coated material is easier to clean than noncoated material because it is less porous; this is especially helpful for patients who require long-term orthosis use—less likely to take on odor and dirt.
- Do not overstretch coated material; this disrupts the coating and may cause the material to inadvertently adhere to itself.

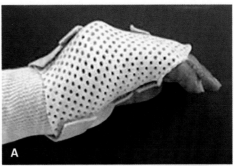
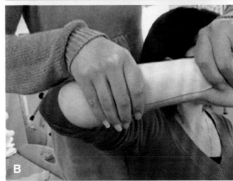

FIGURE 5–8 A, Notice intimate fit achieved with highly drapable material. **B,** A forearm-based ulnar wrist orthosis is molded more easily with assistance of gravity.

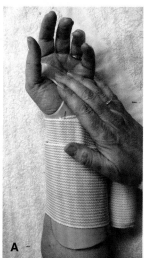

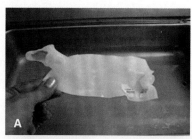

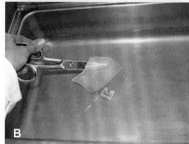

FIGURE 5–9 **A,** Forearm-based wrist orthosis is molded with a proximal wrap to allow hands-on positioning distally. **B,** Rigid material was utilized on this patient with high tone in the wrist and digit flexors.

- The coating may be removed with a solvent or by aggressively scratching the surface with an emery board/sandpaper or awl/scissors if adherence to another piece of material is required.
- Uncoated material adheres to itself when both areas are heated fully and pressed together, which is especially helpful when attaching outriggers or when using an extra piece of material to reinforce a particular area of the orthosis. Using a heat gun to make the thermoplastic slightly tacky can help ensure a strong bond, also be sure that both areas are completely dry.

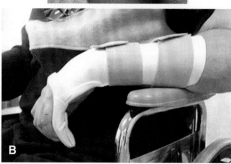

FIGURE 5–10 Demonstration of material memory: material was heated and stretched out **(A)**, then reheated and shrunk back to original shape **(B)**.

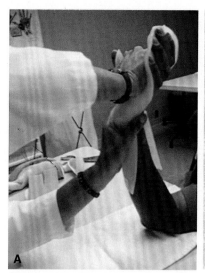

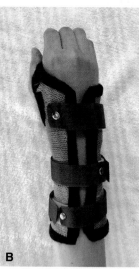

FIGURE 5–11 **A,** When fabricating an orthosis that needs to withstand potentially high forces, such as this serial static wrist and digit mobilization orthosis, choose a material that is rigid (thick and solid). **B,** Wrist orthosis fabricated using Delta-Cast® (Essity) allows for ability to fabricate rigid circumferential designs.

- Use a stockinette liner over the dressing when molding with uncoated material to prevent sticking to dressings and superficial skin.
- When coated material is unavailable, use a wet paper towel or hand lotion between two pieces of uncoated material to prevent adherence (Fig. 5–12B).

Heating and Working Times

Each material has an optimal heating temperature (ranging from 140°F–170°F), **heating time** (ranging from 0.5–2 minutes) and **working time** (from 1–7 minutes). Specific information can be found in manufacturers' catalogs and literature that accompanies sheet material (AliMed, 2019; Chesapeake Medical Products, 2019; DeRoyal Industries, 2019; Kinetec USA 2019; North Coast Medical, 2019; Orfit Industries America, 2019; Performance Health, 2018-2020). The working time refers to the time in which the heated material can be molded onto the body part before the orthosis sets.

- All materials should be partially heated (for approximately 30 seconds) before the specific pattern is cut out. Material is heated partially when lifting the edge with scissors or spatula reveals moderate stiffness with slight bending. This partial heating can save the therapist's thumb from the forceful cutting of hard material.
- Some materials provide a self-sealing edge for a smooth finish after being cut while warm, preventing the need for edge finishing later.
- When making large orthoses, the novice therapist may want to hold one edge of the material while the other edge is partially heated for cutting; this allows the therapist to maintain control of the material at all times.
- Thin or highly perforated materials have a shorter working time; thick, solid materials have a longer working time.
- Elastic and rubber-like materials tend to have longer working times than plastic materials.
- Do not remove the material from the body part too soon or the shape and fit may be lost, causing buckling or ridges to form in the orthosis.
- Materials with longer working times are recommended for complex orthoses requiring multiple joints in specific positions, such as commonly encountered with neurologically involved patients.

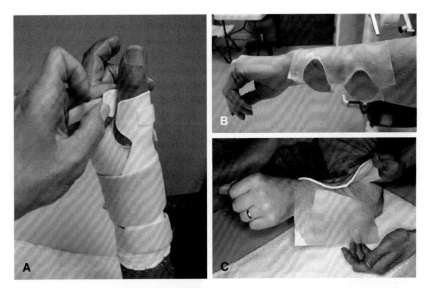

FIGURE 5–12 **A,** Coated material allows overlapped pieces to pop open, which can accommodate, for example, an enlarged thumb IP joint. **B,** A protective forearm immobilization orthosis applied with the pinch-and-pop technique. The edges will be trimmed to form smooth borders. **C,** A wet paper towel placed between uncoated materials prevents adherence.

- Materials with shorter working times are recommended for patients who are unable to hold a specific position for a long period (i.e., pediatric patients).
- Sometimes, it is necessary to hasten the setting time (i.e., for a patient who is in pain). Note that this cannot be done using material with memory because the final fit may be altered.
- Accelerate the cooling by wrapping the material with an elastic wrap that has been soaked in ice water or with a TheraBand® that has been stored in the freezer (Performance Health). Use caution with this technique—wrapping may cause irritation if it causes the edges to dig into the skin.
- Accelerate the cooling by using cold spray or by removing a partially set orthosis and placing it under cold running water. Note that the cold spray technique may irritate the skin or eyes, so do this away from the patient.
- Avoid overheating the material (leaving in water too long, placing in water too hot), which can alter its properties and lead to overstretching, thinning, and material fatigue, which in turn can decrease the rigidity of the completed orthosis. Allow material to cool off on table prior to handling/molding—cold countertops can hasten the cooling process.
- Always dry off any excess water on the material prior to applying to the body part.
- Before applying the material to the patient's body part, check the material's temperature against the therapist's skin.
- Be extra careful to avoid overheating or burning the skin of patients who have any sensory involvement including loss of sensation or skin hypersensitivity (commonly seen after cast removal). Use a stockinette over the body part to minimize heat.

PHYSICAL CHARACTERISTICS

Thickness

Materials are available in several thicknesses, most commonly 1/16″, 3/32″, and 1/8″ thick (Fig. 5–13) (AliMed, 2019; DeRoyal Industries, 2019; Kinetec USA 2019; North Coast Medical, 2019; Performance Health, 2018-2020). Commonly, therapists get in the habit of using 1/8″ material for all orthoses, but this is not always necessary. The therapist may choose a specific thickness based on the orthosis' function. In general, 1/8″ is suitable for arm, forearm, elbow, and wrist orthoses; 3/32″ and 1/16″ are appropriate for

hand-based and pediatric designs. To create the lightest and least bulky device, the therapist should choose the thinnest material possible that provides the required support and rigidity. Thicker materials tend to provide more rigid support. Thinner materials offer a less bulky, lighter weight alternative. When thin materials are used for circumferential orthoses, they can create adequate rigidity if the therapist takes advantage of contouring. For example, circumferential forearm fracture orthoses may be best created with 3/32″ or 1/16″ material instead of 1/8″ material, which creates a bulky orthosis that can impede function. Thinner materials can be cut more easily, which can decrease the strain on the therapist's hands.

Perforations

Almost all thickness and types of material are available in **perforated** and **nonperforated forms**. The density of perforations can range from 1% to 42% (Fig. 5–14A–C) (Kinetec USA 2019; North Coast Medical, 2019; Performance Health, 2018-2020). Perforated materials allow air exchange, which helps decrease the incidence of skin problems such as rash, excessive sweating, and/or maceration (Breger Lee & Buford, 1991, 1992). Orthoses fabricated from perforated materials are lighter in weight and also more flexible, which can make donning/doffing easier with circumferential designs.

The therapist must decide whether providing a lightweight orthosis with increased ventilation is worth the sacrifice in rigidity. This potential downside must be weighed carefully to ensure that the

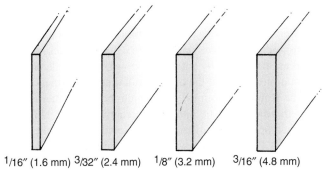

1/16″ (1.6 mm)   3/32″ (2.4 mm)   1/8″ (3.2 mm)   3/16″ (4.8 mm)

FIGURE 5–13 Materials of different thicknesses.

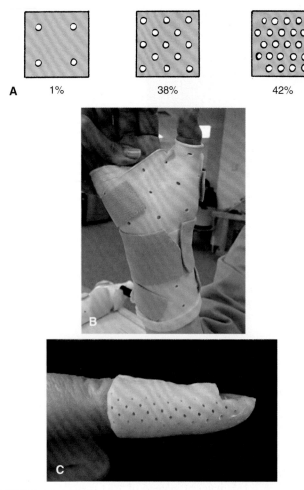

FIGURE 5–14 **A,** Density of perforations. **B,** 1% perforation pattern can be effective in reducing maceration in palm. **C,** 11% perforation in digit orthoses can allow for air exchange and prevent sweating issues.

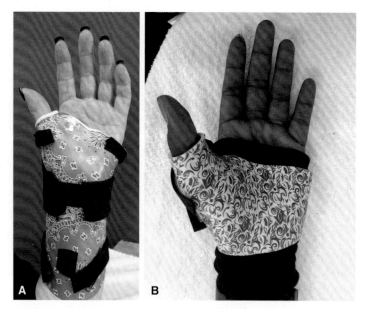

FIGURE 5–15 **A,** Wrist and thumb immobilization orthosis fabricated using patterned material: Rolyan® Imprints® Blue Bandana Polyform® (Performance Health). **B,** Thumb orthosis using custom printed material from Kinetec USA.

orthosis provides an adequate amount of rigidity or support. For example, an orthosis to support a fracture requires a more rigid support than one applied for tendinitis. In most cases, a 3/32″ lightly perforated material in a circumferential design can adequately support a distal radius fracture while allowing air exchange.

Because perforations help decrease the orthosis' weight, they may improve wear compliance. Extra perforated materials may need to be edged with extra-thin material (thermoplastic or soft liner) to provide a smooth, reinforced border. Do not overstretch heated perforated materials because the holes elongate, and the material may thin out unevenly.

Colors

Orthotic materials are available in an assortment of colors. Bright colors may help maximize compliance in a young patient or aid in a quick retrieval among bed linens in a nursing home. On the other hand, some patients may feel the colors draw unwanted attention to themselves and their condition. In these cases, skin tones are the more appropriate choice. Darker colors, such as black, help hide dirt and are best worn by patients who work in an industrial environment or need to wear the orthosis full time. Performance Health offers the Rolyan® Imprints® line, which includes patterns on one side of the thermoplastic and most recently Kinetec USA offers customized printing to further allow personalization of the orthosis (Fig. 5–15A,B). There is a wide selection of patterns which adds to the therapist's creativity and the bonus is that patients appreciate making their orthosis unique.

CATEGORIES

The most commonly used thermoplastic materials can be categorized in and described by the following terms: plastic, rubber or rubber-like, combination plastic and rubber-like, and elastic (Performance Health, 2018-2020). These groupings help the therapist keep track of each type of material and its workable characteristics. Refer to Table 5–1 for current thermoplastic material selections. Thermoplastic materials are traditionally sold in 18″ by 24″ sheets; however, some manufacturers now sell materials in smaller sheets, allowing for easier storage and less need for laborious cutting in the clinic. Label the thermoplastic sheets upon delivery and as the sheet is being cut down so there is no question in the future what type of material it is. Otherwise, as the product gets used, it may be confusing what types of material are left over.

Plastic

Plastic materials are generally highly conformable and have minimal resistance to stretch (i.e., Clinic®, North Coast Medical; Polyform™, Performance Health; Multiform™, Alimed; Excel™, Chesapeake) (Breger Lee & Buford, 1992). These materials are best used with gravity's assistance and by an experienced therapist because the material can be challenging to control. The ability to make minor adjustments in an orthotic pattern by stretching the material can help ensure a better fit. Small orthoses requiring a well-molded precise fit are best made with these materials (Fig. 5–16A). Plastic materials contour nicely when molding over pins or bony prominences.

The therapist may leave fingerprints in the material if he or she uses a too aggressive hands-on approach during the molding process. Gentle handling with smooth, light strokes is the best way to work with these materials. Overheating can make plastic materials too soft, leading to overstretching and making them difficult to control. To minimize overstretching, handle these materials horizontally on pan netting rather than vertically. Plastic materials are not suggested for novice therapists because of the material's high degree of conformability.

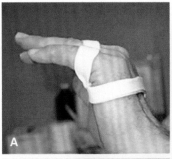
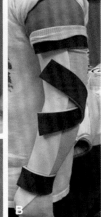
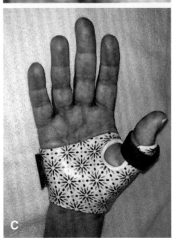

FIGURE 5–16 **A,** An intimate fit can be achieved with plastic materials; note the detail of the contours obtained across the dorsum of the phalanges. **B,** Rubber-like materials tend to mold to the shape of the extremity with less detail. **C,** Blend materials allow for control during the molding process but nice contouring about the crevices in the hand (Kinetec USA custom printed on Manosplint˚ Wisconsin).

Rubber or Rubber-like

Rubber or **rubber-like materials** offer a good degree of control at the expense of conformability owing to their high resistance to stretch (i.e., Manosplint® Carolina, Kinetec USA; Rolyan® Ezeform®, Performance Health; Omega™ Plus, North Coast Medical). These materials do not drape and contour as well as plastic materials; thus, the final fit is less detailed (Fig. 5–16B). Larger orthoses that do not require an intimate fit, such as a wrist/hand immobilization orthosis worn over wound dressings, are best made with these materials. Rubber materials offer a significant degree of control with minimal stretching or fingerprinting. Novice therapists may find these materials easy to work with because it is forgiving and can tolerate repeated handling and manipulation; firm handling is required to achieve a contoured fit. Cut rubber-like materials when still slightly warm to obtain extremely smooth edges.

Combination Plastic and Rubber-like

Perhaps the most versatile fabrication products are those with moderate resistance to stretch or those in the middle of the continuum; **combination plastic and rubber-like materials** tend to offer the best of both worlds in terms of conformity and stretch (i.e., Manosplint® Wisconsin, Kinetec USA; TailorSplint™, Performance Health; Preferred®, North Coast Medical). These "blended" materials can be used for virtually all types of orthoses and are an excellent choice for a multiuse material in the clinic. These materials produce an orthosis with a well-molded fit while allowing the therapist some degree of control during the molding process. Many therapists find these materials to be useful for a wide variety of orthoses, including forearm- and hand-based designs (large and small) (Fig. 5–16C). The specific characteristics depend on the proportions of rubber and plastic in the thermoplastic base.

Elastic

All **elastic materials** have some amount of memory with varying degrees of resistance to stretch (i.e., Aquaplast®, Performance Health; Manosplint® Ohio, Kinetec USA; Prism™, North Coast Medical; and Orfit products). As noted earlier, this characteristic is best used in situations in which there is a need for frequent remolding to accommodate for changes in tissue. Some of these materials are available uncoated, which allows them to adhere to the body part; this may help in achieving a precise, intimate fit by acting as a second pair of hands. The degree of conformability and stretch depends on the specific material's chemical composition.

When pinched together lightly, coated elastic materials can provide a temporary bond that can be popped apart once the orthosis is set. This technique can be helpful when fabricating without the assistance of gravity (Fig. 5–16D). It is easy to determine when most elastic materials are heated fully because they turn transparent (except for some colored elastic materials, which turn opaque). This transparency provides visualization of sites where potential irritation can occur and allows for accommodations of these hot spots during the molding process. Therapists generally deem these materials as quite versatile and use them successfully for a multitude of orthoses.

Elastic materials do have some disadvantages. If the molded orthosis is removed when the material is still slightly warm, the material will continue to set, causing further tightening or shrinking and altering the final fit. Obtaining a well-contoured orthosis with 1/8″ material may be troublesome because of the material's tendency to shrink during its setup time. Elastic materials have a longer setup time than plastic materials and can be frustrating when time efficiency is an issue. In addition, the novice therapist may find it difficult to achieve a smooth edge with these materials. Accurate pattern creation, along with cutting the pattern out while the material is warm, can help therapist to achieve smoother edges.

Precut and Preformed Orthoses

Precut forms can help save time and money as well as decrease material waste. These precut forms come in various material types, thicknesses, perforation patterns, colors, and sizes to satisfy most orthotic fabrication needs (Fig. 5–17A). They are heat pan ready, avoiding the time needed to create and cut out patterns.

Rolyan® AquaForm™ Zippered Splints (Performance Health) and Orfizip®Light (Orfit, Norfolk VA) are thermoplastic precuts with a zipper sewn in for closure, providing the therapist with a valuable option to address a multitude of diagnoses (Fig. 5–17B, C). They are commonly used for fractures and as the base for a mobilization orthosis. Refer to Section 2 for more specific information including fabrication tips.

Preformed orthoses are also available (prefabricated into a specific shape and size); these are offered in a wide range of types, sizes, and materials (Fig. 5–17D). Once heated, most of these can be modified to provide a custom fit. This is a great option for the therapists challenged with fabricating general orthoses in a setting where they do not have either the skills or time to fabricate the orthosis from scratch (i.e., acute care or rehabilitation setting).

Other

Thermoplastics in pellet form are available; these can be used for adaptations of tools and utensils improving function with activities of daily living (Fig. 5–18A). Simply soften them in a cup of hot water and then mold around the item to form a handle. Other sheet material choices currently available include lined materials

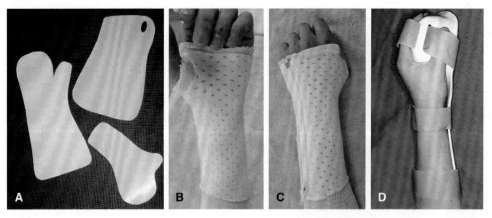

FIGURE 5–17 **A,** Precut orthosis forms. **B and C,** Rolyan® AquaForm™ Zippered Wrist Splint (Performance Health). **D,** Preformed Rolyan® Neutral Position Hand Splint (Patterson Medical).

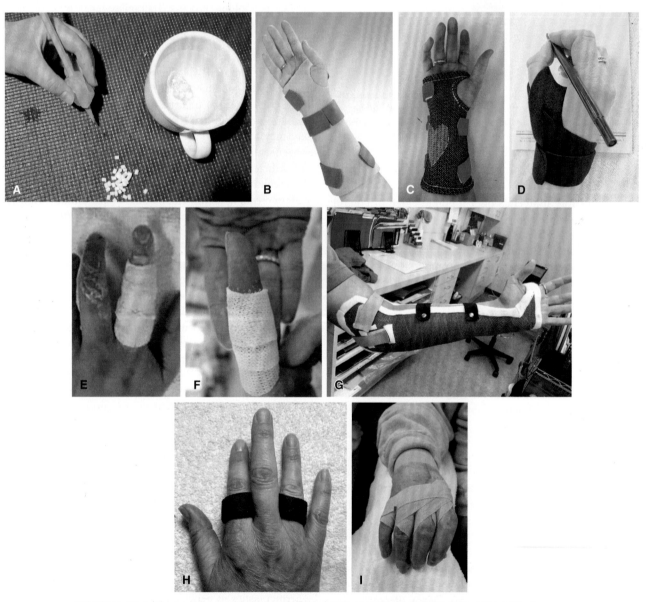

FIGURE 5–18 **A,** Thermo-Pellets™ used to form pencil grip (North Coast Medical). **B,** Fabric-lined OhioF (Kinetec USA). **C,** X-Lite® PLUS used for this wrist orthosis (Allard USA). **D,** Custom neoprene carpometacarpal (CMC) restriction orthosis. Plaster of paris **(E)** and QuickCast 2 (Performance Health) **(F)** to address proximal interphalangeal (PIP) flexion contracture (Performance Health). **G,** Delta-Cast® application to create long arm orthosis to prevent forearm rotation (Essity). **H,** Orficast® is a versatile material—here used for a relative motion orthosis (Orfit). **I,** Kinesio® Tex Tape helps to minimize tendency for metacarpophalangeal (MCP) joints to ulnarly deviate following MCP arthroplasty.

(i.e., Manosplint® OhioF; Kinetec USA) (Fig. 5–18B), mesh-type thermoplastic materials (i.e., X-Lite®, Allard USA) (Fig. 5–18C), and neoprene for soft restrictive orthoses (see Chapter 14) (Fig. 5–18D). Casting techniques provide an option for some forms of orthotic intervention. Casts require the use of plaster of paris (Fig. 5–18E), Delta-Cast® Casting Tape (Essity) (Fig. 5–18F), QuickCast 2 (Performance Health) (Fig. 5–18G), and Orficast® (Orfit) materials (Fig. 5–18H) (see Chapters 11 and 12) (Colditz, 2002). Various taping products are gaining popularity for immobilizing or restricting a joint or body part, including the McConnell Taping method, elastic therapeutic taping (Kinesio® Tex Tape) (see Chapter 13) (Fig. 5–18I). As noted earlier, therapists must be diligent in keeping up with new materials and techniques.

ADDITIONAL EQUIPMENT

STRAPPING MATERIALS

Strapping is used to secure an orthosis to a body part. The proper application of straps is crucial to ensure the orthosis serves the intended purpose. Commonly, therapists focus on molding the thermoplastic material to the patient and obtaining a contoured fit and tend to minimize the importance of strapping as it relates to proper orthosis fit. Careless application of straps can ultimately lead to an ineffective device. Like thermoplastic materials, numerous types of strapping systems are available. As therapists, we must challenge ourselves to look beyond the traditional **hook** and **loop** for specific situations. First, therapists must appreciate the mechanics of orthotic fabrication. The wider the strap, the better the force will be distributed. However, straps should not be so wide that they inhibit full motion. Narrow straps can potentially cause redness and irritation of the underlying soft tissue. When applying straps over bony regions, consider using foam to further distribute the pressure. Be mindful to maximize the mechanical advantage of the orthosis. Use the length of the orthosis when fastening the straps. You can mold the orthosis optimally, yet if the strapping is not secured at the proximal and distal edges, the best possible mechanics may never be realized.

The most common method to secure an orthosis to a body part is with hook-and-loop straps. Velcro® is the most familiar brand name; however, other versions are available. Usually, the adhesive-backed hook strip is attached to the orthosis and the loop strip is wrapped around the body part. Hook-and-loop straps are available in several widths (1/2″–2″) and colors. Precut strapping is convenient, reducing waste and speeding up the fabrication process. Adhesive-backed hook strips are available in precut lengths, which can eliminate sticky scissors. Many patients, especially children, enjoy choosing their own strap colors, and involving the patient can help maximize compliance. Spot heating the adhesive-backed hook before applying it to the orthosis increases adherence and provides a firm attachment; this is an especially helpful technique when using thermoplastics with a protective coating.

When a hook strip is used to secure a circumferential loop strap, the therapist must decide whether to use one or two pieces of hook (Fig. 5–19). A disadvantage of using two smaller pieces is the increased risk of detachment with repeated donning and doffing of the orthosis. Two pieces, however, may better accommodate a bulky forearm, as when applying straps proximally. An advantage of one longer strip of hook material is the increased surface area of attachment, lowering the chance that the strap will come off the orthosis. However, this method requires more hook-and-loop material, which can be costly. Remember to allow enough loop strap to cover the

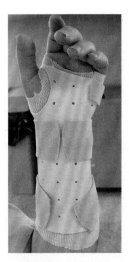

FIGURE 5–19 Methods of applying adhesive-backed hook strips to a wrist orthosis. Using two separate strips proximally to prevent any hook from remaining uncovered and catching on clothing.

hook fully; otherwise, the hook tends to stick to clothing and bedding. Round the edges of both the hook and loop strips to prevent snagging and inadvertent detachment; in addition, rounded edges are more aesthetically pleasing.

In addition to the conventional hook-and-loop material, therapists can use an elasticized loop to secure the orthosis firmly to the patient. Soft foam is also available; they may be more comfortable against the skin than traditional hook-and-loop tape. These materials conform nicely to the contours of the extremity and allow for some fluctuations owing to edema. These straps are not as durable as hook-and-loop material and thus may increase the cost of an orthosis. In specific situations, using these more expensive straps may be the best choice. Specialized strapping may be beneficial in terms of comfort and function. For example, when fabricating an orthosis for a patient with arthritis, soft strapping such as Rolyan® SoftStrap® Strapping Material (Performance Health) may be the optimal choice (Fig. 5–20A). Be aware that these materials have less "repetitions" than traditional loops; just flip the strap over to double the use. For patients using the orthosis during functional use, it may be beneficial to choose an elasticized loop such as RStretch™ (Performance Health) or a neoprene strap (Fig. 5–20B). These stretchable straps accommodate muscle contraction/relaxation better than stiffer loop material. Neoprene straps are versatile, depending on how they are cut from the sheet they can provide a stretch or not. When applying small finger orthoses, consider RThin™ (Performance Health) loop material because its low profile minimizes bulk between the digits (Fig. 5–20C).

Many other strapping systems exist, including hook-and-loop strips combined on one strap. This material works well for patients with limited use of an extremity. For the pediatric population, systems are available that provide the extra strength needed to secure orthoses adequately to active children (i.e., Dual-Lock® Fastening System, Performance Health). D-rings and buckles are options for securing straps that need to control the tension; these are especially beneficial for circumferential orthoses used as fracture bracing.

A rivet can be used to secure one end of the strap permanently to a small area of the orthosis where an adhesive-backed hook strip would be inefficient. A hole punch and blunt-nosed pliers are all that is needed to set these rivets. Riveting one end may also help keep patients (pediatric, geriatric) from losing their straps (Fig. 5–21). Be sure to cover the underside of the rivet with a small piece of lining material or tape to protect the skin; rusting can occur as a result of excessive moisture.

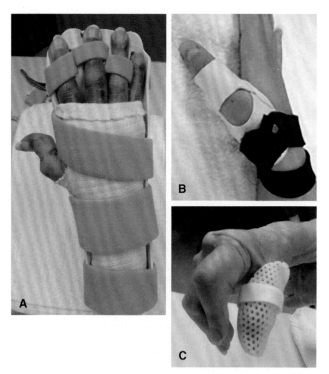

FIGURE 5–20 **A,** Rolyan® SoftStrap® used to secure digits in this wrist and hand immobilization orthosis used after extensor tenosynovectomy. **B,** Neoprene strap used to accommodate muscle movement in this metacarpophalangeal immobilization orthosis during functional use. **C,** Thin loop strapping used for a thumb orthosis.

Therapists must be creative when designing strapping systems for an orthosis, taking into account each patient's unique needs. For example, a patient with severe arthritis may benefit from specialized loops on the straps to ease donning and doffing of the orthosis and the strategic placement of the straps to aid in improving joint alignment. Patient education regarding the proper application of straps is imperative. Taking a photo with a cell phone of the orthosis in place can help with proper application later. Have patients don and doff the orthosis in the clinic to be sure they are confident in proper placement of the straps. The adhesive hook should act as a "road map" for proper placement of loop material. Numbering of the straps may be helpful. Patients should be aware of potential problems associated with improper application such as neurovascular compromise and bony/soft tissue irritation. The strapping should be snug enough to hold the orthosis in place but not so tight it causes tissue irritation. If there is an issue of significant edema,

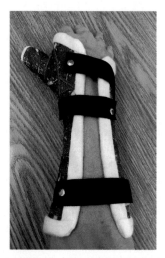

FIGURE 5–21 Rivets applied to secure the straps in this thumb orthosis fabricated with Delta-Cast® (Essity).

and the potential for "window edema" between the straps is present, perhaps using a circumferential wrap may be beneficial while the edema subsides. Proper orthotic strapping is commonly overshadowed by the focus on thermoplastic selection and the molding process itself. Strapping selection is a crucial step in the orthotic fabrication process and can assist in maximizing the effectiveness and final outcome. There are multiple options available, and we need to use critical thinking to challenge ourselves to come up with the optimal strapping solution.

Helpful hints in the form of Clinical and Pattern Pearls are provided throughout Section 2 to highlight where and why straps should be placed in specific areas. Keep the following general principles in mind when considering where to place straps on an orthosis.

- Wider straps offer better force distribution than narrow ones (Bell-Krotoski & Breger-Stanton, 2011; Brand & Hollister, 1999; Fess, Gettle, Philips, & Janson, 2005). Increasing the area of pressure contact helps prevent soft tissue irritation. However, straps should not be so wide that they impair the range of motion at unaffected joints.
- Use self-adhesive foam in conjunction with the strap to prevent uneven pressure distribution and tenderness at bony regions (Fig. 5–22A). Uneven pressure can result from placing a strap across a bony area, such as the ulnar styloid process.
- To make the straps sit flush against the skin, they must be placed at an angle to accommodate the shape of the body part. For example, when applying straps to a forearm, the therapist must take into account the tapered shape of the body part. This is especially applicable when securing an orthosis on a patient with large forearms (Fig. 5–22B).
- Straps should be tight enough to hold the orthosis securely in place but not so tight that circulation is impaired. Pinching the skin against the borders can irritate superficial sensory nerves and should be avoided. Educating the patient regarding signs of neurovascular compromise is imperative.
- Remember to maximize the mechanical advantage of an orthosis by securing straps in specific areas (Brand & Hollister, 1999; Fess et al., 2005). For example, the proximal and distal straps on a long arm orthosis should be placed as close to the edges as possible and the middle strapping should be attached about the axis of elbow to prevent the patient from flexing out of the orthosis (Fig. 5–22C).
- To make the orthosis less likely to be removed by a questionably compliant patient, use a circumferential bandage to secure the device (Fig. 5–22D) or with digit orthoses tape may suffice (Fig. 5–22E).
- If the straps have caused window edema (swelling between the straps), try applying a bias-cut wrap (commercially available nonelasticized material cut on the bias) from distal to proximal as well as elevation to decrease swelling (Fig. 5–22F). This technique provides a more even pressure distribution across the entire area. When the edema subsides, the wrap can be replaced with traditional hook-and-loop strips.
- Soft straps can be fringed to improve pressure distribution, increase comfort, and aid in edema control. Patients should always be told to watch for signs of swelling (especially distal to and between straps), vascular compromise, sensory changes, and improper fit. They should be instructed to loosen the straps appropriately (Fig. 5–22G).
- As a cost-saving measure, consider purchasing 1″ adhesive hook, which should meet all of your fabrication needs. Patients appreciate that this narrow width allows full hook coverage, preventing the hook from sticking to clothes and bedding.

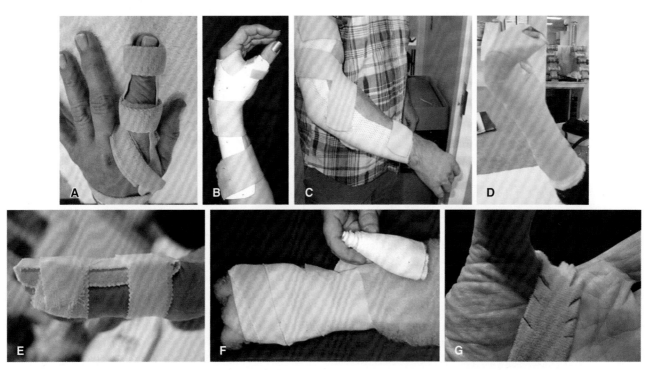

FIGURE 5–22 **A,** Foam placed dorsally across the straps can prevent irritation of bony prominences. **B,** Notice angle of proximal strap to accommodate the bulk of the forearm musculature. **C,** Notice proximal and distal strap placement to maximally secure elbow. **D,** Elasticized wrap used in acutely postoperative patient where edema fluctuations made traditional strapping not appropriate. **E,** Athletic tape can be an effective way to minimize bulk and prevent digit orthoses from falling off. **F,** A bias-cut wrap secures resting support for a patient with severe edema. The lining of Dacron batting helps maintain a dry environment within the orthosis. **G,** Customizing strapping through the webspace and prevent skin irritation issues that commonly occur in this sensitive region.

- To save time, keep on hand a supply of precut hook tabs in the most common lengths.
- To minimize ordering multiple widths, consider keeping 2″ loop strapping in stock and cut it down as needed.
- Keep all scraps of loop material for future use. This will allow for full use of all loop material.
- Ordering multiple colors can allow for ultimate orthosis customization and could aid in orthotic wear compliance.

LINING AND PADDING MATERIALS

Occasionally, therapists find it beneficial to line the inside of an orthosis partially or completely with a **lining material** to improve comfort, especially for older patients with thin, sensitive skin that may get irritated by direct contact with the thermoplastic (Fig. 5–23A,B). Be judicious with adhering permanent linings within an orthosis because they cannot be washed. Linings often become malodorous and discolored from the perspiration that inevitably occurs when airflow is prevented. Skin integrity can be compromised when subjected to a prolonged moist environment; rashes, macerations, or actual skin breakdown may be seen. Adhesive-backed liners are difficult to remove, and frequent changes can be frustrating and expensive. Padding and lining materials are available in various thickness and textures; keeping a few in the clinic's inventory should be sufficient.

Orthotic liners may be permanent (adhesive on one side) or removable (completely separate from the orthosis itself). With most orthoses, use a removable liner, which can be washed to avoid potential hygiene issues that could become problematic with the more permanent types. There are some specific clinical situations when permanently applying a liner within the orthosis may improve the comfort and, likely, the compliance with a wearing schedule. In these cases, choosing a product that can be easily removed and

replaced (low tack) would be advantageous. Possible hygiene issues such as excessive moisture (caused by sweating, wound exudates, etc.) or sloughing of skin can be avoided by changing the liner frequently. Choosing a liner that is "closed cell" (impenetrable by liquid and easy to clean but does not permit air exchange) versus "open cell" (allows the absorption of liquid) can provide an environment that is easily cleansed. Open-cell products are somewhat breathable, absorbing any excess moisture, which could create a potentially unhealthy environment for the affected hand. OhioF is a prelined material available through Kinetec USA that has a permanently attached washable antimicrobial fabric liner (Fig. 5–18B). Excessive moisture is commonly an issue when patients need to wear an orthosis full time in warm, humid climates. Helpful options include using a perforated material to allow increased ventilation (Fig. 5–22C) or using a thin layer of polyester quilting batting (available in craft stores) between the skin and thermoplastic. Removable polyester (Dacron) batting effectively wicks the moisture away from the skin (Fig. 5–22F). Do not use cotton batting or gauze, which allows the wetness to remain against the skin. The batting should be changed at least daily to prevent skin problems.

In terms of removable products, cotton stockinette is the most common and economical product available. These can be removed, washed, and reused, providing a suitable interface between the skin and orthosis. If the patient has a problem with excessive moisture within the orthosis, polypropylene stockinette is an option; it has a wicking action to keep the area dry. For patients with edema, consider providing an elastic sleeve such as TubiGrip™ or SurgiGrip® (Fig. 5–23C) (Performance Health); for those requiring padding, consider TubiPad®. For digit orthoses, cotton stockinette (SurgiTube®) or elasticized wraps (Coban™ or CoFlex®) can be used as a liner; just remember to apply the product to the area prior to molding to allow for extra room within the orthotic design

CHAPTER 5

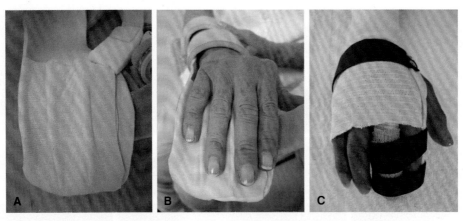

FIGURE 5–23 A and B, Adhesive foam lining is used to form individual troughs so that the fingers can rest within them. **C,** Notice use of removable elasticized sleeve for hand/forearm and digit wrap to address edema.

(Performance Health). For patients who require long-term use of an orthosis or request a thicker liner, the durable Terry-Net™ liner may be the best option (Performance Health). Liners that include the thumb are available for application beneath thumb orthoses. If a sewing machine is accessible in the clinic, thumb components can be sewn into stockinette liners. Instruct patients to change the liner daily, wash by hand, and air dry.

Use orthotic padding material sparingly, if at all. Remember that a well-molded, properly fitting orthosis does not generally require padding. There is no substitute for a well-molded orthosis; therefore, it is not appropriate to apply padding hoping to improve the fit after the molding process. Adding padding after fabrication alters the orthosis fit and can create shear and compression stresses to adjacent areas (Brand & Hollister, 1999; Fess et al., 2005). The increased bulk over the padded area may cause an increase in pressure. On the other hand, padding in orthoses can be beneficial if used correctly. Padding can be valuable over areas where excessive pressure may create potential "hot spots" such as bony prominences or superficial nerves. When applying padding to the thermoplastic, anticipate the potential trouble areas and proactively prepad that region (Fig. 5–24A). Mold the thermoplastic directly over this padding and finish by inverting the padding back into the formed orthosis. If a patient returns to the clinic with complaints of a pressure point, avoid applying padding after the molding process; this can cause a shifting of the orthosis, producing a different pressure point in another region. Instead, prepad the irritated area and heat/remold the entire orthosis. When choosing padding for an orthosis, therapists must consider the thickness as well as the texture. Generally, choose a padding that is as thin as possible but still meets the needs of the patient to protect the area. As an alternative to foam-based products, therapists may find gel padding effective in protecting a sensitive area, especially if there is a scar present (Fig. 5–24B). Padding can be applied not only on the thermoplastic segment of the orthosis but to the strapping system as well. This can be especially helpful when straps traverse over one of those potential "hot spots." Padding incorporated into straps at specific areas can be used to provide gentle feedback to optimally position joints (Fig. 5–24C). This is particularly helpful when immobilizing in the antideformity position: metacarpophalangeal (MCP) joint flexion/proximal interphalangeal (PIP) joint extension. Padding over the PIP joints can aid in maintaining this position. Padding may help prevent or gently stretch joint contractures by imparting a gentle stretch to the tissue: just be sure that the diagnosis allows for this type of stress on the tissue. Alternative products that are helpful in the clinic include Microfoam™ Tape and hook-receptive neoprene (Performance Health). Microfoam™

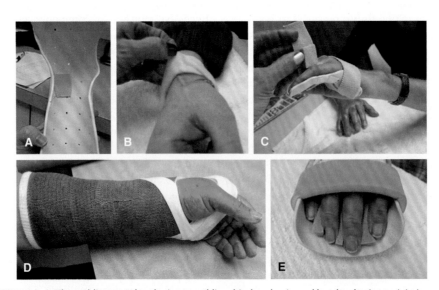

FIGURE 5–24 A, The padding was placed prior to molding this dorsal wrist and hand orthosis to minimize pressure at the distal ulna. **B,** Gel used to protect hypersensitive radial sensory nerve. **C,** Foam adhered to strapping will encourage optimal proximal interphalangeal (PIP) joint position in extension. **D,** Microfoam™ Tape used to line this wrist cast. **E,** Foam cut into triangles adhered to orthosis for separating digits for a patient with arthritis to wear at night.

Tape is a low-tack foam tape that can be applied to pad specific areas of an orthosis, very useful around the first web space (Fig. 5–24D). This tape has a nonskid quality similar to Dycem® that can be helpful in preventing orthosis migration: apply longitudinal strips within the orthosis. Neoprene can be used as an alternative to traditional padding materials. This soft and contouring material is comfortable against the skin: attach within an orthosis via hook or permanently bond to noncoated thermoplastics during the molding process. Foam pieces can also function as finger separators in resting orthoses (Fig. 5–24E).

Scar management techniques can be incorporated directly into the orthotic design by employing the use of gel, Putty Elastomer™, or Otoform™ products (Performance Health). Gel is available in sheets or pads (Fig. 5–24B). Form the heated material over the scar and mold to allow for accommodation of the product within the confines of the orthosis (Fig. 5–25). These products need to be reformed as the scar changes; at which time the orthosis must be remolded to adjust for this alteration in dimension. Using a thermoplastic material that is conducive to frequent reheating, such as one from the elastic group, is the best choice. Some materials on the market have a layer of gel laminated to the thermoplastic material, providing another means of scar management (Silon-STS®, Performance Health).

COMPONENTS

This section presents the orthotic components needed to fabricate a mobilization orthosis (dynamic and static progressive). The specific systems as well as fabrication instructions are discussed in Section 2. Because there are frequent innovations in orthotic fabrication techniques and products, it is important to read current catalogs and journals to stay abreast of what is on the market.

Outrigger Systems

The outrigger portion of an orthosis is an extension from the orthotic base that acts as an anchor to apply a mobilizing force (Fig. 5–26A). **Outrigger systems** must be adjustable devices that allow the therapist to maintain the optimal 90° angle of pull. Each rehabilitation catalog offers numerous outrigger systems to meet specific therapy

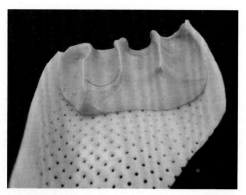

FIGURE 5–25 This volar orthosis has an incorporated scar mold for a patient with contracted volar scars.

needs (AliMed, 2019; North Coast Medical, 2019; Performance Health, 2018-2020) (refer to Appendix A for a complete listing of vendors).

To determine which is the most appropriate option for a given patient, the therapist must carefully consider many factors: the therapist's preference, the patient's unique needs, and product availability. For example, when presented with a patient who needs a digit extension mobilization orthosis, the therapist must determine which design to use: hand or forearm based; single or multiple digits; high or low profile; custom or prefabricated; and static progressive, serial static, or dynamic (Austin, Slamet, Cameron, & Austin, 2004) (Fig. 5–26B). In general, the accessories for a specific system—line guides, pulleys, and proximal attachment devices—can be purchased separately to allow custom-fabricated orthoses.

When a commercial outrigger kit is not appropriate or available, the outrigger can be easily made from wire, rolled thermoplastic, or thermoplastic tubing (see Section 2 for details) (Fig. 5–26C,D). Copper or aluminum wire can be cut with pliers or snips and bent using a vice, pliers, or a bending bar. A small piece of perforated thermoplastic material can be molded to the frame to allow the line to glide through. Thermoplastic tubes can be easily shaped into outriggers after they have been softened in warm water. To attach a custom outrigger to the orthotic base, use a big enough piece of

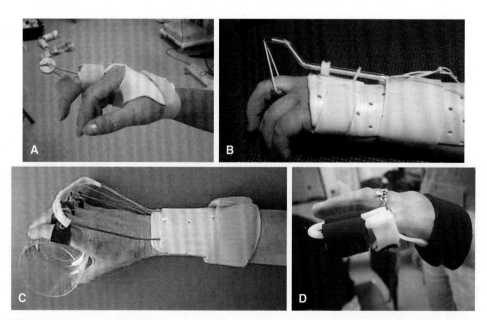

FIGURE 5–26 Outriggers: **(A)** Hand-based proximal interphalangeal (PIP) extension mobilization orthosis with a dorsal Rolyan® Adjustable Outrigger Kit (Performance Health) **(C)**. Metacarpophalangeal (MCP) extension mobilization orthoses using **(B)** Orfitube™ system (Orfit) and **(D)** bent wire with scrap thermoplastic to create pulley system and Rolyan® Aquatubes® heated and formed into outrigger (Performance Health).

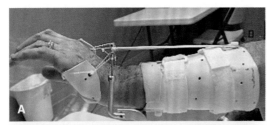
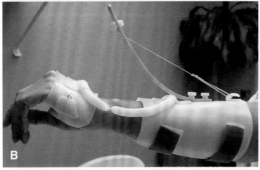

FIGURE 5–27 Wrist extension mobilization orthoses: **(A)** Phoenix Wrist Hinge (Performance Health) and **(B)** custom hinge using Rolyan® Aquatubes® (Performance Health). Also shown is Digitec Outrigger System (Performance Health).

thermoplastic material to adequately cover the proximal portion of the outrigger. The higher the outrigger, the less stable the attachment site; be sure to provide adequate proximal length for attaching to the orthotic base. To form a strong bond, use solvent to remove any coating on the material. If no wire or tubing is available, heat a strip of thermoplastic material and create a rolled tube, which can then be formed into an outrigger.

Hinges

Rehabilitation catalogs offer **hinges** for addressing the wrist and elbow joints. Hinges allow motion in one plane of movement. They are extremely versatile, satisfying various orthotic fabrication needs (Fig. 5–27A). They can be used for immobilization by creating a static situation when locked to prevent motion, restriction by blocking a portion of the available range of motion, and mobilization by using a dynamic component or static line to stretch the joint or soft tissue structures. Hinges are helpful for mobilization orthoses to prevent migration; for example, in a dynamic elbow flexion orthosis, the hinge prevents the proximal and distal cuffs from being drawn together by the rubber band traction. If kits are not available, handmade versions can be fashioned from a crimped piece of thermoplastic tubing or by loosely attaching two pieces of thermoplastic material together with a large rivet or rubber band post (Thomes & Thomes, 1999) (Fig. 5–27B).

Accessories

Fingertip Attachments

Mobilization orthoses of the digits frequently requires a way to apply force directly from the fingertips via a **fingertip attachment**. The options available include fingernail hooks, adhesive-backed hooks, and wrap-on hooks (Trueman, 1998) (Fig. 5–28A,B). Fingernail hooks and adhesive-backed hooks require the use of glue on the nail to provide a secure attachment. To prepare the surface of the nail for a secure bond, scratch with an emery board and then clean with alcohol. The devices are detached by using nail polish remover. Removable wrap-on hooks provide a means of attaching a mobilization force without disrupting the nail; they are lined with a slip-resistant material. Kinesio® Tex Tape can also be trimmed to create a means to attach line to a fingernail (Fig. 5–28C,D). When using these products, be mindful not to compress the digit's neurovascular structures.

Finger Slings and Loops

Finger slings and **loops** can be purchased in various materials, including suede, leather, and soft material, the choice of which depends on preference. For cost containment, use strap material scraps to make custom slings and loops. The small finger can be challenging to fit with a prefabricated sling, commonly needing trimming for both length and width. A sling is an open trough in which each end of the fabric has its own line; those lines may or may not converge. A loop is a closed trough in which the two ends of the fabric converge to a single line (Fig. 5–29A–C). Loops are easier and quicker to apply because only one line needs to be secured, whereas a sling requires two lines. Caution should be taken not to compromise vascularity in the digit when applying finger slings and loops. Slings decrease the compressive forces on the digit. Educate the patient on the signs and symptoms of impaired circulation. See Chapter 4 for details about designing line attachments to minimize compressive and shear forces on the digit (Bell-Krotoski & Breger-Stanton, 2011; Brand & Hollister, 1999; Fess et al., 2005). A digital cuff fabricated from thermoplastic material can also help prevent unnecessary forces under the sling. The same mechanical principles are applicable when designing a mobilization orthosis for the wrist or elbow; the distal cuff is analogous to the finger sling or loop (Fig. 5–27A,B).

Lines

Static **lines**, which connect the distal attachment to the more proximal connection, can be fashioned using nonelastic monofilament or nylon cord (Fig. 5–30A). These materials create a line that is resistant to drag, which is especially important when they are gliding through line guides or pulleys. The length should be sufficient to

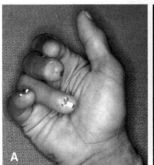
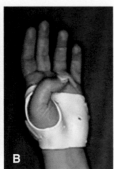
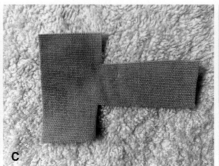
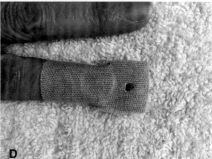

FIGURE 5–28 Fingertip attachments for the application of mobilization forces include **(A)** dress hooks glued to the nails and **(B)** hook material glued to the nails. **C and D,** Therapeutic tape custom cut to include fingertip for force application.

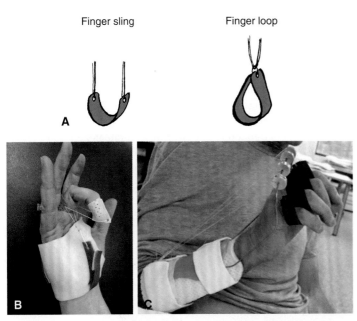

FIGURE 5–29 **A,** Finger sling and finger loop. Homemade using scraps of **(B)** thermoplastic material used for digit flexion mobilization orthosis and **(C)** neoprene soft strapping material for radial nerve palsy orthosis.

allow unobstructed gliding through the pulleys. Because these lines are nonelastic, they can be effectively used for fabricating static progressive orthoses (Schultz-Johnson, 2002a, 2002b). Traditionally, fishing line was used by therapists; however, this can be challenging to manage and keep knots tied because of its smooth texture. Nymo Cord (Performance Health) offers a better option that is easier to handle when knotting and guiding through pulley systems (Fig. 5–30B).

Line Guides

A **line guide** or pulley gives the therapist a means to change the direction of a force. Maximizing the angle of application, ideally at 90°, improves the effectiveness of the orthosis (Bell-Krotoski & Breger-Stanton, 2011; Brand & Hollister, 1999; Fess et al., 2005) (refer to Chapter 4 for details). There are many types of commercially available guides (Fig. 5–31A,B). The therapist can fashion one by using a scrap piece of thermoplastic material and punching a hole in it to allow the line to pass through. Perforated materials are user-friendly; the therapist can easily change the angle of pull by choosing from the many existing holes (Fig. 5–31C,D). Metal

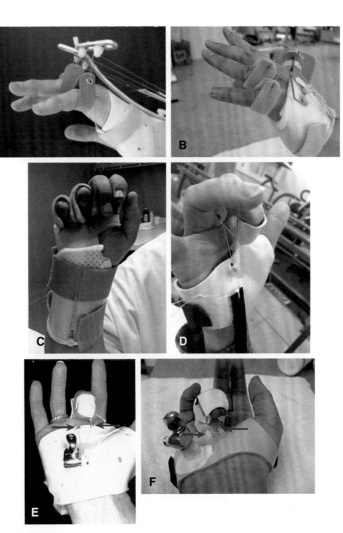

FIGURE 5–31 Pulley systems: **(A)** Digitec Outrigger System is highly adjustable, allowing for easy modification of pulley position (Performance Health). **B,** Phoenix° Adjustable Outrigger Kit with pulleys over proximal phalanges; hand based for metacarpophalangeal (MCP) extension mobilization following laceration of digit extensors over the MCP joints. **C,** Homemade pulley using scrap of perforated thermoplastic material. **D,** After punching small holes, the proximal region of orthosis was heated and pulled out to allow for line to pass in this static progressive digit flexion orthosis. **E,** Safety pins were bent, heated, and embedded into the thermoplastic material to act as line guides for the static progressive force. **F,** Rolyan° Aquatubes° were cut and embedded within this version of a similar orthosis (Splint-Tuner™; North Coast Medical).

eyelets and safety pins offer yet more options; they are inexpensive and can be easily bent, heated, and embedded in the thermoplastic material (Fig. 5–31E). Thermoplastic tubes can also be used to create line guide (Fig. 5–31F).

Line Connectors and Stops

Line connectors provide an alternative to knots for attaching the line to slings or mobilization forces. They allow the therapist to adjust tension in a dynamic orthosis easily by changing the placement of the connector rather than becoming frustrated with tying and retying knots that frequently loosen. Connectors are simply crimped with pliers.

Line stops provide a means to control the available range of motion allowed in a restrictive-type orthosis (Fig. 5–32). Stops are applied to the line proximal to the line guides or pulleys at a specific point determined by the desired motion restricted. They can be removed and reapplied to change the available range. Tape can also be used on the line to restrict the range of motion.

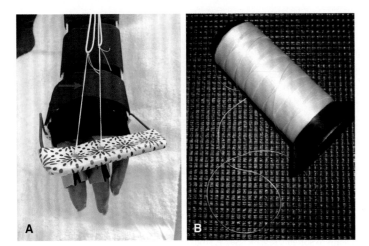

FIGURE 5–30 **A,** A static line is used to attach neoprene finger cuffs to wrapped elastic cord in this digit extension mobilization orthosis. **B,** Spool of Nymo Cord (Performance Health).

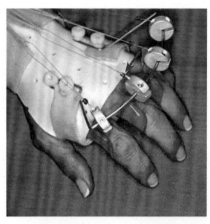

FIGURE 5–32 When rehabilitating an extensor tendon repair, line stops can be used with a dynamic digit extension orthosis to restrict metacarpophalangeal (MCP) flexion (Phoenix Outrigger Kit, Performance Health).

Mobilization Forces

The therapist can apply a **mobilization force** to a body part in several ways. For dynamic orthoses, choose from stretchy forces, such as wrapped elastic cord, graded rubber bands (Fig. 5–33A–C), elastic thread, elasticized loop, pajama elastic, neoprene, elasticized wrap, graded springs/coils, and TheraBand® or TheraTubing® products (Mildenberger, Amadio, & An, 1986) (Fig. 5–33D–I). Replace elastic products frequently to ensure an accurate generation of force on the tissue. These force-generating components may be connected distally by means of a static line. Consider using a force or tension gauge to measure the applied force to prevent the sling from being too aggressive with the tissue.

Static progressive orthoses use a nonelastic means of applying a mobilization force. Turnbuckles can be fashioned to provide this static force. Components such as the MERiT™ (Performance Health) or Splint-Tuner™ (North Coast Medical) provide an

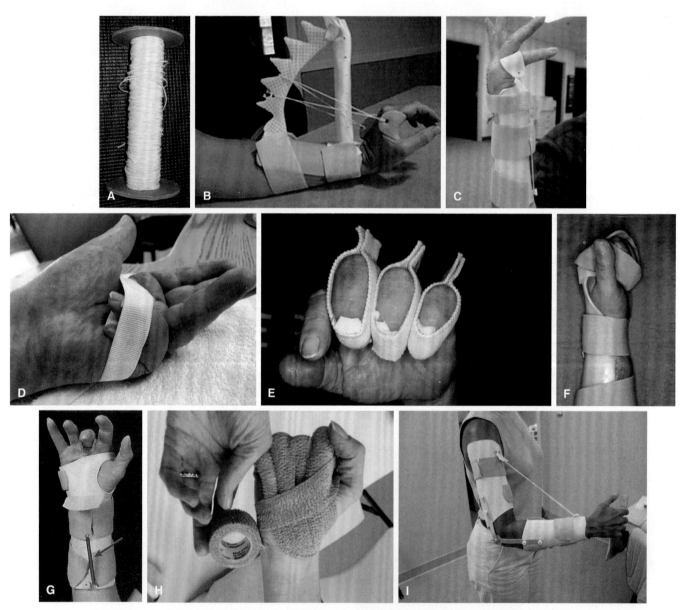

FIGURE 5–33 Dynamic mobilization forces: **(A)** Spool of wrapped elastic cord allows for easy modification of force applied. **B,** Wrist extension mobilization orthosis—"dinosaur design" chosen to allow for maintenance of optimal 90° line of pull. **C,** Simple application of flexion force using rubber band. **D,** Use a safety pin dorsally with pajama elastics to easily create this flexion strap. **E,** Elasticized loop material can be staples dorsally to create this proximal interphalangeal (PIP)/ distal interphalangeal (DIP) strap. Note use of foam to soften stress on nails. **F,** Strap of neoprene material provides final flexion stretch in this digit mobilization orthosis. **G,** Spring coil delivering metacarpophalangeal (MCP) flexion force. **H,** Elasticized wrap used for a quick way to apply general flexion stretch to digits. **I,** Thera-Tube for force application with this elbow flexion mobilization orthosis (Phoenix elbow hinge, Patterson Medical).

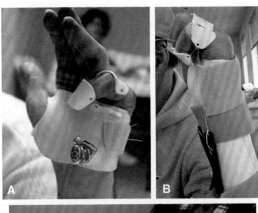

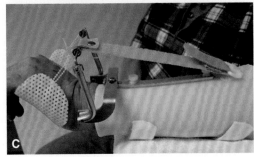

FIGURE 5–34 Static progressive forces: **(A)** MERiT™ (Patterson Medical) and **(B)** homemade using traditional hook-and-loop material allowing for adjustments of static tension. **C,** Hook and loop provide this adjustable static progressive force to address wrist extension deficit—note the use of D-Ring proximally to allow for easy adjustment by patient (Phoenix Wrist Hinge, Performance Health).

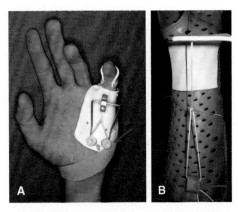

FIGURE 5–35 A, A rubber band post acts as convenient proximal attachment device for this proximal interphalangeal (PIP) flexion orthosis (Phoenix Outrigger, Performance Health). **B,** Homemade hook from scrap thermoplastic material used on this digit flexion mobilization orthosis.

adjustable means of static force application that can be used in a multitude of orthoses (Fig. 5–34A). This thumb screw on the device provides a way to progressively change the static tension. A less costly alternative is to purchase a banjo tuner from a music product supplier. A homemade option includes the use of hook-and-loop material that can be progressively changed to impart a greater stretch. Loop strips allow easy adjustment; the strip is simply attached to a different place on the hook material to alter the tension (Fig. 5–34B). Using a D-Ring in the design allows for ease of adjustability (Fig. 5–34C).

Proximal Attachment Devices

A distally applied dynamic or static force requires a **proximal attachment device** for connecting to the orthosis (Fig. 5–35A,B). Dynamic forces can be attached with rubber band posts or hooks

made from scrap thermoplastic material. Static progressive forces can be secured through the use of adjustable devices as noted earlier.

CONCLUSION

It is imperative for the therapist to keep abreast of current available equipment and materials to provide patients with the most effective orthotic intervention. Therapists with the knowledge and skills required for orthotic fabrication are able to respond to the individual needs of each patient by blending creatively this knowledge base to fabricate the most appropriate orthosis.

CHAPTER REVIEW QUESTIONS

1. Why is having a good pair of scissors so important with orthotic fabrication?
2. What other tools are helpful to have in the clinic for orthotic fabrication?
3. Describe the term *resistance to stretch* and how this relates to the different types of thermoplastic materials.
4. When is using padding or lining material appropriate in an orthosis?
5. What are the best ways to stay abreast of the new component systems available?

6 Fabrication Process

Noelle M. Austin, MS, PT, CHT[*]

CHAPTER OBJECTIVES

After study of this chapter, the reader should be able to:
- Appreciate the importance of therapist-physician communication.
- Name and describe the different segments of a comprehensive upper extremity examination.
- Recognize the importance of evidence-based practice (EBP).
- Develop an understanding of the PROCESS of orthotic fabrication.
- Integrate the results of the examination into a comprehensive treatment plan including the role for orthosis intervention.
- Appreciate the various frames of reference and how they influence orthosis application.

KEY TERMS

Bio-occupational approach

Disabilities of the Arm, Shoulder, and Hand (DASH)

Evidence-based practice

Frames of reference

Goniometers

Grip dynamometers

Numerical Rating Scale (NRS)

Person, Environment, Occupation (PEO) Model

Pinch gauges

PROCESS

Rehabilitative approach

Upper Limb Functional Index (ULFI)

Visual Analog Scale (VAS)

Volumeter

INTRODUCTION

This chapter presents the process of orthotic fabrication, from receiving the physician's orders to issuing the orthosis to the patient. Discussion includes information needed from the physician, items to include on the upper extremity examination, interpretation of the findings, and the establishment of an appropriate intervention plan. Finally, this chapter introduces the unique style of Section 2 of this book, which details a specific approach to orthotic fabrication. This format uses the acronym **PROCESS**, which provides the reader with a systematic method for creating orthoses and makes the description of each orthosis simple to follow and easy to understand. All the chapters in Section 2 follow this format; therefore, it is critical for the reader to be familiar with the PROCESS concept.

REFERRAL

A patient is generally referred to the therapist by a physician for fabrication of an orthosis and/or therapy. The referral should include as much of the following information as possible:

- Patient name
- Diagnosis and/or surgical procedure
- Date of injury and/or date of surgery
- Precautions
- Orthosis specifications
  - Purpose (i.e., immobilization)
  - Type (i.e., immobilization orthosis to rest a body part)
  - Desired joint position(s) (i.e., antideformity position: wrist at 30° extension, metacarpophalangeal [MCP] joints at 40°

flexion, proximal interphalangeal [PIP] joints, and distal interphalangeal [DIP] joints at 0°)
  - Goal (i.e., allow tendons to heal)
  - Wearing schedule (i.e., at all times, except bathing and exercise)

Obtaining a copy of the operative report is extremely helpful, especially for complicated cases in which multiple procedures were performed that require protection in specific positions. Understanding what structures were injured and how they were repaired dictates the postoperative rehabilitation and orthotic management approach. Viewing radiographs and other special studies (i.e., magnetic resonance imaging [MRI], computed tomography [CT] scans, and nerve conduction velocity studies) is also beneficial to gain a greater insight about the patient's condition.

Although the therapist may not always have the opportunity to see test results or operative reports before examining the patient, it remains imperative that the therapist has a full understanding of the diagnosis and prescribed intervention before rendering treatment. If there are questions or concerns, do not hesitate to call the physician's office to receive clarification of orders. When in doubt, be conservative with positioning; orthoses can always be modified once the physician is contacted.

Ideally, therapists should strive to establish a strong relationship with their referring physicians. Appreciate that each doctor has his or her own philosophy on treatment approach. Communicating effectively with the referral source promotes a professional relationship full of mutual respect and trust. Physicians are more apt to return phone calls and respond to requests when they have thoughtful interactions with the therapist. Always organize questions and concerns before speaking with the physician; his or her time is

[*]With additional contributions by: Gary P. Austin, PT, PhD, OCS, FAAOMPT, FAFS; Gail Dadio, OTD, MHSc, OTR/L, CHT, CLT; Pat McKee, MSc, OT Reg (Ont), OT(C).

valuable and often limited. Asking intelligent, relevant questions helps instill confidence in the therapist's skills and provides for optimum patient treatment.

Sometimes general referrals are sent, giving the therapists some latitude to decide on the orthosis to be made. Therapists are then challenged to use their clinical skills to provide patients with the most appropriate device. As the patient's conditions evolve, their orthotic needs most likely change. It then becomes essential for patients to follow up with their doctor to receive an updated referral or signed therapy progress note with new orders that reflect the change in status.

EXAMINATION

The examination provides the basis for all critical thinking and therapy intervention. All patients must be evaluated so the most appropriate orthosis can be chosen. Appendix B includes a sample upper extremity examination. Orthotic fabrication should not be approached as a rote intervention; each patient should be viewed as a unique case, and the therapist should appreciate that no two patients are alike in terms of rehabilitation and orthotic needs despite similar diagnoses. Even when patients are referred for a one-time visit, therapists must perform at least an abbreviated yet comprehensive version of an examination. Therapists are challenged to gather and integrate all the pertinent information that will allow them to make decisions that are in the best interest of the patient.

During the examination process, the therapist not only establishes a rapport with the patient but also gains some insight into the issues of compliance and motivation. Note the resting posture of the injured part and how freely the patient uses or moves the extremity. Addressing signs of neglect early on to prevent long-term disuse is essential. At the other extreme, the overzealous patient should be cautioned when the diagnosis requires complete rest or limited use. Keep in mind that some patients, owing to diagnostic precautions, may not tolerate a complete examination; thus, portions of the examination (range of motion and strength) may not be appropriate to assess (status post multiple flexor tendon repairs). As healing progresses, these segments of the examination should be addressed.

This section briefly reviews the subjective and objective information that the therapist should obtain from the patient as part of the examination process, highlighting some key points related to orthotic application. For more details, see one of the many available upper extremity rehabilitation texts. The sources listed as suggested reading for this chapter offer more in-depth information.

SUBJECTIVE INFORMATION

Age

The therapist must take into consideration the age of the patient because the approach to orthotic fabrication differs for an infant, child, young adult, middle-aged adult, and older patient. For example, when applying orthoses to infants, it is important to be sure that there are no small parts that can potentially loosen and present a choking hazard. Thin thermoplastic material, 3/32″ or 1/16″, generally provides sufficient strength for their small hands. Consider taking advantage of the available hard-to-remove strapping systems when designing a device for a pediatric patient. Compliance of the older child may be enhanced if he or she is given an orthosis that is colored or decorated to the child's taste (Fig. 6–1A). Chapter 24 gives more specific information on addressing the pediatric patient.

A strong, durable material that is easy to clean is generally the appropriate choice for a young athlete. When addressing geriatric

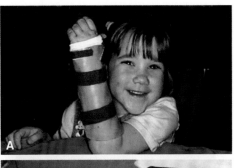

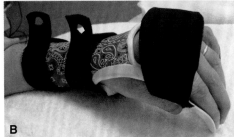

FIGURE 6–1 **A,** Pediatric dorsal wrist and hand immobilization orthosis used after a thumb fracture. **B,** Notice how the soft straps used on this wrist and hand immobilization orthosis have loops dorsally to allow for independent donning and doffing of the device in this elderly patient.

patients who have fragile, sensitive skin, consider using lightweight, perforated materials. Strapping systems for the older population should be constructed to allow for easy, independent donning and doffing. Soft straps that are gentle on the skin and superficial bony prominences may aid in wear compliance (Fig. 6–1B).

Hand Dominance

Hand dominance becomes especially important when considering the functional needs of a patient. Patients may require instruction and specific training on how to modify activities of daily living (ADLs) to compensate for orthosis constraints. Adaptations to the orthosis can be incorporated during fabrication—for example, to provide built-up handles on tools or utensils to be used in combination with the orthosis—to maintain function of the dominant hand (Fig. 6–2).

Past Medical History

Consideration should be given to past medical history, including unrelated medical conditions and how they can influence the present upper extremity diagnosis. Note previous surgeries and any known allergies. Inquire about any previous injuries or surgeries in the affected area. A listing of current conditions and medications

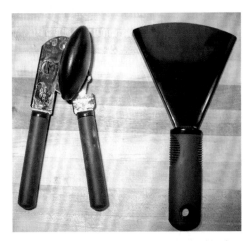

FIGURE 6–2 Large-handled kitchen gadgets can make cooking less stressful for hand joints.

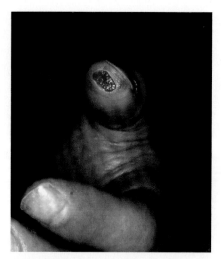

FIGURE 6–3 This diabetic patient unknowingly burned his thumb in the oven and did not realize it because of lack of sensation.

should be obtained for the medical record. For example, a patient with diabetes may suffer from decreased circulation, which can lead to prolonged healing times and sensory changes (Fig. 6–3). This condition mandates frequent and vigilant inspection of the skin under the thermoplastic material and straps to check for skin changes. Chapter 3 provides further information on how specific diseases can affect the healing process. Last, understand that medical problems can mimic or contribute to upper extremity conditions; be sure to conduct a thorough screening starting with reviewing medical history (Goodman, 2010).

History of Present Condition

Questioning the patient regarding the history of the present condition should include factors such as the onset of symptoms, mechanism of injury, previous therapeutic intervention, surgical history, and postoperative management. This information can guide the therapist in making decisions about how to treat the patient most effectively. During the interview process, the therapist should begin to think about the rehabilitation options. However, the therapist must realize that an orthosis is only one part of the treatment regime and is best complemented by other modalities, such as exercise and patient education. For example, a patient with conservatively managed carpal tunnel syndrome may benefit from an orthosis to position the wrist in neutral while sleeping. But if that patient does not make complementary lifestyle changes, such as creating an ergonomic workstation, the symptoms of the syndrome will likely remain problematic. A thorough screening for proximal issues is essential because symptoms originating in the neck and shoulder region can overlap and interact with more distal diagnoses (Yung & Asavasopon, 2010).

SOCIAL AND VOCATIONAL HISTORY

The home environment can affect a patient's ability to comply with a rehabilitation regime. Obtaining information regarding the level of assistance a patient has at home (from family members or other caregivers) becomes pertinent when there is a question about the patient's ability to don and doff the orthosis independently and to follow through with a home program or activity limitations. For example, a patient who is supposed to wear an orthosis full time while acting as the sole caretaker of three children may have difficulty functioning within the constraints of the device. Therapists need to consider the patient as a whole person, not just a diagnosis. Find out if the patient is a smoker because this can impact healing of bone and soft tissue. Document alcohol use as well; this relates to overall general health.

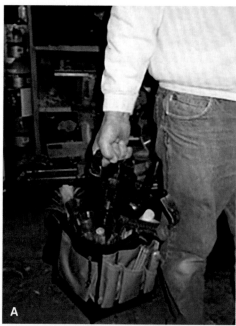

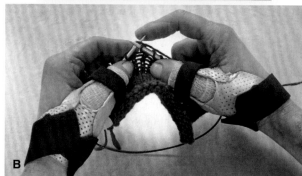

FIGURE 6–4 **A,** Discussing job tasks in detail is imperative to safely return a patient to work. **B,** Bilateral functional hand use with MP joint immobilization orthoses for osteoarthritis.

Interviewing the patient regarding his or her work environment, including work tasks, is also important, especially if the patient must wear the orthosis during work hours (Fig. 6–4A). Functional demands help dictate the material and design of the orthosis. Regarding orthotic selection, for example, thicker materials (1/8″) may be the most appropriate choice for individuals who work at labor-intensive jobs. Adaptations may be needed to allow maximal function. The same is true when considering a patient's avocational interests (Fig. 6–4B). For example, if the patient participates in athletic competition, the orthosis must abide by sports-specific regulations to be acceptable during play. Exterior padding may be required to prevent injury to others.

OBJECTIVE INFORMATION

Functional Level

Discussing the patient's current functional level is important to ascertain how the injury or surgery has affected his or her life. In addition to the detailed history, standardized testing of dexterity and coordination can help the therapist assess functional performance (Apfel, 1990; Jebson, Taylor, Trieschmann, Trotter, & Howard, 1969; McPhee, 1987; Smith, 1973; Tiffin & Asher, 1948; Totten & Flinn-Wagner, 1992). Completion of a simple questionnaire that asks the patient to grade his or her functional ability to complete specific tasks (e.g., no assistance through minimal, moderate, or maximal assistance or unable to complete) is another way to gather information. These data help the therapist establish functional goals and provide a means to mark progress. The **Disabilities of the Arm, Shoulder, and Hand (DASH)** and the **Upper Limb Functional Index (ULFI)** are two commonly used questionnaires to assess functional status (Baltzer, Novak, & McCabe, 2014; Cox, Spaulding, & Kramer, 2006; Gabel, Michener, Burkett, & Neller, 2006; Gabel, Yelland, Melloh, & Burkett, 2009; Lehman, Sindhu, Shechtman, Romero, & Velozo, 2010).

Dexterity refers to the skill or ability to use one's hands for completion of tasks related to ADLs. There are numerous tests available to quantify the level of dexterity, including the Jebsen Taylor Hand Function Test; Purdue Pegboard Test; Nine Hole Peg Test; and Minnesota Rate of Manipulation Tests, Crawford Small Parts Dexterity Test, and O'Connor Pegboard Test to name a few (Desrosiers, Hébert, Bravo, & Dutil, 1995; Fess, 2011; Mathiowetz, Weber, Kashman, & Volland, 1985). These tests of dexterity and coordination can be chosen depending on the individual patient and his or her ability level.

Involve the patient in setting up functional goals. Integrating personal goals into the treatment plan is a great way to maximize compliance. For example, a patient may be discouraged with his or her inability to play the piano after a trigger finger release. Acknowledging this frustration and establishing goals that include the return to playing the piano may make the patient more apt to follow the prescribed treatment regime.

Patients must have a clear understanding of their limitations while wearing an orthosis. For example, a patient who underwent an extensor tendon repair requires full-time immobilization and is thus unable to use that hand during the early stages of healing. This patient may require assistance with tasks such as bathing, dressing, and food preparation. The therapist must fully discuss with the patient the precautions and risks associated with the diagnosis, surgical procedure, and therapy program (including use of orthosis) to maximize compliance and reduce chance of rupture or attenuation of the surgical repair.

Therapists can offer patients helpful hints on how to improve independence and function for ADLs. Simple modifications such as using kitchen utensils with built-up handles can ease the stress and pain of arthritic joints. These modifications can be used simultaneously with an orthosis, or a device can be fabricated for use with a specific functional task. For example, cylindrical foam, elastomer, or thermoplastic material can be used to modify writing utensils.

Pain

The therapist should ask the patient to describe pain in terms of quality, degree, and location (Chapman, Schimek, Colpitts, Gerlach, & Dong, 1985; Echternach, 1993; Melzack, 1975; Schultz-Johnson, 1988a). Changes in degree can be determined by using a scale: **Visual Analog Scale (VAS)** or **Numerical Rating Scale (NRS)**, usually 0 (*no pain*) to 10 (*pain as bad as it can be*) (Sindu, Shechtman, & Tuckey, 2011; Walton, 2015). Mapping out the pain on an illustration of the upper extremity may help define the location. Avoid placing patients with moderate to severe pain in mobilization orthoses. Aggressive mobilization may aggravate pain and increase edema. If mobilization orthoses are ordered for such a patient, contact the physician to discuss any concerns. Oftentimes, waiting a few days can make a big difference in terms of reduction of inflammation and increased tolerance to mobilization. Pain may also influence the choice of materials used; highly drapable materials may be easier to apply because they conform without much hands-on manipulation. Orthoses can be fabricated to accommodate the electrode pads often used to modify pain (transcutaneous electrical nerve stimulation [TENS] or high volt).

Visual Inspection and Palpation

Inspect the affected area and take a note of any masses, swelling, deformities, atrophy, scars, or wounds (Rayan & Ackelman, 2011) (Fig. 6–5A–D). Following visual inspection, begin to gently palpate the region; commence this portion of the examination in an area

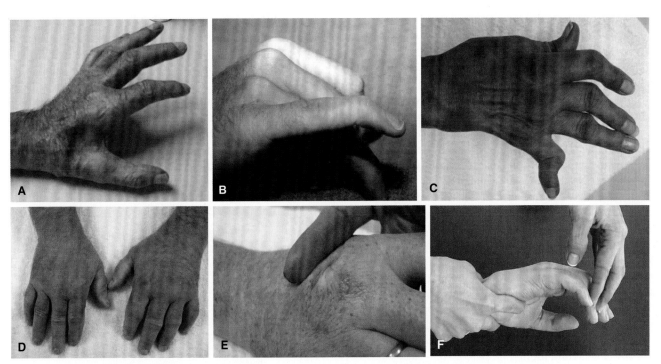

FIGURE 6–5 A, The patient presents with atrophy of first dorsal interossei following prolonged ulnar nerve compression at the elbow. **B,** Lack of terminal tendon function indicated by flexed posture at the distal interphalangeal (DIP) joint. **C,** Significant digit joint deformities—if able, take photo for patient record. **D,** Notice redness at index finger metacarpophalangeal (MCP) joint, generalized edema, flexed posture of PIP joints, and increased hair growth. **E,** Palpation of scar reveals adherence to the underlying tissue. **F,** Gentle passive range of motion (ROM) used to determine soft-tissue extensibility.

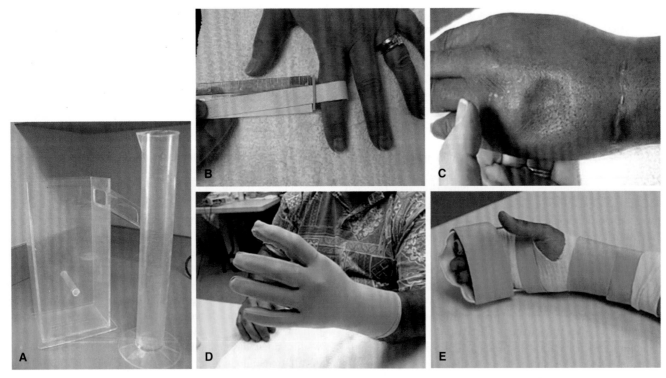

FIGURE 6–6 **A,** A volumeter quantifies edema. Measure the contralateral limb for comparison. **B,** Circumferential measurement of individual digits. **C,** Pitting dorsal hand edema following extensor tendon repair. Edema management may include the use of a compression glove **(D)** and a circumferential elasticized wrap at digit level with elasticized tubular bandage more proximally **(E)**.

away from the focal point (Fig. 6–5E,F). In some clinical situations, physically palpating the area may not be indicated. If applicable, view both extremities simultaneously to compare the two sides. This is an opportune time to gain rapport with the patient, being gentle and confident with this hands-on interaction. In addition, note the posture of the hand and the patient's willingness to move.

Edema

Quantify edema whenever possible by measuring volume or circumference. Use a **volumeter** to measure the volume of the limb or a measuring tape to quantify circumference (Fig. 6–6A,B) (Brand & Wood, 1977; Lavelle, 2015; Schultz-Johnson, 1988b; Villeco, 2011). The therapist must fully describe the quality (e.g., pitting, brawny) and location. In the early stages of healing of an acutely injured or postoperative extremity, edema is frequently an issue that requires therapy intervention (Fig. 6–6C). Edema may be reduced by an orthosis that correctly positions the extremity; compression garments (gloves, elasticized wraps, and sleeves); and education regarding elevation, ice, and exercise (if appropriate) (Fig. 6–6D,E) (Villeco, 2012).

Edema may increase after the use of orthoses, especially with mobilization tissue. Consistent, repeated evaluation provides the therapist with information about how the tissue is tolerating the therapy and orthotic intervention. If the extremity becomes edematous and reactive, the approach should be modified. For example, if edema is aggravated by a mobilization orthosis, consider resting and immobilizing the area for a few days. Once the edema has decreased, cautiously reintroduce the mobilization orthosis, monitoring for any edema response.

Fluctuations in edema should influence the strapping choice. Window-type edema, which occurs between two straps, may be avoided by wrapping the limb circumferentially or by applying a compressive sleeve under the orthosis. Circumferential wraps (e.g., Coban™ or Ace™ wraps), applied distal to proximal, impart an even pressure to an edematous limb. Circumferential orthoses should be used cautiously with patients who have an edematous extremity; if applied too tightly, problematic pooling of edema distal to the orthosis can occur. In select cases, these orthoses may help reduce edema; Chapter 10 provides more information.

Sensibility

Assessing **sensibility** is essential when conducting an upper extremity examination (Bell-Krotoski, 2011; Bell-Krotoski, Weinstein, & Weinstein, 1993; Callahan, 1995; Dellon, 1981; Jerosch-Herald, 2015; Moberg, 1958; Novak, Mackinnon, Williams, & Kelly, 1992; Tan, 1992). Monofilament examination and two-point discrimination testing are the most common methods for evaluating sensation (Fig. 6–7). A monofilament examination, considered a threshold test, is administered by applying graded forces of filaments to the testing area (Bell-Krotoski & Tomancik, 1987). Two-point discrimination, considered an innervation density test, involves the ability to distinguish between two stimuli applied to the skin at

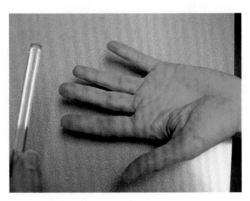

FIGURE 6–7 A monofilament set.

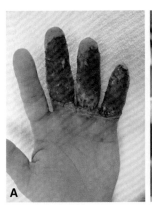
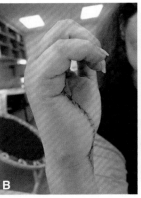
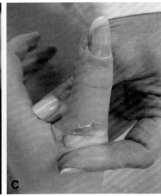

FIGURE 6–8 **A,** Inflammatory stage: burn wound. **B,** Proliferative stage: healing incision after tenolysis. **C,** Scar maturation stage: notice adherent scar.

specific locations (Dellon, 1978; Dellon, Mackinnon, & Crosby, 1987; Mackinnon & Dellon, 1985). Quick screening for light touch may be adequate if the patient has no complaints or signs of nerve involvement.

The therapist must consider impaired sensation in order to provide the patient with a properly fitting orthosis and to prevent tissue irritation. Every effort should be made to increase the surface area of application to disperse the pressures on sensory-impaired regions. When applying an orthosis to a limb with impaired sensation, the therapist must review the precautions with the patient. Any complaints of numbness or paresthesias should be dealt with immediately. Because they lack complete sensory feedback, such patients must learn to perform frequent visual examinations of the affected extremity, looking for any signs of excess pressure.

Soft Tissue and Wound Status

Therapists should assess the soft tissue and wound status. Document any wounds or surgical incisions and quantify with measurements and descriptions (Evans, 1991; McCulloch & Kloth, 1990; Von Der Heyde & Evans, 2011) (Fig. 6–8A–C). Digital photos offer a valuable way to document changes in a wound status. Maceration, rashes, and skin breakdown can result when the skin is subjected to prolonged orthosis wear or excessive moisture. Perforated materials are a good choice for application over wounds because they allow air exchange between the thermoplastic and skin.

Therapists frequently need to be creative when applying orthoses over wound dressings and/or surgical hardware, such as pins or external fixators. To mold material directly over exposed pins, prepad the area and then apply the warm thermoplastic material. Consider using solid, highly drapable material for this type of orthosis. For sensitive scars, gel-lined materials are available. Scars can also be prepadded with gel or a scar management product such as elastomer or Otoform™.

Vascularity

Color and temperature differences between the involved and uninvolved side should also be noted to address the vascular status of the limb. Altered sympathetic response may present with color and temperature changes of the skin. Assessment becomes of extreme importance when vascular structures have been injured or surgically repaired (Ashbell, Kutz, & Kleinert, 1967; Levinsohn, Gordon, & Sessler, 1991) (Fig. 6–9A). Orthoses, straps, or slings that are applied too tightly may impede circulation, manifested by a change

in color and/or temperature (Fig. 6–9B). Wide straps and slings may dissipate pressure on the affected part by increasing the area of force application (Brand & Hollister, 1999; Fess, Gettle, Philips, & Janson, 2005). Chapter 4 provides a more detailed discussion of these concepts.

Circumferential designs are not the best choice for patients who have undergone vascular repair or who have possible vascular compromise. Such orthoses may not provide enough room for fluctuations in edema. When edema increases, the pressure within the device may also increase, leading to impaired circulation.

Range of Motion

Goniometers are used to measure active and passive range of motion (ROM) (Fig. 6–10A,B) (Boone et al., 1978; Cambridge-Keeling, 1995; Dadio & Nolan, 2018; Gibson, 2015; Hamilton & Lachenbruch, 1969). Active ROM provides information about a patient's willingness or ability to move. Gaining insight regarding the soft-tissue and joint status of the musculotendinous unit is important (e.g., tendon adherence, tendon continuity, and nerve innervation). Joint stiffness and musculotendinous tightness can be assessed with passive ROM measurements.

Ongoing evaluation of ROM becomes imperative when introducing an orthosis to mobilize tissue. ROM is a way of measuring gains and provides feedback for the orthotic intervention effort. If no improvements are evident, the regime must be changed accordingly. For example, if no gains are made from use of a dynamic PIP extension orthosis, the therapist should consider changing to a serial static treatment approach or perhaps using both day and night orthoses. ROM measurements can also

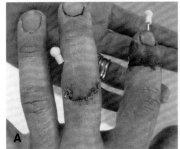
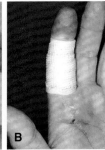

FIGURE 6–9 **A,** Distal interphalangeal (DIP) joint open dislocation with pinning and surgical repair of vascular structures along with terminal tendon. Note dusky appearance distal to injury. **B,** When a circumferential orthosis is applied to a body part, the patient must monitor for any throbbing or color/temperature changes.

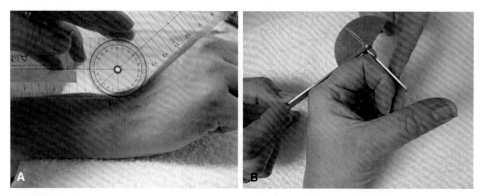

FIGURE 6–10 A, Medium-sized goniometer for measuring the wrist and elbow. **B,** A small finger goniometer is a convenient way to measure the small joints of the hand.

indicate that joints are getting tighter, as is sometimes seen at the MCP joints when a wrist cast extends too far distally, impeding full MCP motion.

Strength

Grip dynamometers, pinch gauges, and manual muscle testing (MMT) provide ways to assess muscle function and nerve innervation (Fig. 6–11A–C) (Bechtol, 1954; Fournier & Bourbonnais, 2015; Hislop & Montgomery, 2007; Kendall, McCreary, & Provance, 2005; Mathiowetz, Volland, Kashman, & Weber, 1985; Mathiowetz, Weber, Volland, & Kashman, 1984; Schectman & Sindhu, 2015; Schmidt & Toews, 1970). Three types of pinch may be tested: lateral or key pinch, three point (three-jaw chuck), and thumb tip to index finger tip (tip pinch) (Fig. 6–12A–F) (Casanova & Grunert, 1989). Quantifying changes in strength is helpful when justifying the need for continued therapy. Repetitive grip testing has been used by therapists to attempt to quantify sincerity of effort (Shechtman, Guiterrez, & Kokendofer, 2005; Sindhu, Shechtman, & Veazie, 2012).

Strength testing may be contraindicated in many cases, depending on the diagnosis and healing timeframe. For example, elbow flexion strength testing should be deferred in the early stages of healing after a biceps tendon repair owing to the high risk of rupture immediately after surgery. Strength can be safely assessed once the physician has approved the initiation of progressive resistive exercise.

MMT provides the means for monitoring recovery from a nerve injury (Dadio & Nolan, 2018; Kendall et al., 2005). As the nerve reinnervates muscles, patients present with higher muscle grades (0 to 5). This change in status alters the therapy and orthotic

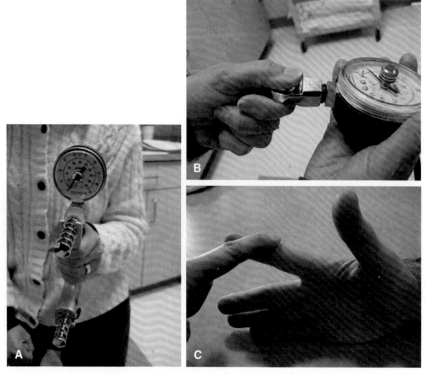

FIGURE 6–11 Grip **(A)** and pinch **(B)** dynamometers. **C,** Manual muscle testing (MMT) testing of first dorsal interossei muscle.

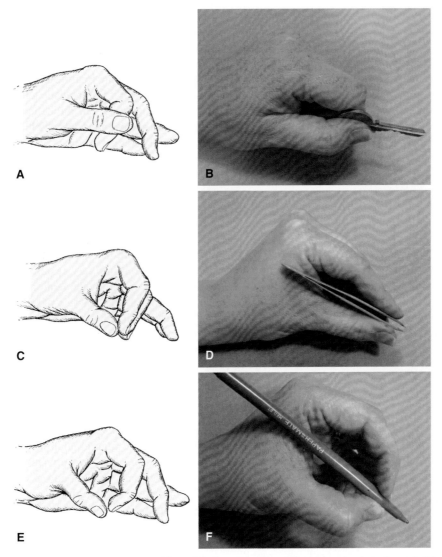

FIGURE 6–12 Three types of pinches: lateral **(A and E)**, three point **(B and C)**, and thumb to index finger tip **(C and D)**.

intervention plans. For example, the orthosis must be modified for a patient with radial nerve palsy once the wrist extensors become innervated. Because the orthosis no longer needs to incorporate the wrist, the therapist should choose a hand-based MCP extension mobilization orthosis to allow the newly innervated wrist extensors to function while regaining strength.

Exercise orthoses can be fabricated to provide resistance to movement through the use of graded rubber bands, wrapped elastic cord, elastic thread, graded springs, and TheraBand® or TheraTubing® products. The patient can use the orthosis for frequent daily exercise sessions to improve strength in the targeted muscle group(s). When treating patients with adherent tendon repairs, adding resistance may aid in improving tendon glide through scar tissue.

Special Testing

Special testing depends on the specific diagnosis (Rayan & Ackelman, 2011) (Fig. 6–13A–C). Not all testing needs to be

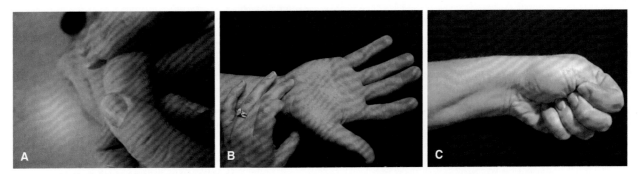

FIGURE 6–13 **A,** Proximal interphalangeal (PIP) joint mobility testing, **B,** Phalen test for carpal tunnel syndrome is positive when the tapping over the median nerve causes distal tingling in the median nerve distribution, and **C,** Finklestein testing for deQuervain tenosynovitis.

completed on each and every patient. The previous parts of the examination, as well as the diagnosis they were referred with, will help guide the therapist regarding which special tests should be completed. For example, with a patient referred with a diagnosis of carpal tunnel syndrome, the examination should include the Phalen test (wrist flexed position for 60 seconds), Tinel test (tapping over volar wrist to elicit distal symptoms), and Durkan compression test (direct pressure over the volar wrist) (Rayan & Ackelman, 2011). To be thorough, the proximal regions, shoulder and neck, should be screened as well to check for any contributory factors.

PROBLEM-SOLVING AND GOAL SETTING

From the findings of the examination and the information gathered from the patient interview, the therapist is able to establish treatment goals. Therapists must appreciate that orthotic intervention is only one way problems can be addressed. The therapist must first define a list of problems. Table 6–1 outlines the problems and corresponding goals for a patient at 1 week post surgery for carpal tunnel release.

Note that for each problem, there is a short- and long-term goal. Although this is a relatively simple example, this method of creating an appropriate treatment plan is applicable to all patients. The critical thinking process allows the therapist to organize the findings of the examination and begin to plan the therapy intervention. The therapist must then prioritize the problems. It can be overwhelming to treat a patient with multiple injuries; setting priorities is mandatory (although sometimes difficult to do). All treatment problems and interventions are interrelated. For example, when edema has been successfully addressed, ROM is usually also improved.

After the problems are defined, the therapist should establish short- and long-term goals. For example, when applying a mobilization orthosis, the therapist should set reasonable short-term ROM goals that can be reached in 1 week; this encourages the patient to follow the wearing schedule and therapy program. Each time the patient reaches a goal, a new goal should be established. As mentioned previously, the patient's own goals should be integrated within the therapy goals (when appropriate).

Therapy intervention is a dynamic process, limited only by the lack of imagination on the part of the therapist. The therapist needs to take the time to interpret the evaluative findings and appreciate that as the patient progresses, the problems and priorities also change, as should the treatment goals. Ideally, all problems should be addressed. But it is unrealistic to think that one treatment modality is going to satisfy all the deficits. A comprehensive treatment plan should be instituted, of which orthotic usage may or may not be a part. Therapists must use critical reasoning skills, based on knowledge and experience, to devise the best treatment regime, taking into account the patient's individual needs. Each time a patient returns to the clinic, he or she should be reevaluated to determine if changes in therapy management must be made. Integrating clinical experience and **evidence-based practice** is crucial when forming a comprehensive treatment plan. Decisions regarding intervention techniques should be based on the best systematic research whenever possible to justify services. Box 6–1 offers an overview of EBP as it relates to orthotic intervention.

In relation to the practice of occupational therapy, **frames of reference** provide the link between theory and practice. Orthotic intervention within the specialty of hand therapy would include the biomechanical and rehabilitative frames (Radomski & Trombley, 2013). These theoretical frames help guide practice in the field of hand therapy and subsequent orthotic intervention, providing therapists with reasons for their treatment based on theory. The profession of occupational therapy applies these approaches of intervention with the goal of returning the patient to their maximal functional ability. The biomechanical approach involves the principles of physics as it relates to human movement, forces, and posture, addressing deficits in ROM, strength, and endurance. The **rehabilitative approach** focuses on getting the patient back to being as independent as possible involving environmental changes and physical adaptations. Box 6–2 provides a more detailed description of this theoretical approach to treatment.

A skilled therapist would never approach two patients in the same way. Therapists need to be responsive to the specific and changing needs of their patients, altering the therapy treatment in response to changes in tissue status. For example, when considering the stage of healing of a particular tissue, therapists must apply the most appropriate orthosis for that stage. An orthosis that is appropriate

TABLE 6–1	**Approach to Goal Setting**		
Therapy Problems	**Short-term Goals (2–3 wk)**	**Long-term Goals (1–2 mo)**
Healing incision	Healed incision.	Soft, mobile scar.
Moderate edema in hand	Minimal edema in order to be able to hold a water bottle to drink.	No edema in hand or wrist to allow unimpeded use of hand while washing and blow drying hair.
Pain level: 2[a]	Pain level: 1	Pain level: 0
Decreased range of motion (ROM) of wrist and digits	Increase ROM of digits to normal and of wrist to 75% in order to use a pen to pay bill and be financially independent.	Normal ROM to return to work as a computer programmer.
Decreased grip and pinch strength	Increase grip to 5 lb and pinch to 2 lb for the ability to cut meat and feed self.	Strength 75% of normal for lifting groceries out of car and transporting to home in order to feed family.
Impaired ability to complete activities of daily living (ADLs)[b]	Independent with minimal modifications for self-care activities and driving a car in order to return to work safely.	Full functional independence for all household tasks inclusive of cleaning and heavier cooking in order to care for self and family without risk of reinjury.

[a]On a scale of 0–10.
[b]Includes self-care, driving, cooking, and cleaning.

BOX 6-1   EVIDENCE-BASED PRACTICE AND ORTHOTIC INTERVENTION

Contribution by Gary P. Austin, PT, PhD, OCS, FAFS, FAAOMPT
Professor and Chair, School of Physical Therapy
Belmont University, Nashville, TN

Evidence-based practice (EBP) has become an important concept in the healthcare industry and currently is the dominant clinical decision-making paradigm. Unfortunately, this term has been subject to overuse, misuse, and misunderstanding. It is important that healthcare providers and consumers understand both what EBP is and is not. Research has shown that "intuition, unsystematic clinical experience, and pathophysiologic rationale are insufficient grounds for clinical decision-making" (Guyatt & Rennie, 2002). EBP is classically defined as "the conscientious, explicit, and judicious use of current best evidence in making decisions about the care of the individual patient. It means integrating individual clinical expertise with the best available external clinical evidence from systematic research" (Sackett, Rosenberg, Gray, Haynes, & Richardson, 1996). Contrary to popular belief, EBP is neither prescriptive, restrictive, inefficient, nor idealistic but rather guided by clinical practice and expertise; individualized/patient-specific; lifelong/career-long; self-directed; problem-based; cost-effective; and time-efficient.

The three pillars of EBP are (1) individual patient values, preferences, and expectations; (2) individual clinical expertise; and (3) clinical evidence. Evidence-based clinical decision-making requires the clinician to evaluate the relevance and significance of all information and subsequent decisions within the context of each patient's unique values, preferences, and expectations. Collaborative decision-making has been demonstrated to positively impact the patient and clinician (Elwyn et al., 2004; Towie, Godolphin, Grams, & Lamarre, 2006), adherence (Wilson et al., 2010), and outcomes (Godolphin, 2009; Mulley, Trimble, & Elwyn, 2012; Stiggelbout et al., 2012). Clinical expertise can be defined as the acquisition of clinical proficiency and judgment through experience and practice and is demonstrated, in part, "by effective and efficient diagnosis and in the more thoughtful identification and compassionate use of individual patients' predicaments, rights, and preferences in making clinical decisions about their care" (Sackett et al., 1996). Clinical experts are able to determine if the available evidence is relevant, and if so, how to best incorporate this information into the decision-making based on the individual patient values and preferences. Clinical

evidence is simply relevant and useful information that enlightens and enhances the clinician's understanding of the individual patient scenario. Evidence comes from various sources, in multiple forms, and variable strength. Clinicians must strive to be aware of and incorporate information based on the well-designed, high-quality studies (e.g., randomized controlled trials). We must take caution not to dismiss weaker forms of evidence because they often provide the best available evidence. When clinicians rely on weak evidence, they acknowledge the risk of administering useless or even harmful interventions. Furthermore, clinicians must be aware of higher quality studies that provide stronger evidence as it is available and subsequently replace the weaker evidence with the higher quality information. Clinical evidence, in all its forms, can serve to both invalidate previously accepted diagnostic tests and interventions and inform the innovation and adoption of new and more powerful, more accurate, more efficacious, and safer techniques (Sackett et al., 1996). Although clinical evidence informs and is informed by clinical practice and expertise, it is not a substitute for individual clinical expertise. Ultimately, clinical practice guidelines are the best source of evidence for clinicians. Although there are numerous clinical practice guidelines available for hand therapists, few are evidence based and much work is needed to summarize and integrate the best available information related to hand therapy and upper extremity orthoses (MacDermid, 2004; Szabo & MacDermid, 2009).

The patient-centered clinical expert effectively integrates the best available clinical information with the unique patient values, such that each patient receives not similar care but uniquely individual care reflective of the vast variability among individual values and presentations. Evidence is necessary, but wholly insufficient, for the efficient and effective management of the individual patient.

The authors have integrated their clinical expertise and the best available and most contemporary evidence into this text. Readers are strongly encouraged to remain abreast of the most current and best available evidence to both inform their developing clinical expertise and to supplement the work of the authors of this text.

for a patient for 1 week may not be the best choice a month or even a week later. In general, immobilization orthoses are appropriate for resting an acutely injured body part; this is followed by a more aggressive approach, such as mobilization orthoses, during the later stages of healing. Refer to Chapter 3 for a more detailed discussion. Taking a client-centered **bio-occupational approach** to orthotic fabrication, described by McKee and Rivard (2011b), involves the appreciation of the patient's unique needs as well as the specific biologic requirements of the involved tissues. This approach results in a functionally relevant orthosis allowing for occupational performance that maximizes the patient's functional use yet provides the affected tissues with the appropriate environment for healing. Box 6–3 provides a clinical example highlighting the main concepts of this unique approach to orthotic fabrication.

PATIENT EDUCATION AND PRECAUTIONS

Educating the patient is essential for deriving the greatest benefit from the use of an orthosis. A sample patient education handout is given in Box 6–4. An opportune time to educate the patient is during a trial wearing of the orthosis (20 to 30 minutes) in the clinic to check for any immediate problems. Patients must understand the purpose of the orthosis, which relates to understanding the diagnosis and treatment approach. The patient and caregiver should be made aware of how to don and doff the orthosis, what to expect and what to look out for while wearing the device, and when and how long to wear it. Taking photos of the orthosis properly in place with cell phones can be very helpful for the patient to have something to refer to later at home.

BOX 6-2   ORTHOTIC INTERVENTION AND OCCUPATIONAL THERAPY: A THEORETICAL FRAMEWORK

Contribution by Gail Dadio, OTD, MHSc, OTR/L, CHT, CLT
Hand Therapist
Connecticut Orthopedics, Milford, CT
Part time Faculty, School of Health Sciences
Quinnipiac University, Hamden, CT

When considering orthotic intervention in the rehabilitative approach, the client's occupational needs should be considered. Occupations are the actions that people take to occupy their time that are meaningful and have purpose for the individuals. Occupations encompass "the active process of living: from the beginning to the end of life, our occupations are all the active processes of looking after ourselves and others, enjoying life, and being socially and economically productive over the lifes pan" (Boyt Schell, Gillen, Scaffa, & Cohn, 2013, p. 3). In occupational therapy practice, there are eight areas that define occupations, including the following:

- ADLs
- Instrumental ADLs
- Education
- Work
- Play
- Leisure
- Social participation
- Sleep

Understanding what the clients do with their time, what occupations they engage in, as well as their impact on society can aid the therapist in formulating an intervention plan that can incorporate a useful/functional orthosis with the clients. In addition, when treating a client with hand injury, the rehabilitative approach can also be combined with the occupational performance approach. The occupational performance, or the **Person, Environment, Occupation (PEO) Model**, is a theoretical frame of reference that can assist the therapist in understanding the clients' functional level, their occupation, and the environment in which they engage in at a certain time in their life span (Strong et al., 1999). The overlap of these three subsets in this model is critical in relation to the fabrication of an orthosis. The PEO model supports the hand therapist in determining how the orthosis may change the clients' functional abilities, affect their occupations, and, ultimately, the overall impact the orthosis may have on their occupational performance in their environment. This systematic approach in analyzing these factors aids the therapist in assessing the therapeutic value of the orthosis as well as assisting in the determination of the specifics of the orthosis. For example, a laborer with an occupation of work returning to his job with a healing wrist fracture can benefit from a custom-fabricated wrist orthosis used for support and protection while working, as compared to the elderly woman with a mild case of osteoarthritis who is engaging in her occupation of leisure, who can benefit from a prefabricated thumb orthosis for support while performing her knitting activities.

The application of the combined rehabilitative and PEO approaches to occupational therapy practice, including the fitting of an orthosis, enables the interrelationship between the therapist and the client in determining a successful outcome to which one can engage in a meaningful occupation in a chosen environment (Strong et al., 1999). This collaborative or client-centered approach

involves the experience and knowledge of the client to facilitate set therapeutic goals with the treating therapist as it relates to the fitting and training of the orthosis (Boyt Schell et al., 2013). "Effective therapy is only as good as the quality of the relationship between the therapist and the consumer" (Boyt Schell et al., 2013, p. 133).

When assessing a client for an orthosis, not only should identification of the client's areas of occupation be determined but also his or her performance skills. This may include assessment of the client's sensory, motor, cognitive, and communication skills, all of which are imperative for compliance with an orthosis. In addition, evaluation of the demands of an activity as it relates to a specific orthosis should be determined to allow full functional mobility of the hand/upper extremity while the client is performing the desired task. Client factors such as his or her values and spiritual beliefs should be respected when assessing for an appropriate orthosis. Because therapists provide holistic interventions, identifying underlying factors that may influence a client's motivation to engage in occupations with an orthosis should be considered (American Occupational Therapy Association [AOTA], 2008).

The "Occupational Therapy Practice Framework: Domain and Process" identifies performance patterns that may affect a client's rehabilitation (AOTA, 2008). Performance patterns such as habits, routines, roles, and rituals may influence the use of an orthosis. For example, the role of a mother with child-rearing can be disrupted or altered with an injury or disability; therefore, assessment of a role change as it relates to the fitting and training of an orthosis should be considered when determining the appropriate orthosis by the hand therapist (Boyt Schell et al., 2013).

Contextual influences are also part of the "Occupational Therapy Practice Framework." Contexts are interrelated conditions that surround the client that may affect the client's performance (AOTA, 2008). Some of these influences include cultural, personal, temporal, physical, virtual, and social. To elaborate on cultural influence, for example, the inability to shake hands during an introduction when wearing an orthosis may alter a client culturally. An example of a personal influence can be a client's inability to return to work while wearing an orthosis. This can affect one's socioeconomic status, thus changing the compliance of the orthosis wearing schedule. The virtual context is another example of an influence that can be affected by the application of an orthosis. In today's environment with a large emphasis on social media such as texting, the inability to communicate because of an orthosis on a client's hand can influence a person contextually.

The fabrication of an orthosis includes evaluation, intervention, and outcomes. Identification of the clients' occupational profile including their diagnosis, concerns, and performance of their occupations should be addressed (AOTA, 2008). An intervention plan regarding the wearing regimen, precautions, and care should be agreed upon prior to implementation of the orthosis. The successful use of an orthosis can support the client's overall health and participation in all of life tasks (AOTA, 2008).

BOX 6–3 BIO-OCCUPATIONAL ORTHOTIC APPROACH

Contribution by Pat McKee, M.Sc., OT Reg. (Ont.), OT(C)
Associate Professor Emeritus, Department of Occupational Science and Occupational Therapy
University of Toronto, Toronto, Canada

Susie, a 29-year-old graduate university student, "always had hand joint problems." She had right (dominant) carpometacarpal (CMC) joint pain that radiated into the first web space, thenar eminence, and second metacarpal and had difficulty with tasks such keyboarding, driving, jar opening, grasping a subway pole, and pen writing.

She was fitted with a custom-molded neoprene-lined thermoplastic, thumb CMC, MP-stabilizing orthosis with IP extension block. It was secured with a stretchy hook-receptive neoprene strap that permitted some CMC and MP mobility while ensuring sufficient stabilization to relieve pain (Fig. 6B–1A–C). Upon donning the orthosis, she immediately noticed she could pick up and grip her laptop computer, with the affected hand only, without pain.

Initially, Susie's gross grasp was 32 and 28 kg with and without the orthosis, respectively, whereas her unaffected hand was 38 kg. After 4 months, gross grasp had increased to 37 kg without the orthosis. Lateral pinch strength was initially 7.5 kg with and without the orthosis and rose to 8.5 kg without the orthosis after 4 months. Susie's worst pain rating decreased from 5/10 to 1/10 and pain frequency reduced from 6.5/10 to 0.25/10 4 months after initiation of orthotic intervention.

Susie wore the orthosis often for about a month, then gradually decreased its use and eventually only wore it for weight-bearing activities such as push-ups. By 4 months, she did not need the orthosis at all, even for weight-bearing through her hand, because of increased hand strength and reduced pain. In addition, she reported little or no difficulty with any tasks. What was most notable was the impact on her mood, sense of control over her life, and ability to engage in physical activities.

In her own words, at 4 months after orthotic fitting, "Orthoses can immediately give a person back much of their function. I didn't realize how much of my life I had abandoned because I wanted to avoid the pain. Much of the activities were leisure based like badminton, basketball, yoga, and Pilates. Since getting the orthosis, I have now lost 35 lb and counting. Having the range of activities to choose from again has been so motivating and provided more chances for successful life changes."

Susie's favorable outcomes were achieved using the client-centered *bio-occupational orthotic approach* (Mckee & Rivard, 2011b), which addresses (1) the person's biologic (anatomical and physiologic) needs and (2) factors that enable participation in activities that are important and meaningful to the person. This approach begins with understanding that an orthosis is "a prefabricated or custom-made device applied to biological structures to optimize *body function and structures*—considering nutrition, length, strength, mobility, and stability—to ultimately promote current or future *activities and participation* in roles important to the individual" (McKee & Rivard, 2011b, p. 1569).

"Body functions and structures" and "activities and participation" are key concepts influencing health, as described in the *International Classification of Functioning, Disability and Health* (ICF) published by the World Health Organization (2002). Sixteen guiding principles, described in the following text, make explicit the professional reasoning of the bio-occupational orthotic approach (Mckee & Rivard, 2011a, 2011b) (see Table 6B–1).

Promote client-centeredness: Susie's therapist worked collaboratively with her using a holistic perspective that considered her unique personal attributes, including age; cognition; affect; physical attributes; and unique context including environment, activity demands, and culture. The therapist engaged Susie the person throughout the assessment, individualized intervention, and monitoring/modification processes.

Consider psychosocial factors: As a child, Susie had been provided with a custom-fitted hand orthosis that she had found too inconvenient and cumbersome to use. Her therapist needed to consider that when Susie came to her hand therapy appointment, negative past experiences could have posed an emotional barrier.

Optimize body function and structures: This goal relates to the ICF's *body function and structures*, acknowledging that orthoses attend to the biologic (physical) causes of impaired function. Susie's orthosis stabilized her thumb CMC and MP joint, thus promoting resorption of lax periarticular structures. In turn, reduced pain, sustained joint stability, and enhanced hand strength and function were achieved.

CHAPTER 6

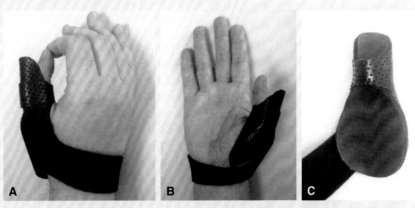

FIGURE 6B–1 Thumb metacarpophalangeal-stabilizing, interphalangeal (IP)-extension-blocking orthosis made from 1/16″ thick thermoplastic bonded to 1/16″ neoprene with a hook-receptive neoprene strap. Note unrestricted thumb IP flexion. A, Dorsal view, (B) volar view, and (C) palmar view of the orthosis showing neoprene lining.

(Continued)

TABLE 6B–1	**Guiding Principles of Bio-Occupational Orthotic Approach**

1. Promote client-centeredness
2. Consider psychosocial factors
3. Optimize body function and structures
4. Enable activity and participation
5. Consider environmental factors
6. Well engineered
7. Monitor and modify
8. Optimize usability
9. Provide choice
10. Optimize comfort
11. Minimize harm
12. Optimize cosmesis
13. Optimize convenience
14. Use a less-is-more approach
15. Provide comprehensive client/caregiver education
16. Evaluate outcomes

From McKee, P., & Rivard, A. (2011a). Biopsychosocial approach to orthotic intervention. Journal of Hand Therapy, 24(2), 155–163 and McKee, P., & Rivard, A. (2011b). Foundations of orthotic intervention. In Skirven T., Osterman L. E., Fedorczyk J., & Amadio P. (Eds.), Rehabilitation of the hand and upper extremity (6th ed., pp. 1565–1580). Philadelphia, PA: Elsevier.

Enable activity and participation: This goal relates to the ICF's *activity and participation*. For Susie, hand pain and reduced grip/pinch strength had caused difficulty with many tasks. With the orthosis, she was immediately able to perform tasks without fear of pain and over time returned to valued leisure and health-enhancing activities.

Consider environmental factors: For Susie, consideration of *environmental factors*, another key construct of the ICF, included her physical and social environments.

Well engineered: Sound design and fabrication features of Susie's orthosis included unrestricted mobility of the wrist joint and thumb interphalangeal (IP) joint flexion, secure bonding of the neoprene to the thermoplastic, and incorporating a stretchy, conforming neoprene strap.

Monitor and modify: Monitoring involves ongoing evaluation and collaboration with the client/caregiver to determine whether the orthosis is meeting biologic and functional/occupational goals. It assists the therapist to identify whether or not the person is wearing the orthosis and, if warranted, to explore reasons for nonuse. Monitoring of Susie's orthotic use revealed that she was experiencing numbness in her ring and small fingers and pain over her pisiform bone. She was advised to fasten the strap more loosely and to reposition the strap to avoid pisiform pressure.

Optimize usability: To enhance the likelihood of orthotic use, ask the question, "Is this orthosis useful to this individual?" A collaborative approach optimized the usability of Susie's orthosis, ensuring that perceived benefits were more compelling than any inconvenience, discomfort, or embarrassment imposed by it. Also, it was easy to don and doff and clean.

Provide choice: Individuals feel included and respected when they are provided with choices. Choices offered to Susie included color of thermoplastic and neoprene and inclusion/exclusion of neoprene lining.

Optimize comfort: Uncomfortable orthoses are unlikely to be used, thus comfort enhances usability. The neoprene lining and stretchy neoprene strap optimized the comfort of Susie's orthosis.

Minimize harm: The orthotic intervention process should ultimately make some positive contribution to the individual's life. If the orthosis fails to achieve its intended outcome, at the very least, it should minimize biologic harm. To be specific, biologic structures must not be compromised by, among other things, pressure points that result in skin breakdown, diminished circulation, or nerve compression. For Susie, monitoring averted biologic harm from excessive compression and inappropriate positioning of the neoprene strap.

Optimize cosmesis: An orthosis becomes a part of the person's personal environment and, like clothing, is seen by others. Furthermore, it is a product of our therapeutic intervention that will be on display, representing our profession and us individually and, as such, should reflect exemplary standards. For Susie "How it looked made a huge difference for me," thus enhancing usability. Efforts to optimize cosmesis should not be viewed as time consuming and unimportant. If not putting in the required time results in the client not wearing the orthosis, then the time used to fabricate it is truly wasted.

Optimize convenience: For Susie, the orthotic solution was optimally convenient—easy to use and clean, secure adherence of hook Velcro®, and secure bonding of neoprene lining.

Use a less-is-more approach: Minimalism in the design of Susie's orthosis included use of thin thermoplastic and neoprene (both 1/16"/1.6 mm thick), a narrow wrist strap, and no unnecessary restriction of joint mobility.

Provide comprehensive client/caregiver education: To optimize usability, the client and/or caregiver should clearly understand the rationale for the orthosis, when to wear it, how to put it on and make adjustments, how to care for it, when and how to contact the therapist, and assurance that client feedback and inquiries are welcome. For Susie, written instructions were provided. She was trained in how to don and doff the orthosis and how to use the strap.

Evaluate outcomes: Evaluation of outcomes (1) fulfills the therapist's basic professional responsibility to assess the orthotic process for the purpose of continuous program improvement and (2) identifies the extent to which biologic and functional goals have been achieved. Susie's therapist evaluated changes in grip and pinch strength, pain, and degree of difficulty with activities.

Orthoses should be comfortable, fabricated from appropriate materials, aesthetically pleasing, and convenient to use. Comfort, cosmesis, and convenience and, thus, usability, are enhanced by applying the guiding principle of less is more. Monitoring and modifying and evaluating outcomes are essential stages in a process that ensures usability of the orthosis while providing evidence of orthotic efficacy and the continuous improvement of practice guidelines.

Orthoses that are thoughtfully designed with client input can make a difference in a person's life by relieving pain, providing joint stabilization, protecting vulnerable tissues, and enabling valued activities and participation. This in turn promotes physical and emotional well-being.

BOX 6–4　　PATIENT EDUCATION HANDOUT

Care and Use of Your Custom Orthosis

The orthosis was custom made for you by: _____

The purpose of the orthosis is to: _____

The orthosis should be worn: _____

- Notify your therapist if you notice the following:
  - Increase in pain
  - Change in swelling: generalized or between straps
  - Discoloration or temperature changes in the fingers
  - Local redness from pressure (at edges or over bony areas)
  - Numbness or tingling in hand or fingers
  - Areas of skin irritation (rash, itching, blotching)
- Do not wear the straps too tight. They should be firm but not tight or causing pain/swelling. They may require adjustments during the day.
- Wear the stockinette beneath the orthosis to help manage perspiration.

MOST IMPORTANTLY: FOLLOW THE WEARING SCHEDULE PRESCRIBED BY YOUR THERAPIST AND PHYSICIAN.

If you are allowed to remove the orthosis during the day, please remember the following:

- Keep your orthosis away from sources of heat (radiators, ovens, direct sunlight in a car).
- Your orthosis may be cleaned with soap/warm water or rubbing alcohol/disinfecting wipes. Be sure to rinse and dry the orthosis well before wearing.
- Straps and sleeves may be washed by hand and allowed to air dry.
- Do not make any adjustments to the orthosis yourself.

If you have any questions or concerns, please call the therapist who made your orthosis. If not available, please ask for the supervisor.

Therapist: _____ Phone: _____

Instructions should be clear regarding what the patient is permitted to do in terms of activities with the orthosis on and off. Teach the patient to monitor for adverse reactions such as skin redness and irritation, circulatory compromise, and nerve compression. Educating the caregivers is mandatory, especially when dispensing an orthosis to a child or an older individual with cognitive or physical impairments.

Proper care of the orthosis is necessary for hygiene and to ensure greatest function. Patients need to wash the orthosis with warm water and soap or rubbing alcohol and replace the liners and strapping when needed. If the orthosis is exposed to heat sources, it may soften and distort; thus, the patient must keep the device away from stoves, radiators, fireplaces, and direct sunlight (e.g., the car dashboard) (Fig. 6–14). Therapists must give the patient and caregiver written instructions along with a means to contact the clinic if any problems or questions arise.

Ideally, schedule the patient for a follow-up visit to check orthosis tolerance and to review the instructions. If patients are not scheduled to return to the clinic, they often do not report problems of discomfort or ineffectiveness. There is nothing worse than getting a phone call from a physician about a patient who has not worn an orthosis because it was not comfortable or, worse yet, was harmful to the patient in some way. If the patient is unable to return to the

clinic for follow-up because he or she lives far away, the therapist should attempt to call the patient to obtain verbal feedback and/or to offer a referral to a facility closer to his or her home, if appropriate.

ORTHOSIS PRICING AND INSURANCE REIMBURSEMENT

Reimbursement for orthotic fabrication depends on the specific insurance carrier and the contracts with the individual facility. Patients should be made aware of their coverage and encouraged to contact their insurance customer service representative for clarification of benefits. The pricing of orthoses depends on the facility and their individual reimbursement policy; there is no universally accepted system. Each facility determines its reimbursement schedule based on several factors. The cost of an orthosis should include fabrication time, thermoplastic materials, strapping, lining and padding, stockinettes, and components.

Cost constraints have forced therapists to be more judicious with orthotic intervention. Less costly options that do not compromise appropriate treatment standards should be offered to patients. For example, perhaps a prefabricated orthosis purchased at a medical-supply store or local pharmacy could serve the same purpose as a custom-fabricated wrist orthosis. Casting may be a less costly option when compared to the price of thermoplastic materials. Homemade outriggers from wire and scrap thermoplastic material may be less expensive than the commercially available component kits. The Clinical/Expert Pearls included in Section 2 note ways to decrease the costs of these devices offering cost-saving ideas to many situations. Therapists should take a proactive role in their state organizations by educating insurance companies to promote and maximize reimbursement of therapy services. Refer to Chapter 1 for additional information.

ORTHOTIC FABRICATION PROCESS

The chapters in Section 2 are organized first by purpose (immobilization, mobilization, and restriction) and then by the body part of origin (digit, hand, forearm, arm). For example, a static wrist

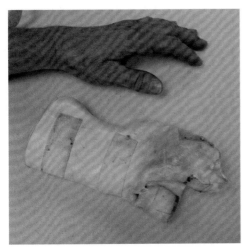

FIGURE 6–14 Flattened orthosis resulting from being left in hot car for a few hours.

support (wrist immobilization orthosis) is described under immobilization (Chapter 1 of Fabrication Manual) and then within the section that focuses on forearm-based orthoses. The description of each orthosis includes common names, alternative options, primary functions, additional functions, and common diagnoses and optimal positions. Positions are suggested as only a guide; the therapist must always be sure to contact the referring physician to determine positioning. Finally, the fabrication process is detailed for each orthosis, using the "PROCESS" concept.

PROCESS

The PROCESS format, used throughout Section 2, provides a highly organized, systematic approach to orthotic fabrication. The PROCESS acronym is defined as follows:

P—Pattern creation

R—Refine pattern

O—Options for materials

C—Cut and heat

E—Evaluate fit while molding

S—Strapping and components

S—Survey completed orthosis

The steps for the fabrication of each orthosis are organized in this manner. Each step consists of a list of information unique to the specific orthosis discussed. The basic principles applicable to all orthoses and a summary are included in the pull-out sleeve at the back of the book. Use the pull-out sleeve as a bookmark when fabricating orthoses and refer to these universal points when fabricating each device. Keep the book open to the appropriate page for handy reference during the fabrication process. Section 2 has been conveniently designed so that the photographs and pattern can be viewed simultaneously to improve comprehension and promote usability.

Clinical and Pattern Pearls are scattered throughout Section 2. These include helpful hints regarding the fabrication process and creative modifications of specific orthoses that the authors have found extremely effective in clinical practice. These tricks of the trade allow the reader to create truly customized orthoses. There is no cookbook method that can be used with every patient. Therapists must individualize their approach according to the specific needs of each patient.

When applying an orthosis on a patient with an injury that does not allow optimal positioning for pattern tracing or molding, the therapist must make modifications. For example, positioning the hand flat on a table is contraindicated for patients recovering from flexor tendon repairs because this position puts the repaired structures at risk for attenuation or rupture. As an appropriate alternative, trace the pattern on the uninvolved extremity. When checking the fit of the pattern, use the uninvolved side, if needed, to eliminate unnecessary movement of the injured extremity. Other positioning techniques include laying a patient on a plinth, using foam arm supports, and getting assistance from another therapist.

The following sections introduce the general instructions for fabricating orthoses.

Pattern Creation (Fig. 6–15A)

- Obtain referral with specific custom orthosis information from the physician.
- Perform upper extremity examination.
- Determine specific needs and decide on the type of orthosis to fabricate.

- Trace the pattern on a paper towel per orthosis diagram and cut it out. Use anatomical landmarks highlighted on the pattern to aid in accurate pattern creation.

Refine Pattern

- Check fit of paper pattern by trying it on patient's extremity (or on unaffected extremity if warranted).
- Mark any areas that need adjustment (i.e., add or delete material).

Options for Material

- Decide on the type of thermoplastic and strapping material.
- Transfer the pattern to thermoplastic material using a wax pencil or pen.

Cut and Heat (Fig. 6–15B,C)

- Partially heat thermoplastic material until soft enough to cut pattern accordingly.
- Place the patient's extremity in desired position and heat thermoplastic material to appropriate temperature.
- Apply any padding to high-risk bony areas before molding.
- Fully heat thermoplastic material, dry water off, and check temperature on your own skin before applying to the patient.

Evaluate Fit while Molding (Fig. 6–15D)

- Mold orthosis to the patient, and remember to
  - Use gravity to assist whenever possible.
  - Incorporate arches.
  - Provide adequate length and width.
  - Evenly distribute pressure while molding.
  - Handle thermoplastic material gently.
- Mark areas to be trimmed with the fingernail edge or pen and carefully remove the orthosis from the patient.
- Trim designated areas.

Strapping and Components (Fig. 6–15E–G)

- Determine optimal means of securing the orthosis to extremity.
- Provide adequate width in strapping and consider foam for key straps to obtain optimal positioning.
- Place the orthosis on the patient's limb and apply appropriate strapping.
- Affix specific components, such as hinges or outriggers, per pattern instructions.

Survey Completed Orthosis (Fig. 6–15H,I)

- Flare edges and round sharp corners of the orthosis. This is best completed by selectively dipping 1 to 2 mm of material's edge into warm water.
- Round corners of strapping.
- Provide the patient with written handouts describing purpose, precautions, proper care, and wearing schedule.
- Instruct in functional use and diagnosis-specific exercise within the orthosis if appropriate.
- Check that patient is able to don and doff the orthosis independently. Patient may benefit from digital photographs of proper orthosis application.
- Provide information on replacements for stockinette, straps, or other items.
- Schedule follow-up visit to reevaluate and modify the orthosis as appropriate.

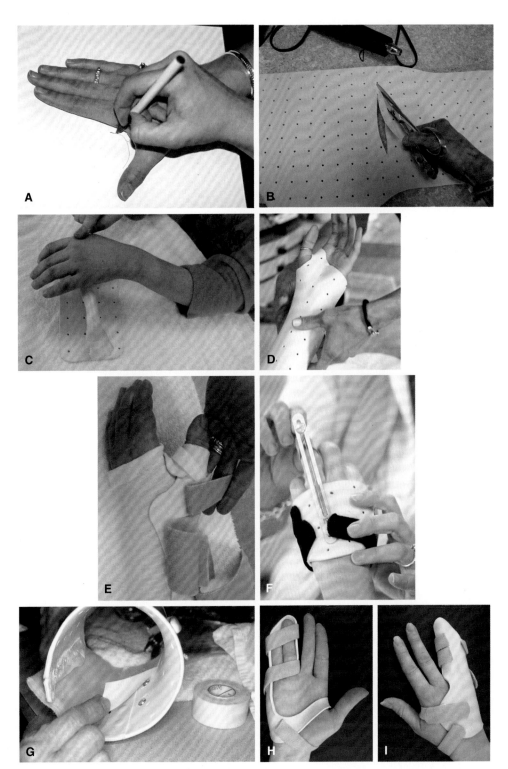

FIGURE 6–15 Orthotic fabrication process: **A,** Drawing pattern onto a paper towel. **B,** Cutting pattern out of thermoplastic material. **C,** Positioning the patient in a gravity-assisted position. **D,** Molding thermoplastic while visualizing creases to allow for distal mobility. **E,** Application of appropriate strapping system including padding for comfort. **F,** Adjusting component system in this mobilization orthosis. **G,** Covering the underside of screws with adhesive tape in this mobilization orthosis. **H and I,** Volar and dorsal views of a completed orthosis, checking for adjacent joint mobility and optimal strap placement.

CONCLUSION

This chapter provides an overview of the orthotic intervention process: from obtaining the physician referral to dispensing the completed orthosis. A comprehensive examination is necessary to gather the information required to make sound clinical decisions regarding specific treatment interventions. The therapist must appreciate the phases of tissue healing and how therapy and orthotic intervention are applied appropriately in order to do no harm. Effective communication with the patient and physician helps maximize the patient's final outcome.

CHAPTER REVIEW QUESTIONS

1. What, ideally, needs to be included in a physician referral?
2. Why is it important to take a medical history?
3. How can pain be measured?
4. What is evidence-based practice and how does it relate to orthotic intervention?
5. Describe the "PROCESS" of orthotic fabrication as described in this chapter.

SECTION 2

Optional Methods

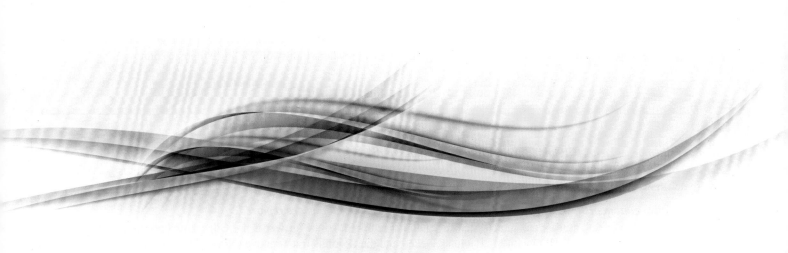

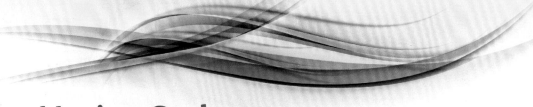

7

Relative Motion Orthoses

Julianne Wright Howell, PT, MS, CHT
Melissa Hirth, B (OT), MSc (OT -Hand & Upper Limb Rehab)

CHAPTER OBJECTIVES

After study of this chapter, the reader should be able to:

- Describe the concept of relative motion
- Be familiar with the term "quadriga effect" as used within the context of relative motion
- Distinguish between relative motion extension and relative motion flexion
- Follow directions to fabricate relative motion orthoses
- Understand that relative motion orthoses encourage early active motion
- Recognize that relative motion orthoses have protective, exercise, or adaptive functions

KEY TERMS

Acute and chronic boutonniere deformity

Early active motion (EAM)

Quadriga effect

Relative motion concept

Relative motion extension (RME) orthosis

Relative motion flexion (RMF) orthosis

Sagittal band injury/repair

Zones IV-VII extensor tendon repair of the fingers

MD NOTE

Wyndell H. Merritt, MD, FACS
Virginia

"Quadriga" is the name the Romans gave their two-wheeled chariot with equidistant reins to control four horses by the charioteer. The "quadriga effect" is a term coined by Verdan (Merritt & Howell, 2020) as a metaphor to bring focus on the complication occurring when the long extensor tendon is sutured to the profundus over an amputation stump causing loss of flexion in the adjacent uninjured fingers. This is due to relative shortening of the injured digit's profundus ("rein"), thereby restricting further contraction of their common muscle ("charioteer"). This anatomic fact can be used to advantage for an increasing variety of hand disorders that Howell and Hirth beautifully outline and classify. This orthotic concept differs from others by utilizing variations of the strong extrinsic muscles with common tendons to control tension on the digital tendons and joints by varying the relationship between MP joint positions. As a consequence, safe immediate active motion and hand functional use is possible following injury or surgical repair. This chapter reviews the distinct improvements in morbidity, allowing hand function during rehabilitation, reducing the need for intensive hand therapy, and allowing significant earlier work return. The authors recognize the increasing array of clinical applications and classify them as "protective, exercise, and adaptive," all of which have the advantage that therapy occurs while doing everyday activities. They focus on this moving target's variations of techniques, without loss of the fundamental concept. The most recent addition of the "protective" utilization has been used with **acute and chronic boutonniere deformity**, which appears to have the potential for a paradigm shift in the management and outcome of this most difficult of the extensor tendon disorders. The variations in construction techniques of their orthoses are comprehensively outlined. It is a well-written and exciting chapter that provides a framework for much more to come.

FAQ

How do I remember which MCP joint position is best for what condition?
Extension of the MCP joint is good for extensor tendons zones IV-VII and the sagittal band. *Flexion* of the MCP joint is good for boutonniere deformity and central slip repairs. Still unsure? Use the RME or RMF pencil test to help yourself think it through.

***Should a relative motion orthosis be used when** all EDC, EIP, and EDM tendons are repaired?*
To levy the "quadriga effect" at least one intact extensor tendon is required, so the answer is no. Other EAM approaches to consider include the Norwich regimen a WHFO with MCP joints blocked and the IP joints free to move (Norwich, Slater/Bynum). If a passive motion approach is feasible, a dynamic outrigger could be useful (Evans).

What can I do to convince a hand surgeon or my colleagues to use relative motion orthoses?

The evidence is convincing for use of RME after long extensor tendon repair, to prepare for your discussion, you can find a great summary of this evidence as well as other relative motion uses with cited references in a scoping review (ref SR). A great visual to demonstrate how relative motion works is to use the "RME/RMF pencil test" or make a relative motion orthosis on the hand surgeon/colleagues.

INTRODUCTION

The **relative motion concept** relies on the relationship that exists between a muscle that is shared by multiple tendons. The extensor digitorum communis (EDC) and flexor digitorum profundus (FDP) are such muscles whereby changing the angle of at least one metacarpophalangeal (MCP) joint relative to the adjacent MCP joints alters the relationship between their respective tendons. When the involved digit's MCP joint is positioned in greater extension or more flexion than the neighboring MCP joints, a "**quadriga effect**" is imposed influencing that digit (Merritt & Howell, 2020). Within the context of relative motion a "quadriga effect" is beneficial in that the length difference created between the tendons sharing a common muscle lessens tendon excursion and muscle force generation. A thorough understanding of the "quadriga effect" and which relative motion orthosis to use are foremost to successful management of many conditions with relative motion orthoses. Relative motion orthoses are static and finger-based and are of two orthotic designs. The **relative motion extension (RME) orthosis** holds the involved MCP joint(s) in greater extension (Fig. 7–1A,B), while the **relative motion flexion (RMF) orthosis** places the involved MCP joint(s) in more flexion (Fig. 7–2A,B). A "quadriga effect" is levied on the EDC and sagittal band with an RME orthosis, while an RMF orthosis imposes a "quadriga effect" on the FDP and its lumbrical

(Merritt & Howell, 2020). Although relative motion orthoses allow a wide range of active finger mobility, at least 15° to 20° of end range of motion is restricted. For these reasons, RME and RMF orthoses are static finger orthoses that function to *both mobilize and restrict* (refer Chapter 1).

LITERATURE SUMMARY OF COMMON DIAGNOSES

The first application of the relative motion concept was used to protect long extensor tendon repairs of the fingers in **zones IV-VII** and **sagittal band repairs** with RME orthoses (Howell, Merritt, & Robinson, 2005; Merritt, 2014; Merritt et al., 2000; Rosenblum & Robinson, 1986). RMF orthoses have recently been introduced to manage acute and chronic boutonniere deformity and, postoperatively, zone III central slip repairs (Hirth, Howell, & O'Brien, 2016; Merritt & Howell, 2020). Today there are many other applications for relative motion orthoses, the most common of which are listed in Table 7–1 (Hirth et al., 2016). Relative motion orthoses are simple, inexpensive, and low profile to fabricate and, when used with early active motion, support immediate functional hand use and earlier return to work (Hirth et al., 2016; Rosenblum & Robinson, 1986).

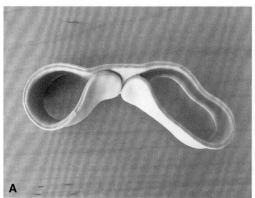
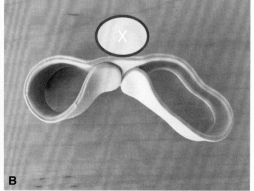

FIGURE 7–1   A and B, RME 4-finger "self-secured" design for left long finger (X).

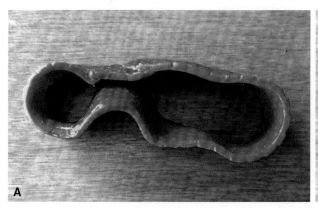
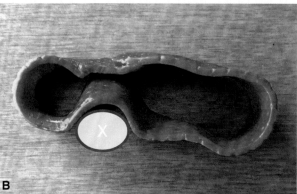

FIGURE 7–2   A and B, RMF 4-finger "self-secured" design for right ring finger (X).

TABLE 7–1	**Common Clinical Indications for Relative Motion Orthoses**	
Orthosis Category	**RME**	**RMF**
Protective	Extensor tendon repair finger zones IV-VII Acute and chronic sagittal band injury/repair MCP joint arthroplasty Tendon transfer Dorsal hand skin graft Trigger finger Hand pain	Acute and chronic Boutonniere deformity Central slip laceration Flexor tendon repair Digital nerve repair Interosseous tear PIP joint arthroplasty Hand pain
Exercise	Address active tendon lag Regain IP joint flexion	Address active tendon lag Regain IP joint extension Regain MCP joint flexion
Adaptive	Improve MCP joint alignment/rheumatoid arthritis imbalances Trigger finger Hand pain	Improve MCP joint alignment/rheumatoid arthritis Ulnar nerve palsy Hand pain

IP, interphalangeal; MCP, metacarpophalangeal; PIP, proximal interphalangeal; RME, relative motion extension; RMF, relative motion flexion.

ZONE IV-VII LONG EXTENSOR TENDON

Relative motion put forth the idea that **early active motion (EAM)** with zones V-VI extensor tendon repairs was safe and practical (Rosenblum & Robinson, 1986). Expanding on this idea of early active motion, the relative motion approach was renamed immediate controlled active motion (ICAM) for EDC repairs as well as extensors indicis proprius and digiti minimi and included zones IV-VII (Howell et al., 2005). Unlike the EDC and FDP that are a single muscle with multiple tendons, the independent long extensors are not. However, RME orthoses have proven effective, probably because the excursions of these independent extensor tendons match those of the common extensor tendons and all share intramuscular and juncturae tendinae connections (Elliott & McGrouther, 1986; Leijnse, Carter, Gupta, & McCabe, 2008).

The relative motion approach (formerly ICAM) requires two orthoses, an RME orthosis and a static custom or prefabricated wrist-hand orthosis (WHO) (Howell et al., 2005; Howell & Peck, 2013). There is evidence that supports the use of only the RME orthosis (RME *orthosis–only* approach) for zones V-VI repair management (Burns, Derby, & Neumeister, 2013; Collocott et al., 2020; Hirth et al., 2011; Svens, Ames, Burford, & Caplash, 2015).

When using the RME *orthosis–only* approach, some have added a static wrist-hand-finger orthosis (WHFO)/resting hand orthosis overnight, with instruction to avoid simultaneous wrist and finger flexion during daytime activity for at least a month (Collocott et al., 2020; Hirth et al., 2011). Others have restricted use of the RME-*only approach* to repairs distal to the juncturae tendinum (zones IV and V) and have implemented the two orthoses approach (RME orthosis and WHO) for extensor tendon repairs proximal to the juncturae tendinum (zone VI) and for all EDM repairs regardless of zone (Svens et al., 2015). The benefits of these additions have not been substantiated (Hirth et al., 2016).

If stiffness is a problem when using the two orthoses approach (RME and WHFO), short arc of wrist motion can be cautiously initiated between 2 and 3 weeks after surgery with the RME orthosis in situ then progressed to simultaneous wrist and finger flexion as described.

Current evidence informs therapists that use of the *RME orthosis–only* approach is safe for zone V repair management, evidence is convincing but incomplete for use of *RME orthosis only* to manage zones IV and VI, and there is no evidence for the use of *RME orthosis only* for zone VII (Burns et al., 2013; Collocott et al., 2020; Hirth et al., 2011; Hirth et al., 2016; Izadpanah et al., 2015; Svens et al., 2015; Turner, 2015). Originally, the relative difference angle for the involved digit's MCP joint was 25° to 30° of greater extension, presently this relative angle of extension is 15° to 20° for extensor tendon repairs in zones IV-VII (Hirth et al., 2016). Both angles have proven safe, with no tendon ruptures reported (Merritt & Howell, 2020). To implement interventions with relative motion, engaging the "quadriga effect" is required; therefore, *at least one EDC, EIP, or EDM must be intact.* Initiating early active motion with RME orthoses varies between 3 and 11 days after tendon repair; less than optimal outcomes may result if starting later (Hirth et al., 2016). Generally, the combination of EAM and relative motion yields "good to excellent" total active motion outcomes, without the need for intensive hand therapy as the hand is being used functionally from the outset (Hirth et al., 2016; Merritt & Howell, 2020). The duration of full-time orthosis wear varies between 4 and 6 weeks, and most clinicians gradually reduce orthosis wear time versus discontinue the orthosis abruptly (Hirth et al., 2016). Once the RME orthosis is fabricated, immediate functional hand use is available for light self-care activities, advancing to medium-duty work around 3 to 6 weeks after surgery, and returning to full unrestricted hand use without the orthosis after 6 to 8 weeks (Hirth et al., 2016). It is understood that many factors influence return to work, including whether or not an orthotic device can be worn on the job; however, the earliest return to work times reported vary between 1 and 21 days after repair (Collocott et al., 2020; Hirth et al., 2016).

CLINICAL PEARL 7–1

Diagnosis Specifics

At least one EDC, EIP, or EDM has to be intact after zone IV-VII repair to safely use the relative motion concept.

CASE 7–1

Long Extensor Tendon Repair (Protective Orthosis)

LE, a 34-year-old cabinet maker, sustained a dorsal laceration to his right dominant hand at work on a piece of sheet metal. Surgical repair was to the EDC tendons in zone V of the ring and small fingers and the MCP joint capsule of the small finger. Three days after surgery, LE attended hand therapy to have an RME orthosis fabricated, which held the ring and small fingers in 20° MCP joint greater extension than the MCP joints of the uninjured index and long fingers (Fig. 7–3). The orthosis was worn full time for 4 weeks, and prescribed exercises while wearing the orthosis included active composite finger flexion, extension, and a hook-fist. Given the acuteness of the injury dorsal hand edema was managed with retrograde massage. LE returned to return to work on modified duties, with permission to use his hand for light-medium tasks, such as assisting his workmates to do the "finishing" touches on installed cabinets. Four weeks post surgery the orthosis was ceased for night wear and worn during the day only for "heavy" tasks, as he was released to full work duties. Edema had resolved and his finger range of motion was minimally restricted. The home exercises focusing on composite active finger extension and MCP joint flexion given 2 weeks earlier, ensured that range of motion had returned to preinjury levels. Eight weeks postoperatively LE was discharged from therapy and the orthosis was no longer required for "heavy" work activities.

ACUTE AND CHRONIC SAGITTAL BAND INJURY AND REPAIR

Active extension of the MCP joint is the role of the long extensor tendon, which in zones IV-V is maintained in its central position over the MCP joint by the deep and superficial fibers of the sagittal band. Disruption of the "ring" formed by the sagittal band, volar plate, flexor tendon sheath, proximal annular pulley, and intermetacarpal ligaments causes the long extensor tendon to dislocate, sublux, or decentralize between the metacarpal heads during finger flexion. Tendon dislocation is often painful, may be transient, or require the digit to be manually lifted back into extension to be reposition. An RME orthosis is a useful tool for managing sagittal band repairs and injuries (Catalano et al., 2006; Merritt, 2014; Merritt & Howell, 2020; Merritt et al., 2000; Peelman, Markiewitz, Kiefhaber, & Stern, 2015). There are various opinions regarding the most effective relative angle of MCP joint extension with some reporting between 25° and 30° while others fabricate the orthosis based on the best angle to eliminate pain and minimize tendon subluxation during active motion (Catalano et al., 2006; Hirth et al., 2016; Merritt & Howell, 2020; Peelman et al., 2015). To protect a repaired or torn sagittal band during healing, the orthosis is worn full time for at least 6 to 8 weeks, and likely an additional 2 to 4 weeks when not repaired. Of course these healing timelines can be lengthened, particularly if when out of the orthosis pain increases (Hirth et al., 2016; Merritt & Howell, 2020). Although the evidence for nonsurgical management is sparse, consensus is that the earlier the intervention, the better the outcomes (Catalano et al., 2006; Peelman et al., 2015).

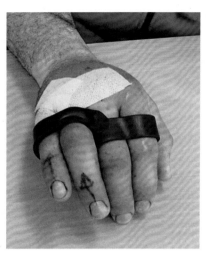

FIGURE 7–3 Case 7–1: RME for long extensor tendon repairs to ring and small fingers.

CASE 7–2

Sagittal Band Injury (Protective and Adaptive Orthosis)

SB, a 30-year-old physical therapist with inflammatory arthritis, attended therapy after suffering progressive pain of the long finger MCP joint and "snapping" of the tendon with strenuous gripping. Disappointed there was no symptomatic improvement after 3 months of orthotic wear (resting hand orthosis full time for 4 weeks, and thereafter nightly along with a daytime volar static hand-based orthosis with the MCP joints blocked and IP joints free), she presented for surgical opinion. Surgery was put "on hold" in favor of a second-hand therapy consult.

SB advised the second therapist that the previous orthoses interfered with hand function and irritated her skin. Local MCP joint effusion, dorsal tenderness, and ulnar subluxation of the EDC tendon with occasional snapping were noted, and a 10-day trial of wearing an RME orthosis recommended. A 3-finger orthosis was fabricated with Orficast™, the angle of MCP joint relative extension determined by the "RME pencil test," and an ulnar block added to prevent ulnar shift of the finger during grip (Fig. 7–4A). The RME orthosis was worn during the day and, if painful, the resting hand orthosis overnight. Returning 10 days later, SB reported there was not enough support from the orthosis during work activities or strenuously gripping. A second 3-finger RME orthosis with an ulnar block was fabricated with a higher profile or greater relative MCP joint (Fig. 7–4B). Three weeks later, SB returned pleased with the higher profile, but asked if another more supportive orthosis could be made for her gym and other sports activities. A third RME orthosis was fabricated, this time a 4-finger design, adding the ring finger in the trough for greater stability (Fig. 7–4C). Learning to modify her grip when not in an orthosis (Fig. 7–4D) and using the correct "protective" orthosis for hand use allowed SB to resolve the sagittal band injury within a further 3 months.

ACUTE AND CHRONIC BOUTONNIERE DEFORMITY

The best treatment of boutonniere deformity is to avoid the deformity by early diagnosis and treatment.

W.H. Merritt (2014)

The most recent application of the relative motion concept is for boutonniere deformity using an RMF orthosis. Under the right conditions, the position of RMF allows for a simultaneously beneficial "quadriga effect" that restores tension in the long extensor and its lateral slips and relaxes the profundus and its lumbrical, so that upon active finger motion, the dynamics of Winslow's Diamond are engaged, correcting the boutonniere deformity (Merritt & Howell, 2020). Taking a closer look at the chain of events that ensue once the injured finger's MCP joint is placed in more relative flexion; this chain starts with relaxing the volar directed pull of lumbrical on the lateral bands, allowing interphalangeal (IP) joint extension via intrinsic input and the lateral slips of the extensor system, of which the latter is now sufficiently tensioned by imposing flexion on the MCP joint. Next in this chain of events is the impact of the RMF position on the dynamics of Winslow's Diamond (Merritt & Howell, 2020). This impact is better understood by reviewing these dynamics under normal conditions. Normally the "diamond" separates and widens during active PIP joint flexion while the EDC tendon relaxes, and then as the intrinsics and EDC muscles contract to extend the PIP joint, the "diamond" relocates dorsally and centrally in a cinching fashion (Merritt & Howell, 2020; Winslow, 1732). After a PIP joint injury, the diamond's normal mechanics are interrupted, resulting in the classic boutonniere deformity. However, when an injured digit with a passively flexible PIP joint is placed in an RMF orthosis and active motion is added, the lateral bands/slips will reposition dorsally and medially once again to extend the PIP joint (Merritt & Howell, 2020). This response is similar to that seen in ulnar nerve palsy, when a dorsal blocking orthosis is used to position the involved digit's MCP joints in more flexion making IP joint extension possible through the lateral slips of the extrinsic long extensor in the absence of intrinsic function. RMF orthoses function in a similar manner when there is complete disruption of the central slip, extensor hood, and triangular ligament, provided the lateral band position remains correctable, and the slack in the EDC is restored by placing the affected MCP joint(s) in at least 15° to 20° more flexion during active range of motion of the digits. Importantly, provided the RMF orthosis is worn, this beneficial "quadriga effect" continues through a wide range of finger motion (Merritt & Howell, 2020).

CHAPTER 7

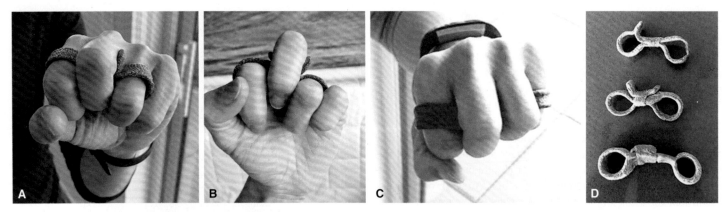

FIGURE 7–4 **A–D,** Case 7–2: Three different RME for long finger: **(A)** 3-finger low profile with ulnar block, **(B)** 3-finger higher profile with ulnar block, **(C)** 4-finger for greater stability needs, and **(D)** comparison of low profile, higher profile, and sport/gym "adaptive RME orthoses." (Sagittal Band injury case report and pictures: courtesy of Lynne Feehan, PhD, PT, CHT.)

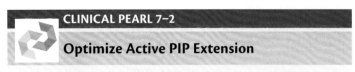

CLINICAL PEARL 7–2

Optimize Active PIP Extension

An RMF orthosis encourages PIP joint extension to discourage boutonniere deformity.

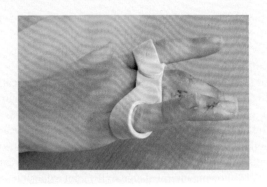

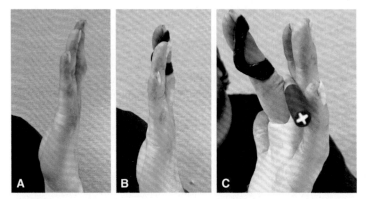

FIGURE 7–5 **A–C,** Acute boutonniere long finger: **(A)** active extensor lag with DIP joint hyperextension due to extrinsic/intrinsic force imbalance, **(B)** an orthosis to block DIP joint hyperextension incompletely corrects active PIP joint extension lag, and **(C)** simulated RMF with "pencil test" rebalances forces.

ACUTE BOUTONNIERE DEFORMITY

As this is the newest application of the relative motion concept, the evidence for the management of acute and chronic boutonniere deformity with an RMF is largely empirical. The likelihood that a boutonniere deformity will be avoided, resolved, or kept from progressing relies on an accurate diagnosis, ruling out other factors that may also contribute to the deformity such as flexor tenosynovitis, volar plate, and pulley injuries (Merritt & Howell, 2020). Furthermore, a satisfactory outcome depends on the patient comprehending the value in wearing an RMF orthosis full time to avoid deformity, as well as committing to wearing the orthosis for at least 6 weeks (acute) or for some indefinitely (chronic) as an "adaptive" orthosis. The ideal patient to use an RMF orthosis is one with a supple PIP joint defined as at least 20° from full passive extension. If the patient's PIP joint is *not supple* a serial cast or a dynamic Capener is required to address the flexion contracture prior to the RMF orthosis (Merritt & Howell, 2020; Merritt et al., 2000). Merritt applies an RMF orthosis immediately after an acute injury when the PIP joint is passively correctable to within 20° from full extension and reports that it takes at least 6 weeks of continuous wear to restore the normal mechanics (Merritt & Howell, 2020). Similarly, if the

PIP joint is passively correctable to within 20° from full extension, but the distal interphalangeal (DIP) joint hyperextends, author JWH combines an RMF orthosis with a dorsal-based finger orthosis to block DIP joint extension until extrinsic/intrinsic balance is restored, usually this requires at least 6 weeks of full-time wear (Merritt & Howell, 2020) (Fig. 7–5A–C). Whenever there is an active PIP extension lag of 25° or more in an acute or chronic PIP joint injury, but the joint can be passively corrected to within 20° from full extension, author JWH adds a short arc motion (SAM) attachment to the RMF orthosis to block PIP joint flexion at 35° until 20° or less from full active extension is obtained (Merritt & Howell, 2020) (Fig. 7–6A,B). As active PIP joint extension improves, indicating that the dynamic requirements of Winslow's Diamond are better, the SAM attachment can be modified by sequentially increasing the amount of active PIP joint flexion allowed. Once (with the RMF orthosis in situ) the mechanics are restored, at least another 6 weeks of full-time wear is recommended (Merritt & Howell, 2020). Others have RMF designs with SAM capability as can be viewed in Figure 7–7A,B and a case study report (Johnson, Swanson, & Manolopoulos, 2019). Patients with generalized finger joint hypermobility may need to wear the RMF orthosis longer for soft tissue healing to stabilize. For some, use of a PIP extension orthosis at night is more comfortable, wearing the RMF orthosis during the day (Merritt & Howell, 2020).

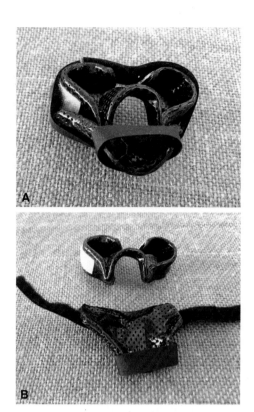

FIGURE 7–6 A–B, 3-Finger RMF orthosis for the long finger with (A) volar SAM attachment to limit PIP joint flexion, and (B) the attachment is removable to modify as more active PIP joint flexion is indicated.

CASE 7–3
Acute Boutonniere Deformity (Protective Orthosis)

AB, a 30-year-old, reports jamming her finger several weeks ago playing basketball, with immediate bruising and swelling. She was informed by the urgent care physician that there was no fracture and instructed to apply ice and buddy tape her finger for a week. After having done this for 1 week she noticed worsening ability to straighten her PIP joint, so was then referred to hand therapy. The PIP joint was bruised and mildly tender to palpation dorsally, active PIP joint extension lacked 20° from full extension and passive 10°. Although it required several attempts at active PIP joint extension in the "RMF pencil test" position, active PIP joint extension matched her passive extension. Residual swelling limited passive/active DIP joint motion to 45°. Contingent on the patient's accurate history, residual dorsal joint tenderness and the results of the pencil test led the hand therapist to be concerned about progression into a boutonniere deformity. She advised daytime use of an RMF orthosis and compression wrap at night. After 2 weeks wearing the RMF orthosis, full active PIP joint extension was attained, DIP joint flexion normalized; however, some local PIP joint tenderness persisted. AB agreed to continue this same intervention for another 2 weeks. On return 2 weeks later, AB had full PIP joint extension without the RMF orthosis and no local joint tenderness. She agreed to therapy discharge with the provision to protectively buddy tape her finger during sports for another month.

CHRONIC BOUTONNIERE DEFORMITY

Historically nonsurgical management of chronic boutonniere deformity has consisted of serial casting and prolonged immobilization with inconsistent results and recurrent deformity (Merritt & Howell, 2020). It is a conundrum as even hand surgeons disagree on which surgery is best or whether surgery improves finger function at all (To

& Watson, 2011). "Excellent" outcome after boutonniere deformity reconstruction is defined as an active PIP joint extension lag of 20° or less; furthermore, no surgical reconstruction is advised when the active lag is 30° or less (Steichen et al., 1982). Consequently, these are the patients sent to hand therapy who have the chronic deformities with varying functional expectations. If approached from a different perspective, these may be the very patients for whom hand therapy intervention may be of more value than surgery. To illustrate this idea, there are some who will have their functional expectations met simply by correcting a fixed-passive PIP joint flexion contracture but have no interest in wearing an RMF orthosis. While others may be willing to wear an RMF orthosis indefinitely "adaptively" to convert an active 45° PIP joint extension lag without the orthosis to an active extension lag of 30° or less, and be encouraged by knowing that dedicated wear of the RMF orthosis will interrupt progression of the deformity. Another category of patient are those sent to therapy to insure that suppleness of PIP joint passive extension and DIP joint flexion have been addressed and the patient is a "good candidate" for the surgical reconstruction needed to correct boutonniere deformity.

CASE 7–4
Chronic Boutonniere Deformity (Protective and Adaptive Orthosis)

Three months after a closed small finger injury involving the right hand, CB, a 65-year-old retiree, attended a hand surgeon's office frustrated with his "bent, painful finger that gets in the way." Assessment shows a chronic boutonniere deformity with compensatory hyperextension of the MCP and DIP joints, and a fixed 70° PIP joint flexion contracture. Finding no suitable surgical intervention, a referral was made to therapy to address the contracture. He was also informed that due to the chronicity of the boutonniere deformity, at least 4 months of therapy was likely.

Serial casting was chosen to reduce the PIP joint contracture, and a daytime RMF orthosis was worn over the cast to block the small finger MCP joint hyperextension. The aim of the RMF orthosis was to utilize the "quadriga effect" to relax the FDP/lumbrical and to restore extrinsic/intrinsic balance. After 4 weeks, active motion improved from 70° from full PIP joint extension to 45° with passive motion to 30°. Keeping the stiff DIP joint out of the cast supported passive/active exercises, resulting in a 25° improvement in total active flexion.

These same interventions were continued for two more weeks (totaling 6 weeks), resulting in complete passive PIP joint extension and 35° from full active extension with the RMF orthosis in situ. With these IP joint motion improvements, casting was stopped and a modified RMF orthosis fabricated to permit SAM limiting PIP joint flexion to 35°. Active and passive PIP joint extensions were encouraged throughout the day with the orthosis in situ, and he wore a nighttime static thermoplastic PIP joint extension orthosis. After 10 more days, active PIP joint extension improved to 30° from full extension indicating SAM motion could be serially increased every 10 days, provided no active extension was lost. After 16 weeks of intervention, active extension was stable at 30° from full extension, passive extension at neutral, and active PIP joint flexion was 70° (Fig. 7–8A,B).

Impressed with CB's results, once again, the hand surgeon felt surgery was unlikely to improve on his nonsurgical outcome. CB opted to self-manage wearing the RMF orthosis "adaptively." He requested a 2-finger design, and while the therapist explained that this would be more like a buddy strap and not provide the same effect as a 3- or 4-finger design, CB insisted he trial this. After 3 months of mostly using the 2-finger orthosis, CB lost PIP extension (Fig. 7–9A,B).

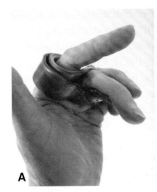
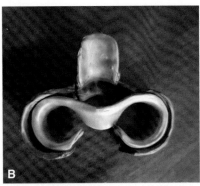
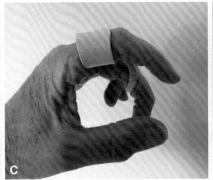
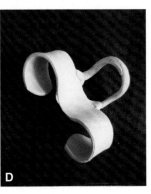

FIGURE 7–7 **A and B,** RMF long finger (gold orthosis). Volar SAM attachment to limit PIP joint flexion (blue orthosis). **C and D,** Alternative design utilizing attached ring volarly to limit flexion. (Orthoses design: courtesy of Gwendolyn van Strien, LPT, MSc.)

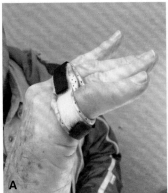
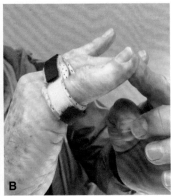

FIGURE 7–8 **A and B,** Case 7–4: RMF 3-finger design for small finger chronic boutonniere. **A,** demonstrating active extension, and **(B)** Demonstrating passive extension.

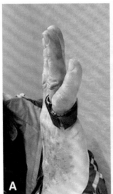
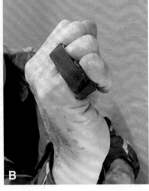

FIGURE 7–9 **A and B,** Case 7–4: "Adaptive" 2-finger RMF orthosis that failed to maintain intrinsic/extrinsic balance in small finger. **A,** Demonstrating *too much* MCP joint hyperextension, and B) *too much* PIP joint flexion; notice loss of PIP joint extension.

PATIENT POPULATION AND DIAGNOSIS FOR BEST USE

It appears that the clinical applications for relative motion orthoses are endless. The numerous conditions for which these orthoses have been utilized are collated in a relative motion scoping review (Hirth et al., 2016). Because the clinical applications were extensive and varied, a classification scheme based on the function of the orthosis as "protective," "exercise," or "adaptive" was suggested by the authors of the review (Hirth et al., 2016).

A relative motion "protective" orthosis as the name suggests protects a healing structure. A relative motion "exercise" orthosis

is implemented with the aim of rebalancing intrinsic/extrinsic muscle forces that contribute to an active tendon lag or shift forces to address stiffness in a distal joint. While a relative motion "adaptive" orthosis would be used to rebalance muscle forces and/or finger alignment to improve hand function or appearance. Table 7–1 provides an overview of common conditions for which relative motion orthoses can be of value. It can be expected that additional uses for the relative motion concept will be developed in the future.

FABRICATION CONCEPTS FOR RELATIVE MOTION ORTHOSES

DEGREE OF RELATIVE EXTENSION OR FLEXION

Essential to the relative motion orthotic design is the ability to maintain the desired "relative" degree of difference between the affected digit's MCP joint(s) and those of the unaffected digit. The recommended "relative degree of MCP joint difference" for a "protective" orthosis varies depending on the condition managed. It is generally accepted that 15° to 20° of relative MCP joint extension difference is required when managing zones IV-VII extensor tendon repairs. The relative degree of difference for sagittal band disruption suggested is 25° to 30°; however, the best angle is the one causing no pain and minimal/no EDC subluxation (Merritt & Howell, 2020). Boutonniere deformity management is still developing with the current suggestion for a relative difference at 20° to 35°, although can be adjusted to achieve the intended response (Merritt & Howell, 2020). As an "exercise" orthosis, the degree of relative MCP joint flexion or extension difference is not as critical as achieving the desired outcome. Quite often when fabricating an "adaptive" orthosis the therapist will need to trial various MCP joint positions and relative motion orthotic designs to determine which best meets the needs for hand function.

FINGERS INCLUDED IN THE ORTHOTIC DESIGN

There are no comparative studies for orthotic design efficacy of 3- or 4-finger relative motion orthoses; the 4-finger design is most often used to manage extensor tendon repairs and a 3-finger design for sagittal band injuries (Hirth et al., 2016). A 4-finger design is advantageous when greater stability is desired or to limit webspace irritation with fragile skin, whereas a 3-finger design can be used to free up fingers, such as the index finger for lateral pinch and typing activities.

CLINICAL PEARL 7–3

4-Finger Design

A 4-finger design will provide more stability than a 3-finger design. In concept, only the injured digits are required to be in the relatively extended or flexed trough/loop, the "balanced" design is a 4-finger design variation used to manage index *and* small finger injuries. Positioning both the index and small fingers in relative MCP joint extension or flexion stabilizes the positions of these joints better keeping the hypermobile border digits under control and the orthosis stays on the hand better (A and B). For lack of a better term, an "unbalanced" design includes only one injured border digit in the relatively flexed or extended position (C-E). In general, the stability and comfort of a "protective" orthosis can be improved simply by adding the adjacent uninjured digit in the design; conditions for which this is helpful include sagittal band injuries and extensor tendon repairs with associated proximal phalanx fracture.

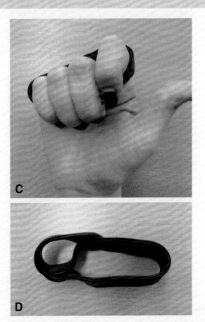

"Self-secured" RME "nonbalanced" option for index finger.

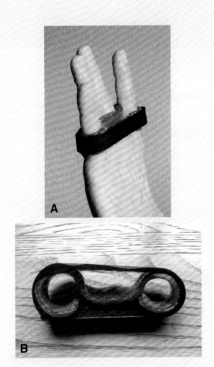

A and B, Hook and loop RME "balanced" option 4-finger open looped design for either an index or small finger.

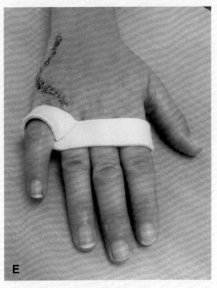

"Self-secured" RME "nonbalanced" option for small finger.

ORTHOTIC MATERIAL SUGGESTIONS

Thermoplastics are preferential when fabricating a "protective" relative motion orthosis, relying on its more firm properties, while a softer material such as neoprene works well for "exercise" and "adaptive" orthoses.

As long as the desired degree of relative MCP joint difference is maintained during motion, practically any thermoplastic or Orficast® can be used. Therapist preference and skill level generally influence thermoplastic selection with some therapists preferring 1.6 mm (1/16″) microperforated highly conforming thermoplastics, while others may be more comfortable using a more rigid 3.2 mm (3/32″) thermoplastic which technically are easier to fabricate. Selecting a solid thermoplastic if the patient is to shower with the orthosis on, as the solid thermoplastic is easier to dry, whereas, because the material is woven between the fingers, perforated thermoplastic

may be preferred in hotter climates or when a lighter, less bulky orthosis is required.

STRAPPING OPTIONS

No strapping is required with a "self-secure" orthotic design option, which is often fabricated with a solid 3.2 mm thermoplastic (Fig. 7–10A,B). Technically this design is easy to fabricate with the added advantages of being easy to dry one-handed after a shower, with no straps to get lost or fastenings that snag clothing. "Hook and loop" strapping is required for the "open looped" orthotic design which can be fabricated with thermoplastic of any thickness. This design is also technically easy to fabricate with the advantage of adjustability for enlarged IP joints or edematous digits, once edema subsides the straps can be snugged (see Fig. 7–6A,B). Of course, for patients who like to customize their orthosis, program adherence

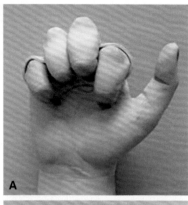

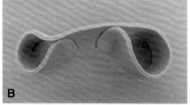

FIGURE 7–10 A and B, Self-secured option, RME for long and ring fingers or RMF "balanced" approach for either index or small fingers. Note the transverse arch in the orthosis design and the "shallow" trough for the long and ring fingers when used as RME.

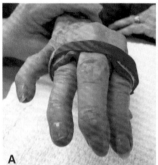

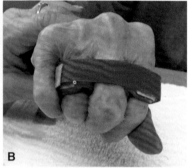

FIGURE 7–11 A and B, Deeper/more conforming trough RME 3-finger design for lateral support of long finger ulnar sagittal band tear. Notice the thermoplastic "hugging" the long finger.

may be optimized when hook and loop or different thermoplastic color choices are available.

TROUGH DESIGN (SHALLOW OR DEEP)

By fabricating a relative motion orthosis with a shallow trough, it is easier technic-wise to provide for a greater degree of relative MCP joint extension or flexion and there is less thermoplastic conformity around potentially fragile skin (Fig. 7–11A,B). While a deeper trough is a bit more demanding as it is woven to conform, it will provide more lateral support such as desired when managing a sagittal band injury or repair.

INSTRUCTION FOR ORTHOTIC FABRICATION

Start with approximately a 1.5 cm wide and 25 cm length strip of thermoplastic. For an *RME* orthosis place the thermoplastic on the *volar surface* of the injured digit(s) and for an *RMF* orthosis place the thermoplastic on the *dorsal aspect* of the injured finger(s). It is important to maintain the transverse arch at the metacarpals, so be careful not to "flatten" the hand while weaving the thermoplastic around the proximal phalanges. For a "self-secured" design, press the thermoplastic into itself. For an "open looped" orthosis, mold the thermoplastic around the outermost radial and ulnar digits, cut the ends in rounded fashion, and then add the hook and loop fastenings.

CLINICAL PEARL 7–4

Positioning

For easier fabrication, ask patients to hold their own injured finger in the desired relative motion position (A)!
Use a pencil to simulate the positions of RME and RMF before fabricating the orthosis (B).

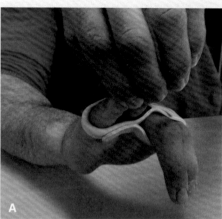

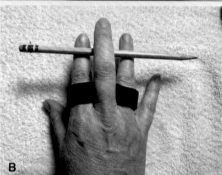

EXERCISE CONSIDERATIONS

Exercise recommendations depend on the clinical condition for which the relative motion orthosis has been prescribed, the results of the clinical evaluation, and the patient's response to the intervention. Functional hand use alone in the RME orthosis is not always enough to sufficiently address tendon excursion or joint stiffness after extensor tendon repair. The addition of a few basic exercises during the initial few postoperative weeks will ensure the anticipated outcomes. Suggested exercises done with the orthosis in situ include composite active finger extension, composite active finger flexion, and a hook fist as displayed in Figure 7–12A–C. These same exercises can be performed when indicated wearing the RME orthosis after sagittal band injury or repair as long as the EDC tendon remains centralized throughout finger motion.

CASE 7–5

Relative Motion Orthoses for "Exercise" to Improve Range of Motion

EO, a 48-year-old marketing manager, sustained a closed midshaft fractured second metacarpal on his right dominant hand. This occurred when his dog suddenly ran toward another dog, with the looped leash crushing his hand. EO was referred to therapy for a thermoplastic orthosis 5 days following the injury. A hand-finger fracture orthosis (HFO) was fabricated immobilizing the MCP joints of the index and long fingers in 70° flexion and the IP joints free to mobilize. Light functional hand use was encouraged while wearing the orthosis, and removal of the orthosis several times daily for active composite finger flexion exercises. Four weeks after injury the orthosis was discarded; however, index MCP joint motion was mildly limited, lacking 10° from full active extension (passive extension was neutral) and limited to 75° of active/passive flexion, compared to his contralateral MCP joint motion of 0°/85°. EO was assigned a home exercise program consisting of active and passive range of motion exercises. Therapy review 2 weeks later demonstrated improved MCP joint extension to neutral but no change in MCP joint flexion. EO reported the tight sensation as well as the stiffness in the MCP joint bothered him. An RMF orthosis was fabricated with the index finger in 30° relative MCP joint flexion compared to his other three fingers. He was advised to wear this as an "exercise" orthosis throughout the day while using his hand functionally. The two aims for the orthosis were to reduce his "extensor index habitus" posture and to harness the force of flexion produced by the other digits to apply a low-load passive flexion force across the index MCP joint. After wearing the RMF orthosis for 2 weeks as prescribed, EO returned to therapy with motion equal to that of the contralateral digit, the RMF orthosis was stopped, and he was discharged a happy patient from therapy.

When using an RMF orthosis to manage a boutonniere deformity or central slip repair, the dynamics of Winslow's Diamond and the "quadriga effect" are activated with active motion. If obtaining end range PIP joint extension is a problem, try adding "place and hold" PIP joint extension exercises. If distal excursion of the lateral bands or stiffness of the DIP joint is problematic, have patients hold their PIP joint in extension while isolated passive/active flexion of the DIP joint is performed.

An "exercise" orthosis requires the therapist to consider the aims of the orthosis as the exercise will happen as patients wear the orthosis and functionally use their hand throughout the day. Before fabricating the orthosis, this is a good opportunity to use the simulated "relative motion pencil test" to be certain the orthosis is meeting your aims (Howell, 2016; Merritt & Howell, 2020). To address a PIP joint extension lag or encourage extension in a stiff PIP joint, try an RMF orthosis. To improve PIP joint flexion, an RME orthosis will block or limit MCP joint motion and direct the force of flexion to the stiff PIP joint aided by the adjacent digits. Relative motion exercise orthoses are practical as the patient simply wears the orthosis while going about daily activities incorporating exercise with routine hand use when the proper relative motion orthosis is selected. A relative motion orthosis worn as an "adaptive" orthosis generally does not require an exercise program, as the orthosis is being used to improve appearance or alignment.

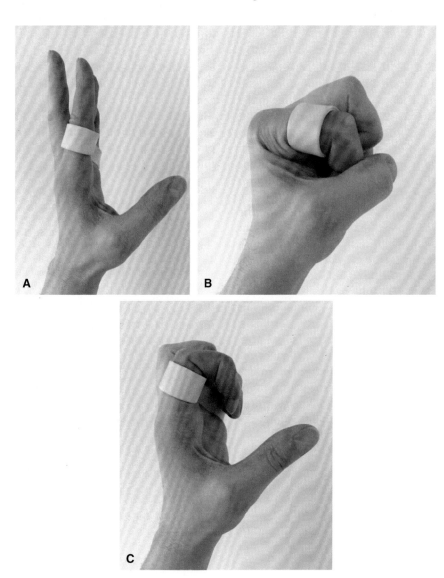

FIGURE 7–12 **A–C,** Active exercises: **(A)** composite finger extension, **(B)** composite finger flexion, and **(C)** hook fist.

CONCLUSION

The authors have presented the use of a finger-based orthosis to position the affected MCP joint(s) in relatively more extension or flexion, to utilize the concept of relative motion for management of a variety of hand conditions in protective, exercise, or adaptive fashion. The easily fabricated orthosis is generally made from a thermoplastic material, is simple in design, and encourages safe hand function. As long-term users of relative motion orthoses, Howell and Hirth have shared their tips for fabrication, rationale, and supporting evidence for clinical use of relative motion orthoses.

FIELD NOTE

Wyndell H. Merritt, MD, FACS
Virginia

In this surgeon's somewhat lengthy career, there have been two notable hand surgery management advances that have experienced slow acceptance, "wide awake" surgery[1] and "relative motion splinting."[2,3] These are related because the first allows convincing evidence verifying the second.[4] For example, temporary use of a single very weak 6-0 nylon suture to repair a long extensor tendon laceration under local anesthesia with epinephrine can easily be seen to remain intact with full active extension and almost full flexion while in a tongue blade simulated relative motion extension orthosis of 15° to 20° greater extension relative to its neighbors. This permits active motion and functional hand use and obviates adhesions.

The relative motion concept differs from other single digit splinting techniques by relying on the strong muscular forces in the forearm accomplished by varying the relationship between adjacent metacarpophalangeal joints. This is possible due to the so-called "quadriga effect," a term coined by Verdan in the 1960s[5] to explain the complication occurring when the flexor profundus tendon is sutured to the extensor digitorum communis over an amputation stump, creating an inability to fully flex the adjacent uninjured digits. "Quadriga" was the Roman name for the two-wheeled chariot used in their Olympics with the Greeks, with the charioteer and equidistant reins controlling the four horses. The charioteer muscles in this metaphor are the extensor digitorum communis, flexor profundi, and lumbrical muscles, with the reins their four tendons. This anatomic fact can be used to increase or abolish tension on these tendons (the "reins") for a variety of conditions, as well outlined in the chapter by Howell and Hirth.[4] They very cleverly subdivide use of the relative motion concept into three categories: protective orthoses, exercise orthoses, and adaptive orthoses. Our greatest experience so far has been protective, with convincing demonstration of its benefit for long extensor repair and acute sagittal band rupture in Howell, Hirth, and O'Brien's scoping review of 375 cases, with no ruptures or chronic pain syndromes reported with this management method clearly providing significantly less morbidity with earlier recovery of range of motion and return to work,[6] and possibly better outcomes. Its protective use in boutonniere deformity is more recent and less well established, but this surgeon's use for acute and chronic boutonniere has been very encouraging. It seems likely that this will produce a paradigm shift in management of chronic boutonniere deformity, which has previously been prolonged PIP immobilization. We have had excellent results with less severe chronic boutonniere deformity, having no more than 45° of fixed deformity following serial casting to neutral and use of relative motion flexion orthoses for 3 months, and after acute boutonniere repairs using relative motion flexion orthoses for 6 weeks. The exercise use of this technique for stiff PIP joints and adaptive orthoses to prevent deformities is evolving rapidly and is promising. The beauty of this technique is that while in the splint, the patients use their hand in daily activities and are constantly performing their own therapy through active use, while retaining function. It is a simple concept that requires a reduced commitment to formal therapy and may someday also prove useful to prevent finger deformities in burns and rheumatoid arthritis patients.

References

1. Lalonde, D. H. (2016). Extensor tendon repair of the finger. In *Wide awake hand surgery* (chap. 35, p. 209). CRC Press, Taylor & Francis Group.
2. Merritt, W. H., Howell, J. W., Tune, R., Saunders, S., & Hardy, M. (2000). Achieving immediate active motion by using the relative motion splinting after long extensor repair and sagittal band ruptures with tendon subluxation. *Operative Techniques in Plastic and Reconstructive Surgery, 7*, 31–37.
3. Hirth, M. J., Howell, J. W., & O'Brien, L. (2016). Relative motion orthoses in the management of various hand conditions: A scoping review. *Journal of Hand Therapy, 29*, 405–432.
4. Merritt, W. H. (2014). Relative motion splint: Active motion after extensor tendon injury and repair. *Journal of Hand Surgery, 39*, 1187–1194.
5. Verdan, C. (1960). Syndrome of the quadriga. *Surgical Clinics of North America, 40*, 425–426.
6. Hirth, M. J., Bennett, K., Mah, E., Farrow, H. C., Cavallo, A. V., Ritz, M., & Findlay, M. W. (2011). Early return to work and improved range of motion with immobilization splinting for zones V and VI extensor tendon repairs. *Hand Therapy, 16*, 86–94.

CHAPTER REVIEW QUESTIONS

1. True or False. The concept of relative motion is based on a relationship created by positioning the MCP joint(s) to affect excursion of multiple tendons shared by a single muscle.

2. Muscle-tendon units that have been demonstrated to be affected by the "quadriga effect" include which of the following? Select all that apply.
   a. (a) Flexor digitorum superficialis, (b) extensor digitorum communis, (c) extensor digiti minimi, (d) extensor digitorum indicis, (e) lumbrical, or (f) flexor digitorum profundus.

3. During RMF orthosis fabrication, on what surface, (a) dorsal or (b) volar of the involved digit is the thermoplastic placed?

4. Match the suggested relative angle of involved MCP joint position with the condition managed. (Select all that apply.)

Angle	Condition
a. 25°-30°	1. Extensor tendon IV-VII repairs
b. 15°-20°	2. Boutonniere deformity
c. 20°-35°	3. Sagittal band injury/repair
d. Best angle to produce the desired effect	4. Active tendon lag due to adhesions

5. True or False. The authors suggest that prior to use of an RMF orthosis, a PIP joint passive contracture of 20° or more with suspected boutonniere deformity be serial casted to reduce the contracture first.

6. In what position of relativity is the affected MCP joint(s) placed when RME is used?

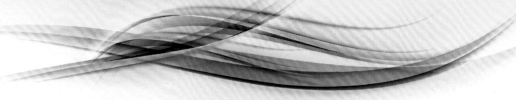

8 Upper Extremity Prosthetics

Debra Ann Latour, OTD, MEd, OTR/L

CHAPTER OBJECTIVES

After study of this chapter, the reader should be able to:
- Differentiate between various levels of upper extremity amputation relative to function.
- Identify the characteristics including the advantages and disadvantages of various upper extremity prosthetic devices.
- Provide examples for therapeutic intervention.
- Explain why individuals with upper limb acquired loss or congenital differences are likely to develop secondary physical and psychosocial conditions.

KEY TERMS

Activity-specific devices
Biofeedback
Body-powered prosthesis
Componentry
Electrodes
Externally powered prosthesis
Harness
Hook elastics
Hybrid prosthesis

Interprofessional
Osseointegration
Overuse syndrome
Passive functional aesthetic device
Pattern recognition
Phantom pain
Phantom sensation
Prosthesis
Prosthosis
Radio-frequency identification (RFID)

Residual limb
Socket
Scapular cutaneous anchor technology
Targeted muscle reinnervation (TMR)
Terminal device (TD)
3D-printed device
Upper limb loss or difference (ULL/D)
Voluntary-closing (V-C)
Voluntary-opening (V-O)

FAQ

How long does it take to receive a prosthesis?

It can take several months from the time of evaluation to delivery of the final, definitive prosthesis. Much of this wait time is due to insurance authorization. A prosthesis is custom-made for each individual; fabrication time for a working prototype can be accomplished within a few days to a few weeks, depending on the level of absence and componentry used.

When is it helpful to start therapy?

Therapy should commence as early as possible. Therapy input to the prosthetic prescription may reveal information about the client and related factors, such as lifestyle, responsibilities, and learning that may be helpful to determine the best options for prosthetic technology and aid in justifying need toward reimbursement.

What to do when the prosthesis breaks?

Notify the prosthetist immediately!

Why is a prosthesis so costly when a 3D device is so inexpensive?

Prosthetic components are like other medical devices in which the unseen costs of product research, development, and protection of the intellectual property are absorbed into the pricing. Comparing to 3D-printed devices seems a bit out of irrelevant: the material used in the AM products are often brittle and not robust. Many require replacement within 2 weeks. Comparatively, a body-powered prosthesis can last years, and even decades with minor repairs.

Will the prosthesis function like a natural hand?

No, it will not function the same as the natural hand but will offer much function. With practice, movements become smooth and almost effortless.

What is meant by "social function"?

We use our hands for many social functions: for example, when we talk, we gesture; we greet each other with a handshake or an embrace. Much of our social presence relates to how we function in public. One of the most common social activities involves eating, so being able to serve oneself, cut food, and pour a drink are forms of social function.

Does the prosthesis ever feel like it is a part of the person? How does the user embody a prosthesis?

Yes, it can become integrated into the user's perception of themselves. It is a complex process that requires time and trust. I often use the analogy that a prosthesis is like getting to know a person. When we first meet, we are acquaintances. We do not "know" each other. As time goes on, we become more familiar with each other, and a friendship likely develops. With more time and experience, we may become best friends. With a prosthesis, we must get to know it, understand how it works, and how it can help us. We learn to take care of it. Over time, we begin to value it and to trust. Hopefully, it becomes our "friend"; at some point, it becomes a part of us, and we identify with its presence on our bodies and in our function.

INTRODUCTION: WHAT IS PROSTHETIC REHABILITATION?

Prosthetic rehabilitation encompasses many factors and is not limited to the training vital to the successful use of prosthetic technology. Whether an individual has lost a limb or is born with a congenital difference, he or she is likely to contemplate using a prosthesis. Some common misconceptions include the following:

- Prosthetic training begins with the delivery of the device to the user.
- A prosthesis has a custom socket, but the other components are standard, similar to an "off-the-shelf" product.
- Individuals with upper limb loss or congenital difference follow the same rehabilitation pathway as other upper extremity injuries or conditions.

The therapist needs to have a clear understanding of the many facets of prosthetic rehabilitation, which include the presentation of the population, the diverse technologies, and the phases of care

(Latour & Vacek, 2019). Refer to Box 8–1 for definitions of key terms used in this specialty. Prosthetic training typically occurs as part of interprofessional collaboration and begins well before the delivery of any technology. The person with limb loss or limb difference needs to prepare in advance of delivery, for successful control and application of this control related to functional activities. A prosthesis typically consists of a custom-made socket that interfaces with other components, such as a forearm, upper arm, joint mechanism, terminal device, and harness to form the prosthesis (Fig. 8–1A–D). Each prosthesis is individually fabricated for its users. Preparation for the device includes:

- Educating regarding the different technology options
- Preparing the residual limb to tolerate the socket, harnessing, and prosthesis weight and length
- Developing adaptive strategies

Individuals with limb loss/difference present differently, even though levels of limb loss may be similar. Individual client factors should be considered in the selection of relevant technology, including all components, and during the various phases of care.

BOX 8–1 DEFINITIONS OF PROSTHETIC KEY TERMS

Activity-specific devices: terminal device intended for a function or types of functions; often oriented to activities of daily living, work, and recreation.

Biofeedback: a training technique by which a person learns how to regulate certain muscle functions; used to develop myoelectric control of the prosthesis.

Body-powered prosthesis: prosthesis that is controlled or powered by body movement.

Componentry: elements that are used to fabricate the prosthesis.

Electrodes: conductors through which muscle electricity is transmitted to control prosthetic technology.

Externally powered prosthesis: prosthesis that is controlled or powered outside of the body; also referred to as myoelectric prosthesis.

Harness: strapping used to suspend or to help to control the prosthesis.

Hook elastics: elastic bands used to control a voluntary-opening terminal device on a body-powered prosthesis.

Hybrid prosthesis: prosthesis with mixed components that are controlled or powered by the body and external to the body.

Interprofessional: refers to the group of individual practitioners from diverse disciplines who collaborate, contribute knowledge, skills, and experiences to offer optimized care for patients/clients.

Osseointegration: the structural link at which human bone and the surface of a synthetic, often titanium-based, implant meet.

Overuse syndrome: type of injury common to the contralateral side among individuals with upper limb acquired loss or congenital difference, caused by repetitive movements or awkward postures; also known as repetitive strain injury (RSI). Symptoms include swelling, pain, and weakness in the affected joints.

Passive functional aesthetic device: static prosthesis that appears to look like a hand; functions include stabilizing, supporting, and social tasks.

Pattern recognition: control requires a set of myoelectric signals, corresponding to possible prosthesis movement, recorded and used to calibrate the control system.

Phantom pain: pain that feels like it is coming from an absent body part; once believed to be psychological, is now recognized that these sensations are real, and originate in the spinal cord and brain.

Phantom sensation: sensation that an amputated or missing limb is still attached.

Prosthesis (px): an artificial device to replace or augment a missing part of the body.

Prosthosis: a hybrid device accessing the qualities and/or functions of a prosthesis and an orthosis for a retained limb with lost/impaired function.

Radio-frequency identification (RFID): a type of wireless communication that typically involves an RFID reader and a tag. The tag has information stored in its memory, and the reader (using an antenna) can read this information.

Residual limb: the remnant limb of a congenital difference or following amputation.

Socket: the part of the prosthetic device that is in contact with the body.

Scapular cutaneous anchor technology: an alternative for the traditional harness.

Targeted muscle reinnervation (TMR): surgical procedure in which residual nerves from the amputated limb are transferred to reinnervate new muscle targets.

Terminal device (TD): component of an upper extremity prosthesis that substitutes for the functions of the hand. There are many types of terminal devices; they may be static or dynamic, accessing voluntary-opening and/or voluntary-closing actions.

3D-printed device: a three-dimensional device that resembles a prosthesis, fabricated from computer-aided manufacturing (CAM); also called additive manufacturing.

Voluntary-closing (V-C): terminal device oriented in the open position; user must actuate to close the device.

Voluntary-opening (V-O): terminal device oriented in the closed position; user must actuate to open the device.

WHAT IS MEANT BY INTERPROFESSIONAL COLLABORATIVE PRACTICE?

The goal of interprofessional (IP) practice is to develop integrated, high-quality, team-oriented healthcare practitioners to provide client-centered care (Nash, Fabius, Skoufalos, Clarke, & Horowitz, 2016). The team that treats individuals with **upper limb loss or difference** (ULL/D) must possess knowledge about the person and understand the diverse upper extremity prosthetic technology to facilitate success.

The team members consist of the client with the ULL/D, family members, physician, prosthetist, hand therapist (occupational or physical), surgeon, case manager, or life care planner, psychologist, and the insurer/reimbursement source (Sheehan & Gondo, 2014; Wijdenes, Brouwers, & van der Sluis, 2016). An IP team approach combines expertise and experience, with members working collaboratively to promote the maximal level of independence for the individual. The primary goal of therapy is to provide the individual with the proper tools and techniques to regain

independence. The best results in upper extremity rehabilitation include IP collaboration and communication (Sheehan & Gondo, 2014; Wijdenes et al., 2016).

Specialized training that is contemporary and reflective of the new technology is often expensive and difficult to access. Courses and support are available directly from some of the manufacturers as well as from continuing education venues such as OccupationalTherapy.com and MedBridgeEducation.com. Information that relates to prosthetic training, as well as adaptive strategies and assistive devices using one hand or feet, can influence how individuals facilitate their maximal level of independence.

SPECIALIZED CARE

Individuals with ULL/D require specialized care, and practitioners addressing the needs of the population should be knowledgeable about the technology, the population, and collaborative dynamics. Box 8–2 offers insight into the questions that clients and practitioners should consider when choosing a prosthetist and therapist for an upper limb prosthesis and its associated training.

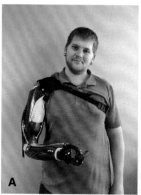 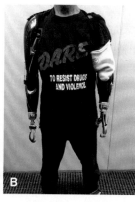 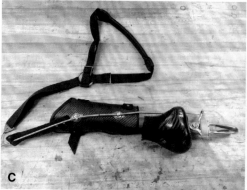 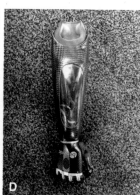

FIGURE 8–1 A, Body-powered prosthesis on user with unilateral loss. The prosthesis is an Ottobock ErgoArm (Duderstadt, Germany) with a Fillauer Quick Disconnect Wrist (Fillauer, LLC. Chattanooga, TN) and a ToughWare V2P™ voluntary-opening hook with shoulder saddle and chest strap (JMS, Neptune, NJ). **B,** This individual with (bilateral loss) is using body-powered technology. The right elbow disarticulation prosthesis features an elbow joint, wrist flexion unit, and voluntary-opening terminal device. The left transradial prosthesis features a wrist flexion unit and voluntary-closing terminal device (Fillauer 400HD Elbow, Sierra Wrist Flexion Units, Fillauer SS-555 as the right hook, and TRS Grip 2S as the left hook). **C,** This body-powered prosthesis features a figure-of-9 harness attached to the cable for control. The forearm is a custom design to accommodate the unique bulbous shape of the residual limb at the distal aspect (Fillauer 5×a voluntary-opening hook). **D,** This is the author's transradial externally powered prosthesis, fabricated with a window to view the inner componentry (Ottobock bebionic hand with COAPT Pattern Recognition Control [Duderstadt, Germany]).

BOX 8-2   QUESTIONS TO ASK PRACTITIONERS

What to Ask a Prosthetist

Are you certified by the American Board for Certification (ABC)?

Do you have a minimum of 5 y of current experience with upper limb prosthetic technology?

Have you fit more than 10 persons with upper limb loss/difference in the past year?

Can you specify what types of externally powered prostheses you have fit in the past 2 y?

Do you work collaboratively with therapists who have extensive experience with upper limb loss/difference?

Will you arrange for (your client) to speak with other clients to discuss their prosthetic experience regarding the care you provide?

Have you received training and certification from prosthetic component manufacturers?

What to Ask a Hand Therapist

Do you have a minimum of 5 y of current experience with upper limb prosthetic technology?

How many individuals with upper limb loss/difference have you worked with in the past year?

Can you specify what types of externally powered prostheses your clients have used during your interventions in the past 2 y?

Do you work collaboratively with a prosthetist who has extensive experience with upper limb loss/difference?

Will you arrange for (your client) to speak with other clients to discuss their prosthetic experience regarding the care you provide?

Have you participated in continuing education directed toward prosthetic rehabilitation?

Are you able to access consultation or mentorship from another therapy practitioner knowledgeable in this area?

Have you received training and certification from prosthetic component manufacturers?

BOX 8-3   TESTS AND MEASURES

Function, Control	Satisfaction Inventories	Pain, QOL
Assessment of Capacity for Myoelectric Control (ACMC)	Child Amputee Prosthetic Project: Prosthetic Satisfaction Inventory (PSI)	Disability of the Arm, Shoulder and Hand Measure (DASH, Quick DASH)
Assisting Hand Assessment (AHA)	OPUS-UEFS Satisfaction Subtest Rehabilitation Institute of Chicago (now Shirley Ryan Ability Lab)	Pizzi Holistic Wellness Assessment (PHWA)
Activities Measure for Upper Limb Amputees (AM-ULA) and Brief-AMULA	Prosthetic Upper Extremity Function Index (PUFI)	SF-36
Box and Blocks Test (BBT) and BBT-Modified	Trinity Amputation and Prosthetic Experience Scales (TAPES)	
Jebsen Standardized Test of Hand Function (JTHF)	McGann Client Feedback Form (MCFF)	
OPUS-Upper Extremity Function Status (UEFS)		
Prosthetic Upper Extremity Function Index (PUFI)		
Southampton Hand Assessment Procedure (SHAP)		
Unilateral Below Elbow Test (U-BET)		
University of New Brunswick Test of Prosthetic Function (UNB)		

This author conducted interviews with leading prosthetists specializing in ULL/D. When asked "What do you wish that therapists engaging in prosthetic rehabilitation knew and would do?" the prosthetists responded that better communication would be an asset, as well as spending more time on functional activities that are meaningful and individualized to the client, rather than general exercises. Several stated that improving awareness of posture, balance, and compensatory posturing is important, particularly as these relate to falls. Strategies should include how to safely fall whether wearing an upper-limb prosthesis or not. Others stated that the use of more relevant outcome measures would help with reporting findings and accessing funding for reimbursement related to the technology and training. Most stated that developing relationships with community therapists would be helpful particularly as hand therapy evaluations offer much information about the client that would be beneficial to the prosthetist as well. Refer to Box 8–3 for resources on specific upper extremity tests and measures.

The Role of the Prosthetist and Hand Therapist

The prosthetist's function is to provide well-fitting prosthetic devices, and the role of the hand therapist is to assist individuals to become independent users of their devices. The therapist can also help determine the most appropriate technology to be provided, to prepare the client to tolerate the device features and to assist the client to develop realistic expectations of the technology (Wijdenes et al., 2016). Unfortunately, only a small number of healthcare providers have extensive knowledge of the rehabilitation of the person with ULL/D, and most therapy practitioners encounter few individuals with upper extremity amputations (Corathers & Janczewski, 2006). Because of high productivity demands, rapidly developing new technologies, and the ever-changing reimbursement requirements, it is challenging for therapy practitioners to remain informed on contemporary prosthetic technology and surgical interventions (Wijdenes et al., 2016).

WHY IS PROSTHETIC REHABILITATION IMPORTANT FOR THE THERAPIST TO UNDERSTAND?

To answer this question, it is because of the numbers! Currently, an estimated 2 million Americans are living with limb loss or difference; approximately 185,000 amputations are occurring in the

United States each year (Amputee-Coalition, n.d.). Individuals with lower limb amputation outnumber those with upper limb loss (ULL) to a 1:4 ratio (Amputee-Coalition, n.d.). There are approximately 2,000 Americans who experience new upper limb amputations at, or proximal to, the wrist (Ziegler-Graham, MacKenzie, Ephraim, Travison, & Brookmeyer, 2008). Loss of one upper extremity at the transradial level (TR) is the second most common amputation.

The most common ULL is a partial amputation of one or more digits. Unfortunately, many individuals with partial hand amputations are lost to follow-up and many do not receive prosthetic technology. Knowledgeable hand therapists could inform the population of prosthetic options that may impact function and quality of life.

According to the literature, 75% of people with amputations use **prostheses** (Nielsen, 2002); however, rejection of a prosthesis occurs frequently. Primary reasons for rejection include a comfortable fit and access to prosthetic training Atkins, 2014). The prosthesis may be abandoned if it is uncomfortable, heavy, or if the wearer has not been properly prepared and trained to use the device (Atkins, 2014). Most prosthetic technology assists to restore participation in meaningful functional activities, as well as to improve body image and cosmesis (Williams, 2011).

Prosthesis use may also help to avert secondary conditions by employing the use of the contralateral limb (Ostlie, Franklin, Skjeldal, Skrondal, & Magnus, 2011). It is likely for individuals with ULL/D to be at risk to experience further impairment due to the overuse of the unaffected side. Pain and musculoskeletal impairment affecting the function of the unaffected arm in individuals with unilateral ULL/D has been well-documented (Burger & Vidmar, 2015; Jones & Davidson, 1999; Ostlie et al., 2011). Gambrell (2008) reviewed literature noting the important responsibility of all team members to prevent the development of an **overuse syndrome** and emphasized practitioner responsibility to educate clients on the likely risk of overuse and methods to limit its impact (Gambrell, 2008).

POPULATION HEALTH

In addition to the increasing population and the need for specialized knowledge, the idea of a population health approach is warranted. Many individuals who experience ULL/D reported that they received little to no information from medical professionals regarding these devices (Amputee-Coalition, n.d.). Contemporary standard medical treatments often exclude psychosocial interventions; however, interventions should address secondary conditions affecting physical and mental health.

A population health approach fosters the goals of wellness, well-being, and preventing disability or further impairment and promotes diverse models of health behavior changes that include educating the client, engaging them in meaningful endeavors that promote beneficial change, and ultimately empowering them. These concepts align well with prosthetic rehabilitation to understand the intervention options and the likelihood of secondary conditions that impact physical and mental health and empower healthier outcomes.

WHAT ARE THE CAUSES OF ACQUIRED LIMB LOSS AND CONGENITAL DIFFERENCE?

There are various causes of limb absence. Among children, the primary cause of limb absence is due to congenital anomaly, with smaller percentages relevant to disease and trauma. What causes the congenital difference is largely unknown, but a common thought is that vascular insufficiency or a vascular event causes anomaly to develop in utero. Among the adult population, 69% of upper limb losses result from trauma with the majority of these due to war (Dillingham, Pezzin, & MacKenzie, 2002). Other causes are a result of disease (27%); only 4% of adult upper limb absence is due to congenital difference (Dillingham et al., 2002). It is projected that the number of individuals living with limb loss will more than double by 2050, primarily due to the increase of vascular disorders (Dillingham et al., 2002; Ziegler-Graham et al., 2008).

DOES THE LEVEL OF LOSS/ DIFFERENCE HAVE AN IMPACT ON FUNCTION AND SATISFACTION?

Current terminology describes the level of amputation in anatomical terms. A loss at the joint level (wrist, elbow, or shoulder) is termed a disarticulation, while a midlevel loss between two joints would be referred to as a transsection, such as transradial (TR) or transhumeral (TH). Figure 8–2 depicts levels of limb absence with the likely prescription for technology components. The level of amputation directly correlates to function loss. A loss at a more proximal level requires more technology; this means that the device will need to hold substantially more weight, and each component will require control and power. Without the device, a person with a higher loss will likely be able to do less with the remnant, or **residual limb**. With a more distal loss, there is likely greater remaining functional ability of the extremity. Because less **componentry** is required, the device will weigh less and therefore less technology to control and power (Williams, 2011). Note that the weight also depends on the type of technology that is chosen to be used and all of its features.

JOINT DISARTICULATIONS

Of greater consequence are joint disarticulations, at or through the shoulder, elbow, or wrist. These levels present with challenges to fit with componentry that offers particular joint function and allows for symmetry to the uninvolved side. For example, if the residual limb is amputated through the elbow (or close to it), there is not enough space for a prosthetic elbow component. The likelihood is that the prosthetic device or the joint area will appear to be asymmetrical to the other side. In this case, one might present with a prosthetic elbow that is a few inches lower than the contralateral limb.

Regardless of level, prostheses help to compensate for lost movements, but limitations will always remain. Consider the steps involved to cut food using a knife and fork as performed by an individual with two hands, and two individuals with unilateral ULL, one at the TH level and the other at the TR level, who are using body-powered prostheses. The person with a TH level of loss will likely need to use a prosthesis with a locking elbow mechanism to secure the joint in a fixed position, while the person with a TR loss can access natural elbow movement for function. In addition, the type of terminal device will influence positioning and grasp of the utensil. Refer to Figure 8–3A,B to appreciate the positioning of a fork in voluntary-opening and voluntary-closing of a terminal device.

TRANSSECTIONAL LOSS

The individual with the TH loss must position and lock the elbow in flexion, and manually rotate the **terminal device** (TD) to the palm-up position with the sound side. The user may have wrist

Prescription guide

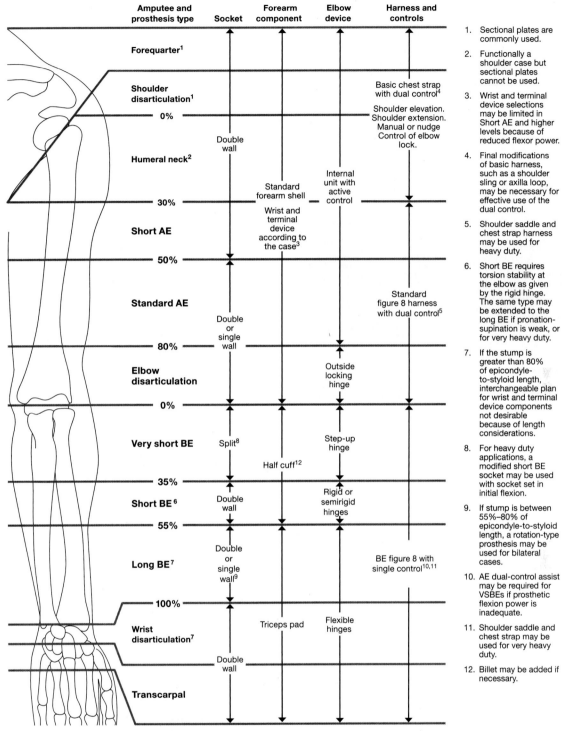

Amputee and prosthesis type	Socket	Forearm component	Elbow device	Harness and controls
Forequarter[1]				
Shoulder disarticulation[1]				Basic chest strap with dual control[4]
0%				Shoulder elevation. Shoulder extension. Manual or nudge Control of elbow lock.
Humeral neck[2]	Double wall		Internal unit with active control	
30%		Standard forearm shell		
Short AE		Wrist and terminal device according to the case[3]		
50%				
Standard AE	Double or single wall			Standard figure 8 harness with dual control[5]
80%				
Elbow disarticulation			Outside locking hinge	
0%				
Very short BE	Split[8]		Step-up hinge	
		Half cuff[12]		
35%	Double wall		Rigid or semirigid hinges	
Short BE[6]				
55%				
Long BE[7]	Double or single wall[9]			BE figure 8 with single control[10,11]
100%				
Wrist disarticulation[7]		Triceps pad	Flexible hinges	
	Double wall			
Transcarpal				

1. Sectional plates are commonly used.
2. Functionally a shoulder case but sectional plates cannot be used.
3. Wrist and terminal device selections may be limited in Short AE and higher levels because of reduced flexor power.
4. Final modifications of basic harness, such as a shoulder sling or axilla loop, may be necessary for effective use of the dual control.
5. Shoulder saddle and chest strap harness may be used for heavy duty.
6. Short BE requires torsion stability at the elbow as given by the rigid hinge. The same type may be extended to the long BE if pronation-supination is weak, or for very heavy duty.
7. If the stump is greater than 80% of epicondyle-to-styloid length, interchangeable plan for wrist and terminal device components not desirable because of length considerations.
8. For heavy duty applications, a modified short BE socket may be used with socket set in initial flexion.
9. If stump is between 55%–80% of epicondyle-to-styloid length, a rotation-type prosthesis may be used for bilateral cases.
10. AE dual-control assist may be required for VSBEs if prosthetic flexion power is inadequate.
11. Shoulder saddle and chest strap may be used for very heavy duty.
12. Billet may be added if necessary.

FIGURE 8-2 Prescription guide with segmental loss descriptors helps guide the therapist to proper selection for prosthetic intervention depending on the level of loss. (Table Courtesy of Fillauer, LLC. Chattanooga, TN.)

technology that allows flexion and extension (improving mid-line access), typically operated manually with the intact hand. Conversely, an individual with TR loss can demonstrate full shoulder and elbow function and may have some forearm movement to complete activities of daily living (ADLs). The ability to flex and extend the elbow, and access forearm movement, offers an advantage. The level of amputation appears to impact function regardless of prosthesis use.

PHANTOM SENSATION AND PHANTOM PAIN

Individuals with amputations often experience **phantom sensation** and/or **phantom pain**. It is important to assure them that phantom sensations and pain are to be expected and are normal. Phantom sensation occurs when the individual feels as if the nonexistent limb is still present and may feel like a tingling sensation. *Phantom*

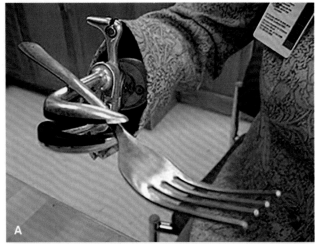

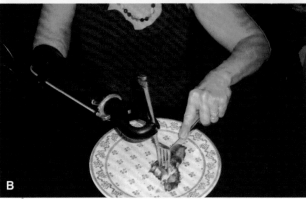

FIGURE 8–3 A, Positioning of a fork in a voluntary-opening of the terminal device (Fillauer, LLC. Chattanooga, TN). **B,** Voluntary-closing of the terminal device (TRS Prosthetics, Boulder, CO). Function is greatly enhanced with proper training of using these terminal devices.

sensation diminishes over time. *Phantom pain* is different from phantom sensation and is not well understood. Commonly an individual will experience phantom pain soon after amputation but the pain will diminish over time. Approximately 80% of individuals with an amputation experience phantom pain (Amputee-Coalition, n.d.). Interventions that may diminish phantom pain include the use of a prosthesis, desensitization, mirror therapy, medications, nerve blocks, and virtual reality activities. Another option is targeted muscle intervention, discussed later in this chapter.

WHAT ARE THE COMPONENTS TO PROSTHETIC TECHNOLOGY AND WHAT IS THEIR FUNCTION?

Before delving into the phases of prosthetic rehabilitation, it is important to fully understand the technology itself, appreciate what it can do, and develop realistic expectations for both the practitioner and the client. Although the prosthesis is technically a replacement for missing anatomy, a single device cannot duplicate the function, reliability, and aesthetic quality provided by the natural human upper limb (Atlas of Amputations and Limb Deficiencies, 2004, 2016).

PROSTHETIC TECHNOLOGY AND FUNCTIONAL ABILITY

Prosthetic technology can improve functional abilities. To many, it is considered to be a "tool," but there is a perspective of embodiment

in which the prosthesis is assimilated into the perception of "self" (Murray, 2005, 2009). Whether the prosthesis is a tool or a perception of self, successful integration depends on a combination of realistic expectations, personal motivation, and specialized training (Bouwsema, Van Der Sluis, & Bongers, 2014).

Each type of prosthesis is fabricated from a selection of diverse componentry that is manufactured from different sources. While some of these components might match well to those created by other manufacturers, some components work only with technology made from the same manufacturer. The experienced prosthetist is well-versed with these limitations and opportunities; they consider these factors when creating the device for each individual. Table 8–1 outlines the basic features, advantages, and disadvantages of each prosthetic option.

THE SOCKET

The socket is probably the most important component of the prosthesis, because it intimately fits over the user's residual limb. This establishes the connection between the prosthesis and the individual's body, and it is through the socket that the user receives "contact" (information such as vibration) with objects to discern some of their features (such as texture, weight, size). The prosthetist fabricates the socket from an exact mold of the residual limb, modifying it to accommodate bony prominences and sensitive areas. Materials such as carbon graphite, flexible thermoplastics, and silicone are used to make a socket that is comfortable, light, and durable (Smith, Michael, & Bowker, 2004; Krajbich & Potter, 2016). Typically, several sockets will be fabricated and trialed in a prototype before the final device is delivered. This helps to increase wearing tolerance and acceptance and facilitates reshaping of the residual limb. Figure 8–4 depicts the socket of a prosthesis.

THE LINERS

Some individuals with ULL/D use liners that offer comfort and/or suspension of the prosthesis. Liners may be a sock or fabricated from materials such as, or similar to, silicone. Some liners incorporate a pin-lock system to keep the prosthesis on the residual limb as illustrated in Figure 8–5. Some individuals prefer a "skin fit" socket, opting not to wear a liner or sock of any sort.

THE HARNESS

The harness suspends the prosthesis and captures power from the body to operate the prosthesis (Smith et al., 2004). The **body-powered prosthesis** always requires harnessing; however, most users complain about harnessing discomfort and it is one of the reasons for prosthetic abandonment. The most common types of harnessing are figure-of-8, figure-of-9, and a chest strap (Fig. 8–6A–C).

The figure-of-8 harness (Fig. 8–6A) typically includes a triceps cuff that supports the posterior upper arm; the harness itself passes over the shoulder, across the back, and under the contralateral shoulder (Smith et al., 2004).

The figure-of-9 harness (Fig. 8–6B) omits the triceps cuff; the harness travels along the dorsum of the extremity and then across the back to the contralateral shoulder. Both the figure-of-8 and the figure-of-9 harness systems have an axilla loop on the sound side that is commonly uncomfortable and can cause numbness and nerve compression, making the user even more susceptible to overuse issues (Smith et al., 2004; Krajbich & Potter, 2016).

TABLE 8–1	Features Versus Advantages and Disadvantages of Prosthetic Options	
Prosthetic Option	**Advantages**	**Disadvantages**
No prosthesis	• Maintain full proprioception, sensation • Ability if technology is in disrepair • No costs for prosthetic technology	• Limited functional ability • Difficult to perform bimanual tasks • Need for assistive devices • May contribute to stigma, awkward social situations • Secondary conditions due to long-term unilateral upper limb (UL) use, adaptive or compensatory strategies
Passive prosthesis	• Lightweight • Minimal (if any) harnessing • No cables • Low maintenance • Static function: support, stabilize, push, type • Typically a hand which offers social function, aesthetic appearance	• No prehension • Difficult to perform bimanual tasks • Likely to discolor • Not robust • Typically a hand which interferes with visual access, may be "klunky"
Activity-specific prosthesis	• Lightweight • Minimal (if any) harnessing • No cables • Static function: support, stabilize, push, pull, may rotate, grasp • Quick to disconnect • Crossover functional purposes • Robust • Reduced maintenance, costs	• Limited relevance to broad range of functions • Need to change TD • May not be aesthetically appealing
Body-powered prosthesis	• Robust construction and function • Reduced maintenance, cost • Easy access to repair • Proprioception • Strong grip force (V-C) • Efficient, ergonomic, and intuitive operation (V-C) • Access to fine motor prehension with hook • Easily reimbursable	• Restrictive/uncomfortable harness • Poor aesthetics • Restrictive functional work area due to harness • Limited grip force (V-O) • Resistance to open V-O • Limited visual access with hand
Externally powered prosthesis	• Less restrictive work area • Social function relative to aesthetic presentation • Increased grip force • Absent or limited use of harnessing • Increased comfort • Contemporary appeal • Interchangeable components	• Battery maintenance • Increased weight • Not robust • Susceptible to damage from moisture, dust, moderate activity • Increased cost • Battery life before recharging is required • Difficult reimbursement

Adapted from Latour, D., & Vacek, K. (2019). Introduction to splinting: A clinical reasoning and problem-solving approach (p. 465). St. Louis, MO: Elsevier Inc.
Note: Prosthetic technology is uniquely fabricated for each user: sockets are custom made to accommodate individual's residual limb; choice of componentry is chosen relative to individual needs, presentation.

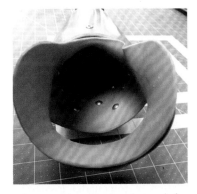

FIGURE 8–4 Externally powered prosthesis socket made from soft silicone materials. The socket is an essential piece of the prosthetic limb, because it is the point of interface between the residual segment and the prosthesis itself. The way it fits on to the residual limb will have a great impact on patient usage and compliance. Therefore, pressure and force distribution must be a focus during fitting and training.

The chest strap (Fig. 8–6C) offers an alternative method of harnessing. This travels across the back, under the contralateral axilla, and across the chest. More information on harnessing and options is found in the body-powered prosthetic section of this chapter.

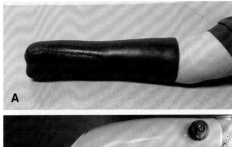
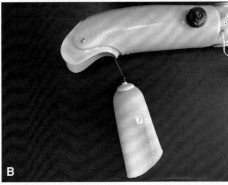

FIGURE 8–5 **A,** Custom silicone liner which plays an important role in proper fit and function of the prosthetic device (Custom Liner manufactured by Handspring Clinical Services, Middletown, NY). **B,** Prosthesis with a pin-lock liner (Iceross® Upper-X Liner with lanyard pull, Ossur, Canada) offers another way to suspend a prosthesis on the residual limb.

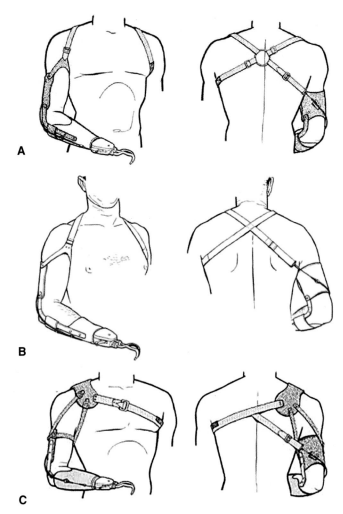

FIGURE 8-6 A, Illustration of the figure-of-8 design and **(B)** the figure-of-9 design. **C,** This image illustrates the chest harnessing strapping system. (Retrieved from www.oandplibrary.org.)

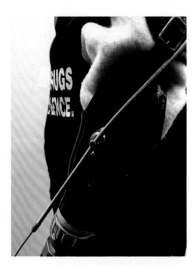

FIGURE 8-7 A cable and forearm prosthesis for an individual with transradial loss; note the position of the cable on the device and as it moves proximally to the triceps cuff. This allows it to actuate the terminal device without interfering with elbow movement.

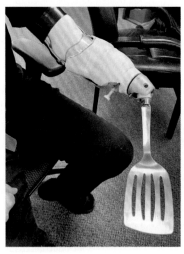

FIGURE 8-8 An activity-specific terminal device with a prototype prosthesis (Texas Assistive Devices, N-Abler V™ Wrist Unit with spatula terminal device, Brazoria, TX).

THE CABLE

The cable helps to access power from body movement to activate the terminal device in a mechanical prosthesis. The cable is routed from the harness through a housing to the terminal device or elbow (Krajbich & Potter, 2016). Cables often break or fray, requiring replacement. Many prosthetists provide a few spare cables to the user for easy and timely repair. More information on cables and cable options can be found in the Body-Powered Prosthesis section (Fig. 8–7).

THE TERMINAL DEVICE

The terminal device (TD) is the distal component and most often appears in the form of a hand or a utilitarian hook. Activity-specific terminal devices may look like tools or have unique features that allow the user to accomplish designated tasks or engage in an activity (Fig. 8–8).

ELBOW COMPONENTS

Elbow components offer flexion and extension and may be body-powered or externally powered. The body-powered options may require a shoulder shrug or ballistic forward flexion to activate, or there may be a pull switch or locking mechanism operated manually by the other hand. Electric options may offer more efficient and less unnatural movement, but these components add weight to the prosthesis.

SHOULDER COMPONENTS

Shoulder joints are also available for body-powered and myoelectric control, but the movements offered are limited to forward flexion/extension and internal/external rotation. The body-powered technology is controlled by a nudge switch or scapular movement. Similar to the elbow technology, the electric shoulder may offer intrinsic control but will add substantial weight to the prosthesis. Cumulatively, the **externally powered prosthesis** for a person with shoulder disarticulation or forequarter loss could weigh 5 to 10 pounds.

PROSTHETIC OPTIONS

There are six general categories of prosthetic options for the person with ULL/D. The options include:

1. no prosthesis
2. **passive functional aesthetic** prosthesis
3. **activity-specific prosthesis**
4. cable-driven body-powered prosthesis

5. externally powered, electrically controlled prosthesis with myoelectric sensors and specialized switches
6. **hybrid prosthesis** that may combine various types of controls

Regardless of the type of prosthesis being used, or not used, acceptance is a key factor to integrated use and success in function. Acceptance is related to the level of the limb absence, realistic functional expectation, socket and harness comfort, the confidence of the prosthetist-provider, and access to a knowledgeable hand therapist. Cosmesis or aesthetic appearance of the technology appears to be a less mitigating factor for most users (Stark, 2020).

NO PROSTHESIS

Wearing no prosthesis is always an option; each person with ULL/D should be instructed to adaptive strategies and assistive devices that enable the independent function in self-care, meal preparation, and home management tasks. For some individuals, not wearing a prosthesis may be the best or the only option. If a patient presents with residual limb hypersensitivity, soft-tissue adhesions, and excessive scarring, they may not be able to tolerate the prosthesis (Meier & Atkins, 2004). Other reasons for prosthetic rejection include limited usefulness, weight, and residual limb and socket discomfort (Hill et al., 2009; Wright, 2009; McFarland, Hubbard Winkler, Heinemann, & Esquenazi, 2010).

The advantages of not wearing a prosthesis include increased proprioceptive and sensory input (Fig. 8–9). Disadvantages include limited functional ability, bimanual task difficulty, and the potential for development of overuse syndrome, nerve entrapment, or vascular damage in the contralateral limb (Jones & Davidson, 1999) (Gambrell, 2008; Ostlie et al., 2011). The reasons some individuals do not wear prostheses can be many, but some of the more common reasons include:

- uninformed or misinformed about prosthesis options
- negative prior experience with prosthetic technology or training
- lack funds or support to justify insurance authorization
- reluctant to undergo surgery for optimal prosthetic fit and reduction of hypersensitivity (Amputee-Coalition, n.d.)

PASSIVE FUNCTIONAL AESTHETIC PROSTHESIS

A passive aesthetic prosthesis is a device that appears to look like the natural hand or digit but is static in nature. In the case of individuals with partial hand loss, a passive prosthesis can be a common option for amputation distal to the elbow because likely they have retained elbow, forearm, and wrist movement. An example of a passive aesthetic digit can be seen in Figure 8–10. This prosthetic offers social function, because it blends in with the other digits and makes the partial digit that is lost, less evident. This can also preserve the function of the residual anatomy, minimizing migration into the space that is no longer occupied (Fig. 8–10A–G).

The passive functional aesthetic terminal device may be a component in a hybrid prosthesis for a person with more proximal loss such as at the TH, shoulder, or forequarter levels.

While these terminal devices may appear to be aesthetic, they also provide some degree of function, such as to support, stabilize, push objects, and offer social function. In addition, digits of a passive prosthesis may be fit with armatures (tiny wires) that

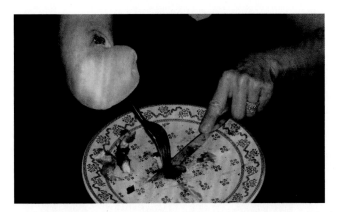

FIGURE 8–9 The task of cutting food is being carried out without a prosthesis.

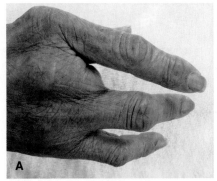 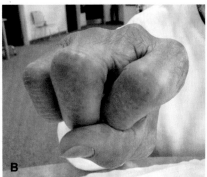

FIGURE 8–10 A, Note the migration of the index finger with the loss of the middle finger (extension). **B,** When digital flexion is attempted, you can appreciate the strain on the radial collateral ligaments of the index finger, and over time, this will lead to instability and discomfort at the index finger metacarpophalangeal (MCP) joint. **C,** A passive aesthetic functional digit, dorsal view; note the creases on the dorsum of the proximal interphalangeal (PIP) joint and the detail to the nail to closely match the adjacent digit; **(D)** volar view. **E,** Light functional movement is shown as the user is making "heart hands." **F and G,** Multiple aesthetic prostheses are used for light functional grasp and release to compensate for the loss of the thumb, index, and middle digits. The aesthetic prostheses also aid in improving cosmetic appearance of the hand (High Definition Silicone Restoration, Prosthetic Artworks LLC. Dingmans Ferry, PA).

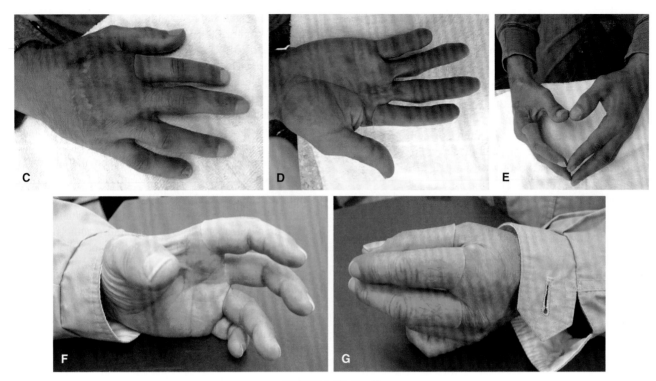

FIGURE 8–10 Cont'd

can be adjusted to assist with activities, such as typing, carrying a lightweight object (wallet or document), or operating the gearshift in an automobile. A passive hand prosthesis is often used as the first prosthesis for children as young as 4 months of age, because it offers symmetry, weight-bearing, and access to the midline. The passive functional aesthetic prosthesis has many benefits including its lighter weight, minimal (if any) harnessing, lack of cables, natural appearance, and low maintenance. Disadvantages include a lack of active grasp and difficulty performing some bimanual tasks (McFarland et al., 2010).

ACTIVITY-SPECIFIC PROSTHESIS

Many individuals are interested in being able to engage in a particular activity or complete a specific task. Sometimes the therapist can fabricate a tool out of thermoplastic or other material that can be attached to a cuff or to the existing TD to serve a specific function. At other times, collaboration with the prosthetist may be necessary to obtain a specific TD or a more individualized/sophisticated adaptation. Activity-specific upper limb prosthetic technology is typically static. The terminal device attaches to the forearm unit at the wrist and allows the function to perform specific activities that may include personal care tasks such as feeding and grooming; instrumental tasks such as cooking, woodworking, and gardening; and diverse recreational activities (TRS, n.d.) (Fig. 8–11A–C).

Crossover Functionality

Some of the devices have "crossover" functions. For example, a device used for bicycling may also be used to grasp the handles of

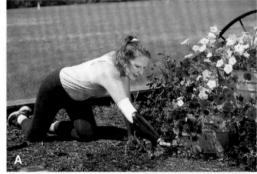

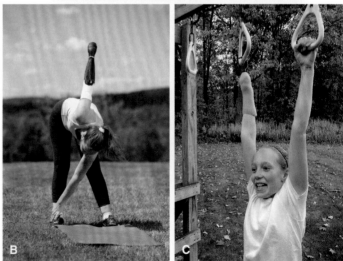

FIGURE 8–11 **A-C,** Activity-specific prosthesis depicting functional envelope (Texas Assistive Devices, N-Abler II™ wrist unit with Hand Cultivator terminal device, Brazoria, TX).

TABLE 8–2	Activity-specific Devices With Crossover Function		
Device	**Action**	**TRS Primary Design Use**	**Crossover**
Criterium Series	• Grasps handles with small to medium diameter • Pivot allows steering, improved control	• Biking (road and flat land)	• Pushing/pulling • Sweeping/raking • Steering
Dragon	• Can secure manage poled style handles through the "donut hole" • Loosely interacts with objects • Allows freedom of movement	• Martial arts	• Home management • Property management • Climbing • Steering
Helix	• Molded, high-performance, polyurethane, "DNA" helical shape • Replicates holding action of the hand in the control of short or long cylindrical handles grips • Unique strength and flexibility; "feels" like the hand and forearm with "reflexive," energy capture, storage and release action.	• Vocational-avocational prosthetic device	• Especially useful in any activity-specific task that uses long handles or "sticks" like lacrosse, hockey (ice, street, and field), raking, shoveling, garden tools. In addition to smaller garden tools, water hose control • Many undiscovered "uses"
ISHI and F-ISHI	• Adjustable grasp • Secure, stable with strap	Archery Fishing	Grooming Holding handled objects
Multi-D	• Adjustable grasp • Secure, stable with strap • Larger • More robust	• Multipurpose	• Home management • Yard work • Holding larger handled objects • Fishing (salt water)
Swinger	Loosely interfaces with objects Allows freedom of movement	Gymnastics	Carrying Climbing Steering Fishing
Raptor	High strength, large "#7"-shaped titanium lifting and supporting terminal device with replaceable, protective tip for cushion and nonmarring applications and greater friction control over surfaces. Unique pivot action increases versatility in lifting, supporting, climbing, etc.	Indoor and outdoor rock and gym climbing	Heavy duty lifting and transport and loading tasks. Handling lifting veneer woods, panels, or similar

Reprinted from TRS Prosthetics. (2019). **TRS high performance prosthetics product catalog.** *Retrieved from https://www.trsprosthetics.com/wp-content/uploads/2019/01/Web-Catalog-JANUARY2019.pdf.*

a shopping cart, stroller, or even a lawnmower, thus enhancing the functional envelope of the technology. Table 8–2 reviews specific devices that offer crossover functions (TRS, n.d.). Activity-specific devices are often robust, lightweight, and offer quick release. The activity-specific prosthesis typically does not require harnessing or cables and requires low maintenance. The activity-specific prosthesis may be suspended with a pin-lock style of a liner (Fig. 8–5B) or a neoprene sleeve.

CABLE DRIVE—BODY-POWERED PROSTHESIS

The **body-powered prosthesis** is a relatively lightweight yet sturdy device that offers prehension. Figure 8–12A–C demonstrates examples of body-actuated prosthetic technology for an individual with partial hand loss. Such technology can offer the function to perform diverse activities necessary for self-care, home management, and navigating the community for work and recreation.

For individuals with more proximal loss, body motion that typically arises from the contralateral shoulder powers the terminal device. Elbow function for individuals with higher level loss may be actuated by a shoulder shrug of the involved limb. These

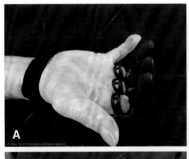
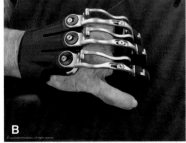
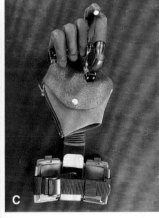

FIGURE 8–12 A and B, Body-actuated partial hand device (Naked Prosthetics MCPDrivers™). **C,** Externally powered partial hand (i-Digits™ Quantum-Ossur, Ossur, Canada).

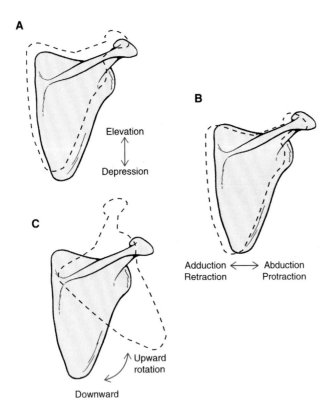

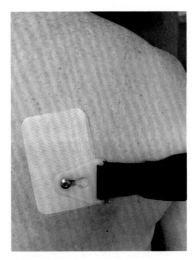

FIGURE 8–14 A scapular cutaneous anchor connected to the prosthesis with transradial application.

FIGURE 8–13 Body motions used to transmit force to the terminal device. Scapula **(A)** elevation/depression; **(B)** abduction/adduction; and **(C)** upward/downward rotation. (From Hamill, J., Knutzen, K., Derrick, T. (2015). *Biomechanical basis of human movement* (4th ed.). Philadelphia, PA: Wolters Kluwer.)

movements create tension in the cable that in turn either opens or closes the terminal device (Fig. 8–13).

The cable attaches to the distal aspect of the prosthesis at the terminal device, travels through housing that stabilizes at the lateral elbow, and attaches to the harness. Body-powered terminal devices may be either utilitarian or handlike in appearance; however, both offer function. Therapists educate individuals with ULL/D to the names of the basic components, such as the type of harness, cable, elbow unit, wrist unit, and TD.

Benefits of a body-powered prosthesis include its access to power, robust function and construction, decreased maintenance and repair costs, and increased proprioceptive input. Disadvantages may include the harness that is restrictive and uncomfortable to many, often a cause of abandonment. Because it traverses across the midline and anchors around the contralateral shoulder, there is potential for nerve entrapment. Furthermore, the harnessing pulls on clothing, giving a skewed aesthetic appearance, and limiting the functional envelope. Body-powered TDs generally weigh less than externally powered prostheses, because they lack the control and battery technology to operate the myoelectric signals and to power the device.

Regardless of harness design, it must be secure enough to activate the TD without impinging on the thoracic outlet or exerting excessive effort, yet permit comfort and free movement of arms including shoulders. Long-term wear and inappropriate fit may cause discomfort or physical damage. The harness limits the functional envelope, which includes the space in front of the user to work at midline, as well to reach to the back (as in tying an apron) and operate the TD. With the body-powered prosthesis,

the function can be limited above the head, behind the back, and near the ground, primarily because of the restricting harness. Contralateral harnessing requires strategic motor planning, as the user must consider the positioning of the intact upper limb for stabilization of the harness to activate the TD, as well as access movement of that limb for task completion (Atkins & Meier, 2011; Krajbich & Potter, 2016).

An alternative to traditional harnessing is the **scapular cutaneous anchor technology** (Latour, 2016). This simple technology adheres to the back using medical-grade hypoallergenic tape, to access scapular power on the same side as the limb loss/difference for control of the prosthesis, eliminating discomfort in the opposite axilla (Fig. 8–14). This increases the functional envelope by permitting function above the head, at the waist, behind the back, and near the ground. The technology allows for more intuitive motor planning, because the power and control are originating ipsilaterally.

The harness and the cable work together to activate the mechanical prosthesis using glenohumeral flexion (Krajbich & Potter, 2016). The TD is the distal component, either a hand or a hook. Most body-powered prosthetic hands open and close in a palmar pinch pattern. The prosthetic hooks offer prehension in a lateral or tip pinch pattern, depending on the positioning of the TD.

Voluntary-Opening and Voluntary-Closing Systems

Hands and hooks are available in two different types of control systems: **voluntary-opening (V-O)** and **voluntary-closing (V-C)**. These are interchangeable as long as they are using the same control system.

Voluntary-Opening

Voluntary-opening devices are positioned in a closed position and the user works to open against the resistance of **hook elastics**. The closure is achieved by relaxing the control and allowing the elastic bands to pull the opened TD into the closed position. Grip strength with V-O technology is dependent upon the number of elastic bands being used. Each elastic band equals approximately 1 to 1.5 pounds of force. However, the user must work against this force to open the TD using the contralateral shoulder as an anchor.

Voluntary-Closing

Voluntary-closing devices are positioned in the open position, resembling the at-rest position similar to the natural hand. The user works to close the device and can regulate the desired grip strength whether a light grasp to hold a child's hand or a stronger grasp to hold a purse. A locking system that conserves energy can be installed for sustained closure. V-C systems appear to offer greater efficiency, because they exert less load on the user to access function, yet offer increased grip strength. New technology is emerging that incorporates the features of both V-O and V-C devices.

Every TD has its advantages and disadvantages. The hand TD may appear to some more aesthetically pleasing, but digits 4 and 5 do not move. The hand is bulky, often occludes vision which in turn impairs function, and is more difficult to keep clean. The hook TD is less bulky, allows for successful fine motor prehension, access to visual input, and is more durable. However, it may be less aesthetically appealing than the handlike TD.

Terminal Gloves

Some hand TDs require a glove, which is a cosmetic covering. Gloves are made of either latex or silicone substances and are removable as well as replaceable. Differences exist between the two types of gloves. Latex gloves are sturdy and come in many different shades. The shade of the glove is matched to the user's skin tone. Latex gloves stain easily but are more durable than silicone gloves. Silicone gloves are custom-fabricated to match the individual features of the user. They are more costly and fragile than latex gloves, tearing easily. Persons who have had an amputation generally prefer the silicone glove because of its lifelike appearance. These gloves are more expensive, and funding for them can be difficult to obtain (Fig. 8–15).

EXTERNALLY POWERED PROSTHESIS (MYOELECTRIC)

The externally powered prosthesis, also called a myoelectric prosthesis, is another prosthetic option. This device operates from the electromyographic (EMG) signal transmitted from the muscles of the residual limb. Beneficial characteristics of a myoelectric prosthesis include an unlimited work area, functional aesthetic

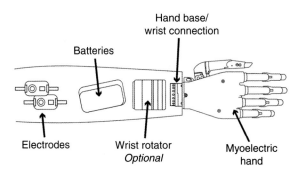

FIGURE 8–16 This diagram illustrates the components of an externally powered prosthesis. (Photo courtesy of Ossur Touch Solutions, Ossur, Canada.)

restoration, increased grip force, elimination of harnessing, increased comfort, interchangeable componentry, and individualized custom fabrication. Myoelectric control is used when possible; however, reimbursement challenges exist related to the terminal device and emerging external control (Corbett, Perreault, & Kuiken, 2011). Disadvantages of a myoelectric prosthesis include increases in weight, cost, maintenance, and risk for damage. The externally powered prosthesis comprises various components, including a socket, forearm shell, **electrodes**, battery, glove, and TD (Fig. 8–16).

Most myoelectric prosthetic devices do not require a harness. However, a harness system is required if it is difficult to fit and maintain contact between the electrodes and the muscle signal, or if the socket is loose because of weight loss or other factors such as a high level of loss. The functional work area is expanded to include the areas above the head, behind the back, and near the ground compared with the body-powered prosthesis, because the harness system is eliminated or minimized. The scapular cutaneous anchor can also be used to secure electrodes and linear transducers; this may be a compelling option, because it does not limit the functional envelope (Latour, 2016).

The externally powered prosthetic socket is unique, because it contains electrodes mounted in the walls of the flexible socket that detect the muscle's EMG signals. The EMG signal stimulates the motor in the prosthesis to produce the desired motion. Prosthetic technology for clients with ULL/D has dramatically changed over the past decade, primarily related to components, socket fabrication, fitting techniques, suspension systems, and sources of power and electronic controls (Esquenazi, Meier, & Sears, 2002). Control systems are determined through team collaboration. Single- or dual-site control systems are available as well as **pattern recognition** and **radio-frequency identification**.

A single-site system is used if the client cannot differentiate and isolate the control of two separate and opposing muscles for electrode sites. This may be beneficial for patients who are cognitively unable to control the dual-site system, such as with young children, or new users (Bouwsema et al., 2014; Brouwers et al., 2014; Egermann, Kasten, & Thomsen, 2008).

A dual-site control system, activated by two separate muscle contractions is often preferred over a single-site system. Electrodes can be embedded in the liner to offer contact, suspension, and comfort. In most other cases, a sock would not be worn, because it would interrupt the connection between the muscle and the electrode. Muscles tend to naturally work together to move arms and hands; the muscles contract in unique ways and generate small amounts of electrical activity called myoelectricity.

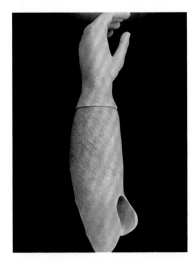

FIGURE 8–15 Prosthesis with passive aesthetic functional glove (i-Limb® Quantum- Ossur, hand covered with a high definition Livingskin™ silicone glove and forearm skin, Ossur, Canada).

Pattern Recognition

The patterns of electrical activity are unique for each movement and can be detected by electrodes placed on the surface of the skin. For those with upper limb loss or difference, remnant muscles can produce these signal patterns; this is termed pattern recognition. Specialized software interprets the signals to control the arm and hand movement of a prosthesis. The command signals can be unique and intuitive to each user the technology provides more efficient and authentic control of multiple prosthetic movements. Pattern recognition works best when it can access multiple myoelectric signals to interpret, so electrode placement is not the same as with conventional single- or dual-site prostheses. The system can read eight myoelectric signals using electrode dome contacts (remote electrodes) and a single wire array to connect them. Pattern recognition requires good skin-electrode contact within the socket and understanding control system, currently being used by individuals with ULL/D at levels proximal to the wrist.

Radio-Frequency Identification

Some externally powered terminal devices can be controlled by using wireless communication known as radio-frequency identification (RFID). This system involves a (RFID) reader and a tag. The tag has information stored in its memory, and the reader can interpret this information. Each tag is programmed with a specific grip pattern and is strategically placed in a location where the person will use the specific grip. This system works well with multiarticulating terminal devices.

Externally powered TDs are available in hand and hook presentations, and these may be V-O or V-C. The standard myoelectric hand offers a basic open-close function with a palmar pinch. Like the body-powered hands, the fourth and fifth digits do not move. Electric hooks are available in different styles and configurations. Most of these devices are not waterproof although some manufacturers offer a protective sleeve. Externally powered TDs have a greater opening range, allowing the ability to grasp objects of larger size. The externally powered prosthesis provides the ability to use prehension capabilities in all planes; the functional work area includes the area above the head, behind the back, and near the ground. Multiarticulating hands are an exciting advancement in technology and offer access to more grip patterns with greater articulation. These hands integrate traditional control systems and with the pattern recognition and RFID control systems.

The Battery

The battery provides the energy for the externally powered prosthesis. Lithium-polymer batteries are much lighter, much smaller, and offer 30% more storage capacity than nickel-cadmium batteries; these improvements have affected the function of externally powered prostheses.

HYBRID PROSTHESIS

Sometimes a person with ULL/D will use a device that consists of components that are a combination of the body-powered and the externally powered, passive, or activity specific. This is more commonly seen in individuals with higher level loss where multiple joints and controls are needed. For example, it is not uncommon for a person with TH loss to use a body-powered or manually operated elbow system with a myoelectric terminal device.

EMERGING TECHNOLOGIES

Emerging technologies are affecting the performance and functional outcome for users of prosthetic devices. One such intervention is **osseointegration.**

OSSEOINTEGRATION

Osseointegration is a surgical procedure defined as "the structural linkage made at the contact point where the human bone and the surface of a synthetic, often titanium-based implant meet". Essentially, a pin is implanted into the end of the bone and extends through the skin to lock into a prosthesis (Fig. 8–17). It has been reported that with an osseointegrated prostheses there is an increase in overall ADL function and an improved perception of disability (Banda, Castillo, & Velez, 2020). The osseointegrated prostheses has been reported to additionally increase tolerance and control to the everyday use of the prosthetic and enhance upper extremity reach (Banda et al., 2020).

TARGETED MUSCLE REINNERVATION

Targeted muscle reinnervation (TMR) is an innovative surgical procedure where residual nerves from the amputated limb are transferred to reinnervate new muscle targets that have otherwise lost function. The results of this procedure work well with pattern recognition and can improve the upper-limb prosthesis control at multiple joints and in the TD (Cheesborough, Smith, Kuiken, & Dumanian, 2015).

TRANSPLANTS OF HANDS

Transplants of hands, much like the toe-to-thumb transplants, have been shown to be an effective alternative to prosthesis use for some candidates (Atkins, 2014). Current research investigating protocol and outcomes is ongoing worldwide. Chapter 27 in this book reviews upper extremity transplantations in great detail.

PARTIAL HAND OPTIONS

Partial hand options have rapidly advanced with new and emerging technologies. Although silicone restoration has been available for decades, both mechanical digits (Fig. 8–12B) (such as Naked Prosthetics, Olympia, WA) and externally powered fingers (Fig. 8–12C) (such as i-Digits™, Ossur America) are gaining attention.

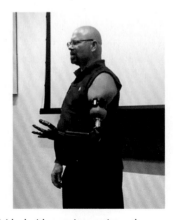

FIGURE 8–17 Individual with osseointegration—the suspension pin is surgically implanted into the bone. Once healed, a prosthesis can be fabricated to integrate to it.

CLINICAL PEARL 8–1

ThumbDriver™, Naked Prosthetics

JY is a 63-year-old man with traumatic amputation of the thumb, index, and middle digits of his left nondominant hand (A). His injury occurred at work while performing his job as a cabinetmaker. After surgery and extensive therapy, JY was evaluated for prosthetic technology and eventually fit with a device that enables him to perform all ADLs and work-related tasks (B and C).

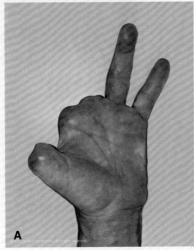

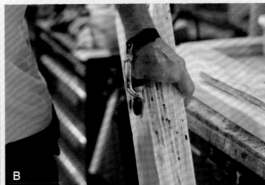

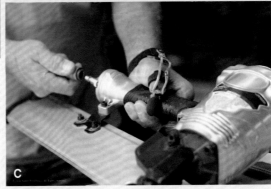

A, Six months post injury and ready for prosthetic fitting and training. **B,** Note the restoration of thumb opposition and strength. **C,** The device (ThumbDriver™, Naked Prosthetics, Olympia, WA) is suspended on and driven by his residual thumb. A mechanism is used to translate MP joint flexion into articulation at the artificial distal phalanx in an intuitive manner. (Photo courtesy of Naked Prosthetics, Olympia, WA.)

CLINICAL PEARL 8–2

MCPDriver™, Naked Prosthetics

NH is a 26-year-old man who sustained five proximal phalanx amputations (A). His injury occurred on the job as a welder. While operating a steel roller, both his hands were pulled into the machine, causing severe crushing injuries and degloving to both hands. He spent a month in the hospital undergoing dozens of surgeries, including skin grafts, joint fusion on his left hand, and an unsuccessful replantation of his right fifth finger. But after months of therapy, NH surpassed expectations and regained some function and range of motion from his residual digits. After extensive surgery and therapy, he was fit and trained in the use of a hand prosthesis for his right hand (MCPDriver™, Naked Prosthetics). NH now uses his device for power grasp and object handling, as well as for fine motor skills such as automotive wiring jobs (B).

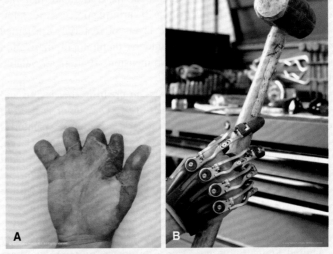

A, Patient at 8 months post injury. **B,** NH is shown wearing an IF–SF IP prosthesis. The power to the IP joints is generated through the intact musculature about the remnants of the metacarpophalangeal (MCP) joints. (CP2A, Photo courtesy of Naked Prosthetics, Olympia, WA. CP2B, MCPDriver™, Photo courtesy of Naked Prosthetics, Olympia, WA.)

CHAPTER 8

CLINICAL PEARL 8–3

PIPDriver™, Naked Prosthetics

JB is a 28-year-old digit amputee who lost half of her index finger at the middle phalanx and suffered injuries to three other digits on her dominant hand in 2017 (A). The amputation was the result of a missing guard in an industrial work setting. Her goal was to get back to work and go back to her main hobbies which included musical instruments and gaming. She was fit with a prosthesis that was powdered by her index finger proximal interphalangeal (PIP) joint (PIPDriver™, Naked Prosthetics). She was able to return to playing double bass and saxophone as well as she did preinjury (B).

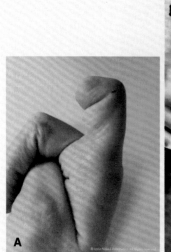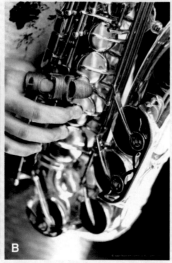

A, JB's injury. **B,** JB playing her instrument. (Photo courtesy of Naked Prosthetics, Olympia, WA.)

3D-PRINTED TECHNOLOGY/ADDITIVE MANUFACTURING

3D-printed technology or **additive manufacturing** (AM) has many pros and cons and has been referred to as "disruptive" because of the impact of reduced costs and decreased time from design to production which in turn has "disturbed" the traditional manufacturing process. The capabilities of the 3D printing process uses additive manufacturing in which single layers of materials are joined together by using heat, additive binders, or photopolymerization and then creates the part in three dimensions (Patterson, Salatin, Janson, Salinas, & Mullins, 2020).

3D printing technologies are used in creating the design and in the manufacturing of the product. The 3D scanner is used in the measurement and the design process, and the 3D printer is used in the actual manufacturing process (Mehmet, Ismail, Harun, & Cigdem, 2020). 3D technology has gained momentum in hand therapy as an alternative to a thermoplastic orthosis and in the creation of patient-specific adaptive equipment. However, in the field of prosthetics there is some skepticism. This technology has proven to be disruptive to the providers and users of prostheses. Prosthetic componentry are medical devices approved by the United States Food and Drug Administration (FDA) and are fit to the user by a prosthetist who has undergone the rigors of academic and clinical preparation as well as national professional certification.

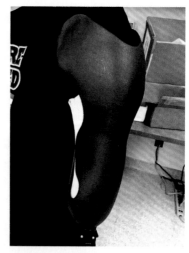

FIGURE 8–18 Custom 3D-printed device (custom fabrication by Handspring Clinical Services, Middletown, NY).

3D-printed devices are not always fabricated or fit by prosthetists. Therapists may be requested to train the user in its use with particular relevance to completing ADLs. The practitioner should check the fit of the device and inspect the functionality. Also, clients should be advised and counseled to issues such as independent donning and doffing, care of the device, and skin inspection. The fabricator of the device should be contacted immediately if there are any problems with the fit or function. Depending on the features of the device, the therapist may utilize different training strategies similar to prosthetic training (Baschuk, 2016) (Fig. 8–18).

PROSTHOSIS

A **prosthosis** is a type of hybrid device that possesses the qualities and functions of a prosthesis and an orthosis for a retained limb with lost or impaired function, such as hemiplegia. These devices may offer support or positioning to the limb as an orthosis, yet have features that offer function, such as a terminal device to offer prehension.

WHAT ARE THE PHASES OF CARE?

The focus of therapy assessment and intervention relates to the client's ability to function and to participate in meaningful occupation (AOTA, 2014). Therapists work with clients throughout the entire prosthetic rehabilitation process, beginning before the delivery of prosthetic technology. Without proper therapy, the benefits of prosthetic use may be limited and the individual may abandon use (Bouwsema et al., 2014; Brouwers et al., 2014). Prosthetic rehabilitation is progressive, with phases designed to build tolerance, skills, and functional applications to address basic ADLs and instrumental ADLs integrating the use of the prosthesis during bilateral activities. This also includes educating the client on proper care and hygiene of the residual limb as well as the prosthesis. It is important for therapy to begin early in the rehabilitation process to facilitate the functional use of the prosthesis (Meier & Atkins, 2004). Table 8–3 provides reviews of these phases.

Prosthetic rehabilitation is categorized into phases of evaluation and intervention (Table 8–3). Each phase contains specific items to evaluate along with typical areas to address; however, areas of overlap exist. Utilize these phases as a guideline and most importantly address the individual client needs.

TABLE 8–3	Phases of Prosthetic Rehabilitation and Intervention Focus
Phase	**Focus**
Preoperative	• Team formulates a plan • Educate client on expectations • Provide adaptive equipment • Practice unilateral strategies
Amputation surgery and dressing	• Surgery • Determine length of residual limb • Wound care • Dressing wound • Pain control
Acute postsurgical	• Pain control • Range of motion, contracture prevention • Wound healing • Emotional support • Address phantom sensation/pain • Transfer hand dominance • Adaptive strategies for activities of daily living (ADLs)
Preprosthetic	• Limb shrinkage and shaping • Increase muscle strength • Foster sense of control • Realistic expectations
Prosthetic prescription and fabrication	• Prosthetic options considered • Practice and preparation for prosthesis biofeedback, simulators • Prosthesis is delivered
Prosthetic training phase	• Prosthetic fitting and training • Desensitization of residual limb • Unilateral independence • Educate client on prosthesis controls, etc.
Community integration	• Purposeful activities relevant to environments, contexts • Participation in meaningful activities and occupations • Bilateral activities
Vocational rehabilitation	• Purposeful activities relevant to environments, contexts • Participation in meaningful activities and occupations • Bilateral activities
Follow-up	• Purposeful activities relevant to environments, contexts • Participation in meaningful activities and occupations • Bilateral activities

The phases include the following:

- Preoperative
- Amputation surgery and dressing
- Acute postsurgical
- Preprosthetic
- Prosthetic prescription and fabrication
- Prosthetic training
- Community integration
- Vocational rehabilitation
- Follow-up for continued skill refinement

PREOPERATIVE PHASE

The assessment and intervention process may begin before the amputation. The specialized IP healthcare team creates a plan and educates the client and family to the surgical procedure and rehabilitation process to ensure realistic expectations. Therapists assess hand dominance and determine the need for adaptive equipment. As clients will eventually use their prostheses with ADLs, assistive devices are provided on a limited basis because it may interfere with transition to prosthesis use. The team explains phantom pain and phantom sensation, as it is common for individuals with acquired ULL to experience these.

AMPUTATION SURGERY AND DRESSING PHASE

Surgeons determine residual limb length before and during the surgery; however, they will often consult with prosthetists and therapists for optimal functional outcomes. Many past limb-salvage techniques have preserved maximal length; however, this can interfere with the best outcome functionally if the amputation occurs at the joint. The surgeon completes myoplastic wound closure covering distal bone with soft tissue. A rigid dressing or removable rigid dressing can assist in controlling pain.

ACUTE POSTSURGICAL PHASE

Pain management, wound healing, and maintaining range of motion are primary postoperative goals. Therapy often incorporates wound care, edema control, limb shaping, contracture prevention, desensitization, and teaching one-handed strategies (Fig. 8–19A–E). Discussions and intervention regarding phantom sensation and phantom pain are ongoing. Functional activity, gentle massage, prosthetic wear, and transcutaneous electric nerve stimulation (TENS) are helpful. Emotional support to the client and family is vital as therapists assist patients to adjust to the amputation.

PREPROSTHETIC PHASE

The primary goals during this phase are to continue to shape the residual limb, increase muscle strength, and restore function and sense of control. Limb shaping and edema control are achieved through compression garments and shrinkers. The residual limb edema can also be managed by wrapping the residual limb in a figure-of-8 pattern. Compression garments or wraps should be worn as much as possible to ensure proper shaping of the residual limb for the best fit of the prosthesis. Other interventions to decrease volume include elevation and retrograde massage. The therapist must reinforce the importance of edema management because of its direct impact on socket fit and comfort (Davidson, Jones, Cornet, & Cittarelli, 2002).

Therapists should educate the client and family to affirm realistic expectations about the technology and the training to use it. Individuals with ULL may assume that they will perform all activities at their prior level of independence and that the prosthesis will function in the same way as the natural hand. Therapists should encourage that the prosthetic device will not replace the natural arm and its abilities, but offer assistance to stabilize, support, and hold objects during bimanual activities; over time, it may be embodied by the user and incorporated into body scheme as an extension of the body. Therapists may use prosthesis simulators to further affirm realistic expectations.

PROSTHETIC PRESCRIPTION AND FABRICATION PHASE

The team collaborates with the client to determine the type of prosthesis that will best meet the client's needs and contexts. The preprosthetic period begins when the individual with

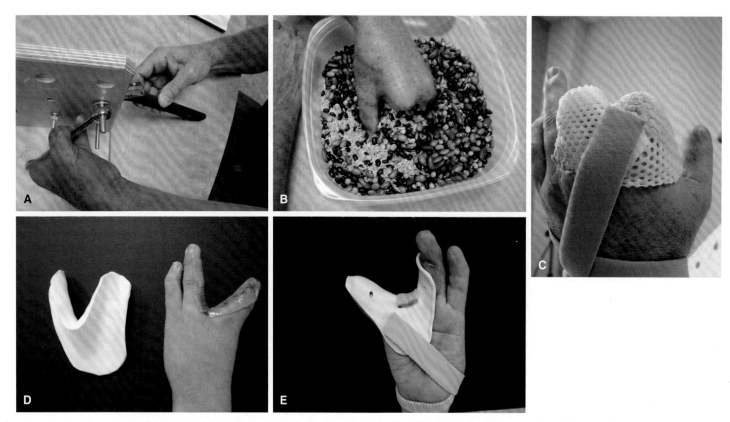

FIGURE 8–19 A, Prior to fitting any device, consider strengthening all intrinsic and extrinsic muscles with functional activities. **B,** Desensitization techniques can be extremely beneficial to prepare the area for prosthetic application. **C,** Elastomer used under an orthosis to help with remodeling scar and maintain web space in preparation for prosthetic evaluation. **D and E,** Use of a silicone gel sleeve and an orthosis to assist with hypersensitivity and maintain wide web space in planning for a functional hand prosthesis.

ULL/D begins an exploration of prosthetic devices. The phase concludes upon prosthetic delivery and overlaps with prosthetic training.

PROSTHETIC TRAINING PHASE

During the prosthetic training phase, therapists address any issues continued from the earlier postsurgical phase. Clients typically see the prosthetist often for fittings and revisions to the socket and the development of the prototype device. Additional goals of therapy include the preparation of the individual to tolerate wearing the prosthesis and using it independently for daily activities using simulator technology. In this way, the individual can become accustomed to the weight and length of the device, the feeling of the socket and the harness, and the functional workings of the components (Latour, 2016). This helps the client to develop a realistic expectation of the prosthesis and its impact on function. In addition to desensitization, maintaining range of motion, eliminating contractures, and unilateral independence, therapists may also engage in electrode placement and training using **biofeedback** and virtual activities.

Clients need to practice muscle contractions in diverse positions, including lying, standing, and sitting to enhance maximal success after delivery of the prosthesis. Collaboration and ongoing communication with the prosthetist are crucial to develop a well-fitting and well-functioning device (Latour, 2016).

Individuals with bilateral ULL/D present with unique challenges. The presentation of the individual may be asymmetrical; differing technology—or no technology—may be utilized. Many individuals with bilateral loss or difference, particularly at a high level (such as shoulder disarticulation), prefer to use their toes to accomplish

dexterous tasks. Clients are educated to donning and doffing strategies, operating switches, replacing batteries, and caring for the prosthesis, as well as inspecting the skin.

COMMUNITY INTEGRATION, VOCATIONAL REHABILITATION, AND FOLLOW-UP PHASES

The three phases of community integration, vocational rehabilitation, and follow-up comprise purposeful activities and participation in meaningful occupation-based activities that include social function. These phases are overlapping yet progressive with skills development toward proficiency, exploration of new methods, and revelation of new needs. Because one prosthesis does not offer the total function of the hand, it is common to pursue other devices at this time. The primary focus of therapy should include bilateral activities for occupational performance. Box 8–4 lists examples of bilateral tasks (McFarland et al., 2010).

PSYCHOLOGICAL AND SOCIAL ISSUES OF CLIENTS WITH AMPUTATIONS

Psychological and/or social issues may arise at any time throughout the rehabilitation process, and after. While it is important to make appropriate referrals to specialists as necessary, it is equally important for practitioners to offer encouragement and support. Davidson (2002) reported that individuals with ULL/D state that they experience far more difficulty dealing with their "social worlds than with their physical worlds." Common issues focus on relationships with family, friends, coworkers, and significant others and handling

BOX 8-4 COMMON BILATERAL ACTIVITIES

Most Common Bilateral Activities

Use a cell phone
Squeeze toothpaste on a toothbrush
Tie shoes
Manage separating fasteners, especially zippers and buttons
Cut food using fork and knife
Open a container
Manage a wallet including removal from pocket or purse and extract currency/cards
Tie a full trash bag closed
Use hand-held tools, such scissors, hammer, screwdriver, or drill
Drive a vehicle

Peel and cut vegetables/fruits
Manage long-handled tools such as a broom, rake, or shovel
Place a plastic garbage bag/liner into a trash can
Remove a full trash bag from the receptacle
Wash dishes in a sink
Dry dishes with a towel
Fold laundry
Push a grocery cart or similar (stroller, wheelbarrow)
Play sports, musical instrument, video or card games
Make a ponytail

awkward social situations in public with strangers. Specific issues may include anger or resentment, posttraumatic stress, body image concerns, loss of sense of wholeness, social isolation, decreased sexual activity, and depression. Murray (2005, 2009) emphasized the importance of psychosocial-emotional health, and Sheehan and Gondo (2014) reported that behavioral health issues are often overlooked and unaddressed for this population.

Family dynamics will likely change when a member experiences limb loss or difference. Because families function as a unit, the ULL/D affects all members in different ways; the common thread is that all perceive loss and adjustment. Fear and anxiety may become overwhelming at times. Family members may worry about how the individual will adjust to his or her changed body. Issues about intimacy and dependency are common concerns. The therapist should encourage a reconnection between the person who has sustained an amputation and his or her partner.

UPPER EXTREMITY PROSTHETIC INTERVENTION FOR CHILDREN

Fitting children with prostheses is considered necessary to maintain and preserve normal development. Early gross motor movements directly involving the hands to balance, support, and stabilize the trunk emerge in children between 4 and 6 months (Cronin & Mandich, 2005; Shaperman, Landsberger, & Setoguchi, 2003). Hanson and Mandacina (2003) correlated that the benefit of the early fitting is the child's immediate acceptance of the prosthetic arm. The most beneficial age range to receive a prosthesis is from 2 months to 2 years (Bouwsema et al., 2014; Egermann et al., 2008; Huinink, Bouwsema, Plettenburg, van der Sluis, & Bongers, 2016; Stark, 2001). Children fitted with prostheses at a young age and who wear their prostheses regularly will demonstrate spontaneous use in daily activities.

Children fitted at later ages are more inclined to use the prosthesis passively or to reject use altogether. Early fitting encourages prosthesis integration with bilateral activities. Children use the prosthesis to practice developmentally relevant activities that require crossing midline, hand position in space, grasping, bilateral tasks, and bringing hands to midline (Bouwsema et al., 2014; Egermann et al., 2008; Huinink et al., 2016).

Family involvement is key to acceptance of the prosthesis, and members should be involved in all aspects of the prosthesis, including its care and understanding its use. Many parents and siblings will use a prosthesis simulator to develop this perception. The family should be educated about the importance and advantages of early and consistent prosthetic use as well as the benefits of therapy to develop skills (Atkins & Meier, 2011; Bouwsema et al., 2014; Egermann et al., 2008).

CONCLUSION

This chapter is meant to give the reader an overview of prosthetic intervention for the hand and upper extremity for those that have an upper limb loss or congenital difference. The chapter reviewed current available types of prostheses and the components necessary for function use and social integration. Through careful study of this chapter, the reader should gain an appreciation for the depth of knowledge that is necessary to properly evaluate, train, and guide this patient population. Refer to resources for both the practitioner (Box 8–5) and patient (Box 8–6) for further information.

BOX 8-5 MANUFACTURER RESOURCES

Manufacturer	Website
COAPT	https://www.coaptengineering.com
COVVI	https://www.covvi.com
College Park Industries	https://www.college-park.com
Fillauer	https://www.fillauer.com
Infinite Biomedical Technologies	https://www.i-biomed.com
Liberating Technologies	http://www.liberatingtech.com
Motion Control	https://www.utaharm.com
Naked Prosthetics	https://www.npdevices.com/
Open Bionics	https://openbionics.com
Ossur	https://www.ossur.com/americas
OttoBock	https://www.ottobockus.com
Pillet	https://www.pillet.com
Steeper	https://www.steepergroup.com/
TASKA	http://www.taskaprosthetics.com/
Texas Assistive Devices	https://www.n-abler.org
Therapeutic Recreational Systems (TRS)	https://www.trsprosthetics.com
TouchBionics	https://www.touchbionics.com

BOX 8–6   POPULATION RESOURCES

Resource	Website
Amplitude	https://livingwithamplitude.com/
Amputee Coalition	https://www.amputee-coalition.org/
Amputee Empowerment Partners	http://www.empoweringamputees.org/
Association of Children's Prosthetic and Orthotic Clinics	https://www.acpoc.org/
Camp No Limits	https://nolimitsfoundation.org/
Handsmart	https://handsmartgroup.org/

Resource	Website
Helping Hands Foundation	http://helpinghandsgroup.org/
Infinitec	http://www.infinitec.org
International Child Amputee Network	http://child-amputee.net/
Lucky Fin Project	https://luckyfinproject.org/
Single-Handed Solutions	http://singlehandedsolutions.blogspot.com/
Skills for Life	http://enhancingskillsforlife.org/

FIELD NOTE: GENERAL INFORMATION–3D PRINTING

Mary Matthews-Brownell OTR/L, MHA, CHT, PTA, CLT
Washington

Why 3D Print an Orthosis?

Have you ever considered 3D printing an orthosis? Depending on various factors, 3D printing for your client could provide some great advantages over traditionally made orthoses. These advantages include:

- a perfectly repeatable design via a digital design file
- a wide array of material choices (color, lightweight, perforations, durability)

The downside currently is the skills it takes to digitally 3D model the orthotic and the required software; these are not typically found in a therapist's clinic. This technology is still the early stages and to the date of this note, there is no upper extremity orthotic design software meant for use by individuals without digital 3D modeling skills.

How Do You Get a 3D Model to Print?

In this author's experience and the examples of 3D-printed sports orthoses found on the internet, an engineer/designer works with a clinician to design the orthosis. To create the digital design there are a few approaches:

- 3D scan the client's upper extremity directly which creates a digital 3D model that can then be used to digitally build the orthosis on top of the extremity (similar to the manual process).
- Manually mold an orthosis from thermoplastic and then 3D scan that orthotic. In this approach, the digital 3D model could be modified with design software to smooth seams, add or remove thickness, or add features like lattices and clasps. The digital design is then exported from the design software in a generic cross-platform 3D model format called stereolithography (STL— similar to a PDF of 3D design).

How Does 3D Printing Work?

The STL file is loaded into the 3D printer software (like the print dialog box in MS Word) where the specific settings for printing that design, on that printer, are finalized before the printer is started. 3D printers run unattended (although they are fun to watch). 3D printers work by stacking many thin layers of material on top of each other. Each layer can have a different 2D profile which allows for an infinite number of created shapes that can be designed.

What Materials Are Available?

Most 3D printers create objects out of a type of plastic and for orthotics this would be the material of choice. There are many different types of plastics that can be utilized, some 3D printers allow for combining different types in one object. This gives the option for hard and flexible plastics in one orthosis or a two-part orthosis can be created out of separate 3D-printed part, each from a different type of plastic.

How Does 3D-Printed Orthotics Complement Thermoplastics and Hand Therapy?

With current thermoplastic materials, the therapist can fabricate and mold the material to the exact specifications needed. After this is complete, the custom thermoplastic orthosis is scanned to become a 3D orthotic. This is done with the help of rehabilitation engineers and orthotists who are knowledgeable in scanning and using 3D printers. The 3D orthotic becomes an exact replica of the custom thermoplastic orthosis; however, it is now replicated with perhaps a material that is lighter, colorful, and more durable and, if lost or damaged, can be exactly duplicated! In addition, the STL file aspect of this process, the therapist can change measurements, which is done with the partnering of a rehabilitation engineer and the skills of a certified hand therapist. The hand therapist understands why there may be a necessary change to a measurement such as to protect joints or tendon reconstruction with the ultimate goal being a guarded and graded recovery with return to functional independence.

3D Example: Protection for Chronic Nerve Pain

Shown in this example is a protective device for this patient's dominant right hand due to chronic nerve pain after small finger amputation (Fig. 8–FN1A). With the orthosis in place, this patient can perform his manual labor job pain free. With the orthosis on, the patient describes that muscle spasms in his right hand are relieved,

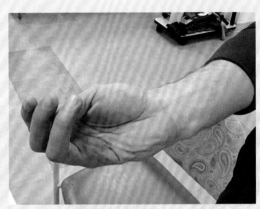

FIGURE 8–FN1A Patient's hand without orthosis—note loss of small finger and raised incision. Muscle spasms in thenar and hypothenar musculature leave him with a nonfunctional and painful hand.

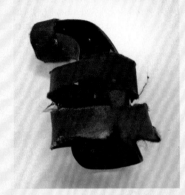

FIGURE 8–FN1B Original thermoplastic orthosis.

which in turn, allows fluid use of his thumb, index, and middle fingers for grasping objects. The original custom thermoplastic orthosis was quickly worn out due to heavy use (Fig. 8–FN1B). Because of the nature of his work demands, he frequently requested this exact orthosis design be replicated as he found it the only way he could perform his job. Most veteran hand therapists can attest that replicating an orthosis is almost impossible. There are always a few small degrees of variance and a wearing time frame that requires

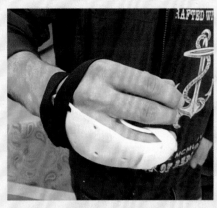

FIGURE 8–FN1C 3D durable option.

adaptability. Thus, a 3D durable option was created which easily replicated, through the 3D file system of the original thermoplastic design, the exact orthosis he had been wearing (Fig. 8–FN1C).

Suggested References

Structure Occipital Scanner. (2019, June 28). Obtained June 28, 2019, from https://structure.io/structure-sensor

Demers, L., Weiss-Lambrou, R., & Ska, B. (1996). Development of the Quebec User Evaluation of Satisfaction with assistive Technology (QUEST). *Assistive Technology: The Official Journal of RESNA, 8*(1), 3–13.

Asanovic, I., Millward, H., & Lewis, A. (2019). Development of a 3D scan posture-correction procedure to facilitate the direct-digital splinting approach. *Virtual and Physical Prototyping, 14*(1), 92–103.

Pyatt, C., Kelly, S., Paterson, A. M., Bibb, R., & Sinclair, M. (2018). Giving patients what they want: Proposing additive manufacture as a method to design and fabricate wrist splints. In Rennie, A. E. W. (Ed.), *Rapid design prototyping and manufacture*, TBC Lancaster University. https://dspace.lboro.ac.uk/2134/35154

Harte, D., & Paterson, A. M. (2018). The fastest field sport in the world: A case report on 3-D printed hurling gloves to help prevent injury. *Journal of Hand Therapy, 31*(3), 398–410. https://dspace.lboro.ac.uk/2134/25781

Short introduction of the Curatio 3D hand scanner developed by Vectory3 and TU Delft. https://www.tudelft.nl/en/ide/research/research-labs/applied-labs/3d-handscanner/

https://youtu.be/saZ-X20j128

Kelly, S., Paterson, A. M., & Bibb, R. J. (2016). A review of wrist splint designs for Additive Manufacture. In Rennie, A. E. (Ed.), Rapid Design Prototyping and Manufacture Conference, Design School, Loughborough University, pp. 29-39.

FIELD NOTE: 3D PRINTING IN HAND THERAPY

Rita M. Patterson, PhD
Texas

Ben Salatin, MS
New Mexico

Robin Janson, OTD, MS, OTR, CHT
Indiana

Sandra P. Salinas, OTR, CHT
Florida

Maria Josette S. Mullins, PT, DPT
Florida

Subtractive manufacturing is a process where material is removed from a piece of wood, metal, or plastic until the desired shape is achieved. Additive manufacturing (3D printing), on the other hand, is a process where individual layers of materials are combined using heat, additive binders, or photopolymerization. Modern 3D printing has evolved from the low-resolution rough parts and lengthy

manufacturing time. Current 3D printing capabilities include the use of a variety of materials from metals to plastics to biologic materials and the ability to fabricate devices with multiple materials at one time. This technology will continue to revolutionize healthcare as already seen with multiple applications being realized due to the COVID-19 pandemic.

CHAPTER 8

For hand therapy, this technology can assist in development of assistive devices, therapeutic equipment, orthotics, orthotic components (e.g., outriggers), and anatomical models, as many 3D designs are available for download from online repositories and requiring little to no customization.

As with all technology, it is anticipated that 3D printing will get easier and more efficient and provide simple, cost-effective treatment solutions that will be mainstream in clinics and hospitals.

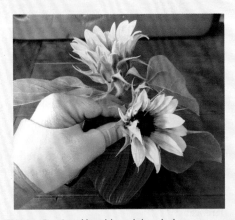

FIGURE 8–FN2A 3D-printed hand-based thumb short opponens orthosis created from a scan. The process of scanning involves obtaining a topographical scan of a patient's hand and then digitally modeling an orthosis onto the scan. Once completed, the computer model of the orthosis is 3D printed. Print time was 4 hours. (Photo credit: Robin Janson. Digital model scan file courtesy of Benjamin Salatin.)

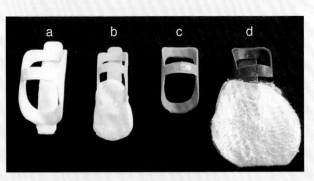

FIGURE 8–FN2C Other examples of 3D-printed orthoses. Proximal interphalangeal extension block—**(a)** white original model, **(b)** yellow pediatric model, **(c)** bright blue final adult model, and **(d)** trigger finger orthosis (model is by "bisquit" of Pinshape).

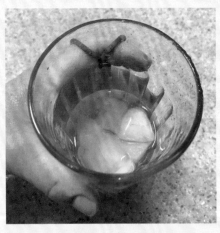

FIGURE 8–FN2B 3D-printed swan-neck orthosis designed with Tinkercad 3D modeling software by custom sizing two torus shapes based on finger measurements and partially overlapping them to make a figure-of-8 shape. The orthosis is 3D printed flat (taking about 7 minutes) and then heated in hot water to soften prior to fitting. Material (PLA) cost of this orthosis is less than .10 cents and may be printed in a variety of colors. (Photo credit: Robin Janson.)

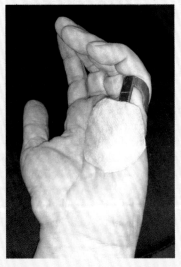

FIGURE 8–FN2D Trigger finger orthosis on a hand using aquaplast beads for the palm and covered in moleskin.

Case Study Section

Case Study RB

The case studies presented here are meant as a teaching guideline only. Treatment and orthosis protocols vary greatly from surgeon to surgeon and from therapist to therapist. The therapist should check with the referring physicians and colleagues to define the preferred treatment and appropriate orthotic intervention.

RB is a young man, aged 28 years at the time of his injury, living with his fiancée and their two daughters (10 and 5 years) in a second-floor apartment. He was employed as a furniture mover and was a passenger in a box truck that was involved in a work-related motor vehicle accident resulting in a rollover. RB experienced a loss of consciousness, requiring extrication that took 30 minutes. Upon removal

from the vehicle, he was found to have near-complete amputation of his right dominant upper limb at the elbow, extreme blood loss, bilateral pulmonary contusions, left popliteal wound, right meniscus tear, bilateral deep vein thromboses, and multiple fractures, including the pelvis, left femur, left proximal fibula, and anterior C1 arch. Emergent care included a massive blood transfusion, wound cleansing, amputation, and subsequent closure of his right upper limb at the elbow joint.

One week later, he underwent skin grafting and femoral intermedullary nailing to the left lower extremity, as well as open reduction to the right lower extremity. He was transferred by ambulance to a hospital closer to home 2 weeks postinjury, where he participated actively in short-term rehabilitation. Efforts included intensive physical therapy to address lower limb range of motion, strengthening, endurance training, and functional ambulation. Hand therapy goals included wound healing, residual limb shaping, desensitization, range of motion, and functional activities of daily living, focusing on self-care and changing hand dominance. RB was discharged after 4 weeks, with limited left leg range of motion, but able to ambulate with a (left) Lofstrand crutch for short distances. He also used a wheelchair, primarily propelling it with his feet.

Collaborative Prosthetic Technology Consult

RB and his fiancée were seen during postinjury week 12 at their home for a collaborative consultation with the prosthetist, hand therapist, and the nurse case manager from the catastrophic care management company engaged by his employer. During the appointment, RB appeared to be lethargic and easily distractible but became more animated and engaged through the consultation. He reported taking medications including gabapentin due to pain that he described as 7/10, as well as phantom pain (8/10) and phantom sensation. The prosthetist showed RB and his fiancée diverse prosthetic technology that would be applicable to his level of loss, and explained the impact of the elbow disarticulation level. Because RB's loss was through the joint, componentry options for elbow movement were limited relative to limb length symmetry in comparison to the left upper limb. Examples of body and external powered prostheses included various terminal devices (TDs). The prosthetist and hand therapist reviewed the functional characteristics of each device and system, emphasizing the "tool" nature of these devices as opposed to the expectation of any technology replacing the complete function of a natural hand. They explained the process of fitting a prosthesis and the importance of a well-fitting socket for optimal functional outcomes.

The prosthetist test fit a soft Alpha Classic® liner to demonstrate the sensation of compression and suspension, which RB appeared to tolerate for the entire session without complaint. RB asked relevant questions and appeared to understand all information presented to him. He expressed his goals that included his desire to overcome his current limitations and dependence on his family. Initial hand therapy assessment revealed a very long, well-healed right upper arm amputation; shape appeared normal; however, dense scarring and some hypersensitivity around the scar tissue appeared evident. RB demonstrated no significant limitations in strength or ROM, although shoulder appeared stiff and may have sustained some injury or postsurgical immobilization. Palpation and cueing revealed adequate voluntary contraction of bicep and triceps muscles for myoelectric control; comprehensive testing will determine precise and optimal location for electrode placement. RB required assistance at varying levels to complete self-care and home management ADLs. He was using his left nondominant hand to complete tasks, but appeared to show awkward fine motor coordination as well as fair endurance. RB desires to become more independent to all ADLs and recreation activities such as cooking and playing basketball and videogames with his children.

Initial Plan

The humeral length will influence the choice of components, eliminating the use of all powered and some hybrid elbows, leaving outside joints as a most likely choice, at least for the hybrid body/external powered variant. A body-powered system with multiple TDs and possibly activity-specific TDs would be useful as well. An externally powered system will allow for multiple TDs to maximize

grasping potential and possibly electronic wrist rotation. Further discussion with rehab team will better define prosthetic and TD choices, but two devices are likely at the outset, which will include variants that enhance function and appearance. In preparation for a prosthesis, RB will be seen for preparatory intervention that includes provision of a shrinker and/or rigid preparatory dressing (per physician), as well as hand therapy for continued training in transfer of hand dominance, endurance and energy conservation/joint protection for left upper limb, and desensitization, soft-tissue mobility, and endurance for right upper limb.

The long-term plan is that RB will benefit from multiple prosthetic devices to facilitate independent function. Upon successful use of the body-powered device, RB will benefit from externally powered and activity-specific devices. These technologies will be pursued following input from the client and the team (physician, community hand therapy, case manager).

Collaborative Prosthetic Technology Delivery 1

RB was seen 6 weeks post consultation for expedited delivery of his body-powered prosthesis with collaborative intervention from prosthetist and hand therapist over a 5-day period (Fig. 8–20A,B). His prosthesis includes outside locking hinges to offer elbow joint function as well as a symmetrical presentation in length to his left upper limb. It includes V-C and V-O hands and hooks to accommodate the diverse activities.

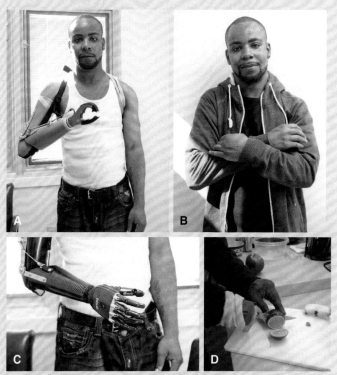

FIGURE 8–20 A, Body-powered elbow disarticulation prosthesis with voluntary-closing terminal device (Fillauer outside locking elbow joints, Fillauer Quick Disconnect wrist unit and TRS Grip 2 voluntary-closing terminal device). **B,** Elbow disarticulation prosthesis with passive aesthetic functional terminal device (Prosthetic ArtWorks). Note the cosmetic appearance of the right hand. **C,** Hybrid prosthesis with multiarticulating terminal device. Shown is a Fillauer outside locking elbow joints with a Motion Control Electric Wrist Rotator (Fillauer LLC, Chattanooga, TN) and an Ottobock bebionic hand (Duderstadt, Germany). **D,** Body-powered elbow disarticulation prosthesis with activity-specific terminal device (Texas Assistive Devices Paring Knife terminal device, Brazoria, TX).

Initial training with prosthetist and hand therapist included the following:

1. education to care of the prosthesis
2. provision of a progressive wear schedule to build up tolerance
3. instruction, demonstration, and practice to don and to doff the technology independently
4. instruction, demonstration, and practice to work the elbow control for flexion and extension
5. instruction, demonstration, and practice to control the different terminal devices via repetitive skills drills and basic functional tasks in diverse positions and at different heights
6. discussion regarding social function and managing awkward situations in public

The team communicated with the physician, case manager, and the community hand therapy practitioner regarding the client's progress and offered recommendations for a continued plan of care. He will be seen as needed by the collaborative prosthetic team, but will receive ongoing intervention from the community hand therapy to develop skills to complete functional tasks toward independence per the plan of care.

Collaborative Prosthetic Technology Consultation and Delivery 2

RB was seen 8 months later for collaborative prosthetic team follow-up and to determine next steps. RB is wearing and using his device actively on a daily basis for approximately 8 to 10 hours per day. He is independent to most self-care tasks and many home management tasks. He would like to attend a job training program; however, the current technology is limiting for some bimanual fine motor tasks, such as typing, telephone use, and tool manipulation. Upon evaluation and full-team consideration, RB will receive a hybrid prosthesis with outside locking hinges at the elbow and an externally powered multiarticulated hand for the terminal device. Preparatory intervention includes biofeedback to further develop the existing myosignals and building tolerance to the increased weight of the device.

RB was seen 6 weeks post consultation 2 for expedited delivery of the hybrid-powered prosthesis with collaborative intervention from prosthetist and hand therapist over a 5-day period (Fig. 8–20C). Initial collaborative training relative to this device included education to care of the prosthesis; a progressive wear schedule to build up tolerance; instruction, demonstration, and practice to don and to doff the technology independently; instruction, demonstration, and practice to control the terminal device via repetitive skills drills and basic functional tasks in diverse positions and at different heights; and extensive discussion and practice to develop social functional skills and to manage awkward situations in community, education, and work environments.

Collaborative Prosthetic Technology Consultation and Delivery 3

RB presented to the collaborative prosthetic team 1 year later for follow-up and to determine next steps. He has not been able to secure employment; however, he cares for his children so his partner can work, and he volunteers with Amputee Coalition as a presenter at Limb Loss Days in his geographic region and offers peer support to individuals with newly acquired upper limb loss. He continues to find value from both of his prostheses but would like to engage more in being able to work out, cook (especially barbecue), and play sports with his children. He was seen approximately 4 weeks following the consultation for delivery of an activity-specific prosthesis with a variety of terminal devices that allow crossover function to recreation activities (Fig. 8–20D). RB was educated to the care of these devices, ability to don and doff the device and to switch out the TDs and to use them during different tasks.

Case Study MT

MT is a young woman, aged 30 years at the time of her injury, living alone in a high-rise apartment in a vibrant metropolitan city. She was employed as senior associate in a private equity firm. Unfortunately, she was injured in a work-related boating accident that resulted in an acquired loss of her nondominant hand. MT was air-lifted from the accident scene to the hospital where reattachment surgery was performed. Unfortunately, rejection occurred and 3 days later surgeons amputated the limb at the transradial level. She was discharged from the hospital at the beginning of week 3 (postinjury), following several surgeries. Her parents and sister decided to stay with her during her first few weeks at home. MT was seen for outpatient hand therapy intervention that included wound healing, edema control, ADLs with adaptive one-handed strategies, and assistive devices.

Initial Plan

Her hospital team, driven by her case manager and hand therapist initiated education to prosthetic technology by setting up a consultation with a prosthetist during the third week posttrauma. The prosthetist showed MT diverse prosthetic technology relevant to her level of loss, and explained the methods of control, benefits, and challenges of each. The prosthetist and hand therapist reviewed the functional characteristics of each device and system, emphasizing the "tool" nature of these devices as opposed to the expectation of any technology replacing the complete function of a natural hand. They explained the process of fitting a prosthesis and the importance of a well-fitting socket for optimal functional outcomes.

MT'S first full-team meeting that included her family, as well as the hospital and community practitioners was held 2 months following her injury. It was determined that she would benefit most from a functional passive aesthetic device as well as an externally-powered multiarticulating hand. The passive device would offer social function and static ability to type, support, stabilize, and push objects. The articulated hand would be helpful during many bimanual activities for self-care, home management, and work-related tasks. It became evident that MT would benefit from ongoing hand therapy to prepare her for the prosthesis via desensitization, core strengthening, and biofeedback to exercise EMG signals for improved control and endurance.

Collaborative Prosthetic Technology Delivery 1

MT was seen 3 months following her accident for intensive collaborative delivery and prosthetic training. She received initial prosthetic training from the prosthetist and hand therapist for both prototype devices that included education to care of the prosthesis; a progressive wear schedule to build up tolerance; instruction, demonstration, and practice to don and to doff the technology independently; instruction, demonstration, and practice to control the multiarticulated terminal device via repetitive skills drills and basic functional tasks in diverse positions and at different heights; and extensive discussion and practice to develop social functional skills and to manage awkward situations in community, education, and work environments (Fig. 8–21A–F).

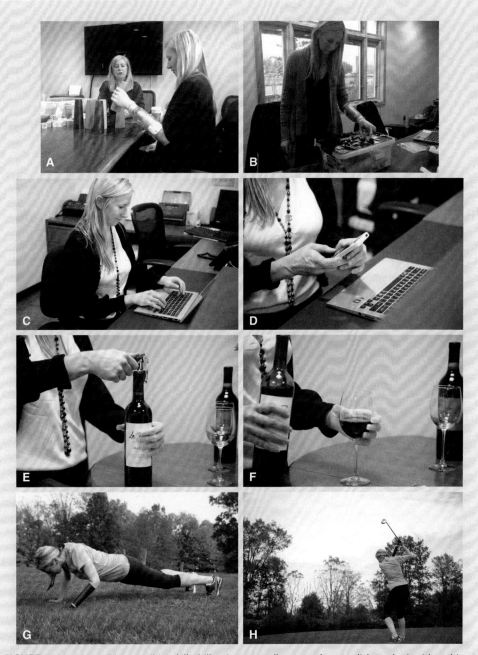

FIGURE 8–21 A, Practicing repetitive skills drills using externally powered transradial prosthesis with multiarticulating terminal device (i-Limb˚ Quantum- Ossur, Ossur, Canada). **B,** With this skill drill, the patient is using an externally powered transradial prosthesis with multiarticulating terminal device. **C,** Eser shown here typing using transradial prosthesis with passive aesthetic functional terminal device (Livingskin™). **D,** Managing cellphone using transradial prosthesis with passive aesthetic functional terminal device. **E,** Opening of a wine bottle using externally powered transradial prosthesis with multiarticulating terminal device. **F,** Stabilizing a wineglass using externally powered transradial prosthesis with multiarticulating terminal device. **G,** Performing push-ups using transradial prosthesis with activity-specific terminal device (TRS Shroom Tumbler terminal device). **H,** Golfing using transradial prosthesis with activity-specific terminal device (TRS EAGLE FLEX terminal device, Fillauer LLC, Chattanooga, TN).

MT took these prototype devices home for a 4-week period to determine fit and function and make recommendations for revisions. During this time, she participated in hand therapy at the outpatient department to further practice skill drills and functional training. She met with the prosthetist at the end of the month to turn the prototype devices to permanent status.

Collaborative Prosthetic Technology Consultation and Delivery 2

MT was seen 10 months later for collaborative prosthetic team follow-up and to determine next steps. She is wearing and using her

devices actively on a daily basis for approximately 10 to 12 hours per day. MT uses the passive aesthetic prosthesis primarily when meeting with clients because of the social function it provides, and that it allows the focus of such meetings to remain client-centered rather than on MT's injury. She uses the externally powered device at home to manage her self-care, most home management tasks, and community living activities such as shopping and banking. Unfortunately, her current technology is not amenable to the recreational activities that MT enjoyed previously such as yoga, pilates, kayaking, and bicycling. The team determined that MT would benefit from additional technology that would meet the robust demands of specific activities. She was seen approximately 4 weeks following the consultation for delivery of an activity-specific prosthesis with a variety of terminal devices that allow crossover function to recreation activities (Fig. 8–21G,H). MT was educated to the care of these devices, to don and doff the device, and to switch out the TDs and to use them during different tasks.

Collaborative Prosthetic Technology Consultation and Delivery 3

MT was seen recently, approximately 4 years from the time of her injury. She is actively using all of her prosthetic technology and presented for repair and replacement of some devices. She stated that she has resumed all previous activities, continues to work full-time, and is planning her wedding. She needs a replacement passive functional aesthetic device to wear for this happy occasion!

CHAPTER REVIEW QUESTIONS

1. Name three basic components of a prosthesis.
2. At what stage would you consider prosthetic intervention?
3. Explain why socket fit is crucial to the user's success in prosthetic function.
4. Name three reasons for prosthetic rejection.
5. Explain one of the new innovations in prosthetic technology control.

ACKNOWLEDGMENTS

The author is grateful for the assistance of Ms. Nancy Vang, OTS, graduate assistant and entry-level OTD student, Division of Occupational Therapy, Western New England University, Springfield, MA, in the preparation of this document. Most images in this chapter are a courtesy of Handspring Clinical Services, and Single-Handed Solutions, LLC.

9

Prefabricated Orthoses[a]

Jamie McMillan, OTR, CHT

CHAPTER OBJECTIVES

After study of this chapter, the reader should be able to:

- Appreciate the various prefabricated devices that are available to address the multitude of upper extremity diagnoses.
- Understand what factors should be considered when choosing between a prefabricated and a custom orthosis.
- Understand basic coding/billing for prefabricated orthoses.
- Give examples of modifications for customization of prefabricated orthoses to address specific patient needs.
- Recognize the various companies that offer prefabricated orthoses.

KEY TERMS

Continuous passive motion (CPM) machine   **Dynamic and static progressive orthoses**   **Prefabricated orthoses**

INTRODUCTION

Healthcare delivery is fluid and ever-changing. As therapists, we must be willing to recognize those changes and make necessary adjustments along the way. One area of practice that has changed rather significantly in recent years is orthotic delivery. This chapter is going to specifically discuss the changes and advancements related to prefabricated orthoses options and how they fit in to our treatment armamentarium. Reimbursements have changed, productivity is often under a microscope, and documentation has become more cumbersome. Concurrently, protocols are evolving; we are oftentimes immobilizing less and moving sooner and fewer casts are being applied. Lastly, our payors are changing; insurance companies are far more finicky as to what they will and will not cover, deductibles are getting higher, patients are experiencing more out-of-pocket expenses, and they are acutely more aware of where their healthcare dollars are going. The collision of these circumstances has made prefabricated orthoses an emerging topic for hand therapists. It is hard to dispute, regardless of our personal preferences, prefabricated orthoses are becoming more prevalent in the practice of hand therapy.

This chapter outlines the considerations related to the use of **prefabricated orthoses** and includes information on how to become an educated consumer on the availability and application of these orthoses. Some of the commonly used and currently available orthoses are reviewed. Prefabricated orthoses can sometimes be used creatively for purposes other than what they were originally intended for; suggestions for these alternative uses are also provided.

CONSIDERATIONS FOR FITTING ORTHOSES

There are several issues to consider before choosing either a custom-made or a prefabricated orthosis. The skill of the therapist is sometimes a determining factor for using prefabricated devices. That is, some therapists custom fabricate orthoses only occasionally; therefore, they either do not have the skills to make the prescribed orthosis or it would not be an efficient use of their time to do so. Similarly, the setting in which a therapist works might dictate the choice of orthoses; those practicing in home healthcare settings without the necessary equipment for custom fabrication may find that prefabricated options are a welcome solution. In addition, one or any combination of the following factors may affect the decision-making process to select the most appropriate orthosis for a patient:

- Specifics of the diagnosis
- Patient needs and preferences
- Time constraints
- Appropriateness and availability of the material
- Ease of application
- Cost-effectiveness

SPECIFICS OF THE DIAGNOSIS

In assessing the patient's needs, one must consider what the best solution is for the immediate situation. The therapist must clearly understand the patient's diagnosis and current status. Does the

---

[a]This chapter is based on the first edition chapter written by Janet Cope, MS, CAS, OTR/L and second edition chapter written by Rebecca Harris, MS, OTR/L, CHT.

patient have a fracture with open wounds and a painful, edematous hand? Does the patient have an external fixator, pins, or other external hardware? Will the patient have specific needs for managing scar tissue? Certain circumstances will require customized orthotic fabrication; in other instances, prefabricated orthoses may be a better choice. Does the patient require rigid immobilization, or would a soft support suffice? For example, a patient with rheumatoid arthritis may use a prefabricated neoprene orthosis to minimize ulnar deviation of the digits during the day and a custom thermoplastic resting orthosis at night (Dell & Dell, 1996).

PATIENT NEEDS AND PREFERENCES

The therapist and patient need to negotiate a safe and reasonable orthosis regimen for optimal outcomes. "Poor compliance to splint wear is a common complaint of clinicians, a complaint that may stem, in part, from a flaw in prescription practices" (Pagnotta, Korner-Bitensky, Mazer, Baron, & Wood-Dauphinee, 2005). Patients are unlikely to wear an orthosis that interferes consistently with their daily activities, however much they require the device, unless time is taken to review rationale and potential outcomes and complications. Patient education and involvement in the plan of care generally increases compliance.

The therapist must consider the needs and desires of the patient. Can the patient wait for the prefabricated orthosis to be ordered if it is not a stocked item? What kind of insurance coverage does the patient have? Will the orthosis be covered? What is the potential responsibility of the patient? The patient's requirements in both the home and work setting should be considered. For example, someone who is a heavy laborer may require a rigid orthosis that is easily washable for work but may be more comfortable in a soft prefabricated orthosis for home. Several other considerations are age, cognitive status, skin integrity, and other current or previous injuries to the involved or uninvolved extremity. The cosmesis and comfort of the orthosis should be considered. If the patient finds the devices uncomfortable or "unattractive," compliance is likely to be affected.

TIME CONSTRAINTS

Time can be a major factor for all organizations and therapists. Today's demand for increased patient caseloads influences how much time the therapist has with each patient. The therapist must evaluate the need and weigh the benefits of a custom-made orthosis versus a prefabricated device. Is it more appropriate to use a prefabricated orthosis and to spend the remaining available time performing hands-on intervention and instruction/education or to fabricate a custom orthosis, limiting the one-on-one time? The therapist must decide what will be the most beneficial to the patient.

APPROPRIATENESS AND AVAILABILITY OF THE MATERIAL

The type of prefabricated orthosis selected or the material used to fabricate a custom-made orthosis can affect patient comfort, tissue healing, and level of support or immobilization. Comfort is an important issue and is directly related to consistent wearing patterns (Rossi, 1988). Patients who have prominent bony structures may be more comfortable in an orthosis that is fabricated from a soft or semirigid material that is not prone to cause discomfort. Thermoplastic is rigid and can be uncomfortable when constant use is required.

Thermoplastic material may be the most appropriate material to use if the patient is required to have his or her hands in water or soil frequently during the day. Thermoplastic material is easy to clean and tolerates moisture better than most fabric-based materials. However, there are patients who perspire and are thus prone to tissue maceration when solid thermoplastic materials are used; a moisture wicking, breathable fabric-based orthosis may be better suited for these patients.

Adjustments can be simple to make on prefabricated orthoses with malleable metal inserts. No equipment is necessary, and the orthosis can be modified at the patient's bedside or in the home when necessary. A thermoplastic orthosis requires a heating source and patient compliance in positioning while the material is molded; this may not always be possible.

EASE OF APPLICATION

Ease of independent application by the patient is an important factor to consider when developing an orthotic intervention plan. The therapist must determine the simplest solution for the patient's requirements. A prefabricated digit extension mobilization orthosis may be easier for patients to apply than a more complicated custom device, while serial static casting might be the simplest solution for other patients.

If the patient has several impairments (e.g., multiple joint contractures or injuries) that need to be addressed with various orthoses, these issues should be prioritized. The therapist must determine the feasibility of the orthotic plan for the patient; an individual who lives alone must be able to don and doff the device(s) independently. Immobilization of healing structures may be the most important issue to be addressed but increasing function may be deemed most important by the patient. Balancing these demands is essential when considering solutions to meet patient goals.

COST-EFFECTIVENESS

When evaluating the patient's needs, the therapist must consider all of the cost-related variables. Is the orthosis going to be worn for a short period of time or will it be required on a more permanent basis? Will the patient's insurance pay for a prefabricated or custommade orthosis? The insurance carrier may or may not cover either type of orthosis. What is the potential out-of-pocket responsibility of the patient for either device? In some situations, the prefabricated orthosis may be more affordable to the patient without compromising the quality of treatment. It is appropriate to educate the patient regarding the options and to include him or her in the decision-making process. In some cases, the patient may require several orthoses, worn alternately throughout the day and night. Some of these orthoses may be custom-made and others prefabricated.

EDUCATED DECISION-MAKING

An educated decision must be made each time an orthosis is selected for a patient. There is a wide variety of materials, components, and prefabricated orthoses available for almost every situation. It is challenging to keep abreast of all of the available prefabricated orthoses, but there are many ways to stay informed.

To keep up with new trends, therapists can attend upper extremity continuing education events, including lectures and hands-on labs on successful orthotic interventions. Larger conferences frequently feature vendor booths that allow therapists to investigate new materials and prefabricated orthoses. Therapists can try orthoses on and gain information directly from the manufacturers. Vendors are eager to provide in-service training, offer product samples, and help with specific patient problem-solving. Company representatives are often therapists who have decided to enter the equipment provision aspect of the business; they are integral to the development of new product lines and improvements of existing ones. In working with therapists all over the country, they collect valuable information on trends and helpful hints and are willing to share the tips they have learned.

Catalogs and websites provide an expansive amount of information regarding orthotic selection, fitting, and therapy intervention. Updated frequently, they enable the therapist to stay abreast of therapy trends. See Appendix A for a list of vendors and rehabilitation companies along with contact information.

Therapists can also review articles in therapy and surgery publications to gain a better understanding of the theoretical basis behind the decision-making for the application of orthoses. There are various treatment options available to treat every patient's diagnosis; what is best for one patient may not be ideal for the next. A custom orthosis might meet the biomechanical issues but may cause problems for the patient in the areas of maintaining skin integrity or comfort (Rossi, 1988). Solutions to many orthotic-related problems can be found by reviewing current literature.

BASIC CODING AND BILLING PRINCIPLES FOR PREFABRICATED ORTHOSES

Billing for a prefabricated orthosis is very similar to billing for a custom orthosis; L-Codes are used to bill both. There are separate L-Codes for custom versus prefabricated, but the overall definitions are congruent; using acronyms to describe what joints are included (E, W, H, F), noting if it is an immobilization or mobilization brace, and, lastly, a prefabricated brace can be either "custom" or "off the shelf" (Table 9–1). The last nuance, "custom" versus "off the shelf" is relatively new and has caused some confusion; however, both are prefabricated. Prefabricated "custom" requires customization

such as bending, molding, and trimming and is fit by a person with expertise. Prefabricated "off the shelf" can be applied right out of the box, by anyone. The difference between prefabricated "custom" and prefabricated "off the shelf" is where the term "split code" comes from. Customize when you can and document it. After all, you are a person of expertise!

With prefabricated braces, there is one extra tool that you can utilize to determine the most appropriate billing code. While it seems that should be "easy" in theory, it is not always cut and dry. Manufacturers of upper extremity orthoses have the option to submit their products to PDAC for code determination. PDAC stands for Pricing, Data Analysis, and Coding and is a contractor to CMS that maintains the Durable Medical Equipment Coding System (DMECS). PDAC is responsible for providing suppliers and manufacturers with assistance in determining which HCPCS code should be used to describe durable medical equipment, prosthetics, and orthoses for the purpose of billing Medicare. Some manufacturers voluntarily submit upper extremity products to PDAC so they can confidently stand behind the billing codes associated with the products they release. Because it is not required by Medicare to submit upper extremity products to PDAC, many manufacturers opt out of the process and rather put a *suggested* code on their label. Every product that has a PDAC determined code has a PDAC letter as documentation of the determination that is available on the PDAC website or through the product manufacturer. That PDAC letter can be very helpful when seeking reimbursement or filing an appeal following denial.

PREFABRICATED ORTHOSES FOR THE UPPER EXTREMITY

This section, which presents a review of various prefabricated orthoses, is organized according to where on the upper extremity

TABLE 9–1	Commonly Used L-Codes for Prefabricated Upper Extremity Orthoses	
L-Code	**Abbreviated Definition**	**Product Examples**
L3670	Shoulder orthosis (SO), acromio/clavicular (canvas and webbing type), prefabricated, off the shelf	Shoulder immobilizer Shoulder abduction sling
L3760	Elbow orthosis (EO), with adjustable position locking joint(s), prefabricated, item that has been trimmed, bent, molded, assembled, or otherwise customized to fit a specific patient by an individual with expertise	Hinged elbow brace
L3762	Elbow orthosis (EO), rigid, without joints, includes soft interface material, prefabricated, off the shelf	Cubital tunnel brace Elbow immobilizer
L3908	Wrist hand orthosis (WHO), wrist extension control cock-up, nonmolded, prefabricated, off the shelf	Carpal tunnel brace Wrist orthosis
L3807	Wrist hand finger orthosis (WHFO), without joint(s), prefabricated item that has been trimmed, bent, molded, assembled, or otherwise customized to fit a specific patient by an individual with expertise	Forearm-based thumb spica Forearm-based ulnar gutter Forearm-based resting hand
L3924	Hand finger orthosis, without joints (HFO), may include soft interface, straps, prefabricated, off the shelf	Hand-based thumb spica Hand-based ulnar gutter
L3927	Finger orthosis (FO), proximal interphalangeal (PIP)/distal interphalangeal (DIP), without joint/spring, extension/flexion (e.g., static or ring type), may include soft interface material, prefabricated, off the shelf	Mallet finger orthosis Oval 8/silver ring
L3925	Finger orthosis (FO), proximal interphalangeal (PIP)/distal interphalangeal (DIP), nontorsion joint/spring, extension/flexion, may include soft interface material, prefabricated, off the shelf	LMB Joint jack

Commonly used upper extremity orthoses that are typically cash items:
   1. Counterforce straps
   2. Prefabricated neoprene wrist wraps
   3. Prefabricated neoprene sleeves
   4. Prefabricated soft thumb supports
   5. DRUJ supports
   6. Dynamic PIP extension orthoses

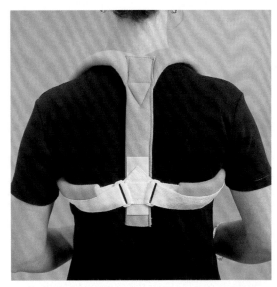

FIGURE 9–1 The Rolyan® Clavicle Posture Support. Observe the patient for 20 minutes after applying a clavicle brace to ensure proper fit. Monitor for any signs of neurovascular compression—numbness, tingling, coolness, or pain in the extremity—and readjust as needed. (Photo courtesy of Performance Health, Warrenville, IL.)

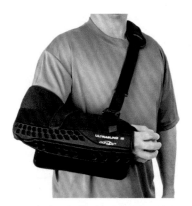

FIGURE 9–2 The Don Joy® Ultrasling® III provides shoulder immobilization for rotator cuff repairs, capsular shifts, Bankart repairs, glenohumeral dislocations/subluxation, and soft-tissue repairs/strains. The De-Rotation Strap hook prevents internal rotation by securely holding the arm in neutral position. (Photo courtesy of DJO® Global, Dallas, TX.)

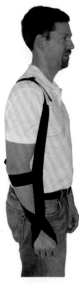

FIGURE 9–3 GivMohr® sling is a positioning device for the flaccid upper extremity. Target populations include individuals who are ambulatory or potentially ambulatory. This sling was developed in a collaborative effort between Victoria Givler, OTR and Paul Mohr, PT in response to the lack of appropriate support devices available. (Photo courtesy of GivMohr® Corporation, Albuquerque, NM.)

the orthosis is to be applied. For each region, various prefabricated orthoses are presented, and comparisons are made to highlight specific fitting issues. This discussion is not meant to be inclusive of all available prefabricated orthoses; each manufacturer has versions of the commonly used prefabricated orthoses, and available products are too numerous to mention all. We recommend a thorough review and update of billing rules, insurance coverage, and proper coding (if applicable) of these prefabricated orthoses be conducted in order to stay compliant and ethical with reimbursement (refer to Chapter 1 for additional information). **Static progressive orthoses, dynamic orthoses,** and **continuous passive motion (CPM) machines** will be discussed in separate sections.

SHOULDER AND UPPER ARM ORTHOSES

The diagnoses commonly treated with prefabricated orthoses at the shoulder and upper arm are clavicle, scapula, and humerus fractures; humeral head dislocations or subluxations; and rotator cuff injuries and surgical repairs. The types of prefabricated orthoses used to treat these conditions are shoulder orthoses (SO) of varying designs including clavicle orthoses, slings, shoulder immobilization orthoses, and upper limb fracture orthoses.

Clavicle Orthoses

Clavicle orthoses are available in a limited variety from most of the major rehabilitation suppliers (Fig. 9–1). Some providers also stock pediatric sizes. When fitting a patient with a clavicle orthosis, a key point to evaluate is an appropriate fit through the axilla. The strap system should be adequately padded and not create increased pressure on the brachial plexus and artery. A loose fit will likely allow for a flexed cervical posture and is not appropriate for proper clavicular stabilization. The patient should be able to relax the shoulders while good cervical and thoracic posture is sustained. Slings/shoulder immobilizers may also be used for managing clavicle fractures. Discuss options and preferences with the referring physician.

Sling/Shoulder Immobilizer

Many of the commonly known and used slings and shoulder immobilizers are very similar in design. The primary difference in many is that a sling consists of the sling body and a single strap

that traverses the shoulder/neck to provide upward support to the affected arm/shoulder. A shoulder immobilizer provides the same support as a sling with additional immobilization of the extremity with a swath/waist strap to prevent the arm from moving away from the body. A sling is typically not reimbursable by insurance, while a shoulder immobilizer is most times a covered item.

There are a wide array of sling and shoulder immobilizers available that stabilize healing structures about the shoulder (e.g., rotator cuff, capsule, ligaments, bone, neurovascular, and other shoulder surgeries). For certain postsurgical protocols, an abduction pillow will be worn in conjunction with the shoulder immobilizer to place the glenohumeral joint in the desired position for optimal healing (Fig. 9–2). Patients with a stable humeral fracture may wear a sling for support and comfort; it should be removed regularly throughout the day for appropriate exercise (Colditz, 1995). There are devices that are designed to specifically provide support and properly position the hemiplegic shoulder. Hemiplegic arm slings are recommended for patients who have hemiplegia or a subluxating humeral head. There are several versions of the hemiplegic sling that have been used for many years; however, the GivMohr® Sling (GivMohr®

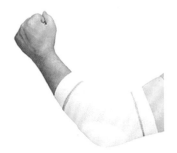

FIGURE 9–6 When fitting a patient with an elbow protector such as the Norco™ Elbow/Heel Protector shown, measure the distance circumferentially around the patient's elbow flexion crease, keeping in mind that the protector is intended to fit snugly. (Photo courtesy of North Coast Medical, Morgan Hill, CA.)

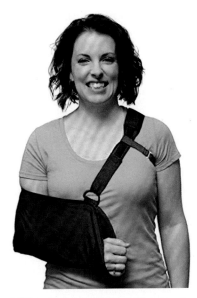

FIGURE 9–4 The Off-Your-Neck Arm Sling provides a way to rest the entire upper extremity. It has a patent pending Neck Relief Strap that relieves discomfort and unnecessary tension on the neck. (Photo courtesy of RangeMaster® Shoulder Therapy, Spokane, WA.)

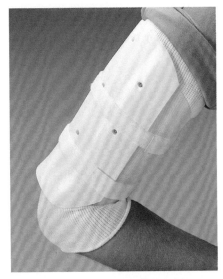

FIGURE 9–5 The circumferential Rolyan® Preformed Humerus Brace allows elbow and forearm motion while providing good immobilization and support to the healing fracture. (Photo courtesy of Performance Health, Warrenville, IL.)

Humeral Fracture Orthoses

A prefabricated humeral fracture orthosis is used to stabilize a fracture in the upper arm while allowing elbow motion. The orthosis promotes fracture healing by compressing the soft tissue in the arm to limit fracture motion. It is imperative that the straps and plastic shell stay tight over the humerus to allow for proper healing. A nonarticular design, which permits shoulder and elbow motion, may be chosen for midshaft fractures (Fig. 9–5) (Sarmiento & Latta, 2006). There are also designs that include a shoulder cap that extends over the deltoid for select cases.

ELBOW AND FOREARM ORTHOSES

The elbow is a complex and challenging joint to position properly and comfortably because it is composed of bony prominences and superficial nerves surrounded by forceful muscles. Some of the prefabricated elbow orthoses (EO) that are available include protectors/sleeves, proximal forearm braces (counterforce braces), hinged elbow orthoses, and elbow immobilization orthoses. Supination/pronation orthoses that have their effect on both the proximal and distal radioulnar joints (DRUJs) are also included in this section.

Elbow Protector/Sleeve

Elbow protectors can be used for a variety of indications but are commonly dispensed before and after surgery for patients with cubital tunnel syndrome (ulnar neuropathy) or bursitis. One available option incorporates a silicone gel pad insert to help reduce shock/vibration and provide light compression and protection from impact (Fig. 9–6). Neoprene compression sleeves may be used to treat ulnar neuropathies, muscle strains, or arthritis of the elbow by providing gentle compression, warmth, and support (Fig. 9–7). The sleeve should fit snugly but not so tightly as to increase or induce any neurologic symptoms (tingling, pain, or numbness distally). It should be noted that some elbow sleeves do not meet the definition of an orthosis and are considered a supply.

Proximal Forearm Orthosis (Counterforce Brace)

Counterforce straps and sleeves which are frequently used to treat medial and lateral elbow pain/epicondylosis come in various options (Fig. 9–8A). Many have padded regions that create a compressive force to the forearm muscles in an effort to change the fulcrum from the epicondyle to the muscle bellies, creating a psuedoattachment (Anderson & Rutt, 1992). This facilitates the muscles to work from across the padded strap rather than directly at the epicondyle, allowing the muscle insertion to rest and heal. They also help reduce the intensity of the muscle contraction, which may reduce pain. When treating a patient with lateral elbow pain/epicondylosis, apply the

Corporation, Albuquerque, NM) is an option that offers proprioceptive input in its design with the added benefit of reducing shoulder subluxation (Dieruf, Poole, Gregory, Rodriguez, & Spizman, 2005) (Fig. 9–3). The therapist must carefully monitor patients who are using slings to ensure that they are removing the sling and exercising the injured extremity, as recommended, to prevent complications of edema and stiffness in distal extremity.

Patients who have undergone hand surgery also may be issued a simple sling to be worn for comfort and protection of the upper extremity during the early phases of healing (Fig. 9–4). Selection of an appropriate sling is contingent on the patient's diagnosis. Patient education with this population is key to minimize the potential ill effects of dependent positioning of the hand: edema and stiffness. Appropriate exercises should be regularly performed to prevent undue stiffness of the proximal joints (stiff elbow or frozen shoulder), and occasional sling removal is important to prevent onset of neck issues.

pad over the forearm extensors about two finger widths distal to the lateral epicondyle. With the elbow in extension, have the patient make a tight fist and then secure the strap firmly. Make sure to have the patient grasp, extend the wrist, and flex the elbow to check for comfort; pain at the lateral elbow should be diminished with the brace properly applied. Caution the patient not to secure the strap too tightly because the radial nerve is vulnerable to compression in this region (radial tunnel) with these particular braces (Aulicino, 1995; Kleinert & Mehta, 1996). Educate regarding the signs of compression which include pain in the radial tunnel region with referral into the dorsoradial aspect of the hand.

Many of the straps and sleeves designed for the treatment of lateral elbow pain/epicondylosis can also be used in the treatment of medial elbow pain/epicondylosis by rotating the pad to apply pressure on the medial forearm muscles. Some sleeves and straps can be used to treat patients who are diagnosed with both medial and lateral elbow pain/epicondylosis. These devices are designed to apply compression to both the extensor and the flexor muscle groups simultaneously (Fig. 9–8B,C).

Hinged Elbow Orthoses

Prefabricated hinged orthoses can be used for restricting range of motion (ROM) in one or both directions or to restrict motion in either direction (Fig. 9–9). For example, when treating a patient with a distal biceps tendon repair, initially the brace can be locked to restrict full elbow extension, thereby preventing tension on the repaired tendon, while allowing for a full flexion arc. As healing progresses, the extension restriction can be modified to allow progressively greater extension. Hinged elbow braces are also commonly used to provide varus/valgus support to the elbow while allowing for ROM in the flexion/extension plane. A variety of hinged elbow braces are available that include antihyperextension straps as well, frequently used for athletes who are returning to sport after injury.

Elbow Immobilization Orthoses

Prefabricated elbow orthoses are available to statically position the elbow joint. Night positioning has long been considered a staple of conservative treatment for cubital tunnel syndrome; however, its efficacy is dependent on elbow position and patient compliance (Shah, Calfee, Gelberman, & Goldfarb, 2013). Keeping the elbow out of hyperflexion for prolonged periods of time (i.e., during sleep) decreases tension and inflammation of the nerve. There are a variety of prefabricated braces on the market that immobilize the elbow: anterior or posterior designs (Fig. 9–10A). Other indications for an elbow immobilization orthosis may include but are not limited to dislocation, fracture, and arthritis. The Tiny Cast-Away™ (Hely & Weber®, Dallas, TX) (Fig. 9–10B) is rigid but made from soft materials that are well tolerated by children, and hygiene is more manageable for caregivers than a cast. While a custom-fabricated orthosis is also a reasonable solution for these patients, it can be challenging to have children hold still in the required position for the duration of the molding process with thermoplastics.

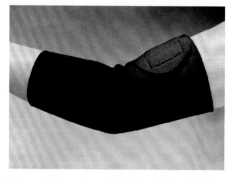

FIGURE 9–7 After applying a circumferential orthosis such as this Comfort Cool® Open Elbow Support, monitor the patient for a short time, watching for any signs of neurologic symptoms: numbness and tingling. (Photo courtesy of North Coast Medical, Morgan Hill, CA.)

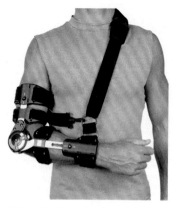

FIGURE 9–9 Innovator X® Post-Op Elbow has one of the most user-friendly hinges in postop bracing, increasing patient satisfaction and compliance. (Photo courtesy of Össur® Americas, Inc., Reykjavik, Iceland.)

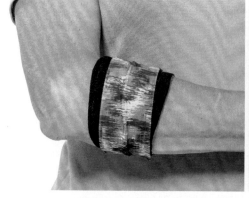
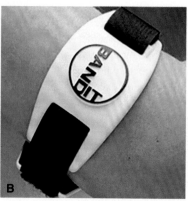
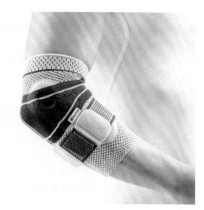

A   B   C

FIGURE 9–8 A, The Elbow POP™ Splint should reduce the patient's pain; adjust the amount of compression applied as needed to increase patient comfort. (Photo courtesy of 3-Point Products®, Stevensville, MD.) **B,** The BandIT® Tennis Elbow Strap is useful for treating medial or lateral epicondylitis. The unique design compresses across the flexor, extensor, and supinator muscles and allows movement without compromising circulation. (Photo courtesy of North Coast Medical.) **C,** The user-friendly EpiTrain® elbow sleeve combines the benefits of a compressive elbow sleeve with a tennis elbow brace. (Photo courtesy of Bauerfeind® USA, Inc., Atlanta, GA.)

Supination/Pronation Orthoses

Immobilization of forearm rotation is commonly managed by a sugar tong or Muenster-type orthosis. The MTC Fracture Brace™ (Hely & Weber®) is a prefabricated option that allows for functional elbow ROM while immobilizing supination/pronation (Fig. 9–11). The brace is comprised of an elbow and a forearm component, and the therapist can choose the position of immobilization of the forearm based on the diagnosis. Fabrication of a custom design can take significant time, requires a large piece of thermoplastic, and can be challenging to mold.

A tone and positioning (TAP) orthosis is a simple and comfortable alternative to a custom-molded supination/pronation orthosis. The Comfort Cool® Pronation-Supination Splints (North Coast Medical, Morgan Hill CA) provide a gentle, low-load supination or pronation stretch to aid in increasing functional hand position (Fig. 9–12). This device, although originally developed for patients with neurological conditions, can be beneficial in facilitating supination or pronation ROM if the tissue at the forearm and wrist is not too dense (soft-end feel). This orthosis is not capable of delivering the torque required for patients with hard-end feel or long-standing limitations in ROM.

WRIST ORTHOSES

The wrist is made up of several joints that allow multidirectional movement, which can be complicated to support properly. When immobilization is the goal of an orthosis, it is essential to provide adequate support to the wrist in all planes of motion. Prefabricated orthoses used for treating diagnoses at the wrist are wrist hand orthoses (WHO) which cross the wrist joint, leaving the digits free, and wrist hand finger orthoses (WHFO) which cross the wrist joint and include at least one digit.

Wrist Hand Orthoses

There are several issues to consider when fitting a patient with a prefabricated WHO including clearance of the distal palmar crease/thenar eminence and comfort at the first web space. Proximal fit at the forearm should be ensured to reduce migration, digital movement should be observed, and appropriate wrist position is important.

Adequate distal clearance is necessary for unrestricted grasp and pinch activities. The patient should be able to flex all fingers fully and comfortably with little or no interference from the distal portion of the wrist support. Be mindful when fitting these devices, if they do not extend far enough distally, the wrist will not be immobilized adequately. Patients with large forearms and narrow wrists have inherent problems with distal migration of wrist orthoses and improper fit. The Titan Wrist™ Lacing Wrist Orthosis (Hely & Weber®) is a prefabricated WHO that addresses common problems associated with prefabricated wrist braces; the web space strap is padded, contoured, and adjustable to avoid irritation in a highly vulnerable area. Also, there is a movable dorsal stay pod that allows for

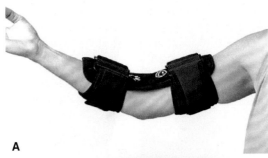

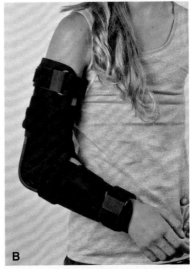

FIGURE 9–10 **A,** The Cubital Comfort™ Brace is an anterior brace designed to avoid pressure along the ulnar nerve while immobilizing the elbow in the desired position which is customizable. **B,** Tiny Cast-Away™ is a pediatric specific rigid elbow brace designed to be a cast replacement or a cast step-down option. (Photos courtesy of Hely & Weber®, Dallas, TX.)

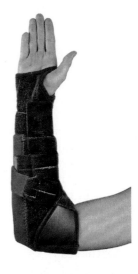

FIGURE 9–11 MTC Fracture Brace™ is a therapist-designed orthosis used to control forearm rotation; commonly used for TFCC injuries/repairs, postop ulnar shortening procedures, and other pathologies of the DRUJ. DRUJ, distal radioulnar joint; TFCC, triangular fibrocartilage complex. (Photo courtesy of Hely & Weber®, Dallas, TX.)

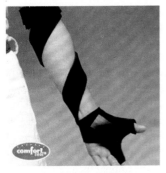

FIGURE 9–12 The Comfort Cool® Pronation-Supination Splint is made of neoprene and applied in either supination or pronation, to patients of all age groups. The neoprene strap can be used with the included glove component or with a custom-fabricated thermoplastic wrist support. (Photo courtesy of North Coast Medical, Morgan Hill, CA.)

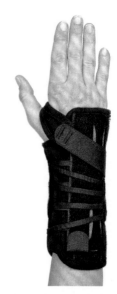

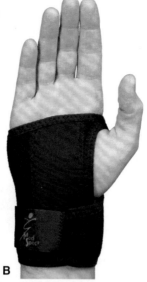

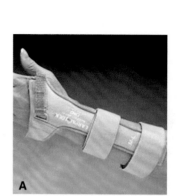

FIGURE 9–13 The Titan Wrist™ Lacing Wrist Orthosis allows for adjustability in fit and rigidity making it customizable to fit each patient. (Photo courtesy of Hely & Weber®, Dallas, TX.)

FIGURE 9–14 **A,** The Carpal Lock® dorsal-based wrist orthosis positions the wrist in neutral, allowing unrestricted digital motions. (Photo courtesy of North Coast Medical, Morgan Hill, CA.) **B,** The GelFlex® Wrist orthosis provides scar management within the design ideal for postoperative patients. (Photo courtesy of Medical Specialties, Inc., Charlotte, NC.)

sizing adjustments within the brace providing an excellent fit (Fig. 9–13). If a prefabricated orthosis is unable to provide the patient with adequate support or fit, a custom-fabricated orthosis may be indicated.

The actual position of the wrist should be visualized while the prefabricated orthosis is on the patient and adjusted appropriately as per the specific diagnosis. For example, a patient with a wrist sprain is usually positioned for comfort, whereas an individual with a distal radius fracture is often positioned in 20° to 30° wrist extension after cast removal. If the patient is unable to obtain the desired range of extension, a prefabricated orthosis with a malleable metal or thermoplastic insert can be molded to the appropriate degree of wrist extension and later modified.

Carpal Tunnel Syndrome

Prefabricated volar wrist supports are commonly prescribed to patients with carpal tunnel syndrome as a conservative method of treatment (Keith et al., 2009). Patients should be immobilized in a neutral wrist position to provide maximum space at the carpal tunnel and reduce compression on the median nerve (Brininger et al., 2007) (Fig. 9–14A).

For patients with postoperative scar hypersensitivity, the Med Spec GelFlex® Wrist Brace (Medical Specialties, Inc., Charlotte, NC) has a gel pad on the volar aspect of the brace to provide gentle, conforming compression to the incision site (Fig. 9–14B). The gel is formulated with medical-grade mineral oil aiding in scar maturation. The single volar stay gives gentle feedback to prevent extreme joint positions following surgery.

Arthritis

Volar wrist supports (Fig. 9–15) afford mobility at the hand and digits; they are frequently prescribed for people with arthritis as a means to rest the affected wrist joint. Although wrist supports can be beneficial, patient compliance for wearing them is relatively low (Pagnotta, et al., 2005). Patient concerns regarding wrist supports (whether prefabricated or custom) include comfort, interference with activities, appearance, cost, and reduced freedom of movement.

When treating patients with arthritis, the therapist needs to clearly define all relevant issues and goals to help determine which regimen best suits the needs of the patient (see Chapter 17 for more details).

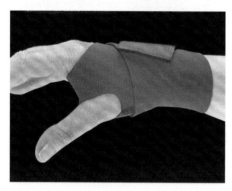

FIGURE 9–15 The thumb hole of this AliMed® Neoprene Wrist/Hand Wrap can easily be modified by simply trimming with scissors. (Photo courtesy of AliMed®, Dedham, MA.)

Some patients have problems with hyperhidrosis and prefer a light, breathable fabric orthosis, whereas others find orthoses that help keep the area warm to be helpful. Patients who are working or physically active tend to prefer the least restrictive orthosis. Patients may not tolerate metacarpophalangeal (MCP) support during the day but will use a wrist/hand/finger orthosis (WHFO) to comfortably position the hand while sleeping (Fig. 9–16).

Ulnar-Sided Wrist Pain

Ulnar-sided wrist pain is a common problem that can be a result of injury to bone, cartilage, ligaments, or tendons. Common causes include fracture, triangular fibrocartilage complex (TFCC) injury, or ulnar impaction syndrome. Diagnosis can be difficult, and therefore treating ulnar-sided wrist pain can be challenging. In recent years, several orthoses have been developed to specifically address this problem (Fig. 9–17A–C)

Wrist Hand Finger Orthoses

Individuals with various diagnoses may require a WHFO for day and/or night use. Orthoses that meet the definition for WHFO include resting hand orthoses, immobilizing orthoses, and forearm-based dynamic gloves.

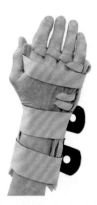

FIGURE 9–16 This forearm-based orthosis called the Comforter™ Splint has extra padding and is intended for night use; target patient populations include those with arthritis or neurological dysfunction. (Photo courtesy of 3-Point Products®, Stevensville, MD.)

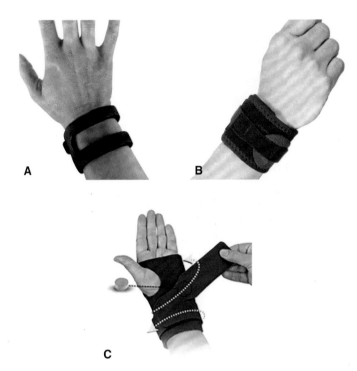

A

B

C

FIGURE 9–17 A, The WristWidget® is designed to address ulnar-sided wrist pain due to a TFCC (triangular fibrocartilage complex) tear. When suspecting a TFCC injury—performing a weight-bearing test can help further define the extent of injury and assist in developing an intervention plan. (Photo courtesy of WristWidget®.) **B,** "Squeeze" ulnar compression wrap treats ulnar-sided wrist pain through focal point compression to avoid the tourniquet effect of circumferential wraps. (Photo courtesy of Hely & Weber®, Dallas, TX.) **C,** Comfort Cool® Ulnar Booster™ is specifically for those experiencing ulnar-sided wrist pain and midcarpal instability; designed to realign and stabilize the carpal bones while depressing the ulnar styloid. (Photo courtesy of North Coast Medical, Morgan Hill, CA.)

Resting Hand Orthoses

There are several designs available for the treatment of patients with diagnoses such as arthritis, burns, nerve palsies, crush injuries, and spasticity. The approach can be volar, dorsal, or circumferential. There are soft versions that provide a gentle, continuous stretch to spastic muscles and more rigid plastic orthoses that provide immobilization (Wallen & O'Flaherty, 1990). The SaeboStretch (Saebo Inc., Charlotte, NC) orthosis is an example of a flexible prefabricated WHFO that provides support used for patients with mild to moderate increased tone (Fig. 9–18A). To address issues such as decreased functional use, increased tone, and contractures in the pediatric population, Comfy™ Hand Orthoses (Lenjoy Medical

Engineering, Inc., Gardena, CA) offer various options that are terry cloth lined in multiple colors (Fig. 9–18B). The Benik Corporation W-700 series (Benik, Silverdale, WA) offers patients with radial nerve palsy several options for wrist and/or digit support in a low-profile design (Fig. 9–18C). See Chapter 20 for more details about the neurologically involved patient.

Immobilizing Orthoses

Forearm-based thumb orthoses (Fig. 9–19A,B) are frequently used as an immobilizing orthosis for diagnoses such as carpometacarpal (CMC) arthroplasty, DeQuervain's, and healing fractures. There are a variety of prefabricated options available from low-profile designs that restrict motion to more substantial options with various features to meet specific patient needs. Additionally, forearm-based radial/ulnar gutter style orthoses are frequently used to treat metacarpal fractures.

Dynamic Gloves

For patients with peripheral nerve injury, the Robinson InRigger Gloves (AliMed®, Dedham, MA) provide dynamic digit extension dorsally for the wrist and digits while allowing full finger flexion for function (Fig. 9–20A,B).

HAND FINGER ORTHOSES

Because the hand is unique, the therapist is faced with many challenges in balancing the medically necessary restrictions with the patient's need for functional use. Some of the prefabricated hand finger orthoses (HFO) include immobilizing orthoses, thumb restrictors, and ulnar deviation orthoses.

Immobilization Orthoses

At times, it is necessary to rigidly immobilize the patient's thumb or finger, and there are various prefabricated and preformed immobilization orthoses available for this purpose.

The thumb is responsible for approximately 40% of hand function (Swanson & de Groot Swanson, 1990). When supporting a patient's thumb, the therapist must consider that the thumb is involved in all tasks requiring grasping, pinching, stabilizing an object, or requiring sensory information to operate (King, 1992). The therapist can be extremely challenged to find an orthosis, prefabricated or custom made, which is comfortable and functional while providing the proper support and positioning for the thumb joints. A painful CMC joint can limit pinch or grip and severely impair hand function. An ideal orthosis for osteoarthritis at the CMC joint is one that stabilizes the joint in midpalmar/radial abduction, restricts adduction, and allows for full flexion at the IP joint (Melvin, 1995). The Push® MetaGrip® (BraceLab, Raleigh, NC) immobilizes and supports the CMC joint (MP and IP joints free). This device is adjustable, extremely durable, available in multiple sizes, can be cleaned in a washing machine, and will not lose shape in the heat (Colditz & Koekebakker, 2010) (Fig. 9–21A,B).

The EXOS® Hand-Based Ulnar Gutter (DJO® Global, Dallas, TX) (Fig. 9–21C) is used to immobilize fractures to the fourth or fifth metacarpals or proximal phalanges. This molded orthosis is designed to provide a custom fit and allows for the fabricator to obtain up to 70° of MCP flexion of the fourth and fifth digits.

Thumb Restriction Orthoses

Neoprene thumb orthoses (either prefabricated or custom) can provide warmth and support to the thumb (see Chapter 14 for details). Custom-made thermoplastic orthoses for CMC arthritis are quite effective in immobilizing the thumb joint in a position of rest.

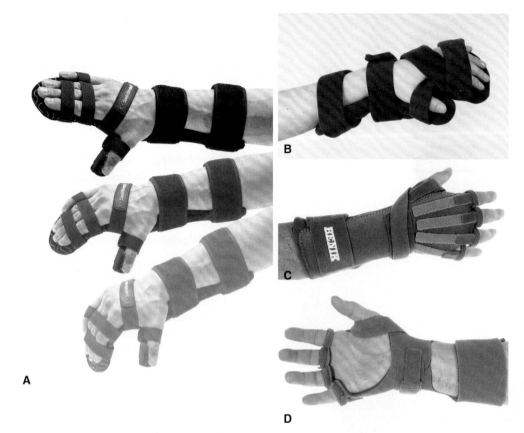

FIGURE 9–18 **A,** The SaeboStretch is recommended for patients with neurologic conditions such as mild to moderate spasticity. (Photo courtesy of Saebo, Inc., Charlotte, NC.) **B,** This Comfy™ Resting Hand Orthosis with finger separators is washable and easily modified to obtain a custom fit. Many options are available including thumb and dorsal-based designs. (Photo courtesy of Comfy Splints, Gardena, CA.) **C and D,** The Benik W711 Radial Nerve Splint is a low-profile forearm-based option helpful for those patients requiring long-term orthotic management. Note that this device is also offered in a hand-based design for patients without wrist involvement. (Photos courtesy of Benik Corporation, Silverdale, WA.)

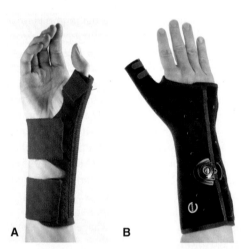

FIGURE 9–19 **A,** The Target Hitchhiker Thumb Orthosis allows IP joint motion while immobilizing the wrist and thumb MP/CMC joints. (Photo courtesy of Corflex®, Manchester, NH.) **B,** The Long Thumb Spica Fracture Brace from EXOS® (distributed by DJO® Global) provides an alternative to casting or a circumferential orthosis. This unique prefabricated device allows for a customizable fit by dry heating the precut form and molding it directly to the patient. The unique BOA® closure system provides adjustable compression to accommodate for edema changes and patient comfort. This orthosis can be washed or worn while bathing or swimming without risk of skin maceration due to perforations and unique material characteristics. (Photo courtesy of DJO® Global, Dallas, TX.)

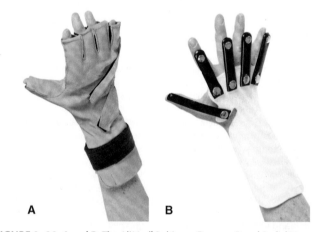

FIGURE 9–20 **A and B,** The AliMed® Robinson Forearm-Based Radial Nerve Splint provides a low-profile and inexpensive alternative to managing this challenging population, also available in hand and forearm-based designs. (Photos courtesy of AliMed®, Dedham, MA.)

Unfortunately, this immobilization orthosis can significantly hinder normal hand function and is often bothersome to the patient's skin and bony prominences. Patients often complain that the orthoses are uncomfortable and interfere with their daily routines. The CMC Controller Plus™ (Hely & Weber®) is designed to counter the classic deformity that occurs with CMC arthritis by utilizing a small aluminum stay that helps lift the metacarpal head, with a sling strap

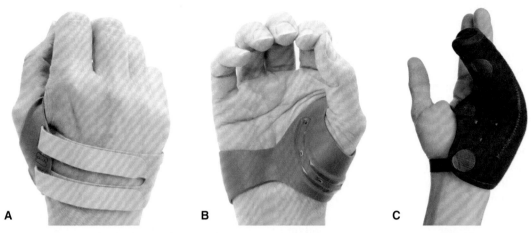

FIGURE 9-21 **A and B,** The Push' MetaGrip' allows for maximum thumb and hand function while still offering optimal CMC joint positioning. An aluminum insert is adjustable to fit the individual patient. (Photos courtesy of BraceLab, Raleigh, NC.) **C,** The EXOS' Hand-Based Ulnar Gutter Brace is a sized orthosis that uses convection heat to mold and achieve a custom fit. CMC, carpometacarpal. (Photo courtesy of DJO® Global.)

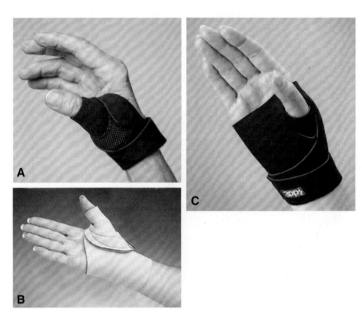

FIGURE 9-22 **A,** CMC Controller Plus™ is a hybrid approach to pain relief and positioning—malleable stay supports the metacarpal head and assist strap allows for easy application. (Photo courtesy of Hely & Weber®, Dallas, TX.) **B,** The neoprene material of the Comfort Cool' Thumb CMC Restriction orthosis provides the joint warmth, gentle support, and protection. A version of this design is available that includes a moldable thermoplastic piece to provide a rigid stay at the CMC joint. (Photo courtesy of North Coast Medical, Morgan Hill, CA.) **C,** The 3pp' ThumSling' NP provides adjustable compression and support about the thumb. Note that a longer version including the wrist is also available. (Photo courtesy of 3-Point Products®, Stevensville, MD.)

that captures and seats the metacarpal base, opening the web space (Fig. 9-22A). The Comfort Cool® Thumb CMC Restriction Splint (North Coast Medical) is another functional orthosis commonly used for CMC dysfunction including instability and arthritis (Fig. 9-22B). A version of this design is available that includes a moldable thermoplastic piece to provide a rigid stay at the CMC joint. The 3pp® ThumSling NP (3-Point Products®, Stevensville, MD) is designed to stabilize the CMC joint while allowing some mobility (Fig. 9-22C).

MCP Joint Deviation Orthoses

The therapist should closely follow patients who have rheumatoid arthritis and are using supportive devices to slow the progression of carpal collapse and the resulting ulnar deviation at the MCP joints

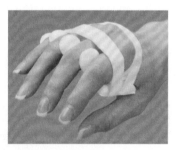

FIGURE 9-23 An LMB Soft Core Ulnar Deviation Splint is worn to support the MCP joints in extension and prevent radial deviation, which enables the patient to better perform functional grasp activities. (Photo courtesy of DeRoyal', Powell, TN.)

(Dell & Dell, 1996). Patients with an ulnar drift may benefit from being supported with an ulnar deviation orthosis (Fig. 9-23). Short and long versions of this orthosis and other suggested prefabricated orthoses for this population are reviewed in Chapter 17.

FINGER ORTHOSES

There are a variety of prefabricated finger orthoses (FO) available to address numerous pathologies common to the digit. Prefabricated finger orthoses are divided into two categories: immobilization (without joint, ring type) and mobilization (nontorsion joint/spring).

PIP/DIP Joint Immobilization Orthoses

A common injury to the finger that requires immobilization is a boutonniere deformity or the disruption of the central slip (portion of extensor mechanism as it inserts onto the base of the middle phalanx) (Palchik et al., 1990). Aronowitz and Leddy (1998) treat all patients with acute boutonniere deformities with a device that positions the PIP in extension, leaving the distal interphalangeal (DIP) free to move actively or passively. Oval-8® (3-Point Products®) and SilverRing™ Boutonniere Splint (Silver Ring Splint Company, Charlottesville, VA) may be used for the correction of a boutonniere deformity and offer a more cosmetic solution for long-term deformity (Fig. 9-24A,C). Active and passive ROM at the DIP joint, while extension is passively maintained at the PIP joint, facilitate optimal anatomic positioning of the lateral bands.

Swan-neck deformity, hyperextension of the PIP joint and flexion of the DIP joint, is commonly seen in patients who have rheumatoid arthritis or chronic volar plate injuries at the PIP joint. Orthotic selection will typically include a restriction orthosis; application aims to prevent hyperextension of the PIP joint while allowing for full flexion. These devices prevent the often painful "snapping" of the lateral bands as they slide dorsally when the PIP joint goes into hyperextension. The Oval-8® from 3-Point Products® (Fig. 9–24B) and the SilverRing™ Swan Neck Splint from Silver Ring Company (Fig. 9–24D) offer a low-profile, attractive, and extremely effective option to maximize function of the digit with this chronic deformity.

Mallet finger, the disruption of the terminal tendon at its attachment on the distal phalanx, requires a rigid DIP extension orthosis. The goal of treatment is to immobilize the DIP joint, allowing the terminal tendon to scar down during an uninterrupted period of 6 to 8 weeks (Alexy & De Carlo, 1988). One concern for the treating therapist and physician is maintaining tissue integrity on the dorsum of the DIP joint during this required immobilization period. Prefabricated options include Auerbach Mallet Splint (Hely & Weber®) and Stax Splints (North Coast Medical) (Fig. 9–25A,B). The Auerbach Mallet Splint can be worn volar or dorsal, and the rigid stay is malleable so that the

position can be adjusted. A benefit of the clear plastic Stax Splint is visualization of the vulnerable skin on the dorsum of the finger. One limitation is that alterations in position of DIP joint are not possible. Garberman, Diao, and Peimer (1994) report that as long as the injured digit is continuously kept immobilized in extension for 6 to 10 weeks, the type of orthosis used is insignificant in the successful outcome of mallet finger deformity. Although an AlumoFoam® splint is an accessible solution for the treatment of mallet finger for many, it does not meet the code definition to be considered an orthosis and therefore is not billable by L-Code. Rather, it is a splint and would be considered a supply. Keep in mind that due to the variability in patient presentation, a custom-fabricated orthosis may be the most appropriate option for some patients.

PIP/DIP Mobilization Orthosis: Dynamic and Static Progressive

There are various digit-based spring-loaded (dynamic) PIP extension mobilization orthoses available to address PIP joint flexion contractures. The amount of padding, length, and ability to alter force depend on the design. The LMB Spring Finger Extension

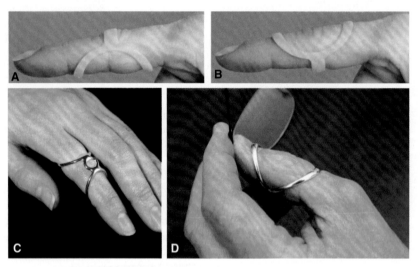

FIGURE 9–24 A and B, Oval-8® Finger Splints may be used for management of a more chronic boutonniere **(A)** or swan-neck deformities **(B)**; they are offered in multiple sizes and can be modified with a heat gun. (Photos courtesy of 3-Point Products®, Stevensville, MD.) **C,** SilverRing™ Boutonniere Splint blocks flexion, deviation, and extreme hyperextension. **D,** SilverRing™ Swan Neck Splint blocks hyperextension while allowing finger flexion for function. (Photos courtesy of Silver Ring Splint Company.)

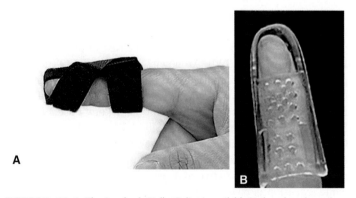

FIGURE 9–25 A, The Auerbach Mallet Splint is available in three lengths and can be used for any aspect of digital immobilization. (Photo courtesy of Hely & Weber®, Dallas, TX.) **B,** The Open-Air™ Stax Finger Splint is perforated, allowing air circulation and decreasing the likelihood of tissue maceration. (Photo courtesy of North Coast Medical, Morgan Hill, CA.)

Assist (DeRoyal® Industries, Powell, TN) is one example of this common orthosis (Fig. 9–26A). These come in various lengths; be sure to properly fit the device to the digit watching for any undue stress on adjacent joints.

Digit extension neoprene sleeves, such as the AliMed® Dynamic Digit Extensor Tube™ (AliMed®), can also be used to treat patients with PIP joint flexion contractures that have a soft-end feel (Fig. 9–26B). Patients may tolerate wearing this orthosis longer because the heat generated by wearing a neoprene material can increase tissue extensibility and blood flow while decreasing joint stiffness, pain, and muscle spasms (Michlovitz, 1990). Patients should be instructed in tissue monitoring because maceration of the skin can occur owing to excessive perspiration (Clark, 1997).

Other PIP joint mobilization orthoses include variations of the Bunnell™ Safety Pin Splint (Tiburon Medical Enterprises) that provide a dynamic force via a spring coil (Fig. 9–26C). A Rolyan® Sof-Stretch Coil Extension Splint (Capener) (Performance Health) may

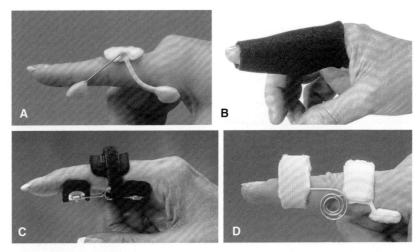

FIGURE 9–26 **A,** The LMB Spring Finger Extension Assist can be adjusted to provide more force (straighten orthosis) or less force (squeezing pads together) to the PIP joint. The lateral wires can also be pulled out slightly to accommodate edema. (Photo courtesy of DeRoyal®, Powell, TN.) **B,** The AliMed® Dynamic Digit Extensor Tube™ is made of neoprene and applies a low-tension load to the PIP joint into extension. This "banana-shaped" device is comfortable to wear and comes in various sizes. (Photo courtesy of AliMed®, Dedham, MA.) **C,** The Bunnell™ Safety Pin Splint can be utilized to address PIP joint flexion contractures. (Photo courtesy of Tiburon Medical Enterprises, Inc., San Jacinto, CA.) **D,** Rolyan® Sof-Stretch Coil Extension Splint (Capener) can be used to position the PIP in extension. (Photo courtesy of Performance Health, Warrenville, IL.)

also be used in the treatment of boutonniere injuries postoperatively and PIP joint flexion contractures (Fig. 9–26D) (Capener, 1967; Colditz, 1990; Iselin, 1997; Prosser, 1996). In an investigation by Prosser (1996), patients reported that the low-profile Capener Splint was easy to wear during the workday. Patients are more likely to use a comfortable, low-profile orthosis, thus spending more time in the device. Time spent at total end range is a significant factor; the greater the wearing time, the greater gains made in treating a PIP flexion contracture (Flowers & LaStayo, 1994; Prosser, 1996).

SUPPLIES

There are many supplies often used in the hand therapy clinic that do not meet the code definition of an orthosis. They are still valuable tools that therapists depend on to help achieve patient goals.

Elasticized wraps, such as Coban™ and CoFlex® (Performance Health), can also be applied to address limited passive flexion of the digits. This reusable wrap is self-adherent, making it easy to apply, hold in place, and reuse. The 2″ to 4″ rolls are useful for wrapping all fingers into flexion if limited motion is consistent across the digits. The 1″ rolls are best used when the fingers require individual levels of stretch. Many manufacturers have a version of this elastic wrap. The thinner wraps are useful for applying a stretch wrap to the digits and then dipping in paraffin because the wax can seep into contact with the fingers fairly readily. The thicker wraps are best for gentle edema wrapping because they provide support to a swollen, painful finger.

PIP/DIP flexion wraps are fabricated and sold by many companies to provide a flexion stretch to the PIP and DIP joints simultaneously or separately (Fig. 9–27A,B). However, the therapist can easily fabricate this simple wrap with 3/4″ pajama elastic forming an adjustable loop. Patients can readily increase the tension by sewing, stapling, or securing a safety pin to make the loop tighter and impart a greater stretch.

The flexion glove is a staple found in most hand therapy clinics (Fig. 9–27C). It can be used alone or in conjunction with a volar wrist support to prevent the wrist from collapsing into flexion when a flexion force is applied to stiff digits. The patient can easily apply the glove and adjust it to a comfortable level of stretch independently. Consider customization of the glove by converting the

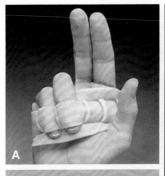

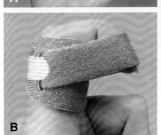

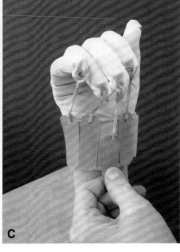

FIGURE 9–27 **A,** The Norco™ Cinch Strap provides a flexion stretch for combined MCP and PIP limitations. (Photo courtesy of North Coast Medical, Morgan Hill, CA.) **B,** The 3pp® Final Flexion Wrap™ also addresses digit extension contractures: simple to use, adjustable, and offers a flexible comfortable material. This device can also be used for other issues—refer to Table 9–1. (Photo courtesy of 3-Point Products®, Stevensville, MD.) **C,** The Finger Flexion Glove produces digit and thumb flexion stretch by providing dynamic traction to the MCP, PIP, and DIP joints via rubber bands.

force applied from dynamic to static progressive by replacing the rubber bands with static line for those patients not responding to the dynamic stretch.

Various types of gloves are available, including short-fingered work gloves, bicycle gloves, and weight-training gloves, which are used to protect the hand from vibration, cold, contact stress, or repetitive work activities (Fig. 9–28A). People who use wheelchairs frequently wear palmar-padded gloves to increase their ability to grasp and decrease the wear and tear on their hands.

For patients with significant scarring to either the dorsal or the volar surface of the hand, the Bio-Form® Pressure Glove (North Coast Medical) can help control edema and hypertrophic scarring (Fig. 9–28B). This glove is available with or without open fingertips, which can provide opportunity for vascular monitoring and

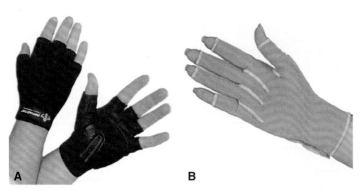

A   **B**

FIGURE 9–28 **A,** Impacto˚ Gloves come in various sizes and lengths; they are often helpful for patients managing multiple trigger fingers by padding the palm and preventing the ability to fully flex the digits. (Photo courtesy of Impacto, Ontario, Canada.) **B,** The Bio-Form˚ Pressure Glove helps reduce edema, provides compression to scar tissue, and allows monitoring of vascularity. (Photo courtesy of North Coast Medical, Morgan Hill, CA.)

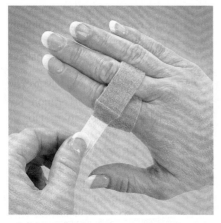

FIGURE 9–29 The 3pp˚ Buddy Loops˚ are one example of prefabricated buddy straps, commonly used to ease the transition out of an immobilization orthosis. (Photo courtesy of 3-Point Products˚, Stevensville, MD.)

sensory input. For scar management alone, fully lined silicone gloves are available. For edema alone, various compression gloves, such as Isotoner® gloves, are available from most medical suppliers.

Buddy straps are readily available in different forms from most major medical supplier and are used to treat many finger injuries including fractures, dislocations, sprains, and extensor tendon injuries (Fig. 9–29) (Alexy & De Carlo, 1988). These straps can be prefabricated or custom-made and are easily adjusted to fit to swollen or slender fingers (see Buddy Strap fabrication in Fabrication Manual Chapter 4, Nonarticular Orthoses).

AlumoFoam® splints come in a variety of sizes and shapes and can be a quick option to immobilize a finger for a variety of indications. The material is lightweight, sturdy, and malleable for bending/molding to achieve desired immobilization position. Simply trim to the correct size and secure in place with elastic bandage or tape. They are most commonly used for finger fractures, strains/sprains, cuts, fingertip and nail bed injuries, and mallet finger injuries (Fig. 9–30).

OTHER DEVICES

CONTINUOUS PASSIVE MOTION MACHINES

Continuous passive motion (CPM) machines can be used during initial phases of rehabilitation following surgery or trauma. The goals of early rehabilitation are pain control, decrease swelling/inflammation, and provide passive ROM in a specific plane of motion while protecting the injured/repaired tissues. The CPM device moves the joint through

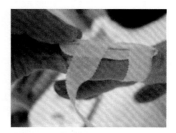

FIGURE 9–30 AlumoFoam˚ secured with tape. Applying the tape obliquely to the volar fingertip and then crossing it over the dorsum of the device provide maximum distribution of pressure and secure the distal phalanx in good extension while the terminal tendon is healing.

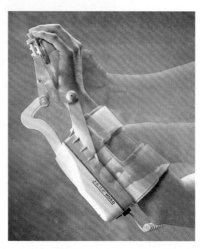

FIGURE 9–31 The JACE™ W550 Wrist CPM Machine allows for control of end-range stretching including programmable tension and time parameters. (Photo courtesy of JACE™ Systems, Cherry Hill, NJ.)

a controlled ROM; the exact range is specific to each individual, but, in most cases, the ROM is increased over time. This section is organized by each joint of the upper extremity that CPMs can be utilized for.

Shoulder

A shoulder CPM machine can be used for treating postoperative shoulders to prevent joint and soft-tissue contractures. The Optiflex® S Shoulder CPM (Chattanooga, Vista, CA) is an example that is universal for left or right upper extremity use and has a memory chip card to store data for patients.

Elbow

An elbow CPM machine may be used to increase ROM, prevent joint contracture, or to decrease pain. The Artromot™ E2 Compact Elbow CPM (Chattanooga) provides anatomical motion for the elbow and enhances patient comfort and compliance. The device addresses full ROM limitations of flexion and extension at the elbow and supination and pronation of the forearm.

Wrist

Wrist CPM machines may be used to aid in increasing ROM at the radiocarpal joint. The JACE™ W550 Wrist (JACE™ Systems, Cherry Hill, NJ) (Fig. 9–31) is a lightweight, portable CPM that is capable of performing full ROM of the wrist in flexion/extension and radial/ulnar deviation. The device will "warm-up" the wrist with limited ROM as the treatment session begins and slowly increases to the full ROM programmed over time.

Hand Finger

CPM machines may be used to treat patients with stiff edematous fingers, a common complication of many injuries of the upper extremity. The CPM can be used to facilitate gentle ROM throughout the fingers or can be used to achieve increased motion at a specific joint. Note that obtaining full DIP flexion is a challenge when applying these devices. Furthermore, the unaffected joints often compensate by maximally flexing, thus decreasing the force aimed at the target joints. For example, when addressing tight PIP joints, the MCP joints may hyperflex, thus prohibiting optimal stretch at the PIP joints. The Vector1 (Lantz Medical) is an example of hand/finger CPM machine (Fig. 9–32) that allows for comprehensive finger ROM with specific ROM considerations for each digit. Early goals for rehabilitation of patients with hand burn injuries include restored soft-tissue coverage and "rapid advancement of active ROM" at the MCP joints (Barillo et al., 1997). Patients with burns who are unable to flex the MCP joints to at least 70° and those who are unable to flex the digits actively secondary to the side effects of medication, may use a CPM for 4 to 8 hours during the day and possibly while they sleep. The therapist should carefully monitor the use of a CPM machine, and the settings should be checked frequently.

STATIC PROGRESSIVE AND DYNAMIC DEVICES

Following prolonged immobilization or trauma, the connective tissue surrounding joints can become shortened resulting in joint contracture. When typical ROM progress is not being made with therapy alone, an increase of therapeutic end-range stretch can be an effective solution. Static progressive and dynamic devices are designed to provide low intensity and prolonged stretch to shortened connective tissues at their end range to achieve permanent tissue elongation. Both treatment techniques are used to permanently lengthen shortened connective tissue and restore joint function. Static progressive and dynamic devices are most effective when used in conjunction with formal therapy. Although they share a common end goal of permanent remodeling of joint tissues, each does so with a different approach and protocol. In this section, popular static progressive and dynamic orthoses will be discussed for each joint of the upper extremity. Please refer to Chapter 15 for further information.

Static progressive stretching involves using inelastic components to stretch and hold the tissue at a constant length near end ROM, applying a stress-relaxation load. The tissue resistance decreases over time, and the force is then increased incrementally throughout the treatment session, lengthening the tissues. Dynamic devices use elastic or spring-loaded tension to apply a constant, low-load stretch on the joint at or near end joint ROM over a prolonged period of time to elongate the shortened tissues. The soft tissue responds to the prolonged force and remodels; this is called creep (Schwartz, 2016).

According to Joint Active Systems® (JAS®) (Effingham, IL), a leader in the industry, numerous published peer-reviewed studies support a protocol of three 30-minute sessions per day for optimal results using a static progressive stretching device. Alternatively, suggested wearing protocols for dynamic devices range from 3 to 12 hours of continuous use per day. Ultimately, the wearing schedule for either device should be customized by the therapist to each patient based on their individual needs and response to treatment.

A number of factors should be considered when choosing what mobilization device would be most beneficial for a particular patient. Patient compliance, pain tolerance, and independence with donning/doffing and performing adjustments, all might affect which device would be most appropriate. Using the Modified Weeks Test is an objective way to determine which type of orthoses to prescribe. First, a PROM measurement is taken of the affected joint. Heat is then applied for 15 to 20 minutes followed by manual or mechanical mobilization of the joint. PROM is remeasured. If a gain of approximately 10° is achieved, a dynamic brace is indicated. If the gain is 5° or less, a static progressive device is chosen (Flowers, 1994).

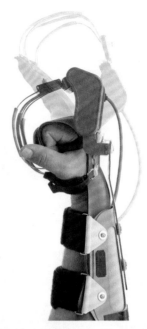

FIGURE 9–32 The Vector1 Hand CPM has an easy-to-apply glove design that allows for individualization of each digit. Setup is quick; device is lightweight and easy to operate. (Photo courtesy of Lantz Medical, Indianapolis, IN.)

Shoulder

Stress relaxation and static progressive stretch may be used to nonoperatively restore ROM for adhesive capsulitis and other injuries that result in shoulder stiffness. Using a static progressive stretch orthosis compared to physical therapy alone produced significant improvement in all planes of ROM (Ibrahim et al., 2012). The Stat-A-Dyne Shoulder (Lantz Medical) can perform static or dynamic stretch in full shoulder external/internal rotation and abduction/adduction ROM.

Elbow/Forearm

Stiffness secondary to fractures and dislocations at the elbow can be treated with various prefabricated static progressive and dynamic elbow orthoses that provide a corrective force to the tissue. Devices such as the Elbow Extension or Flexion Dynasplint® System (Dynasplint® Systems, Severna Park, MD) and Progress™ Elbow Hinge Orthosis (North Coast Medical, Morgan Hill, CA) have neoprene or foam cuffs with malleable metal attachments both proximal and distal to the elbow. These orthoses are flexible and comfortable for the patient and can be easily adjusted when there is a decrease in bandages or edema. Patients can wear this type of orthosis with the load adjusted to provide a gentle stretch for sleep or intermittent daytime use. The application of a gentle stretch over a long period of time improves tissue extensibility and yields permanent tissue lengthening (Bonutti, Windau, Ables, & Miller, 1994). To maintain the gains in ROM, the orthosis can be locked at a specific end range if desired, providing a means of static progressive positioning. Dynasplint® Systems offers these orthoses in pediatric and infant sizes as well as adult sizes; separate units for extension and flexion are required.

JAS® has developed a static progressive orthosis that can be used to treat limitations of forearm supination and pronation in a single device. Similarly, they have a separate unit that addresses both elbow flexion and extension contractures (Fig. 9–33). The device has proximal and distal cuffs, which can be adjusted to fit various limb lengths, and a load-adjustable hinge centered at the olecranon. Patients with spinal cord injuries at C5–C6 frequently develop elbow flexion contractures and may benefit from this type of orthosis. Mackie Elbow Brace (Ortho Innovations, Rochester, MN) offers a static progressive stretch in either flexion or extension in the same

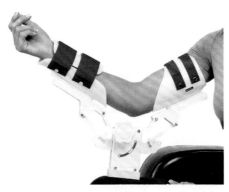

FIGURE 9–33 The JAS' SPS Elbow can be used to address either flexion or extension contractures at the elbow. The patient can easily don this orthosis and adjust the tension until a stretch is felt. (Photo courtesy of Joint Active Systems', Effingham, IL.)

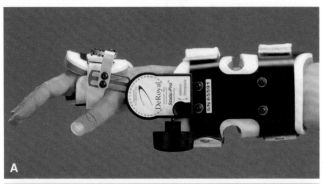

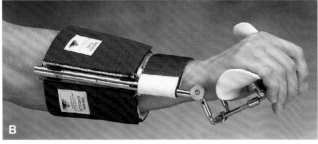

FIGURE 9–34 **A,** The Static-Pro' Wrist offers a static progressive stretch at the joint's end range. (Photo courtesy of DeRoyal', Powell, TN.) **B,** This Dynamic Wrist Extension Splint provides a stretch in one direction only; multiple units are required to address multiple areas of stiffness. These units can be rented or purchased. (Photo courtesy of Dynasplint' Systems, Inc., Severna Park, MD.)

unit. The Stat-A-Dyne™ ESP from Lantz Medical (Indianapolis, IN) allows for addressing elbow flexion/extension and supination/pronation limitations either with a static progressive or dynamic approach all in one device.

Wrist

Prefabricated dynamic and static progressive wrist orthoses are commonly prescribed to increase wrist ROM. The JAS® SPS Wrist (Joint Active Systems) is designed to increase wrist flexion and extension. The Static-Pro® Wrist Orthosis (DeRoyal®) provides an alternative for wrist flexion and extension mobilization (Fig. 9–34A). Dynasplint® Systems also offers Dynamic Wrist Splints for wrist extension and flexion orthoses in both adult and pediatric sizes (Fig. 9–34B).

Hand Finger

Various prefabricated static progressive and dynamic finger orthoses are available to address stiffness (see Chapter 15 for more detailed information). Full ROM at the PIP joints is imperative for hand function; therefore, both dynamic and static progressive PIP orthoses are commonly used in the clinic. A loss of extension at this joint can limit a person's ability to release objects, extend digit to prepare to grasp larger objects, or collect change with an open palm. A loss of flexion at this joint can severely limit the ability to grasp objects or even shake hands (Prosser, 1996). The Stat-A-Dyne® WHFO uniquely provides for full ROM in both wrist and digit extension and flexion (Lantz Medical) (Fig. 9–35A,B). Other PIP joint mobilization devices include the Dynasplint® Systems PIP Extension unit and the JAS® EZ Finger (which offers extension and flexion within a single device) (Joint Active Systems®).

PREFABRICATED ORTHOSES ADAPTATIONS

Keeping abreast of all of the information on available orthotic materials, components, and prefabricated options is both challenging and interesting. Therapists must be able to use all available resources to best meet the needs of their patients. Sometimes, this means adapting prefabricated orthoses for purposes other than what they were originally intended to do. Table 9–2 provides a few creative ways to use prefabricated orthoses.

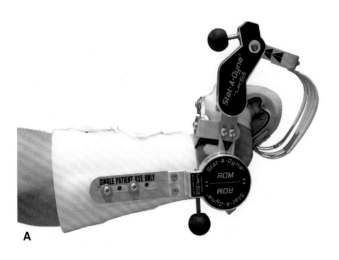

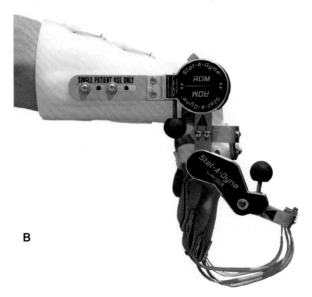

FIGURE 9–35 **A and B,** The Stat-A-Dyne™ WHFO provides the therapist with the ability to isolate the tissue stretched by positioning the wrist and digits accordingly. This device also allows for a synergistic stretch into a functional grasp and release pattern as shown. (Photos courtesy of Lantz Medical, Indianapolis, IN.)

TABLE 9-2	**Creative Uses of Prefabricated Orthoses**			
Prefabricated Orthosis	**Intended Use**	**Expanded Use**	**Adaptations**	
MTC Fracture Brace™ (Photo courtesy of Hely & Weber®)	Immobilize forearm rotation	Static progressive orthosis	Lock forearm at end range of supination or pronation; progress as tolerated to address rotation ROM deficits	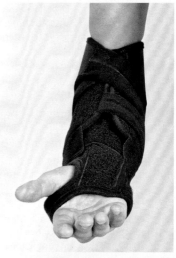
Wrist orthosis	Wrist support	Act as base for digit mobilization for radial nerve palsy or MCP joint stiffness	Add finger loops around proximal phalanx of involved digits. To address loss of active digit extension attach to hook dorsally—radial nerve palsy (A); to address lack of passive MCP flexion attach to hook volarly—MCP extension contracture (B)	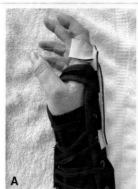 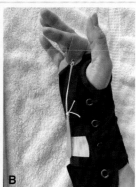
Padded palmar work gloves (or as an alternative padded biking/ weight lifting glove) (various)	Reduce shock and vibration in hand	Reduce MCP flexion in trigger finger; reduce impact at A1 pulley region	Patient wears glove to sleep preventing composite digit flexion and for functional use during day to relatively build up handles of tools	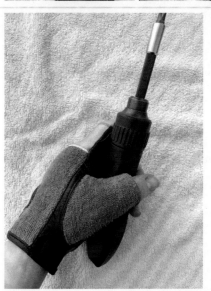
3M Coban™ Self-Adherent Wrap (Performance Health)	Edema control	Digit flexion stretch	Apply to individual digit or all digits in full fist position; may also wrap hand and then utilize paraffin to combine stretch and heat modality	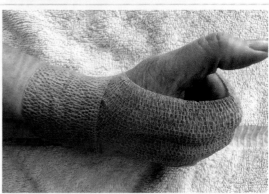

(Continued)

TABLE 9–2	**Creative Uses of Prefabricated Orthoses** (Continued)			
Prefabricated Orthosis	**Intended Use**	**Expanded Use**	**Adaptations**	
Finger Flexion Glove (North Coast Medical)	Digit flexion stretch via dynamic traction (rubber bands)	Digit flexion stretch via static progressive approach (static line)	Remove rubber bands and replace with static line/ segments of loop strapping—to attach to hook proximally—will allow for adjustment as tissue allows	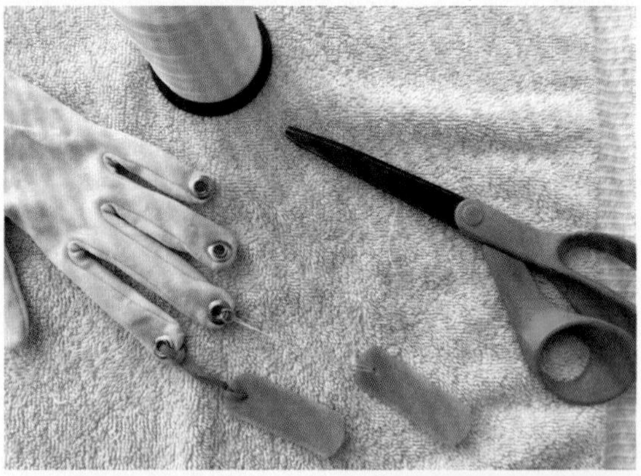
Isotoner® glove (A) (or as alternative use generic garden glove (B)) (Performance Health)	Edema reduction	As flexion mobilization glove (may utilize in combination with volar wrist orthosis) to prevent compensatory wrist flexion	Punch holes at tips and attach rubber bands (dynamic) or static line/ loop strapping (static progressive) to apply flexion force	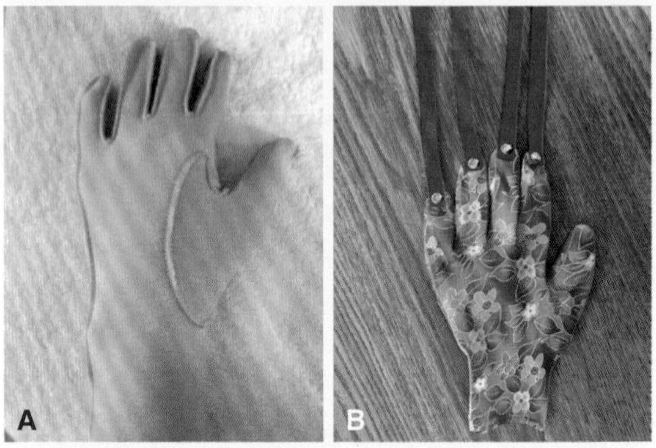
Reverse finger knuckle bender (Performance Health)	PIP extension	FDP or FPL resistance exercise tool	Move orthosis to distal phalanx and instruct patient to pull actively through resistance of rubber band—adjust resistance accordingly	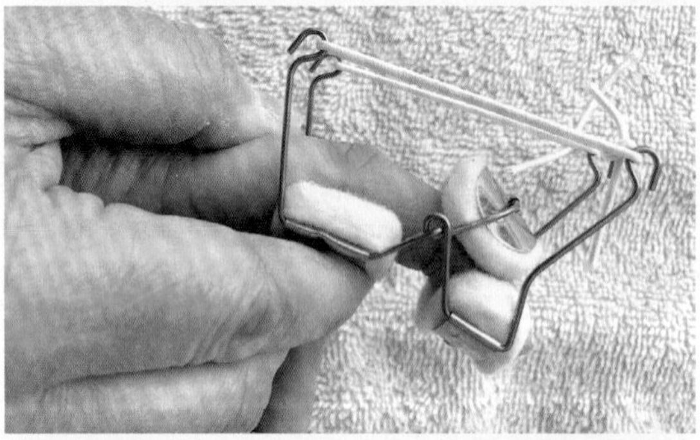
LMB Spring Finger Extension Assist (DeRoyal®)	PIP extension	Increase tissue extensibility	Use in combination with paraffin/hot pack to combine stretch and heat modality	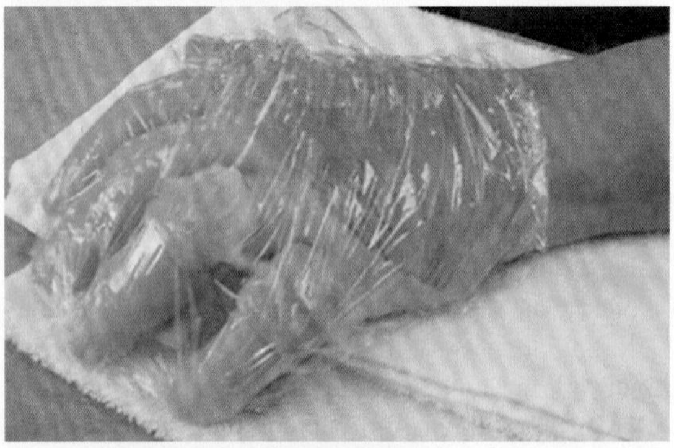
Dynamic Digit Extensor Tube™ (Alimed®)	PIP extension	Increase PIP extension	Add thermoplastic piece volarly (Orficast shown here); may be applied directly against skin or adhere to outside of tube	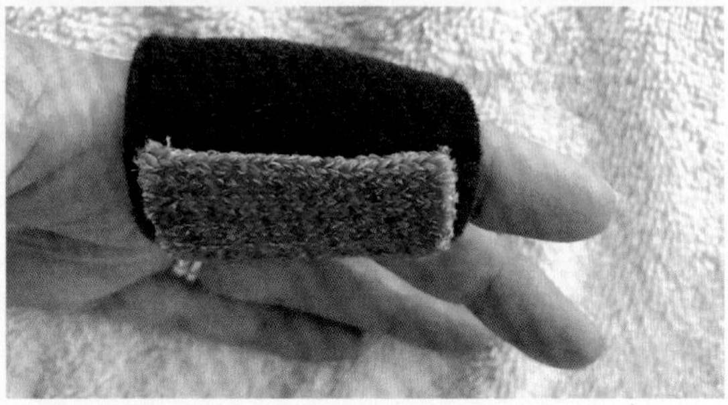

TABLE 9–2	Creative Uses of Prefabricated Orthoses (Continued)			
Prefabricated Orthosis	Intended Use	Expanded Use	Adaptations	
Oval-8˚ Finger Splints (3-Point Products˚)	PIP extension	Isolated DIP flexion	Clear DIP proximally, use as exercise blocking orthosis to promot FDP glide	
Exam Glove (various)	Personal protective equipment	Digit flexion stretch	Cut off a single finger and the distal end, apply as a loop/cinch around the distal and proximal phalanges to impart end-range stretch	
Rolyan Digit Finger Sleeve (Performance Health)	Edema reduction	As strapping alternative—may be helpful to prevent "window edema" between traditional strapping	Choose size that provides appropriate amount of compression to digit, accommodating for orthosis	
Silipad™ Digital Cap (North Coast Medical)	Scar management	As strapping alternative—may be helpful to prevent "window edema" between traditional strapping	Choose size that provides appropriate amount of compression to digit, accommodating for orthosis	

CONCLUSION

Prefabricated orthoses play an integral part in the practice of upper extremity therapy. The therapist should carefully evaluate each patient and then determine which type of orthosis is most appropriate. When determining what orthosis to use, the therapist must consider the biomechanical goals, requirements for the treatment of a specific diagnosis, and, most important, the patient's goals. Sometimes, a custom-made orthosis is necessary; and at other times, a prefabricated orthosis is the better choice.

CHAPTER REVIEW QUESTIONS

1. What factors should be considered when choosing between a prefabricated and a custom orthosis?
2. Give an example of a modification that can be made to a prefabricated orthosis in order to address a specific patient need.
3. What diagnoses would be most appropriate for a prefabricated orthosis? Which would not?
4. How can a therapist keep abreast on the wide variety of prefabricated orthoses available?
5. Give two examples of prefabricated mobilization orthoses and their function, advantages, and disadvantages.

CHAPTER 9

10 Casting[a]

MaryLynn A. Jacobs, MBA, MS, OTR/L, CHT

CHAPTER OBJECTIVES

After study of this chapter, the reader should be able to:
- Define and discuss key concepts and terms related to casting.
- Identify key factors to consider when selecting the most appropriate cast technique.
- Appreciate the material choices available for casting the joints of the upper extremity.
- Understand the various applications for casting a joint or body part.
- Describe the most common diagnoses or conditions that would be appropriate for the casting techniques presented.
- Explain the general precautions relative to the use of the various casting materials.

KEY TERMS

Bivalved

Casting motion to mobilize stiffness (CMMS)

Cylindrical

Drop-out cast

Fiberglass casting materials

Plaster of Paris (POP)

Serial stati

Soft casting materials

Univalved

INTRODUCTION

Casting is the circumferential application of rigid or semirigid material to a part of the body. Casting is one choice in the initial step of nonsurgical management of hand injury (Catalano, Barron, Glickel, & Minhas, 2018). The materials used include **plaster of Paris (POP)**, rigid or soft casting tape, and digit casting tapes. These tapes function similar to, but are not the same as, thermoplastic tapes such as Orficast® (Orfit) and QuickCast (Performance Health). In this chapter, the reader will find some examples with the use of thermoplastic tapes that can be used as an alternative. Pictures of these thermoplastic tapes are included and briefly reviewed because many practitioners still associate these tapes as a casting product. The subsequent chapters—Chapter 11—will go into greater detail about the specifics of the materials, their function, and level of performance.

Often, the cast has no opening for removal, but it can be **univalved** or **bivalved** to allow the cast wearer to remove and reapply it. Serial stretchers, often made of POP, incorporate half the extremity circumference (Tribuzi, 1990). A **drop-out cast** is circumferential on one side of a joint and incorporates half the extremity circumference on the other side. This design blocks joint motion in one direction but allows motion in another; thus, the patient may use active motion to help resolve a passive limitation but cannot regress to a prior posture (Hill & Yasukawa, 1999; Flinn & Craven, 2014). Although the cast, drop-out cast, and serial stretcher have no moving parts and are often considered immobilization orthoses, they can provide or augment the functions of a mobilization orthosis (Bell-Krotoski, 1987, 2011). Colditz (2011) describes the use of casting materials for the mobilization of chronically stiff joint(s). This concept is reviewed briefly in this chapter but in greater detail in Chapter 15 (Box 10–1).

INDICATIONS FOR USE

Clinicians find casting to be a powerful weapon in their treatment arsenals. The casting technique helps solve several challenging problems that the therapist frequently identifies during the patient evaluation. Because casting provides optimal pressure distribution and a cast usually remains on 24 hours per day, the patient population for casting often includes those with sensory, motivation, and cognitive problems (Bell-Krotoski, 1987, 2011). Cast immobilization is also shown to be slightly more effectual than the traditional approaches (immobilization and mobilization removable orthoses) most likely due to the casts' greater capacity to reduce edema (Tocco et al., 2013). Casting maintains the maximum tolerable end-range position and thus maximizes end-range time. As described by Flowers and LaStayo (1994), (2012), the greater the end-range time, the faster the contracted tissue lengthens, and passive range of motion (PROM) increases.

INDICATIONS FOR CASTING INCLUDE THE FOLLOWING:

- **Swollen, painful proximal interphalangeal (PIP) joints**—common after joint dislocation and joint reconstruction (Bell-Krotoski, 1995, 2011; Colditz, 2002)
- **Acute, closed central slip avulsion without fracture** (Colditz, 2002; Coons & Green, 1995; Evans, 2011; Rosenthal & Elhassan, 2011; Schneider & Smith, 1987)

---

[a]This chapter is based on the first-edition chapter written by Karen Schultz, MS, OTR/L, FAOTA, CHT.

BOX 10–1   TYPES OF CASTS

Univalved cast: opened only on one side normally to increase space secondary to edema or discomfort; can be secured with hook-and-loop or a circumferential wrap (Fig. 10–12A).

Bivalved cast: cut on both sides for easy removal; can be secured with hook-and-loop or a circumferential wrap (Fig. 10–12B).

Drop-out cast: part of the extremity can be moved within the cast; restricts motion in one or more directions (Fig. 10–12C).

Cylindrical cast: typical circumferential fracture cast needs to be removed using a saw (Fig. 10–12D).

Plaster slab/stretcher cast: these incorporate half the surface/circumference of the body part; most often used to give rigid support to a joint and used with a circumferential wrap or to apply a stretch to extrinsic tendons and tight tissues (Fig. 10–12E).

- **Acute, closed terminal extensor tendon rupture or avulsion** (Brzezienski & Schneider, 1995; Rosenthal & Elhassan, 2011; Catalano et al, 2018)
- **Extrinsic muscle-tendon unit tightness**—a sequelae to protective positioning and common after many types of injuries, including extensive soft-tissue injury to the hand or wrist, crush injury, tendon and nerve laceration, replantation, and fracture (Colditz, 2002; Tribuzi, 1990; Catalano et al, 2018)
- **Hard end feel contractures of any joint**—may be secondary to fracture; amputation; dislocation; tendon rupture, laceration, or repair; nerve repair; volar plate avulsion; and burn (Bell-Krotoski, 1995; Colditz, 2002; Schultz-Johnson, 1992, 1999; Tribuzi, 1990)
- **Muscle-tendon unit imbalance at a joint**—may be the result of ulnar nerve palsy, arthritis, tendon avulsion, or tendon laceration and repair (Bell-Krotoski, 1987; Ugurlu & Ozdogan, 2016)
- **Proximal joint loss of PROM**—improvement requires long lever arms via a mobilizing orthosis (Bell-Krotoski, 1987; Colditz, 2002)
- **Chronically stiff hand**—casting motion to mobilize stiffness (CMMS) (Colditz, 2000a, 2000b, 2002, 2011)
- **Compliance problems** (Bell-Krotoski, 2011; Colditz, 2011; Sailer & Salibury-Milan, 2000)
- **Loss of PROM owing to spasticity** (Goga-Eppenstein, Hill, Seifert, & Yasukawa, 1999; Midgley, 2016)

CASTS CAN BE USED FOR VARIOUS PURPOSES, INCLUDING THE FOLLOWING:

- To rest and/or protect a joint, especially when edema needs to be controlled (Bell-Krotoski, 1995; 2011)
- To coapt acutely ruptured tendons or bony avulsion and to immobilize the part to allow anatomical healing (Brzezienski & Schneider, 1995; Coons & Green, 1995; Schneider & Smith, 1987; Catalano et al., 2018)
- To increase PROM by holding articular and periarticular structures at the maximum tolerable length for long periods of time, remodeling tissue (Flowers & LaStayo, 1994, 2012; Glasgow, Tooth, Fleming, & Hockey, 2012)
- To transfer a muscle-tendon unit force to adjacent joints (Bell-Krotoski, 1987; Colditz, 2011)
- To rebalance flexor and extensor mechanisms at the PIP joint (Bell-Krotoski, 1987)
- To increase the effective lever arm and thus the force at a proximal joint when distal joints are casted (Bell-Krotoski, 1987)
- To act as a base for mobilizing orthoses when distributing pressure and minimizing migration are essential
- To mobilize multiple joints by casting specific joints in positions of function and allowing self-mobilization of noncasted joints via active range of motion (AROM) (Colditz, 2000a, 2000b, 2011)
- To mobilize a joint by blocking motion in one direction and allowing motion in another (Goga-Eppenstein et al., 1999)
- To decrease tone and increase soft-tissue length in spastic extremities (Colditz, 2002, 2011; Flinn & Craven, 2014)

SWOLLEN, PAINFUL PIP JOINTS

After joint dislocation or reconstruction, the PIP joint may require rest in the maximum available extension (Fig. 10–1A,B). This position reduces the incidence of PIP flexion contractures, assists in controlling edema, and places the joint structures in the optimal position to regain function. Dorsal dislocations or fracture dislocations are exceptions and require an orthosis to block extension in order to protect the healing volar structures (Baltera, Hastings, Sachar, & Jitprapaikulsarn, 2010; Lubahn, 1988). A cast reduces edema and provides excellent pressure distribution (Tocco et al., 2013). The hard shell offers protection from external forces. However, the cast may stress the PIP joint during removal, even if it is soaked first to soften it. Thus, for highly acute joint involvement that results in extreme tenderness, the therapist may need to choose another form of orthotic intervention other than casting.

ACUTE, CLOSED CENTRAL SLIP AVULSION AND ZONE III EXTENSOR TENDON REPAIR

Casting is one treatment method for acute, closed central slip avulsion and zone III extensor tendon repair (Fig. 10–3A–C) (Evans, 1995, 2011; Rosenthal & Elhassan, 2011; Catalano et al., 2018). The sooner this injury is identified and treated, the better. However, even weeks and months after injury, if the finger still appears to be inflamed, the tendon may still benefit from a period of undisturbed extension in a cast. When the tendon is allowed to rest in the stress-free, shortened position, it may heal without surgical intervention. Positioning the finger with the PIP in neutral and the distal interphalangeal (DIP) left free coapts the ends of the torn central slip and allows the rebalancing of the extensor mechanism at the DIP joint. It also helps elongate the oblique retinacular ligament (ORL) and improve DIP flexion. Evans (1995), (2011) adds a nail hook and rubber band to the cast with a proximal rubber band attachment on the volar side of the cast to increase DIP flexion in the finger with a tight ORL. Another option to consider when the digit presents with a tight ORL (instead of a nail hook) may be to use a strip of elastic therapeutic tape or a soft Microfoam™ tape to apply gentle flexion force. To use this approach, start on the dorsal proximal surface of the cast and direct the tape over the DIP joint with gentle pressure ending on the volar proximal surface of the cast (Fig. 10–2D,E).

Ideally, if the finger demonstrates full PIP extension, the cast is left in place for approximately 6 weeks. If the finger has developed a flexion contracture, then the PIP needs to be serially casted until full extension is reached. Once the PIP flexion contracture is resolved, the 6-week period of immobilization commences. Some clinicians recommend starting small arc–guarded active motion at 3 weeks; however, this must be done with great care and with a responsible patient (Evans, 1995), (2011). If the patient flexes the PIP abruptly during this time, the therapist can assume that the continuity of the central slip has been compromised, and the 6 weeks of extension must begin again. Making this information clear to the patient facilitates compliance. At the 6-week point, the patient is gradually weaned from the cast and can begin wearing a removable orthosis. Discontinuing extension positioning abruptly can compromise the end result.

EXTRINSIC MUSCLE-TENDON UNIT TIGHTNESS

Extrinsic muscle-tendon unit tightness occurs after many types of injuries, including extensive soft-tissue injury to the hand or wrist, crush injury, tendon and nerve laceration, replantation, and fracture. It can also be a sequela to protective positioning. The therapist has many treatment options for minimizing the muscle-tendon unit shortening, one being the POP stretcher, which can be very effective if constructed well (Fig. 10–3).

The advantage of plaster lies primarily in its extreme rigidity. The initial plaster costs little. However, if the patient requires many serial stretchers, the price of the material added to the cost of setup and cleanup may equal or even exceed the cost of thermoplastic material. The **serial static** treatment process necessarily involves progression of the orthosis' shape to position the tissue at ever-greater lengths. Although plaster cannot be remolded the way thermoplastic material (elastic based) can, it often gives superior results. The type of thermoplastic material that can withstand frequent remolding is often not rigid enough to maintain the joint at end range. Highly rigid thermoplastics cannot tolerate frequent remolding and must be discarded for new material. Reinforcing the thermoplastic requires effort each time the orthosis is revised. With a minimum of practice, therapists can fabricate POP stretchers efficiently and cost effectively.

Another essential advantage is POP's superior drape and ability to distribute pressure. When pressure is distributed well along the skin surface, the patient can withstand higher forces (Brand, 1988). The limitations in the amount of force that can be generated in an orthosis are related to skin tolerance because this is usually the weak link in force delivery. However, if the force is well distributed, the target tissue can often withstand higher loads (Brand, Hollister, Giurintano, & Thompson, 1999a). It is theorized that higher loads may have the potential to increase tissue length faster. Thus, plaster provides the opportunity to increase PROM faster than materials that are less conforming and less efficient at distributing the load.

HARD END FEEL JOINT CONTRACTURES

Brand (1988) was the first clinician to use serial casting on hard end feel contractures of the PIP joints (see Chapter 15 for details). Since then, therapists all over the world have used this technique on PIP joints and other joints of the upper extremity with great success (Fig. 10–4). Serial casting positions shortened tissue at maximum length but not beyond it, the way mobilizing orthoses with elastic traction tend to do. This positioning applies a mechanical stress to tissue, causing it to remodel in a longer form. Clinical experience has shown that almost any contracture involving live tissue, even one that is years old, will benefit from serial casting. Serial casting has been shown to be an effective treatment modality to address dense flexion contractures in the PIP joints of patients with arthritis (Ugurlu & Ozdogan, 2016). Notable exceptions are Dupuytren's disease and contractures caused by fibrotic tissue (see Chapter 15 for details). Heterotopic ossification and exostosis do not respond to casting.

Tissue that has been overstretched will shorten when placed on slack for a significant duration in a cast. Clinical experience suggests that tissue remodeling to increase length occurs more rapidly than remodeling to shorten overstretched tissue. In the case of a PIP flexion contracture, the cast may reestablish enough length in the palmar tissues to allow full passive PIP extension. However, the overstretched dorsal hood extensor mechanism often will not be able to accomplish full active extension; thus, surgery may be necessary (Catalano et al., 2018). The surgical procedure creates an inflammatory response in the extensor hood. If immobilized long enough (usually 3–4 weeks) to allow collagen cross-linking to form and then mobilized at just the right speed, extension and flexion may be restored at 8 to 10 weeks post surgery without reproducing the previous extensor lag. The patient will not be a candidate for the extensor procedure until the flexion contracture resolves.

MUSCLE-TENDON UNIT IMBALANCE

Addressing the AROM and PROM limitations induced by nerve injury, Bell-Krotoski (1987) noted that casting can help "rebalance externally what has become imbalanced internally by a selective muscle loss." After paralysis of the hand's intrinsic muscles, an imbalance of the extensor mechanism—overpull of the proximal phalanx by the extensor digitorum communis (EDC) into extension and absent translational forces of the intrinsics on the dorsal hood—prevents the fingers from being fully extended at the interphalangeal (IP) joints (Fig. 10–5A). In addition, the metacarpophalangeal (MCP) joints lose their primary flexor, and these joints flex only after flexion of the IP joints by the flexor digitorum superficialis (FDS) and flexor digitorum profundus (FDP).

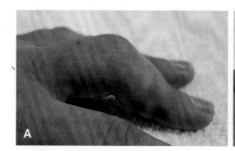
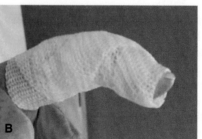

FIGURE 10–1 A, Central slip disruption following a blunt trauma to the dorsal PIP joint, resulting in an inability to actively extend the PIP joint. Note the posturing of the DIP joint into hyperextension. **B,** Initial cast includes the PIP in extension with the DIP flexed to overcome the strong tendency to revert back into the deformity.

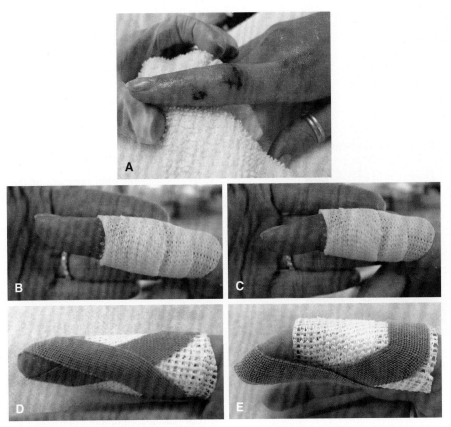

FIGURE 10–2 **A,** A lacerated and repaired zone III extensor tendon injury is managed in much the same way as a closed central slip avulsion. **B,** The PIP is positioned in full extension, and the DIP is free to move. **C,** Note the tight ORL with attempts at flexing the DIP joint with the PIP extended. **D and E,** Elastic therapeutic tape is applied to impart a gentle dynamic flexion stretch to ORL. The amount of tension applied can be easily adjusted by the patient.

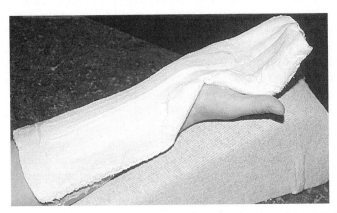

FIGURE 10–3 A POP stretcher is used to lengthen the muscle-tendon unit itself as well as any muscle-tendon unit adhesions.

Bell-Krotoski (1987) explained that casting of the IP joints into extension allows the fingers to be brought into full extension by the EDC and into flexion at the MCP joints by the FDS and FDP (Fig. 10–5B,C). Thus, casting allows external rebalancing of the fingers and can be used temporarily before and after intrinsic replacement surgery in lieu of dynamic mobilization. The hyperextension in the intrinsic minus hand commonly present at the MCP joint does not usually continue after the casts are applied because the primary flexion of the MCP joint has been restored.

Another example is using the material to place the thumb metacarpal in a functional (palmar abduction) to address the weakened thenar muscles from a nerve injury or compression such as carpal tunnel syndrome (Fig. 10–6A). The abductor pollicis brevis (APB) is a very powerful and important muscle about the thumb innervated by the median nerve. Strengthening this muscle is a challenge secondary to the strong compensatory pull of the thumb extrinsic muscles. To assist in blocking these extrinsic muscle-tendon units, simply cast the thumb IP joint in extension. This will help isolate the action of thumb palmar abduction by isolating the APB muscle. The patient can then work on thenar activation or strengthening (Fig. 10–6B,C).

Casts can also be used as an exercise tool to facilitate movement. To improve tendon glide and joint motion, provide the patient with DIP and PIP casts to apply during exercise sessions (Fig. 10–7A, B). These are a helpful addition to a home program to maximize glide and joint motion.

LENGTHENING LEVER ARMS

Occasionally, the therapist identifies a situation in which a contracture requires the use of higher force levels. In such cases, the physics of levers may help deliver the force. Casting is an excellent method for stabilizing a joint to increase mechanical advantage. As described in Chapter 4 the farther away the sling or loop is placed from the affected joint, the higher the force that the orthosis can generate. For example, when an orthosis is fabricated to increase MCP joint flexion, the sling can be placed distal to the stabilized PIP to increase the force at the MCP. Without PIP stabilization, the distally placed sling will instead act on both the PIP and the MCP. This stabilizing technique is especially desirable for small fingers—the short proximal phalanxes result in a decreased mechanical advantage (Fig. 10–8A,B). The therapist who uses long lever arms must first take note of joint stability and then closely listen to the patient for complaints of joint pain (Brand et al., 1999b). The examples in Figure 10–8C–E are excellent, real-life representations of how one can take advantage of casting to maximize lever arms (Fig. 10–8C–G).

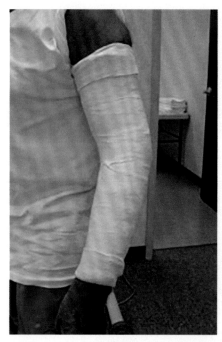

FIGURE 10–4 Serial static approach to improve elbow extension using POP. Note the generous length proximally and distally to maximize pressure distribution and patient comfort.

CHRONICALLY STIFF HAND

Effectively treating chronic stiffness of multiple joints of the hand and upper extremity can seem overwhelming. Strategically casting specific "looser" joints of the hand while leaving stiffer joints free for mobilization via AROM has proven effective when other approaches have failed (Colditz, 2000a, 2000b, 2002, 2011).

Hand therapists have been taught to fabricate mobilization devices that increase joint motion in one direction, but cautioned that gains in one direction should never be at the expense of losing motion in the opposite direction. An additional principle taught is that immobilization of *any* joint that is not absolutely necessary to be within the orthosis should be avoided. Colditz (2000b), (2002), (2011) makes the exception with her approach: **casting motion to mobilize stiffness (CMMS)**. She describes a process of using circumferential casting to recover motion in the hand with multiple chronically stiff joints (Fig. 10–9). This technique requires careful molding of a *POP* cast to immobilize proximal joints so as to focus

and redirect all the power of active movement to the targeted "stiff" distal joints (Bell-Krotoski, 2011; Colditz, 2011). Active movement of the distal joints is possible in both directions of flexion and extension, reestablishing differential glide of the soft-tissue layers necessary for normal joint motion. This technique has been successful in managing stiffness, edema, and tissue fibrosis (Midgley, 2016). The reader is referred to Chapter 15 which covers CMMS in greater detail.

The advantages of CMMS are the following:

- The consistent light pressure of the cast and the active motion within the circumferential cast facilitate lymphatic flow, thus mobilizing chronic edema.
- The patients are able to focus active motion on the stiffest joints, which they have previously been unable to effectively move to gain joint range.
- The targeted, repetitive active movement of the stiff joint(s) enables cortical reintegration and recreates functional movement patterns.
- POP is inexpensive, therapy visits are fewer and less frequent (decrease in copayments), and cast changes are infrequent because the cast is left in place for prolonged periods to allow retention of joint movement gained (Colditz, 2000a, 2000b, 2011).
- There is a brief immobilization period from this casting protocol that unfortunately contributes to functional losses, but these losses are temporary and reversible (Midgley, 2016).

COMPLIANCE PROBLEMS

Motivation, cognition, family demands, and maturity can each affect compliance. Therapists and physicians need to recognize that a fairly high percentage of patients are not fully compliant when issued a removable orthosis (Sanford, Barlow, & Lewis, 2008). When compliance becomes a major concern in patient treatment, the therapist/physician should consider a circumferential, nonremovable cast (Colditz, 2011). This will offer the best opportunity for achieving treatment goals because it requires no judgment or cooperation. The patient needs to only keep the cast on and in good condition. If a caregiver is involved, then the clinician must instruct the caregiver to watch for signs of cast intolerance, vascular compromise, and how to remove the cast. The cast eliminates difficulties that result from donning and doffing the orthosis improperly and inconsistently.

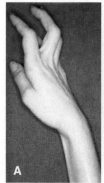
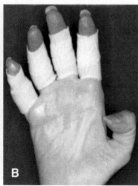
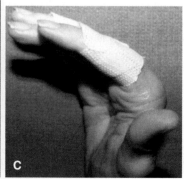

FIGURE 10–5 **A,** Combined ulnar and medium nerve injury leading to intrinsic paralysis and an imbalance of the extensor mechanism prevents the fingers from being fully extended at the PIP joints. Casting of the PIP joints into extension allows the MCP joints to be brought into full extension by the EDC **(B)** and full flexion by the FDS and FDP **(C).**

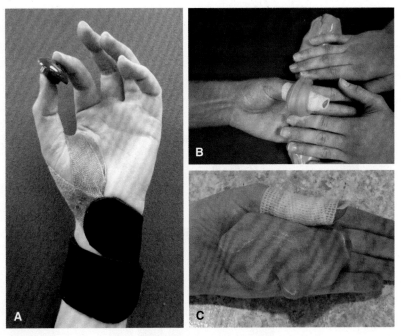

FIGURE 10–6 **A,** Orficast® tape used to position the thumb out of the palm with a patient (although POP and QuickCast can also be used) demonstrating loss of thenar muscle function after median nerve injury; tape adheres directly to neoprene strap, securing orthosis around the wrist. Exercise orthoses: **(B)** Thumb IP extension immobilization cast assists in redirecting the power of thumb palmar abduction to the APB muscle and MP flexion to the flexor pollicis brevis (FPB) muscle **(C)**.

CASTING FOR CENTRAL NERVOUS SYSTEM DISORDERS

Traumatic brain injury, stroke, and cerebral palsy commonly result in muscle tone and muscle synergy disorders that create joint contractures (see Chapter 23 for more information). Because patients with these disorders often lack the cognitive and sensory awareness to monitor their own status, their orthoses must distribute pressure optimally or harm to skin and joints can result (Schultz-Johnson, 1999). A frequently used technique to increase PROM for central nervous system (CNS) disorders is serial casting (Colditz, 2011; Goga-Eppenstein et al., 1999). For many years, casting for upper limbs has been a recommended intervention for stroke patients with spasticity. Despite limited research and lack of evidence to fully support this treatment option, benefits of casting have been noted in the literature (Flinn & Craven, 2014). The circumferential design provides even pressure distribution, edema control, and scar remodeling via pressure. Because the ROM problems confronting these patients are mostly owing to hypertonicity of muscle in consistent patterns, the clinician usually does not need to worry about losing motion in the opposite direction from the cast goal.

The therapist must carefully consider the number of joints incorporated into the cast, since hypertonicity controlled at one joint may increase tone at adjacent joints. For example, if an elbow cast does not control the wrist, flexor tone (now controlled at the elbow) may increase at the wrist, causing dramatic wrist flexion posture and potential median nerve compression against the distal volar end of the cast.

CNS CASTING MATERIALS

Many therapists use synthetic casting tape lined with cast padding to treat spasticity because it is strong yet lightweight. Some therapists still favor plaster, especially for use around the fingers, thumb, and palm, because it conforms well and allows air exchange (Fig. 10–10).

FABRICATION

Casting an adult, especially one in an agitated state, most often requires additional positioning assistance. The patient's joint is placed in a tolerable position—usually a submaximal position for the joint—while the clinician applies the casting material. All plaster casting materials heat the extremity during fabrication, which in turn can warm soft-tissue structures, making the extremity more flexible. If the cast fabricator takes advantage of the increased PROM, the joint position obtained during casting may be too extreme for the patient to tolerate. Therefore, caution should be

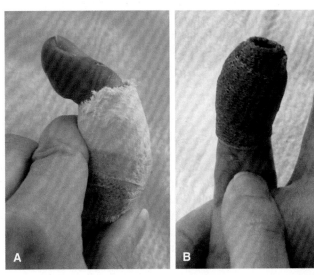

FIGURE 10–7 Blocking casts can assist with home program; PIP cast for encouraging DIP/FDP glide **(A)** and DIP cast for PIP/FDS glide **(B)**.

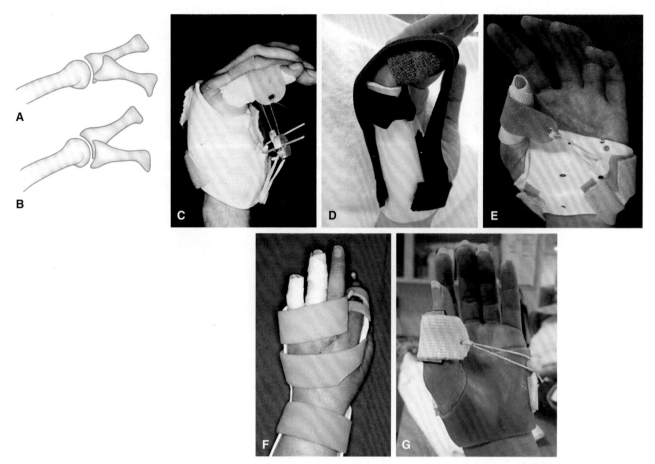

FIGURE 10–8 Applying stress to a joint can result in undesirable tilting (**A**) or desirable gliding (**B**). **C,** This PIP casting technique can be used when an MCP extension contracture and a PIP flexion contracture coexist. **D,** The small-finger (SF) DIP joint is casted in order to increase the lever arm for better mechanical advantage when applying dynamic stretch to the PIP joint via the strip of neoprene. **E,** Adding this thumb IP joint cast allows for isolated stretch at MP joint. **F,** Adding circumferential casts to the IP joints to prevent contractures while allowing healing of adjacent tissues. **G,** A thermoplastic tape can be used as an effective sling to guide motion. Note the soft neoprene adhered under sling.

taken during fabrication not to overstress the tissue. As the joint/tissue position progresses, some swelling may occur; should this happen, reassess cast position, cast tightness, and any other conditions that may have caused this. If the edema is due to dependent positioning, then simple elevation may suffice.

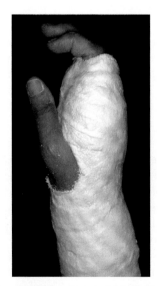

FIGURE 10–9 Wrist and MCP extension cast fabricated from POP used to encourage motion at the IP joints.

PRECAUTIONS

Casting for patients with CNS injuries has its own set of precautions and concerns. The clinician must frequently check for signs of cast intolerance by looking for color and temperature changes, swelling, and subtle signs of discomfort. To avoid the possibility of cast-caused trunk abrasions, the therapist may choose to cover the cast with a soft material or wrap, such as Moleskin, stockinette, or an Ace™ wrap. The clinician must instruct the family and/or nursing staff to be sure that the patient does not put things into the cast. Taping the cast's edges prevents this possibility. All caregivers must remember to keep the cast dry.

CNS CAST REGIMEN

Particularly important with this patient population is to not initiate casting on a Friday if the patient cannot be checked over the weekend. If the setting permits, the therapist should check the first cast a patient receives several times a day. In an outpatient facility, the therapist must make sure that the patient and/or caregiver understand all precautions. If the patient does well, the cast can be left in place 3 to 6 days, after which it is removed. If it is clear that the patient has tolerated casting well, then the clinician may immediately replace the cast and leave it on for up to 2 weeks or as the medical doctor (MD) recommends. Careful monitoring must continue.

Casting over a prolonged period can lead to muscle atrophy. Although considered a contraindication or negative side effect in the primarily orthopedic patient, in the patient with CNS dysfunction,

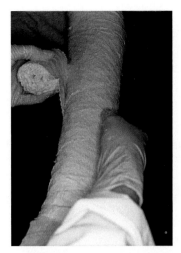

FIGURE 10–10 POP being used to fabricate an elbow cast to combat spasticity in a patient with a neurologically involved upper limb.

this loss of muscle strength is considered a goal. The atrophy helps reduce flexion posture and subsequent joint contracture (see Chapter 23 for detailed information).

CASTING MATERIALS AND EQUIPMENT

PLASTER OF PARIS

Therapists have used gauze impregnated with POP to cast finger contractures, especially PIP flexion contractures (Fig. 10–11) based on the work of Paul Brand, MD. Plaster is the material first used by Dr. Paul Brand for patients with Hansen disease in India and then in the United States (Wilson, 1965). Brand developed a technique of applying POP casts that imparted a gentle stretch to the tissue as it was being applied. He slowly and serially corrected the clubfoot deformity that many patients with Hansen disease presented with. Through his work and documentation, hand therapists have fruitfully used this technique for smaller joints of the hand and upper extremity. Every clinician is encouraged to read his book, *Clinical Mechanics of the Hand* (Brand, 1985; Brand & Hollister, 1993), and a letter he wrote shortly before his death to the *Journal of Hand Therapy*, "Lessons from Hot Feet" (Brand, 2002). Plaster has been one of the preferred materials of choice because it is readily available, inexpensive, breathable, friendly to skin and wounds, and accurately conforming. Patients can be instructed in how to remove and apply plaster for use in a home program.

POP's primary disadvantage is that it is vulnerable to moisture. POP softens and loses its strength when exposed to water. Plaster is heavier and often thicker than thermoplastic. Although POP is messy to apply, the practiced therapist can develop a system to

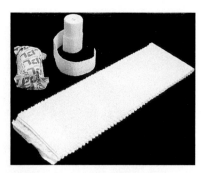

FIGURE 10–11 POP comes in rolls and sheets of various widths.

minimize cleanup. When POP and water mix, an exothermic chemical reaction takes place. Cases of burns caused by the application of POP have been reported; thus, the therapist must observe the patient carefully for this possible complication (discussed in detail later in this chapter) (Becker, 1978; Grazer, 1979; Haasch, 1964; Kaplan, 1981; Lovell & Staniforth, 1981; Schultze, 1967; Staniforth, 1980) (Box 10–2).

FIBERGLASS (RIGID)

With the advent of **fiberglass casting materials** (gauze impregnated with a water-activated resin), therapists have been able to take advantage of its lightweight quality to make larger casts and be creative with its properties (Fig. 10–12A–F). Fiberglass is rigid, durable, and lightweight, making it a good alternative for casting large joints. It is available in bright colors and all sorts of patterns. A few available products for rigid immobilization include Scotchcast™ Plus Casting Tape (3M™, St. Paul, MN), Cellacast® Xtra Cast Tapes (Performance Health), and Delta-Lite® (Essity, Charlotte, NC). These materials can be used for serial casting of wrists and elbows; however, they are not an option for casting fingers. Unfortunately, the skin does not tolerate the chemicals in the fiberglass and such casts require padding; thus, finger casts are too bulky and nonconforming. Fiberglass casts must be removed with a cast saw, and it also has a shorter shelf life than plaster (Box 10–3).

SOFT CASTING (SEMIRIGID)

Application of a soft cast offers an alternative to traditional rigid casting when some degree of mobility is indicated. Commonly available products include Scotchcast™ Soft Cast (3M™, St. Paul, MN), Cellacast® Soft Cast tape (Lohmann & Rauscher, Topeka, KS), and Delta-Cast® Soft (Essity). This category of soft materials is unique in the world of casting materials. They remain somewhat flexible and never set rigidly, as does their fiberglass and POP counterparts. These characteristics offer two major advantages. First, because they never become rigid, soft casting tapes can be used for patients who will benefit from slightly flexible immobilization.

BOX 10–2   WHY CONSIDER PLASTER OVER THERMOPLASTICS?

- Excellent conformability, thus decreases the possibility of pressure sores
- Absorbs perspiration due to its porous nature
- Generates neutral warmth, which allows for gentle stretching as it sets
- Cutaneous stretch receptors rapidly adapt to the change in length with serial casting

- Provides more even skin pressure (cylindrical)
- Aids in edema reduction because of the circumferential "snug" application
- Can be made as nonremovable; changed only by therapist
- Extremely cost-effective

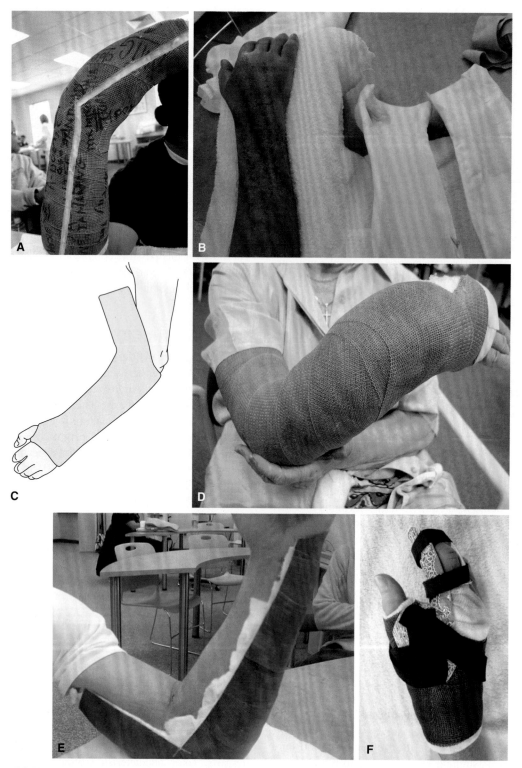

FIGURE 10–12 Cast types: univalved forearm and hand cast **(A)**, bivalved wrist cast **(B)**, drop-out cast **(C)**, cylindrical long arm cast **(D)**, posterior elbow slab/cast **(E)**, and a short arm cast used in combination with a custom molded thermoplastic orthosis—applied to prevent digit flexion and thumb adduction contractures. The neoprene strapping "grabs" onto the cast material quite well and contributes to stability and adherence of the additional material **(F)**. (Photo (C) borrowed from Deshaies, L. D. (2008). Upper extremity orthoses. In Radomski M. V., & Trombly Latham C. A. (Eds.), *Occupational therapy for physical dysfunction* (pp. 440). Philadelphia, PA: Lippincott Williams & Wilkins.)

Second, they do not require a cast saw for removal, so they can be used for patients who cannot tolerate a cast saw or who may need to remove the cast when away from the facility. This material cannot be made into a bivalved cast. This is applied directly on the skin or over light stockinette; no padding is necessary underneath the material. The soft cast material has no shelf life once the package is opened; any cast material not used must be discarded. Other materials such as thermoplastics or a plaster slab can be creatively incorporated into the cast orthosis to increase overall rigidity or block a direction of motion.

Soft casting is a great transition modality from a hard cast to semirigid one. Soft casting is often used with athletes for return to sport with the appropriate padding on the outside of the orthosis (see Chapter 22 for greater detail). Increasing the layers increases the durability and rigidity; however, this makes the cast heavier and bulkier. The overall setting time for this material is approximately

BOX 10-3   PLASTER VERSUS FIBERGLASS

Plaster
- Longer drying time
- More prone to indentations that can lead to breakdown
- Stronger
- Heavier
- Less costly

Fiberglass
- Shorter drying time
- Higher risk of splintering
- Harder
- Lighter
- More resistant to dirt
- More durable
- More costly

5 to 6 minutes. If univalved or upon permanent removal, a cast spreader is used to open the cast. Once open, the borders are lined with a Moleskin or Moleskin-like material to decrease irritation from possible rough edges. Securing the cast on the extremity can be done with any type of circumferential wrap. During contact sports, the athlete will need to have additional padding to protect opposing players.

DELTA-CAST® CONFORMABLE: FUNCTIONAL CAST THERAPY

Gaining popularity is the concept of **functional cast therapy (FCT)**, formerly referred to as focused rigidity casting (FRC), based on the premise that using a device that allows functional use while providing protection and stabilization to the injured structure(s) prevents many of the harmful consequences of prolonged immobilization. The editors of this book have dedicated an entire chapter to functional cast therapy (Chapter 12), so the reader is referred to that chapter for detailed information of indications and instructions in use.

The theory is that an early return to function helps minimize muscle atrophy and joint stiffness and improves circulation to the healing area. These orthoses are made from Delta-Cast® Conformable Casting Tape (Essity), a knitted, elastic, polyester fabric, imbedded with a clear resin. This product can be used as an alternative to traditional thermoplastic orthoses; it may allow for increased function and more comfort than a traditional fiberglass cast. Due to a three-way stretch, Delta-Cast® Conformable provides for a smooth, contoured application resisting wrinkling around the wrist and digits (Fig. 10–13A). The cast is applied over a terry cloth stockinette, removed with simple bandage scissors, and edged with felt. The number of layers determines whether the final cast will be flexible or rigid. A zip-cutting stick, a flexible thin barrier that is slid under the cast exactly where it is to be cut off with bandage scissors, is used to avoid harming the patient because there is minimal padding between skin and cast. These washable casts are ultimately secured to the area with hook-and-loop closure (Fig. 10–13B). Indications for use are similar to all other casting materials, commonly used as an alternative to an immobilization orthosis or circumferential cast.

Some benefits of Delta-Cast® are as follows (refer to Chapter 12 for more detail):

- Latex- and fiberglass-free formulation
- Durable—same device can be used throughout all phases of healing
- Fit may be adjusted by trimming if edema changes
- Easy to trim and remove with bandage scissors using zip stick—no cast saw required
- Washable (device can be hand-washed and then dried with a hair dryer or air dried)

- Multidirectional (three-way) stretch providing wrinkle-free application
- Excellent conformability and good rigidity
- Smooth finish, which helps to increase patient comfort
- Working time: 0 to 3 minutes; setting time: 3 to 20 minutes
- Available in various widths 1″ to 4″

DIGIT THERMOPLASTIC TAPES

QuickCast 2 and **Orficast®** are two types of thermoplastic taping options currently available for digit management. Although both names imply that these are "cast materials" in actuality, they are considered a thermoplastic tape due to the material properties. The editors of this book have chosen to include QuickCast 2 in this chapter since many practicing clinicians continue to assume this as a "cast" material. Orficast® material has grown in material selection beyond a tape into an entire product line that warrants its own chapter. Refer to Chapter 11 for complete information on the product line.

Both of these thermoplastic tapes have become very popular in hand therapy, offering the therapist a means to make a low-profile, circumferential digit orthosis quickly and with excellent conformability (Fig. 10–14A–D). The slight tackiness of these materials helps to obtain maximal contouring. QuickCast 2 is an elastic fiberglass mesh, impregnated with heat-softened thermoplastic. The material shrinks when it is heated with a hair dryer or heat gun (on low). Laminated tapes can also be used creatively to assist in adhering components onto a thermoplastic base or to reinforce a thin weaker area of an orthosis. Once heated, the individual strips can be applied either directly onto the skin or over some type of light cotton stockinette. For a firm cast, only one or two layers of tape are required; the more layers that are applied, the more rigid the final cast will be (less airflow, more bulky). Not only do these circumferential orthoses create a comfortable fit, but, because the material is so thin as compared to POP, they also allow the therapist to cast adjacent fingers without forcing them into extreme abduction. These thermoplastic tapes set up quickly, several minutes faster than plaster or fiberglass, making it a time-efficient material. The setup and cleanup for a QuickCast orthosis is minimal compared to plaster. The therapist does not need to wear any gloves during application. A finger cast made from these thermoplastic tapes can sometimes be removed (discussed later in this chapter), reheated, and reused as long as there has not been excessive wear, and it does not have to be cut off the finger. This is in sharp contrast to plaster, where the therapist must discard these casting materials after removal. The therapist can create univalve finger casts to make them removable with Serial Cast Scissors. The short blades, with blunt ends, are contoured for safety when cutting close to the skin, and the proportionally long handles provide excellent mechanical advantage.

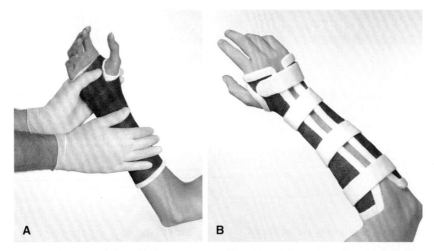

FIGURE 10–13 Delta-Cast® Conformable Casting Tape used for FCT technique: circumferential application requires gloves to protect hands **(A)** and final device shown with hook-and-loop closure **(B)**. FCT, functional cast therapy. (Photos courtesy of Essity, Charlotte, NC.)

CLINICAL EXAMPLE: SERIAL STATIC PIP JOINT EXTENSION ORTHOSIS

ACTIVATION OF QUICKCAST 2

The most common method to activate QuickCast 2 tape is to use a hair dryer that is long nosed, 1,600 W with high airflow. This type of dryer heats the tape effectively and quickly. It is important that it is long nosed because the dryer will not shut off when hot air is funneled back into the end. Short-nosed dryers shut down when hot air returns into the nose, which often occurs when heating QuickCast 2. The tape is placed on a towel or silicone surface so that when the airflow is applied, it will not "fly" off the surface. The activation time is approximately 60 seconds. The working time is approximately 30 seconds, which may be challenging for a clinician that is not familiar with this material. However, with handling experience, this working time should be sufficient. (**Caution:** manufacturer recommends to NOT use a heat gun with QuickCast 2—although some therapists use heat gun on low setting to activate this material.)

Casts fabricated from QuickCast 2, if in good condition, can be gently unwrapped, reheated, and reapplied. The reader is referred to the manufacturers' instructions for more detailed information on the specific properties, advantages, and areas for caution for the material. Overheating of the material will cause breakdown of the material itself. Patients can expose their fingers to water with this material; however, they must dry the cast thoroughly to prevent skin maceration or softening of the cast. The patient can dry the cast with a towel or hair dryer on a low setting. Patients should use caution with getting casts wet whenever possible due to the potential loss of cast rigidity and joint position.

MATERIALS AND METHODS

Making a tape cast requires the following materials:

- QuickCast 2 tape
- Activation source: hair dryer
- Serial Cast Scissors (Performance Health)
- Towel
- Spray bottle with water (optional)
- Petroleum jelly (optional)
- Cast padding (optional)
- Tincture of benzoin (or similar; optional)

To begin the cast fabrication process, cut the length of the tape needed for the finger. The length depends on the length and circumference of the finger and the number of joints involved (Fig. 10–15A). The finger cast requires only a single layer of material with about 1/8″ overlap.

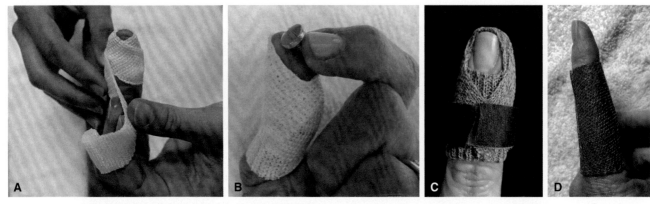

FIGURE 10–14 **A,** Note the pliability of heated QuickCast being used to treat a mallet finger injury. **B,** QuickCast 2 used to fabricate this thumb IP immobilization orthosis following a terminal tendon injury, leaving the tip free for sensory input. **C,** Orficast molded to DIP joint addressing a mallet finger injury—secured with hook/loop strapping. **D,** Orficast conforms well to create a smooth PIP immobilization orthosis after a central tendon injury.

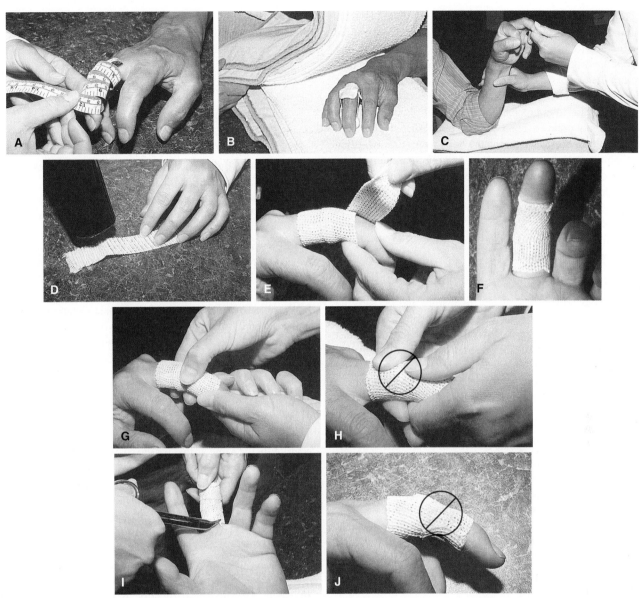

FIGURE 10–15 **Steps for fabricating a QuickCast 2 finger cast. A,** Estimate the amount of tape needed by spiraling a cloth dressmaker's tape around the finger in the same configuration as the planned cast. **B,** Heat in combination with a digit extension mobilization orthosis to precondition the finger to gain maximum PROM just before casting. **C,** Extend the patient's PIP joint using axial traction. **D,** Hold the dryer above the QuickCast tape, which will shrink as it becomes soft and hot. Keep the dryer steady; avoid moving it back and forth. **E,** Keeping the tape stretched cautiously, wrap all the way around the proximal phalanx once and then begin to spiral distally, wrapping once for each layer and overlapping the previous layer. **F,** Wrap the finger so the DIP joint is free to move. **G,** Use a continuous rotary motion to conform the material closely to the finger and obtain an optimal fit. **H,** To avoid point pressure, do not poke at the cast with your fingertips; instead, use the length of your fingers for maximal pressure distribution. **I,** Use the Serial Cast Scissors to contour and smooth the edges. **J,** If there are any indentations, the cast must be removed and remade.

Preconditioning the Finger

The cast results are more rapidly achieved and of greater magnitude when the joint is preconditioned or stretched out just before casting (Flowers & LaStayo, 2012; Glasgow et al., 2012). The therapist should use one of the following techniques to gain maximum PROM just before casting: compression and/or massage for edema reduction, heat and stretch, joint mobilization, active and passive exercise, and therapeutic activities (Fig. 10–15B).

Position and Technique

Before making the cast, decide on patient and finger positions. Practice with the patient. Be sure the patient understands the materials, technique, and rationale for cast application. Position the finger as follows:

1. Remove any rings from the finger to be casted.
2. Seat the patient, placing the elbow of the affected extremity on a firm but padded surface.
3. Have the patient (or an assistant) hold the finger to be casted at the distal phalanx, leaving the DIP crease free, and then pull the finger using axial traction while the patient (or an assistant) pulls the hand away from the traction force by extending the wrist or bending the elbow (Fig. 10–15C). The force must take the PIP joint to maximum available extension without causing pain.
4. Activate the cut tape (Fig. 10–15D), and when softened, pick it up and stretch it back to maximum length.
5. Sustain the traction force until the cast is set.

Take note that with QuickCast 2, after the tape is applied on stretch to the finger, it will not significantly shrink back down and overcompress the finger. The tape may be tacky; therefore, the therapist should moisten his or her hands with water to prevent the tape from sticking and to make the material easier to work with. Taking care to avoid the fragile skin of the finger web space, place the tape as far proximally as possible on the proximal phalanx. Keeping the tape cautiously stretched, wrap it all the way around the proximal phalanx making sure to appreciate the individual oblique angle of the proximal digital creases. Then begin to spiral distally, overlapping each wrap by about 1/8″ over the previous wrap (Fig. 10–15E). If the DIP joint is to be left free to move, end approximately 1/16″ proximal to the DIP joint flexion crease, but extend the cast fully to the DIP joint dorsally (Fig. 10–15F). Once the tape has been applied to the entire finger, use a continuous rotary motion of the fingers to "screw" the material down onto the digit (Fig. 10–15G). **Caution:** Avoid point pressure against the tape at all times (Fig. 10–15H). Keep fingers moving on the cast tape.

Check and Revision

Inspect the palmar joint crease at the MCP joint and be sure the patient can flex the MCP without the proximal-palmar end of the cast pressing into the joint crease. If this occurs, use the Serial Cast Scissors to carve out some of the material and allow unimpeded movement (Fig. 10–15I). Next, check the DIP crease to be sure that the DIP joint can fully flex. Again, either push the material away from the crease or use the Serial Cast Scissors to trim the cast if needed. Finally, check the web spaces and contour or trim as needed. The Serial Cast Scissors present minimal risk to the patient's skin. All of the edges must be smooth to prevent skin irritation. Observe the cast closely for any signs of indentation along the substance of the cast. If any indentation is evident, remove the cast and start over (Fig. 10–15J).

If the cast appears unsatisfactory, simply unwind the material—this is an option even a few minutes after the cast is completed. After the tape is off the finger, simply repeat the heating process and reapply the same material. Unwinding the material becomes more challenging once the tape is fully hardened. The cast will set up in approximately 1 minute or less. **Caution:** Do not use the hair dryer (or heat gun) to reheat the tape when it is on the finger. The heat can cause great discomfort and may burn the tissue.

Occasionally, the cylindrical thermoplastic cast will become loose enough that it may slide off the finger, especially after the first few applications. This may be due to a decrease in edema and/or a loosening of the tape due to body heat and extended wear. If the cast comes off at a time where the patient cannot come back to the clinic for remolding, the patient should always be instructed on how to keep the cast on in these situations. Microfoam™ tape, Coban™, paper tape, and similar self-adherent–type wraps can be applied to both the proximal portion/border of the cast and exposed skin in order to anchor the cast on the finger. This should be sufficient enough to hold the cast in place until the patient can return to the clinic.

USING PLASTER OF PARIS

Materials and Preparation

Making a PIP extension cast from POP requires the following materials (Fig. 10–16):

- POP rolls cut into 2 1/2″ strips, folded in half
- Hot water
- Small clean bowl
- Serial Cast Scissors
- Tissue
- Petroleum jelly
- Cast padding (optional)
- Drapes or towels to protect work surfaces and patient's clothes

For best results, use 3″-wide POP folded in half and then trimmed to a 1 1/4″ width. Choose the fastest setting plaster obtainable and one that has a fine texture and, in the end, creates a smooth, strong cast that sets quickly. There are numerous products on the market that have these qualities; one example is Gypsona® (Essity).

Prepare the clinic for POP application and gather the required materials and equipment needed. To protect surfaces from plaster drippings, cover them with disposable waterproof covers. Place drapes over the patient's clothing. The therapist may wish to wear an apron. The therapist and patient should remove watches and rings.

Fill a small clean bowl with hot water. The hotter the water, the faster the plaster will set. Cut the length of POP needed for the finger; the length depends on the length and circumference of the finger and the number of joints involved. Estimate the amount of POP needed by spiraling a cloth dressmaker's tape around the finger in the same configuration as planned to make the cast and then double the length (Fig. 10–17A). Remember that each layer of the cast requires two wraps of POP, and each layer overlaps the preceding one by 50% or 3/4″.

Method

Precondition the finger as described for making a finger cast earlier in the previous section (Fig. 10–15B). Positioning for POP casting is virtually the same as that for the casting tapes (Fig. 10–15C), with a few exceptions.

To begin the cast fabrication process, coat the finger with petroleum jelly (Fig. 10–17A), which protects against the drying effects of the plaster. Dip the length of plaster into the water, and then run the POP between two fingers to remove excess water (Fig. 10–17B). Taking care to avoid the fragile skin of the finger web space, place the tape as far proximally as possible on the proximal phalanx. Wrap all the way around the proximal phalanx twice and then begin to spiral distally, wrapping twice for each layer and overlapping the previous layer halfway or by about 3/4″ (Fig. 10–17C). To allow the DIP joint to move freely, end approximately 1/16″ proximal to the DIP joint flexion crease but extend the cast fully to the DIP joint dorsally (Fig. 10–17D). Once the material is applied to the entire finger, use a continuous rotary motion of the fingers to coax the material down onto the finger (Fig. 10–17E). **Caution:** Avoid point pressure against the material at all times (Fig. 10–17F).

Check and Revision

Once the POP has been applied and with traction sustained on the finger, check the cast. Inspect the palmar joint crease at the MCP joint and be sure the patient can flex the MCP without the proximal-palmar end of the cast pressing into the joint crease. If this occurs, push or roll the damp plaster back away from the crease or use the Serial Cast Scissors to carve out some of the material to allow unimpeded movement. Next, check the DIP crease to be sure that the DIP joint can fully flex. Again, either push or roll the damp plaster back away from the crease or trim the cast if needed. Finally, check the web spaces and contour or trim as needed (Fig. 10–17G). The Serial Cast Scissors pose a minimal risk to the patient's skin. Of course, under optimal conditions, the cast will not need trimming. Observe the cast closely for any signs of indentation along the substance of the cast. If indentation is evident, remove the cast and start over (Fig. 10–17H).

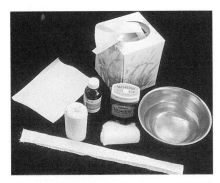

FIGURE 10–16 Materials and equipment needed to fabricate a POP finger cast.

If the cast appears unsatisfactory after making it, the therapist can remove the plaster and begin again with a clean bowl; clean water; and new plaster, petroleum jelly, and tissue. It may be possible to raise the end of the POP cast and unwind it. The patient may soak the POP cast off in very warm water. Alternatively, Serial Cast Scissors can be used to cut into the plaster either at the proximal or distal end to help remove it.

HELPFUL TECHNIQUES FOR FINGER CASTING

Cast Removal

Both the patient and the therapist must be familiar with techniques for cast removal. The patient should leave the clinic only after indicating a clear understanding of how to remove the cast. The patient must be instructed that the cast cannot be removed with a cast saw because there is no padding.

If the patient's contracture is approximately 30° or less, then the patient will most likely be able to pull the cast off. For patients with unstable MCP joints (such as with rheumatic disease), the proximal phalanx will need to be stabilized before pulling off the cast. If the joint is too tender for this removal technique, if the joint is quite swollen, or if the contracture is more severe, then the cast removal is more involved.

Unwinding

For the first few casts, mark the distal end of the tape with a pen; this will help with cast removal in an emergency and help assure the patient that he or she can unwind the cast (Fig. 10–18A). The patient can immerse the casted finger in the warmest tolerable water to soften the material and unwind the cast (Fig. 10–18B). The patient should soak the cast in the warmest water tolerable for 5 minutes or longer. Once the distal flap of the casting material is raised, it is possible to unwrap the cast. This "unwinding" can be challenging; however, it is frequently done with QuickCast 2 tape in order for the piece to be reused. It may need to be resoaked several times before the cast can be removed. If the tape has served its purpose, it can simply be cut off with the Serial Cast Scissors. The therapist or patient can soak the cast to soften it partially and then use Serial Cast Scissors to cut it off.

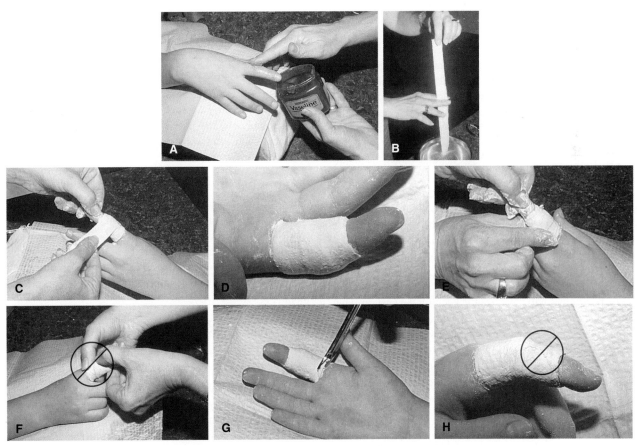

FIGURE 10–17 Steps for fabricating a POP finger cast. A, The lubricating process helps protect the finger from the drying effects of the POP. **B,** Squeeze to remove excess water. **C,** Wrap all the way around the proximal phalanx twice and then spiral distally, wrapping twice for each layer and overlapping the previous layer. **D,** To allow the DIP joint to move freely, end just short of the DIP flexion crease. **E,** Use a continuous rotary motion to closely form the material to the finger and obtain optimal fit. **F,** To avoid point pressure, do not poke at the cast with your fingertips; instead, use the length of your fingers for maximal pressure distribution. **G,** Use the Serial Cast Scissors to contour and smooth the edges. **H,** If there are any indentations, the cast must be removed and remade.

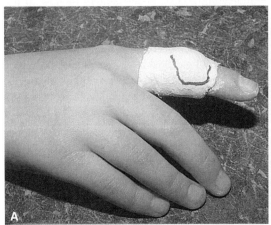 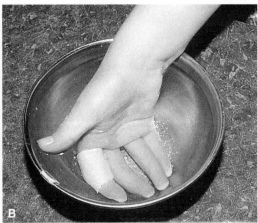

FIGURE 10–18 **A,** Mark the end of the cast to ease removal. **B,** Remove the cast by soaking it in warm water.

Paraffin

Another technique that may be used when the purpose of the cast is to be used intermittently (such as for just night wear or exercise sessions) is to apply one layer of paraffin to the finger prior to cast application. This technique can be used with all digit circumferential materials detailed in this chapter. The paraffin seeps through the porous holes in the tape/plaster, making for a smooth nonabrasive surface for the digit to slide within. This technique may also be used for those with fragile or sensitive skin (Fig. 10–19A,B). The distal and proximal borders of a circumferential cast can also be dipped in order to provide a smooth surface, maximizing comfort during wear and donning/doffing (Fig. 10–19C).

Cutting

The therapist may choose one of two approaches to cut the cast for removal. Bell-Krotoski (1987, 2011) described a window technique by which the dorsal aspect of the cast is cut out along the proximal phalanx. With this section of the cast removed, the patient can usually slip the cast off (Fig. 10–20A). The other option is to create a univalve in the cast with a longitudinal cut along either the radial/palmar or the ulnar/palmar border using the small Serial Cast Scissors shown in Figure 10–20D (Fig. 10–20B–D). The location for these cuts has two advantages. The palmar skin has more subcutaneous padding than the dorsal skin, and the volar approach avoids the PIP condyles. Cutting over a bony prominence usually creates discomfort for the patient. Either the window or the univalve approach can be used to make the cast removable for intermittent wear.

Securing the Cast in Place

Occasionally, the patient will have trouble keeping the cast on. This occurs rarely but is most frequently seen with very small fingers that are approaching full extension and fingers that were edematous when the cast was applied and have since lost volume. When presented with this problem, the cast maker must be certain that the cast was applied properly. Three techniques are helpful for maintaining cast position on the finger when the proper casting technique does not result in a secure cast:

1. **Circumferential wraps.** The patient can wrap the cast and adjacent skin with self-adherent wraps, such as Coban™, or with various adhesive tapes such as Microfoam™ tape, elastic therapeutic tape, paper tape, or athletic tape. The wrap can be applied around the cast and proximal (Fig. 10–21A–C). The type of wrap chosen will depend on how the patient intends to use the digit with the cast on.

2. **Additional tape material.** The therapist can cut an additional piece of material, laminate it to the proximal end of the cast, and continue wrapping through the first web space and around the palm (Fig. 10–22). DIP casts can be secured proximally to the digit with circumferential wraps as described previously or creatively positioned with a thin rolled piece of additional material (Fig. 10–23).

3. **Preparing skin.** Tincture of Benzoin, Tuf Skin Taping Base (Performance Health), and Skincote™ Protective Prep Pads (Performance Health) are products that create a tacky surface on the skin. A tiny amount of these can be dabbed on the skin before applying the cast. The products can be removed with rubbing alcohol when desired. Applying these products will assist in keeping the cast in place.

Protecting Adjacent Fingers

Sometimes, the finger adjacent to the casted finger becomes irritated from rubbing against the cast. To prevent this or to relieve it once it occurs, the patient may cover the cast with Moleskin, a bandage (such as a Band-Aid®), finger stockinette, or light Coban™ wrap (Performance Health).

Reinforcing the Cast

After the casting process is complete and it is apparent that the rigidity is not enough to hold the joint position, the cast can be reinforced with additional material. Heating and applying an additional strip of the casting material circumferentially can work, but this increases the overall bulk of the cast. If this is a concern, instead a scrap piece of thermoplastic can be added to the cast for reinforcement (Fig. 10–24A,B).

PRECAUTIONS FOR FINGER CASTING

Material Tolerance

If the patient does not tolerate the cast tape directly against the skin or if additional padding is desired, one or more layers of tubular finger bandage may be applied to the finger before making the cast. In the case of wounds or the use of padding, the patient must avoid getting the finger wet. Techniques for keeping the finger dry in a cast range from putting a plastic bag around the whole hand, using a "finger cot" to cover the digit (available at local drugstores) or cutting a finger from a surgical glove and placing it over the cast (Fig. 10–25).

Hand therapists' reports of POP intolerance are minimal; however, the therapist should be aware that increasing the dipping water

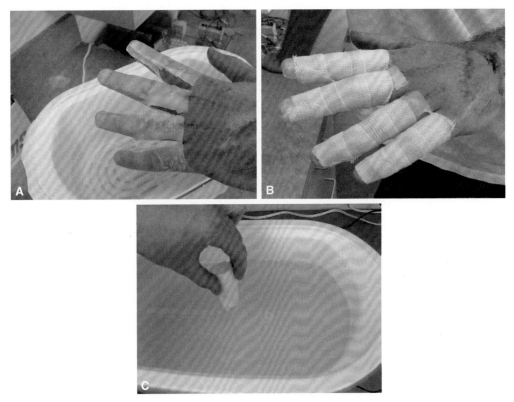

FIGURE 10–19 **A and B,** One layer of paraffin wax can be applied to the fingers prior to casting tape application (works with QuickCast 2, Orficast®, and POP). The paraffin will, in turn, make the casts easy to remove and provide a smooth gliding surface for repeated donning/doffing. Caution should be taken as to not apply the warmed tape material until wax is fully dry. These casts are being used as exercise orthoses in order to isolate and encourage MCP extension/flexion. **C,** The proximal and distal borders of the cast are being lightly dipped in paraffin to smooth out irregular/sharp and potentially irritating edges.

temperature for the POP material and increasing the number of layers of POP applied can significantly increase the temperature within the setting cast (Conroy, Ward, & Fraser, 2007). Covering the POP with a towel or pillow while the material is setting can significantly increase the internal temperature (Gannaway & Hunter, 1983; Lavalette, Pope, & Dickerson, 1982) (Boxes 10–4 and 10–5).

Casting Over Wounds

Each clinician must use personal judgment when the finger still has open wounds. POP casts can be applied over open wounds and over dressings and are generally tolerated well. The nature of the POP material assists in absorbing wound drainage (Colditz, 2002, 2011). QuickCast 2 can be applied over open wounds that

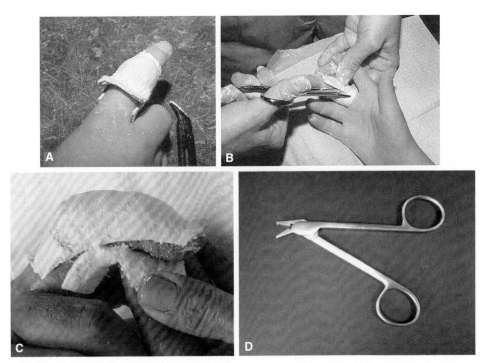

FIGURE 10–20 Window **(A)** and univalve **(B)** cutting techniques for cast removal. **C,** Gently pull apart material to remove the cast. **D,** Splint Cast Trimmers (Performance Health).

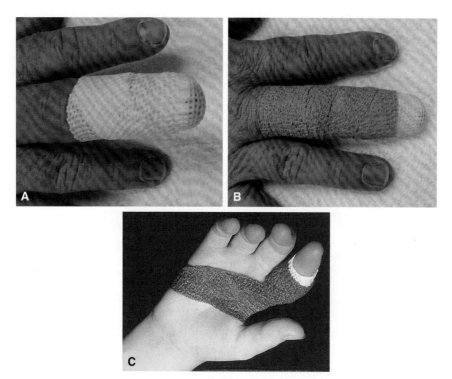

FIGURE 10-21 **A and B,** QuickCast 2 DIP extension orthosis with Coban™ applied on the cast and then onto the proximal phalanx to prevent slippage. **C,** For securing a PIP cast, Coban™ (or similar material) can be wrapped around the cast and anchored through the palm.

are dressed (Brand & Yancey, 1997). The thinner the dressing the better, in order to gain the most benefits from the conforming properties of the material and even pressure distribution. A layer or two of petroleum gauze such as Xeroform™ (Patterson Medical, 3M™, St. Paul, MN) may be all that is needed. The person applying the cast must take care to keep the dressing in place during cast application. Casts can be used to secure scar management products to an area of the hand. Elastomer™ (Performance Health) products adhere into the fabric of the casting tapes (Fig. 10–26).

Indications for Cast Removal

The therapist must thoroughly instruct the patient in symptoms that signal an ill-fitting cast. A poorly made cast can compromise nerve, vascular structures, and/or skin. The symptoms that signal pressure on a nerve are tingling, numbness, and unusual pain. Point pressure directly against a digital nerve can cause a neuropraxia. The symptoms that signal vascular compromise are tingling, numbness, unusual pain, color change, unusual coolness, and persistent throbbing. The symptoms that signal skin compromise from sharp edges are unusual pain and red skin just proximal or distal to the cast. Excess pressure can produce significant redness over the affected area, commonly seen at the PIP joint dorsally.

Sensory Compromise

Casting the patient with sensory compromise places an even greater responsibility on the therapist to make a well-fitting cast. The patient with numbness will not have the primary signal (pain) to warn that the cast is causing problems. However, it is helpful to know that Brand's (1988) initial casting population suffered extreme sensory compromise from Hansen's disease but did extremely well with POP casting. It is precisely the pressure-distributing nature of the circumferential cast that makes it appropriate for this at-risk population. Placing a three-point pressure orthosis on a numb part is often not an option that can be considered. Still, the therapist must

strongly emphasize the potential risks to the patient and teach him or her to inspect the skin regularly to check for problems that the nervous system may miss.

Vascular Compromise

When the cast is completed, the therapist must inspect the color of the fingertip. It may appear slightly darker red than the adjacent fingers or can change color so much as to appear purplish, which indicates difficulty with venous outflow (Fig. 10–27). The finger may also become white or dusky, indicating difficulty with arterial inflow. The patient must remain in the clinic until the color of the finger normalizes. This usually happens within 5 to 10 minutes; however, it may take more than 20 minutes before vascular tone normalizes for vascular outflow difficulty. Usually, the discoloration occurs in a patient who is receiving a first cast, and the problem does not recur. The person applying the cast must use judgment to determine whether the color of the finger means that the cast should be left on or removed and redone. A sustained color change can signal that focused pressure against major arteries or veins exists and must be relieved.

Skin Tolerance

If the patient presents initially with erythema of the dorsal aspect of the PIP joint or develops this over a period of time in the cast, the cast will need to be reapplied using a better cast distribution technique or protective padding prior to application (Fig. 10–28A,B). Vascular compromise dorsally, if not dealt with, can cause skin breakdown. Bell-Krotoski (1987, 2011) described a technique using clouds, or wisps, of cast padding to protect vulnerable tissue (Fig. 10–28B). To make the cloud, pull a small fluff of cast padding from the roll. Apply petroleum jelly over the area where the padding will go to keep the cloud in place during cast fabrication. With the padding over the dorsum of the PIP, the normal casting procedure can begin. The therapist must be sure that the padding stays in place during cast fabrication. Bulkier approaches to padding the cast usually do

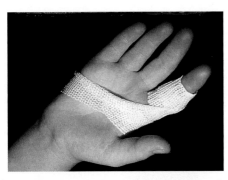

FIGURE 10-22 Another technique for securing a finger cast includes using additional casting material attached to the cast and wrapped through the web space and palm.

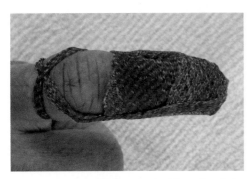

FIGURE 10-23 To secure this DIP cast, a proximal "strap" made from thinly rolled Orficast® tape was used; however, QuickCast or POP can also be used.

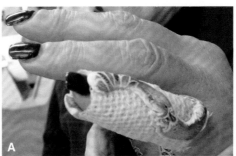

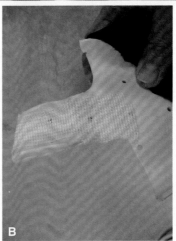

FIGURE 10-24 A, Thermoplastic material can be adhered directly to the casting tape to improve rigidity in an area without increasing the bulk of the orthosis. **B,** A strip of laminated tape can be used to reinforce weakened or thin areas of an orthosis—here applied to MCP joint region.

not have a satisfactory result (Bell-Krotoski, 1987, 2011). Sharp cast edges—proximally or distally—can also compromise skin integrity regardless of the type of casting material or thermoplastic tape used (Fig. 10–28C). Another issue regarding tissue integrity is when maceration occurs beneath the cast if the patient gets the finger wet. This persistent moisture can eventually cause itching and skin breakdown if not addressed with a period of "drying out" and a prompt cast change (Fig. 10–28D).

Skin Lubrication

Popular is the application of petroleum jelly (or like lubricants) to the skin before POP cast application. As mentioned, petroleum jelly helps lubricate the skin under the moisture-robbing plaster. It also helps secure small amounts of padding. As described earlier, a single layer of paraffin can also be considered before casting with POP or QuickCast 2. A layer of paraffin fully cooled can be used under the application of these casts. The paraffin allows for easy removal and a very light coating against the skin to soften the harshness the materials may have on a sensitive skin. However, if the paraffin is not allowed to cool and POP (with its heating qualities) is applied, the skin under this material may become reddened and severely irritated. Caution and sound clinical judgment should be used (Fig. 10–19A,B). Paraffin can also be used to coat irregular edges on a cast that is intended to be removable (Fig. 10–19C).

CASTING REGIMEN

Frequencies of cast changes vary with the characteristics of the patient. Diagnosis, severity and duration of contracture, and wound and sensory status all help determine the number of times a week or month a patient will be seen for a cast change (Flowers & LaStayo, 2012; Midgley, 2016). The issues of geography, financial status,

patient schedule, and motivation usually have more impact on the regimen than the medical factors.

Some patients seem to benefit from less frequent cast changes, whereas others have the best results with frequent cast changes. Theoretically, the more frequent cast changes will have better results because a new end range is captured with each cast change, enhancing the mechanical signal to the tissue to remodel.

CLINICAL EXAMPLE: SERIAL STATIC POP STRETCHER FOR MODIFYING SCAR TISSUE

MATERIALS AND PREPARATION

The materials needed to make a POP stretcher are as follows (Fig. 10–29):

- Approximately 10 plies of POP cut from rolls or strips
- Stockinette
- Additional POP strips for finishing
- Hot water
- Clean bowl
- Bandage scissors
- Tissues
- Drapes to protect work surfaces and patient's clothes
- Finger loops of vinyl with line attached or flexible surgical drain tubing
- Cast padding (optional)
- Draped arm wedge (optional)
- Banding metal, thermoplastic strips, or additional POP strips for reinforcement (optional)

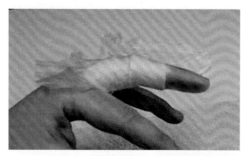

FIGURE 10–25 To keep a finger cast dry, use a plastic bag or a surgical glove.

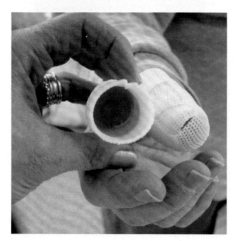

FIGURE 10–26 The cast provides the means of holding the scar mold in place.

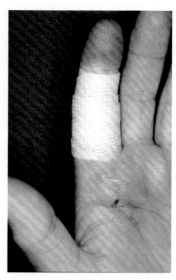

FIGURE 10–27 Vascular compromise noted distally worsens with attempts at DIP flexion.

Position and Technique

Before making the POP orthosis, decide on patient and joint positions. Practice with the patient. Be sure the patient understands the materials, technique, and rationale for cast application. Position the patient and prepare the tissue as follows:

1. Clean and dry the area of the arm to be covered.
2. Seat the patient and place the affected extremity on a firm but padded surface (a foam wedge is excellent) with the forearm supinated and position the joints as desired.
3. Start with the wrist in neutral and place the MCP and IP joints in maximum available extension; once the fingers demonstrate full passive extension, begin progressing the wrist into extension while maintaining digit extension until full composite extension is achieved.
4. To position the fingers, especially if the flexor tightness varies significantly between digits, place vinyl finger slings or loops with line attached or place flexible surgical drain tubing over the fingertips and have the patient or an assistant place the fingers under traction into maximum tolerable extension (Fig. 10–30E). **Caution:** Avoid point pressure at all times.

Applying the Plaster of Paris Stretcher

As the process begins, keep in mind that even with extra-fast-setting plaster, the therapist will have adequate time to contour the POP to the arm. The POP will set in 3 to 5 minutes. Tribuzi (1990) described the application of padding or stockinette before applying the POP. However, this author has never used an interface between the POP and the skin in the fabricating process and has never encountered a complication.

Using care to fully saturate all of the POP, all the strips are immersed as a group into the water. Remove the POP as a unit and gently squeeze along the length of the strips to remove excess water (Fig. 10–30F). The wet plaster is then placed on the patient's arm and over the fingers (or fingers in the slings, if used). Using all of the POP layers as a single unit, mold the POP to the arm, carefully contouring the forearm, palm, fingers, and spaces between the fingers (Fig. 10–30G). No pressure need be applied to the POP. The person positioning the fingers controls the finger and wrist joint angles, and the person forming the stretcher simply follows the shape and position of the hand and arm.

The number of initial POP strips depends on the size of the arm to be managed. The hotter the water, the faster the plaster will set, but be careful not to burn the patient. Finger loops are especially necessary if flexor tightness differs significantly among the digits. The optional arm wedge may be foam or solid.

Prepare the clinic for POP application. Gather the required materials and equipment. To protect surfaces from plaster drippings, cover them with disposable, waterproof covers. Both the therapist and patient will want to protect their clothing with drapes or aprons and should remove watches and rings.

Determine the amount of POP required for the stretcher (Fig. 10–30A,B) by measuring the greatest width of the extremity, generally the palm or proximal forearm. Be sure to include the drape of the material halfway down the forearm or palm in the measurement. Measure the length from the longest fingertip to two-thirds of the way up the forearm to determine POP strip length. Round the corners of the plaster lay the plaster down on the hand to determine the location of the thenar eminence (Fig. 10–30C). Cut a slit in the plaster at the midway point of the thenar eminence. This will be turned back to leave the thumb free, and the overlap will reinforce this thinner part of the orthosis (Fig. 10–30D). Finally, fill a large clean bowl with hot water.

METHOD

Tissue Preconditioning

As for finger casting, gains in PROM of the forearm are more rapid and of a greater magnitude if the tissue is preconditioned or stretched out just before orthosis application (Schultz-Johnson, 2003). Methods of preconditioning were discussed earlier in this chapter. Note that patients with sensory compromise may not be candidates for tissue preconditioning.

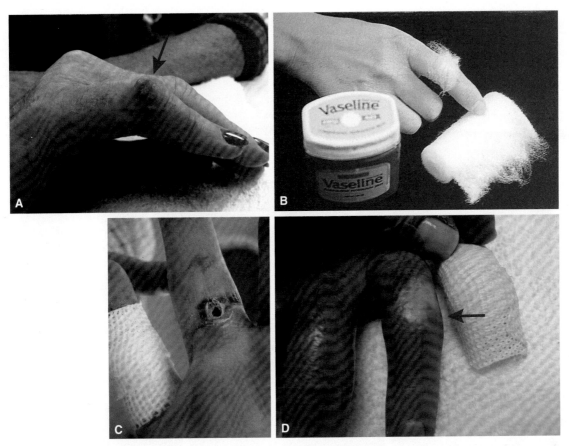

FIGURE 10–28 A, Note significant redness overlying the PIP joint after cast removal. **B,** A minimalist approach to padding relieves pressure over the PIP in the cast. Petroleum jelly helps stabilize the wisp of padding. **C,** Tissue breakdown from the proximal edge of a finger cast. **D,** Area of maceration on the dorsum of the digit after cast moisture was retained under the cast for a few days.

When the POP is set, remove it from the arm. Although the plaster is dry on the surface, it is still wet in the deeper layers and will still be soft enough to smooth edges by hand or with plaster scissors. At this point, the therapist may add any reinforcement desired to increase the rigidity of the orthosis. Thermoplastic and banding metal are both effective reinforcement materials. The reinforcement bar should extend over most of the length of the stretcher (Fig. 10–30H). Additional strips of POP secure the reinforcements to the POP base.

Securing the Plaster of Paris Stretcher

Once the final POP stretcher revisions are made, the patient puts it on and wraps it into place with an elasticized bandage. The therapist must carefully instruct the patient in proper wrapping technique to avoid vascular compromise. To start the wrap, the patient tucks the end of the wrap in between the index finger and POP stretcher and

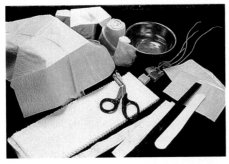

FIGURE 10–29 Materials and equipment needed to fabricate a POP stretcher.

then starts wrapping proximally in a Figure-8 or spiral fashion (Fig. 10–30I,J). D-ring hook-and-loop straps may be added to reinforce the wrist or finger position (Fig. 10–30K).

If the arm underwent preconditioning before stretcher fabrication, the therapist must instruct the patient in cast application when the lengthened tissue returns to its shorter length. When first applied, the arm will not fit perfectly into the stretcher. The wrap will have to be readjusted over time as the patient wears the stretcher and tissue once again lengthens. Some patients do not tolerate this readjustment process well. For them, avoid tissue preconditioning. Patients with sensory compromise are not candidates for the readjustment period because pressure distribution is poor and the risk of skin injury is high.

Check and Revision

Check the stretcher for sharp edges, cracks, and pressure areas. Sharp edges can be rounded with the application of hot water. A pair of sharp plaster scissors is also effective. Should cracks appear in the plaster, apply warm water to the cracked area, and add two or more strips of plaster. These strips do not need to be the length of the whole orthosis but must be long enough to adhere well and give adequate reinforcement.

PRECAUTIONS FOR POP STRETCHER

Material Properties

Care must be taken to avoid stressing the POP before it has fully set. It takes several hours before the POP will have its full strength. After the initial exothermic heat reaction, the plaster will be quite

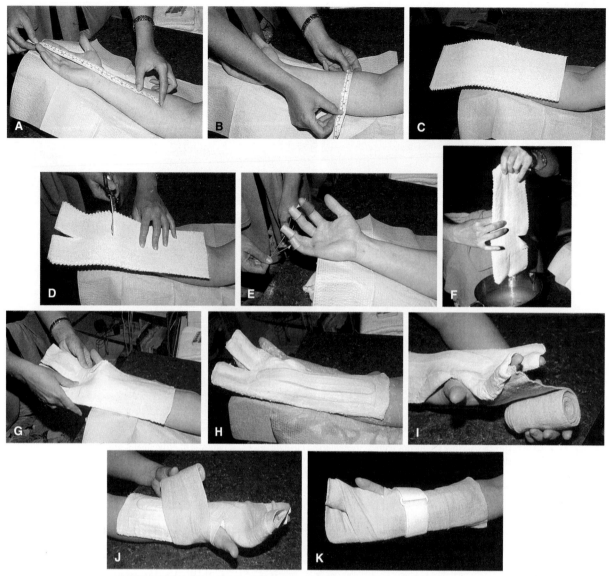

FIGURE 10–30 Steps of applying a forearm POP stretcher. A and B, Determine the appropriate plaster dimensions by measuring the length and greatest width of the extremity. **C,** Check that the plaster is of the proper dimensions. **D,** Cut a slit in the plaster at the midway point of the thenar eminence. If the range of motion of the fingers differs significantly, cut the plaster longitudinally between the fingers to position the fingers at different angles. **E,** This traction maneuver maximizes the stretch on the affected tissue. The fingers may be stretched individually as well. **F,** Immerse the plaster in water for 5 to 10 seconds and remove any excess water. **G,** Gently mold the POP to the arm, avoiding point pressure. **H,** If reinforcement is desired, contour the plastic or metal to the stretcher and cover it with two or three layers of POP to secure it in place. **I and J,** Tuck the end of the wrap in between the index finger and POP stretcher and wrap proximally. The tips of the digits are left uncovered so a patient with diminished sensation can check color and temperature. **K,** D-ring hook-and-loop straps help secure the stretcher in position and distribute the pressure.

cold for the next few hours until it fully dries. Some patients may find this uncomfortable. However, providing the patient with a stockinette (preferably polypropylene) may resolve this problem. Tolerance to the material was discussed in detail earlier in this chapter (Box 10–4).

As always, the patient must have a thorough understanding of the signs and symptoms that indicate orthosis removal. Vascular, dermal, and neurologic symptoms were discussed earlier in this chapter (Box 10–5).

Skin Lubrication

POP wicks moisture from the skin and can be very drying. Having the patient wear a stockinette as an interface between the arm and the POP can improve skin lubrication. Patients who wear a POP stretcher may need to apply a skin lubricant more frequently.

Pressure Areas

The patient must be instructed to check for the deep red marks in the skin that indicate pressure areas and to report these to the therapist. Teach the patient to attempt to resolve pressure areas with repositioning the stretcher, adjusting the wraps and straps, or inserting small temporary bits of tissue or cotton. Pressure problems that do not respond to these interventions indicate that the stretcher cannot be worn until the therapist can make the appropriate revisions.

Casting Over Wounds

Casting over wounds was discussed in detail earlier in this chapter. Plastic wrap placed over a dressing protects the dressing during stretcher formation and will keep it free from POP and moisture. Clinical experience suggests that POP aids wound healing. Experts have noted that POP wicks away exudate when it

BOX 10-4 PLASTER OF PARIS CONTRAINDICATIONS

- Severe heterotrophic ossification (HO)
- Skeletal muscle rigidity because it may increase their tightness
- Excessively edematous extremity
- Impaired circulation
- Partial or complete sensory loss in the involved area

- Pathologic inflammatory conditions, including arthritis
- Poor compliance/attendance as an outpatient
- Metastatic disease due to the risk of fracturing with serial casting
- A claustrophobic patient (Colditz, 2011, pp. 894–921)

---

is applied either directly to the wound or over a light dressing. Although some clinicians may fear that the wound will stick to the plaster, the adherence aids in wound healing because it prevents shear stress (the greatest enemy to wound healing) (Bell-Krotoski, 2011; Colditz, 2002).

Thermal Effects of POP

When POP and water mix, an exothermic chemical reaction takes place. The literature does report cases of thermal burns with the application of POP bandages (Becker, 1978; Grazer, 1979; Haasch, 1964; Kaplan, 1981; Schultze, 1967; Mahler, Pedowitz, Byrne, & Gershuni, 1996). When working with plaster, therapists should keep this thermal effect in mind. Tribuzi (1990) noted that casts reach maximum temperature in 5 to 15 minutes after application. Tribuzi listed several variables that may increase the temperature of the exothermic reaction, including the following:

- High room temperature
- High humidity
- Cast thickness of more than eight plies
- Undersaturation or oversaturation with water
- Use of fast-setting plaster
- Dipping temperature
- Inadequate ventilation during the drying period

Inadequate ventilation can occur from overwrapping the freshly applied plaster with cotton or elastic bandages, covering the plaster with blankets, or placing the cast or orthosis near a pillow or mattress (Johnson and Johnson Orthopedic Division, 1985; Kaplan, 1981; Lavalette et al., 1982).

Bell-Krotoski (1995), (2011) postulates that these injuries may actually be caused by pressure from an improperly applied POP rather than from heat. When working with plaster, the clinician must always use clean water because the plaster residue left in the dipping container from previous casts is thought to act as an accelerator and increase the exothermic reaction. In addition, shards of set plaster can accidently be incorporated into the orthosis and cause irritation and discomfort.

Although Tribuzi (1990) noted that POP should never be applied directly to the skin, Bell-Krotoski (2011) and others state that there is no contraindication to this practice (Bell-Krotoski, 2011; Brand & Yancey, 1997; Colditz, 2002; Tribuzi, 1990). Certainly, any time a clinician would like to include cast padding to a circumferential plaster cast, the padding must be placed first. A cast saw cannot be used if there is no padding under the cast.

STRETCHER REGIMEN

Deciding when to fabricate a new stretcher is easier than deciding how frequently to change a serial cast because the extremity demonstrates what it needs. When a patient is consistently able to lift out of the stretcher by 5° at the target joint(s), the time has come for a new stretcher.

It is the responsibility of the therapist to assess the characteristics of each patient to determine a safe and effective wearing schedule. As with any removable orthosis, the patient should initially wear the orthosis for a trial period of 20 to 30 minutes to determine skin tolerance. Once tolerance is established, the patient can gradually increase time in the orthosis. Nighttime tolerance is a goal. This achieves 6 to 8 hours of end-range positioning and then leaves the extremity free during the day for exercise. When the goal is stretcher wear during sleep, the therapist may want to decrease the amount of stretch placed on the tissue during stretcher fabrication or may avoid preconditioning before fabrication.

For the patient who cannot sleep while wearing the stretcher, the therapist must achieve a balance between stretcher wear, activities of daily living, and exercise. Remember that the more the patient wears the stretcher, the faster the patient will reach the therapeutic goals. A minimum amount of time in the stretcher (which depends on the individual patient) must occur for the stretcher to affect tissue change (see Chapter 15 for details) (Flowers & LaStayo, 2012; Flowers & Michlovitz, 1988; Glasgow et al., 2012). The therapist may consider combining other orthoses or POP finger casts with stretchers. Applying the finger orthosis or casts before stretcher fabrication may help achieve optimal IP joint position.

BOX 10-5 CAST PRECAUTIONS

Monitor cast in clinic for any of the issues noted below and then instruct the patient in home observation every 2 hours. The following are issues to watch for:

- Pain
- Edema proximal or distal to the casted segment
- Sensory changes
- Circulatory changes—check pulse points distally

- Increased or decreased movement in cast
- Skin integrity
- Severe itching
- Cracks, dents, or softening of cast

If any of these occur, cast must be removed and application reassessed.

CONCLUSION

Casting is a powerful treatment technique that has the ability to provide outcomes that no other orthotic intervention can offer. The circumferential approach has many benefits, including improved pressure distribution and minimized shear and migration. Casting offers an efficient and effective means to decrease contractures, including those with a hard end feel. Even patients with cognitive and sensory impairment can benefit from casting. Future studies continue to be necessary to examine the impact of using casting to manage upper limb impairments, especially for those patients with wrist and hand spasticity, and to assess the efficacy of those casts not widely adopted in current practice such as inhibitory and drop-out casts (Flinn & Craven, 2014).

As with any treatment approach, the therapist must carefully consider the nature of the problem before applying the cast. Patients with PROM limitations owing to soft-tissue abnormalities that will not respond to low-load, prolonged stress should not receive a cast. Joint limitation caused by heterotopic ossification, exostosis, or loose body will also not benefit from casting. The circumferential design of the cast allows mobilization of a joint that might not be a candidate for conventional orthotic management, for example, in the case of some forms of joint instability and acute inflammation. However, avascular necrosis, infection, unstable fracture, marked demineralization, myositis ossificans, and stress across healing structures without adequate blood supply or tensile strength to withstand tensile stress remain contraindications to cast application.

The family of casting products continues to increase, offering patients and clinicians even more options. Keeping current and familiar with the characteristics of each new product helps the therapist choose the material that best meets the patient's needs. This chapter reviewed only a few of these materials, and the reader is encouraged to read Chapters 11, 12, and 19 to stay abreast of all casting options that are made available. Circumferential and noncircumferential casting techniques to serially increase PROM require skills that are unique to this modality. Continued innovation in the use of casting will benefit patients in new and effective ways.

CHAPTER REVIEW QUESTIONS

1. Name three of the most common indications for casting.
2. Explain the material choice and rationale for use of a cast for zone III extensor tendon injuries.
3. Give a clinical example of a serial static mobilization orthosis using two types of cast material. What is the injury and why did you choose this material?
4. What are the general precautions of POP casting and how is the plaster removed?
5. What are the some creative uses and techniques that can be done with thermoplastic tapes?

ACKNOWLEDGMENT FROM SECOND EDITION

A very warm thank you to Karen Schultz MS OTR CHT FAOTA who laid the foundation for this chapter 20 years ago. It's with your work that we continue to grow and learn!

Sincere thanks to Judy Colditz, OTR/L, CHT, FAOTA, for her guidance with integrating information on casting motion to mobilize stiffness (CMMS) and Deborah Schwartz, OTD, OTR/L, CHT, for her insight regarding the use of Orficast® from Orfit Industries.

ACKNOWLEDGMENTS FROM THE FIRST EDITION

Many thanks to Trudy Hackencamp, OTR/L, CHT, for the information she provided regarding casting spasticity. Thanks also to Judy Bell-Krotoski for our many discussions over the years regarding the use of POP and serial casting of fingers. Finally, thanks to Jessica Hawkins, my patient of many years, who has worn more casts than anyone can count and has given me invaluable feedback.

11 Orficast® and Orficast® More

Deborah A. Schwartz, OTD, OTR/L, CHT

CHAPTER OBJECTIVES

After study of this chapter, the reader should be able to:
• Understand the unique properties of a knitted thermoplastic material.
• Understand the clinical reasoning process for selecting this material over alternate sheet materials to fabricate an orthosis for a client.
• Describe the goals of orthotic fabrication using Orficast® and Orficast® More products.
• Detail the steps required to activate the material, mold an orthosis, and attach hook and loop strapping.
• Describe the necessary steps to fabricate three to five specific orthoses for immobilization using Orficast® and/or Orficast® More materials.
• Recognize additional nonorthotic uses for Orficast®.

KEY TERMS
Orficast®
Orficast® More

FAQ

How Do You Remove an Orficast® Orthosis From a Finger?
Orthoses from Orficast® can be slipped off the finger if the orthosis is not made too tight. They can also be cut off with small curved scissors. The client can soak the orthosis in warm water until is completely wet, in which case it, should allow for cutting with the scissors or the ability to pull the orthosis off the finger. If the orthosis is made too tightly around an enlarged IP joint of the thumb, a small triangle can be cut away from the dorsal portion of the orthosis and left open or filled in with additional Orficast® material.

How Do You Attach Hook and Loop Strapping to an Orficast® Orthosis?
See section on attaching strapping.

Can an Orficast® Orthosis Get Wet?
An Orficast® orthosis can get wet, and it will not change the shape of the orthosis. However, it does take a while to dry out completely, so it might be better to remove for showers and bathing or place a bag around the orthosis.

How Long Will It Take to Dry Completely?
It really depends on how much water was left in the material during the fabrication process and the surrounding humidity. It should dry out within an hour or so.

INTRODUCTION

Clinicians well versed in orthotic fabrication will do well to keep abreast of new innovations and advances in the realm of thermoplastic materials and other resources for orthotic fabrication. Manufacturers of thermoplastic materials are constantly striving to introduce novel versions of their high-quality materials in order to meet all the needs and demands of the market, and there are many major advances in this area. The original materials available for orthotic fabrication nearly 50 years ago were not considered low enough in temperature to place directly on a client's extremity. Today's low-temperature thermoplastic materials are easy to mold and remold, can be placed directly on a client's extremity, and have many different characteristics which, when used correctly, can ease the clinician's fabrication process and be more comfortable for the client. Selection of the appropriate thermoplastic material for any client must be done with thoughtful consideration of the specific diagnosis, the correct positioning for that diagnosis, the size of the client's extremity, and, perhaps, a bit of clinician preference.

ORFICAST® AND ORFICAST® MORE

Orficast® is a knitted thermoplastic material comprised of thermoplastic threads knitted together with a nylon cross weave. This unique construction creates a soft fabric–like material that when activated by immersion in hot water (160°F–165°F) is stretchy, moldable, and conforming. Activation by the dry heat of a heat gun is possible but not recommended for orthotic fabrication. The dry heat from a heat gun makes the product very sticky and is helpful at adhering the straps and/or hook to the orthosis. Dry heat activation in a specialized oven is possible for orthotic fabrication as it offers effective and even activation of all of the thermoplastic material at the same time. As the material cools, it hardens and captures the shape of the anatomy that it covers. The thermoplastic threads have memory so the material can be stretched lengthwise and will revert back to their original length when reheated. The nylon threads do not have memory. Any stretching of the material to widen it will not allow for reverting back to the original width. It is important to understand that the feature of memory (reversion back to an original length or size) in a thermoplastic material is not automatic. It will not occur if components of the material are well adhered together or have been cut. Materials with memory require specific handling; the clinician should allow the material to harden in place before removal. If a material with memory has been stretched to enlarge the size and left to harden, it will return to its original size when reheated. All thermoplastic materials will become softened and flattened when reimmersed in heated water, but only products with memory will revert to their original size as well.

Orficast® and **Orficast® More** are thermoplastic materials that come rolled up in a small box, not in a sheet (Fig. 11–1). Simply pull out the material from the slot opening and cut as much is needed.

Orficast® was introduced to the therapy market in boxes containing either 1″ or 2.5″ widths of material in lengths of nearly 10 ft (3 m). The ease of use is evident in the packaging as clinicians only need to cut various lengths of material to fabricate simple finger and thumb orthoses. Orficast® is easy to store in the clinic as each box takes up little space and can be placed on the counter. Orficast® More was introduced as a thermoplastic material several years later in a wider and thicker format. The increased number of thermoplastic threads of material and the wider versions offer clinicians increased rigidity of the product with wider material pieces for multiple orthotic interventions including hand, forearm, and even foot and ankle applications. Orficast® More products are similarly packaged in boxes of increasing sizes to accommodate the different widths. All of these products are available in black and blue with more colors to come in the future. Tables 11–1 and 11–2 outline the features and benefits of Orficast®.

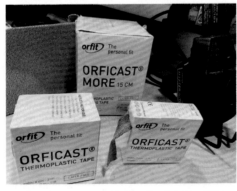

FIGURE 11–1 Boxes of Orficast® and Orficast® More.

TABLE 11–1	Features of Orficast® and Orficast® More
Packaging	Comes in a various-sized small boxes for easy storage
Size/length	Orficast®: Available in 1″ or 2.5″ widths × 10′ length Orficast® More: Available in 2.5″, 5″, and 6″ widths × 10′ length
Colors	All widths available in blue and black
Method of activation	Minimal time needed for full immersion in heated water (160°F–165°F) Activation by dry heat is possible but not recommended (makes the product very sticky)
Material characteristics	Moderate memory lengthwise along thermoplastic threads High conformability and drape with stretch Minimal to moderate rigidity—depends on number of layers and overlap

OVERVIEW OF USE

Orficast® and Orficast® More are relatively easy to use, but general guidelines for best usage and practice should be followed. A strip of Orficast® can be easily cut in the desired length for the given orthosis. The material is placed in the splint pan or a bowl of heated water (160°F–165°F) and allowed to thoroughly heat up. The material is removed from the hot water and briefly dried on a towel. Use the heel of the hand to pat it dry quickly on both sides. The heat from the hot water allows for the moldability and adherence of the product to itself, but avoid dripping hot water on the client during the fabrication process. Over time, the clinician will learn just how much hot water to remove to prevent dripping and also maintain enough heat in the product for molding. If all of the moisture is removed and the product has dried before beginning the application, it will simply become hard and stiff and not moldable at all and/or not adhere to itself.

TABLE 11–2	Benefits of Orficast® and Orficast® More
Packaging	Nearly 10 feet of rolled material in either 1″ or 2.5″ widths (Orficast®) Nearly 10 feet of rolled material in either 2.5″, 5″, or 6″ widths (Orficast® More)
Types of orthoses	Any finger or thumb orthosis can be made from Orficast® Any thumb- and/or hand-based orthoses can be made from Orficast® More Radial- and ulnar-based orthoses can be made from Orficast® More
Time factor	Quick activation time—about 40 s in water heated to 160°F–165°F Quick hardening time—about 1 min after positioning as desired
Pattern making	No pattern needed. Can use variations of a wrap and pinch method of orthotic fabrication
Weight and feel	Lightweight product for increased client comfort and compliance Feels like a fabric, not plastic
Ventilation	Well-ventilated product which allows skin to breathe

FINGER PIP EXTENSION ORTHOSIS WITH PINCH METHOD (ORFICAST® MORE 2.5″) (FIG. 11–5)

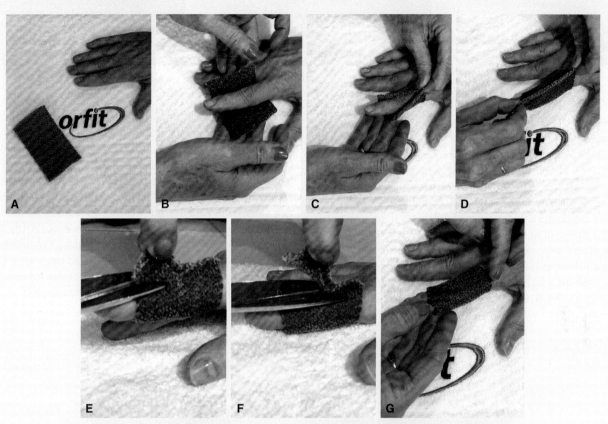

FIGURE 11–5 A, Cut a piece of Orficast® More 2.5″ about 4″ long or 6-7″ piece of Orficast® 2.5″and fold in half width wise and activate. **B,** Place directly underneath the finger. **C,** Bring both sides of the material together dorsally and pinch firmly. **D,** Create an evenly pinched seam on the dorsum of the finger. **E,** While the material is warm, pull it upward and cut underneath, creating a flat well-bonded seam. **F,** Continue to pull upward and cut the entire seam. **G,** Check to see that the edges of the seam are well adhered and the orthosis fits snugly on the finger in the desired position; trim material away to allow DIP flexion.

Swan Neck Deformity

The swan neck deformity is characterized by hyperextension of the PIP joint and flexion of the DIP joint. The deformity might be rigid or flexible but can lead to difficulty flexing the PIP joint for grasping objects. Rigid swan neck deformities may require surgical intervention (Lalonde, 2015). Orthoses that block hyperextension of the PIP joint are known as anti–swan neck orthoses, and there are many commercial types available as well as methods for custom orthotic fabrication (van de Giesen et al., 2010). The orthotic design offers three-point pressure to the proximal and middle phalanges and the volar PIP joint (Fig. 11–6A–C). While blocking full extension at the PIP joint, the orthosis should not limit full PIP flexion. The orthosis also contributes to lateral stability of the joint (Spicka, Macleod, Adams, & Metcalf, 2009).

For the oval ring design (Fig. 11–6B), *take a strip of Orficast® 1″ about 6″ long, activate and roll lengthwise creating a narrow tubular shape. Beginning at the finger's medial side of the PIP joint, create an oval covering the entire length of the proximal and middle phalanges. The finger must be in maximum flexion throughout the process. Connect the material at the starting point, then pull the remaining material underneath the flexed PIP joint and attach to the opposite side of the PIP joint. Wait until hardened before removing and keep the finger in PIP flexion.*

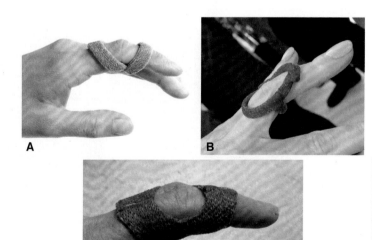

FIGURE 11–6 A–C, Three versions of the anti–swan neck orthosis. **A,** Figure-of-8 method. **B,** Oval ring method. **C,** Pinch method.

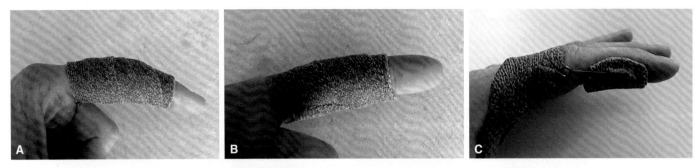

FIGURE 11–7 **A and B,** PIP extension orthosis. **C,** Dynamic extension orthosis for PIP flexion contractures.

PIP Flexion Contracture

Flexion contractures of the PIP joint are a common sequela from injuries and/or surgery of the fingers and/or hand (Farzad, Arazpour, Shafiee, Layeghi, & Schwartz, 2019). The periarticular structures of the joint tend to shorten, especially when there is prolonged edema or prolonged immobilization (Boccolari & Tocco, 2009). Orthotic fabrication is an intervention to help remodel the soft-tissue structures and place the PIP joint in maximum extension. Serial static orthotic fabrication refers to the practice of remolding or remaking an orthosis in maximum PIP extension to match the evolving condition of the contracture, with the goal of eventually reaching and maintaining full extension (Fig. 11–7A,B) (Tuffaha & Lee, 2018). Each orthosis may

be worn by the client for a week or so, and then a new orthosis might be applied after a treatment session of heat and stretching. Another option for the client is to wear a dynamic extension orthosis with coils placed at the PIP joint (Fig. 11–7C) (Valdes, Boyd, Povlak, & Szelwach, 2018). Clinical recommendations from a recent systematic review of orthotic interventions for PIP flexion contractures suggest that clients will benefit from wearing an orthosis for at least 6 hours per day for a total of 8 to 17 weeks (Valdes et al., 2018). In addition, the force from the orthosis should be low enough so that the client can feel slight tension, but no pain. The total end-range time (TERT) that the orthosis is worn by the client is a key factor in regaining full range of motion with orthotic intervention (Flowers & LaStayo, 2012).

PIP EXTENSION ORTHOSIS WITH WRAP METHOD (ORFICAST® 1″) (FIG. 11–8)

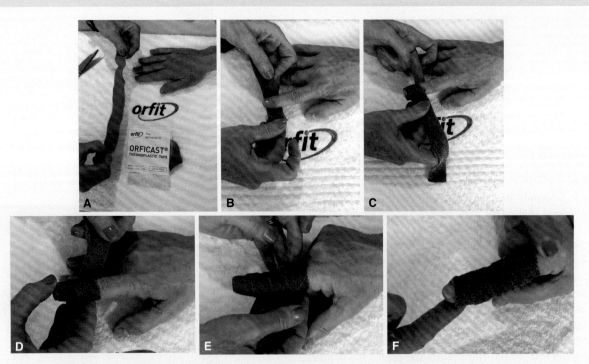

FIGURE 11–8 **A,** Cut a strip of Orficast® 1″ about 8″ long. **B,** Activate the material and wrap around the distal finger edge. **C,** Anchor the material to itself. **D,** Continue to wrap the material around the finger at an angle, overlapping the material 50% each wrap stretching slightly for increased conformity. **E,** Stretch the end of the material at the proximal edge of the finger and make sure the corners are well adhered to the material underneath. Take time to smooth all of the layers together. At the end of the finger, make sure the corners of the Orficast® are firmly pressed and bonded to the material underneath, and no corners can be pulled off. **F,** Check the positioning of the finger. Once the material is firmly bonded together, place the MCP joint in flexion and place a small amount of stress toward PIP extension. Keep the desired position and let the material harden. Determine whether to leave as is on the finger or remove for additional trimming and attaching straps.

Relative Motion Orthosis

Acute sagittal band injuries at the level of the metacarpophalangeal (MCP) joint can be treated conservatively using a relative motion extension orthosis (Lutz et al., 2015). This orthosis typically wraps around three or four fingers but holds the affected finger in 15° to 20° more MCP joint extension than the adjacent fingers (Fig. 11–9A,B). Full range of motion is permitted while wearing this orthosis which limits tension on the involved MCP joint structures (Hirth, Howell and O'Brien, 2016; Merritt, 2014). This orthosis also helps elicit active PIP flexion in clients with PIP flexion contractures. Relative motion flexion orthosis places the MCP joint of the involved finger in relatively flexed potion to elicit active PIP extension (Fig. 11–9C,D).

The relative motion orthosis can be made from Orficast® 1″ (three layers is recommended); Orficast® 2.5″ wide (fold in half on into thirds lengthwise); and/or Orficast® More 2.5″ (fold in half lengthwise). Use enough material so that after folding as indicated, the length is long enough to wrap around the indicated three or four fingers. Before beginning to fabricate this relative motion extension orthosis, position in pronation and place a pencil underneath the intended finger's proximal phalanx as a reference. Remove the pencil and place the activated Orficast® in the same position, leaving enough material on each side to wrap around the adjacent finger's proximal phalanx. Supinate the hand and wrap the material around each adjacent finger's proximal phalanx, creating rings. Press the ends together firmly over the involved finger's proximal phalanx on the volar surface and press down, making sure to hold the adjacent fingers close together. Let gravity assist in the process and press the involved finger into more MCP extension by pressing the proximal phalanx downward. The orthosis should be easy to don and doff. If one of the finger rings is too tight, simply reheat quickly and stretch out.

Trigger Finger Orthosis

Trigger finger or "digital stenosing tenosynovitis" is a condition in which the flexor tendon of the involved finger "triggers" or "snaps" as the client flexes or extends.

Inflammation of the flexor tendon and/or its surrounding tendon sheath can lead to swelling or the formation of a flexor tendon nodule preventing the normal gliding of the tendon underneath the finger pulley(s). The A1 pulley (located at the MCP joint) is most frequently involved (Colbourn, Heath, Manary, & Pacifico, 2008). Research indicates that wearing a flexion-blocking orthosis for the PIP or MCP joints can decrease the triggering of a single isolated trigger finger, and symptoms can be resolved with 6 to 10 weeks of orthotic wear (Fig. 11–10) (Colburn et al., 2008; Lunsford, Valdes, & Hengy, 2017; Valdes, 2012).

A simple MCP flexion–blocking orthosis can be made with an 8″ strip of Orficast® 1″. Activate the material and pat dry. Starting with one end of the Orficast®, wrap around the specific finger's proximal phalanx, and then, on the volar surface, fold the material so that it goes into the palm. Fold back on itself around the level of the distal palmar crease and bring the material up to the PIP joint. Then fold again on itself creating three layers of material in front of the MCP joint. Trim all layers at the level of the distal palmar crease. Make sure the client can fully flex the PIP joint and make sure all layers of material are well bonded together and trimmed.

Buddy Tapes

An injury to the collateral ligament of the PIP joint may occur as a result of lateral force to the involved joint resulting in pain and possibly joint laxity. Buddy tapes are utilized to secure the injured finger to its adjacent finger for protection and support (Fig. 11–11) (Feldscher, 2010; Freiberg, Pollard, Macdonald, & Duncan, 2006; Leggit & Meko, 2006).

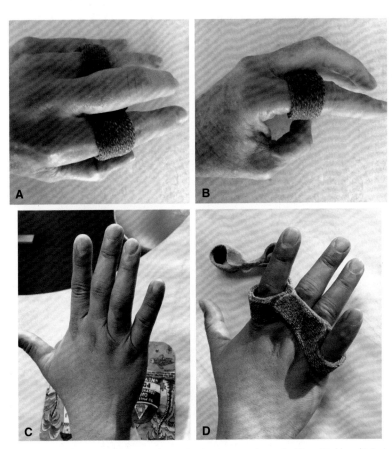

FIGURE 11–9 **A and B,** Relative motion extension orthosis—commonly used with sagittal band injuries. **C,** Relative motion flexion orthosis for the middle and ring fingers—notice PIP flexion contractures. **D,** Active extension with orthosis.

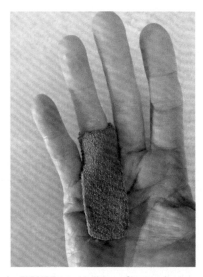

FIGURE 11–10 Trigger finger orthosis.

*Buddy tapes can easily be fabricated using two strips of Orficast®
1" × 5": folding it lengthwise after activation, wrapping one proximally around the proximal phalanges and the second one distal to
the joint around the middle phalanges.*

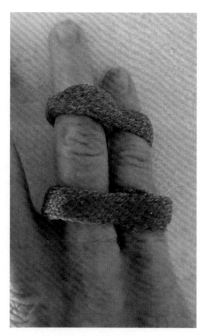

FIGURE 11–11 Buddy tapes.

APPLICATION TIPS FOR ADDING STRAPS TO ORFICAST® AND ORFICAST® MORE ORTHOSES (FIG. 11–12)

Since the orthosis may still be wet or damp when it is time to apply straps, use these tips to help adhere the loop and hook:

1. Prepare two pieces of Orficast® 1" × 2", a small piece of adhesive backed hook and a longer piece of loop strapping.
2. Using dry heat from the heat gun, heat up one piece of Orficast® and the adhesive side of the hook and press together. The Orficast® acts as an interface (Fig. 11–12A).
3. Trim the excess Orficast® and adhere to the orthosis using dry heat on both the orthosis and the prepared hook. Fold over the excess Orficast® as a border (Fig. 11–12B).

4. Heat the second strip of Orficast® and wrap around one end of the loop strapping. Trim corners.
5. Heat the orthosis and the prepared end of the loop strap with dry heat and press together (Fig. 11–12C).
6. Alternatively, heat a thin strip of Orficast® and use as binding tape around the edges of the hook and the loop after these have been bonded to the orthosis (Fig. 11–12D).

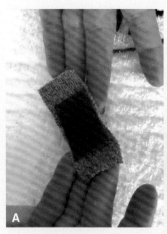
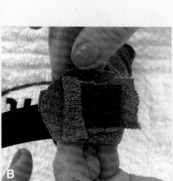
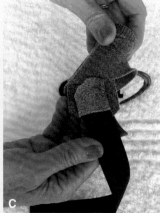
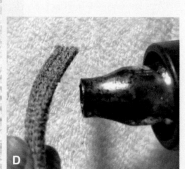

FIGURE 11–12

COMMON CONDITIONS OF THE THUMB

Orficast® and Orficast® More can be used to fabricate well-fitting and conforming orthoses for the thumb. Hand-based thumb orthoses (short opponens) for the carpometacarpal (CMC) and MCP joints can be made from Orficast® 2.5″ width and also from Orficast® More in either 2.5, 5″ or 6″ widths. These types of orthoses (rigid or semirigid) offer a degree of stabilization for thumb diagnoses with rheumatoid arthritis and/or osteoarthritis and help to stabilize the first metacarpal bone in a better anatomical position. The finished product is thin enough to fit under many types of gloves including those for athletes, gardening, workman's gloves, and even gloves used by dental hygienists and surgeons.

Basal Joint Arthritis

Multiple studies have demonstrated that an orthosis for either osteo-arthritis or rheumatoid arthritis of the thumb can improve hand function and decrease pain (Valdes & Marik, 2010; Beasley, 2012). A variety of orthotic options are available to the clinician: an ortho-sis may immobilize both the CMC and MP joints, while another approach is to immobilize and support the CMC joint alone (Fig. 11–13A–C). Both types of orthoses may offer relief (Cantero-Téllez et al., 2018). A recent study suggests that the user's view of their orthosis and its purpose as either a joint stabilizer, a tool for heavy tasks, a healer of arthritis, or other similar characteristics can have an effect on the user's compliance and wearing schedule (Grüschke, Reinders-Messelink, van der Vegt, & van der Sluis, 2018).

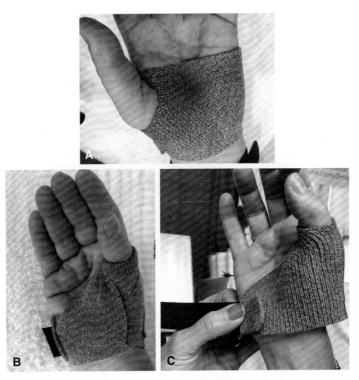

FIGURE 11–13 A, Thumb CMC orthosis without MP joint. **B,** Thumb CMC and MP orthosis from Orficast® 2.5″. **C,** Thumb CMC and MP orthosis from Orficast® More 6″.

THUMB ORTHOSIS WITH WRAP METHOD (ORFICAST® 2.5″) (FIG. 11–14)

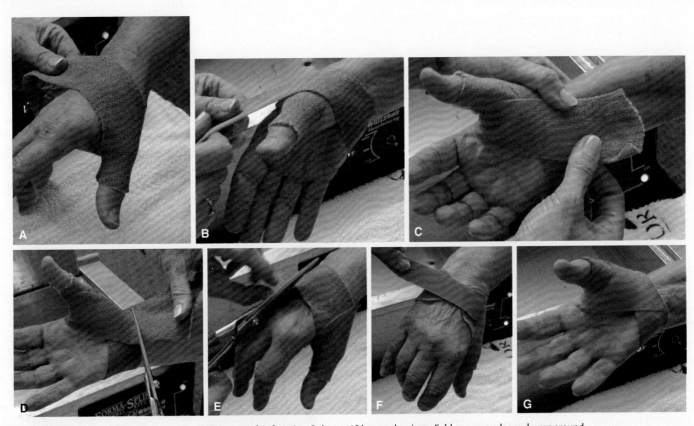

FIGURE 11–14 A, Cut a strip of Orficast® 2.5″ about 12″ long and activate. Fold over one edge and wrap around the thumb lengthwise, just under the IP joint with the remainder placed around the dorsal radial side of the wrist and forearm. **B,** Wrap around the dorsal hand and then the palm, leaving the wrist crease free of material. Bring the Orficast through the first web space, from the dorsum to the palm. **C,** Overlap the thenar muscles and press all layers of the material together firmly. **D,** Let the material harden and trim away any excess in the front. **E,** Cut the back of the orthosis. **F,** Attach hook and loop straps. **G,** Check the fit and make sure the IP joint can flex.

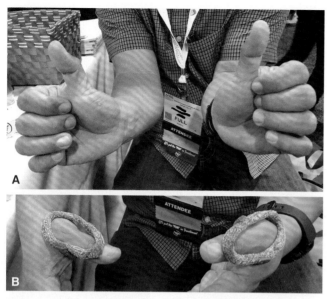

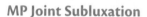

FIGURE 11–15 **A,** Client with MP joint subluxation. **B,** Anti–swan neck for thumb MP joint.

MP Joint Subluxation

A simple orthosis made from a strip of rolled Orficast® and formed in an oval design can also help prevent hyperextension of the thumb MP joint as this may become painful when a pinch is attempted (Fig. 11–15A,B). The orthosis must be fabricated while maintaining the MP joint in maximum flexion.

First Web Spacer

Orficast® materials can easily be molded to create a first web spacer orthosis (Fig. 11–16). This type of orthosis prevents adduction

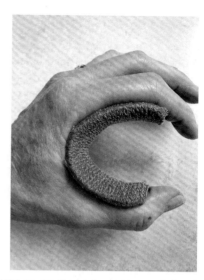

FIGURE 11–16 Thumb first web spacer Orficast® More.

contractures of the first web space that might result after an injury to the thumb or median nerve. A simple rectangle of Orficast® 2.5″ folded, or Orficast® More 2.5″, 5″, or 6″ wide material is molded into the first web space and extended from the index finger proximally to the thumb IP joint crease distally. The device positions and maintains the thumb in maximum abduction. This orthosis is typically prescribed for night use and can be adjusted periodically to increased tissue length over time. However, a shorter version of this orthosis may also help clients with functional pinch by maintaining an open web space when there is significant muscle weakness, especially for clients with amyotrophic lateral scoliosis (ALS) (Tanaka, Horaiya, Akagi, & Kihoin, 2014).

HELPFUL HINTS

1. Always make sure all layers are adhered firmly together. If a corner of material has started to unravel on the side of the orthosis, use the dry heat from a heat gun to secure.
2. An orthosis around the finger that appears to be too tight to slide off can be soaked in warm water until softened. Then try again to slide off or use small curved scissors to cut through the material.

3. Use the heat gun to help with attachment of hook and loop strapping to a wet orthosis. Either use additional Orficast® that has been dry heated as binding around the edges of the hook material or place underneath.
4. A hair dryer on a cool setting can be used to speed up the drying process. Excessive heat will cause the material to lose its shape.

HAND-BASED ORTHOSES

Gutter-Type Orthoses for Metacarpal and/or Phalangeal Fractures

A review of clinical treatments for metacarpal fractures (head and/or neck) found that stable fractures and also unstable fractures treated with open reduction internal fixation (ORIF) can be protected with a hand-based dorsal orthosis, with the MCP joints in 70° of flexion (Fig. 11–17A,B) (Midgley & Toemen, 2011). Placing the MCP joints in flexion helps to control the force of the extensor digitorum communis (EDC) from pulling on the fracture fragments. The orthosis should allow clients to flex and extend their PIP and DIP joints if not contraindicated. The orthosis should be worn for 2 weeks if the fracture was considered stable, and, for fractures treated surgically, the orthosis should be worn for a total of 4 weeks (Toemen & Midgley, 2010).

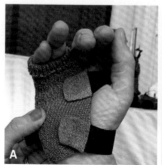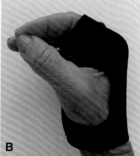

FIGURE 11–17 **A,** Ulnar gutter for small-finger metacarpal fracture. **B,** Radial gutter for index-finger metacarpal fracture.

ULNAR GUTTER ORTHOSIS (ORFICAST® MORE 5″) (FIG. 11–18)

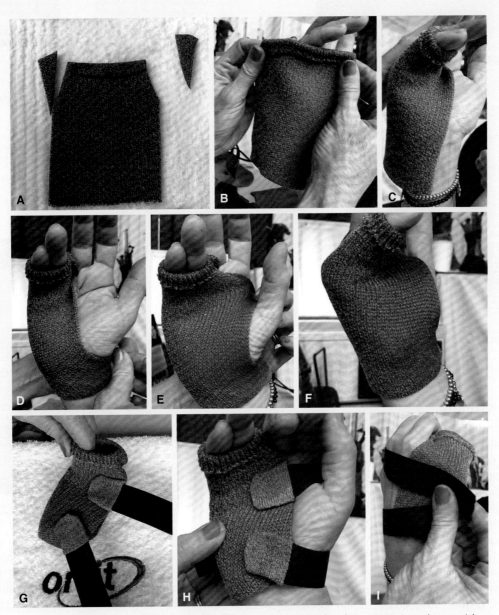

FIGURE 11–18 A, Trim two triangles away from a 6″ × 6″ square of Orficast® More. **B,** Activate the material and fold over the edge. Wrap around the ulnar portion of the hand with the rolled edge just proximal to the PIP joints of the ring and little fingers. Overlap the corners inside the web space between the ring and middle fingers. **C,** Place the MCP joints in flexion. **D,** Pull the proximal corners together at the radial border of the wrist to help the material stretch and conform. **F,** Check the positioning of the fingers. **E,** Stretch the material together through the first web space. **F,** Check the positioning of the fingers. Open all pinched material, remove the orthosis, and trim away the pinched areas. Let the orthosis clear the wrist. **G,** Attach two Velcro loop straps directly to the volar surface using the tips on adhering loop strapping as outlined. **H,** Check the strap placement through the first web and at the wrist level. **I,** Place hook on the dorsal surface of the orthosis.

Anticlaw Orthosis

The anticlaw orthosis is used for individuals with damage to the ulnar nerve that results in loss of the intrinsic muscles (Fig. 11–19A,B). The intrinsic muscles contribute to MCP flexion and PIP/DIP extension. Without the intrinsic muscle function, individuals typically display a deformity known as the claw hand, where the MCP joints of the ring and little fingers hyperextend and the PIP/DIP joints flex. The anticlaw orthosis positions the MCP joints in flexion and transfers the power of movement to the distal PIP and DIP joints, helping to achieve extension while limiting the hyperextension of the MCP joints (Seu & Pasqualetto, 2012; Sousa & Macedo, 2016).

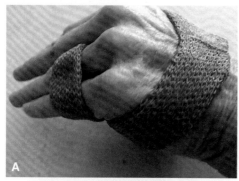

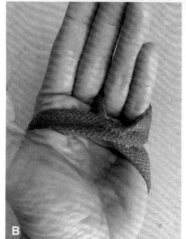

FIGURE 11–19 **A and B**: Anti–ulnar claw orthosis.

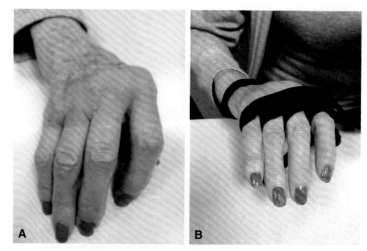

FIGURE 11–20 **A,** Client with ulnar drift. **B,** Anti–ulnar drift orthosis.

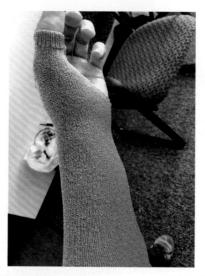

FIGURE 11–21 Wrist/thumb orthosis using Orficast® More.

Anti–Ulnar Drift Orthosis

MCP ulnar drift is a common deformity seen mostly in clients with rheumatoid arthritis (RA). Many factors can contribute to the development of ulnar drift over time and include synovitis, stretching, or attenuation of the joint capsule and radial collateral ligaments with subsequent subluxation of the extensor digitorum ulnarly, destruction of the metacarpal head, and volar dislocation of the proximal phalanx. Many activities of daily living (ADLs) also contribute ulnar- and volar-deviating forces across the MCP joints, such as gripping, lateral pinching activities, and writing tasks. The anti–ulnar drift orthosis can help to position the fingers for more effective grasp (Fig. 11–20A,B). It is important to note that this orthosis can only be used when the fingers can be corrected into normal alignment passively. If there is a fixed deformity, the orthosis will not be of much use. Special attention should be directed to all involved structures including the metacarpals as well as the metacarpal joints (Beasley, 2012).

FOREARM-BASED ORTHOSES WITH ORFICAST MORE

The relatively increased width and number of thermoplastic threads in Orficast® More 5″ and 6″ allow for the fabrication of longer and wider orthoses which can be molded around larger body parts, such as the wrist and forearm. While the material is not rigid enough in one layer to completely immobilize the wrist in a standard volar or dorsal wrist cock-up style, it does provide support when fabricated in a double layer; circumferentially as a wrist immobilization orthosis; or as a radial or ulnar gutter immobilization orthosis. One such example is a wrist/thumb (long opponens) orthosis placed on the radial forearm (Fig. 11–21).

The long opponens orthosis is appropriate for clients with DeQuervain's syndrome. Huisstede et al. (2014) describes a Delphi consensus strategy which was used to create a multidisciplinary treatment guideline for clients with DeQuervain's disease. In the sessions, clinicians and surgeons agreed that clients should receive both a home program and an additional treatment to alleviate the inflammation of the abductor pollicis longus (APL) and the extensor pollicis brevis (EPB) in the first dorsal compartment. The additional treatment could be an orthosis which includes the wrist and thumb MCP joint, nonsteroidal anti-inflammatory medications, an injection, or a combination of these treatments and/or surgery.

LONG OPPONENS ORTHOSIS (ORFICAST® MORE 6″) (FIG. 11–22)

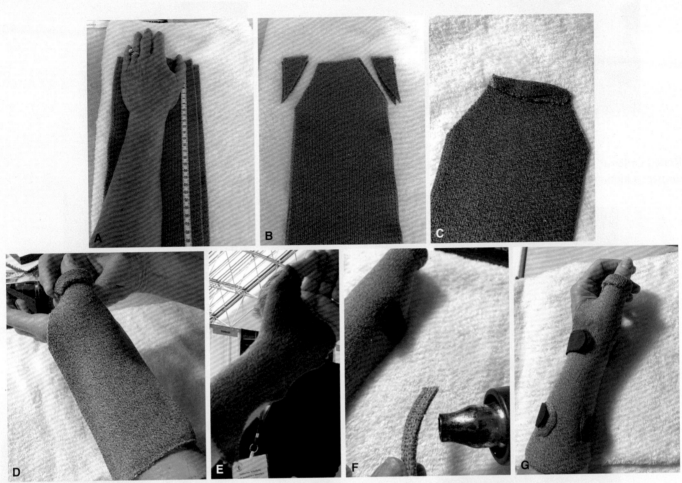

FIGURE 11–22 A, Measure a long rectangle of Orficast® More 6″ about 10″ long. **B,** Trim away two triangles of material and activate. **C,** Fold over the distal edge. **D,** Wrap around the radial side of the thumb and overlap the material underneath the IP joint. **E,** Stretch the material to the ulnar side and pinch at the level of the distal palmar crease, the proximal forearm, and the wrist, creating three pinches in total to help the material conform. Open the pinched areas and reclose them and let the material harden. Remove the orthosis, trim the sides. **F,** Attach loop straps and hook with reinforcement material as described. **G,** Strap with either two or three straps.

CREATIVE USES OF ORFICAST® MATERIALS

1. Increase the size of the end of the loop strap for ease in pinching for a client with arthritis and limited pinch (Fig. 11–23)

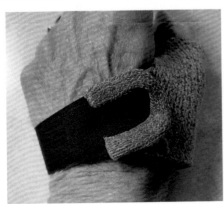

FIGURE 11–23

2. Help with adherence of outrigger attachments (wires and coils) (Fig. 11–24)

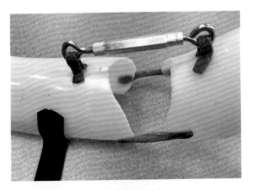

FIGURE 11–24

3. Rolled Orficast® hinges placed at the joint axis level access allow motion for dynamic and static progressive orthoses (Fig. 11–25)

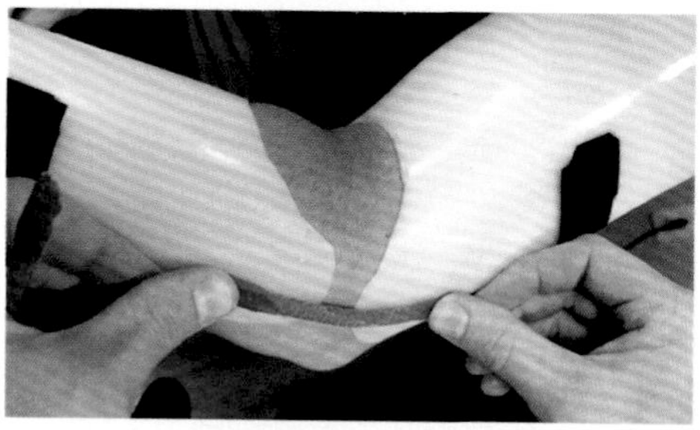

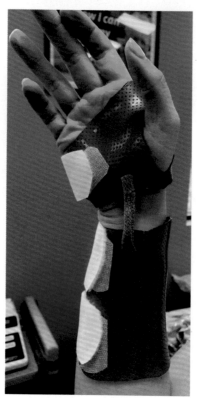

FIGURE 11–25

4. Rolled Orficast® can also be placed to block motion as in a dart thrower's motion orthosis (Fig. 11–26)

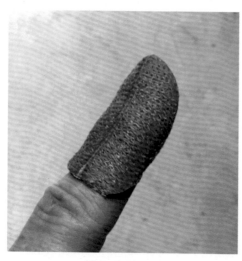

FIGURE 11–26

5. Orficast® can be made into finger caps for protection (Fig. 11–27)

FIGURE 11–27

6. Orficast® can be made into finger cuffs for mobilization orthoses (Fig. 11–28)

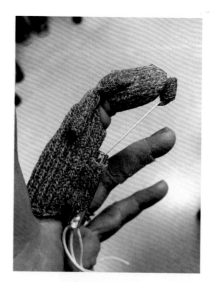

FIGURE 11–28

7. Orficast® can be used as finger separators in a resting orthosis (Fig. 11–29A,B)

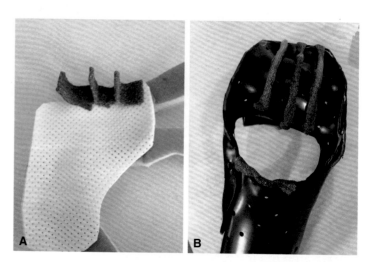

FIGURE 11–29

CHAPTER REVIEW QUESTIONS

1. What are Orficast® and Orficast® More? Are they considered casting materials or a thermoplastic material?
2. List a minimum of three creative uses for this product.
3. Name three diagnoses that could benefit from the use of this material.
4. What temperature should the water be heated to thoroughly heat up the material to make it pliable to apply to the body segment?
5. True or false?
   a. Multiple layers will add to rigidity.
   b. Multiple layers will increase airflow.
   c. Orficast® and Orficast® More are recommended for larger and more rigid orthoses.

RESOURCES

Please check out the following online resources for valuable information and multiple instructional videos:

www.orfit.com

https://www.orfit.com/physical-rehabilitation/blog/

https://www.youtube.com/results?search_query=orficast

https://www.facebook.com/groups/Orfit.splinting/?ref=bookmarks

DISTRIBUTORS

Orficast® and Orficast® More products are available from the following distributors:

Fabrication Enterprises at https://www.fab-ent.com

North Coast Medical at https://www.ncmedical.com

Performance Health at https://www.performancehealth.com

12 Delta-Cast®

Janine Thomas, OTR/L, CHT, COMT

CHAPTER OBJECTIVES

After study of this chapter, the reader should be able to:

- Understand the clinical reasoning process for selecting Delta-Cast® Conformable/Prints or Delta-Cast® Soft to fabricate an orthosis for a patient.
- Report the properties and characteristics of Delta-Cast® Conformable/Prints and Delta-Cast® Soft as it relates to safe and effective application.
- Develop the clinical reasoning skills and techniques required to reproduce the orthoses described in this chapter.
- Appreciate the unique characteristics and opportunity for creative alternatives in orthotic management.

KEY TERMS

Functional Cast Therapy (FCT)
Delta-Cast® Conformable
Delta-Cast® Orthoses

Delta-Cast® Prints
Delta-Cast® Soft
Terry-Net™ Stockinette

Terry-Net™ Adhesive Fleece Edger
Terry-Net™ Adhesive Padding
Zip Stick or cutting strip

FAQ

How do you modify a Delta-Cast® orthosis if the patient's edema decreases?

The Delta-Cast® orthosis can be modified by trimming down the edges, decreasing the circumference allowing for an improved fit with decreased edema. (Please note that a segment of fleece edger will need to be applied.) The edges can also be overlapped to accommodate for decreased edema.

Can the orthosis get wet in the shower or be used for swimming?

Yes—this material can get wet without risking changes occurring to the fit. The orthosis will need to be removed and air dried (which can take several hours) or dried with a hair dryer. Essity suggests that the orthosis may be dried in the dryer, but it has been our experience that this may affect the orthosis more negatively when it comes to sustainability since the fleece edger can be disrupted causing it to come away from cast material.

How do you clean an orthosis made from Delta-Cast® Conformable tape?

These orthoses can be hand washed in warm soapy water, rinsed, and dried as noted above. They may also be placed on the top rack of dishwasher per Essity, but note that this may also disrupt the adherence of the fleece edger.

Can an orthosis made with Delta Soft also be washed?

Delta Soft has water-resistant qualities.

Can the material be cut while it is still tacky?

No. When the material is still tacky, it is still conformable and setting. If you cut the orthosis while tacky, you may compromise the final form and fit.

Where can Delta-Cast® products be obtained?

Essity.com, Performance Health, North Coast Medical

Contact your local Essity Medical representative or customer service at 1-800-552-1157 for further information.

INTRODUCTION

The purpose of this chapter is to educate and expose the reader to Functional Cast Therapy as it relates to the use of the Delta-Cast® Conformable, Delta-Cast® Prints, and Delta-Cast® Soft products for the fabrication of custom orthoses in the realm of hand therapy. Delta-Cast® products have been used in orthopedic care for many years, and there are a variety of products; the uses and opportunities to be creative in the fabrication of custom orthoses are limitless. Delta-Cast® is supplied by Essity, formally known as BSN Medical.

Delta-Cast® Conformable, Delta-Cast® Prints, and Delta-Cast® Soft are fiberglass-free materials made from a multidirectional elasticized polyester substrate. The polyester nature of the cast tape allows for conformability and wrinkle-free application as well as a smooth finish with soft edges that improve patient compliance, comfort, and satisfaction. Variance in the three substrates will affect the rigidity and elongation of the material. Therapists should become familiar and skilled in the application of Delta-Cast® Conformable before using Delta-Cast® Prints or Delta-Cast® Soft.

Delta-Cast® Conformable, Prints, and Soft are lightweight, breathable materials offering an alternative to traditional thermoplastic orthoses for a variety of diagnoses, as well as to traditional rigid fiberglass casts for fracture management. An orthosis fabricated from Delta-Cast® Conformable, Prints, or Soft allows for early mobility and function and can reduce complications related to rigid immobilization such as muscle atrophy and joint stiffness. Orthoses will maintain their form over time and can be customized to meet the patient's specific needs (degree of rigidity) by varying the number of layers and allowing for unrestricted motion in unaffected joints. This lightweight semirigid orthosis will provide support to the injured region and allow for the ability to complete hygiene, self-care, and ROM (if appropriate) since it is removeable.

This chapter is focused on the use of Delta-Cast® Conformable and Prints. Delta-Cast® Soft is a newer product to the market and has been found useful in pediatric settings since it can be removed without scissors by peeling apart the layers if needed. Delta-Cast® Soft is also being used in applications by athletic trainers for quick provision of support or protection to an area; the fabricated device can be removed and reapplied as needed. Use in the hand therapy clinic includes serial casting, to improve compliance by supplying a nonremovable orthosis and for fractures with the addition of a rigid stay to protect a healing region. The reinforcement strips can be fabricated from Delta Conformable as described in the application process below. When using this product for serial casting, traditional cast circumferential padding can be used.

OVERVIEW OF THE PROCESS

When using Delta-Cast® products, it is helpful to be organized, having the required materials and supplies ready. The working time for applying and molding an orthosis with Delta-Cast® Conformable and Prints is approximately 3 to 5 minutes and a full 20 minutes until the product reaches maximal rigidity. Fabricating the orthosis according to the steps listed in the application process will ensure patient comfort during initial removal of formed orthosis and ultimately allow the patient to don/doff the orthosis independently.

PRECAUTIONS/CONTRAINDICATIONS

All products provided by Essity for the application of a conformable orthosis are latex free. When modifying application using non-Essity products, be sure to check for presence of latex. Keep in mind that when using Delta-Cast® to fabricate orthoses for stabilization in a circumferential manner, the patient may have difficulty donning/doffing the orthosis independently; they will likely require assistance to avoid motion of the involved region. Preplanning for optimal opening and strapping can aid in this maneuver.

BENEFITS OF FUNCTIONAL CAST THERAPY

- Improved patient compliance and comfort—able to apply soft-cushioned padding throughout design.
- Addition of personality and color to orthoses increases patient compliance.
- No pattern making or hot water required.
- Circumferential support allowing for edema management that can be progressed from the use of circumferential wrapping (using cohesive bandage or elasticized wraps) to the use of traditional hook and loop strapping. Circumferential wrapping can also be helpful with patients when wear compliance may be an issue.
- X-ray translucency allowing orthosis to remain in place during examination.
- No cast saw required—cutoff easily with standard bandage scissors.
- Wrapping technique is easy to learn, allowing the therapist plenty of time to position the patient appropriately during the setting process.
- Does not lose shape under extreme heat conditions.
- Decreased need for follow-up adjustments since straps can be tightened/loosened per patient comfort to accommodate for edema fluctuations. This is especially helpful in the acute postoperative healing phase when fluctuating edema may be present.
- Lightweight and durable.
- Minimal material waste during fabrication.
- Circumferential application with excellent conformability allows for intimate fit for patients with significant joint deformity or external fixation of fractures.
- Perforation in material allows for air exchange leading to less skin maceration and maximal comfort.

SUGGESTED POPULATIONS/DIAGNOSES

Delta-Cast® Conformable, Prints, and Soft can be used with as much versatility and creativity as thermoplastic materials. Communication with the referring physician is important if they are not familiar with this fabrication technique. These materials can be used for immobilization, restriction, and mobilization orthoses (serial static casting using Delta-Cast® Soft, and base for dynamic or static progressive orthoses).

The most common diagnoses for Delta-Cast® orthoses are humerus fractures (midshaft and distal), proximal and distal radius/ulna fractures, fourth/fifth metacarpal fractures, and diagnoses requiring immobilization of the thumb (i.e., fractures, DeQuervain, CMC arthritis/arthroplasty). With elbow orthosis, therapists are commonly intimidated to fabricate these large devices out of thermoplastic material due to the large piece of material required, challenging with patient positioning and padding commonly required in this bony region. Using this circumferential application technique is easier for both the patient and therapist in regard to positioning, and the therapist is able to prepad the region making for a very comfortable final design. Utilizing this product line when addressing fractures requiring external pins allows for orthoses that protect pin area easing patient's anxiety common with this fracture management technique. This can be much easier than fabricating a two-part orthosis out of thermoplastic material including a protective "clamshell" dorsally.

Functional Cast Therapy is a useful alternative in the following patient situations:

- Claustrophobia with inability to tolerate a nonremoveable traditional cast.
- Fear of cast saw in pediatric population.
- Athletes to return safely back to the game with a low-profile protective orthosis that is strong and washable.
- Patients who work in extreme heat environments.

INSTRUCTIONS IN APPLYING DELTA-CAST®

ZONES OF RIGIDITY

Consider the goal of your orthosis, the area of injury, and where stabilization is required prior to application. Be mindful that the benefit of Functional Cast Therapy is to provide stabilization to the injured area while allowing flexibility both proximally and distally in order to promote muscle function, blood flow, and prevent unnecessary joint stiffness (Fig. 12–1).

EXPERT PEARL 12–1

Application Tips
AMANDA HALL, PT, MPT, PCS, ATP
Washington, DC

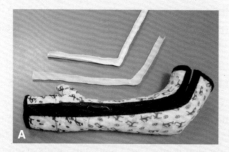

1. Thermoplastic materials can be used to make custom cutting strips for circumferential application. Heat a 1 to 2″ strip of scrap thermoplastic material into a trough shape. This allows for safe use of bandage scissors to cut through circumferentially applied Delta-Cast Conformable. **(A)**

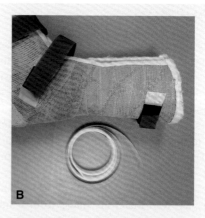

2. To prevent strap failure due to adhesive backing coming off over time, use scrap pieces of thermoplastic material to secure the edges of adhesive hook. With a heat gun, warm piece of thermoplastic material, overlapping the edge of the hook onto the orthosis. Rub it into both the hook and the porous cast material, forming a strong bond. Aquaplast Ultra Thin Edging Material (Performance Health) can also be used—shown here. **(B)**

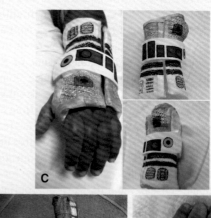

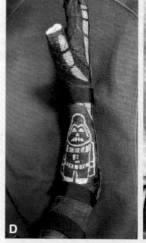
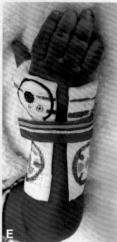

3. Compliance is improved by incorporating aesthetics into orthotic design. Use commercially available duct tapes to finish edges to add color or patterns. A rainbow of loop strapping colors are available (Performance Health). Delta-Cast Conformable can easily be personalized with permanent markers, paint pens, or acrylic paint **(C-E).**

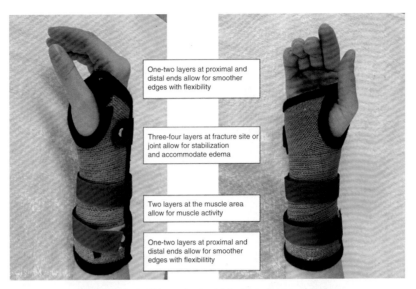

One-two layers at proximal and distal ends allow for smoother edges with flexibility

Three-four layers at fracture site or joint allow for stabilization and accommodate edema

Two layers at the muscle area allow for muscle activity

One-two layers at proximal and distal ends allow for smoother edges with flexibilitity

FIGURE 12–1 Wrist orthosis with indicated zones of rigidity.

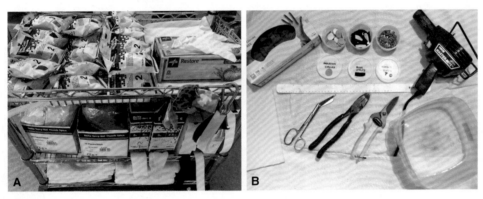

FIGURE 12–2 **A,** Metal cart on wheels housing all supplies required to fabricate using Delta-Cast products. Notice the samples of casting and strapping materials hanging from the front to aid in the process of patient color selection. **B,** Tools and accessories also needed for fabrication process.

CASTING STATION SETUP

To maximize time efficiency with application of Delta-Cast® orthosis, having an organized station is key (Fig. 12–2A,B). In clinical practice, application of these orthoses is often as a work in, and this allows for quick setup with all required items to be moved easily between hand tables. A brief history can be obtained from the patient, while the application is taking place. Prior to the step-by-step process described below, allow your patient time to pick their color or print of cast tape and loop material. Explain to your patient that it will appear that you are placing them in a cast but that you will be cutting it along the strip, removing it, and applying hook/loop straps to make it a removable orthosis. This allows for improved understanding of the application process as well as decreasing patient anxiety.

MATERIALS NEEDED

- Delta-Cast® tape 2″ and 3″
- Zip Stick (cutting strip)
- Bandage scissors
- Delta Terry-Net™ stockinette 2″ and 3″
- Delta Terry-Net™ Thumb Spica sleeves 2″ and 3″
- Terry-Net™ Adhesive Foam
- Terry-Net™ Adhesive Fleece Edger
- 1″ Adhesive hook

ADDITIONAL SUPPLIES

- Towel or gown to protect patient's clothing
- Gloves
- Water basin
- Heat gun
- Speedy rivets (medium)
- Hole punch
- Blunt nose pliers
- Wax pencil or marker

CARE OF ORTHOSIS/PATIENT INSTRUCTION

Instruct the patient in appropriate care of orthosis. A written handout should include the following information:

1. Orthosis precautions: to include any redness, swelling, or pain related to the orthosis. Patient should contact the Hand Therapy clinic immediately to schedule a return appointment to prevent further irritation.
2. Orthosis wearing schedule: Can they remove the orthosis for showers or protective skin care with hand washing in the sink?
3. Orthosis care: Orthoses fabricated from Delta-Cast® can be hand washed with soapy water. They will require several hours to dry or can be dried with a hair dryer on a cool setting.

STEP-BY-STEP APPLICATION (FIG. 12−3A−S)

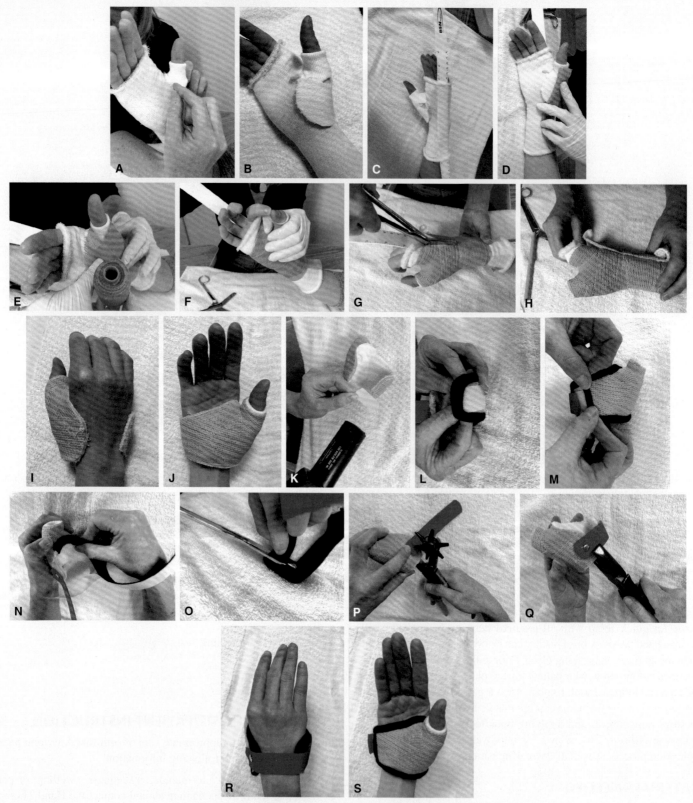

FIGURE 12−3 A-S, Fabrication process: hand-based thumb orthosis.

1. Stockinette

Cut the Delta Terry-Net™ stockinette—this is a unique polyester material that is conforming and soft providing the cushioned inside of the finished orthosis. This stockinette becomes the "liner" of the finished orthosis—the casting material should NOT come in contact with the patient's skin. Avoid any creases after application.

Clinical Pearls

- The length of the Terry-Net™ stockinette should be greater than the length of the region being covered, longer than one would think—to allow for shrinkage.
- If the patient has a fresh incision or a wound with active bleeding/drainage, use a traditional stockinette sleeve (or two to accommodate for any edema) beneath the Terry-Net™ stockinette to keep the permanent liner of the orthosis clean. Wound bandages should be applied first and then the Terry-Net™ stockinette over this to provide ample room in final device.
- Cut a small thumb hole in vertical fashion on the fold of the stockinette to prevent the hole from over stretching (Fig. 12–4). This allows for material application around the thumb preventing contact of the tape with the skin.
- A thumb spica Terry-Net™ stockinette should be used for all thumb orthoses—roll at distal thumb to create soft edge (Fig. 12–3A).
- When fabricating nonarticular orthoses such as a humeral fracture or forearm cuff, apply two layers of the Terry-Net™ stockinette to allow for overlap of the edges increasing the circumferential nature of the orthosis. The layer in contact with the skin will be removed; the second layer will become the liner of the orthosis. This extra room allows for circumferential adjustability.
- For patients with hypersensitive skin, turn the Terry-Net™ stockinette inside out to provide a smoother surface in contact with the skin.

2. Padding and Zip Stick

Apply padding to all bony prominences (olecranon, epicondyles at elbow, radial/ulnar styloid processes, dorsal metacarpophalangeal (MCP) joints, thumb CMC joint) (Fig. 12–5). Also apply padding to the first web space and any incisions (Figs. 12–3B, 12–6, and 12–7). Place the cutting strip **inside** the Terry-Net™ liner directly against the patient's skin—be sure to plan this placement carefully considering where

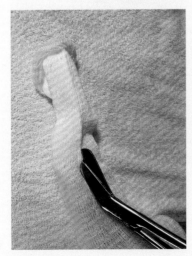

FIGURE 12–4 Make a small hole—this will stretch when applied to the patient.

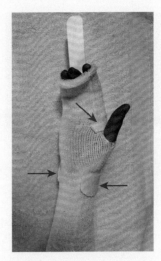

FIGURE 12–5 Prepadding bony regions can prevent irritation of this susceptible areas.

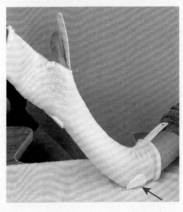

FIGURE 12–6 May use padding that comes with this system or traditional padding commonly used with thermoplastic orthoses: Terry-Net Foam liner shown here.

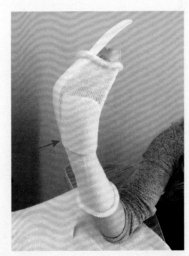

FIGURE 12–7 Padding applied over fifth metacarpal fracture incision to increase comfort in design.

stability is needed and optimal opening for easy donning and doffing (Fig. 12–3C). Remembering to utilize the Zip Stick is critical—once the cast material has been fully applied and set, it is nearly impossible to insert cutting strip at that point during the fabrication process!

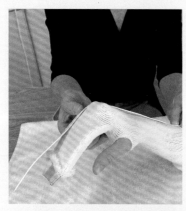

FIGURE 12-8 Zip Stick placed under stockinette directly against skin—this was bent to accommodate for metacarpophalangeal (MCP) flexed position.

Clinical Pearls

- The Zip Stick is bendable to allow for molding over flexed joints (Fig. 12-8).
- Thermoplastic "domes" can be used to mold over percutaneous pins creating a protective bubble (Figs. 12-9A and 12-10A,B).
- Thermoplastic digit extension piece can be used to ensure proximal interphalangeal (PIP)/distal interphalangeal (DIP) joint extension position during the molding process (Fig. 12-9B,C).
- With Delta-Cast® Soft, no additional padding is required due to the intimate fit of this soft material.

3. Cast Material Molding

Don gloves and open the Delta-Cast® package. Do not handle material without gloves, otherwise, the material residue will stick to your hands which is difficult to remove. Submerge the roll in room temperature water for approximately 3 seconds. There is no need to squeeze out all the extra water prior to application.

Clinical Pearls

- Cold water slows curing rate, warm water will speed it up decreasing the working time.
- Squeezing out the water after dipping speeds curing rate. Allowing it to remain wet will increase the time you have to position joints during application.
- Delta-Cast® Soft can be applied dry or wet.

Consider where rigidity is required. Reinforcement segments of cast material are applied prior to fully wrapping the extremity.

Clinical Pearls

- Wrist orthosis: Cut a piece of cast tape double length from proximal volar forearm to DPC—position it volarly (Fig. 12-11).
- Thumb orthosis: Cut a piece of cast tape double the length of rigidity region—most commonly radial aspect of thumb (Fig. 12-3D).
- Elbow orthosis: Place a doubled strip along the posterior elbow. This will allow for stability and coverage, therefore preventing the orthosis from becoming too thick on the anterior side which can make it difficult to cut off as well as for the patient to don and doff later (Fig. 12-12).

Begin circumferential application of cast tape, overlapping 50% of the previous layer. Three to four layers are needed in areas where more rigidity is required (remembering that the reinforcement strips will provide two layers) and two to three layers proximal and distal to allow for flexibility during functional muscle activity.

Clinical Pearls

- Ensure to position the beginning of the roll to allow for easy unraveling of the cast tape (Fig. 12-3E).
- Trim material to allow it to sit flush against the targeted region and prevent wrinkles—especially helpful when traversing through the first web space (Fig. 12-13A,B).

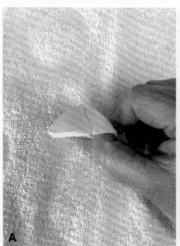
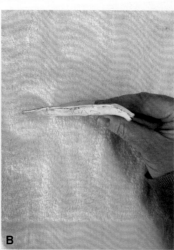
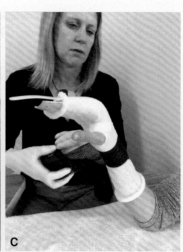

FIGURE 12-9 A, Premake multiple sizes of these protective domes to be used during the molding process. **B and C,** Notice use of thermoplastic piece UNDER the stockinette—this is removed after fabrication process and does not become a part of the final orthosis.

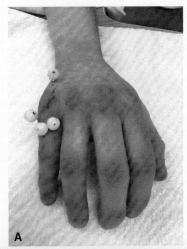

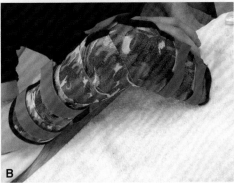

FIGURE 12-10 **A,** Pins to address fifth metacarpal fracture. **B,** Orthosis fabricated using dome to provide protective bubble over this sensitive area.

You will have approximately 2 to 3 minutes to mold the orthosis for a custom fit once the region is fully wrapped with casting material. Pay close attention to smoothing out any wrinkles. Keep your hands moving as the material sets to prevent unwanted pressure areas. Wetting your gloves prior to completion of molding will allow for improved lamination of the different layers of material and provide a smooth finish. Be careful

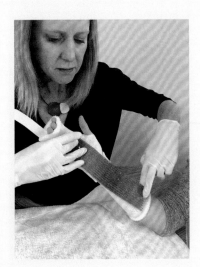

FIGURE 12-11 This doubled reinforcement strip provides required rigidity in key portion of orthosis.

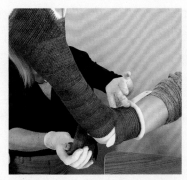

FIGURE 12-12 Minimizing bulk of cast material volarly at elbow crease will make it easier to cut off after the material has set. The more layers that are applied in this region, the harder to cut through and remove due to flexed angle.

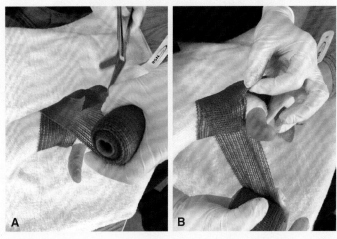

FIGURE 12-13 **A,** Trimming of material prior to pulling through first web space. **B,** Notice how therapist gently tugs material on either side of thumb to lay it flat against skin.

not to use too much water as this may increase the dampness of stockinette beneath slowing completion of orthosis and could effect adhesion of hook (Fig. 12-3F).

Explain to the patient that they will experience warmth as the material sets up and that it may feel tight which will be relieved when it is cut off and modified to a removable orthosis.

4. Cast Removal and Trimming

When the tape is no longer wet or tacky, the orthosis can be removed by carefully cutting along the Zip Stick using designated bandage scissors (Fig. 12-3G). Be mindful to follow the Zip Stick path to avoid digging edge of bandage scissors into the patient's limb.

Clinical Pearls

- Gently squeeze the orthosis together to "open up" the area above the cutting strip creating more space to ease this process of cast removal (Fig. 12-14).
- You may need to change the way you are approaching the intended opening by starting proximal versus distal or vice versa—especially when cutting and opening up at the volar elbow region.

With the orthosis back on the patient, use a marking pen or wax pencil to indicate areas to be trimmed (Fig. 12-3H). Cut along all edges marked to create desired orthosis dimensions (Fig. 12-3I,J). Most

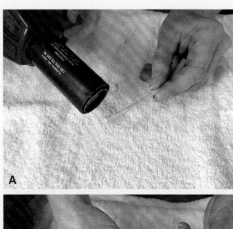

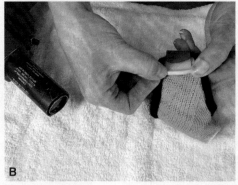

FIGURE 12-15 A, Heating of scrap strip of thermoplastic with heat gun. **B,** Application at edge of adhesive hook.

importantly, reapply to patient to ensure a good fit with full clearance for ROM of all unaffected joints. This step is critical because once the edging material is applied, adjusting any borders can be time consuming. Determine locations of adhesive hook application to obtain optimal strapping and mark with wax pencil.

5. Strapping and Edging

Remove from the patient and begin final stages of orthosis fabrication. Apply adhesive hook to designated areas first. Note that Essity offers specific Terry-Net™ adhesive hook and stretch loop—but traditional products used with thermoplastics also work well.

Clinical Pearls

- Allowing the material to be completely dried will improve adherence of adhesive hook.
- Use the heat gun to further activate adhesive on hook segments. Utilizing an extra sticky adhesive is ideal to prevent loosening during wear (Fig. 12–3K).
- Place hook close to the edge of orthosis so that the fleece edger secures it on one end—keep segments as long as possible to provide maximal adhesive coverage (Fig. 12–3L).
- Use a small piece of fleece edger on the other edge to secure to orthosis (Fig. 12–3M). A scrap piece of thermoplastic material can also be used since thermoplastics can stick to the cast material (Fig. 12–15A,B).
- For patients who are unable to tolerate the segment traversing the first web space, utilize a piece of soft loop material instead by riveting on the palmar aspect of orthosis and attaching to hook dorsally.

Apply the Delta Fleece lining to the edges of the orthosis.

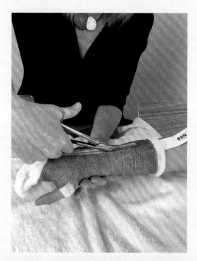

FIGURE 12-14 This tends to make patients feel less fearful during the cutting process.

Clinical Pearls

- Ideally, application of the fleece edger in one continuous piece will prevent multiple edges which can lead to these segments lifting away after continuous orthosis use (Fig. 12–3N). This can become a cosmetic issue causing patients to return for new edging. For new users of this product, it is recommended applying one length of fleece edger at a time since it can be tricky to complete in one piece. This material's adhesive is very tacky—making it challenging to cut and adhere without having it adhere to itself—this process improves with practice.
- Adhere edging to itself at borders and trim to create a smooth border (Fig. 12–16).
- Cut edges that overlap to decrease bulk and improve patient comfort (Fig. 12–3O).
- When rounding corners while edging—cut small segmental darts to allow it to sit flush—helpful when lining the thumb hole of wrist orthosis.
- As mentioned previously, be sure to overlap the edging onto the adhesive hook pieces to further secure to orthosis.

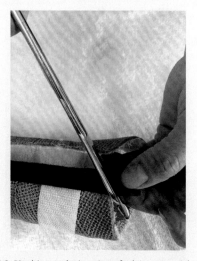

FIGURE 12-16 Pinching and trimming of edging material at the end of orthosis.

Apply loop strapping—traditional or elastic-based such as neoprene or elastic loop (Fig. 12–3P). Choice of application will be determined by the function of the orthosis and the patient's ability to don/doff. If requiring an adjustable circumferential application, strapping can be applied in opposing directions (Fig. 12–17A,B).

6. Final Fitting

Reapply to the patient to ensure comfort and appropriate fit (Fig. 12–3Q,R). Have the patient and/or family member don and doff the orthosis while they are in the clinic so that you can ensure ease of performance as well as appropriate fit. Be sure to give a written handout regarding orthosis care and wearing schedule. Another helpful tip is to have them take a photo of orthosis in place to ensure appropriate application at home.

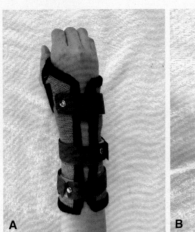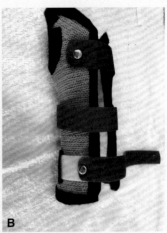

FIGURE 12–17 A, Alternating riveted straps to provide ability to modify circumferential pressure. **B,** Notice application of rivet over the adhesive hook further secure hook onto cast material. Rivets also add the bonus of minimizing strap loss!

EXPERT PEARL 12–2

Application Tips
MICHELLE COIL, MOT, OTR, CHT, PYT, CEAS
Texas

1. For the novice fabricator, practice wrapping techniques using an ace wrap. This is a great way to get familiar with unrolling the tape on an extremity without using cast tape.

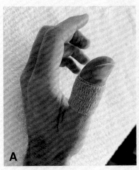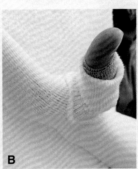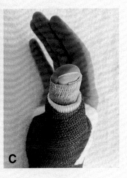

2. Use Coban around the thumb IP joint before fabricating a thumb functional cast. Then remove after fabrication to help accommodate a larger thumb IP joint and prevent the cast from "getting stuck" on the patient making don/doffing easier. This will also accommodate for any swelling that may occur. **(A-C)**
3. When making a thumb orthosis, fold the stockinette over the reinforcement piece before cast tape application. This will ensure you will clear the thumb IP, and it prevents you from having to use liner around the thumb IP opening which will make it narrower.
4. Strapping

- Heat backing of adhesive hook before applying to cast. This will activate the glue to help adhere.
- Use a long piece of loop strapping and have the patient remove the strap in the center of the hook to avoid pulling up on the ends.
- Use the edges of the fleece liner to help smaller pieces of hook adhere to the cast.
- Place hook on the cast while still damp to allow the glue to activate while the cast is curing. Only perform this technique if you know exactly where the hook/loop is going prior to cutting the cast off.

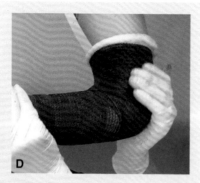

5. Molding

- Do not squeeze all the excess water out of the material after dunking—the extra water gives a little more working time!
- Keep a water bottle nearby to spritz the cast material to slow curing time and to help get wrinkles out.
- If you can see the white stockinette after material application through the perforations, that means the cast is too thin ("white is not right") **(D)**.

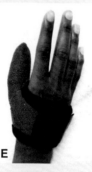

6. Do not be afraid to cut the reinforcement piece to accommodate smaller digits like this hand-based thumb cast. The hand surgeon ordered a hand-based thumb tip protector—covering the distal phalanx so the patient could get back to playing on the football field. **(E)**

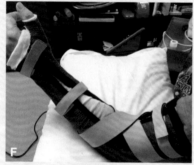

7. Criss-cross strapping at the elbow crease for a long arm. Use one long loop strap, apply the center of the strap over the posterior upper arm, criss-cross at the elbow crease, then attach the two end pieces just distal to the olecranon **(F)**.

CREATIVE USES OF DELTA-CAST® CONFORMABLE IN HAND THERAPY

This patient underwent a flexor tendon repair. A Delta-Cast® Print material was used for her dorsal block orthosis at 5 days postop. Due to poor compliance with her home exercise program (HEP), she developed stiffness in all digits. Her dorsal blocking splint (DBS) was later modified to provide static progressive flexion mobilization of her digits. The padded nature of the orthosis allowed for comfort of the MCP joints while promoting composite digit flexion to the DPC (Fig. 12–18A,B).

Delta-Cast® Prints/Conformable is an excellent material for elbow orthoses. This patient required a static progressive elbow flexion orthosis. The circumferential nature of the proximal and distal cuffs decreased pressure areas by maximizing pressure distribution, improving comfort and compliance. The use of the Phoenix elbow hinge prevented migration of the cuffs. The patient was also able to lock into maximum extension at night. The fleece edger was used to secure the D-ring and fed through a slit in the Delta-Cast® which provided excellent fixation (Fig. 12–19A,B).

This patient sustained a fourth and fifth proximal phalanx fracture. With postoperative stiffness, she required a mobilization

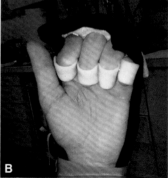
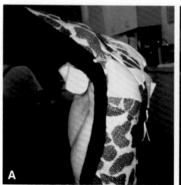

FIGURE 12–18 A and B, Combined PIP/DIP static progressive flexion orthosis. Delta-Cast prints pattern in Camo shown here.

TABLE 12–1 Common Delta-Cast Orthoses

Orthosis Design	Common Indications	Clinical Pearls
Hand-based thumb orthosis **HFO: L3913** 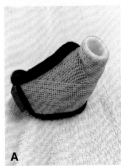 A B	• Thumb Fx • Thumb dislocation • Capsule/ligament injuries (UCL or RCL) • Soft-tissue injuries • Tendon injury/repair • CMC OA or s/p arthroplasty • Positioning orthosis	• Option to easily include IP joint if desired by starting wrap at tip—this can be modified later in healing if desired to free IP joint for motion. • Fold over stockinette at distal edge of thumb to create soft border (Fig. 12–3A). • When applying tape through first web space, cut vertically into tape to allow for decreased bulk and to avoid creases (Fig. 12–13A,B). • Padding in first web space and over CMC joint will improve comfort (Fig. 12–3B).
Forearm-based thumb orthosis **WHFO: L3808** 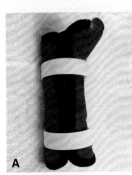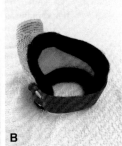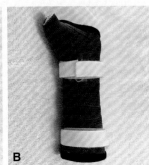 A B	• Thumb Fx (scaphoid, Bennett) • Capsule/ligament injuries • Soft-tissue injuries • Tendon injury/repair • CMC OA or s/p arthroplasty • Positioning orthosis	• Option to easily include IP joint if desired by starting wrap at tip—this can be modified later in healing if desired to free IP joint for motion. • When applying tape through first web space, cut vertically into tape to allow for decreased bulk and to avoid creases. • Pad radial/ulnar styloids, first web space, and over the CMC joint to improve comfort (Fig. 12–5).
Wrist orthosis **WHO: L3906** 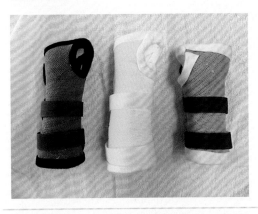	• Fractures of distal radius and/or ulna • Wrist ligament injury/sprain	• Padding in first web space will improve comfort. • If patient is unable to tolerate the segment through web space, replace with soft loop strap. • Pad radial/ulnar styloids, first web space, and over the CMC joint to improve comfort (Fig. 12–5).

Forearm-based wrist/digit (radial gutter) orthosis
WHFO: L3808
Hand-based digit (radial gutter) orthosis
HFO: L3913 (Not shown)
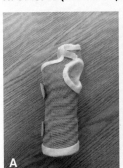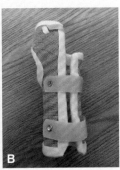
A   B
	• Forearm-based:
	  • Second and third metacarpal fractures
	  • Flexor and extensor tendon repairs
	  • Lacerations/soft-tissue injuries
	• Hand-based:
	  • Second and third MC shaft/neck fractures
	  • Proximal and middle phalanx fractures
		• Padding over fracture site may improve comfort (Fig. 12–7).
		• Thermoplastic digit extension piece will aid in positioning MCPs in flexion and maintain PIP/DIP extension during fabrication process (Fig. 12–9B,C).
		• Use thermoplastic domes to mold over pin sites (Figs. 12–9A and 12–10A,B).
		• Padding between digits can improve comfort and decrease likelihood of skin maceration.

(Continued)

TABLE 12–1 Common Delta-Cast Orthoses (Continued)

Orthosis Design	Common Indications	Clinical Pearls

Forearm-based wrist/digit (ulnar gutter) orthosis
WHFO: L3808
Hand-based digit (ulnar gutter) orthosis
HFO: L3913 (Not shown)
 	
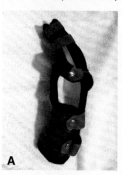 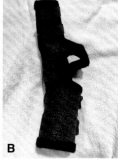
A B
	• Forearm-based:
	  • Fourth and fifth metacarpal fractures
	  • Flexor and extensor tendon repairs
	  • Soft-tissue injuries
	• Hand-based:
	  • Fourth and fifth MC shaft/neck fractures, proximal and middle phalanx
	  • Proximal and middle phalanx fractures
		• Padding over fracture site may improve comfort (Fig. 12–7).
		• Thermoplastic digit extension piece will aid in positioning MCPs in flexion and maintain PIP/DIP extension during fabrication process (Fig. 12–7B,C).
		• Use thermoplastic domes to mold over pin sites (Figs. 12–7A and 12–10A,B).
		• Padding between digits can improve comfort and decrease likelihood of skin maceration.

Elbow orthosis **EO: L3702** 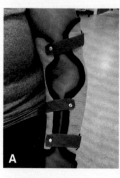 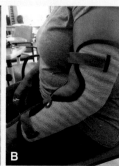 A B	• Distal humerus fracture (epicondyles, capitulum) • Olecranon fracture • Radial head fracture • Elbow dislocation • Cubital tunnel syndrome • Elbow ligament injuries	• One-two layers of padding over epicondyles and olecranon (Fig. 12–6). • Figure-8 wrapping proximal and distal to elbow crease will allow for coverage and decrease bulk at anterior elbow easing removal from patient (Fig. 12–12).
Elbow/forearm restriction orthosis (Muenster/Sugar Tong) **EWHFO: L3763** 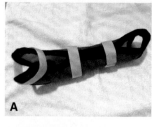 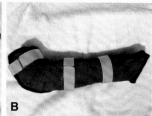 A B	• Midshaft radius/ulna fractures • Elbow dislocations • Elbow ligament injuries • TFCC injury	• One-two layers of padding over epicondyles and olecranon (Fig. 12–6). • Figure-8 wrapping proximal and distal to elbow crease will allow for coverage and decrease bulk at anterior elbow easing removal from patient (Fig. 12–12).
Humeral orthosis **SO: L3671** 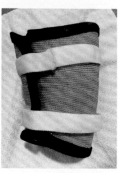	• Humerus shaft fractures	• Double layer of Terry-Net™ stockinette to allow for circumferential adjustability.

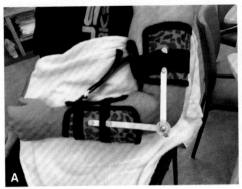
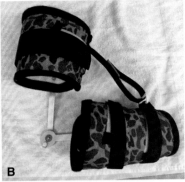

FIGURE 12–19 **A and B,** Due to material flexibility, patient was able to don/doff independently.

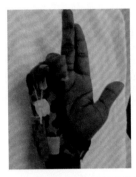

FIGURE 12–20 Pulley in palm adhered to cast material using scrap piece of thermoplastic that was dry heated via a heat gun to maximize adherence.

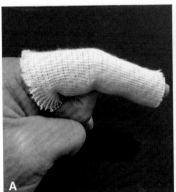
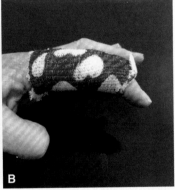

FIGURE 12–21 **A and B,** DIP allowed to move in this PIP cast fabricated from Delta-Cast Soft.

orthosis to improve small-finger MCP joint flexion and ring-finger PIP/DIP joint flexion. Her initial immobilization orthosis was modified to a static progressive mobilization orthosis. Thermoplastic adheres well to the Delta-Cast® material when heated with a heat gun allowing for creative applications for static progressive mobilization (Fig. 12–20).

Delta-Cast® Soft can be used for serial casting of a digit. Application of stockinette beneath the Delta-Cast® Soft will protect the skin. Delta-Cast® Soft can be easily removed by peeling decreasing time in the clinic for changes as no soaking is required. Delta-Cast® Soft has water-resistant qualities and can get wet when bathing. It will need to be dried with a hair dryer following bathing to protect skin integrity (Fig. 12–21A,B).

CONCLUSION

Delta-Cast® materials provide unique and patient-friendly options for custom orthoses based on the characteristics described in this chapter. Delta-Cast® Conformable, Prints, and Soft can be used in the conservative management of arthritis, in orthopedic care, both conservative and postoperative management, and additionally for the management of neurological conditions and in the pediatric population.

Take the information and clinical pearls provided and be creative, experiment, and explore the possibilities of this versatile material providing your patients with another option in the realm of orthotic intervention.

CHAPTER REVIEW QUESTIONS

1. Explain the benefits of using Delta-Cast® products for fabrication of a custom orthosis versus traditional thermoplastic material.
2. Give two examples of modifications to a Delta-Cast® Conformable orthosis that can be made to accommodate for decreased edema.
3. What can you do to increase the rigidity of segments of the orthosis?
4. Which Delta-Cast® product is recommended for serial casting?

13 Taping Techniques[a]

Kimberly Gross, MEd, OTR/L, CHT, CKTP, CDTI

CHAPTER OBJECTIVES

After study of this chapter, the reader will be able to:
- Distinguish characteristics of tapes commonly used for therapeutic intervention.
- Appreciate popular taping methods: athletic taping, McConnell taping, elastic therapeutic taping (previously known as Kinesio taping method), and Dynamic taping.
- List the commonly encountered injuries for each taping application.
- Describe the similarities and differences between each taping application and the specific goals for each type of tape.
- Understand the precautions and contraindications for each taping technique.

KEY TERMS

Anchor	Elastic therapeutic taping	Spray adherent
Athletic taping	Dynamic taping	Recoil
Correction technique	Figure-8 or locking strip	Paper-off
Kinesiology taping	"I," "Y," "X," FAN, and buttonhole cuts	Prewraps
	McConnell taping	Undertapes

INTRODUCTION

Therapeutic taping has become an excellent option after the acute phase of injury to provide support for healing tissue while allowing safe range of motion (ROM) which increases compliance, function, quality of tissue repair, and improved healing time (Cyr & Ross, 1998). From sports medicine and athletic training to professional athletes and the Olympic arena, strapping and/or taping techniques have been successfully used for pain reduction associated with edema, early protected return to activity (Ewalt, 2010; Hilfrank, 1991; Ozer, Senbursa, Baltaci, & Hayran, 2009), and scar modification (Atkinson, McKenna, Barnett, McGrath, & Rudd, 2005; Niessen, Spauwen, Robinson, Fidler, & Kon, 1998; Reiffel, 1995). Taping is not applicable for conditions requiring the protection of rigid devices, but it may be incorporated along the recovery continuum to allow for protected mobilization or to assist in neuromuscular retraining (Bennell, Duncan, & Cowan, 2006; Hsu, Chen, Lin, Wang, & Shih, 2009; Jaraczewska & Long, 2006; McConnell, Donnelly, Hamner, Dunne, & Besier, 2011; McConnell & McIntosh, 2009; Ozer et al., 2009; Salsich, Brechter, Farwell, & Powers, 2002; Yasukawa, Patel, & Sisung, 2006). Therapeutic taping should be used as a complement to a comprehensive rehabilitation program. Taping is a cost-effective treatment that can be taught to clients or family members to carry over the effects of treatment at home. Formal training is recommended to ensure proper use of the techniques described in this chapter.

TAPING MATERIALS

There are many types of nonelastic (rigid) and **elastic therapeutic tapes** (tapes with elastic properties, adhesive properties, and recoil ability) available on the market, each with their own indications, characteristics, and functional applications (Table 13–1). This chapter provides a brief overview of taping methods and application techniques for nonelastic tapes, including **athletic taping** and **McConnell taping**, and elastic tapes, including **Kinesiology taping** (originally known as the Kinesio taping method) and **Dynamic taping** (Fig. 13–1). With the rapid expansion of elastic therapeutic tapes, the reader is encouraged to stay abreast of new products. Table 13–2 compares these distinctly different taping methods and provides a summary of their features. It is important to learn the similarities and differences of the tapes to make the most appropriate therapeutic choice for the client. These tapes should not be confused with bandages or cohesive circumferential wraps that do not adhere directly to the skin such as Coban™, **prewrap**, or **undertape**.

TAPING PRECAUTIONS

All adhesives pose a risk. Although these risks are small, there are some general precautions to be aware of to reduce the risk of injury:

- Avoid taping a client with thin, frail skin.
- Clients with vascular compromise should not be taped circumferentially.

---

[a]This chapter is based on the 1st edition and 2nd edition chapters written by Ruth Coopee OTR/L, CHT, CLT, LMT.

TABLE 13–1	Commonly Used Materials and Functions
Skin tougheners Adhesive sprays	These are applied to the skin in either a pad or spray method before taping to improve adhesion of tape to the skin and decrease chemical tape irritations. Tougheners have an additional astringent to prepare the skin. Note that these products can also cause irritation if used for prolonged periods.
Undertapes	An adhesive backed, nonelastic material used as a base to which a sports tape is applied. It also serves as a light padding to protect skin or bony areas and prevent skin blisters and cuts.
Prewraps	Similar to undertape, except that it does not have an adhesive backing; it is composed of a fine, porous polyester foam material that has a slight stretch to help conform to contours. It provides increased padding to skin and bony areas but requires a spray adherent to increase skin contact.
Adhesive tapes	Rated by the number of vertical fibers per inch, this relates to tensile strength and weight; available in 1/2″, 10″, 1 1/2″, and 2″ widths; often referred to as "white tape," zinc oxide, or linen tape. They are not elastic and provide a high degree of joint support and immobilization.
Kinesiology tape	Dependent on the percentage of elastic stretch to allow for controlled movement in a joint and functional muscle support; rated by percentage of elastic stretch or recoil. Increasing popularity of this method with athletes has led to development of a larger choice of products, some with higher elastic recoil. Caution should be exercised with these products because they are intended for the young healthy athlete. Higher recoil will increase shearing forces on the skin and may lead to blister formation or tissue injury.
Dynamic tape	A high recoil elastic tape that aims to modify movement patterns, modify tissue load, decrease pain, and increase function by improving biomechanics.

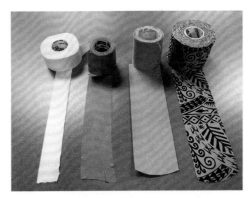

FIGURE 13–1 **Tape comparison.** Athletic tape, McConnell tape, Elastic therapeutic tape, and Dynamic tape.

This is beneficial to provide support for injuries and restrict forces that would apply stress to injured tissue. Athletic tape can also support and protect a weakened muscle by limiting tendon excursion and allowing tissues to rest. Depending on the technique of application, athletic taping can provide minimal-to-moderate constraint of healing tissues while allowing joint motion for controlled, protected healing. Encapsulating acutely injured joint structures assists in edema control via compression and active muscle pumping. Athletic tapes should be considered for use during the continuum of care for its rigid and supportive properties (Arnheim & Prentice, 2000).

GOALS OF ATHLETIC TAPING

- Support and protect weakened joint structures.
- Limit harmful movement and assist in planes of movement.
- Provide a progressive method to achieve pain-free functional movement.
- Allow for movement of an injured part to improve circulation and healing.
- Assist in controlling edema.
- Prevent worsening of injury and muscle atrophy.
- Improve kinesthetic awareness in an acutely injured joint.
- Allow early return to function.

INDICATIONS FOR USE

Athletic taping is cost effective and most often used in the treatment of sprains, strains, subluxations, and dislocations with ligament tears or ruptures resulting in unidirectional or multidirectional instability (Ewalt, 2010; Kaneko & Takasaki, 1996; Ozer et al., 2009). When a thorough medical evaluation determines it appropriate and if applied properly, taping creates a rigid support and provides for maximal soft tissue control. This technique is particularly effective in the conservative management of subacute injuries.

TECHNIQUE

The manner in which the tape is applied determines the degree of mobility that will be allowed across a joint. Table 13–3 lists common techniques and methods used in athletic taping (Arnheim & Prentice, 2000; Austin et al., 1994). The skin should be cleansed of all oils, perspiration, hair, and old adhesive. A **spray adherent** or skin toughener can be used to create a microscopic layer to protect the skin from tape irritants and increase the adhesive quality of the tape. Prewrap is applied to the skin to prevent skin breakdown from the highly adhesive athletic tape (Fig. 13–3). The prewrap is porous and has a soft light foam texture. It eliminates or minimizes the need to shave hair prior to taping. Prewrap (i.e., M-Wrap by

- Avoid taping over cuts or open wounds.
- Avoid areas with sunburn or other skin conditions that would cause pain with removal.
- Children and clients with cognition deficits should be evaluated for comprehension of the tape use and care.
- Special consideration should be given to a client with insensate skin or diabetic neuropathy.

ATHLETIC TAPING

GENERAL PRINCIPLES

The field of athletic training started in 1888 shortly followed by the invention of **Athletic tape** in 1893 by Dr. Virgil Gibney. He coined the term "Gibney Basketweave Technique" (Fig. 13–2) which is the athletic tape application using a crossed pattern when taping across joints (Wilkerson, 2002). The main function of athletic taping is to restrict or immobilize specific joint structures while allowing for some degree of active movement (Arnheim & Prentice, 2000; Austin, Gwynn-Brett, & Marshall, 1994). Multiple layers of nonelastic adhesive tape are applied across a joint to provide rigid stability.

TABLE 13–2	**Comparison Chart**			
Method	**Athletic**	**McConnell**	**Kinesiology**	**Dynamic**
Materials	Adhesive spray Prewrap (i.e., M-Wrap by Mueller) Padding adhesive tape	Undertape (i.e., Cover-Roll') Brown adhesive tape (i.e., Leukotape')	(Many brands) Kinesio' Tex tape Balance Tex tape KT tape PerformTex tape Rock tape	Dynamic tape Adhesive spray
Evaluation	Muscle Joint Soft tissue	Analysis of structural alignment and dysfunctional biomechanics	Analysis of muscle, soft tissue, and fascial dysfunction and its relationship to pathology	Analysis of muscle, soft tissue, strength of muscle contraction, nerve function, joint biomechanics
Indications	Joint injury Ligament injuries grades 1–3 Muscle injury Rigid yet flexible protection	Postural reeducation Muscle retraining Joint alignment	Scar and soft tissue modification Relieves myofascial pain Edema reduction Muscle support and reeducation Joint support (correction) Postural reeducation Increase circulation	Joint alignment Force contribution to assist weak muscles Modify movement patterns Absorb muscle load Reduce pain
Technique/ methodology	Provides a progressive amount of support and immobilization to healing tissues and prevents reinjury while allowing continued participation in activity	Passively repositions soft tissue and "holds" bony structures into proper alignment to retrain and restore normal static and dynamic functional biomechanics	An elastic tape used to facilitate the neurosensory and physiologic mechanisms of skin and muscle, affecting soft tissue, fascia, and muscle tension while modifying functional biomechanics and reducing pain	Biomechanically manages tissue load by using a high recoil material to manage load, assist or resist motion, and improve joint positioning. Neurophysiological effects of relieving pain.
Advantages	Maximum support to healing structures	Provides support to very weak structures and allows full range of motion	Gentle approach to treatment of myofascial pain and soft tissue injuries allows full range of motion	Provides external load management for optimal muscle and tissue function
Disadvantages	Tape trauma and irritation Needs to be replaced and checked often for maximum support Patient false dependency	Tape trauma and irritation Pulling of the tape may be "pain" restrictive in exercise Not appropriate for grade 3 injuries	Complexity Tape allergy Not appropriate for injuries requiring rigid immobilization	Complexity Tape allergy Can cause mechanical irritation with improper taping application Not appropriate for frail skin

Mueller, Prairie du Sac, WI) can also be applied to protect bony prominences, soft skin creases, or superficial nerves and arteries. Tape anchors are applied proximal and distal to the joint being taped as shown in Figure 13–4A.

The joint is placed in a well-supported and unstressed position. Depending on the degree of injury, the target joint is taped in either an anatomical neutral position or placed in a slack position to restrict movement stress on healing structures. The amount of support and joint restriction is dictated by the degree of injury and is achieved by the technique and tension applied during taping (Fig. 13–4B). The joint should be evaluated on completion to determine if there is adequate restriction of motion. There should be no pain. Inspection must include evaluation for distal patency and assessment of surrounding tissue to ensure there is no occlusion or impairment of circulatory or lymphatic function (Fig. 13–4C). Taping may be used for a particular event or may stay in place for up to 5 days. The taping becomes progressively looser with activity and should be evaluated regularly so the joint does not become vulnerable.

If possible, teach the patient how to apply the tape. The tape may also be used only for specific events and need to be taped frequently. Athletic tape and prewrap are inexpensive and available commercially in pharmacies or online (Fig. 13–3). The patient instructions should include directions for periodic evaluations to ensure proper support and appropriate timing for replacement. The patient

should remove the tape immediately if there is an increase in pain or adverse vascular signs. Athletic taping can achieve immobilization, support and/or restriction through the quality of the material, the specific technique used, the tension applied by the tape, and the number of layers used to restrict movement. Keeping this in mind will assist in customization for individual needs and diagnosis.

Tape removal should always be performed carefully so as not to damage or accidently tear the skin. Blunt-ended bandage scissors are used on the opposite side of the injury to tunnel under the tape and slowly ease the tape off of the skin. Slowly cut and gently peel the tape away by pressing down on the exposed skin while drawing the tape parallel to the surface of the skin following the hair growth. Do not pull up on the tape because this may tear the skin and cause subcutaneous hemorrhaging. Close inspection and evaluation of the skin is imperative for preventing breakdown from adhesives, chronic shearing forces, or tape irritation.

PRECAUTIONS

- Examination of circulation and tape performance should be completed after application and throughout the day.
- Inspection of the skin between tapings is necessary to check for possible skin breakdown in the form of maceration, blister formation, or rash; taping should be suspended or discontinued if these signs are noticed.

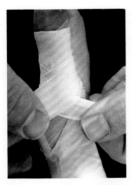

FIGURE 13-2 Gibney Basketweave design with athletic tape.

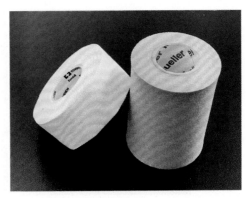

FIGURE 13-3 Prewrap and athletic tape.

- Do not tape over abrasions, blisters, lacerations, or cuts.
- Decreased sensibility from a disease process, ice application or edema may mask tissue response and alter sensation of pain during taping, resulting in injury.
- Do not use ice or heat prior to taping, particularly in the subacute phase. Reduction in interstitial tissue volume from the ice application may create a progressive tightening of the taping as the tissue warms up. Conversely, tissue volumes may decrease after heat application, resulting in reduction of support.
- Improper application can aggravate an existing injury or create a new one.

HELPFUL HINTS

- Place joint in position to be stabilized or protected.
- Overlap at least half the width of the underlying tape strip to prevent separation.
- Avoid using a continuous roll. Apply only one turn around a joint then tear. Continuous wrapping increases tension and becomes constrictive.
- Smooth and mold each strip as it is laid on the skin, allowing it to flow around the natural contours of body. This is more difficult with heavier, stiffer tapes.
- Maximum control is achieved by (1) the amount of tension applied to the tape (if elasticized tape) and (2) the position the joint is in if using a traditional nonelasticized tape.
- Do not tape immediately after application of heat or cold; wait until the tissue returns to normal temperature.

TABLE 13–3	**Techniques and Methods Used in Athletic Taping**
Anchor	Circumferential pieces of tape placed proximal and distal to the injury form a base to attach tape strip ends; may use elastic tape if room for muscle expansion is needed.
Stirrup	A U-shaped loop of nonelastic tape used to create lateral stability (ankle or carpometacarpal [CMC] joint).
Vertical strips	Tension is applied as the tape is attached moving from the distal to the proximal anchor. Increased stability of the affected joint is achieved through joint compression and fascial restriction.
"Butterfly" or check reins	Multiple strips of tape are applied at angles to each other with the apex at the joint to limit movement in unidirectional or multidirectional planes (X or star). A variation of this technique to inhibit abduction in the fingers is applied with anchors to adjacent digits. The tape between the anchors is twisted onto itself to create a "rein"-limiting movement.
Locks	A smooth roll application with increased tension at key points of support and reinforce joint stability yet allow protected functional movement (Figure-8 with cross-point at the support point).
Figure-8 or locking strip	Used to complete a taping, covers open areas, and tape strip ends while adding stability.
Closing up (in) Cover-up	Strips of tape are applied to cover all open areas and finish taping job. This increases durability and provides consistent coverage to prevent blisters and constriction with focal edema.
Strip method	One strip of tape is laid down in a specific direction with highly controlled tension from one anchor to the other.
Smooth roll method	Refers to the use of one single continuous uninterrupted piece of tape; it may begin and end at the same anchor as with joint locks.

> **CLINICAL PEARL 13–1**
>
> ## Use of Prewrap During Fabrication
>
> Prewrap can be used during orthosis fabrication to protect frail skin, hypersensitive skin, or to hold padding in place. Thermoplastic material that has a coating will not stick to prewrap. This is a great option for padding bony prominences during fabrication to create a bump out of the material.

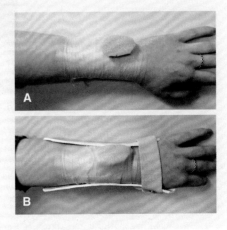

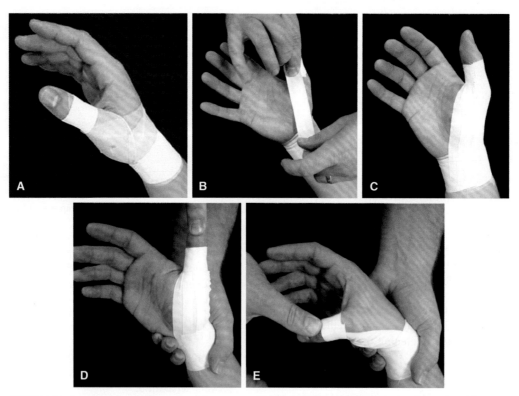

FIGURE 13–4 Athletic taping for a thumb hyperextension injury. A, Apply prewrap and anchor strips with special attention to form a secure anchor but avoiding compression of vascular and nerve tissue. **B,** Position and maintain the MP joint in desired degree of MP flexion and begin to apply multiple strips of tape volarly from the proximal anchor to the distal anchor per photo. **C,** Add anchor strips to proximal and distal borders. **D,** Check for restriction of extension. **E,** Notice unrestricted MP flexion in final taping.

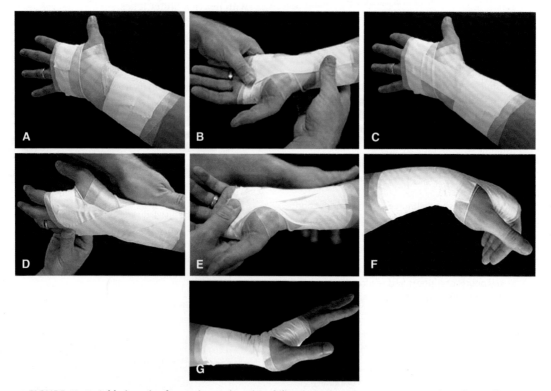

FIGURE 13–5 Athletic taping for a wrist sprain or instability. A, Apply undertape or prewrap circumferentially to protect the forearm; place white tape anchors around the proximal forearm and at the metacarpals. The skin may be further protected with an adhesive spray or prep pad. **B and C,** Place the wrist in neutral position (unless otherwise indicated) and apply a strip of white tape, with tension, from the distal anchor to the proximal anchor both dorsal and volar. To provide more support or restriction to extension, another strip may be placed, overlapping and parallel to the longitudinal piece along the ulnar aspect. **D,** Apply 2 strips, with tension, from the distal anchor (dorsal and volar), forming an X to support the radial aspect of the wrist. **E,** Repeat this process on volar and ulnar aspects of the wrist. Note the positions of the X supports. (Additional X supports may be added to further limit motion, if necessary.) Complete the taping by applying a top anchor strip to secure the distal ends. Close in the forearm by applying overlapping circumferential strips, moving distal to proximal. **F and G,** Final taping with restriction in flexion and extension noted.

CLINICAL EXAMPLES OF ATHLETIC TAPING

Thumb MP Joint Hyperextension Injury

Athletic taping can be used for thumb volar plate sprain or hyperextension injury (Fig. 13–4A–E) to prevent hyperextension at the metacarpophalengeal (MP) joint while still allowing the MP joint to flex. After taping, check for appropriate restriction of thumb MP extension with unrestricted flexion (Fig. 13–4D). For both the volar plate and ligaments surrounding the thumb MP, consideration should be given to avoid undue stress to injured structures during this taping procedure. Instruct the patient in self-evaluation of the taping with attention to vascular changes distally to the anchor. The patient should replace the tape if gapping, loosening, or vascular changes is noted. The patient should remove the tape immediately with pain, numbness, or vascular changes. The tape should be replaced in 2 to 3 days depending on the activity level of the patient. When placing the strips, be sure to overlap tape strips to prevent gapping.

Wrist Sprain and Instability

The materials required for wrist stability taping are 1 1/2″ to 2″ wide white adhesive or linen tape and prewrap (Fig. 13–5A–G). If additional support is needed, a dorsal X taping may be used before closing in. After taping, check for appropriate application and motion restriction. Apply additional tape as necessary to provide maximum protection to the structures that require more stability. Tape strips are placed on tension to provide support but should not be so constrictive as to impinge on the skin or vascular structures. A backup orthosis may be necessary to protect the wrist between tapings or as needed.

MCCONNELL TAPING

GENERAL PRINCIPLES

This taping method developed in 1984 by Jenny McConnell, an Australian physical therapist, was initially used for the conservative management of patellofemoral pain (Bennell et al., 2006; Derasari, Brindle, Alter, & Sheehan, 2010; Pfeiffer et al., 2004; Salsich et al., 2002; Tremain, 1996). Later, she successfully expanded her philosophy and treatment techniques to include the spine and upper extremity (McConnell et al., 2011; McConnell & McIntosh, 2009). The McConnell technique involves an extensive muscle evaluation, analysis of individual biomechanics, and posture. Treatment of structural misalignment in conjunction with poor movement patterns is addressed through a comprehensive rehabilitation program. The rigid tape serves to assist in the physical reeducation of the body. McConnell taping is applied *not* to restrict normal movement but *to* facilitate proper joint alignment, muscular function, and biomechanics.

GOALS OF MCCONNELL TAPING

- Position a joint into more appropriate alignment.
- Increase stability of a joint (ligament support).
- Correct articular orientation by inhibiting short, tight muscles.
- Facilitate firing capacity of weak, lengthened, or overstretched muscles.
- Enhance muscle retraining by balancing tissue length/tension relationship.
- Assist in both static and dynamic neuromuscular reeducation.

INDICATIONS FOR USE

McConnell taping is used to directly control fascia and establish proper structural alignment for improved muscular recruitment and neuromuscular retraining. Proper analysis of the underlying pathology is essential to maximize the effectiveness of this method, which focuses on reestablishing a proper length/tension relationship and motor control. The following issues respond well to McConnell taping: subluxation, unidirectional or multidirectional instability, impingement, postinjury or postoperative retraining, overuse, and poor alignment (Bennell et al., 2006; Derasari et al., 2010; McConnell et al., 2011; McConnell & McIntosh, 2009; Pfeiffer et al., 2004; Salsich et al., 2002; Tremain, 1996).

TECHNIQUE

A thorough evaluation is completed to determine the pathologic mechanisms involved and how best to correct them. Specific taping materials are used in this technique owing to their tensile strength and durability. First, a white adhesive undertape (such as Cover-Roll®) is applied to the skin without tension (Fig. 13–6A). This provides a protective bed for application of a heavyweight working brown adhesive tape (which is sold

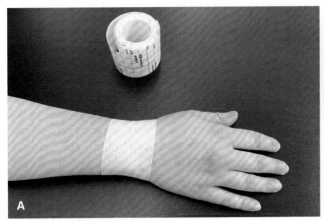
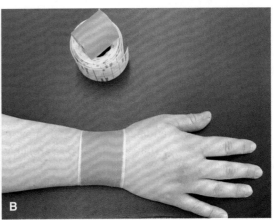

FIGURE 13–6 **Undertape. A,** Undertape is applied prior to applying McConnell tape. **B,** McConnell taping with undertape to protect the skin from the strong adhesive of the McConnell tape.

by many different names and brands such as Leukotape® (Fig. 13–6B). The undertape is extremely important because it protects the skin from shearing forces and the strong holding adhesive of the McConnell tape.

Taping with a vertical strip pattern gains control of muscle tissue and fascia. If applied correctly, there should be an immediate reduction in pain and no restriction of normal movement. Taping should be completed before exercise to allow proper pain-free exercise performance. The tape uses the surrounding fascia to hold the joint in a corrected, tension-free position. To treat shortened tissues or inhibit overactive muscles, the goal is to create a multidirectional stretching force to the muscle belly or shortened tissue. The working tape is applied with tension, perpendicular to the alignment of muscle fibers, and with downward force to create a lateral stretch while providing a compressive stretch to the muscle and fascia. To treat lengthened or weak muscles, the tape is used to draw the fascia or muscle proximally to passively shorten the fibers. This provides support through somatosensory feedback and prevents overstretch. To ensure proper joint and bone alignment during application of McConnell tape, the desired position is maintained manually by the nontaping hand or an assistant. The tape will then maintain the body in the proper position to assist in neuromuscular and postural reeducation. The tape may remain in place for 1 to 3 days before replacement is necessary. Remove the tape as described earlier for athletic tape. The skin should be evaluated and cleansed thoroughly before reapplication.

PRECAUTIONS

During application, care should be taken not to apply strong tension because this can create shearing forces to adjacent as well as target tissues. When taping the shoulder, be careful not to compress the brachial plexus as it crosses the humerus. Remember, the patient should experience immediate improvement and reduction in pain; if the patient experiences an increase in pain, the tape should be removed immediately. It is important to have received training by a certified instructor, which will improve effectiveness and proficiency in the technique.

HELPFUL HINTS

- A skin toughener may be helpful in reducing skin irritation.
- The tape should improve symptoms immediately.
- If there is no change in symptoms, discontinue use.

CLINICAL EXAMPLES OF MCCONNELL TAPING

Shoulder Subluxation

When taping for a shoulder subluxation (Fig. 13–7A,B), the goal is to realign the glenohumeral head. Use a spray adherent or skin toughener to protect the skin from irritation, if necessary. McConnell taping for the shoulder may cause increased irritation depending on the condition of the muscle carrying the weight of the arm. This taping does not address multidirectional instability, only the anterior subluxation commonly seen in patients who have undergone cerebrovascular accidents (CVAs). The vertical strip serves to support the weight of the arm and provides upward lift of the humerus, and the transverse strip supports the humeral head in the glenoid serving as a reinforcement of the anterior ligaments. When applying the vertical working tape, avoid pulling straight up, which may create additional stress to the skin. Rather, move parallel to the skin and gently taking up

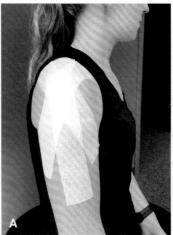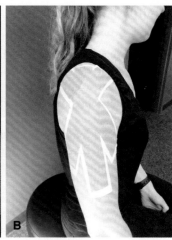

FIGURE 13–7 McConnell taping for shoulder subluxation. A, Apply the vertical undertape over the anterior surface of the upper arm beginning distal to the deltoid insertion and ending just medial to the scapula. Apply the anterior and posterior undertape following the anterior and posterior deltoid muscles. **B,** When applying the brown adhesive tape on top of the undertape, use the nonworking hand to approximate the head of the humerus superio-posteriorly while applying the working tape to provide numeral head stabilization.

the slack, observing the skin on the edges for signs of excess tension. If the patient experiences increased pain or paresthesia, remove the tape immediately. This taping may stay in place for 3 to 4 days depending on the patient's age, overall medical condition, diagnosis, and skin condition. The technique shown here may not be appropriate and will not replace a sling or outside supportive device for heavy extremities or large subluxations of 2 cm or greater.

Use caution with all shoulder tapings employing nonelastic tape. Excess force and pressure can have adverse effects on joint and soft tissue structures. This technique should be combined with a comprehensive strengthening program for the muscles affecting the joint to provide extrinsic stability and prevent further damage or stretching of supporting ligaments and joint structures. McConnell taping for shoulder subluxation also works well for anterior instability because the tape strips create a perpendicular capsular support. In this case, a shorter vertical strip may be used to avoid upward compressive forces that may result in subacromial impingement.

Lateral Epicondylitis

Lateral epicondylitis can be treated with McConnell taping. Use a spray adherent or skin toughener, if necessary, to protect the skin from irritation (Fig. 13–8A). The materials required are brown heavyweight adhesive tape and an undertape cut into 1″ strips. The taping technique shown uses a diamond unloading pattern to shift the fascia and soft tissue restrictions away from the lateral epicondyle (Fig. 13–8B). The patient should experience immediate decrease or relief of symptoms after taping. The taping can remain in place for 2 to 3 days before needing to be replaced. Be careful to maintain the adhesive tape on the undertape to prevent skin contact and irritation on removal. The taping for lateral epicondylitis should be combined with a comprehensive stretching and strengthening program for the upper extremity, focusing on the forearm extensors. Do not pull up on the tape, rather glide the fascia parallel to the skin. When the taping has been completed, there will be a puckering and lifting of the skin over the lateral epicondyle.

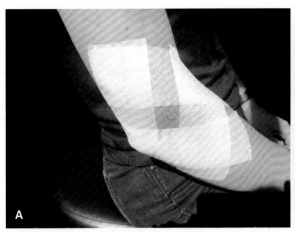
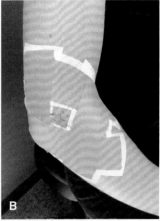

FIGURE 13-8 **McConnell taping for lateral epicondylitis (right elbow, lateral view). A,** Place the undertape in a diamond configuration to surround the area of pain (noted with marker). **B,** Attach the brown tape at the inferior anterior section of the diamond starting at the inferior apex. Stretch the fascia superior and anterior along the course of the undertape and attach it at the anterior apex of the diamond. Repeat the process, placing the tape in the direction of the inferior posterior aspect of the diamond. Repeat, placing the tape at the posterior superior aspect of the diamond. Place the last tape at the anterior superior aspect to complete the diamond pattern unloading the lateral epicondyle.

ELASTIC THERAPEUTIC TAPE

GENERAL PRINCIPLES

Elastic therapeutic taping (ETT) is a broad term that encompasses any tape that has elastic properties that are applied to the body for therapeutic intervention. Elastic therapeutic tapes have elastic properties, adhesives to apply directly to the skin and recoil ability. Coban™ can be considered an ETT due to its ability to stretch and stick to itself, but as it does not anchor to the skin, it is more commonly considered a circumferential dressing. Kinesiology tape is the most widely used and is effective in treating many acute and chronic orthopedic and complex conditions. ETT is most commonly used to treat injured tissue resulting from poor postural habits, subluxations, sprains, impingement syndromes, complex regional pain syndromes, fibromyalgia, overuse, edema, scar adhesions, and muscle dysfunctions (González-Iglesias, Fernández-de-Las-Peñas, Cleland, Huijbregts, & Del Rosario Gutiérrez-Vega, 2009; Hsu et al., 2009; Jaraczewska & Long, 2006; Kalichman, Vered, & Volchek, 2010; Kase, Wallis, & Kase, 2003; Kase, Hashimotom, & Okane, 1996; Kaya, Zinnuroglu, & Tugcu, 2011; Liu, Chen, Lin, Huang, & Sun, 2007; Murray & Husk, 2001; Paoloni et al., 2011; Schneider, Rhea, & Bay, 2010; Slupik, Dwornick, Bialoszewski, & Zych, 2007; Thelen, Dauber, & Stoneman, 2008; Yasukawa ea al., 2006). Dynamic tape, which we will discuss later in this chapter, is the most recently developed ETT. It has a high elastic recoil that adheres to the skin and creates a spring-like rebound to reduce load on injured tissue. We will discuss the methodology and common uses for both Kinesiology tape and Dynamic tape in the following sections.

ELASTIC THERAPEUTIC TAPING—KINESIOLOGY TAPE

GENERAL PRINCIPLES

Kinesiotape (the original kinesiology tape) was developed by a Japanese chiropractor, Dr. Kenso Kase, in 1973. After chiropractic training in the United States, Dr. Kase returned to Japan and specialized in rehabilitation and therapeutic medicine. Intrigued with conservative management of treating traumatized soft tissue, he used sports tape to assist in soft tissue control. Not satisfied with the stiff restriction of athletic tapes, he developed an elastic tape that would work with the flexibility of muscle, fascia, and skin to facilitate healing. Since the development of the original Kinesiotape, kinesiology taping has evolved into a mainstream therapeutic intervention tool used by therapists, physicians, athletic trainers, chiropractors, high school and collegiate coaches, professional athletes, and the general population.

 CLINICAL PEARL 13-2

Taping for Joint Position

Kinesiology tape can be used to manually correct or assist alignment of a joint. The kinesiology tape is realigning the distal interphalangeal (DIP) into neutral after a ligament injury. In this case, the circumferential orthosis is fabricated over the tape allowing the therapist to use both hands during the fabrication process.

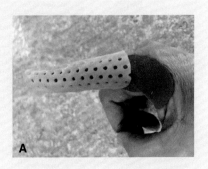

Kinesiology tape can be used to position joints over an orthosis or cast during the healing process.

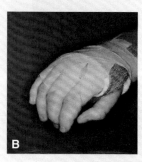

CLINICAL PEARL 13–3

Taping for Dynamic Assist

The kinesiology tape is applied with a 50% stretch to assist the orthosis in wrist and digital extension post radial nerve injury. The additional extension assist complements the wrist/digit extension mobilization orthosis by decreasing potential shearing forces from the tape alone and lessens the distal migration of the orthosis.

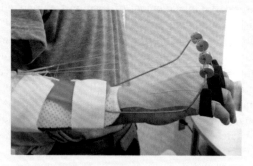

CLINICAL PEARL 13–4

Mobilization With Kinesiology Tape

Tabs can be added to the kinesiology tape to assist in myofascial release, soft tissue and scar mobilization, and lymphatic drainage. The tab is created using an "I" cut and folding a 1-inch section in half onto itself. Attach both ends with no stretch on top of the therapeutic tape. Now, the client can hold the tab and mobilize the underlying tissue.

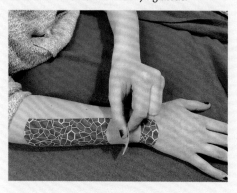

GOALS OF KINESIOLOGY TAPE

* Decrease pain and abnormal sensation in skin and muscle.
* Reduce edema and inflammation.
* Normalize muscle tone and abnormality of fascia involved in pathology.
* Support a weakened muscle in movement (expanding effects) by preventing overstretch and reducing fatigue.
* Reduce spasm or over contraction of a shortened muscle.
* Improve ROM.
* Provide muscle and proprioceptive reeducation.
* Reestablish muscular balance to correct misalignment of a joint.
* Support normal joint alignment for rehabilitation.
* Prevent injuries in exercise or activities of daily living (ADLs).
* Improve kinesthetic awareness of proper posture and structural alignment.
* Increase circulation.

INDICATIONS FOR USE

Proper application of the tape does not restrict soft tissue movement as do conventional adhesive tapes such as athletic and McConnell tapes, but rather relies on the movement of skin for multilevel effects. The tape, when applied with stretch, will **recoil** creating convolutions in the skin thereby increasing the interstitial space. The tape, in combination with proper application, has multisystemic effects on vascular, lymphatic, soft tissue, joint, and muscular dysfunctions (Kaya et al., 2011; Shim, Lee, & Lee, 2003). A thorough and comprehensive understanding of pathology and its relationship to muscle physiology and kinesiology is essential to the success of this form of taping. An evaluation of muscle, fascia, soft tissue continuity, and structure is completed to determine the causal factors of the pathology.

The elastic recoil of the tape is used to provide support to weak muscles and encourages full joint range (Fig. 13–10). The movement of taped skin and soft tissue creates a massaging effect that promotes lymph and blood flow (Shim et al., 2003), decreasing pressure on mechanoreceptors, thus reducing pain and edema. Sensory receptors located in the skin also act on ascending and descending neurologic pathways to reduce pain and assist in control of muscle tension via Golgi tendon organ input (Leonard, 1998). The application may specifically address sensory receptors in the skin, lymphatic movement for edema and circulation, muscle tension control, or joint support. An advanced application skill, the **correction technique**, can be used to offer support to a target ligament. In this taping application, the center portion of the tape is stretched to 75% and then placed straight onto the involved joint/ligament structure. This allows the elastic properties of the tape to recoil, pulling the fascia to the center of the tape.

PRODUCT VARIATIONS

Over the past 10 years, there has been a significant increase in media exposure and commercial availability of kinesiology tape. Kinesiology tape is commonly used by professional athletes for injury recovery and injury prevention. With this increase of media exposure, there is an ever-expanding market with manufacturers developing and producing tapes with higher elastic recoils, specialty prints, adhesive patterns, and stronger adhesives (Fig. 13–9). When tapes from different manufacturers are compared, there are differences in tension (Selva et al., 2019), adherence (Matheus, Zile, Matheus, Lemos, Carregaro and Shimano, 2017), maximum elongation before rupture (Boonkerd & Limroongreungrat, 2016), recoil force, tenacity (Selva, Pardoners, Aquado, Montava, Gil-Santos, Barrios, 2019), and adherence assays (Matheus et al., 2017). More research is needed to define tape properties among the continuum of taping manufacturers. It is important to become familiar with the brand properties you are using

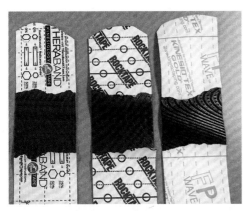

FIGURE 13–9 **Various manufacturers of kinesiology tape.** From left to right; Kinesiotape, Rock Tape, and Theraband brand. Notice the different patterns of adhesive and backings. The printed backing provides cut guidelines in 1/2 inch or 1-inch increments.

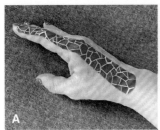 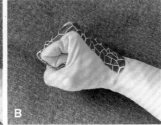

FIGURE 13–10 **A,** This client is taped with kinesiology tape to assist in index finger extension. **B,** Notice the client can still fully flex the index finger.

and recommending to clients. With all therapeutic interventions, it is strongly recommended to get training by a certified instructor and use clinical judgment skills when taping clients.

PATIENT EDUCATION

Elastic therapeutic taping is used to complement a rehabilitation program and can easily be taught to patients, family members, or other caregivers for continued application in chronic conditions or for specific situations in self-management (Jaraczewska & Long, 2006; Yasukawa et al., 2006) (Fig. 13–10A,B). Lateral epicondylitis

is a common chronic condition that can benefit from kinesiology tape. There are taping methods and suggestions available for common diagnosis online from the Kinesio taping Association, Rock Tape, KT Tape, Theraband, Youtube, and many more. Some chronic conditions require creativity and persistence to find the right taping method for the client and the symptomology (Fig. 13–11A–C). It is important when educating a client that the taping patterns are simple, reproducible, and comfortable while maintaining the anatomical goal of the taping technique.

- The patient or caregiver should be given verbal and written instructions for application, ordering information, and how to care for the kinesiology tape.
- Directions should be modified based on comprehension level.
- Most kinesiology tape has preprinted sections on the back of the tape ranging from 1/2-inch to 1-inch sections. This can be used to measure the proper length of the tape for home use.
- The provider should demonstrate how to properly self-tape with specific attention to the amount of tape pull and using no stretch on the anchors. There is a tendency to overstretch the tape in hopes of better results, but this is not accurate and should be discussed.
- Have the client demonstrate the taping technique prior to leaving the clinic.
- Always educate the client on tape precautions allowing them to remove the tape if they notice itching, increased pain, or a rash developing.

PROPERTIES OF TAPE AND TECHNIQUE OF APPLICATION

Elastic tape combined with proper application affects the superficial fascial structures in the skin and creates a lifting effect in resting tissue thereby reducing subcutaneous interstitial pressure, improving lymphatic drainage and edema reduction (Kase et al., 2003). During normal movement, there is a constant tactile stimulus to low-threshold cutaneous mechanoreceptors of the skin (Murray & Husk, 2001). This stimulates muscle, decreases pain, and enhances proprioception for neuromuscular reeducation. The elastic recoil of the tape also provides support to weak muscles, reducing fatigue. The thickness and weight of the tape is approximately the same as skin.

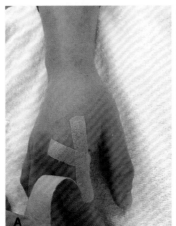 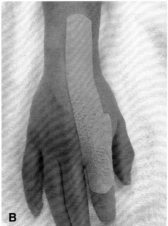 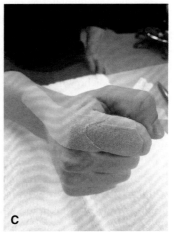

FIGURE 13–11 **Taping for extensor tendon subluxation.** This client is a 26-year-old male with a history of ECU subluxation that is exacerbated while snowboarding. A custom orthosis was trialed, but it was too restrictive and cumbersome to fit under his glove. **A,** Two 1/2 inch "I" strips are taped with 50% stretch to support the collateral ligament and sagittal band of the MP joint. **B,** A 1-inch "I" cut was then applied along the extensor tendon at 25%. The tendon still slightly subluxed; therefore, a second 1-inch "I" cut was applied with a buttonhole anchor along the extensor tendon for reinforcement. **C,** He is able to fully flex with no subluxation, and it is able to fit inside the ski glove. He was able to reproduce this taping on himself. Creativity, trial and error, and persistence can lead to successful treatment interventions with taping.

It stretches in the longitudinal axis only up to 140% of its resting length (Halseth, McChesney, DeBeliso, Vaughn, & Lien, 2004). The tape is made of woven cotton fabric and has no latex or medicinal properties in the tape. An acrylic, heat-activated adhesive forms a pattern with perforations to allow for passage of perspiration and air. The tape is available in 2″ and 3″ widths with multiple colors and designs available. Most tapes are "water resistant" using a light paraffin spray coating to increase wearing time when exposed to perspiration or water. The tape may be worn for up to 4 days (or longer depending on the patient's skin qualities and area of body part application), and the patient is able to shower with the tape in place. The digits, thumb, and volar palm of the hand can be challenging in terms of prolonged adherence partially due to exposure to water and other liquids and may require a spray adhesive for adherence. Care should be taken when drying as not to roll up the edges of the tape, this is why it is important to round the edge of the tape. After water exposure, the tape is dried by dabbing the tape with a dry terry cloth (or absorbent) towel or paper towel to wick the moisture from the tape.

A thorough evaluation should be performed as the specific taping technique and methods used in Kinesiology taping (Table 13–4) are determined by the target fascia and tissue to be treated. The most commonly used cuts are the "Y"- and "I"-shaped cuts from 2″-wide tape. The "X," "buttonhole," and "fan" cuts are also important to learn as they each have specific functions. Table 13–5 describes the proper tape tension as described by the Kinesio taping Association. Most kinesthetic tapes come with a 10% to 25% stretch on the paper backing. **Paper-off** refers to pulling off the paper backing as the tape is applied to the skin (Fig. 13–12A). Tissue involved with the pathology should be taped following the tension guidelines for optimal results.

The direction of application (i.e., origin to insertion or insertion to origin) has determined to not alter the effects of the tape (Lemos et al., 2018; Choi & Lee, 2018; Serrao et al., 2016). When researching tape methods, you will find a variety of successful taping techniques for the same diagnosis. Anatomical knowledge, listening to the client's symptomology, completing a thorough evaluation and understanding of the tapes properties and capabilities will allow you to become an innovative and successful taping practitioner.

After application, rub the tape to activate the heat-sensitive glue. The tape may be applied over fine hair, but more coarse hair should be clipped short with scissors or shaved (Fig. 13–12B). Once rubbed to activate the glue, the tape may not be reapplied. For best adherence, it should be applied 20 to 30 minutes before strenuous activity to better tolerate perspiration. It is not necessary to use an adhesive spray before application, except when applying the tape to moist tissue areas, the palm, or naturally oily skin that requires an added layer of adhesive. Athletes who will be training and sweating profusely and water athletes may benefit from the use of an adhesive spray applied prior to tape application.

To remove the tape, it is best to start at the proximal end and work distally, moving with the direction of hair growth. Brushing the tape briskly while rolling it onto itself is most effective for overstimulating sensory receptors and decreasing discomfort. To reduce trauma to the skin, a thin, viscous oil (such as olive oil) may be rubbed and absorbed into the tape to loosen the adhesive prior to removal.

PRECAUTIONS

- Do not overstretch the tape. Only correction tapings should have stretch above 50%.
- Proper application will decrease pain, improper application will increase pain.

- Do not tape a client with adhesive allergies. A skin test can be performed for clients that report sensitivity to adhesives (Fig. 13–13).
- Application of a skin barrier or spray adherent may prevent irritation.
- Application of dry heat (such as a hair dryer) to the adhesive prior to application will activate the adhesive and increase bonding to difficult areas such as the palm. This technique will not work to reattach the tape because small cellular debris limits adhesion.
- Evaluate prior to initial application and reevaluate prior to each application as symptomatology can change between tapings. It is not uncommon to alter tapings from one treatment to another in response to the changes and individual needs of the patient.
- Formal training from an experienced and certified instructor is highly recommended to obtain optimal results.

TABLE 13–4	Techniques and Methods Used in Kinesio Taping	
"I" or single strip cut	May be used on all muscles across a joint in a correction technique or to encourage rotation; it is applied moving along the center of the muscle. A 10 width is used for a small muscle.	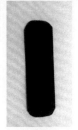
"Y" cut	Used to surround multiple or a large muscle belly; the base of the letter is used as the anchor. The separation of the ends or tails assists in changing the tension of the tissue between, lifting it to increase lymphatic flow.	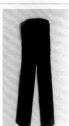
"X" cut	Used to stabilize at a joint for treatment of rhomboidal-shaped muscle or in a correction technique.	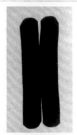
"Fan" cut	Used primarily for edema reduction; the anchor serving as the drawing point to which you want the lymph to drain toward.	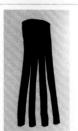
"Buttonhole" cut	Used as an anchor in forearm tapings to prevent rolling; athletic or bandage tape may be used to secure the short end if using partial hand coverage as illustrated in lateral epicondylitis taping.	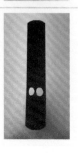

TABLE 13–5   Proper Tape Tension

No tension	There should be no "pull" at the anchor or end of the tape. Very gentle stretch needed to stimulate the lymphatic system. Can be used with the Fan cut for edema and lymphedema.	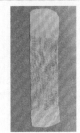 Note the visual change at the anchor ends where there is 0% stretch, versus the middle where the tension is 75%-100% tension.
10%-25%	"Pull-off" paper stretch is the most effective tension for muscle taping.	
25%-50%	Tape may be slightly stretched if applied to nonstretched skin (i.e., joint contracture or contraindications to joint movement).	
50%-75%	Tape is applied with all elastic stretch taken out only when using a "correction" technique (i.e., adhesive scars).	

HELPFUL HINTS

- Move through an ROM before applying the tape to maximize tissue movement.
- Clean the skin of any oils or lotions and dry thoroughly.
- Long or coarse forearm hair, it may need to be shaved or trimmed to ensure adhesive contact. Shave the hair only where the tape is to be applied (Fig. 13–12B).

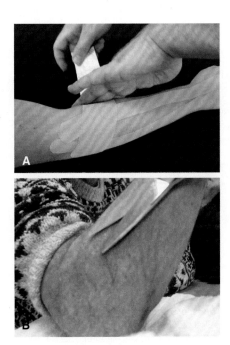

FIGURE 13–12 A, To **paper off**, pull the paper off with the hand on the same side as the tape while following along with the opposite hand to adhere tape to the skin. The tape comes on the paper backing with a 20%–25% stretch applied making this technique popular for muscular tapings. **B,** Trimming hair prior to tape application can ease comfort of tape removal.

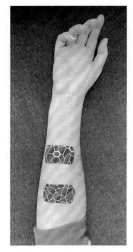

FIGURE 13–13 Allergy skin test trial. Manufacturers use different adhesive compositions. Do not assume if the client did not breakout from one brand that all brands are safe to use. Allergic responses to the adhesive are seen as a blister-type rash or hives. Apply two pieces of tape approximately 1–2 inches in length to the volar forearm where the skin tends to be more sensitive. Do not use any tension to rule out rash development from overstretching. Have the client remove the first piece 4–6 hours after application, and if there is no reaction, remove the second piece at 24 hours. Have the client remove all tape immediately should any itching or pain occur during the trial.

- Apply the anchor of the tape securely (minimum of 1″) without tension while the body is in neutral position. There should be an anchor at each end of the tape with NO tension.
- Be sure of proper placement prior to smoothing down the tape; work from the center outward to prevent lifting of the ends.
- Round the edges of the tape to prevent snagging on clothes. Rub to create friction heat to secure.
- Consider taking photos/video with phone to ensure proper home application.

CLINICAL EXAMPLES OF KINESIO TAPING

Lateral Epicondylitis

Kinesio taping for lateral epicondylitis addresses the tight forearm extensor muscles by applying the tape to the forearm extensors and to assist the overused supinator muscle (Fig. 13–14A–C). The technique requires 2″-wide Y-cut tape for the extensors and an "I" cut for the supinator. A 1½″ to 2″ end is needed to provide a secure anchor proximal to the lateral epicondyle and distally over the dorsal wrist. This is a common taping method for lateral epicondylitis; however, several other application patterns do exist. The patient should experience rapid relief of symptoms.

Mallet Finger

Tension can be varied depending on the stage of healing. An acute mallet finger needs to be immobilized. Kinesiology tape (Fig. 13–15A,B) is a good option when weaning from a rigid orthosis. Start with moderate tension and decrease tape tension with each taping until weaning is complete. Kinesiology tape can be used for post-op mallet repairs. The cross above the DIP joint will also function as a scar mobilization technique. Clinical judgment is required to evaluate the stability of the healing and appropriate tension applied to effectively protect the healing structures.

DeQuervain's Tenosynovitis

The target tissues for Kinesio taping for DeQuervain's tenosynovitis (Fig. 13–16A–D) are the inflamed extensor pollicis brevis and abductor pollicis longus. Retinacular ligament taping uses a

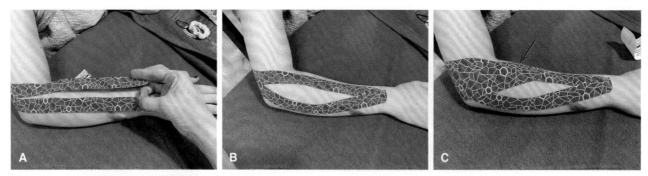

FIGURE 13–14 **Elastic therapeutic taping for lateral epicondylitis. A,** Measure the length of the tape from the lateral epicondyle to the wrist. Cut into a Y pattern leaving 1–2 inches for the anchor. Apply the anchor just proximal to the lateral epicondyle. **B,** Paper off along the borders of the extensor wad with distal anchor at the dorsal wrist. **C,** Measure the second piece the length of the supinator. Anchor the tape just proximal to the first piece of tape. Paper off with a 25% pull over the supinator.

correction technique to lift the skin and fascia over the first dorsal compartment and carpometacarpal (CMC) joint, reducing edema and improving vascular flow. The materials required are a 2″-wide Y-cut tape measured from the IP of the thumb to the origin of the abductor pollicis longus, a 2″-wide I-cut tape. The wrap around the thumb often needs to be reinforced. Tell the client to use a Band-Aid or elastic wrap such as Coban to keep the edges in place. This taping is also effective for relieving associated sensory radial nerve signs and provides support to the CMC joint, reducing pain, and associated edema with use of the "lifting strip" at the retinacular ligament.

Edema Management

The target tissue for Kinesio taping for edema management is tight flexor and extensor muscles that inhibit lymphatic flow (Fig. 13–17A). The movement of the fascia during normal activity also assists in lymph drainage, causing decompression and space correction. In theory, the elastic recoil demonstrated by the tape once applied to the overextended skin lifts the connective tissue fibers. This contributes to improved lymphatic mobility and secondarily decreases pressure on the underlying structures, which in turn may aid in lessening pain. When worn, the stretch properties of the tape during dynamic movement functions

much like a soft tissue massage by increasing blood flow and decreasing edema. Several techniques can be used. Shown in Figure 13–17A is a technique utilizing a length of 2″ tape material cut into the fan shape. This technique is effective for treating postoperative pain and edema, but caution should be taken when addressing acutely healing tissues. The taping should be combined with active motion because this creates movement and massaging of the skin to improve lymphatic return. Technique shown in Figure 13–17B–G is another popular taping pattern for edema management.

Scar Management

The target tissue for Kinesio taping in scar management (Fig. 13–18A–D) is adherent scars or those incision areas that may be at risk for adherence such as the dorsum of the MP joints or the radial styloid area. The application of the tape over an adherent scar can gently "lift" or lightly "pull" the skin and underlying soft tissue away from the structure to which it is fixed or adhered. This taping

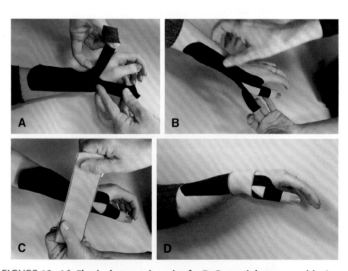

FIGURE 13–16 **Elastic therapeutic taping for DeQuervain's tenosynovitis. A,** Cut two 1-inch "I" cuts approximately 5 inches long. Anchor the first piece with no stretch on the dorsal side of the MP joint. Wrap around the MP joint with a 25% pull leading it over the CMC. **B,** Repeat this taping around the MP joint in the opposite direction paying special attention to having no stretch at the anchor of the tape to avoid occlusion of the blood vessels to the thumb. **C,** Cut a 2″ section of tape approximately 3/4 circumference of the wrist. Anchor the tape on the dorsal ulnar side of the wrist. Over the area of the most pain, increase the pull to 50% and paper off leaving the last inch to anchor with no stretch. **D,** Completed taping.

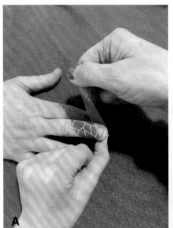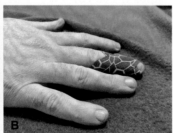

FIGURE 13–15 **Elastic therapeutic taping for mallet finger. A,** Anchor tape on the volar distal phalanx. **B,** Pull tape with 75% pull over the dorsal DIP joint in a crisscross pattern and anchor tape to the lateral and medial sides of the finger to not impede motion at the PIP joint. Decrease tension as the tensile strength progresses.

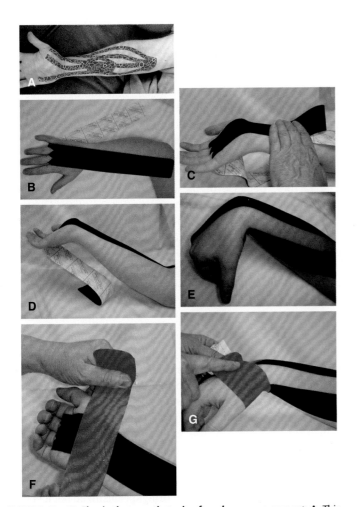

FIGURE 13-17 **Elastic therapeutic taping for edema management. A,** This taping requires a "Fan" cut. If the edema is global, tape the client on the volar and dorsal sides of the forearm. The anchor (uncut portion) should have no stretch. The tails should have 5%–10% stretch. The tape should follow the lymphatic system and end at a major drain site (epitrochlear or axillary nodes). The will create a gentle lifting and massaging effect to stimulate the lymphatic system. Use multiple pieces as necessary to follow the line of drainage. **B, Alternative edema management technique**: Place buttonhole cut tape through the middle and ring fingers. **C,** With the wrist in maximum extension, apply the tape to the volar surface of the hand to the wrist. **D,** Apply the tape over the flexor muscle mass, ending at the medial epicondyle. **E,** Move the wrist into maximum flexion. Apply the tape over the dorsum of the hand, wrist, and extensor muscles, ending at the lateral epicondyle. **F,** Place the wrist in gravity-assisted extension and apply a correction tape (all out stretch) perpendicular to the first taping. **G,** Then move the wrist into flexion and apply the tape without stretch tension to the edge of the dorsal strip to prevent circumferential restriction.

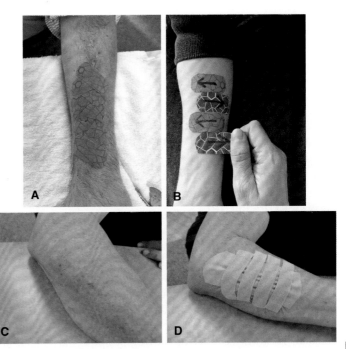

FIGURE 13-18 **Taping for adherent scar. A,** Traditional X pattern with 50% pull crisscross over the scar. **B,** Alternating lateral pull in opposing directions to create cross friction of the scar. **C,** Adherent surgical scar. **D,** Strip placement was changed at each therapy visit to provide the tissue with various tensions to improve soft tissue mobility.

can also be used to prevent adhesions. The traditional X pattern can be alternated with the zipper technique to glide the tissue in a different line of pull. By keeping the tape on, the movement of the fascia under the tape during normal activity creates a gentle shear stress, which in turn may aide in facilitating gentle independent gliding of the tissue. This would be considered a correction technique because the tape is stretched beyond the pull-off paper tension. Caution should be taken with application over acutely healing tissues or with clients that have frail skin.

Carpometacarpal Osteoarthritis

Traditionally this tape application is used for CMC osteoarthritis (OA) as it supports the radial side of the wrist, CMC joint, and thumb (Fig. 13–19A–D). This tape application is also beneficial to treat symptoms present with texting thumb, radial-sided wrist pain, and MP joint instability. The length and direction of

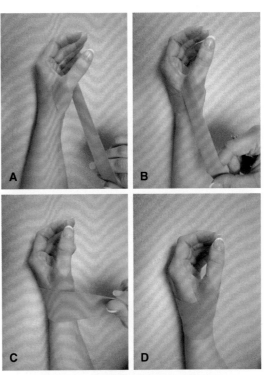

FIGURE 13-19 **Taping for first CMC osteoarthritis.** To begin, cut two 1-inch "I" cuts approximately 4 inches long and one 2-inch "I" cut 5 inches long. **A,** Anchor the first 1-inch "I" cut on the ulnar border of the thumb MP joint with no stretch. Apply 25% stretch around the MP volarly anchoring on the dorsal wrist. **B,** The second 1-inch "I" cut will be wrapped in the opposite direction with the anchor applied at the radial side of the MP joint wrapping volarly around the MP joint and anchoring at the base of the MCP joint. **C,** The 2-inch piece will be anchored on the ulnar styloid with no pull. Apply a 25% stretch over the first CMC joint and paper off around the wrist leaving no stretch on the ends to avoid forming a tourniquet on the client. **D,** The completed taping should feel supportive to the first CMC and MP joints with a lessening of symptoms.

the tape can be adjusted depending on the symptoms present. Consider the integrity of the radial wrist extensors and precaution to avoid irritation of the dorsal radial sensory nerve by overstretching the tape.

ELASTIC THERAPEUTIC TAPING—BIOMECHANICAL TAPING/DYNAMIC TAPE

GENERAL PRINCIPLES

Dynamic tape (Fig. 13–20) was developed in 2010 by Ryan Kendrick, MPhtySt, BPhty, a musculoskeletal physiotherapist from Australia. Kendrick specializes in working with high-level athletes and found their injuries were commonly sustained from excess load demand placed on muscle and tendon tissue. The tissue's inability to control the load demand led to injury. Kendrick began experimented with products to externally manage the load demand. He theorizes that optimizing position, movement, and tissue loading are necessary for tissue repair and pain management (Kendrick interview, 2019). He experimented with high recoil materials such as TheraBand, elastic bands, and bicycle tires strapped to the skin to help unload muscle tissue. Finding success with this technique of unloading tissue, he proceeded to develop a low-profile tape that would have a high recoil and deceleration effect to unload tissue.

Dynamic tape comes in either 2- or 3-inch width and has a tattoo pattern printed on the tape. It is latex free and has an adhesive side and a nonadhesive side which is comprised of a Nylon/Lycra blend. The tape has a four-way stretch with no end point with similar properties to a rubber band or a bungee cord. It has a strong recoil that applies an external force to the kinetic chain. The further you stretch it, the stronger the recoil force is. For example, when a bungee jumper initiates a fall, they will decelerate on the way down as the recoil force builds, then the load absorbs and creates a spring back in the opposite direction as the force is reinjected into the kinetic chain. As the energy is used, the jumper will start to fall again and the cycle is repeated. Dynamic tape has these same properties of decelerating motion, absorbing load and transferring the energy back into the kinetic chain. Table 13–6 describes the Dynamic tape options and properties available.

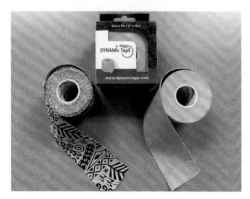

FIGURE 13–20 Dynamic tape materials.

Dynamic tape is primarily used for its biomechanical properties but does have some positive effects with respect to pain management. Pain is highly subjective with both internal and external factors effecting pain perception. Environmental, genetic, social, cultural, psychosocial, and biological factors all contribute to the individual's perception of pain (Moayedi & Davis, 2013). Tissue injury can range from minor to major and painless to painful (McNeil & Penderson, 2016). Pain results from a complex interplay between sensory information from anatomical structures, nervous system processing, and psychosocial factors. Because of these factors, the same anatomical injury can have drastic differences in pain perception. Dynamic tape is not primarily used as a neurophysiological treatment but has shown positive neurophysiological effects generated from the skin contact and should be considered when evaluating a client post taping for the effectiveness of the application. The tape should be removed immediately if there is any increase of pain or discomfort.

INDICATIONS FOR USE

Biomechanically, the tape can be used in the absence of pain when nerve injury is causing limited muscle contractions. For example, radial nerve palsy or weakness following a tendon repair or transfer causes weak or absent wrist and/or finger extension. The client is able to pull against the tape into flexion while it builds force and then springs back assisting extension (Fig. 13–21). Dynamic tape can also be used to modify gross movement patterns or accessory motions where that movement is known to increase load on a target structure. This will improve the movement patterns and decrease pain that is caused by the firing of sensitized nociceptors. For example, taping a client's MCP joints into radial deviation following changes due to osteoarthritis may decrease joint pain and assist in realigning the joint(s) into a more functional pattern of movement.

GOALS/AIMS OF DYNAMIC TAPING

1. Modifying load/soft tissue offloading

This is used to reduce the load on injured or overloaded muscle tissue. This allows the client/athlete to reduce the workload of the tissue without necessarily compromising technique. This can also contribute to pain reduction by reducing stimulation of the sensitized nociceptors. The tissue is manually gathered from all directions and held in place with the tape recoil. See lateral epicondylitis offloading in clinical examples (Fig. 13–29C–E).

2. Improve position or modify movement patterns

This approach applies to changing the movement pattern without particular attention to the forces leading to the motion. Changing the kinematics of motion can increase stability, improve ease of motion, correct deformity or unwanted motion. See clinical example for MCP ulnar drift (Fig. 13–27B).

3. Force contribution

This approach is used to contribute force to tissue that requires assistance for proper function. This approach is used following a radial nerve injury or tendon injury to provide external force to contribute to motion. See clinical example for wrist and finger extensors (Fig. 13–25A–D).

TABLE 13–6 Dynamic Tape Properties

	Color	Properties	Uses
Dynamic Tape Original	Black pattern on Beige tape	Most commonly used Good resistance and recoil Reduces the work of injured, overloaded, or fatigued tissue Functional assist for weak or absent muscle function	Musculotendinous units Functional muscle tapings following nerve injury or weakness Long multi-joint tapings
Dynamic Tape Original	Beige pattern on Beige tape	Preferred for more sensitive skin Slightly less recoil More discreet for lighter skin tones	Same as above when less recoil is desired
Dynamic Tape ECO	Gray pattern on black tape	Made from recycled plastic bottles Less recoil and more resistance than the DT original Provides firm resistance and minimal movement	Ligament tapings Stability tapings Single joint applications Joint positioning tapings

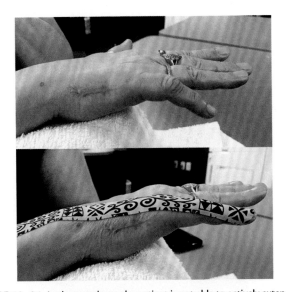

FIGURE 13–21 In the top photo, the patient is not able to actively extend the small finger due to scar adhesion over the dorsal MCP joint and atrophy from extended nonuse. In the bottom photo, Dynamic tape was applied, and the patient has full functional range of motion.

4. Force closure

Form closure applies to the joint stability via the anatomical structure. If the form closure is compromised it becomes an unstable joint. The tape can be used circumferentially to externally to force close the joint. See clinical examples for swan-neck deformity (Fig. 13–28F,G).

FUNDAMENTALS OF BIOMECHANICAL TAPING

In order to mechanically affect the tissue, there are three critical factors that must be applied. These include the following:

1. Crossing a joint or joints.
2. Apply the tape in a shortened position. The joint should be placed in a shortened position when taping so the tape will decelerate motion and unload the underlying tissue. The tape does not need to be stretched when applied. The recoil of the tape when applied to a shortened joint will produce the desired recoil effect (Fig. 13–22).
3. Get good purchase on the levers. It is imperative to have large anchors to provide good purchase to apply appropriate force on the tissue.

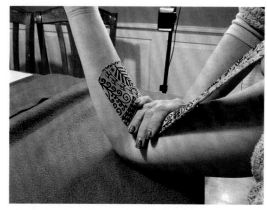

FIGURE 13–22 During this taping for the bicep, the elbow is flexed to place the joint in a shortened position. Notice there is a wide anchor to provide adequate purchase on the lever arm.

POWER BANDS

Some conditions or clients may require more elastic energy. The clinician can use a 3″. tape rather than a 2″ tape for this technique. The elastic force can be increased by layering the tape.

The power bands are a good option to provide increased recoil rather than using multiple strips that crisscross over the skin which can create shearing between the layers of tape causing mechanical irritation. Multiple layers of the Dynamic Tape Original will increase the recoil effect. Multiple layers of Dynamic Tape Eco will increase the resistance and force closure ability (Fig. 13–23).

TECHNIQUE AND APPLICATION

Evaluate the patient for appropriateness of Dynamic tape. Determine what the aim of the taping is to distinguish between original or Eco tape and whether a single layer or power band should be applied. Once this has been evaluated and determined, follow the steps below:

1. Make sure the skin is clean and free from oils. Soap and water are the best to clean the skin. Rubbing alcohol or hand sanitizer can break down the adhesive.
2. Excessive hair will need to be removed prior to application to ensure appropriate adhesion.
3. Round the corners of the tape so it does not catch on fabrics.
4. Create an anchor point three to four finger widths long. The anchor should have no tension.
5. Apply the anchor with no resistance. The anchor should be at least three fingers wide. Bring the joint you are crossing into a shortened position.
6. Continue to hold the anchor and apply the tape with the opposite hand paying attention NOT TO STRETCH THE TAPE—simply take up the slack. If the tape narrows, you have too much stretch applied. The tape tension is created by the position of the joint not the tension applied to the tape. Create a three to four finger sized anchor at the other end.
7. Post taping, evaluate the desired axis of rotation, line of pull, position of the joint, and leverage achieved.
8. If you have the desired result and the client has no increased pain, irritation, or itching sensations, press the tape down thoroughly paying special attention to areas that overlap or are curved.
9. Hold the tape in place for 30 to 60 seconds to activate the adhesive. Dynamic tape is pressure activated.
10. The tape can be worn up to 5 days.

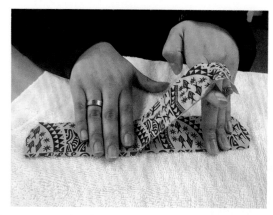

FIGURE 13–23 **Power bands.** Cut several pieces to be the same length. Place one strip on a firm surface and spray the fabric side with adhesive spray. Remove the backing of the second piece and lay it over the first piece with no stretch. Trim and round the adhered tape strips ends. Add a third layer in the same manner if needed. This forms a "power band" and should only be applied to strong healthy skin. As the power band has more recoil, the anchor points should be at least 3 inches in length.

PRECAUTIONS/CONTRAINDICATIONS

- Allergic reactions can occur from an allergy to the tape's adhesive. This is very rare and will occur within 30 minutes of application. Remove the tape immediately and clean off the adhesive with soap and water to stop the reaction from continuing. Antihistamines or hydrocortisone may be used if needed.
- Contact dermatitis can develop if moisture is trapped under the tape. This is also rare as the tape is perforated but should be discussed as a precaution.
- Mechanical irritation (Fig. 13–24A,B) is the most common reaction due to application error. It is caused by excess shearing on the skin from applying too much tension on the tape or not providing a large enough anchor. Mechanical irritations can lead to blistering if the tape is not removed at the first signs of irritation.

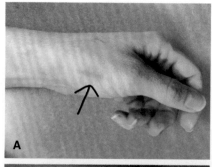

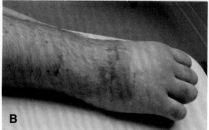

FIGURE 13–24 **Mechanical irritation. A and B,** Notice the red marks (arrow) that were created by tape shearing. This indicates the tape had too much tension where it overlapped with another piece creating a sheering effect on the skin with motion.

- Do not tape over frail, damaged or sunburnt skin, or insensate skin.
- **Tell the client to remove the tape immediately if they have any itching, burning, stinging, irritation, numbness, tingling, or increased pain.**
- Patient information sheets can be downloaded on the Dynamic tape website.

HELPFUL HINTS

- Dynamic tape training by an accredited practitioner is recommended prior to application on a client.
- Avoid excessive overlapping of the tape as it will cause shearing which can lead to mechanical irritation.

- The tape needs time to create a strong bond. Wait 1 hour before swimming or vigorous exercise.
- Adhesive spray can be used to protect the skin and increase the bond between tape layers and skin.
- The stronger the tension spring desired, the larger the anchor needs to be.
- Circumferential applications should be applied at an angle to prevent nerve and capillary compression.
- Remove the tape in the direction of the hair growth by holding the skin and pulling with the hair growth.
- Do not remove Dynamic tape when wet. Coconut oil or other natural oils can be used to decrease the adhesive bond before removal.

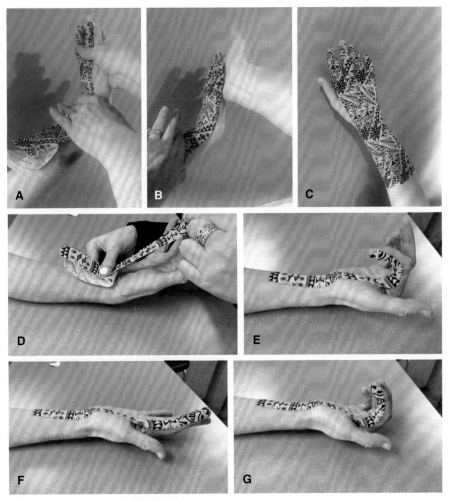

FIGURE 13–25 **Radial nerve injury/extensor weakness. A,** A Y-cut can be used for the IF/MF and RF/SF. Split a 2-inch piece of tape in half to accommodate the fingers. Alternately, each finger can be taped individually with special attention to places the tape overlaps to prevent irritation from shearing. **B,** Anchor the tape at the distal phalanx while holding the client in wrist and finger extension. **C,** Apply the tape distal to proximal with the joint in the shortened position. Hold the tape in place for 30–60 seconds as pressure will adhere the tape to the skin. **D,** The completed taping will passively extend the fingers with relaxation of the flexor musculature. **E,** The finger flexors can be taped in the same fashion. A spray adhesive should be applied to the palm as the tape does not adhere as well to the skin on the palm. Anchor at the distal phalange. **F,** Flex the fingers and wrist. **G,** Adhere the tape distally to proximally along the palm. **H,** Hold the tape in place for 30–60 seconds to adhere the tape. Completed taping.

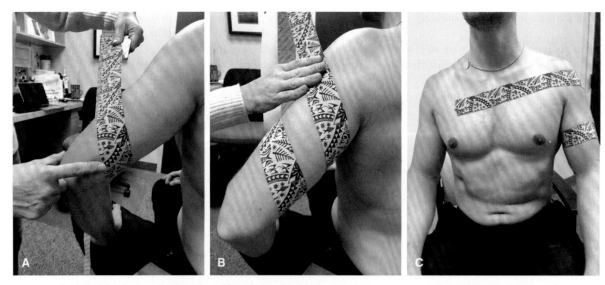

FIGURE 13−26 Anterior shoulder subluxation. A, Anchor the tape on the dorsal upper arm angled toward the body. **B,** Place the arm in internal rotation. Without stretching the tape, spiral superiorly at approximately 45° to avoid circulation compromise. **C,** Depending on the amount of desired recoil, the arm can be horizontally abducted to increase the resistance of external rotation. Cross over the front of the glenohumeral joint and finish on the contralateral side. The tape angle over the glenohumeral joint can be altered to achieve the desired degree of force and resistance.

CLINICAL EXAMPLES OF DYNAMIC TAPING

Wrist and Finger Extensors

This taping can be used to treat lateral epicondylitis, wrist drop, radial nerve injury, extensor tendon injury or repair, tendon transfers, or adherent extensor tendons (Fig. 13–25A–D). This taping technique will assist the forearm extensor muscles my mimicking their action and lifting the fingers. This reduces the load of the extensor muscles. Depending on the level of weakness or nerve damage, a power strip may need to be applied to produce enough power to lift the wrist and fingers. The power strip should extend the entire length of the tape. Remember, the greater the force is, the larger the anchor needs to be.

Shoulder Anterior Instability

This application (Fig. 13–26A–C) can be used to prevent anterior shoulder subluxation. When the patient externally rotates and horizontally abducts into the position of apprehension, the tape will recoil providing external sensory input and biomechanically pulling the shoulder back into internal rotation and adduction to decrease the risk of subluxation.

MCP Ulnar Drift

This taping (Fig. 13–27A,B) is used to mechanically correct joint positioning following a ligament injury. This technique will realign the MCP joint while still allowing for full ROM. This diagnosis is often seen in elderly clientele with arthritis. Use clinical judgment to determine the proper tape to use. Often, older skin is frail and at risk for mechanical irritation due to the increased glide of the skin and decreased thickness. Consider choosing the type of tape carefully with the patient population.

Mallet Finger/Swan-Neck Deformity

This taping (Fig. 13–28A–G) can be used after the rigid immobilization stage of recovery from a mallet injury or surgery. If the client has a swan-neck deformity, the taping should be extended through the proximal interphalangeal (PIP) joint to prevent hyperextension. This taping may need to be repeated throughout the day depending on the amount of hand washing and use. This taping can be applied in a reversed manner to address boutonnière deformity.

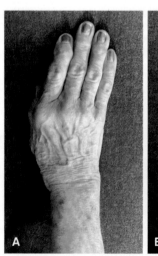
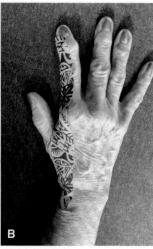

FIGURE 13−27 MCP Ulnar drift. A, This taping is a mechanical joint correction to realign the MP joint. Notice the amount of ulnar deviation in the resting position. **B,** Passively position the joint into as much radial deviation as tolerated. Anchor the tape at the radial side of the distal phalange. Stretch the tape until it has no slack and anchor the proximal end along the radial side of the metacarpal bone. A second smaller piece can be used to correct the distal interphalangeal (DIP) joint. The tape can then be held in place for 30–60 seconds to adhere the tape. Upon completion, the client should be able to fully flex without pain.

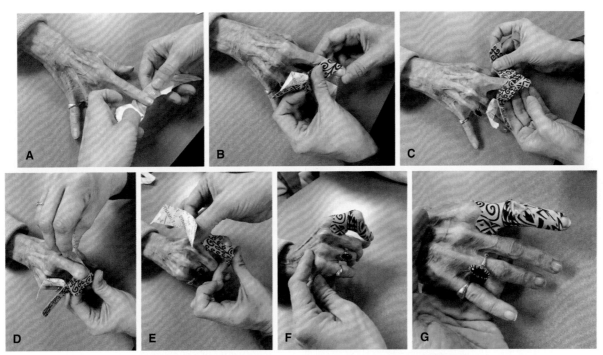

FIGURE 13-28 Mallet/swan-neck deformity. A, Anchor a 1″ piece on the dorsal distal phalange. **B,** Hold the DIP in as much hyperextension available and wrap the tape medially across the dorsal DIP to hold the DIP in extension. **C,** Repeat laterally. **D,** If the proximal interphalangeal (PIP) joint is involved (swan-neck deformity) extend the taping through the PIP joint. Flex the PIP joint and place the tape along the medial border of the PIP and cross over the proximal phalange. **E,** Repeat on the lateral side. **F,** Hold the tape in place for 30–60 seconds to adhere the tape. Completed taping. **G,** The finger is able to actively fully extend with some effort.

Medial or Lateral Elbow Soft Tissue Offloading

This taping is used to unload the musculotendinous origin as well as offload the injured tissue. The taping can be used medially or laterally with the lateral taping (Fig. 13–29A–E) being displayed.

It is important to evaluate for areas of tension where the tapes cross to avoid sheering of the tissues. If any discomfort is felt, gently pull the skin out from under the tape until the tension is relieved.

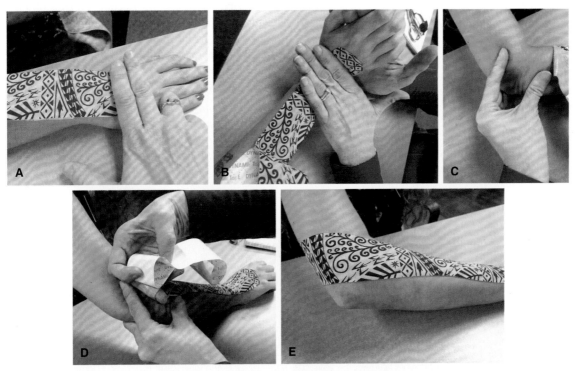

FIGURE 13-29 Lateral epicondylitis. A, The anchor should be two–three fingers wide. **B,** Unload the forearm extensors by placing the joint in a shortened position, the tape should be applied distally to proximally toward the epicondyle. **C,** The tissue around the epicondyle should be unloaded by pinching the tissue toward the epicondyle. **D,** Place the tape over the unloaded tissue. **E,** Hold the tape in place for 30–60 seconds to adhere the tape. Completed taping.

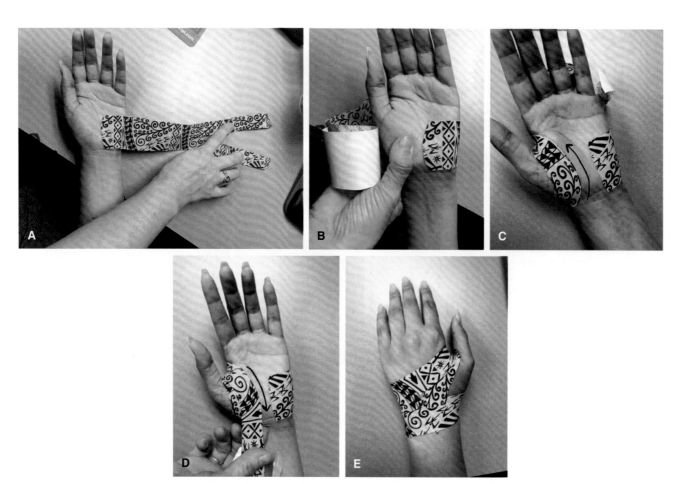

FIGURE 13–30 **Carpal tunnel. A.** Anchor a Y-cut at the ulnar border of the carpal tunnel. **B,** Wrap the tape around the dorsum of the hand. **C,** Take the proximal cut of the Y and wrap in between the webspace while holding the thumb in ABD and extension. **D,** Use the other tab to wrap around the CMC joint and then distally up through the webspace reinforcing the thumb position in ABD and extension. **E,** Hold the tape in place for 30–60 seconds to adhere the tape. Completed taping.

Carpal Tunnel

This taping (Fig. 13–30A–E) mechanically opens the carpal tunnel. Evaluate the tape as it crossed through the webspace and along the dorsal hand. This is an area that has an increased risk for irritation due to the natural wrinkles in the webspace and thinner skin on the dorsal hand. Symptoms should decrease immediately. If there is any increase in symptoms, remove the tape immediately. Figure 13–31A,B shows an optional application technique.

Carpometacarpal Joint

This taping (Fig. 13–32A–E) is used for CMC arthritis, laxity, post-op arthroplasty, or texting thumb. This taping opens the webspace and realigns the CMC joint. Pay attention to the areas of tape that overlap. If the client complains of a pulling sensation, gently pull the skin out from under the tape to relieve the pressure. This taping should immediately reduce symptoms. If any pain or discomfort increases, remove the tape.

WEBSITES

Dynamic Taping. www.dynamictape.co.
Kinesio Taping. www.kinesiotaping.com.
McConnell Institute. www.mcconnell-institute.com.
Nicholas Institute of Sports Medicine and Athletic Trauma. www.nismat.org.

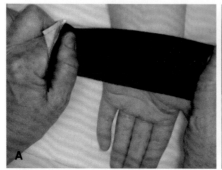
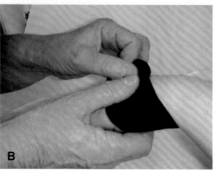

FIGURE 13–31 **Carpal tunnel. A,** Position the hand in tolerable wrist extension. Apply correction tape ("1"-cut tape with all stretch taken out of the center and applied directly down onto the area) over the transverse carpal ligament. **B,** Move the wrist into relaxed flexion and apply the ends without tension (shown here with KT Tape).

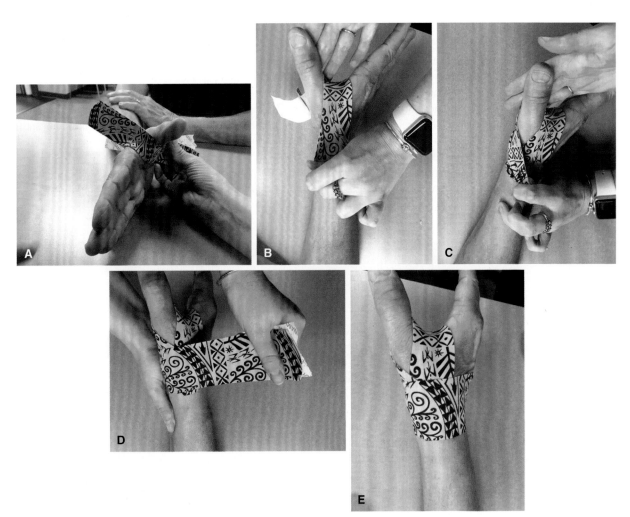

FIGURE 13–32 CMC joint. A powerband or the Eco tape approximately 1 1/2″ should be used for this taping to increase the stability and support for the CMC joint. **A,** Anchor the tape to the volar MP joint. **B,** Mobilize the thumb into extension and ABD to open the webspace. Adhere the tape between the webspace through the dorsum of the hand. **C,** Wrap the other side around the thumb midmetacarpal overlapping the dorsal hand piece. This will support the CMC in place. **D,** A second 2″ piece should be anchored on the ulnar border of the carpal tunnel and wrapped around the CMC joint onto the dorsal radial border of the wrist. **E,** Hold the tape in place for 30–60 seconds to adhere the tape. Completed taping.

PerformTex. www.performtex.com.
Rock Tape. www.rocktape.com.
SpiderTech. www.spidertech.com.
Taping Supplies. www.medco-athletics.com.
Theratape Company. www.theratape.com.

CONCLUSION

The use and application of any of these methods is only limited by the creative skills of those trained to apply these tapes. Training is recommended for each technique to provide proficiency and improve comprehension of the underlying mechanisms and associated therapeutic programs prior to application to clientele. The clinician must have an extensive clinical knowledge of anatomy, kinesiology, and the physiology of healing to determine if taping is indicated and, if so, to determine the best choice of technique and material. Note that each patient and injury is unique and requires a comprehensive evaluation by the physician and therapist before therapy intervention (Austin et al., 1994). The evaluation should include knowledge of the physical demands and requirements of the patient, the structure(s) involved, the degree of injury, and the stage of healing.

Patients using taping techniques should be closely monitored. Frequent reevaluation of the injured body part, healing process, tension, and tape placement as well as the taping materials themselves is essential to maximize the success of taping as a method of treatment. Inspection of the completed taping should be conducted to ensure proper support and proper taping application. Patients are at risk for significant harm if they return to activity with inadequate support or limitation of movement. Therefore, sound professional clinical judgment and proper diagnosis are imperative to ensure a positive outcome. Treatment may also include instruction of proper tape application and removal by the patient, family member, or other caregiver. It is important to educate the patient about the precautions and to stress the necessity of frequent monitoring of the body part for changes in skin integrity and neurovascular and lymphatic function.

Taping is not for every patient or therapist and should be employed with caution and sound clinical judgment. In addition, taping should not be viewed as a replacement for traditional forms of orthotic management because it holds a special place in upper extremity rehabilitation. The advantages of soft tissue support and increased joint mobility that taping provides place it in a class of its own. Athletic taping has had a longer history and is supported by more clinical research studies than the other taping methods. The effectiveness of McConnell taping and elastic therapeutic taping to date has been primarily the result of years of anecdotal reports, clinical experience, and individual case reports. These, along with growing research studies, support the effects of these taping techniques.

Websites provide information on educational opportunities and links or resources for obtaining taping supplies. Some sites offer instructional vignettes to assist the novice. The limitations found with the application of orthoses may also be found with taping. For example, patients may not want to wear the tape in public or may object to wearing the tape for a prolonged period of time. Patients may become frustrated when learning to handle and manage the

tape. A strong patient-therapist educational base is important; but as with all new skills, it takes time and practice to develop proficiency. The growing use of taping to treat injuries is rapidly evolving. Clinicians should master these taping techniques and add them as an additional tool to further enhance a patient's treatment possibilities. Taping is an expanding area of practice and, as with all modalities, should be performed by a skilled clinician and only a part of a comprehensive rehabilitation program. Clinicians should stay abreast of new tapes and products as they enter the market because this will allow opportunities for further study in developing unique taping applications to address specific populations.

FIELD NOTE: THE ART OF KINESIO TAPING

Alison Taylor OTR/L, CHT, CKTP, CKTI
Texas

The ART of Kinesio taping does not just involve putting a piece of tape on a patient, but rather a thorough assessment of the six physiological systems that can influence pain that include skin, fascia, circulatory lymphatic, muscle, joint, and tendon.[1] By understanding these systems and how they influence pain, we can assist our patients on the road to recovery faster.

The Kinesio taping method was invented By Dr. Kenzo Kase in 1979 and has become an essential piece of the treatment plan for many hand therapists. If we listen to the descriptions of pain reported by our patients, we can accurately target which system needs to be addressed.

Where taping is therapeutic, it is also diagnostic. The information provided by the tape will make you look closer at the influence of joint alignment, muscle imbalance, origins and insertions, and the superficial sensory system. This in itself helps us progress in our assessment skills and may provide use with answers on how to treat some common but allusive diagnoses.

The 4 S's (skin, scar, swelling, and sensation) are areas we touch on in our treatments but are more influential on pain than we realize. The complexity of the skin, especially the epidermis or the "Outer Brain," will never be truly understood. By using the lightest taping, 0% to 20% tension, we can effectively influence this level and change the patient's outcomes (Fig. A,B).

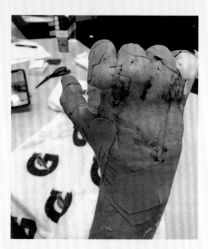

FIGURE B Complex hand injuries require complex taping. Taping for joint alignment, scar and skin movement, and nerve length.

Scar is something that is a significant contributor to pain. And the concept of changing scar after several years is unexpected. But by understanding taping and its influence on tissue movement and "lift", you can effectively remodel scar tissue. If the patient always moves in the same movement pattern, you will never change a scar; however, if you change the superficial tissue layers by the application of tape, you can subsequently influence the deeper layers, as demonstrated by Dr. Jean Claude Guimberteau.[2]

Kinesio taping is most recognized for its ability to move or channel fluid.[3] Pictures of bruises that have quickly disappeared are both dramatic and exciting. By changing pressure gradients and directing or "channeling" fluid to a healthier lymphatic location, we can prevent the influence of chronic swelling on tissues. This in itself will reduce pain and allow the patient to move faster through the recovery process (Fig. C,D).

The superficial sensory system has a great influence on the body; its feedback loop will allow or prevent motion. This system is responsible for perception and kinesthesia; it registers touch, vibration, temperature, pressure, and direction through a massive neural network. That as well as other sensory influences like the visual motor system, allow our patients to interact with the environment.[4,3] Studies show

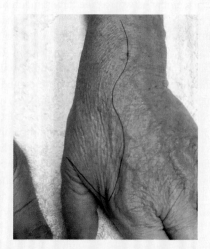

FIGURE A Skin pattern demonstrating impairment in the superficial branch of the radial nerve (SBRN).

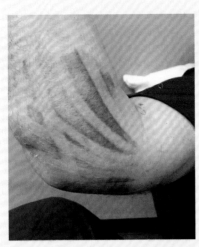

FIGURE C High- and low-pressure gradients with FAN taping, at 20% tension, demonstrates channeling of fluid (bruising).

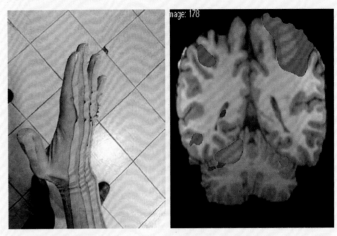

FIGURE E AND F Images borrowed with permission by Dr. Gustavo Mendoza MD, CKTI 2015. Study presented in KT 1 to 2 Lecture series 2,016.

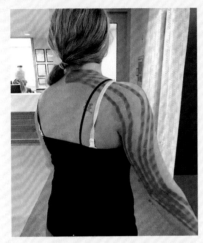

FIGURE D Fan taping to move fluid out of the limb from distal to proximal.

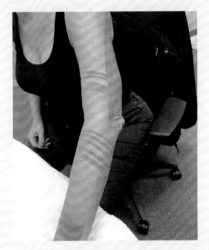

FIGURE G Taping for triceps for elbow joint approximation and serial taping for fascia can be beneficial.

that 0% tension with Kinesiotape, has a major influence on cortical perception. This means by applying tape to a flaccid, amputated, or injured limb, we can influence the brain and effectively start to retrain the patient to integrate both sides of the body.

Study demonstrating cortical imaging post finger taping with 0% tension. Red is resting level; blue is imaging after Kinesiotape was applied; and pink indicates overlap of cortical activity.

The influence of muscle and joint taping cannot go unmentioned since this is one of the greatest examples of Kinesio taping. By assessing kinematics during painful motion such as elbow pain with lifting or wrist pain with weight bearing, we can assess if joint alignment and muscle imbalance is creating a cycle of pain[5,6] (Fig. E,F).

Mechanical corrections of the radial head and posterior elbow during painful elbow activities have shown to be effective in the rehabilitation of lateral and medial epicondylitis[5] (Fig. G).

Joint corrections of the pisiform and the proximal carpal row also demonstrate a positive influence on the mechanics of the wrist in resisted and weightbearing activities (Fig. H). Taping in a similar pattern can assist in the recovery from with DeQuervain's tenosynovitis, TFCC injuries and SL repairs.

But most exciting is taping for the fingers, and the correction of soft tissue and joint "faults." By correcting joint positions, moving fluid,

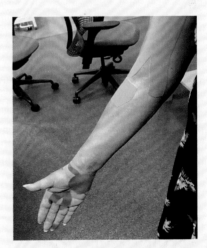

FIGURE H Muscle and joint corrections along the whole chain are required for complex hand issues.

mobilizing scar, and addressing soft tissue, we can help our patient navigate back to health quicker. Kinesio taping offers a treatment like no other to influence all these systems and rewards the patient and therapist when pain is eliminated, and ROM is improved which at times can be unexplainable (Fig. I,J).

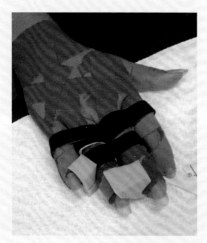

FIGURE I Creative alignment corrections of the fingers with tape and wedges.

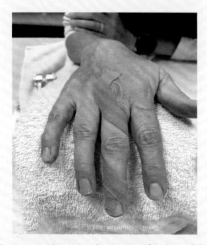

FIGURE J Alignment and rotational correction for the middle finger.

The tape is designed to do what the therapist's hands do, and no other modality allows the patient to "take you home with them." We therefore have a great tool in our toolbox that will help change our outcomes and progress our knowledge of the body and the influence of pain.

References

1. Kase, K., Wallis, J., Kase, T. (2003). *Clinical therapeutical applications of the kinesio taping method.* Tokyo, Japan: Ken Ikai Co Ltd.
2. Wong, R., Geyer, S., Weninger, W., Guimberteau, J. C., Wong, J. K. (2016). The dynamic anatomy and patterning of skin. *Experimental Dermatology*, 25(2), 92–98.
3. Williams, S., Whatman, C., Hume, P.A., Sheerin, K. (2012). Kinesio taping in treatment and prevention of sports injuries: A meta-analysis of the evidence for its effectiveness. *Sports Med*, 94, 2315–2328.
4. Hagert, E. (2010). Proprioception of the wrist joint: A review of current concepts and possible implications on the rehabilitation of the wrist. *The Journal of Hand Therapy*, 23, 2–17.
5. Amro, A., Diener, I., Bdair, W. O., Hameda, I. S., Shalabi, A. I., & Ilyyan, D. I. (2010). The effects of mulligan mobilization with movement and taping techniques on pain, grip strength, and functioning patients with lateral epicondylitis. *Hong Kong Physiotherapy Journal*, 28, 19–23.
6. Villafañe, J.H., & Valdes, K. (2015). Mobilization with movement and elastic tape application for the conservative management of carpometacarpal joint osteoarthritis. *Journal of Hand Therapy*, 28, 82–84.

 FIELD NOTE

Tissues do not fail because of pain; they fail because of load. If the load applied to a tissue exceeds its capacity to accommodate that load, pathology or damage can result. This can occur due to a single high force such as a fracture, from repeated subthreshold loads with inadequate adaptation or recovery periods resulting in a stress fracture or tendinopathy, or due to sustained loading where submaximal load is maintained for prolonged periods. While the mechanism may not be purely mechanical in some cases, load is a key driver of the pathology. If the load is modified and managed, the tissue will be able to heal.

Ryan Kendrick *MPhtySt, BPhty* (Developer/Owner of Dynamic Tape, 2020).

CHAPTER REVIEW QUESTIONS

1. What are the popular taping methods discussed in this chapter and how do they differ?
2. For what injuries is athletic taping most often used? Give three specific examples.
3. Before the application of athletic tape and McConnell taping, are there any additional procedures that must be done?
4. Name a minimum of three indications of use for elastic therapeutic taping.
5. What is a power strip and when is it appropriate to use?
6. What are the precautions for each taping technique?

ACKNOWLEDGMENT

Special thanks to Ryan Kendrick, MPhtySt, BPhty, for his help in the Dynamic tape portion of this chapter and Kevin Auffrey, ATC, for his input, guidance, and many photographs of the three athletic taping techniques reviewed in this chapter.

14 Neoprene Orthoses

Sabrina Cassella, MEd, OTR/L, CHT

CHAPTER OBJECTIVES

After study of this chapter, the reader should be able to:
- Describe the history and evolution of neoprene materials and its unique application within the field of upper extremity rehabilitation.
- Appreciate the properties and characteristics of neoprene materials.
- Understand the use of neoprene for joint positioning, mobilizing tissue, and in creating functional orthoses.
- Develop the clinical reasoning skills and techniques required to reproduce the orthoses described.
- Appreciate the innovative characteristics and boundless possibilities that neoprene offers the clinician when faced with alternative orthotic management.

KEY TERMS

Breathoprene
Comfortprene
Contact dermatitis
Direction of stretch

Hook receptive
Latex allergies
Neoplush
Neoprene
Polychloropene

Prickly heat (maliaria rubra)
Seam tape
Unbroken loop

INTRODUCTION

This chapter is written to inspire and stimulate the creative use of **neoprene** material in daily practice. Threaded throughout this chapter, the reader will find highlights from the first and second editions blended with new and innovative uses of neoprene. Within this chapter, it is unrealistic to include all of the possibilities that can be made with this versatile material. It is the intent of the author to provide a frame of reference and, in doing so, inspire the reader's imagination and creative thought. This chapter is predominately based on experience because there is little research available on custom neoprene orthotic fabrication. Throughout this chapter, the reader will find case studies and clinical pearls that portray the innovative process of using this unique and adaptable material. The content encompasses the results after trial and error, patient feedback, physician support, and collegial contributions.

The goal is to keep it simple by using materials commonly found in the average hand therapy clinic. There is no cookbook approach to making a neoprene orthosis especially because there is little need for pattern usage. The historical use of neoprene, quick and easy alternative fabrication techniques, and a host of strapping methods will be discussed. The scope of orthotic management with neoprene is vast, owing only to one's creative imagination and the complete understanding of the underlying diagnoses to which these devices are applied.

HISTORY OF NEOPRENE

Neoprene was invented by DuPont scientists in 1930 to provide an alternative to natural rubber as the demand and price for this resource increased. It was the first synthetic rubber product ever created and also goes by the name **polychloroprene**. Neoprene is a synthetic, latex-free polymer, making it an excellent option for the growing number of people with **latex allergies**. During World War II, all the available neoprene went toward war efforts to make products like tires, hoses, and fan belts. Neoprene is still used today for products such as wet suits, automobile tires, and the soft coating around exercise weights (American Chemistry Council, 2012; Colditz, 1999; Trujillo & Amini. 2013).

Neoprene conforms and drapes, making it easy to work with. This unique orthotic fabrication alternative can offer support to the incorporated joint(s) while still allowing for some mobility (Colditz, 1999). There are many neoprene products available on the market. Besides traditional neoprene, there are also neoprene-like products such as **Breathoprene™**, **Neoplush™**, and **Comfortprene™**. The reader is referred to the resource section for a current list of neoprene suppliers and products.

CHARACTERISTICS OF NEOPRENE

There are many characteristics of neoprene that make it an excellent choice for orthotic fabrication.

- Neoprene is available in various thicknesses ranging from 1.5 to 6.0 mm (or 1/16″–1/8″). These measurements pertain to the rubber core and do not take into account thickness of the material added by backings, such as nylon knit or loop (Colditz, 1999).
- Neoprene is more resistant to water, oils, and heat than natural rubber (American Chemistry Council, 2012).

- Traditional neoprene is nonperforated, which makes it an excellent insulator. Perforated options may help patients who tend to sweat readily or for use during athletic competition.
- Neoprene is elastic in nature. Neoprene's rubber core has equal stretch in all directions. The laminated top layers, commonly nylon knit, terry cloth, or loop material, can affect the direction of stretch (Colditz, 1999).
- Neoprene can be directly adhered to thermoplastic materials and tapes.
- Custom neoprene orthoses can be fabricated to immobilize, mobilize, or restrict motion.
- The "wetsuit" properties of neoprene also allow patients to wear the strapping or orthosis during "sweat or wet" activities. This characteristic may increase wear compliance and patient satisfaction.
- Neoprene can be easily cut/trimmed without risk of fraying edges and material breakdown.

DIRECTION OF STRETCH

The **direction of stretch** should be considered when deciding the goal of the orthosis. If the desired goal is to *restrict* motion, then the direction with the *least* degree of stretch would be applied to the target joint. If support *during motion* is the goal, then the direction of *most* stretch is applied around the joint (Colditz, 1999).

MOBILIZATION FORCE

With escalating costs and decreasing reimbursements for many therapy services, fabrication of mobilization orthoses can be an expensive treatment option. Based on the elastic properties of neoprene, the material can be used as a "dynamic" force in the fabrication of mobilization orthoses instead of using traditional rubber bands. "Orthoses made of neoprene material have the advantage of being pliable and at the same time can be constructed as dynamic orthoses" (Punsola-Izard, Rouzaud, Thomas, Lluch, & Garcia-Elias, 2001).

TYPES OF LAYERS

The following are types and characteristics of the laminated top layers commonly found on neoprene.

Unbroken Loop (Defined in This Chapter as "Hook Receptive")

- Feels similar to loop strapping material; readily attaches to hook material
- Adds bulk to the neoprene (is thick)
- Reduces the amount of stretch and drape
- Offers maximum durability for exterior or interior linings
- Feels cushiony, fuzzy, and warm against the skin
- Takes no time to add fasteners (use hook strap directly anywhere)
- Allows quick application of supportive straps for any orthosis

Nylon

- Adds no bulk to the neoprene (is thin)
- Allows full stretch and drape
- Provides moderate durability of exterior or interior linings
- Does not have ability to directly attach to hook or loop material
- Takes time to add fasteners such as rivets
- Feels slick and cool against the skin

Terry Cloth

- Adds no bulk to the neoprene (is thin)
- Allows full stretch and drape
- Provides maximum durability for interior linings (rarely used on exterior)
- Takes minimal time to add fasteners (use hook strap for short term, iron-on fasteners for permanent use)
- Feels soft and cool against the skin

PRECAUTIONS AND CARE OF NEOPRENE

Although it is rare, there are reported cases of allergic **contact dermatitis** (ACD) and **prickly heat (miliaria rubra)** caused by neoprene use (Colditz, 1999; Stern, Callinan, Mark, Schousboe, & Yutterberg, 1998). When dispensing a prefabricated or custom neoprene orthosis, it is important to instruct patients to frequently monitor skin integrity. The warm compressive qualities of neoprene may be very inviting to some patients, but for others, it may be intolerable. Caution should be used when dispensing these orthoses for use during strenuous exercise, heavy manual labor, or for use in very warm climates. Skin breakdown and maceration may become problematic (Colditz, 1999).

To reduce the risk of skin irritation, the orthosis should be frequently hand-washed with mild soapy water or machine washed in a gentle cycle with all hook and loop fastened (Colditz, 1999). Neoprene orthoses should be thoroughly air dried before reapplication to prevent skin breakdown and irritation. Patients wearing neoprene straps during wet activities such as swimming will require a second set of straps to allow complete drying of wet straps prior to reapplication. Wearing stockinette sleeves under a neoprene orthosis may help to absorb sweat but will not act as a barrier to ACD (Stern et al., 1998). Neoprene that has perforations may be useful in minimizing issues related to sweat and perspiration by allowing greater air exchange.

WHY CHOOSE A CUSTOM VERSUS PREFABRICATED NEOPRENE ORTHOSIS?

Custom options allow flexibility to make adjustments and alterations based on specific patient needs and evaluation findings. Patterns or designs can be adjusted and easily modified to accommodate the special requirements of each patient. By considering the alternative fastening techniques described in this chapter, fabrication time for these custom neoprene orthoses can be significantly reduced.

The traditional fabrication of custom-made neoprene orthoses required sewing or the use of iron-on seam tape and glue (this technique is found in Appendix A). This process was lengthy and depended on clinics to be equipped with a sewing machine, iron, or special dowels to accommodate for using seam tape. In a fast-paced rehabilitation setting, this option may be impractical for some therapists due to time constraints, thus making a prefabricated neoprene orthosis the desired alternative. Proper fit of prefabricated devices can be challenging as well as costly in that most clinics do not have the resources to stock all the necessary inventory of types and sizes available. The fabrication techniques described in this chapter offer another alternative and cost-effective way to customize these soft orthoses without the use of a sewing machine, seam tape, special iron, or glues.

CREATIVE FABRICATION AND FASTENING TECHNIQUES

The following are the fabrication and fastening techniques used by this author. Many of the tools and supplies used are common items found in a hand therapy clinic setting.

Fabrication Supplies

- Neoprene material (preferably hook receptive)
- Scissors
- Rivets (various sizes from small to large)
- Blunt-nosed pliers
- Quality hole punch
- Spot heat gun
- Adhesive-backed foam or Moleskin-type material
- Adhesive-backed hook
- Solvent (optional)

There are several options to consider for fastening and creating a custom neoprene orthosis. The techniques described attempt to keep the fabrication process simple with no sewing, gluing, or seam tape required. Strong hook receptive backing on neoprene has decreased the need to sew or iron-on strap attachments (Beasley, 2011).

Attaching Neoprene to Thermoplastic

Adhesive Hook

- Apply adhesive tab to desired location on thermoplastic orthosis.
- Place trimmed and previously fitted neoprene strap.

Rivet (A–E)

- To prevent removal of strap, a speedy rivet can be used in combination with the adhesive hook (the addition of adhesive hook assists in "grabbing" the loops on the neoprene material and

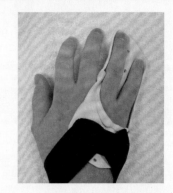

Neoprene is a nice option for functional orthoses, allowing muscle movement beneath the strapping as seen in this digit immobilization orthosis.

prevents the hole in the neoprene from stretching out and eventually popping up and over the rivet).
- Using a hole punch, make a small hole through all three layers of material (thermoplastic, adhesive hook, and neoprene).
- A rivet can then be placed through this hole and set with blunt-nosed pliers.
- Homemade rivets can be easily made using small scrap pieces of thermoplastic (refer to clinical pearl list for this option).

Direct Adherence (A–E)

- When using a coated thermoplastic material, apply solvent to desired area.
- Using a heat gun, warm thermoplastic material for 5 to 10 seconds until area is tacky but does not lose shape.

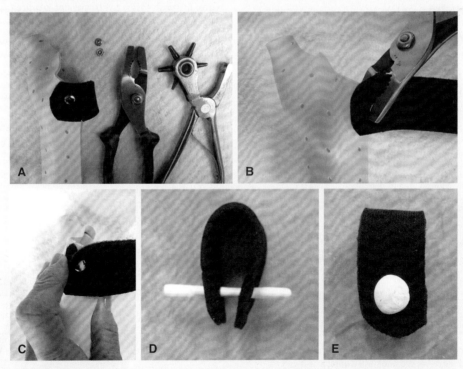

A, The materials required for riveting through thermoplastic and neoprene. **B,** Securing rivet through thermoplastic. **C,** Rivet in place through neoprene and adhesive hook. **D,** A small piece of thermoplastic is heated and rolled into a thin tube. Using the rivet punch, a hole is placed into neoprene material where it is to be connected. Push thermoplastic tube through holes and "hyperheat" each end using a heat gun. **E,** Flatten warmed material into a wide, round surface maintaining gentle pressure until material hardens over the neoprene material.

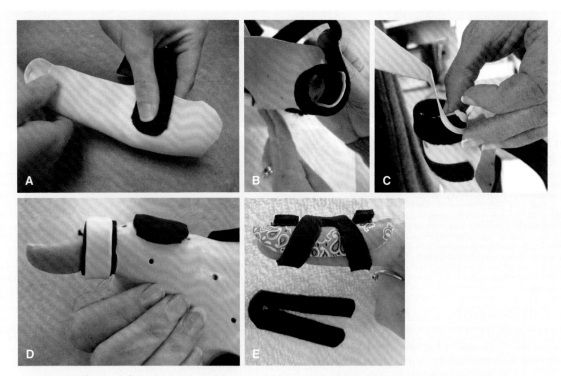

A, Direct adherence of neoprene to thermoplastic material. **B,** A piece of neoprene can be used as a volar support to the thumb proximal phalanx within an immobilization orthosis. **C,** A rivet or thermoplastic strip can be added for extra reinforcement. **D,** A ring of thermoplastic can be adhered over neoprene if increased stabilization of the thumb is necessary. This is an excellent alternative for those patients who do not tolerate thermoplastic against skin. **E,** This concept can be applied to other digits as shown in this PIP extension immobilization orthosis. The neoprene provides a flexible, bivalved strap to secure the orthosis while maintaining PIP extension.

- Place and hold neoprene to this area for 15 to 20 seconds with good prolonged compression.
- If necessary, for added security, the fabricator can add an additional piece of thermoplastic material over the top of the adhered strap. This will be applied over the strap borders and onto the thermoplastic base.

Attaching Neoprene to Neoprene
Heated Hook Material (A,B)

- Using a heat gun, hyperheat the precut length of adhesive-backed hook for 5 to 10 seconds until edges begin to curl.
- Place hook on desired location of neoprene and apply moderate pressure, paying special attention to the edges to ensure a good bond.

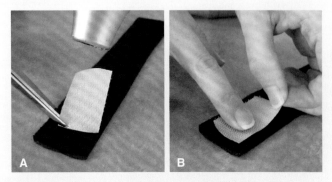

A, Hyperheat adhesive hook to apply to neoprene. Scissors or pliers can be used to hold a piece of adhesive-backed hook while using a heat gun to activate the adhesive. Hold the tab approximately 2″ from heat gun for 5 to 10 seconds. This method is intended to hyperheat the adhesive backing. The warm "tacky" glue should then penetrate and seep into and between the fabric fibers of the neoprene, further securing the hook onto the neoprene. **B,** Applying pressure to secure adhesive hook.

- This technique can work alone or can be used in conjunction with rivets for a more secure application (see instructions in the following text).

Rivets (for Use as a Closure)

Note: *In most cases, rivets are not required with the use of a highly adhesive-backed hook (described in* chapter 5). *The following use is described as an additional option for the fabricator in cases where excessive force or pull is required that exceeds the strength of the adhesive-backed adhesive.*

- Using a heat gun, hyperheat the precut length of adhesive-backed hook for 5 to 10 seconds.
- Place hook on desired location of neoprene and apply moderate pressure, paying special attention to the edges to ensure a good bond.
- Using a hole punch, create small holes for rivets on the edges of hook. Consider application of a rivet where there is likely the most force or pull from neoprene or application of the orthoses or strap. The rivets should be of adequate size; a rivet that is "too

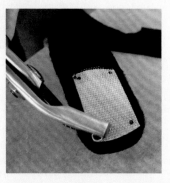

Securing rivet through adhesive hook and neoprene.

large" may lead to irritation of the skin against the rivet. Consider Moleskin or similar type padding over the rivet that is in direct contact with the skin.

- Place a rivet through each hole and secure with blunt-nosed pliers.

Rivets With Hook, Foam, or Moleskin (to Act as a Washer)

- In cases where rivets are attached to neoprene without adhesive hook, it is recommended to apply foam, a small piece of adhesive hook, or Moleskin-type material to the neoprene at the area where the rivet will be applied.
- This will in turn function as a "washer," preventing the material from pulling through the riveted area after repeated use.
- The author has found that using this technique disperses the pressure of the rivet head, therefore increasing the life span of the custom orthosis.

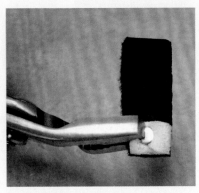

Securing rivet using a foam "washer."

CREATIVE USES OF NEOPRENE

A wide variety of conditions exist that may benefit from soft neoprene orthoses. Many patients prefer soft orthoses, which may improve orthosis wear compliance, and often these soft devices are more easily tolerated versus thermoplastic ones (Beasley, 2011). Custom orthoses can promote independence with daily activities, help decrease pain and stress on joints, and facilitate patients returning to self-care/work following injury or surgery. Custom neoprene orthoses can be flexible or semiflexible, depending on the fabrication techniques chosen and the addition of thermoplastic stays or supports (Beasley, 2011). Therapists are only limited by their own imagination! The following are examples of how the author has used neoprene for patients with a wide variety of diagnoses.

THUMB AND DIGITS

Interphalangeal Joints

Using small or scrap pieces of 1/16″ or 3/32″ neoprene material, custom orthoses can be fabricated for the digits. Patients following digital nerve repairs or amputations may benefit from custom neoprene digit sleeves. These patients often present with hypersensitivity to touch and/or vibration and temperature intolerance. Custom digit sleeves can offer protection while still allowing flexibility to incorporate the affected digit in activities (Fig. 14–1). Buddy strapping can be helpful following collateral ligament repairs, complex fractures, tendon repairs, or arthroplasty to encourage or maintain proper digital alignment (Beasley, 2011) (Fig. 14–2A,B).

To mobilize the proximal interphalangeal (PIP) joints, distal interphalangeal (DIP) joints, and intrinsics, dynamic PIP/DIP straps can be made using a safety pin or staple for closure or simply adhering it onto itself (Fig. 14–3A,B). This allows for a gentle progression of stretch as a patient's range of motion (ROM) improves.

A gentle composite stretch is being applied to the extrinsic extensors by applying a dynamic stretch via neoprene distally to the PIP and DIP joints. Note the strip of Microfoam Tape that is applied to the volar aspect of the neoprene strap in order to apply an antiskid property to the strap (Fig. 14–3C). Immobilizing the metacarpophalangeal (MCP) joints in extension, in combination with PIP/DIP mobilization straps, will provide an isolated stretch to the intrinsic muscles. This simple approach allows for an easy, quick, and inexpensive alternative to traditional mobilization orthoses (Fig. 14–3D).

First Carpometacarpal Joint

Patients with first carpometacarpal (CMC) joint osteoarthritis (OA) can benefit from pain relief with the use of a properly constructed neoprene orthosis (Beasley, 2011). Traditionally, patients with thumb OA are prescribed hard thermoplastic thumb orthoses. Many patients are intolerant of this option and/or have difficulty using these for daily activities including work-related tasks. Orthoses are commonly used to decrease pain and joint stress, minimize deformities, and provide support (Beasley, 2012). Studies have shown that patients with CMC and MCP joint OA prefer soft neoprene orthoses when compared with the traditional hard plastic option (Weiss, LaStayo, Mills, & Bramlet, 2004). Patients with MCP

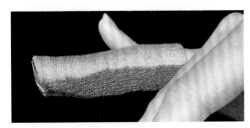

FIGURE 14–1 Digit sleeve using Orficast™ Tape for closure of the neoprene material. This was fabricated to provide gentle digit extension. This same orthosis can be made using a thin strip of thermoplastic for closure.

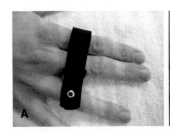
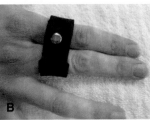

FIGURE 14–2 A, A proximal phalanx orthosis (Buddy strap) showing adhesive hook riveted to neoprene. Strap was fabricated with hook receptive backing facing away from skin. **B,** Orthosis/Buddy strap shown applied to a patient.

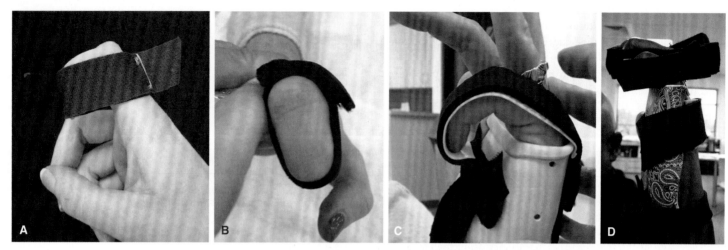

FIGURE 14-3 A, Traditional PIP/DIP orthosis utilizing nylon-backed neoprene and a safety pin. **B,** Simple neoprene and adhesive hook for a low-profile PIP/DIP strap. **C,** Composite isolated digit flexion with a gentle neoprene flexion stress. Note the strap is lined with Microfoam tape to prevent the neoprene from "slipping" off the digit. **D,** MCP extension immobilization orthosis combined with PIP/DIP mobilization straps for isolated intrinsic stretching.

and/or CMC joint OA may benefit from a soft, flexible support to complete the simplest activities of daily living (ADLs) (Leonard, 1995). The author of this chapter has had great success using custom neoprene orthoses for this patient population as an alternative to, or in conjunction with, traditional thermoplastic devices. Patient feedback supports the use of orthoses during all activities with improved comfort and pain relief. Patients that need to wear gloves at work report that a glove can be easily applied over this low-profile orthosis. A strip of thermoplastic or thermoplastic tape can be added to increase the stability of the first CMC joint. Another option can be to bivalue the terminal strap to have top section traverse through the web space and the bottom section pass beneath the first CMC both ending up on the radial dorsal portion of the hand.

Additionally, a trial with 11 patients utilizing a custom neoprene orthosis with thermoplastic stabilization showed decrease in pain after 30 days. After 90 days with the use of this custom option, pinch and grip strength improved (Bani et al., 2014).

CUSTOM NEOPRENE FIRST CMC ORTHOSIS

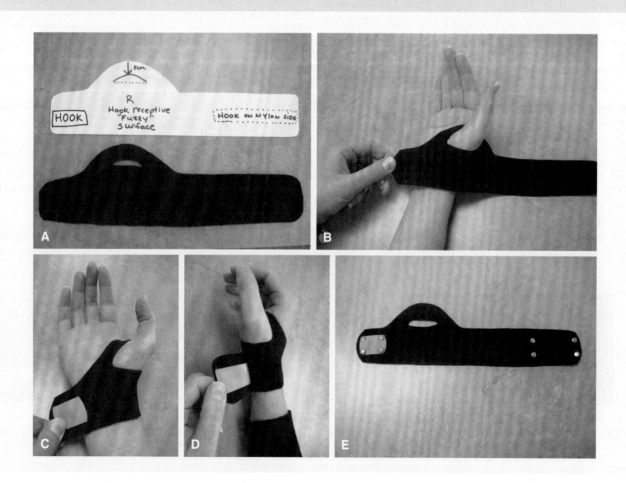

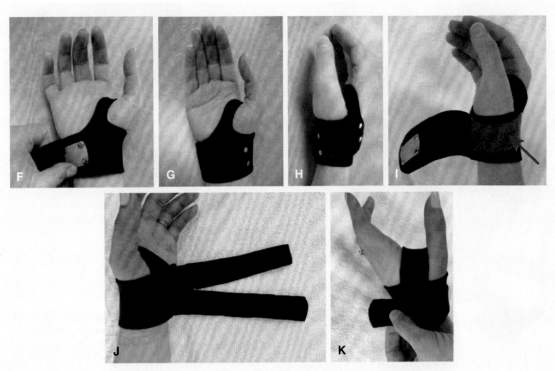

A, Create pattern as shown, being attentive to which hand, right or left, the orthosis is being fabricated for. One generic template can be used, making adjustments for wrist and hand size; orthosis pattern demonstrated here is for right hand. Note that for clarity of this pattern fabrication, the soft hook receptive side will be termed the *fuzzy* side. This becomes important when attaching the closures. Trace pattern using school chalk onto the fuzzy side of the neoprene. Cut out pattern from neoprene. Mark and center the thumb placement by measuring approximately 2 cm from the apex of the pattern. The shape of the thumb opening should follow the general curve of the neoprene pattern. Fold material in half to line up traced thumb marking and cut along this line. This cut should resemble a thin crescent moon shape rather than an oval or a circle. **B,** Place neoprene on the patient to assess size (nylon surface should be against skin). Check for fit of thumb opening, adjusting as needed. Ideally, the orthosis should rest on the midshaft of the first metacarpal. **C,** Trim the volar ulnar arm (ulnar tablike piece) of the neoprene material to end at the midulnar border of the hand. Cut a piece of adhesive hook approximately 4 cm in length (make sure to round corners to reduce lifting of borders). Apply the adhesive hook on the ulnar tab of the neoprene (fuzzy side). The placement of this adhesive hook acts as a catch to maintain proper position of the "wrap around" nature of the orthosis. **D,** Next, address the dorsal radial arm of the material by gently pulling it around the dorsum of the hand to meet the "ulnar tab." Once the dorsal strap has met this "tab" continue to wrap in a radial dorsal direction as shown. This is the time to measure for the length of this segment. Trim any excess that may go beyond the head of the second metacarpal. Cut a piece of adhesive hook approximately 7 cm in length. This piece of adhesive hook should begin approximately at the flexor carpi radialis (FCR) insertion and end at the midshaft of the second metacarpal. Attach this piece of adhesive hook to the nylon side of the radial segment as shown. **E,** Ensure orthosis fits patient comfortably and the adhesive hook pieces are correctly placed. Using a rivet punch, make holes on all four corners of each piece of adhesive hook. This helps to prevent lifting of the corners of the adhesive hook for longevity of the orthosis. If irritation occurs with rivets placed at the ulnar tab, consider applying two rivets at each end instead of the four described here. Placement of rivets: Radial arm: Ensure that the cap segment (not stem) of the rivet is on the **opposite** side of the material that the adhesive hook lies on. Ulnar arm: The stem segment should be placed against the skin with the cap segment on the **same** side of the material that the adhesive hook lies on (as the cap segment may irritate the skin). **F,** With the forearm supinated as shown, apply neoprene material through thumb opening. The descriptions that follows is for patient instruction on proper application of the orthosis. Pull the ulnar arm of the neoprene toward the pisiform, simultaneously grab the radial arm, and pull in a volar ulnar direction, aiming to meet the adhesive hook on the ulnar tab. Once connected, continue to wrap across the volar wrist, capturing the radial thumb column and terminating about the midshaft of the second metacarpal. **G,** Volar view of completed orthosis. **H,** Radial view of completed orthosis. **I,** In this neoprene thumb orthosis, the Orficast Tape provides additional stabilization to the first CMC joint. Other materials such as uncoated thermoplastic material (sticky) or Quickcast tape can be added to an area where extra support is desired. **J,** Alternate design of this custom orthosis for the patient requiring greater 1st web space abduction. **K,** Follow steps A-C. Cut length of the radial arm longitudinally as shown and wrap through first web space. Adhesive hook is applied to distal ends of radial arm tabs for closure. Length and width can be modified specific to patient needs and amount of abduction deformity that may be present.

For patients with rheumatoid arthritis (RA), neoprene orthoses can ease stress on joints when manipulating objects and prevent further advancement of joint deformity. The patient with RA often experiences inflammation, pain, and sensitivity about the affected joints (Beasley, 2011). Studies have shown that the use of a stabilizing orthosis to reduce joint mobility during times of acute inflammation can decrease joint friction and prevent excessive joint loading (Beasley, 2012). In a study by Callinan and Mathiowetz (1996), it was found that 57% of patients with RA preferred soft orthosis options as compared to those fabricated from traditional rigid thermoplastic materials. Compliance with the use of soft orthoses was 82% compared to 67% with hard orthoses (Fig. 14–4A–D).

Nerve Injury

Following nerve repair, patients require an orthosis to help maintain proper joint positioning and facilitate functional use of the involved extremity while awaiting nerve return. This is often referred to as antideformity orthotic management. The author has used neoprene to create some alternative options to traditional orthotic fabrication techniques for this patient population.

Ulnar Nerve

Some patients have difficulty tolerating thermoplastic MCP extension restriction orthoses (traditionally termed *anticlaw orthoses*)—a well-accepted protocol following ulnar nerve repair.

This soft alternative is best for people with more subtle clawing of ulnar digits as seen with high ulnar nerve lesions (refer to Chapter 20 for more detail). Thermoplastic reinforcement can be added to the neoprene, over the dorsal digits, to improve pressure distribution and offer increased stability if necessary (Fig. 14–5A,B).

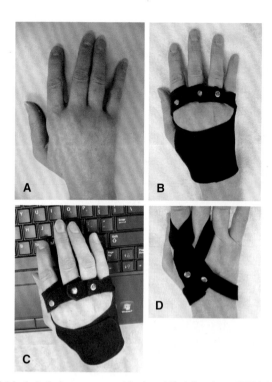

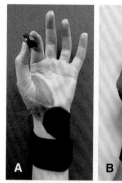

FIGURE 14–6 **A,** Opposition strap using Orficast Tape adhered to neoprene. **B,** This thumb abduction/opposition strap is being used 6 weeks after median nerve repair to improve functional position of the thumb column for prehension.

Radial Nerve

Fabricating custom orthoses for patients with radial nerve or posterior interosseous nerve palsies can be challenging.

Traditional functional custom orthoses may be bulky and oftentimes consuming to fabricate, also requiring frequent adjustments and repairs. Orthoses can be fabricated using neoprene alone or in conjunction with a thermoplastic material to provide a low-profile option for these often-frustrated patients. Because of neoprene's elastic properties, the dynamic force it imparts can be used to support the weakened digit and/or wrist extensors. In the radial nerve injured hand, this can translate to a low-profile design, assisting the weakened or absent extensors while allowing unimpeded wrist and/or digital flexion (Fig. 14–7A–F).

WRIST AND HAND
Wrist Instability

From simple wrist irritation to complex instability issues, many patients can benefit from custom wrist neoprene orthoses. Simple circumferential wrist wraps can be fabricated with 1/16″ neoprene to provide light support and compression for patients, including athletes or workers with mild wrist pain or discomfort (Beasley, 2011) (Fig. 14–8A,B). Ulnar-sided wrist pain is a commonly reported symptom by patients after wrist injury. Ulnar variance and/or triangular-fibrocartilage complex (TFCC) injuries are a common cause of this pain. TFCC tears can cause changes to the relationship of the radius an ulna creating a positive ulnar variance (Shim, Im, Lee, Kang, & Cho, 2019). One option that is relatively low profile and has shown effectiveness is the use of a WristWidget™. A custom neoprene option that simulates this concept has been used by this author with reported success. The soft neoprene edge about ulnar head and customizable width assists with the ease of use with sport and work activities. The neoprene material allows for use in wet activities such as swimming.

Patients experiencing wrist instabilities may require more support to decrease pain during active ROM, especially with forearm rotation. This can be accomplished with a thicker 3/32″ neoprene or neoprene combined/adhered to thermoplastic material. As noted by Beasley (2011), foam padding can be strategically added to help increase compression provided by these soft orthoses.

FIGURE 14–4 **A,** Patient presents with ulnar drift deformity at MCP joints from RA. **B,** Custom-fabricated neoprene orthosis demonstrating improved digit alignment. **C,** Patient using orthosis during functional activity. **D,** A similar design for a patient requiring only index- and middle-finger realignment.

Median Nerve

Following median nerve repair, opposition straps are commonly fabricated to assist in maintaining a wide first web space and thumb opposition/palmar abduction. This orientation places the thumb in a functional position for pinching and fine motor activities (refer to Chapter 20 for more detail). The authors have used a combination of Orficast™ adhered to neoprene to increase and maintain the pull into opposition, creating proper purchase about the first CMC joint (refer to Chapter 11 for more details) (Fig. 14–6A,B). These designs can be modified to meet the needs of other neurologic diagnoses including post–cerebrovascular accident (CVA) and spinal cord injuries.

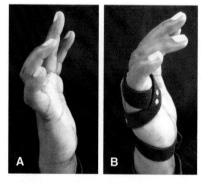

FIGURE 14–5 **A,** Patient with a claw deformity following a high ulnar nerve injury waiting return after motor nerve grafting. **B,** Custom neoprene MCP extension restriction orthosis.

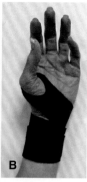

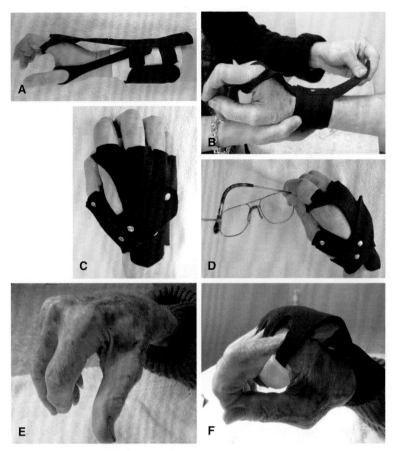

FIGURE 14–7 A, Using a thermoplastic forearm cuff, neoprene is attached to provide both dynamic wrist, thumb and digit extension. **B,** Dynamic distal forearm-based composite light wrist and digit extension orthosis for patient with returning radial nerve palsy. **C,** Dynamic hand-based digit and thumb extension orthosis for a patient with posterior interosseous nerve (PIN) palsy. **D,** Patient demonstrating functional pinch using custom orthosis. **E,** Patient presenting with loss of extensor digitorum communis (EDC). **F,** Custom orthosis fabricated with foam applied over the dorsum of the MCPs to promote functional pinch and gentle digit extension.

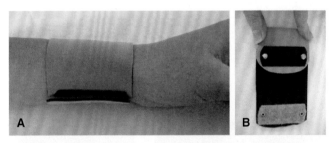

FIGURE 14–8 A, Simple circumferential wrist orthosis fabricated from nylon-backed neoprene. **B,** Adhesive hook and adhesive loop riveted to material for closure.

CUSTOM NEOPRENE WRIST WRAP

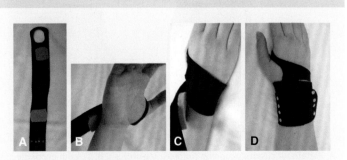

A, Pattern for custom wrist wrap. **B,** Application of wrist wrap with dorsal to volar pull aligning foam pad over ulnar head. **C,** Second foam pad placed over same location for increased pressure volarly to stabilize ulnar wrist. **D,** Completed wrist wrap with riveted adhesive hook for closure.

Wrist and Thumb

For patients with a combination of thumb and wrist pain, a custom neoprene orthosis can be designed to provide dynamic support and compression allowing earlier return to previously painful activities. De Quervain tenosynovitis is a common diagnosis resulting in thumb and radial wrist pain. A neoprene orthosis can be created to assist in dynamic thumb extension. These soft devices can be especially welcoming to those who are sensitive over the first dorsal compartment. Thermoplastic material or casting tape "struts" can be simply adhered to the neoprene material giving it additional reinforcement to decrease the load on the inflamed tendons. Due to neoprene's elastic nature, it can provide compression and support for repetitive motions for populations like musicians or new mothers (Beasley, 2011) (Fig. 14–9).

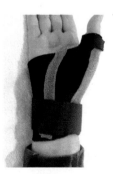

FIGURE 14–9 Custom wrist and thumb orthosis fabricated for an active patient with a history of mild CMC OA and de Quervain tenosynovitis who requires support to engage in recreational activities such as kayaking and golf. Notice the Orficast™ Tape adhered to provide rigidity and extra support to the design.

FOREARM

Many patients following wrist or elbow fractures have difficulty regaining forearm rotation. Straps made from neoprene can be used to provide a dynamic passive stretch into supination and/or pronation. These straps can be used alone or in combination with a distal thermoplastic component (such as a forearm-based wrist immobilization orthosis) to better isolate forearm rotation and distribute forces directed to the forearm.

CUSTOM NEOPRENE FOREARM SUPINATION/PRONATION ORTHOSIS

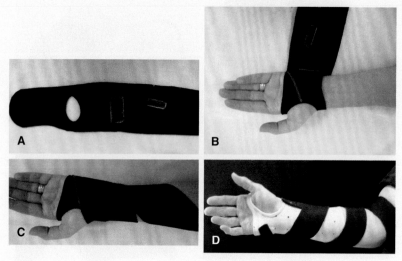

A, Pattern for forearm supination mobilization orthosis. **B,** Orthosis application with chalk outline for the angle of pull across palm and hook to prevent neoprene from separating. **C,** Showing proximal application of orthosis on patient. **D,** Patient status after open reduction internal fixation (ORIF) for a distal radius fracture using a supination mobilization orthosis combined with a wrist immobilization orthosis. Combining this forearm rotation strap with an immobilization orthosis allows for supination (or pronation) forces to be isolated to the forearm.

ELBOW

Proximal Forearm Straps

A common condition seen among manual laborers and athletes is medial and/or lateral epicondylitis involving the proximal insertions of the wrist muscles. Counterforce braces/orthoses have been used to help disperse force and strain on the involved tendons for many years. In application of these devices, caution has been promoted to avoid compression of radial nerve over the supinator muscle (Carin, Borkholder, Hill, & Fess, 2004). Custom neoprene orthoses allow for these proximal devices to be fabricated with optimal fit, taking into consideration the size of the arm, location of pain, and where the patient feels the greatest amount of relief when compression is applied. Foam or silicone inserts can be used under the orthosis to increase the specificity of the force being applied. Similar straps can be fabricated to treat bicep or triceps tendonitis as well.

Elbow Sleeves/Straps

Custom elbow sleeves can be used to protect sensitive structures about the forearm and elbow. Padding can be added to provide cushioning over bony prominences, soft tissues, or nerves that are irritated. Patients with cubital tunnel often complain of pain during activities; protective padding of the medial elbow may offer some relief (Beasley, 2011).

Many patients who undergo an ulnar shortening osteotomy experience extreme sensitivity over hardware. The plate often needs to remain in place until there is evidence of complete bony healing. Patients may find relief and protection from a custom elbow/forearm sleeve combined with silicone or foam padding placed over the sensitive region to relieve pressure and function as a barrier to external forces (Fig. 14–10A,B). This may help patients to resume

CUSTOM NEOPRENE COUNTER FORCE ORTHOSIS

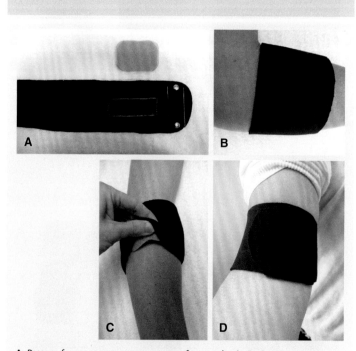

A, Pattern for custom neoprene counterforce orthosis. **B,** Custom neoprene counterforce orthosis on patient. **C,** Foam applied over proximal extensor carpi radialis brevis (ECRB) muscle belly to provide counterforce. **D,** Similar pattern used for patient with distal bicep tendonitis, using hook-backed silicone as counterforce to prevent distal migration of orthosis.

CUSTOM ELBOW ORTHOSIS

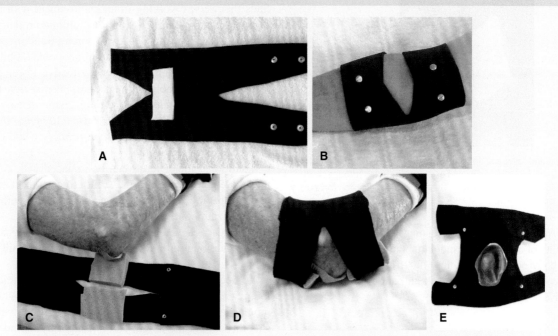

A, Pattern for custom elbow orthosis/sleeve with foam padding placed over the cubital tunnel. **B,** Elbow orthosis shown on patient. **C,** A patient with scleroderma with chronic olecranon ulcer using custom neoprene orthosis to reduce pressure and facilitate healing. **D,** Custom orthosis shown on the patient. **E,** Gelbodies™ silicone insert used in custom neoprene elbow sleeve to pad olecranon.

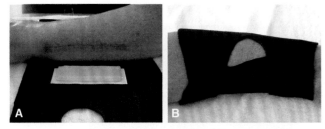

FIGURE 14–10 A, Sensitive ulnar forearm scar following ulnar shortening osteotomy with custom orthosis and silicone insert for protection and scar management. **B,** Orthosis shown on patient.

daily activities or return to work sooner. A clinician may encounter a patient who has a sensitive scar after carpal tunnel release, trigger finger release, or a nerve repair. These patients often have pain with grasping and weight-bearing through the affected wrist and hand. Silicone gel sheeting or elastomer molds can be held in place using neoprene over the affected area providing protection and improved tolerance to temperature and vibration (Beasley, 2011).

CREATIVE NEOPRENE STRAPPING WITH CUSTOM THERMOPLASTIC ORTHOSES

Neoprene's soft elastic nature makes it a comfortable and conforming strapping option. Elastic materials are helpful in maintaining more constant and consistent pressure as patients move and function during ADLs and work tasks, allowing muscles to contract and relax beneath the straps (Beasley, 2011). The author has experienced that the life span and durability of neoprene straps is far greater than the traditional loop or hook receptive strapping products available. Neoprene allows for creative and custom strapping options with minimal to no fraying and

material breakdown. For example, straps can be cut extra wide to more evenly distribute pressure over an edematous hand or wrist. Custom neoprene straps can be split to increase orthosis stability or increase conformity about joints and/or bony prominences (Fig. 14–11A–E).

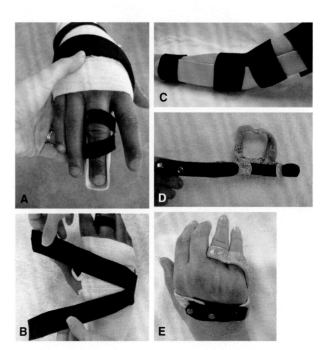

FIGURE 14–11 A, Split strap maintaining PIP extension stabilizing both proximal and middle phalanges. **B,** Bivalved neoprene strap providing stabilization through first web space and around wrist to prevent migration of orthosis. **C,** Large neoprene strap placed over anterior elbow to maintain elbow positioning within orthosis. Strap is split on both sides to increase contour about the elbow. **D,** Traditional MCP extension restriction (anticlaw) orthosis with single neoprene strap pulled through holes in thermoplastic; strap is weaved through neoprene similar to buddy strap design described earlier. **E,** Shown on patient with strap closed.

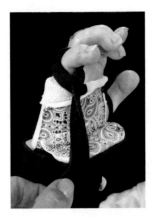

FIGURE 14-12 Soft and "dynamic" finger loop option has been created for this patient with scleroderma by weaving one end of a neoprene strap through small slit in the distal end forming a "loop or sling." Then a gentle MCP flexion force is applied to mobilize the MCP joint.

These characteristics make it a great strapping option and may help to maintain stability of a custom thermoplastic orthosis while patients engage in their daily activities. Colditz (1999) noted that neoprene straps are an excellent option for people with pain, hypersensitivity, edema, or sensitive bony prominences.

MOBILIZATION OPTIONS

Dynamic mobilization options are widely used to address ROM and subsequent functional deficits in patients. Traditional options can be cumbersome for a patient to apply thus contributing to a decrease in compliance and anticipated outcome. Traditional options can also be challenging to fabricate for the less experienced clinician who finds themselves working in an environment with little resources. Components for traditional options (aluminum outriggers and pulley systems) can be quite costly to purchase and for some clinics and situations, cost prohibitive. Custom neoprene mobilization options provide an opportunity for a cost-effective lower profile orthosis that is easily adjustable by the patient. *Please note that traditional rules apply for timelines of healing, tissue density, and end feel. Experience and skill is suggested when applying this technique to ensure force is applied most appropriately while considering the above factors.*

Traditional finger loops can be replaced with custom neoprene loops. Neoprene provides the ability to custom fit each finger loop to meet specific patient (width and angle) needs with the fabrication of mobilization orthoses (Fig. 14–12).

Neoprene can be used to apply a gentle dynamic stretch to a targeted joint or multiple joints with a mobilization orthosis (Fig. 14–13A–H).

A piece of neoprene can be used as a dynamic "low-profile" mobilization force when attached to a base with a homemade thermoplastic outrigger. The strip of neoprene is cut with several small slits throughout the length and is caught by the hook. This allows for the patient to control the progression of the dynamic stretch being applied to the tissue (Fig. 14–14).

Neoprene strapping can be used to mobilize the digits and thumb while the patient is immobilized or casted (Fig. 14–15A,B).

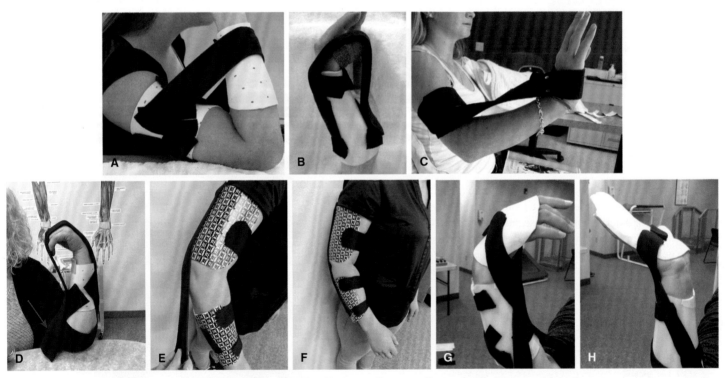

FIGURE 14-13 A, Elbow flexion mobilization orthosis using forearm and humeral cuff with neoprene strap for a patient following open reduction internal fixation (ORIF) of an olecranon fracture. **B,** Dynamic PIP flexion mobilization orthosis with a DIP extension immobilization cast in order for the flexion forces to be solely directed to the PIP joint. **C,** Dynamic wrist extension and elbow flexion mobilization orthosis following an elbow joint debridement in this college gymnast. **D,** Composite wrist and digit flexion mobilization orthosis following wrist fracture. **E,** Elbow extension mobilization orthosis using forearm and humeral cuff with neoprene strap to assist with regaining terminal extension of elbow following open reduction internal fixation (ORIF) of an olecranon fracture. **F,** Humeral and forearm cuffs can be lined with neoprene that has the nylon layer removed to expose rubber core to reduce migration of mobilization orthosis. **G,** Wrist flexion. **H,** Composite wrist/hand/thumb extension.

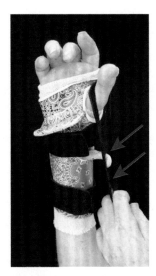

FIGURE 14–14 Strap used within an immobilization orthosis for progressive thumb web space mobilization.

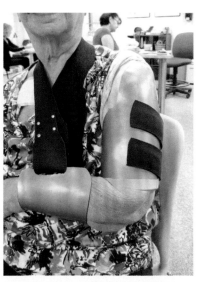

FIGURE 14–16 Custom "cuff and collar" sling for patient following humeral fracture.

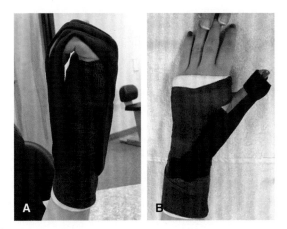

FIGURE 14–15 A, Strapping used as to gain composite flexion while patient still in cast. Adhesive hook can be adhered directly to fiberglass cast. **B,** Finger loop strapping can be used to provide gentle stretch to an adhered flexor pollicis longus (FPL) tendon.

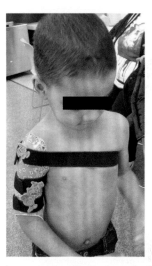

FIGURE 14–17 Strap shown on a Sarmiento-type orthosis to stabilize proximal border of orthosis and prevent migration. The brace is adorned with stickers for increased compliance and acceptance of orthosis.

ALTERNATE USES

Neoprene allows for many other creative uses in a therapy clinic.

- Neoprene can also be used to fabricate custom slings and/or supports for patients with proximal upper extremity fractures or pathologies (Fig. 14–16).
- Straps can be used to stabilize a nonarticular orthosis such as a humeral fracture brace owing to gentle expansion and contraction of tissues with movement (Fig. 14–17).
- Patients experiencing limited hand function may encounter other challenges in their daily life, such as donning and doffing orthotic devices. Creative uses of neoprene can help provide solutions for previously difficult tasks (Fig. 14–18).
- Prefabricated orthoses can be customized to meet individual patient needs. For example, a prefabricated neoprene thumb and hand orthosis can be quickly converted with a custom neoprene strap to incorporate the wrist for a patient with de Quervain tenosynovitis who requires a flexible wrist support to return to work (Fig. 14–19A–C).

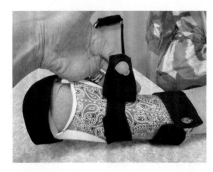

FIGURE 14–18 Neoprene loops added to this custom-made dorsal-volar wrist/hand immobilization orthosis for a patient with increased flexor tone. The loops within the straps provide for ease of donning and doffing when bilateral dexterity and outside assistance is limited.

- Nylon layer can be removed revealing the rubber core of the neoprene material to be used as an antiskid layer. Hook-receptive side of neoprene can be adhered directly to thermoplastic by hyperheating the thermoplastic and attaching it (Fig. 14–20A–C).

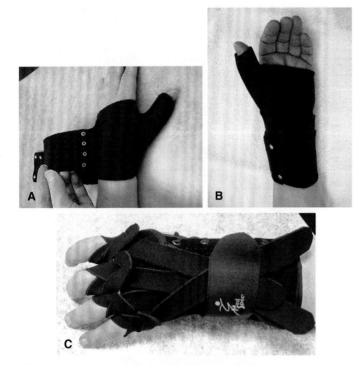

FIGURE 14–19 A, Neoprene strap riveted to a prefabricated neoprene hand and thumb orthosis. **B,** Illustrates completed design with additional custom wrist support. **C,** Neoprene "dynamic" MCP extension loops added to a prefabricated wrist immobilization orthosis for a patient with a radial nerve injury. Note how a "slit" in the distal end of the neoprene straps allows for the proximal end to feed through and form a "sling" to assist in MCP extension yet allow functional flexion. The straps attach to the hook on the proximal border of the orthosis. Dynamic finger extension loops added to prefabricated wrist immobilization orthosis for patient with radial nerve palsy.

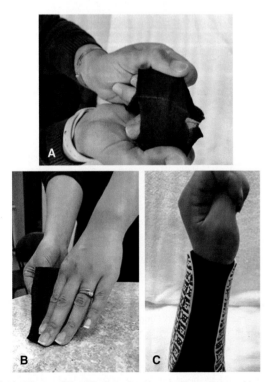

FIGURE 14–20 A and B, Nylon layer is stripped off revealing a rubber core that can act as a nonskid surface. **C,** An ulna osteotomy protective orthosis using a lining of neoprene where the nylon layer has been removed and used against the skin to assist with prevention of distal migration.

CONCLUSION

Neoprene is a versatile material used as a soft orthosis option based on its characteristics as described in this chapter. The use of neoprene as an orthotic material is appropriate for a wide variety of patients including those with arthritis, neurologic conditions, and orthopedic diagnoses to name a few. The author has only touched the surface of orthotic fabrication possibilities with neoprene; it is up to therapists to use these tips, practice their skills, and tap into their creativity to fabricate a truly custom device to meet the needs of their unique patient.

Case Study Section

The case studies presented here are meant as a teaching guideline only. Treatment and orthosis protocols vary greatly from surgeon to surgeon and from therapist to therapist. The therapist should check with the referring physicians and colleagues to define the preferred treatment and appropriate orthotic intervention.

Case Study 1: Rheumatoid Arthritis

A 47-year-old female patient presents with RA affecting bilateral hand and wrists, with pronounced symptoms in the right hand (Fig.14–4A). All digits present with ulnar drift at the MCP joints, with radial side of index MCP joint being acutely tender to palpation. Her wrist and hands are most painful at work as an administrative assistant with activities such as typing, sorting papers, and opening binder clips. She reports increased pain with home tasks such as gardening and cleaning. Bilateral custom immobilization orthoses were fabricated for night use (resting orthoses). A trial of Kinesio® Tape was applied to her right hand to aid in passively realigning her second- and third-digit MCP joints into radial deviation. This helped determine if a custom neoprene orthosis would be of benefit. Patient reported increased lateral stability (during lateral prehension activities) and decreased pain with the use of this tape. It was therefore concluded that a custom, more permanent strapping system should be devised to replicate the positioning offered by the Kinesio® Tape.

A custom neoprene ulnar drift orthosis was created (Fig. 14–4B). The orthosis was fabricated for all digits and was helpful in realigning the digits (specifically the proximal phalanges) during active use. The patient reports that the neoprene orthosis reduces her pain and increases her function with work and home tasks that were previously bothersome (Fig. 14–4C).

Prior to fabrication of such an orthosis, consider factors such as the following:

- Number of digits requiring support within the orthosis
- Amount of force required to realign the digit and whether force can be generated with neoprene alone or with an added piece of rigid thermoplastic
- Type of closure best suited for the patient for easy donning and doffing of orthosis (i.e., permanent closure vs. adjustable tabs with adhesive hook)

Case Study 2: Ulnar Instability

An 18-year-old female softball pitcher presented with a peripheral TFCC tear requiring surgical intervention. The patient requested to continue playing in order to finish the softball season. Her physician agreed and referred her for fabrication of a custom neoprene wrist wrap to support the ulnar wrist while she plays. The patient reported that she had significantly reduced pain with the use of the neoprene device, allowing her the chance to finish her season. The patient went on to have a TFCC repair and continues to use the neoprene orthosis for support to reduce the impact stress on the ulnar wrist while pitching.

Case Study 3: Wrist Fracture

A right-dominant 32-year-old mother of two tripped and fell down her front steps sustaining an intra-articular distal radius fracture (Barton fracture). She underwent open reduction and internal fixation. She was originally seen in the clinic before cast removal for digital ROM due to limitations noted at recent MD follow-up. Neoprene strapping was used to provide a gentle dynamic force to address the extrinsic and flexor limitations of the digits and thumb. The extra tacky adhesive hook adheres directly to the fiberglass casting and was used as the anchor point for the strapping (Fig. 14–15A,B). Post cast immobilization, she was placed into a custom thermoplastic circumferential "zipper" orthosis for additional protection. She began a guarded graded therapy program. Despite previous addressing of the extrinsics, there was continued wrist and digit soft-tissue limitations. Her wrist was very stiff wrist along with extremely tight extrinsic flexors and extensors of all digits and her thumb. A custom option of thermoplastic and neoprene was fabricated to address both extrinsic flexor and extensor limitations (Fig. 14–13D). This option allowed for ease of donning/doffing and compliance with wear schedule due to her line of work. Tension was progressed in the clinic and subsequently by the patient at home. She wore this option for approximately 4 weeks two to three times daily. Functional improvements were made for ADL's as well as the patient was able to return to practicing yoga.

Case Study 4: Elbow Fracture

An 18-year-old female athlete suffered a displaced olecranon fracture after falling down her college dorm stairs. She underwent open reduction internal fixation (ORIF) and was treated with immobilization for 2 weeks. She was referred to therapy after 4 weeks for gentle active ROM (AROM) of her elbow and forearm. Her AROM was as follows at initial evaluation: Elbow extension/flexion—50/110. Forearm supination/pronation—75/70. After 2 weeks of therapy, she followed up with her MD who referred her back to therapy for more progressive ROM. Forearm limitations were resolved. Two weeks later, with therapeutic intervention, elbow flexion progressed. However, terminal elbow extension continued to be problematic for this active patient. A custom orthosis of neoprene and thermoplastic materials was fabricated to address this 35-degree deficit (Fig. 14–13E,F). The patient was very compliant with this low-profile design. After 3 weeks of wear, two times per day (increasing wearing times per tolerance and balancing with total elbow ROM), she was able to regain the remaining degrees necessary to return to tennis.

CHAPTER REVIEW QUESTIONS

1. Describe the various types of neoprene materials that a clinician can choose from.
2. Why is the unbroken loop side of the neoprene important?
3. What are the advantages of a custom neoprene orthosis versus a prefabricated neoprene orthosis?
4. Give two examples of a diagnosis and neoprene orthosis management. Describe the advantages of the neoprene versus a thermoplastic orthosis in these two cases.
5. Give an example of two ways to apply adhesive-backed hook to a piece of neoprene material?

Orthotic Intervention for Specific Diagnoses and Populations

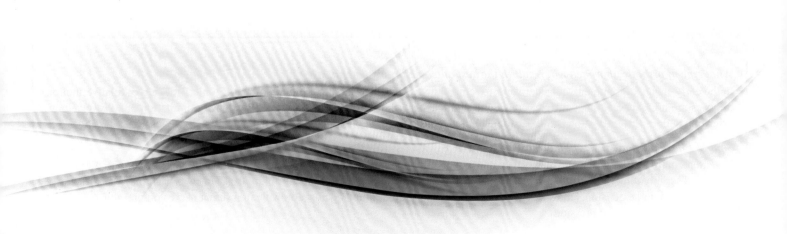

15 Stiffness[a]

Gary Solomon, MS, OTR/L, CHT

CHAPTER OBJECTIVES

After study of this chapter, the reader should be able to:
- Understand the causes and contributing factors to why segments of the upper extremity become stiff.
- Explain the common patterns of contractures that occur in the upper extremity after injury.
- Describe the various designs of orthoses that can be used in managing the stiff extremity.
- Become familiar with the preventative use that orthoses can play in managing common diagnoses that can lead to stiffness.
- Give examples of each type of mobilizing orthosis and the rationale for their use.

KEY TERMS

Adaptive shortening
Adhesion
Casting motion to mobilize stiffness (CMMS)
Dynamic orthoses
Extrinsic tightness
Hard end feel

Intrinsic tightness
Joint stiffness
Low-load, prolonged stress (LLPS)
Mobilization orthosis
Plaster of paris
Relative motion orthoses
Scar formation

Serial static orthoses
Static progressive orthoses
Soft end feel
Springy end feel
Stress
Torque-angle range of motion

We should regard the hand as a mobile organ and never let it stiffen. It must move to survive.

Sterling Bunnell, 1947

MD NOTE

Ajay K. Balaram, MD
Illinois

As a hand surgeon, I depend on hand therapists to mitigate the effects of trauma and surgical intervention to restore range of motion and function for my patients. Advances in fracture fixation as well as tendon and nerve repair provide opportunities for controlled early motion under a therapists' guidance. As a result, we are able to see substantially better range of motion and functional outcomes. When joints do demonstrate stiffness, therapists are able to fabricate a number of different orthoses to restore joint mobility. In my practice, we use a variety of interventions from a simple relative motion orthosis to a complex turnbuckle orthosis to restore motion. The type of intervention is as a result of collaboration between surgeon and therapist and dependent on the type of surgery and/or skeletal stability. This collaborative approach enables us to provide creative solutions to maximize range of motion even after significant traumatic injury.

FAQ

What type of orthotic approach will result in the best outcome for my patient, what factors should I consider?
In the early stages of treatment, consider ways to redirect active forces to facilitate motion of a stiff joint. Blocking or relative motion orthoses are a great place to start. Also consider a night static orthosis for issues such as PIP extension limitation or wrist or elbow extension deficit. If joint motion continues to be limited, consider supplementing with a dynamic or static progressive orthosis.

Should I have my patient wear an orthosis at night?
Research continues to support the importance of the total end range time (TERT) concept. A static orthosis positioning a joint at end range and serially remolded as motion improves is an excellent and effective approach for night use. This approach may be particularly effective for digital extension, elbow extension, and wrist extension. Caution against elbow flexion (ulnar nerve compression) and wrist flexion (median nerve compression).

---

[a]Based on 1st edition by Karen Schultz, MS, OTR/L, FAOTA, CHT and 2nd edition by MaryLynn Jacobs, MBA, MS OTR/L, CHT.

How much tension should I apply through an orthosis in order not to cause more harm?

Tension on an orthosis should be set at where a patient perceives a very gentle stretch. If a patient tends to be too aggressive, alternative static progressive components such as Velcro hook and loop strategically positioned may limit a patient's ability to go beyond recommended limits.

How will persistent edema affect my patient's stiffness?

Edema causes "drag" which significantly increases the work which must be done to move a joint through its range of motion. Although edema is often measured and identified as a "problem" upon evaluation, early and consistent management is a key component to decreasing stiffness. Light consistent compression, early motion within safe parameters, elevation, as well as simple manual techniques are important keys to limiting joint stiffness following acute injury.

INTRODUCTION

Dr. Paul Brand, in his influential book *Clinical Mechanics of the Hand*, compares the hand to a simple machine. A "motor" or muscle generates a force and pulls on a "cable" which transmits the force. The force acts on its end point, and feedback is instantaneously provided back to the "motor" with information to correctly calibrate the amount of force to achieve the desired task. This "machine" works on an environment where external forces may create resistance or "drag" which interfere with the mechanics of the machine. When problems occur with muscle, tendon, or nerve, or an increase in drag develops from edema, scar, or collagen disorganization, stiffness of the hand is often the result.

In the 1999 keynote address at the American Association of Hand Surgeons, Seminar on Joint Stiffness, Hardy noted that, although the profession has made great strides in hand surgery and rehabilitation, joint stiffness continues to remain a challenge (Hardy, 1999). **Stiffness**, the loss of normal passive range of motion (PROM) and active range of motion (AROM), remains one of the most common reasons for visiting an upper extremity specialist (Copeland, 1997; Means, Saunders, & Graham, 2011). Although the clinician has many weapons in the therapy armamentarium for improving ROM, orthotic intervention is one of the most powerful.

But how do clinicians know when to apply an orthosis and what type will offer the best outcome for the patient? To find the answer, therapists combine a thorough understanding of the diagnosis with a comprehensive evaluation. The clinician also needs the well-honed ability to see into the future. This does not suggest the ability to be clairvoyant but rather states the importance of knowing according to the tissues affected, the predictable effects of position, edema, the progression of wound healing (see Chapter 3 for more information), cortical reintegration, and the potential contractures.

The reader should keep in mind that although this chapter reviews several orthotic approaches in the mobilization of stiff tissues—dynamic, serial static, static progressive, orthoses to redirect active force including relative motion, blocking, and casting motion to mobilize stiffness (CMMS)—there is yet no agreed-on optimal approach (Michlovitz, Harris, & Watkins, 2004).

This chapter describes how the therapist applies knowledge of wound healing and of the unique anatomy and mechanics of the hand to predict and avoid or to evaluate and treat stiffness. After reviewing the nature and cause of stiffness, the effect of an orthosis to help restore movement is presented. Table 15–1 summarizes the common contractures seen in the upper extremity.

PATHOLOGY OF JOINT STIFFNESS

Trauma, especially in conjunction with necessary prolonged immobilization, often results in decreased tissue elasticity and PROM (Akeson, Ameil, Avel, Garfin, & Woo, 1987; Akeson et al., 1977; Akeson, Ameil, & Woo, 1980; Ameil, Woo, Harwood, & Akeson, 1982; Colditz, 2011; Enneking & Horowitz, 1972). This loss of joint flexibility has two major sources: **scar formation** and **adaptive shortening** (Flowers & Michlovitz, 1988). Both create formidable barriers to motion.

Following traumatic injury, the healing process has three distinct phases (Glasgow, Tooth, & Fleming, 2010). Initially there is an acute inflammatory response, followed by collagen being deposited (fibroplasia phase) and then remodeling. During the initial inflammatory phase, immobilization may either be required, or self-immobilization occurs due to pain and edema. Glasgow et al. (2010) describe the following process of collagen deposition during the Fibroplasia phase. "If continued immobilization is required during fibroplasia, detrimental changes within the joint commence. These include disorganization of cellular and fibrillar components of ligaments and the joint capsule, the development of adhesions between the folds of synovial lining, formation of fibrofatty connective tissue within the joint space, atrophy of cartilage and osteoporosis" (Glasgow et al., 2010). During the remodeling phase, tensile load of forces during movement of the structures of a joint allow disorganized collagen to be replaced, remodeled, and strengthened based upon the forces and elasticity required. If a joint is unable to move through full motion, collagen will continue to lay down in a shortened position, and a contracture may become permanent.

Formed to repair tissue defects, scar is deposited not only between discontinuous structures but also in uninjured tissues surrounding the wound. All wounded and some nonwounded structures become attached, resulting in the one wound/one scar phenomenon (Peacock, 1984) (Fig. 15–1) (Box 15–1). An **adhesion**, the pathologic attachment of one structure to another via scar, limits the excursion of articular and periarticular structures, restricting useful joint motion. As the scar matures over time, it contracts and becomes denser (Akeson et al., 1980; Frank, Ameil, Woo, & Akeson, 1985).

ADAPTIVE SHORTENING

Inflamed tissue undergoes remodeling in a shortened form when it is immobilized in a slack position and deprived of constant stress in the form of motion (Brand, 1985). Brand (1985) theorized that this adaptive shortening occurs when lack of stress signals the body to reduce tissue constituents, creating structures with less length. Inadequate tissue length limits joint motion. Both scar and normal tissue may become adaptively shortened and contribute to loss of motion.

STRESS AND RESTORATION OF PASSIVE RANGE OF MOTION

To reverse the motion-robbing effects of scar and adaptive shortening, the clinician faces the challenge of changing the length and

TABLE 15–1	Comparison of Orthotic Passive Mobilization Approaches		
Characteristic	**Dynamic**	**Serial Static**	**Static Progressive**
Force and ROM adjustment	• Establishes elastic tension that places tissue at maximum length • Some difficult controlling amount of force consistently • Patient can pull against the dynamic force, shortening the tissue on an intermittent basis, which thwarts the purpose of the orthosis (to hold the tissue at its maximum length for long periods of time)[a]	• Creates constant tension and joint positioning • End-range position with tolerable tension is easily achieved • Patient cannot move from the end range established by the clinician; orthosis holds tissue at its current maximum length	• Static progressive tension and joint positioning are infinitely adjustable • Always possible to establish a static tension that places tissue at maximum length but not beyond it • As tissue remodels into a longer form, orthosis can immediately be adjusted to capture increased length and PROM • Patient remains at end range until orthosis is readjusted to optimize the combination of ROM and tension
Tension	• Dynamic component continues to shorten even when tissue has reached the end of its available length. Improper tension may cause microtears and increased scar • Microtears, in turn, undergo the normal phases of wound healing • As the scar matures, it contracts and further limits PROM	• Holds the tissue at maximum length and does not stress beyond it	• If tension properly set, holds the tissue at maximum length and does not stress beyond it. Improper use may cause micro-tears and increased scar
Force control	• Springs and elastics deform over time • Neither clinician nor patient has control of forces	• Clinician has control over forces	• Clinician can maintain control over forces or instruct patient in proper use, so the patient has control • Patient education regarding being overly aggressive important
Orthosis tolerance and time dose	• Because dynamic component continues to shorten, it frequently stresses tissue beyond its available length, leading to poor orthosis tolerance and the inability to wear the orthosis for as many hours as required to achieve permanent length change[a]	• Appropriate stress fosters consistent orthosis wear, resulting in tissue growth and reorganization in a longer form and creating a permanent length change	• Appropriate stress fosters consistent orthosis wear, resulting in tissue growth and reorganization in a longer form and creating a permanent length change
Orthosis tolerance and sleep	• Because patient often cannot tolerate the orthosis during sleep, the orthosis must be worn during the day, which interferes with functional use of the hand • If the dynamic force is light enough to allow sleep, it probably is not taking the joint to end range	• Patient can tolerate the orthosis during sleep, minimizing need for daytime wear	• Patient may be able to tolerate the orthosis during sleep if only minimal end-range tension
Joint end feel	• Improves PROM in joints with soft end feel but is ineffective for hard end-feel joints	• Improves ROM of soft end-feel joints faster than do dynamic orthoses • Improves PROM in joints with soft or hard end feel[a,b]	• Improves ROM of soft end-feel joints faster than do dynamic orthoses • Improves PROM in joints with soft or hard end feel[a,b]
Efficiency	• May require increased time compared with other approaches	• Highly effective in increasing PROM, especially for patients with compliance and sensory problems	• Increases PROM faster than any other approach and, sometimes, when no other treatment approach is successful[c]

[a]Bell-KrotoskiJ. A. (1987). *Plaster casting for the remodeling of soft tissue.* In Fess E. E. & Phillips C. (Eds.), **Hand splinting: Principles and methods (2nd ed., pp. 453–454).** St. Louis, MO: Mosby; Bell-Krotoski J. A. (2011). *Tissue remodeling and contracture correction using serial plaster casting and orthotic positioning.* In Hunter J. M., Mackin E. J., & Callahan A. D. (Eds.), Rehabilitation of the hand: Surgery and therapy (6th ed., pp. 1599–1609). St. Louis, MO: Mosby, and Fess E. E. (2011). **Orthosis for mobilization of joints: Principles and methods (6th ed., pp. 1588–1598).** St Louis, MO: Mosby.

[b]Fess E. E. & Phillips C. (Eds.) (1987). **Hand splinting: Principles and methods (2nd ed.).** St. Louis, MO: Mosby.

[c]Bonutti P. M., Windau J. E., Ables B. A., & Miller B. G. (1994). *Static progressive stretch to re-establish elbow range of motion.* **Clinical Orthopedics and Related Research, 303,** 128–134.

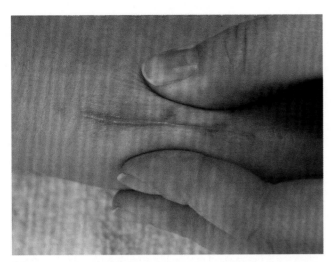

FIGURE 15–1 Adherent incision along the ulnar aspect of the hand interferes with tissue mobility and tendon excursion.

BOX 15–1 COMMON CONTRACTURES OF THE UPPER EXTREMITY

Joint	Contracture
DIP	Flexion or extension (decreased flexion or extension)
PIP	Flexion (decreased extension)
MCP	Extension (decreased flexion)
Thumb MP	Flexion (decreased extension)
Thumb CMC	Adduction (decreased abduction)
Wrist	Flexion and ulnar deviation (decreased extension and radial deviation)
Forearm	Pronation (decreased supination)
Elbow	Flexion (decreased extension)
Shoulder	Decreased flexion, abduction, and external rotation

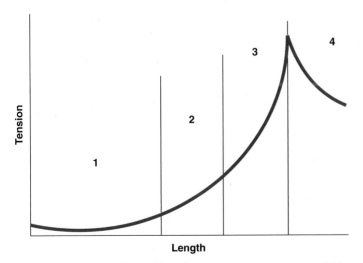

FIGURE 15–2 The four phases of the soft-tissue response to stress. 1 = unfolding, 2 = alignment, 3 = stiffening, 4 = failure. (Glasgow C., Tooth L. R., Fleming J. (2010). Mobilizing the stiff hand: Combining theory and evidence to improve clinical outcomes. *Journal of Hand Therapy*, 23, 392–401.)

density of the adhesions and shortened tissue. To achieve the desired length change, the clinician controls the environmental demands on the tissue and applies the mechanical stimulus of **stress**. Living tissue, including scar, will reorganize and change in response to stress.

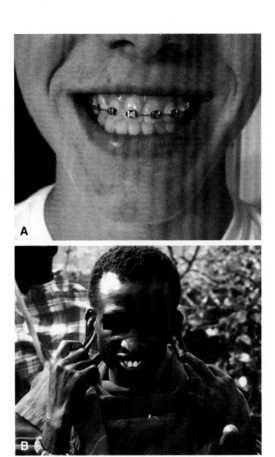

FIGURE 15–3 **A,** The theory of low-load, prolonged stress (LLPS) is applied in the practice of orthodontia. **B,** The elongated earlobes of this African man are the result of LLPS owing to the lifelong use of graded ear dowels.

The scientific community has not yet quantified the exact amount of stress required to stimulate change in tissue length. Research supports the hypothesis that the longer tissue remains at maximum tolerable length, the more it will increase in length (Cyr & Ross, 1998; Flowers & LaStayo, 1994, 2012; Glasgow, Tooth, Fleming, & Hockey, 2012; Glasgow, Tooth, Fleming, & Peters, 2011). Typically, the clinician employs experience and data from repeated evaluation to determine optimal stress loads. In addition to intensity, the clinician must also consider the effect of the variables' duration and frequency because they mediate total stress delivery (Flowers & LaStayo, 2012; Flowers & Michlovitz, 1988; Glasgow et al., 2012, 2011).

OPTIMAL STRESS APPLICATION: DELIVERY APPROACH

Low levels of applied stress initially result in the unfolding of collagen fibers. As more stress is applied, collagen fibers elongate and fibers realign. As further stress is applied, the fibers will reach an end tension and stiffen, and further stress beyond that point results in tissue failure (Glasgow et al., 2010). This principle is essential for clinicians to understand in order to provide the correct amount of stress to improve motion without resulting in tissue failure (Fig. 15–2).

Clinical experience, observation of some cultures' success at altering the body's configuration, and the orthodontic and orthopedic literature also support the use of **low-load, prolonged stress (LLPS)** over any other combination of load and stress for achieving permanent increase in tissue length and, therefore, in PROM (Arem & Madden, 1976; Flowers & LaStayo, 1994, 2012; Glasgow et al., 2012; Glasgow et al., 2011; Hotchkiss, 1995, n.d.; Light, Nuzik, Personius, & Barstrom, 1984) (Fig. 15–3A,B). Clinically, low-load, brief stress (LLBS); high-load, brief stress (HLBS); and high-load, prolonged stress (HLPS) have failed to demonstrate effectiveness in producing permanent length change. LLPS works by providing a mechanical stimulus that causes scar to remodel biologically into a permanently lengthened form.

LOW-LOAD, PROLONGED STRESS

The clinician has several options for applying LLPS to tissue. However, the most powerful LLPS technique of the longest duration is orthotic intervention. An orthosis maintains the tissue elongation gained during therapy, a home program, and functional use of the hand. Using low tension, it maintains the newly gained length over long periods of time. Brand (1985) theorizes that the application of mechanical stress via an orthosis signals contracted tissue to grow or add cells while the body absorbs redundant tissue. In the clinic, therapists note that an orthosis applied at end range brings about increases in PROM much more quickly than LLBS and exercise (Fig. 15–4A,B). Sometimes an orthosis creates increases in PROM that were previously unavailable by any approach short of surgery. McKee, Hannah, and Priganc (2012) caution the clinician that the duration of immobilization at end ranges may impair the nutrition of tissues and undesirably compresses articular cartilage. This is something the clinician should consider when using any orthotic intervention.

The decision to use a custom versus a prefabricated LLPS orthosis should be made based on a number of factors. However, for this patient population, it can be a challenge to replace a custom fabricated orthosis with a prefabricated one because so many factors have to be considered. No one stiff joint is the same as another. The hand therapy specialist possesses the knowledge base and the technical skill to create or prescribe the best orthosis to meet the specific goals of the patient.

EXPERT PEARL 15–1

Waiting...For Tissue to Grow
HandLab: Clinical Pearls

JUDY C. COLDITZ, OT/L, CHT, FAOTA
North Carolina

Doctors Brand and Hollister in the definitive text, *Clinical Mecha1nics of the Hand*, explain the difference between "creep" and "growth."[1] To paraphrase:

When composite cadaveric tissue (skin, for example) is stretched, it lengthens. Even if the tissue is not taken to the point of rupture, it will not return to its original length because it has undergone "creep." Creep is a gradual but permanent lengthening of the tissue due of slippage of short collagen fibers.

Because human cadaveric tissue responds this way to the stress applied, one might assume the same type of stress (stretch) needs to be applied to living tissue to create permanent change. But living tissue undergoes microscopic tearing of the fibers and cells, resulting in inflammation and small hemorrhages which leads to fibrosis that limits tissue mobility even more.

Living tissue held at its easy elastic limit, however, will activate the collagen fibers to turnover in a way that modifies the cross-linking of the fibers, allowing greater length. There is no creep or inflammation but rather a response that can be called "growth." Growth is unique to living tissue.

Growing Tissue

A symbol of status for the women of the Mursi tribe in the Omo Valley of southern Ethiopia is a large hole in the lip, created by inserting increasing diameter disks slowly over a long period of time. In Western cultures, silicone balloon expanders are placed under the skin near an area of tissue to be repaired. Slowly over time the balloon is ailed with salt water, causing the skin to stretch and grow so it is large enough for the planned procedure.

In both of these examples, the element of time and the consistency of low stretch creates the tissue response of growth.

Clinical Suggestions

With the concept of tissue "growth" as a background, here are some clinical suggestions to consider:

- Frequency of Serial Cast Changes
  Customary teaching about the application of serial casts to resolve flexion contractures of the small joints of the hand encourages changing the cast every few days. Clinical experience reveals that the first one or two casts usually brings about significant improvement, but there is diminishing response to continued cast changes over time. When the time between cast changes is increased, a significant improvement in both range of motion and quality of motion is noted, even with the most stubborn joints. When the cast is left on for longer intervals, often the active range of motion is greater than the maximum passive motion at the time of cast application.
  Why are increased intervals more effective? If one continues to change the cast every few days, the tissue response cannot keep pace. In other words, there is not enough time for the tissue to grow. A change of the first cast (or two) within a few days works well and slowly increasing the time between casts as the casting continues results in an improved response to each cast. If examination of the joint reveals a hard end feel, one knows immediately the intervals need to be longer to allow the collagen cross-linking to be modified so more motion is possible. These longer intervals, in addition to decreasing resistance to motion, also appear to minimize/eliminate any inflammatory response. The concept is to avoid pushing the joint to change and to give the tissue time and opportunity to make its own change.

- Exercise Frequency
  The more acute and inflamed the tissues, the more rest is needed, with exercises needing to be intermittent throughout the day but with a minimal number of repetitions. When a trigger finger or tendinitis develops during hand rehabilitation, excessive exercising is usually the culprit.
  It is logical to increase the frequency of exercise sessions before increasing the number of repetitions. Observation of the tissue response to the exercise will signal when the tissue is, or is not, ready for more exercise. Perhaps it is helpful to explain rest and exercise to patients this way: "If you moved your uninjured hand all day, it would be sore and swollen. Even uninjured tissues need a balance of movement and rest. Your injured hand needs more rest than exercise in the beginning. As you progress, your hand will tell you when your exercises are excessive by responding with increased pain, swelling and/or inflammation. You want to sneak into more exercise and not be excessive. A good guideline is to not move your injured hand more than your uninjured hand would easily tolerate."

- Tissue Maturity
  In many cases our patient treatment has a time limit imposed by third party payors (especially in the United States). This discharge deadline may cause us to urge tissues to reach their maximum pliability before that date. Regardless of treatment, tissue maturity following injury requires approximately 1 year, assuring that our patients continue to improve after discharge (especially when discharge is only after a few months since injury.) For a less experienced therapist to become comfortable with a less-than-full result when the patient is discharged, it may be helpful to ask the patient to return for an unofficial visit a year after the injury to simply allow the therapist to see the final result. Being assured that time for tissue maturation brings continued improvement allows us to be more tolerant of discharging a patient when less than total motion is present.

Brand P. W., Hollister A. M. (1999). *Clinical mechanics of the hand.* 3rd ed. St. Louis, MO: Mosby, Inc.

Clinical Pearls reprinted with permission from Clinician's Classroom at BraceLab.com written by Judy Colditz OT/L CHT FAOTA, copyright HandLab/BraceLab, Raleigh NC. No. 31, August 2014.

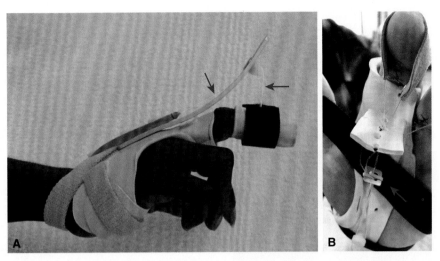

FIGURE 15–4 A, A proximal PIP extension mobilization orthosis (dynamic approach) using the Digitec outrigger system is applied with tension generated through a rubber band. Note the exact 90° angle of pull between the monofilament and the middle phalanx (arrow). Also note that if tension generated through the rubber band is too much, this patient may develop a pressure area at the dorsum of the PIP joint (arrow). This orthosis design can also be used as an exercise orthosis (with lighter rubber band tension), to generate resistance against the rubber band, facilitating PIP flexion. **B,** A PIP flexion mobilization orthosis using light "dynamic" rubber band tension. A tension adjustable finger loop (arrow) enables the clinician to easily set a safe amount of tension which can be tolerated for a long period of time.

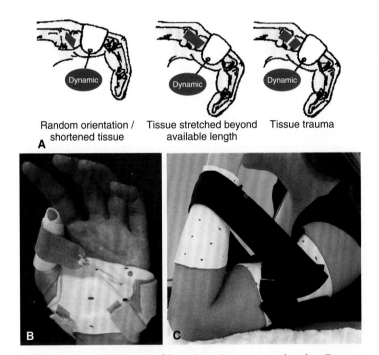

FIGURE 15–5 A, With the use of dynamic tension, care must be taken. Too much stress in healing tissues can promote increased inflammation and tissue damage. A dynamic orthosis generates tension as long as the elastic component can contract, even when the shortened tissue reaches the end of its elastic limit; thus, tissue trauma can result. **B,** A hand-based thumb MP mobilization orthosis is shown using light dynamic rubber band tension. The IP joint is casted in extension to best redirect the forces of flexion directly to the MP joint. **C,** Gentle elbow flexion mobilization is assisted with a wide custom cut neoprene strap.

CHARACTERISTICS OF APPROACHES IN ORTHOTIC INTERVENTION

When increasing PROM is the goal of the orthosis, the clinician may choose one of the three passive mobilization approaches: **dynamic**, **serial static**, or **static progressive**.

Orthoses can also be used to mechanically redirect ACTIVE motion force toward a stiff joint during active motion in order to improve joint stiffness. Examples of these orthoses are relative motion orthoses, blocking orthoses, and the technique of casting motion to mobilize stiffness **(CMMS)** which Colditz (2011) has described as

active redirection for management of the *chronically* stiff hand that is not responding to a more standard therapy approach.

DYNAMIC ORTHOSES

Dynamic orthoses have self-adjusting resilient or elastic components—such as spring wire, rubber bands, or springs—that create "a mobilizing force on a segment, resulting in passive or passive-assisted motion of a joint or successive joints" (Fess, 2011; Fess & Phillips, 1987; Glasgow et al., 2011) (Fig. 15–4A,B). In addition, dynamic orthoses allow active-resisted motion in the direction opposite of their line of pull (Fig. 15–4A). The dynamic tension generated continues as long as the elastic component can contract, even when the shortened tissue reaches the end of its elastic limit. Care must be taken to set tension lightly and educate patient on emphasizing light stretch in order to avoid trauma to tissues (Fig 15–5A–C). Glasgow et al. (2012 and 2011) found that with dynamic intervention, the most important predictors of outcome were the following:

- Degree of pretreatment stiffness
- Type of deficit (flexion improves faster than extension)
- Length of time since injury (<12 weeks) the dynamic orthosis was applied
- Amount of time throughout the day the device was worn

STATIC PROGRESSIVE ORTHOSES

Static progressive orthotic intervention involves the use of inelastic components, such as hook-and-loop strapping, static lines, progressive hinges, turnbuckles, and screws. These components allow progressive changes in joint position as PROM changes without needing to change the structure of the orthosis. Only the line of pull must be changed as PROM progresses. A static progressive orthosis holds shortened tissue at its maximum length (Fig. 15–6A–D). Because the components lack the elasticity of those used in a dynamic approach, the appropriately set tension of the orthosis does not continue to stress tissue beyond its current maximum length limit (Schultz-Johnson, 1992).

SERIAL STATIC ORTHOSES

Serial static orthotic intervention differs from a static progressive approach in that the clinician must remold the orthosis to accommodate increases in mobility. Proximal interphalangeal

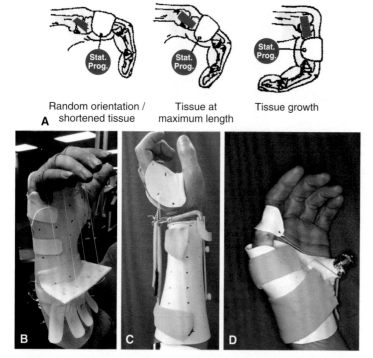

FIGURE 15–6 **A,** Because static progressive components lack the elasticity of those used for dynamic orthotic intervention, the appropriately set tension of the orthoses does not stress tissue beyond its current maximum length limit. Tissue lengthening occurs without tissue trauma. **B,** Static progressive stretch created with the use off a static line and hook and loop for a static progressive MCP flexion mobilization orthosis. **C,** Wrist extension using a Phoenix Wrist Hinge (Performance Health) and simple static hook-and-loop closures to create the static progressive approach, **D,** Thumb IP flexion mobilization orthosis using a MERiT⁻ component.

(PIP) serial casts and serial wrist extension orthoses exemplify this approach. The clinician establishes the tension of the orthosis to maximum tolerable end range. Therefore, the orthosis does not continue to stress tissue beyond its current maximum length limit (Schultz-Johnson, 1992). No change in joint position occurs until the clinician modifies the orthosis. Flowers and LaStayo (1994), (2012) have gathered data to substantiate Dr. Paul Brand's suggestion that a joint held in a lengthened position for a significant period of time will adapt to that length, causing growth of connective tissue about the joint. They have shown that the most effective form of stress delivery is to maximize the length of time that stress is delivered. Although their research was on the PIP joint, they propose that this principle could be applied to other synovial joints of the body (Flowers & LaStayo, 2012) (Fig. 15–7A–F).

RELATIVE MOTION ORTHOSES

While the restoration of PROM demonstrates the potential for improved function, the restoration of AROM is the desired end result. Relative motion orthoses (RMO) are important tools to restore proper force mechanics and balance to improve functional hand use. The orthoses act to redirect force toward the IP joints to either facilitate restoration of flexion or extension. Published uses of relative motion orthosis to restore movement include successful intervention for PIP flexion and extension lags (PROM > AROM) as well as PIP joint stiffness due to a number of hand pathologies (Hirth, Howell, O'Brien 2016) (Fig. 15–8A,B). Chapter 7 describes these in great detail.

BLOCKING ORTHOSES

Blocking orthoses can provide an excellent tool for rebalancing forces in the hand and facilitating IP joint flexion. By blocking the MCP joints in extension, flexion forces are redirected to facilitate PIP and distal interphalangeal (DIP) flexion allowing patients to improve joint stiffness and flexor digitorum superficialis (FDS) and flexor digitorum profundus (FDP) gliding. The use of a blocking orthosis should be considered when isolated MCP motion is relatively normal; however, PIP motion is limited (Fig. 15–9A,B). The external support of the MCP joints in extension creates a simple tool for patients to use to redirect active force to the limited joint(s).

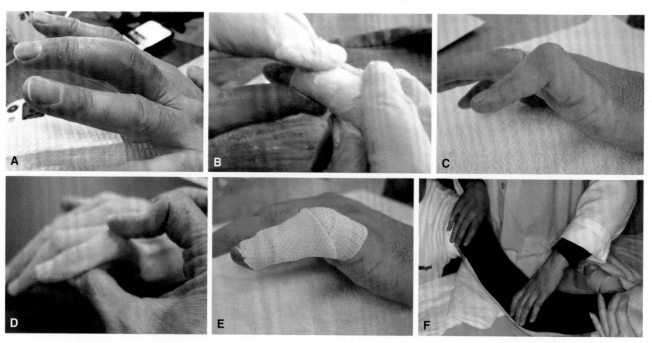

FIGURE 15–7 **A,** Proximal interphalangeal (PIP) flexion contracture and **(B)** serial static extension mobilization orthosis (serial cast) using plaster of paris (POP)—note the gentle extension pressure applied as the circumferential orthosis is being applied. **C and D,** Dense small finger (SF) PIP flexion contracture noted via the gentle passive extension **(D). E,** Application of a thermoplastic tape (QuickCast2, Performance Health) to statically place the joint into extension to allow the tissue/joint to accommodate to new length. **F,** An example of a serial static approach to gain elbow extension. Using an elastic-based material allows for frequent remolding as the tissues and joints respond.

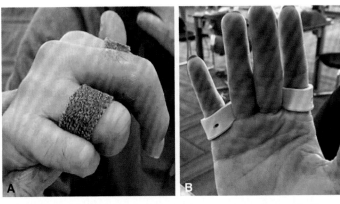

FIGURE 15–8 **A,** Middle finger relative motion extension orthosis to facilitate proximal interphalangeal (PIP)/ distal interphalangeal (DIP) flexion places the MCP joint in relative extension to other digits. **B,** A middle and ring finger relative motion flexion orthosis to facilitate PIP extension places the MCP joints involved in relative flexion to other digits. Both of these relative motion orthoses assist to address joint stiffness by facilitating motion.

CASTING MOTION TO MOBILIZE STIFFNESS

Colditz (2000), (2002), (2011) describes use of a nonremovable cast to direct *active* motion only toward the stiffest joints. The cast is used for the chronically stiff hand (Fig. 15–10A, B). (*Chronic* is defined as hard end-feel joint motion regardless of time since injury.) This technique is referred to as CMMS. Colditz (2011) purports this technique "simultaneously mobilizes stiff joints, reduces edema, and generates a new pattern of motion to revive the cortical representation of normal motion" (Colditz, 2011). The reader is encouraged to further study CMMS (Colditz, 2011) and make this approach an option for management of the chronically stiff hand. In this technique, a carefully molded cast from **plaster of paris** (POP) is applied. It is important to use a "highly compliant material" (Colditz, 2000), such as POP, to obtain an intimate fit and allow for prolonged wear with minimal risk of soft-tissue irritation. Immobilizing the proximal joints, including the wrist when the goal is mobilizing the digits, is necessary in order to focus and redirect all the power of movement to the targeted distal joints (Bell-Krotoski, 2011; Colditz, 2011). Chapter 10 reviews the application of POP in detail.

Advantages of CMMS (Colditz, 2011)

- Circumferential nature and light pressure applied by the cast aids in mobilization of edema.
- Joint motion is possible in both flexion and extension.
- Targeted repeated movement facilitates cortical integration.

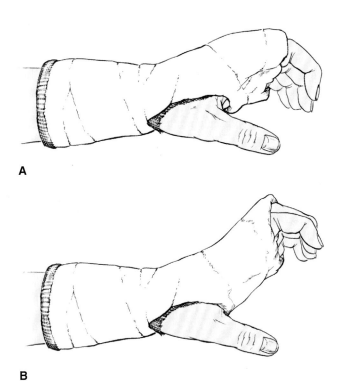

FIGURE 15–10 **A,** A circumferential wrist and MCP extension orthosis (without hood) isolates the proximal interphalangeal (IP) joints for active flexion and extension. **B,** This intrinsic stretching cast positions the MCP joints in full extension to encourage lengthening of the tight intrinsic muscles. (Photos courtesy of Judy C. Colditz).

- Cost of POP material is low.
- Therapy visits and cast changes are less frequent than with traditional therapy methods.

Challenges of CMMS (Colditz, 2011)

- Determined optimal cast design (decided by deficits in tightness and altered patterns of movement)
- Precise application of the cast (refer to Chapter 10)
- Adequate amount of time in the cast
- How to wean from the cast and not lose gains made

INDICATIONS FOR ORTHOSIS APPROACH

Orthosis Algorithm

As a foundation for making the choice among the approaches for orthotic intervention, clinicians have developed an algorithm that matches the type of orthosis with the phase of wound healing (Fig. 15–11).

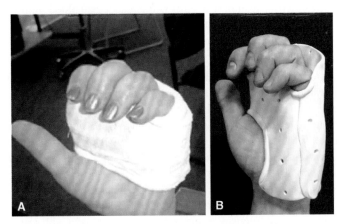

FIGURE 15–9 A blocking orthosis made with plaster of paris **(A)** and thermoplastic material **(B)**. Other recommended materials include Orficast (Chapter 11) and Delta-Cast (Chapter 12).

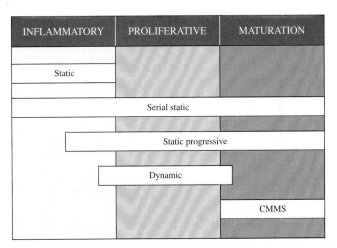

INFLAMMATORY	PROLIFERATIVE	MATURATION
Static		
Serial static		
Static progressive		
Dynamic		
		CMMS

FIGURE 15–11 Algorithm for matching the type of orthosis with the phase of wound healing.

This algorithm serves as a guideline only; therapists must choose the approach that best suits each patient's many characteristics, keeping in mind also the benefits of relative motion orthoses, and blocking orthoses. The CMMS approach may also be an option for the chronically stiff hand.

Based on this algorithm, many clinicians have delayed using the static progressive approach until the later phases of wound healing, because they consider it a high-load generator. This is a misconception. A static progressive force generator has a wide range of load application from extremely low to extremely high. Because the static progressive force generators are infinitely adjustable, the range of force is more diverse than that achievable from a rubber band or spring. Thus, any tissue that can tolerate dynamic traction can tolerate static progressive traction. In addition, tissues that cannot tolerate dynamic orthotic intervention may tolerate static progressive traction. It is up to the clinician to establish the correct amount of tension or load for the given tissue and to set up the orthosis appropriately (Schultz-Johnson, 2000). Table 15–1 compares the approaches (Schultz-Johnson, 2000).

End Feel

A soft end-feel joint indicates either (1) relatively young scar tissue that has not yet formed significant cross-linking or (2) transient physiologic changes that have occurred, such as swelling or malnourished cartilage. A joint contracture has been produced which has a soft and spongy end range of motion. At this point, the body still has to work to absorb the abnormal cells in the area in order for that joint to regain normal motion (Bell-Krotoski, 1987), (2011). A hard end-feel joint indicates mature scar tissue with advanced cross-linking, the presence of a check rein, or the absorption of tissue required for normal passive

motion (e.g., a PIP flexion contracture when the body absorbs volar skin and joint capsule) (Fig. 15–12A) (Bell-Krotoski, 1987), (2011).

Assessment of **torque-angle range of motion (TAROM)**, the quantification of the amount of torque force required to gain a certain amount of PROM at a joint, helps the therapist decide what type of orthosis will resolve the patient's PROM limitations (Roberson & Giurintano, 1995). If a joint requires a significant amount of torque to gain maximum PROM and the torque-angle curve has a rapidly rising slope, then the joint will have a **hard end feel** (Fig. 15–12A). Serial static or static progressive intervention is probably the only means to increase PROM. However, if a joint requires only a low amount of torque to gain maximum PROM and the torque-angle curve has a slowly rising slope, then the joint will have a **soft** or **springy end feel** (Fig. 15–12B). A soft end-feel joint can benefit from serial static, static progressive, or dynamic orthotic intervention.

The analysis of the duration and nature of the contracture, coupled with the information gained from TAROM measurements, helps the therapist select the appropriate orthosis. McKee et al. (2012) have suggested that although static approaches to managing joint stiffness achieve positive outcomes in tissue lengthening, one should appreciate that continued joint immobilization may impair nutrition to tissues and adversely compress articular cartilage (McKee et al., 2012).

CONTRAINDICATIONS TO ORTHOTIC INTERVENTION

Just as it is important to know the indications for mobilizing orthoses and for approaches that match a given problem, it is important to know the contraindications for orthoses that seek to mobilize joints.

COMMON CONTRAINDICATIONS INCLUDE THE FOLLOWING

- Joint instability
- Avascular necrosis
- Neurovascular deficiencies
- Acute inflammation
- Infection
- Unstable fractures
- Marked demineralization
- Myositis ossificans
- Heterotopic ossification
- Exostosis formation
- Loose body in joint
- Stress across healing structures without adequate blood supply or tensile strength to withstand tensile stress
- Patients with claustrophobia
- Patients with altered mental status

In addition, special diagnostic categories that are most always contraindications to mobilizing orthoses require special comment: Dupuytren contracture and motion loss due to irradiation.

Dupuytren contracture does not respond to LLPS (Abbott, Denney, Burke, & MGrouther, 1987; Sampson et al., 1992). Owing to its nature, Dupuytren tissue, made up of myofibroblasts, does not remodel in the same way as normal tissue or scar. Only in the post–medical intervention period (surgery or injection/manipulation) will Dupuytren contracture respond to orthotic intervention, because the intervention removes the unresponsive tissue and replaces some of it with scar.

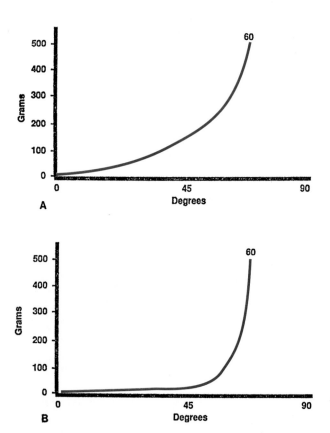

FIGURE 15–12 A, A hard end-feel joint requires a significant amount of torque to gain maximum passive range of motion (PROM) and has a torque-angle curve with a rapidly rising slope. **B,** A soft end-feel joint requires only a low amount of torque to gain maximum PROM and has a torque-angle curve with a slowly rising slope.

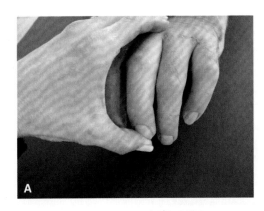

FIGURE 15-13 A, Limited passive range of motion (PROM) noted at the interphalangeal (IP) joints secondary to stiffness from immobilization after fracture dislocation of the middle finger (MF) proximal interphalangeal (PIP) joint. **B,** The accordion phenomenon is caused by scar formation between the folds, leading to decreased PROM.

Irradiated tissue does not usually respond to LLPS. The tissue is mostly fibrotic and does not possess the same viscoelastic properties as normal connective tissue. It lacks the live cells required to respond to the mechanical stimulus and to reorganize.

Whenever the clinician applies an orthosis—and especially when any doubt about orthosis appropriateness or tolerance exists—the therapist must rigorously check for the following signs that indicate a problem with this device:

- Pain (dolor)
- Heat (calor)
- Redness (rubor)

- Edema
- Decreased ROM
- Decreased strength
- Decreased sensation

If any of these symptoms and signs is seen, the therapist must thoroughly check the orthosis for fit and pressure distribution. It is important for the clinician to rethink the rationale for orthosis application to be certain of its appropriateness.

CAUSES OF JOINT STIFFNESS

When discussing joint stiffness, the nature of the limitation in joint PROM must be addressed. Changes in the soft-tissue structures surrounding a joint, the periarticular structures (e.g., ligament, joint capsule, volar plate, and sagittal bands), can cause such motion limitation. Changes in the structure of the articular surfaces of the bones forming the joint can also lead to loss of PROM (Fig. 15–13A). The relationship of adjacent bones to one another also affects arc and ease of motion.

As noted, periarticular structures may adaptively shorten when positioned on slack for a significant period of time; inflammation hastens this process. Arem and Madden (1976) described how periarticular structures may fold upon themselves, like an accordion, and become stuck in that position when scar forms between these folds (Fig. 15–13B). Spot-welding of periarticular structures may also occur during scar formation when the scar attaches the normally mobile tissue to less mobile tissue. This leads to a decrease in extensibility and glide.

PRECIPITATING CONDITIONS FOR STIFFNESS
Edema

When not managed, edema will progress to the infiltration of tissue spaces, become brawny and pitting, and eventually lead to fibrosis (Villeco, 2011) (Fig. 15–14A–D). In the worst scenario, edema will disrupt blood and nutrition to vital tissues. Therefore, intervention of the edematous hand is paramount.

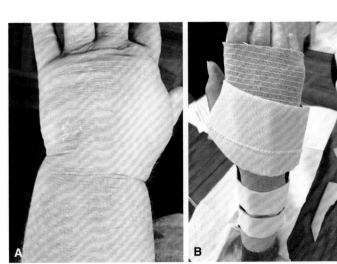

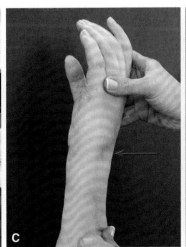

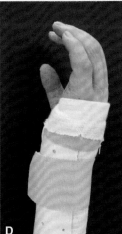

FIGURE 15-14 A, Note the pitting and brawny edema on the dorsum of the hand. **B,** This wrist immobilization orthosis with elastic stockinette and wide straps aids in reducing edema along with active hourly digital range of motion (ROM) and other edema management techniques. **C,** Pitting edema (via the finger indent, arrow) on the dorsum of the hand. **D,** Orthosis with compression sleeve worn beneath to manage edema.

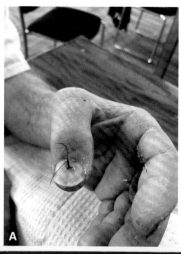

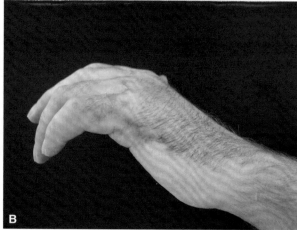

FIGURE 15–15 **A and B,** Position of ease with wrist slightly flexed, MCP joints extended, and interphalangeal (IP) joints flexed.

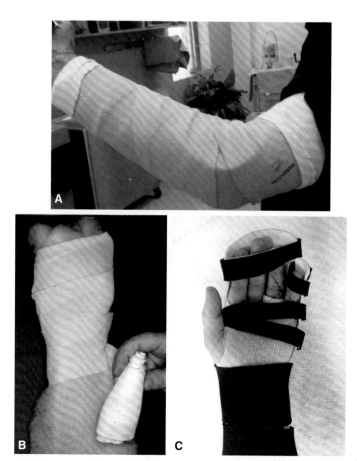

FIGURE 15–16 **A,** An elasticized wrap is used to hold this elbow flexion mobilization orthosis (serial static approach) in place to evenly distribute pressure and manage edema. **B,** Dacron (quilting) batting can be added as a layer between the circumferential wrap and the tissue in order to enhance moisture absorption. **C,** At the forearm, soft wide neoprene straps are used in this wrist/hand extension restriction orthosis post-flexor tendon repair. Note the bivalued straps about the digits. Neoprene is conforming and will not fray when cut.

In the presence of diffuse edema, the hand assumes the position of ease: wrist flexed, metacarpophalangeal (MCP) joints extended, and interphalangeal (IP) joints flexed (Grigsby deLinde & Miles, 1995). This position minimizes tension on the dorsal skin of the hand, on the ligaments, and on the periarticular structures. When the edema remains and the hand is left untreated, the wrist loses extension, the MCPs develop extension contractures, and the IPs develop flexion contractures (Fig. 15–15A,B). Orthotic intervention provides the desired extremity posture. Traditional strapping applied to the edematous hand may obstruct lymphatic flow and cause "window" edema or pooling of edema proximal and distal to the strap placement (Villeco, 2011). This warns the clinician that the placement of the strap is causing harm (Colditz, 2011). Strategic fabrication of the orthosis, such as a circumferential design, may better assist in even pressure distribution. Gentle circumferential compression wrapping or wide soft straps are another alternative for light distribution of pressure. Both of these techniques can effectively hold an orthosis in place while assisting in edema control (Fig. 15–16A–C). Once edema subsides, the wide straps or wraps can be replaced with traditional strapping methods if necessary.

The position of choice for minimizing or preventing hand stiffness and deformity is called the antideformity position (Fig. 15–17A–C) (Box 15–2): wrist in 20° to 25° extension, if available; maximum tolerated MCP flexion; and maximum tolerated

IP extension. Even if the PROM limitations do not permit the initial orthosis to secure the desired position, serial adjustments to the orthosis should generally accomplish the goal.

Intrinsic Tightness

Injury or disease can create tightness or scarring of the intrinsic hand muscles. Intrinsic tightness causes loss of simultaneous MCP extension and IP flexion. When these movements are impaired, the clinician should perform a test of intrinsic length (Fig. 15–18A,B). If intrinsic tightness is present, the PIP joint will have greater passive flexion when the MCP is positioned in flexion, and the PIP will have less passive flexion when the MCP is positioned in extension. If intrinsic tightness is noted, the therapist begins the appropriate orthosis and exercise regimen to increase composite MCP extension and IP flexion.

Severe intrinsic tightness may even create an imbalance that results in swan-neck deformity at the PIP and DIP joints (Melvin, 1989). Loss of intrinsic function can result in loss of the intermetacarpal movement, as described earlier. When intrinsic muscles become fibrotic, they may become resistant to orthotic intervention and exercises geared to increase their length. It is possible that fibrotic tissue lacks an adequate number of living cells to respond to tension stimuli and to reorganize in a manner conducive to length increase.

EXPERT PEARL 15-2

Adustable Digit Flexion Strap

MARY ANNE DYKSTRA, OTR/L, CHT
Illinois

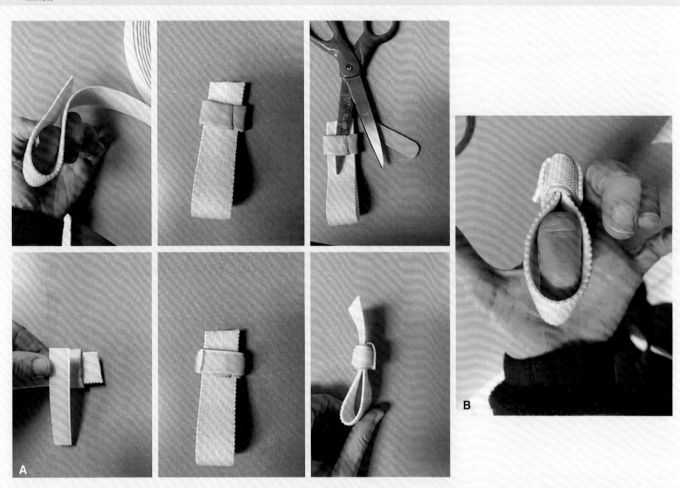

Choose hook receptive elastic (must have loop material on both sides if you would like both sides adjustable). Cut off enough elastic to go around the finger in a claw position as well as 1 inch on each side to lay down/adjust the material as motion improves. Fold in half and wrap thermoplastic material 1 inch below cut ends. Fuse the thermoplastic material ends together, and while warm, wrap the hook circumferentially around the orthosis material. Place scissors in one or both sides under orthosis material to fee any elastic from orthosis material. Slide the elastic through to assure it remains adjustable. To make one side adjustable, embed one side of elastic into the thermoplastic material to leave one "mobile" side.

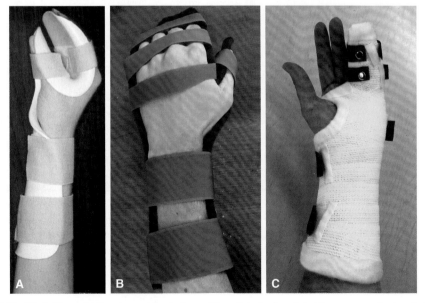

FIGURE 15–17 A, The antideformity position is the position of choice for minimizing or preventing hand stiffness and deformity. **B,** Volar view of a similar hand immobilization orthosis that is positioning the digits in slight abduction and the thumb in mid-radial/mid-palmar abduction. **C,** Ulnar-based design including ring and small fingers to address fifth metacarpal fracture—orthosis fabricated using Delta-Cast˚.

BOX 15–2	INTRINSIC/EXTRINSIC STIFFNESS	
	MCP Extended	**MCP Flexed**
Intrinsic tightness	PIP passive flexion decreased	PIP passive flexion increased
Extrinsic tightness (dorsal structure)	PIP passive flexion increased	PIP passive flexion decreased
Joint stiffness	PIP motion unchanged	PIP motion unchanged

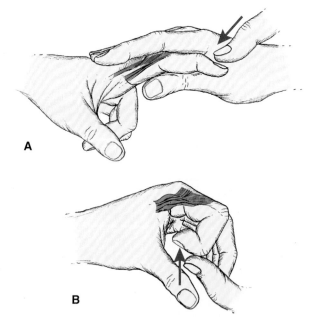

A

B

FIGURE 15–18 **A and B,** The intrinsic tightness test. Note the loss of simultaneous MCP extension and interphalangeal (IP) flexion.

Extrinsic Tightness

Extrinsic tightness can occur in either the flexor/pronator or extensor forearm muscles. Extrinsic extensor tightness condition leads to the loss of composite finger flexion (MCPs and IPs simultaneously) or the loss of composite finger flexion combined with wrist flexion (Fig. 15–19A,B). Just the reverse is true for extrinsic flexor tightness; it creates the loss of composite finger extension (MCPs and IPs simultaneously) or the loss of composite finger extension combined with wrist extension. When extrinsic tightness is not improving with range of motion and stretching activities, composite extension or flexion orthotic intervention is often necessary to increase motion.

EXPERT PEARL 15–3

Dynamic PIP Extension Mobilization Orthosis
MICHELE AUCH, OTR/L,CHT
Illinois

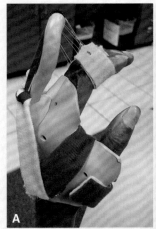
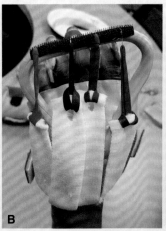
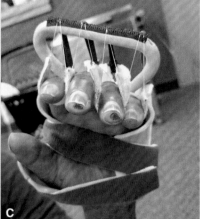
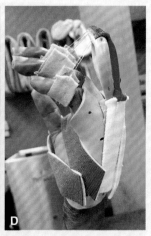

Hand-based design with homemade components: (1) slings made from Moleskin, (2) rolled thermoplastic formed into outrigger to obtain optimal line of pull, (3) hook adhered to top of outrigger to prevent line slippage, and (4) rubber bands distally connected to elastic loop attached to hook proximally on orthosis providing adjustable dynamic stretch.

EXPERT PEARL 15–4

Static Progressive Composite Finger Flexion Orthosis

BOB PHILLIPS, OTR/L, CHT
Georgia

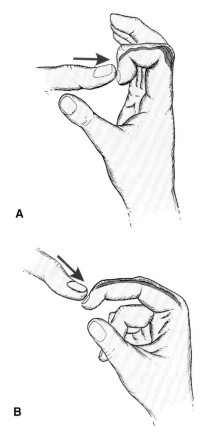

Design is used for overall finger stiffness. The slings are fabricated and threaded to give the IPs a flexion force. The line is pulled toward the scaphoid tubercle through hooks at the distal palmar crease to pull the MCPs into flexion.

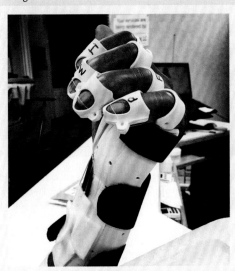

A

B

FIGURE 15–19 A and B, The extrinsic tightness test. Note the loss of composite finger flexion.

Joint Stiffness

With pure joint stiffness, the passive joint motion will be the same no matter what the position of the proximal and distal joints are. It is essential to differentiate the cause of joint motion loss in order to determine the correct orthosis to resolve the problem.

EXPERT PEARL 15–5

Why I Avoid Passive Flexion of the DIP Joint
HandLab: Clinical Pearls

JUDY C. COLDITZ, OT/L, CHT, FAOTA
North Carolina

At every splinting course I teach, one or more participants ask about construction of a composite finger flexion splint. My answer is always the same: I have made one of these in my career and cannot imagine making another!!!!! Many of you will be shocked by my statement...let me see if I can explain.

DIP Joint: Intrinsic Extension Versus Extrinsic Flexion

Extension of the distal interphalangeal (DIP) joint is primarily driven by intrinsic finger muscles via a complex blending of tendinous fibers as they cross the metacarpophalangeal (MCP) and proximal interphalangeal (PIP) joints before reaching the DIP joint. Extension is an intricate coordinated movement, without significant force. Unlike intrinsically powered DIP joint extension, DIP joint flexion is powered by a strong extrinsic flexor: the flexor digitorum profundus (FDP). The FDP provides both a robust muscle belly and an unrestrained single tendon which passes under a mechanically efficient pulley system. Simply stated: Force available for DIP joint flexion is much greater than the force available for DIP joint extension. So why favor the stronger motion with splinting? The FDP has the power to mobilize the DIP joint into flexion.

Normal Coordinated Motion of PIP and DIP Joints

The complex anatomy of the dorsal apparatus mandates that two adjacent distal joints of different sizes move in a coordinated manner. The lateral/volar movement of the lateral bands at the PIP joint during flexion provides enough length to allow DIP joint flexion. Therefore, working to gain isolated DIP joint flexion is illogical since it does not reflect normal coordinated joint motion. (A clear exception is DIP joint flexion with PIP joint extension to resolve a chronic boutonniere deformity.)

Composite Flexion Splinting

Splints which pull both finger IP joints into flexion simultaneously always move the joint with less resistance before moving the more resistive joint. So the joint most needing mobilizing gets the least influence!!! In my opinion a better way to regain flexion of the IP joints is to block the MCP joints in extension (preventing flexion) so the extrinsic flexor muscles can more effectively move the IP joints actively (active hook). Even if the DIP joint is stiff in extension and DIP joint flexion is initially impossible, if the FDP can be actively recruited it will in time mobilize the DIP joint.

The effect of FDP muscle contraction at the DIP joint can be enhanced by taping a small exercise splint on the dorsum of the DIP joint to hold the DIP joint in slight flexion while allowing full flexion. (See figures.) With this splint in place, the patient more easily focuses on initiating active finger flexion at the DIP joint. (This is also a useful exercise when working to regain excursion of FDP in zones 1 and 2 and maximum FDP/FDS differential excursion in zone 2.) Gains in passive DIP joint flexion can be made by recruiting the FDP actively, although therapists do not commonly think active motion can compel passive gains.

If one feels passive DIP and PIP joint flexion (splinting) is required, applying a specific passive force to the tighter joint while holding the other joint flexed with a static line will provide more precise flexion mobilization of the more limited joint. Holding the MCP joints in extension will still be helpful in mobilizing the IP joints actively.

(Continued)

Why I Avoid Passive Flexion of the DIP Joint

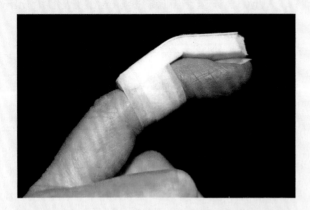

A small splint applied to block the DIP joint in flexion but allow further flexion encourages active flexion of that joint when the PIP joint flexes.

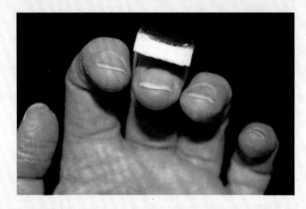

The blocking splint encourages active DIP joint flexion when the other DIP joints are flexing.

The Hidden Restraint: Interosseous Muscle Tightness

Any finger with limited IP joint motion easily develops adaptive shortening of the interosseous muscles (commonly called intrinsic tightness) and may develop lumbrical muscle adaptive shortening. This muscle tightness will continue to prevent full active IP joint flexion even when the IP joints have regained full passive flexion. This tightness (often subtle) must be addressed before full finger flexion can be regained. Elongation of both the interosseous and lumbrical muscles is achieved by blocking the MCP joints in extension and encouraging active IP joint flexion (hook fist).

Conclusion

Harnessing the power of the FDP can mobilize the DIP joint into flexion and passive flexion/splinting of the DIP joint is not needed. Regaining the active hook is the best way to regain full active finger flexion, including the DIP joint.

Clinical Pearls reprinted with permission from Clinician's Classroom at BraceLab.com written by Judy Colditz OT/L CHT FAOTA, copyright HandLab/BraceLab, Raleigh NC. February 2011, No. 12.

ORTHOSES TO ADDRESS INTRINSIC TIGHTNESS

Orthoses to address intrinsic tightness emphasize MCP extension combined with IP joint flexion. If the patient is unable to assume the position of MCP extension with IP flexion, there are several orthotic options including a **blocking orthosis** and an **intrinsic stretch** orthosis (Fig. 15–20A–F). As the patient progresses, if MCP hyperflexion occurs when attempting to make a full fist, but IP flexion is limited, a **relative motion** orthosis may be helpful to achieve end-range motion and restore balance (Fig. 15–21G) (see Chapter 7 for greater detail).

PIP/DIP Stretching
ALISON TAYLOR, OTR/L, CHT, CKTP, CKTI
Texas

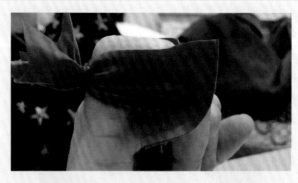

Use a CLX TheraBand and two elastic bands to create a quick Intrinsic stretching device (known as a "GUPPY"). To adjust the direction of the lateral stretch—the seam of the CLX band can be placed on either side of the finger.

Static Progressive Finger Flexion Orthosis
ERFAN SHAFIEE, OT, HAND THERAPIST
Canada

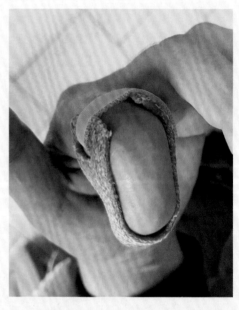

Simple and quick orthosis using Orficast to accomplish full passive PIP and DIP joint flexion by maximizing total end-range time. The force of flexion can be easily adjusted by patient.

ORTHOSES TO ADDRESS EXTRINSIC TIGHTNESS

Orthoses to address extrinsic tightness span multiple joints and act in the same direction. If a patient is able to demonstrate a good hook fist (intrinsic minus position), but the IP joint flexion is limited when the MCP joints are flexed, then an effective orthosis will provide a flexion force acting in a composite manner (Fig. 15–21A–G). The same concept is true for extension—if the IP joints cannot extend as much when the MCP joint is extended, then an orthosis to be effective must act over multiple joints in an extension direction (Fig. 15–22A–C). Serial static orthoses may also be utilized for night use to compliment daytime intermittent stretching—most commonly used when addressing long flexor tightness.

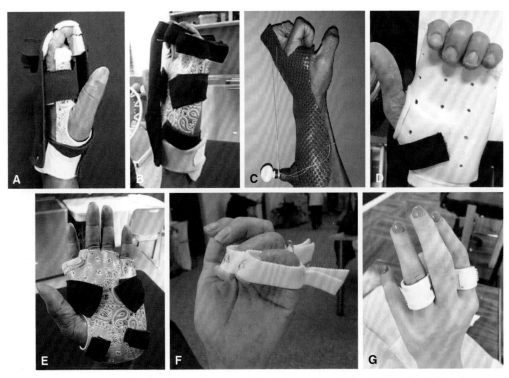

FIGURE 15–20 Management of **intrinsic** tightness. **A,** The MCP extension position in this orthosis allows for focused flexion stress to tight intrinsic muscles. In **(A)** the index finger (IF) demonstrates a greater flexion loss and therefore is managed with a gentle composite flexion strap. **B,** A neoprene proximal interphalangeal (PIP)/distal interphalangeal (DIP) strap is used to gain interphalangeal (IP) flexion in other digits. **C,** Static progressive intrinsic mobilization orthosis—combined PIP flexion and MCP extension. **D and E,** Blocking orthosis—MCP is held extended while the patient is instructed to perform active IP flexion. Note in **(E)** full clearance of PIP flexion crease to allow unrestricted motion. **F,** PIP/DIP strap shown for composite ring finger (RF) and small finger (SF) IP flexion—made from elastic strapping and foam. The patient can rest their hand palm down on table to achieve an intrinsic stretch. **G,** Middle finger relative motion extension orthosis to redirect flexion forces to IP joints.

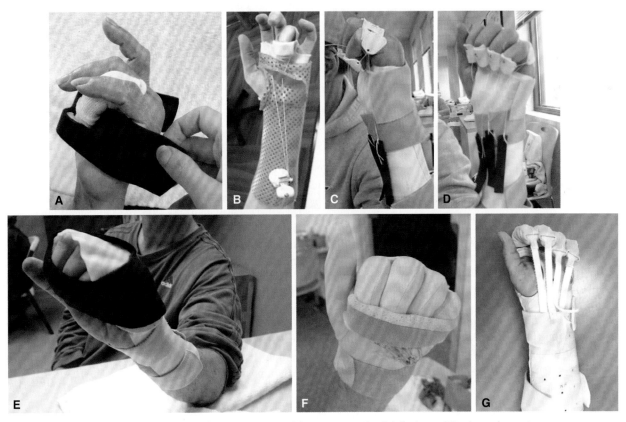

FIGURE 15–21 Management of extrinsic **extensor** tightness: composite digit flexion mobilization orthoses: **A,** Dynamic approach using a neoprene strap. **B,** Static progressive composite digital flexion utilizing individual cuffs for MCP and interphalangeal (IP) flexion and banjo tuner. **C and D,** Volar static progressive approach with monofilament lines and hook/loop adjustments proximally. **E,** Composite MCP/proximal interphalangeal (PIP)/distal interphalangeal (DIP) flexion strap used for gentle extrinsic stretch status post extensor tenolysis. **F and G,** Composite flexion stretch can be achieved using a flexion glove: **F,** shows optional DIP strap with foam to stretch DIP joints and **(G)** the use of wrist orthosis in combination with glove to prevent compensatory wrist flexion.

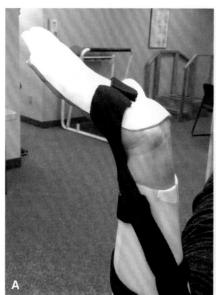
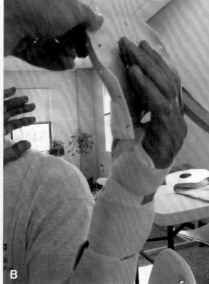
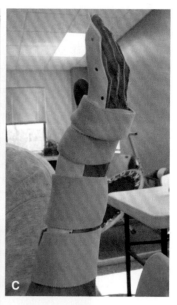

FIGURE 15–22 Management of extrinsic **flexor** tightness: composite digit extension mobilization orthoses: **A,** Composite wrist/hand extension mobilization orthosis utilizing soft neoprene strapping as the elasticized force. **B and C,** Simple management of tight extrinsic flexor tendons can be the intermittent use of a separate digit orthosis that is molded directly over a wrist extension orthosis. This allows the patient to remove the orthosis for functional use and reapply either at night or at times when function is not necessary.

ORTHOSES TO ADDRESS JOINT STIFFNESS

Orthoses to address joint stiffness emphasize targeted intervention at the affected joint. In the presence of isolated PIP joint stiffness with flexion limited, effective orthoses block the MCP joint in full extension as a flexion force is targeted directly to the PIP joint (Fig. 15–4B). With limited PIP extension, a static progressive orthosis would stabilize the MCP joint in a flexed position and an extension force is again targeted directly toward the PIP joint (Fig. 15–4A). Other options may be isolated serial casting for the PIP joint or a mobilization orthosis (Fig. 15–7B,E). Blocking and relative motion orthoses also work to facilitate restoration of active ROM and function by redirecting muscle force and tendon pull toward the stiff joint (Fig. 15–8A,B).

STIFFNESS AT SPECIFIC JOINTS

THE METACARPOPHALANGEAL JOINTS

Problems at the MCP joint rarely result in loss of extension. Even when the joint has been held in flexion for years by Dupuytren fascial contracture, surgical release of the fascia most often readily returns the joint to extension. Injuries involving the soft tissue crossing the MCP crease at a 90° angle or involving most soft tissue in this location (e.g., burns, degloving injuries, and palmar skin graft) create loss of extension (Fig. 15–23A,B). However, restoration of soft-tissue length restores normal motion. With rheumatic disease, the patient may lose passive MCP extension owing to multiple factors, including loss of joint capsule and ligament integrity, intrinsic tightness, and ulnar subluxation of the extensor digitorum communis (EDC) (Alter, Feldon, & Terrono, 2011; Melvin, 1989). Loss of flexion at the MCP joint creates significant clinical challenge and functional loss. Diagnoses associated with this problem are any injury causing generalized edema of the hand, intrinsic paralysis, crush injury, metacarpal and proximal phalanx fractures, dorsal or circumferential burns, and a zone V extensor tendon injury. Each of these injuries results in the sustained extension of the MCP joint, often in the presence of edema, inflammation, and scar formation. The MCP joint's unique anatomy predisposes it to the extension contracture.

The collateral ligaments of the MCP joint are slack in extension and taut in flexion (Chase, 1989; Rosenthal & Elhassan, 2011) (Fig. 15–23C). When the ligaments are allowed to remain slack, especially in the presence of inflammation and scar formation, they can fall prey to the accordion phenomenon, adaptive shortening, or both. Like the volar plate of the PIP, these collateral ligaments are dense and recalcitrant to lengthening. A well-established MCP extension contracture may require significant end-range time to change length and increase PROM.

In the case of isolated joint stiffness, intervention focuses on LLPS isolating the MCP joint. To restore flexion, the angle of pull should be perpendicular to the proximal phalanx at end range and in the direction of the scaphoid (Fig. 15–23D–F). Check for extrinsic tightness prior to making a decision on orthoses to restore motion. If extrinsic tightness is present, then intervention focuses on composite flexion.

EXPERT PEARL 15-8

Digit Foam Wedges
ALISON TAYLOR, OTR/L, CHT, CKTP, CKTI
Texas

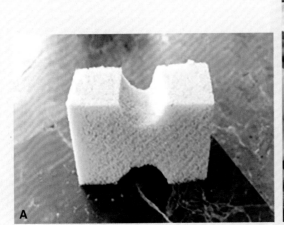

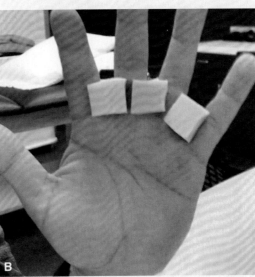

Placing foam wedges between the fingers to help space and align the metacarpals may help reduce pain and restore balance to the intrinsics/interossei in the hand. They assist in abduction of the fingers and help correct soft-tissue shortening of the adductors.

EXPERT PEARL 15-9

Finger Dividers
DEBBIE FISHER, MS, OTR, CHT
Texas

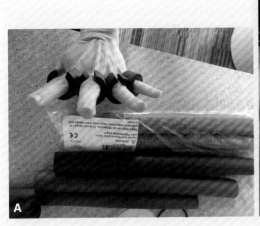

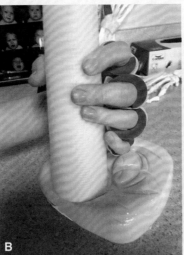

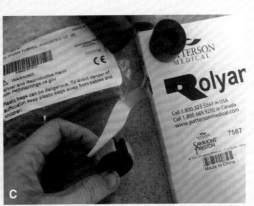

Created from foam tubing to maximize finger abduction and assist with decreasing hand stiffness. Cut tubes to fit between the MCP and PIP joints without restricting finger flexion and extension. If needed, adhesive hook and thin strapping further secure on hand.

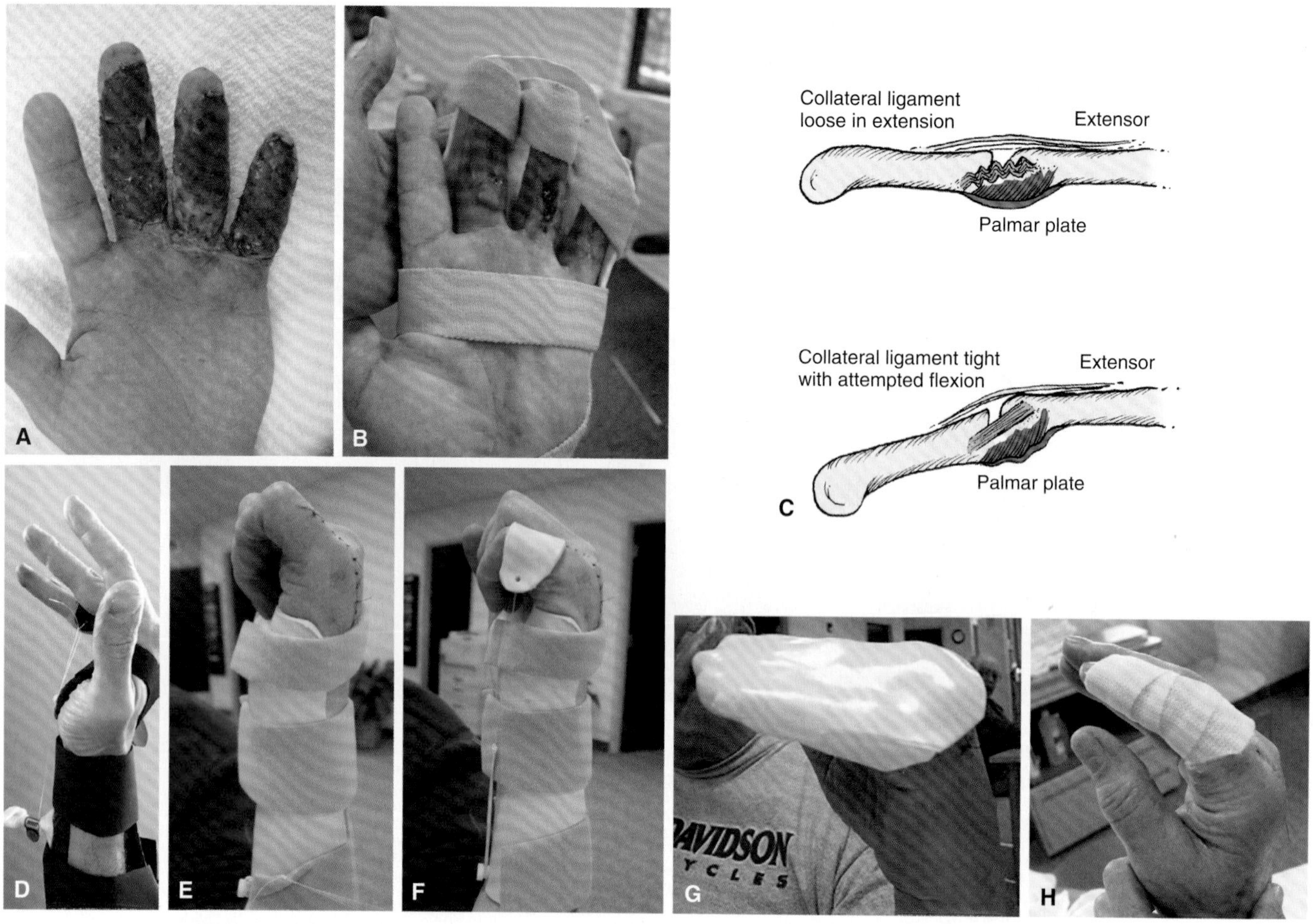

FIGURE 15-23 A and B, Third-degree burns of the volar surface of the hands. The healing wound is being kept in extension via the orthosis to prevent contracture. The patient takes this off for gentle exercises in flexion and extension. **C,** Collateral ligaments about the MCP joints are loose in extension, and with attempted flexion, they become tight. **D,** Static progressive approach to increase MCP flexion via a banjo tuner. **E and F,** Dynamic (rubber band tension) MCP flexion mobilization post capsular release; note the adequate clearance of the distal palmar crease. **G,** Digit extension "flipper" used as an exercise device to encourage active flexion at the MCP joints. This directs the force of flexion to the MCP joints, preventing compensatory flexion distally. **H,** To address individual digit, consider using a circumferentially designed orthosis to block motion distally during active MCP flexion.

THE THUMB METACARPOPHALANGEAL JOINT

Trauma to the thumb often causes stiffness at the MP joint. The diagnoses of fracture, collateral ligament injury, tendon injury, and nerve injury—all frequently present with loss of MP flexion (Fig. 15–24A,B). The problem with restoring thumb MP flexion mirrors those of contracture at the finger but does not have the same primary cause. The collateral ligaments of the thumb have a different architecture than those of the finger MCPs (Imaeda, An, & Cooney, 1992; Kapandji, 1982; Melone, Beldner, & Basuk, 2000). The loss of flexion seems to originate with joint swelling, which may be worsened by dorsal adhesions.

The thumb MP may lose extension with the loss of extensor pollicis brevis (EPB) continuity and losing of the extensor expansion. This imbalance creates a dynamic similar to that of the finger boutonniere deformity. Left untreated, the IP joint of the thumb loses flexion and assumes a hyperextended position. Over time, a fixed deformity can result. A grade 3 tear of either the ulnar or the radial collateral ligament of the thumb MP can lead to MP joint instability with subsequent subluxation and the creation of a flexion contracture.

Rheumatic disease can create various thumb contractures. Rheumatoid arthritis, lupus, and similar diseases can create the Nalebuff type 1 thumb, characterized by MP flexion and IP hyperextension (Fig. 15–24C). The appearance is similar to the boutonniere deformity of the finger. This occurs as a result of chronic synovitis of the thumb MP joint, intrinsic muscle tightness, weakening or attenuation of the EPB, and ulnovolar displacement of the EPL (Melvin, 1989). The joint deformities are further emphasized by the natural tendency to use the thumb for pinch. Clinicians most commonly use orthoses to prevent this deformity (Fig. 15–24D,E). However, aggressive disease or late treatment may present the clinician with the need to address this deformity.

In contrast, the stiffness problem commonly associated with osteoarthritis is the Nalebuff type 2 thumb (Fig. 15–24F). The condition associated with this classification is carpometacarpal (CMC) synovitis of the joint, which stretches the joint capsule and allows the joint to sublux or dislocate in adduction. This adducted posture results in shortening of the adductor pollicis muscles and web space. MP hyperextension develops with attempts to abduct the contracted first metacarpal (Melvin, 1989). Once this deformity exists, an orthosis will not improve it. A thumb MP extension restriction orthosis minimizes the hyperextension and may prevent it from getting worse (Fig. 15–24G,H). Such an orthosis may also help distribute forces in a biomechanically sound way that will unload the CMC joint. The main role for orthosis management for MP hyperextension secondary to CMC instability is prevention.

Thumb/Finger Jux-A-Cisor
LISA RAY, OTR/L, CHT
Virginia

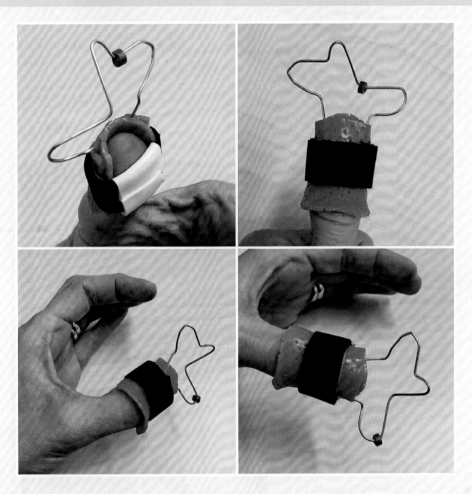

1/16″ thermoplastic utilized; dorsally based with loop strap volarly; paper clip easily formed into random maze with needle nose pliers and attached with scrap piece of thermoplastic. Utilize a washer or bead to complete. Also shown is a Microfoam tape on strap to prevent slippage.

THUMB CARPOMETACARPAL JOINT

Stiffness of the thumb adductor occurs for a variety of reasons including edema, immobilization, and disuse following upper extremity injury, degenerative joint disease, or nerve injury. Restoration of palmar abduction can also be achieved with the use of a web spacer which is gradually expanded in a serial static method or a static progressive approach can be taken if the injury is longstanding (Fig. 15–25A–F).

The carpometacarpal (CMC) joint of the thumb has a unique saddle architecture that renders it highly mobile (Kapandji, 1982). The thumb is critical to hand function and is a frequently used and overused joint. Many people experience thumb CMC arthritis as a result of overuse, trauma, or a multijoint disease. Pelligrini, Olcott, and Hollenberg (1993) hypothesized that over time, overuse, or trauma compromises the ligament system supporting the joint. This allows the joint surfaces to lose congruency, which leads to friction that wears away the cartilage, creating CMC arthritis. Osteoarthritis often first presents at the basal joint of the thumb. This disease has an insidious onset, and the cause and the cure are yet unknown. Refer to Chapter 17 for greater detail on this patient population.

With the loss of the median innervated thumb musculature, the thumb is unable to abduct in the palmar plane. Without the ability to lengthen the thumb adductor, the muscle shortens, producing a first web space contracture. In the case of combined ulnar and median paralysis, the ulnar innervated thumb adductor ceases to function and often becomes fibrotic (Fig. 15–25C). This speeds up the formation of a first web space contracture. Clinicians use web space orthosis intervention to protect the length and width of this web space (Brandsma, 1993) (Fig. 15–25A).

PROXIMAL INTERPHALANGEAL JOINT

As noted, periarticular structures may adaptively shorten when positioned on slack for a significant period of time; inflammation hastens this process. Arem and Madden (1976) described how periarticular structures may fold upon themselves, like an accordion, and become stuck in that position when scar forms between these folds. Spotwelding of periarticular structures may also occur during scar formation when the scar attaches the normally mobile tissue to less mobile tissue. This leads to a decrease in extensibility and glide.

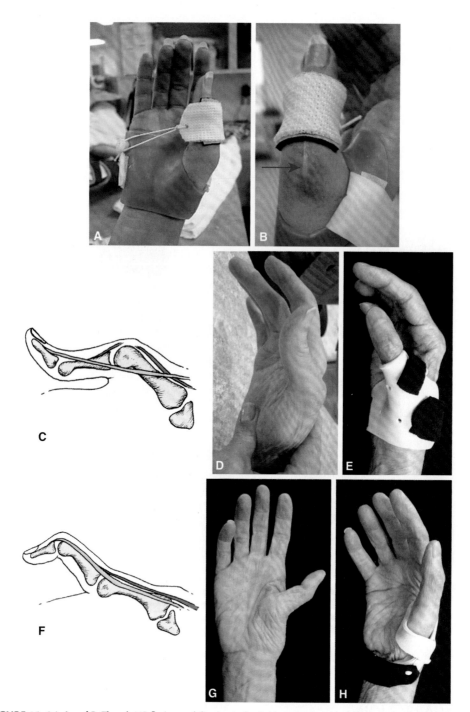

FIGURE 15–24 A and B, Thumb MP flexion mobilization orthosis. Note the dorsal incision over the thumb MP joint. The sling is fabricated with QuickCast 2 lined with soft neoprene material. The width and depth is intentionally wide and deep in order to provide greater pressure distribution and comfort. **C and D,** Often seen in rheumatic disease, thumb contractures can occur due to ligament rupture combined with longstanding posturing (MP flexion and gradual interphalangeal [IP] hyperextension). This deformity (Nalebuff type 1) is further exacerbated by the natural tendency for lateral pinch. **E,** Orthosis management for MP flexion and IP hyperextension. **F–H,** MP hyperextension and IP flexion (Nalebuff type 2 thumb) results in severe adduction of the thumb. If left untreated, the thumb will become stiff in this position; however, as noted in **(H)** this patient was able to be passively corrected and the thumb now lies in a functional position.

The PIP joint can become stiff in either flexion or extension; however, it is the PIP flexion contracture that is the most challenging to resolve for the following reasons (Valdes et al., 2019; Glasgow et al., 2012; Lluch, 1997; Sokolow, 1997):

- Tendency for the volar plate to shorten or fold on itself after trauma
- Prevalence of a flexed finger posture in the position of ease and during function
- Vulnerability of the extensor mechanism (it is thin, superficial, and intimate with the underlying bone)

- Length loss caused by proximal phalanx fractures, leading to redundancy in extensor mechanism length and causing lack of full active extension
- Extensor hood attenuation from prolonged positioning in flexion, rendering the mechanism too long to provide full extension even when the contracture has resolved (Brandsma, 1993)
- Density of the PIP volar plate, making it prone to adaptive shortening, and the thickness of the structure, making its lengthening difficult

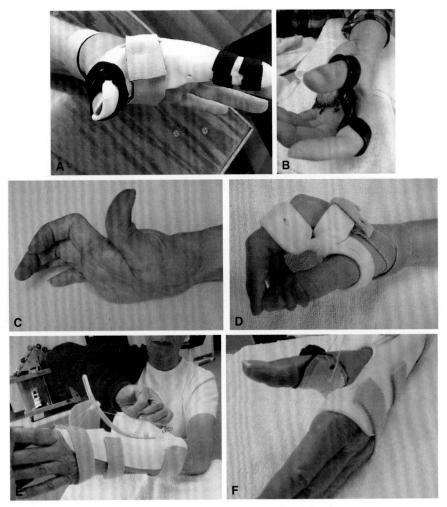

FIGURE 15–25 **A and B,** Two different designs for thumb web spacers/abduction mobilization orthoses using a serial static approach. These can be remolded as the tissue accommodates. **C,** With paralysis of the intrinsics post median and ulnar nerve injury, there is a loss of the arches in the hand. **D,** An MCP extension restriction (with thumb opposition) orthosis applied to this hand to better balance and harness the functioning muscle-tendon units. This position helps to minimize the development of unwanted joint contractures, and tendon and ligament shortening. **E and F,** A patient is able to adjust the tension with this static progressive carpometacarpal (CMC) abduction mobilization orthosis. Shown using the MERiT™ static progressive component and the Digitec outrigger system (Performance Health).

PIP joints are usually held in flexion, and hands are used in flexion. When a patient uses his or her hands for normal function during the day, the PIP joints are frequently in some degree of flexion. The position of comfort and rest is flexion. In the face of pain and edema, the PIPs are held in flexion to place the periarticular structures on slack. During sleep, the PIP joints assume a flexed position.

Many types of trauma (fracture, tendon injury) to the finger cause the extensor mechanism to become adherent to the bone and skin. This adhesion of the dorsal hood creates loss of excursion. Without full excursion, the PIP joint cannot actively assume full extension (Mannarino, 1992; Rosenthal & Elhassan, 2011). When a PIP joint is unable to extend, the volar structures adaptively shorten, causing a flexion contracture (Figure 15–26A). Mild PIP extension ROM limitations can often be remedied with the use of a relative motion orthosis and a night extension orthosis. Flexion contractures with harder end feel

often require serial casting or orthoses providing low load prolonged stretch (Fig. 15–26B–G). In order to resolve a flexion contracture of the PIP joint, best current evidence based on systematic review suggests PIP extension orthoses should position the joint at end range for at least 6 hours per day and force should be low enough, so the patient feels tension but no pain (Valdes et al., 2019).

Loss of PIP PROM in flexion can result from many of the factors described earlier. A fracture or dislocation that requires prolonged immobilization can result in significant adhesion at the joint. This extra tissue can create a physical block to motion that only surgical excision of the scar tissue can improve (Cannon, 2011; Means et al., 2011). Relative motion orthoses or blocking can be helpful as part of a home program to improve joint AROM and tendon gliding. Static progressive or dynamic flexion orthoses isolating the PIP joint are also helpful to restore full PIP ROM (Fig.15–27A–E).

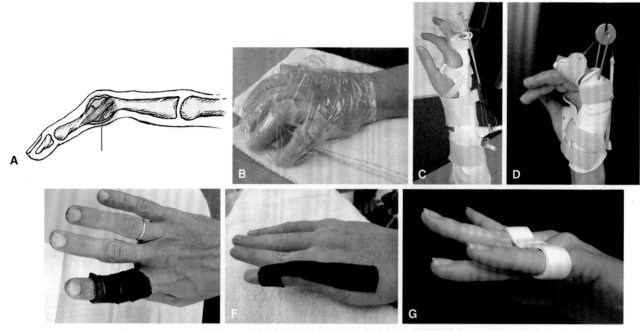

FIGURE 15–26 Proximal interphalangeal (PIP) extension mobilization options: **A,** PIP flexion contracture with shortening of volar plate (arrow). **B,** Prefabricated dynamic PIP extension orthoses used in combination with paraffin to provide heat and stretch simultaneously. **C,** Forearm-based static progressive PIP extension orthosis. **D,** Hand-based dynamic PIP extension orthosis. **E,** Circumferential serial static PIP extension orthosis. **F,** Therapeutic taping to assist with active extension efforts commonly worn with relative motion orthosis. **G,** Middle finger relative motion flexion orthosis worn to encourage PIP extension.

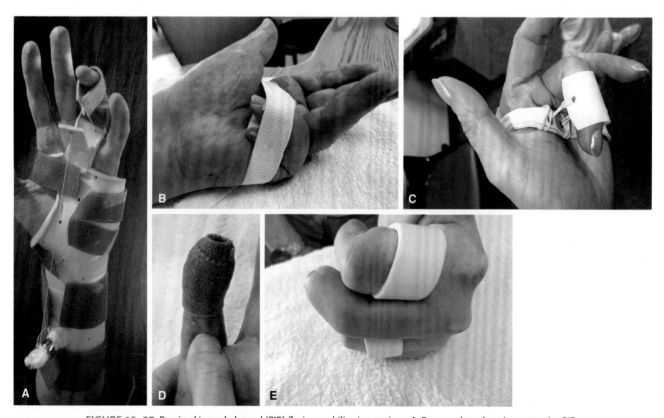

FIGURE 15–27 Proximal interphalangeal (PIP) flexion mobilization options: **A,** Forearm-based static progressive PIP flexion orthosis. **B,** Simple dynamic strap utilizing pajama elastic. **C,** Dynamic cuff using rubber band tension to exert flexion force. **D,** Distal interphalangeal (DIP) cast worn during exercise to direct force to flexion to PIP joint. **E,** Relative motion extension orthosis worn to encourage PIP flexion in middle finger after amputation.

How Long Should I Serial Cast a Finger?

HandLab: Clinical Pearls

JUDY C. COLDITZ, OT/L, CHT, FAOTA
North Carolina

Digital serial casting is nearly always my first choice for treatment of stubborn PIP joint flexion contractures. In addition to contracture resolution, digital edema resolves and inflamed joints become quiescent. In my experience, serial casting is usually more effective than the other approaches to regaining PIP joint extension.

My clinical training taught me to change the serial cast every 2 to 3 days, which I did for many years. But a few years ago my practice setting changed and I was working part-time seeing patients who had driven many hours for treatment. These were patients with chronic contractures whose PIP joint had been unresponsive to other treatment approaches. When I applied a serial cast to a patient's finger it was difficult for me to ask him/her to drive the long distance again 2 days later to have the cast changed. So I increased the intervals between cast changes, with the interval sometimes being as long as 2 weeks because of a variety of circumstances!!! Keep in mind the cast was not removable.

What I discovered to my amazement as these intervals increased, was that not only was passive PIP joint extension greater and had less resistance, but nearly always active PIP extension exceeded the measurements of passive PIP extension at the previous visit. It was as if I had given the tissue long enough to dramatically change, removing resistance to motion. When I was changing the cast every 2 to 3 days, my measurements had shown a dramatic improvement with the first one or two cast changes, but the response diminished as I continued the 2 to 3 day intervals.

Now I have evolved to a different timeline for serial casting for PIP joint flexion contractures. If I am seeing a patient fairly soon after an injury and only a couple of casts are needed, I might still change the cast every 2 to 3 days. But if I am seeing a patient who has a chronic PIP joint flexion contracture I would change the serial cast every 2 to 3 days only once or twice, and then I would increase the time of cast application. In other words, the longer I am casting the patient the more I increase the intervals. I have no set formula for this as I have no way of determining the optimum number of days of immobilization extension. But I think about the length of time since the initial injury and the passive resistance to PIP joint extension and the greater both of these are, the longer the interval I choose between cast changes.

In my opinion, continuing the 2 to 3 day interval over many cast changes often "pushes" the joint to move faster than the tissues are able to "grow" to accommodate the new position. I feel we need to be more respectful of the readiness of the tissue to respond. Flowers and Lastayo's article (*Journal of Hand Therapy*, 7(3), 150–157;1994) proved that 6 days of wearing a serial cast is more effective than 3 days with a variety of PIP joint injuries.

Many therapists are concerned that increased intervals of PIP joint extension casting will lose flexion. Although one may see diminished flexion ability immediately upon cast removal, it is my experience that this is very short-lived and loss of flexion is not a reason to retain short cast intervals in most cases. The flexors are much more powerful!!!

NOTE: For greater mechanical efficiency on those stubborn joints or really short little fingers, you may want to alter the usual casting technique. (See www.HandLab.com for article by Judy Colditz.) I no longer use a splinting material insert because it can cause maceration, but I add a small roll of plaster of Paris longitudinally on the proximal volar piece to reinforce it before wrapping the entire digit.

Clinical Pearls reprinted with permission from Clinician's Classroom at BraceLab.com written by Judy Colditz OT/L CHT FAOTA, copyright HandLab/BraceLab, Raleigh NC. June 2011, No. 14.

Exercise Orthosis

ANDREA MOSER, OT
Austria

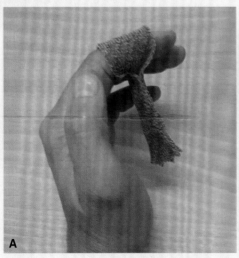

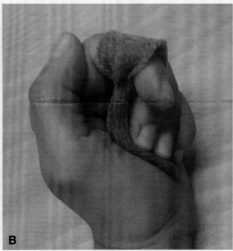

Fabricated with Orficast blocking PIP joint to improve isolated DIP movement.

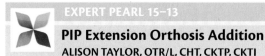

PIP Extension Orthosis Addition
ALISON TAYLOR, OTR/L, CHT, CKTP, CKTI
Texas

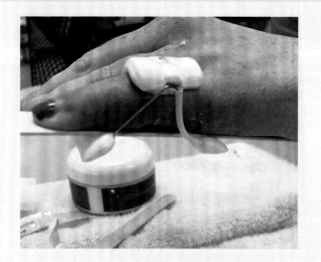

A prefabricated dynamic PIP extension orthosis is commonly used by hand therapists to help provide a slow progressive stretch and to help lengthen contracted tissue. Adding a tongue depressor between the finger and the orthosis can maximize the distribution of force from the DIP to the palm resulting in a more comfortable stretch.

DISTAL INTERPHALANGEAL JOINT

The DIP joint is vulnerable to stiffness in both flexion and extension. The DIP presents a unique challenge in that once the joint becomes stiff, the short length of the distal phalanx offers little in

terms of a lever arm to torque the joint into the desired ROM. The joint is unique in that the motor sensors surrounding the joint are singular and do not have the redundancy that is available at the other joints of the hand. Thus, if one of the motors becomes injured or ineffective, stiffness is likely to result.

The DIP has a dense volar plate that can become folded and adherent in scar in the presence of inflammation. Although some loss of DIP extension might be considered desirable in the face of lost flexor excursion, the resulting extreme flexion contractures can be disfiguring and disabling.

If loss of extension at the DIP is the sequela from a zone 1 or zone 2 flexor tendon repair, the therapist must respect the time for tendon healing but should begin to extend the DIP as soon as the type of repair and the health and cooperation of the patient permit. Progressive isolated DIP extension orthotic intervention improves PROM and minimizes stress on the flexor tendon. However, even though such an orthosis attempts to extend only one joint in the series that the FDP affects, intervention so close to the repair can lead to attenuation or rupture.

Oblique retinacular ligament (ORL) tightness is a common cause of a passive DIP flexion deficit (Fig. 15–28A–D). With a diagnosis of a PIP central slip injury, the therapist must include a program of DIP flexion to prevent ORL tightness. To restore active DIP flexion, a circumferential PIP joint immobilization orthosis can be used for exercise to promote FDP gliding and DIP AROM; this is a device that can be dispensed to be used on an independent basis as part of a home exercise program.

The inability to extend the DIP joint, left untreated, may lead to DIP flexion contractures (Fig. 15–29A–F). Serial static DIP extension orthoses are often safe and effective to restore DIP extension.

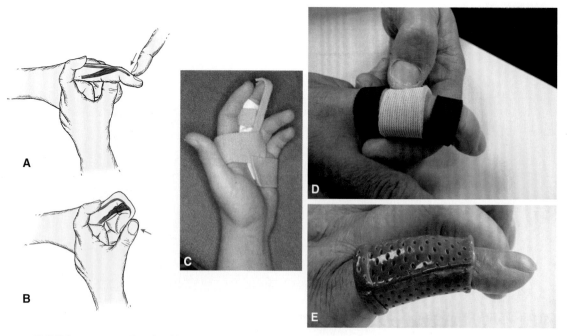

FIGURE 15–28 A and B, The oblique retinacular ligament (ORL) tightness test. Note the lack of isolated distal interphalangeal (DIP) flexion. **C,** DIP flexion mobilization orthosis using strapping material to provide static progressive stretch. **D,** Proximal interphalangeal (PIP) immobilization orthosis supporting full extension permits isolated DIP flexion. **E,** PIP circumferential extension orthosis with DIP free to permit active and passive range of motion (ROM).

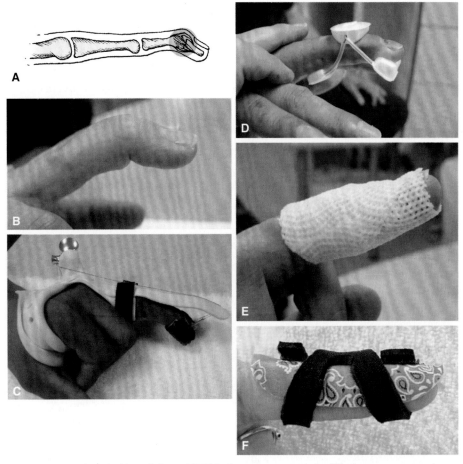

FIGURE 15–29 **A and B,** Distal interphalangeal (DIP) flexion contractures can be difficult to manage secondary to the short lever arm of the distal phalanx and are often combined with proximal interphalangeal (PIP) joint tightness/contractures. **C,** Hand-based static progressive DIP extension orthosis providing simultaneous extension forces to the PIP and DIP joints. **D,** Prefabricated dynamic extension mobilization orthosis; note the use of small size to isolate the DIP joint. **E,** Serial static approach using QuickCast 2. **F,** Dorsal-based digit extension orthosis may be used at night for extension positioning.

EXPERT PEARL 15–14

Dynamic DIP Orthosis
ALFRED NINJA, OTR/L, CHT
Kenya

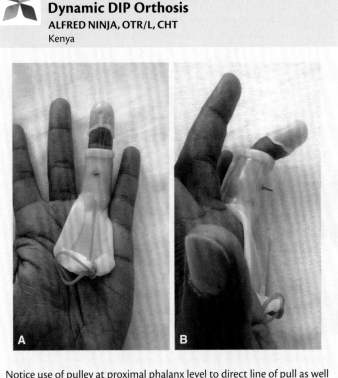

Notice use of pulley at proximal phalanx level to direct line of pull as well as full clearance of DIP joint to allow unrestricted motion.

WRIST JOINT

Unlike the joints discussed so far, the wrist is not generally predisposed to any particular patterns of motion loss. The wrist consists of a complex of joints and contains multiple articulations. As with other joints, stiffness here can arise from intra-articular or extra-articular pathology. Some causes of stiffness at this level are unique to this joint (Saffar, 1997):

- Certain types of idiopathic arthritis (gout)
- Avascular necrosis of the lunate
- Volkmann ischemic contracture (produces wrist flexion)
- Ligamentous injury and carpal instability, including carpal collapse
- Carpal nonunion, especially of the scaphoid

Trauma and its sequelae are the most common causes of lost wrist ROM. The position of the wrist during immobilization often predetermines the direction of stiffness.

The most common type of wrist fracture, the Colles, requires reduction of the wrist in a flexed, ulnarly deviated, and pronated position to align the dorsally displaced distal fragment with the proximal radius (Frykman & Kropp, 1995). The patient remains in the cast for many weeks and often cannot attain a neutral wrist or forearm even after weeks out of the cast. The direction of wrist stiffness is always the opposite of the position in which the patient was casted. Thus, for the common Colles fracture, the patient lacks extension, radial deviation, and supination.

Soft-tissue scarring in the forearm can also limit wrist PROM. When extrinsic flexor and/or extensor muscle-tendon units become adherent to either bone or surrounding less mobile soft tissue, wrist PROM suffers. In the case of predominantly dorsal extensor scarring, wrist flexion decreases. When volar flexor scarring occurs, the wrist loses extension. It is important to note that if these extrinsic problems can be addressed early (as discussed earlier) and if the wrist is spared involvement in inflammation and scar formation, then the wrist complex itself remains healthy and true stiffness of the joint will not result. The clinician has many choices available for mobilization of the stiff wrist.

The patient with carpal instability may undergo surgery—for example, partial fusion, ligament repair, or wrist capsulodesis—to restore stability and decrease pain. In this case, wrist stiffness is iatrogenically introduced; the patient trades some motion to have a stable, pain-free wrist. However, these patients remain immobilized postoperatively for a long duration and frequently come out of the cast with little or no motion. The careful and strategic application of passive treatment, including guarded, graded orthotic mobilization after surgery to restore carpal stability, can result in a more rapid return to motion and function that is both safe and comfortable. Static progressive orthoses can be very useful to restore wrist extension (Fig. 15–31A–D). It is important to exercise caution with the use of wrist flexion orthoses as prolonged flexion positioning may result in median nerve irritation and compression.

Static Progressive Wrist Extension Orthosis
ALFRED NINJA, OTR/L, CHT
Kenya

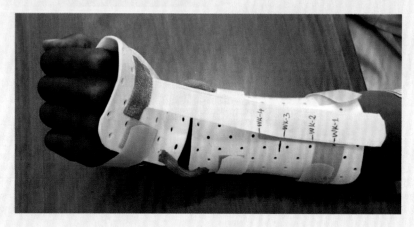

To gradually increase wrist range of motion, use Orficast tape as hinges (4 cm - dry heat - roll - dry heat attachment sites on proximal and distal segments). To monitor progress, mark weekly on the strap dorsally as shown.

Preventing Orthosis Migration
JEANINE BEASLEY, EDD, OTR, CHT, FAOTA
Michigan

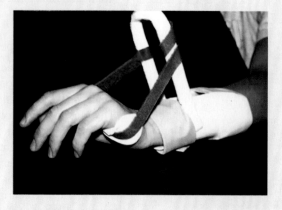

Distal slippage with a static progressive wrist extension orthosis can limit wrist motion. Placing the outrigger base volar and the outrigger dorsal prevents the orthosis base from blocking wrist extension. Incorporating and adhering to a wearing schedule (30 minutes three times a day) can be a challenge. Linking this to meals, television shows, or other daily activities can help assure compliance.

EXPERT PEARL 15-17

Wrist/Forearm Jux-A-Cisor
LISA RAY, OTR/L, CHT
Virginia

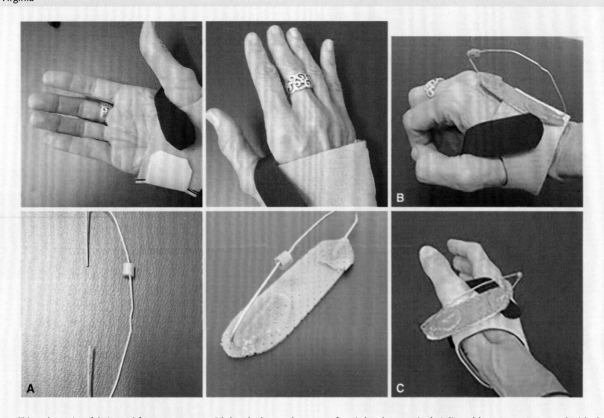

Soft "universal" hand portion fabricated from neoprene with hook closure (outer surface is hook receptive). Adjustable maze constructed with thermoplastic, large paper clip and bead. There is hook attached to back of thermoplastic and can be moved around the neoprene to obtain the desired motion (wrist extension/flexion or supination/pronation).

EXPERT PEARL 15-18

Wrist Mobilization Orthosis
MICHELE AUCH, OTR/L,CHT
Illinois

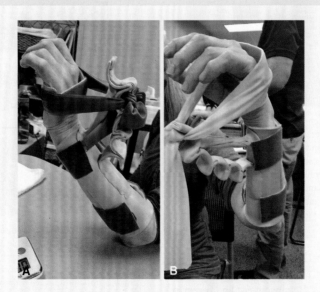

Static progressive wrist orthosis made from scrap materials—can be a more economical alternative versus commercial options. This can easily convert from extension to flexion. Dycem added to inner forearm piece to prevent migration. May be necessary to superglue the outrigger to the forearm base for strength. The exercise band strengths were chosen based on patient's perceived stretch on wrist.

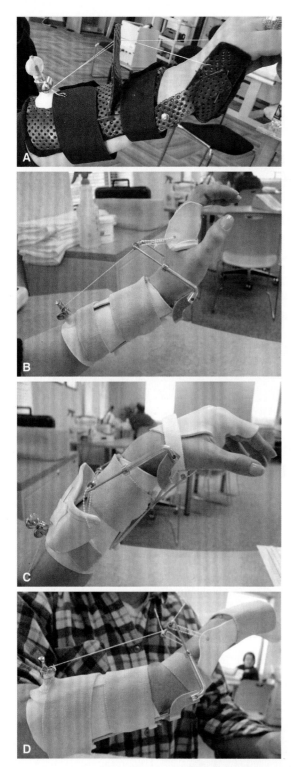

FIGURE 15–30 **A,** Static progressive wrist extension orthosis using the banjo tuner component. Note homemade hinge prevents compressive forces at wrist and orthosis migration during mobilization. **B and C,** Combination orthosis using a static progressive approach for gaining wrist extension and a dynamic approach for mobilizing into flexion (shown Phoenix wrist hinge, Performance Health and MERiT™ component). **D,** Composite wrist and hand static progressive extension mobilization to address a combination of joint and extrinsic flexor tightness.

FOREARM

As for the wrist, a common cause of lost forearm PROM is trauma, and the position of the forearm during a period of immobilization usually dictates the direction of stiffness. Because wrist and forearm fractures are often reduced in pronation, loss of supination is more common than the loss of pronation. However, clinical experience shows that with severe forearm fractures and complex fractures of the distal radioulnar joint (DRUJ) or the proximal radioulnar joint (PRUJ), the patient often loses rotation in both directions.

Although fractures commonly cause loss of forearm motion, soft-tissue injury (with or without fracture) can also cause PROM limitation. Injury to the triangular fibrocartilage complex (TFCC) limits rotation and tends to affect supination more than pronation. Adaptive shortening or scarring of the interosseus ligament prevents the normal rotation of the radius (Fig. 15–31A–E) (Stanley, 1997). Injury to other periarticular soft tissues, such as the supinator muscle or either of the pronator muscles, can limit forearm rotation.

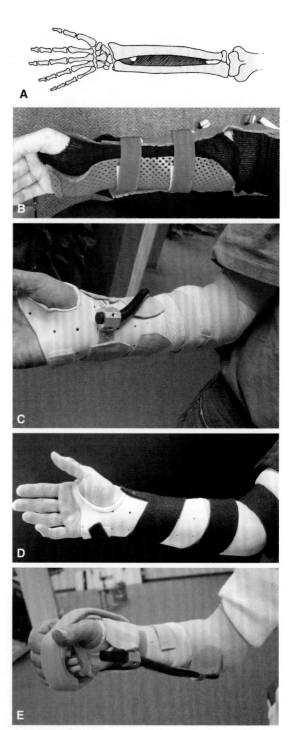

FIGURE 15–31 **A,** The dense interosseus ligament joins and stabilizes the radius and ulna along their entire course. **B,** Static progressive orthosis to restore forearm supination. While there are a number of commercially available orthoses to restore supination, fabrication of a thermoplastic orthosis which uses hook and strapping to create a static progressive rotation force can be simple and effective. **C,** A forearm rotation kit can be used to impart a supination (or pronation) force onto the forearm (shown is the Rolyan® Forearm Rotation kit, Performance Health). **D,** Neoprene can be an effective "dynamic" force to provide a low-load, prolonged stress (LLPS) to the forearm. Note the incorporation of the wrist immobilization orthosis in order to effectively hone-in on pure forearm rotation. **E,** A forearm pronation mobilization orthosis combined with a loop strap providing a simultaneous MCP/proximal interphalangeal (PIP) flexion for tight extrinsic extensors.

"Colello Splint"
CERI PULHAM, OT, CHT
Australia

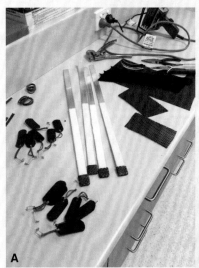

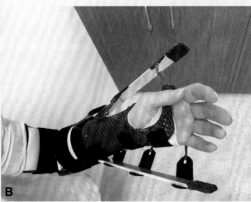

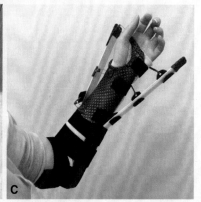

Fabricated with separate elbow-based and forearm-based components made from 2.4 mm perforated Aquaplast, 1.6 × 20 mm aluminum bar with elastic bands/Velcro to provide supination stretch. Can be used to stretch forearm into pronation as well.

ELBOW JOINT

There are a number of factors cited in the literature contributing to elbow stiffness (Dávila & Johnston-Jones, 2006). They include the severity of the trauma, intra-articular involvement, and the duration of immobilization. Following injury, the capsule can thicken as much as 3 to 4 mm. After injury, capsular thickening and contracture of the capsule develop within days. Galley, Richards, and O'Driscoll (1993) studied the effect of intra-articular effusions to explain the early development of flexion contracture from trauma. This condition causes the joint to assume a position of flexion to maximize capacity and minimize pressure. Hotchkiss (1995) describes how the uninjured elbow joint has a thin and usually transparent capsule that leaves adequate clearance for full flexion and extension. However, after trauma, the capsule thickens and limits both flexion and extension as a doorstop and a tether.

Delay in instituting active motion contributes to stiffness, especially in the elbow; therefore, if early on, the injury can be managed with a restriction orthosis, this is preferable (Fig. 15–32A) (Morrey, 2000; Morrey & Nirschl, 2000). These orthoses can be designed to allow a safe degree of motion yet stabilize the intended area as to minimize stiffness (Morrey, 2000).

For the treatment of elbow stiffness, orthotic intervention can be successful as long as the motion limitation is not the result of intrinsic factors such as joint incongruity, heterotopic bone, or a mechanical block (Dávila & Johnston-Jones, 2006). To restore elbow flexion, static progressive orthoses may also be used (Fig. 15–32B,C). If elbow flexion is <110° (Szekeres, 2006), a hinge is needed to prevent compressive forces to the elbow joint. To restore extension, static progressive and serial static night orthoses may be used to achieve adequate end-range time (Fig. 15–32D,E).

If both directions are limited, consider use of static progressive flexion during the day and a serial static extension orthosis for nighttime use.

The medial and lateral collateral ligaments are often injured in elbow fractures and have a propensity toward calcification (Thompson & Garcia, 1967). The brachialis muscle is broad and lies directly on the capsule as it crosses the elbow joint. It is highly vascular, has no tendinous portion at this point, and thus bleeds in response to trauma. Hematoma has been implicated as an inciting cause of heterotopic ossification and subsequent capsular contracture (Glynn & Neibauer, 1976; Husband & Hastings, 1990; Urbaniak, Hansen, Beissinger, & Aitken, 1985). Both the anterior and the posterior capsule often contract. Heterotopic ossification is not amenable to orthotic management.

Ectopic ossification about the elbow can result from various local or systemic insults, including direct injury, neural axis trauma, burns, and genetic disorders (Viola & Hasting, 2000). The most common cause of elbow ectopic ossification is direct elbow trauma (Green & McCoy, 1979). Pathologic bone formation at the elbow level forms an unyielding block to motion and is generally not amenable to orthosis management and ROM treatment. As stated earlier, ectopic ossification is a contraindication for a mobilization orthosis.

Dynamic Orthosis for Elbow Flexion
ANA CANDICE COELHO, PT
Brazil

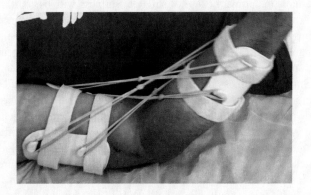

Hooks for elastic bands made on the orthosis itself prevent the hooks from coming off.

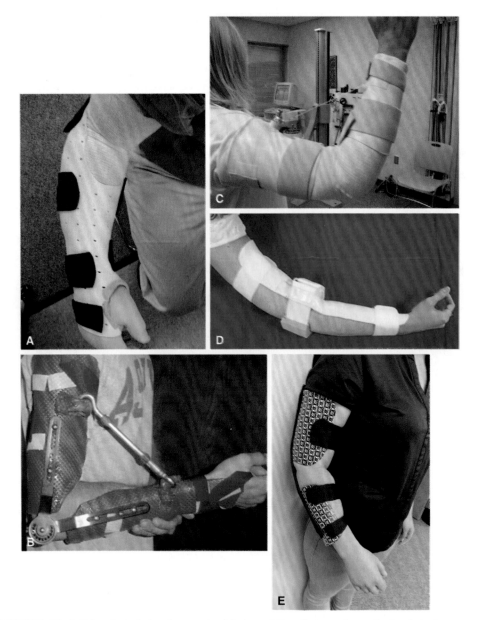

FIGURE 15–32 A, This orthosis design allows nearly a full plane of elbow flexion and extension but limits forearm rotation. **B,** Static progressive elbow flexion orthosis utilizing a hinge to mitigate compressive forces and a turnbuckle to generate static progressive tension. **C,** Elbow flexion mobilization orthosis utilizing a static progressive approach with the MERiT™ component. **D,** Elbow extension orthosis fabricated at the patient's end range with space added anteriorly to allow gentle stretch. **E,** A dynamic elbow extension orthosis utilizing neoprene to impart a gentle dynamic force.

SHOULDER JOINT

Like the wrist, the shoulder is a complex joint made up of several articulations: glenohumeral joint, acromioclavicular joint, scapulothoracic joint, and sternoclavicular joint. According to Copeland (1997), trauma is the primary cause of shoulder stiffness with osteoarthritis, and rheumatoid arthritis is a close second. Other rarer inflammatory arthropathies can contribute to shoulder motion problems. Soft-tissue inflammation, especially rotator cuff tendonitis with impingement and subacromial bursitis, may result in permanent motion loss.

Shoulder stiffness has some causes unique to the glenohumeral complex. Primary frozen shoulder, or adhesive capsulitis, has no known cause. Copeland (1997) emphasizes the need for a general systemic assessment as part of the comprehensive shoulder stiffness examination to rule out contributions from remote sites, including Pancoast tumor, myocardial infarction, esophagitis, subphrenic abscess, cholecystitis, and gastric ulcer. Shoulder PROM loss may also result from shoulder immobilization. This immobilization may occur as treatment for primary shoulder pathology or may happen as the result of sling immobilization or self-treatment during recovery

from injury to the distal joints. Copeland (1997) notes that of all the upper extremity joints, the shoulder most frequently responds to decreased movement with rapid onset of stiffness.

The shoulder demonstrates patterns of motion limitation. Impingement syndrome usually results in loss of elevation, abduction, and horizontal abduction. Cyriax (1978) described the capsular pattern, with loss of elevation and external rotation greater than internal rotation. The clinician frequently encounters this capsular pattern after sling immobilization.

Because shoulder orthoses are often bulky, heavy, and difficult to fabricate and fit, clinicians and patients rarely chose a shoulder orthosis as the first line of treatment. Commercially available static progressive orthoses may be considered to restore shoulder motion. The reader is referred to Chapter 9 for this information.

Many of the diagnosis treated by the hand therapist result in specific patterns of stiffness. While it is recommended that the reader refer to the chapter discussing specific diagnosis, Table 15–2 provides a summary of common stiffness patterns related to several diagnoses as well as recommendations for orthosis intervention should stiffness occur.

TABLE 15–2	**Common Patterns of Stiffness and Orthoses Recommendations by Diagnosis**	
Diagnosis	**Common Complications**	**Orthosis Recommendations**
Extensor tendon injury	• Zones I and II tendon disruptions can result in • DIP flexion contracture • Swan-neck deformity • Zones III or IV tendon disruption can cause • PIP flexion contracture • PIP extension contracture • PIP extension lag • Imbalances at the IP joints • Boutonniere deformity • DIP hyperextension deformity and loss of flexion at the DIP • Adhesions can limit wrist, thumb MP, MCP, and IP flexion, leading to one or more joint extension contractures (see Chapters 18 and 19 for further information)	• Orthosis to address DIP flexion contracture: • Serial static casting or orthosis • PIP extension block (figure-of 8 design) • Orthosis to address limited PIP flexion: • Relative motion orthosis (MCP in relative extension) • MCP blocking orthosis • Static progressive orthosis; MCP joint in full extension as a flexion force is targeted to the PIP joint • Orthosis to address limited PIP extension: • Static progressive orthosis; MCP joint in a flexed position and an extension force targeted toward the PIP joint • Relative motion orthosis—MCP in relative flexion • Hard end-feel PIP contracture: • Serial casting • Low-load prolonged stress (LLPS) for at least 6 hours a day
Flexor tendon injury	• Zone II flexor tendon lacerations: • Stiffness can be caused by • Inflammation, edema, and scar synthesis • Formation of IP flexion contractures • Flexor tendon injury in other zones may also cause IP flexion contractures	• Soft end-feel joint contracture: • Relative motion orthosis for exercise • Night extension orthosis • Hard end-feel joint contracture: • Serial casting • Static progressive orthosis • LLPS for at least 6 hours a day
Fractures	• Fractures cause joint stiffness via several mechanisms: • Edema and inflammation • Normal reflex arc and the patient's normal response to pain limit active motion at the joint • Structures that glide over bone may become trapped in the scar callus that heals the bone • This may lead to extrinsic tightness • Ability to restore and maintain joint motion is severely compromised • Common joint stiffness issues seen in distal radius fractures: • Limited flexion of the wrist • Limited extension of the wrist • Limited forearm rotation (supination and/or pronation) • Limited thumb ROM at the MP or IP joint • Common joint stiffness issues seen in phalanx fracture: • Limited flexion at the MCP, PIP, or DIP joint • Limited extension at the MCP, PIP, or DIP joint	• In the case of isolated joint stiffness: • Focus on LLPS isolating the targeted joint • Check for extrinsic tightness prior to making a decision on orthoses to restore motion • To address extrinsic tightness: • Composite extension or flexion static progressive orthosis • Orthoses to address extrinsic tightness span multiple joints and act in the same direction • To address MCP, PIP, or DIP stiffness: • Forearm or hand-based static progressive orthosis targeted in the desired direction at a 90-degree angle of the affected joint
Ligament injuries/ dislocations	• Sprains directly compromises structures supporting the joint and ligament injuries tend to heal slowly owing to poor vascularity often leading to stiff joints • Edema and pain severely limit motion • Dislocations of the PIP joint: • At the PIP joint and/or DIP joint • Stiffness and flexion contractures • Chronic edema limiting joint arc of motion • Volar dislocation common complications: • Boutonniere deformity • Dorsal dislocation common complications: • Swan-neck deformity	• If joint stiffness contractures occur: • Static progressive or dynamic orthoses targeting affected joint in the opposing direction of the contracture • Serial static orthoses • Blocking and relative motion orthoses to redirect force • To address swan-neck deformity: • Figure-of-8 blocking PIP extension • To address boutonniere deformity: • Serial casting of the PIP joint, static progressive tension targeted to flexion of the DIP with extension of the PIP
Median nerve injury	• The primary complications that occur following a median nerve injury include • Difficulty or inability to pronate the forearm or flex the wrist • Tingling and/or numbness, grip weakness • Inability to oppose the thumb • These complications can cause predictable patterns of stiffness without appropriate orthosis intervention	• Orthosis to address thumb • Web spacer for first web space adduction contracture • Hand-based thumb CMC/opponens orthosis for ADL

(Continued)

TABLE 15–2	Common Patterns of Stiffness and Orthoses Recommendations by Diagnosis (Continued)	
Diagnosis	**Common Complications**	**Orthosis Recommendations**

Ulnar nerve injuries	• Common complications following ulnar nerve injuries:
	  • Sustained flexion of the IP joints and hyperextension of the MCP joint
	  • IP flexion contractures
	  • Lack of functional MCP flexion
	  • Loss of ulnar finger metacarpal rotation and results in the loss of the cupping function of the palm
	  • Intrinsic muscles can become fibrotic, losing the transverse metacarpal arc. The palm assumes a narrow and flattened appearance, a sign of intermetacarpal contractures
	• Claw deformity ("ulnar claw")
	  • Loss of lumbrical's function
	  • Hyperextension at the MCP joints and flexion of the PIP and DIP joints of the fourth and fifth fingers
		• Edema or inflammation can indicate the need for an IP extension immobilization orthosis to prevent contracture
		• Established IP flexion or MCP extension contractures require a static progressive mobilizing orthosis targeting the affected joint
		• Anticlaw orthosis:
		  • Positioning the MCP joints of fourth and fifth fingers into flexion, transmitting force distally to extend the PIP joints

Radial nerve injury	• Radial nerve injuries can cause loss of innervation to
	  • Brachioradialis and supinator muscles
	  • All wrist extensors
	  • Extrinsic finger extensors
	  • Extrinsic thumb abductors
	• Deformity observed with radial nerve injuries is commonly referred to as "wrist drop"
		• Orthosis to address wrist drop:
		  • Orthosis that maintains a tenodesis pattern of the hand to allow function during the healing of the nerve (radial nerve tenodesis orthosis)
		  • Resting orthosis with wrist/MCP extension for night positioning

Burn injury	• Partial-thickness burns cause joint stiffness primarily via adaptive shortening of periarticular structures • Tight skin positions these structures on slack in the presence of inflammation, edema, and scar formation. Healing scar contracts, pulling the joints along with it • Skin damage across motion creases is the most likely to create joint stiffness (Chapter 25 provides more details) • Full-thickness burns can also damage tendon. The loss of active motion, coupled with the adaptive shortening, creates a powerful mechanism for joint stiffness	• The orthosis should not only prevent primary joint contracture but also protect vulnerable tendon structures such as the central slip of the extensor hood mechanism (dorsum of the PIP)

OTHER CONDITIONS LEADING TO STIFFNESS

There are many conditions and disease processes that lead to stiffness. The reader is encouraged to reference the other chapters within this text to get specific information on stiffness for a specific patient population.

PSYCHOPATHOLOGY

No discussion of stiffness is complete without addressing the contribution that psychopathology can make to PROM loss. The problems take many forms, including but not limited to the following:

• Contribution to causing an accident (Hirschfeld & Behan, 1963)
• Self-inflicted wound (Wallace & Fitzmorris, 1978)
• Noncompliance with postinjury care
• Clenched fist syndrome (Vranceanu, 2011)
• Refusal to move a joint via nonfunctional cocontraction (Simmons & Vasile, 1980)
• Refusal to move a joint for a significant period of time (Brand, 1988)
• Secondary gain issues (Vranceanu, 2011)

Improving PROM in a patient with these tendencies usually involves some form of psychotherapy. The patient perceives attempts to increase motion as undesirable and will resist. Empathy and skilled communication are paramount along with a supportive and consistent multidisciplinary team approach (Vranceanu, 2011).

BURN INJURY

Partial-thickness burns cause joint stiffness primarily via adaptive shortening of periarticular structures. Tight skin positions these structures on slack in the presence of inflammation, edema, and scar formation. Healing scar contracts, pulling the joints along with it (Fig. 15–23A,B). Skin damage across motion creases is the most likely to create joint stiffness (Chapter 25 provides more details). Full-thickness burns can also damage tendon. The loss of active motion, coupled with the adaptive shortening, creates a powerful mechanism for joint stiffness. The clinician must be aware of the tendon's vulnerability to thermal injury. The orthosis should not only prevent primary joint contracture but also protect vulnerable tendon structures such as the central slip of the extensor hood mechanism (dorsum of the PIP) (Grigsby deLinde & Miles, 1995).

FRACTURE

Fracture causes joint stiffness via several mechanisms. For example, as discussed early in this chapter, edema and inflammation accompany most injuries, fractures included. Cartilage defects also produce loss of PROM, which occurs in a predictable cascade of increased friction, leading to inflammation that in turn creates pain and edema. The normal reflex arc and the patient's normal response to pain limit active motion at the joint. When the joint fails to go through its full arc of motion, periarticular structures shorten; and eventually, the joint will lose motion.

A fracture may produce loose bodies in an adjacent joint (Raney, Brashear, & Shands, 1971). A loose body limits joint motion mechanically. If the loose body persists and the joint limitation is sustained, the periarticular structures may adaptively shorten, causing joint stiffness.

Structures that glide over bone may become trapped in the scar callus that heals the bone. This may lead to extrinsic tightness or may involve a prime joint mover, such as a wrist extensor. When this occurs, the muscle-tendon unit does not have adequate excursion, and the ability to restore and maintain joint motion is severely compromised (see Chapter 16 for details).

LIGAMENT INJURY OR DISLOCATION

A sprain directly compromises structures supporting the joint. Ligament injuries tend to heal slowly owing to poor vascularity (Levine, 1992). They also tend to be painful for months and even years after they are healed. Clinical experience shows that edema after ligament injury of the small IP and MCP joints tends to linger much longer than for other types of injuries (Mannarino, 1992). The edema and pain severely limit motion. The therapist must fabricate an orthosis carefully to prevent joint contracture and balance this with carefully guided exercise. Once a joint contracture establishes itself, the therapist must carefully note sprain classification, swelling, color, and temperature to avoid aggravating the joint while attempting to restore motion.

INFECTION

As part of the initial evaluation of a trauma patient with wounds or percutaneous pins, the therapist should obtain information about the patient's risk for infection. When risk factors are present, the therapist must be on constant alert for signs of infection. Infection causes an acute and severe inflammatory reaction. Edema always accompanies infection and is the primary reason that infection frequently results in stiffness (see Chapter 3 for detailed information). Some organisms not only trigger inflammatory reactions but also produce toxins that destroy tissue. Frequently, infection management involves immobilization of the involved part, which contributes to joint stiffness. Sepsis has the capacity to turn a good surgical result into a poor one because of its motion-robbing effects (Nathan & Taras, 1995).

DIABETES

The patient with diabetes has a greater risk for hand stiffness as commonly seen with chronic stenosing tenosynovitis, also known as trigger finger (Means et al., 2011). The patient may present with the involved digit locked in either flexion or extension due to long-standing tenosynovitis. Over time, a PIP joint flexion or extension contracture may develop interfering with simple activities of daily living (ADLs) and life tasks. Conservative treatment is aimed at edema reduction and serially casting the digit in the desired direction of correction. Surgical intervention is a last resort, because these patients may have a greater risk for postoperative complications secondary to the complexity of the disease process.

PARALYSIS

Paralysis of the primary IP extensor and MCP flexor occurs with loss of ulnar or combined ulnar and median nerve motor function. This leads to sustained flexion of the IP joints and hyperextension of the MCP joint as the patient attempts to straighten the fingers with only the extrinsic extensor digitorum communis (EDC) (Brand & Hollister, 1999). Over time, this unopposed flexion alone can produce IP flexion contractures owing to adaptive shortening. The hyperextension at the MCP joint further facilitates the loss of IP flexion and subsequent contracture. Left to the whims of the extrinsic flexor, the MCP joint flexes only after both IP joints have done so. The combination of MCP hyperextension (when the patient attempts to open the palm for function) and lack of functional MCP flexion facilitate the loss of MCP flexion.

The presence of edema and/or of inflammation often hastens the contracture. When the therapist notes loss of ulnar or combined ulnar and median nerve function, the treatment plan must immediately include MCP flexion orthotic intervention. With the MCP joint flexed, the power of the EDC transfers to the IP joint and reestablishes active IP joint extension (Brandsma, 1993). Edema or inflammation indicates the need for an IP extension immobilization orthosis to prevent contracture. Established IP flexion or MCP extension contractures require a mobilizing orthosis to increase PROM (see Chapter 20, for details).

Loss of the ulnar nerve innervated intrinsic muscles produces the loss of ulnar finger metacarpal rotation and results in the loss of the cupping function of the palm. When the metacarpals remain immobile and the intrinsic muscles become fibrotic, the transverse metacarpal arch is lost. The palm assumes a narrow and flattened appearance, a sign of intermetacarpal contractures. Orthoses that incorporate the palm must be carefully contoured to preserve the metacarpal arch (Malick, 1972).

CONCLUSION

The stiff joint continues to be one of the great challenges in hand surgery and rehabilitation. With unique anatomy, each joint presents its patterns of response to injury and disease. Understanding the tendencies for a joint to respond to trauma and disease in a certain way helps the therapist predict problems with stiffness and often provides the opportunity to prevent loss of motion. To work toward the goals of either preventing stiffness or minimizing the duration of stiffness, therapists must continue to study the nature of stiffness at the molecular, histologic, and joint complex levels.

FIELD NOTE

Robyn Midgley, BSc (Hons) OT, AHT (BAHT), ECHT (EFSHT)
South Africa

Viscoelastic Behavior of Connective Tissue

Stiffness of the hand is not an increased rigidity of the tissues themselves[1] but a constraint created by cross-linking of the previously elastic configuration of the collagen fibers.[2]

Collagen is a hard, insoluble, and fibrous protein that is found in the extracellular matrix. The word collagen is derived from Kola meaning Glue and Gen meaning producing. Collagen is the glue that keeps our tissues together.

In the dermis, a fibrous network of cells called fibroblasts are present, which play a critical role in wound healing. They produce both collagen and elastin. Collagen provides most of the tensile strength of the tissue in the hand. It can be considered to be stronger than steel. Elastin, like collagen, is a protein which is a major constituent of the extracellular matrix of connective tissue. It is a linearly elastic material that changes with deformation and has very small relaxation effects. Collagen fibers themselves are inelastic, but movement between the collagen fibers imparts elasticity to the tissue.

When an injury occurs, collagen proliferation is accelerated, resulting in the formation of a disorganized layer of collagen that may adhere to skin and restrict the mobility of ligaments, tendons, or joint capsules.[3]

Normal hand motion occurs when these strong, dense connective tissue structures glide relative to one another.[4] Stiffness is caused by the fixation of the tissue layers so that the usual elastic relational motion is restricted by cross-links binding the collagen fibers together.[2, 4-9]

Because of the viscoelastic behavior of connective tissue, as a force is applied, there is elastic behavior up to a certain point (the yield point), and then as additional constant force (creep) is applied, there is further displacement. Removal of the force results in partial return to the initial displacement (relaxation). This viscoelastic response can be appreciated in the stiff hand's temporary response to stretch. This is the key to understanding how to resolve joint stiffness in the hand and why LLPS is the most effective way of resolving digital stiffness long term. The CMMS technique provides the most appropriate LLPS stress and is the treatment of choice for the stiff hand. The change in tissue length and mobility through the use of the CMMS technique is superior to that which can be achieved through the use of mobilization orthoses. Furthermore, once the therapist knows how to apply the CMMS technique, the correct amount of stress will be applied without cause for concern.

Active Motion Resolves Joint Stiffness

The primary motor cortex contains an organized map of motor movement representations, including the hand.

Plasticity is an increase in the cortical area representing the skin surface engaged in the task; therefore, heavily practiced behavior causes cortical plasticity by increasing the size of the muscle groups' representation in the brain. Without attention, plasticity is severely limited.[10]

In the chronically stiff hand, joint stiffness is a result of increased collagen cross-linking. The brief, intermittent nature of passive motion combined with little or no engagement of the somatosensory motor cortex renders passive joint motion ineffective and should be avoided. Furthermore, any forceful stretches result in tissue damage and should also be avoided.[6, 11] Increasing passive motion does not increase active motion. However, increasing active motion, will increase passive motion. There is also no need to apply resistance to joint motion in order to have an effect on joint stiffness.

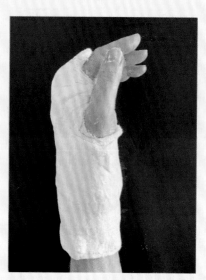

Active motion through the use of the CMMS technique

Treat Multiple Problems Simultaneously

When an injury to a part of the hand occurs, the entire hand responds to the injury. Previously uninjured structures, undergo the same response to trauma, including fibroplasia, increased collagen turnover, and remodeling. One of the greatest challenges therefore is to preserve the integrity of the uninjured structures. The stiff hand becomes immobilized by edema and tissue adherence. This results in the development of a maladapted movement pattern. As this is occurring, the motor and sensory cortical representation of normal, synergistic motion diminishes and is replaced by a maladaptive pattern instead. When abnormal patterns of movement are repeated over time, they give way to changes in the motor cortex.[12] Resolution of joint stiffness is therefore both a mechanical and cerebral challenge. The sooner the abnormal pattern is interrupted the better. Treatment of the multiple problems that are arising in the stiff hand should not occur independently, but rather simultaneously. Time is of the essence when treating the stiff hand. A delay in the appropriate treatment will rob the hand of the possibility of a full return to function. The CMMS technique is the only technique that adequately addresses multiple problems simultaneously, while reestablishing a normal pattern of motion. One need not wait for chronic stiffness to develop before applying the CMMS technique. The technique should be applied as soon as it becomes evident that traditional therapeutic techniques are ineffective. The presence of wounds should not delay the application of the technique. Caution is only warranted in the presence of infection.

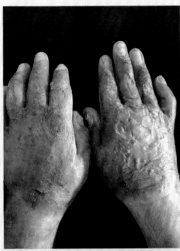

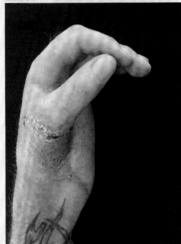

mobilize the stiff hand. The ability to transform a newly stiff hand to a functional and mobile one is dependent on therapist skill. The therapist must be able to critically evaluate the stiff hand and determine which anatomical structures are limiting motion. The type of stress applied and the facilitation of adequate joint motion through selective immobilization of proximal joints in order to facilitate distal motion in a desired pattern and range is paramount to a successful outcome. Skilled therapists blend programs to achieve desirable results. At times the therapist may need to let go of achieving multiple treatment goals and solely focus on one goal, for example, immobilize the MCP joints in order to facilitate digital flexion and extension. On another occasion, one may need to achieve multiple goals simultaneously, for example, reduce edema, facilitate joint motion, and reestablish a normal pattern of motion.

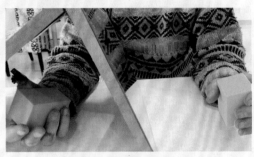

Intrinsic and Extrinsic Joint Tightness

One must always assume that in the presence of joint stiffness, intrinsic tightness is present. Full active range of motion can never be restored if intrinsic or extrinsic tightness is present. The design of the CMMS cast is determined by the pattern of motion and location of tightness. The position for immobilizing proximal joints is not arbitrary. It is determined by the location of intrinsic or extrinsic tightness and knowledge of biomechanical principles. There is no need to fear immobilizing the MCP joints in extension as the interosseous muscles are the prime MCP joint flexor muscle(s). When casting is discontinued, MCP joint flexion can easily be regained without further specific intervention toward mobilizing the MCP joints into flexion. The only exception is if there is the presence of specific dorsal adherence resulting from dorsal trauma. Dorsal tissue adherence will prevent MCPJ flexion and will require slow, prolonged stretch into flexion combined with active motion to resolve the tissue adherence and restore joint motion. Joint positioning combined with movement equals results.

Fibroproliferative Conditions

Fibroproliferative conditions such as Dupuytren disease do not respond well to aggressive therapy. Evidence suggests that overzealous splinting and exercise can increase flare-up and advance the disease process.[13] CMMS has been used effectively to resolve postoperative complications following Dupuytren fasciectomy.[14] Digital flexion has been restored without the need to apply a mechanical force in the form of splinting and without the risk of losing PIP joint (PIPJ) extension. The application of a cast promotes the release of PIPJ tightness as motion of the PIPJ is facilitated in both directions. Scar tissue adherence and edema is reduced so that joint motion can be restored.

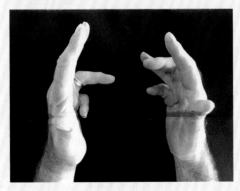

Dupuytren disease

Combined Treatment Techniques

Restoring joint motion in the injured hand demands a respect for tissue response and the healing continuum. It is up to the therapist to choose the type and timing of the intervention to successfully

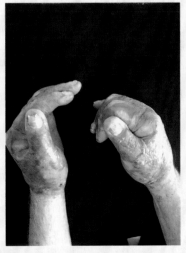

Intrinsic and extrinsic joint tightness

(Continued)

Long-Term Gains Require Slow Weaning

The most common mistake that therapists make is to discontinue casting too soon. It is exciting for the patient to make rapid gains in restoring joint motion, but it can be equally disheartening if the stiffness returns because a weaning period was not introduced. Patients must demonstrate the desired pattern of motion for 2 weeks within a bivalve cast before the cast can be discontinued. A weaning period through the use of a bivalve (removable cast) is essential to avoid joint stiffness returning.

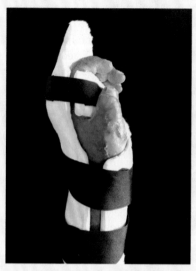

Bivalve cast for cast weaning

References

Watson N. (1994). What is Stiffness? *Journal of Hand Therapy*, 7(3), 147–149.

Frank C., Akeson W. H., Woo S. L., Amiel D., Coutts R. D. (1984). Physiology and therapeutic value of passive joint motion. *Clinical Orthopaedics and Related Research*, 185, 113–125.

Merritt W. H. (1998). Written on behalf of the stiff finger. *Journal of Hand Therapy*, 11(2), 74–79.

Madden J. W. (1976). Wound healing: The biological basis of hand surgery. *Clinics in Plastic Surgery*, 3(1), 3–11.

AkesonAmiel W. H.D., Abel M. F., Garfin S. R., Woo S. L. (1987). Effects of immobilisation on joints. *Clinical Orthopaedics and Related Research*, 219, 28–37.

Brand P. W., Hollister A. (1999). *Clinical Mechanics of the Hand*. St Louis: Mosby.

Grauer D., Kabo J., Dorey F. J., Meals R. A. (1987). The effects of intermittent passive exercise on joint stiffness following periarticular fracture in rabbits. *Clinical Orthopaedics and Related Research*, 220, 259–265.

Meals R. (1993). Posttraumatic limb swelling and joint stifness are not casually related experimental observations in rabbits. *Clinical Orthopaedics and Related Research*, 287, 292–303.

Peacock E. E. (1990). *Wound Healing*. Philadelphia, PA: W.B. Saunders.

Blake D. T., Byl N. N., Merzenich M. M. (2002). Representation of the hand in the cerebral cortex. *Behavioural Brain Research*, 135(1–2), 179–184.

Namba R. S., Kabo J. M., Dorey F. J., Meals R. A. (1991). Continuous passive motion versus immobilization. *Clinical Orthopaedics and Related Research*, 267, 218–223.

Classen J., Liepert J., Wise S. (1998). Modulation of associative human motor cortical plasticity by attention. *Journal of Neurophysiology*, 79(2), 1117–1123.

Evans R. B., Dell P. C., Fiolkowski P. (2002). A clinical report of the effect of mechanical stress on functional results after fasciectomy for Dupuytren's contracture. *Journal of Hand Therapy*, 15, 331–341

Midgley R. (2010). Use of casting motion to mobilize stiffness to regain digital flexion following Dupuytren's fasceictomy. *Hand Therapy*, 15(2), 45–51.

Case Study Section

The case studies presented here are meant as a teaching guideline only. Treatment and orthosis protocols vary greatly from surgeon to surgeon and from therapist to therapist. The therapist should check with the referring physicians and colleagues to define the preferred treatment and appropriate orthotic intervention.

Case Study 1: Hand Crush Injury

MM is a 27-year-old right-dominant male baker who sustained a crush injury to his right hand when it went into a baguette-making machine. His index finger (IF) and middle finger (MF) were crushed up to the proximal phalanx and his thumb was crushed up to the CMC joint. His ring and small fingers were generally unaffected. He had small superficial lacerations on the affected fingers and thumb that were healing well.

He was referred 10 days postinjury with a diagnosis of right crush injury with MF and thumb distal phalanx tuft fractures and a chip fracture of the MF middle phalanx. He presented with moderate edema and hematoma under the nails of the IF, MF, and thumb. He was generally hypersensitive and unwilling to move his hand, apparently owing to pain. His hand postured with his affected fingers in MCP extension, PIP flexion, and DIP in neutral. His thumb MP postured in hyperflexion with the IP joint in slight hyperextension. This thumb posture suggested an undiagnosed soft tissue injury at his thumb MP joint that would affect active and passive MP extension. This concern was shared with the treating physician and patient. A subsequent radiograph revealed a mild subluxation of the thumb MP joint, confirming the diagnosis of a grade 2 to 3 sprain and extensor mechanism compromise.

The therapist discussed the treatment priorities with MM and the rationale for them. MM was told that most physicians and patients prioritize regaining finger IP flexion. However, the therapist's clinical experience supported prioritizing extension. The

patient did demonstrate FDP function, and so prognosis for gaining flexion was excellent. MM learned that if the extensor mechanism was left attenuated over the flexed IP joint, it would almost certainly be permanently lengthened and would never be able to provide full extension again. This would sentence MM to lifelong PIP flexion contractures. MM agreed to the plan.

MM's initial orthosis focused on providing a safe position, with the finger MCPs in maximum tolerable flexion and the IPs in maximum tolerable extension (Fig. 15–33A). The thumb was placed in maximum tolerable abduction with the MP in maximum tolerable extension and the IP neutral. The patient received a custom, volar, hand-based orthosis made of 1/8″ combination rubber and plastic material. This type of thermoplastic provides a rigid orthosis owing to its plastic content while allowing for easier modification because of the rubber content. In conjunction with his orthosis program, the patient was provided with a comprehensive home program of edema control, gentle ROM to the fingers and thumb IP, and desensitization. The orthosis was progressed at each subsequent treatment session to achieve the goal of 75° finger MCP flexion, 0° IP extension, 50° thumb abduction, and 0° thumb MP extension. He rapidly achieved his finger MCP flexion and thumb abduction goals. He progressed in finger PIP and thumb MP extension.

Once the diagnosis of thumb soft-tissue injury was confirmed, the patient was placed in a circumferential, hand-based thumb orthosis made of 1″ QuickCast 2 tape without a liner to allow MM to bathe and wash his hands (Fig. 15–33B). When fabricating such a cast without a liner, extreme care must be taken to keep all parts of the cast smooth and all edges trimmed or folded back on themselves.

For the PIPs, MM received custom gutter orthoses fabricated of 1/16″ thermoplastic with a 1″ strap directly over the PIPs (Fig.

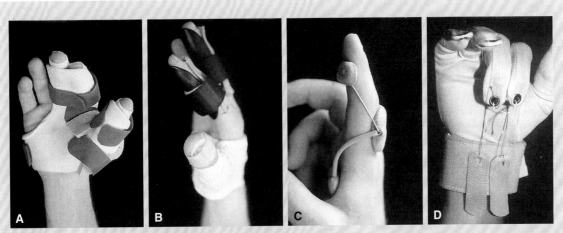

FIGURE 15–33 **A,** Hand-based index finger (IF), middle finger (MF), and thumb immobilization orthosis in the safe position. **B,** Hand-based QuickCast 2 thumb cast and with custom gutter orthoses and 1″ strap directly over the proximal interphalangeal (PIP) joints. **C,** Prefabricated PIP extension mobilization orthosis. The dynamic force is applied through the spring-loaded design of this orthosis. The patient was taught how to adjust the tension. **D,** Static lines provide a static progressive approach to composite flexion of the fingers. Commercially purchased flexion gloves come packaged with rubber bands; however, static line can easily be substituted.

15–33B). The contours of the gutter orthoses were straight volarly at the PIP, and the patient was instructed to tighten the loop strap gradually until the finger met the orthosis. The patient was also provided with a prefabricated PIP extension mobilization orthosis to be used intermittently as tolerated (Fig. 15–33C). MM achieved neutral PIPs 1 week after receiving the new PIP orthosis regimen. It is important to note that during the 7 to 10 days of therapy, MM would not have tolerated the extension forces he was able to tolerate when switched to the gutter/spring orthosis combination.

After achieving neutral extension at the PIPs, the patient received a flexion glove (Fig. 15–33D). The therapist replaced the rubber bands with static line to allow MM to use a static progressive approach to stretch composite flexion of the fingers. MM was instructed to focus on flexion but to return to the gutter orthoses intermittently if he began to lose extension; 2 days later, the patient had increased his flexion by 40° at the PIPs. He could still extend fully.

The thumb cast was changed every other day until the MP reached neutral, for a total of three casts. It should be noted that significant pressure had to be applied to achieve maximum thumb MP extension. Initially, the patient would not have tolerated this degree of force. It should also be noted that after application of each thumb cast, the thumb tip turned a deep red. The patient was asked to remain in the clinic until the color normalized, which it did for every cast.

MM was then placed in a final QuickCast 2 thumb cast that included a rigid dorsal stay made of QuickCast 2; it positioned the thumb MP in anatomical neutral. This orthosis remained in place for 6 weeks, at which time the thumb extensor mechanism was evaluated for competence and a radiograph was taken to confirm anatomical alignment.

Case Study 2: Elbow Capsulotomy and Osteotomy

LS is a 23-year-old college student who sustained a left intra-articular fracture of the humerus, ulna, and radius in a motor vehicle accident. She initially underwent an open reduction and internal fixation (ORIF) but did not have functional ROM after diligent therapy. She then underwent a subsequent manipulation under anesthesia (MUA). This too failed to yield functional motion. She then underwent two osteotomy and soft-tissue releases with the most recent 2 days before presentation. She was referred for fabrication of a custom elbow orthosis to allow her to position herself alternately at maximum extension and maximum flexion.

LS presented with a minimal dressing and a compression sleeve. Her drain was discontinued the same day she arrived for therapy.

She demonstrated 135° of flexion and 10° of extension. Her goal was to maintain this mobility, which proved difficult after the previous surgeries.

A static progressive elbow orthosis (MERiT™ SPS elbow extension kit) was chosen to meet the goals for this patient (Fig. 15–34A,B). The orthosis was fabricated using a circumferential approach the humeral cuff and 1/16″ Aquaplast T for the forearm cuff. The orthosis involved an

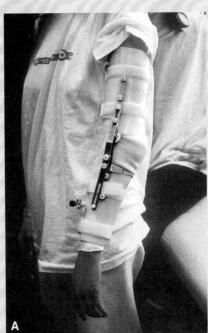

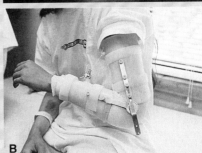

FIGURE 15–34 A static progressive orthosis allows the patient to position herself at maximum extension **(A)** and maximum flexion **(B).** Shown is a MERiT™ Static Progressive elbow extension kit.

elbow hinge and an extension outrigger adjusted to provide a 90° angle of pull. The MERiT™ kit, mounted to the forearm cuff, generated tension, which LS could control after receiving thorough instructions about use and precautions. The orthosis line was done in a three-part fashion, with one line attached to the MERiT™ component and a bra hook, one line attached to the extension outrigger and a bra loop, and the last line attached to the humeral cuff and a bra loop. This allowed the MERiT™ kit to attach alternately to the flexion or extension component.

LS immediately grasped the function and use of the orthosis and stated that she was pleased. She was instructed in precautions for skin pressure areas and was taught to monitor the sensation of the ulnar innervated digits while positioned in flexion. Her goal was to wear the orthosis for as many hours as possible during the day, alternating between flexion and extension.

Because LS lived a long distance from the clinic, she was referred to another rehabilitation facility for ongoing therapy. A 3-month follow-up visit revealed she had maintained her excellent ROM.

Additional case studies can be found on the companion web site on thePoint.

CHAPTER REVIEW QUESTIONS

1. Describe three reasons why the upper extremity may become stiff.
2. Give one example of a diagnosis with the most appropriate mobilization orthosis choice and the rationale for use.
3. Briefly describe casting motion to mobilize stiffness (CMMS) and offer an example of when a clinician would consider this treatment.
4. Give an example of three types of different mobilization orthoses (offer an appropriate diagnosis for each type of device).
5. Describe what low-load, prolonged stress (LLPS) is and why this is important clinically.

16 Fractures[a]

Jennifer Stephens Chisar, PT, MS, CHT
Nancy Chee, OTD, OTR/L, CHT

CHAPTER OBJECTIVES

After study of this chapter, the reader should be able to:
- Describe the upper extremity fractures hand therapists commonly treat.
- Understand the importance of properly positioning joints acutely to prevent contractures often seen in the later healing stages.
- Appreciate the issues and complications related to fracture management of the nonoperative and postoperative patient.
- Give examples and indications for the various materials and closure systems used to fabricate fracture orthoses.
- Understand the role, options, and design choices for managing upper extremity fractures.

KEY TERMS

Barton fracture
Bennett fracture
Boxer fracture
Chauffeur fracture
Colles fracture
Distal radius fractures
Essex-Lopresti injuries

Galeazzi fracture
Gamekeeper thumb
Humeral fractures
Metacarpal fractures
Monteggia fracture
Phalanx fractures
Pilon fractures
PIP joint fractures or dislocations

Radial head fractures
Rolando fracture
Scaphoid fractures
Skier thumb
Smith fracture
Terrible triad

MD NOTE

Gregory M. Buncke, MD
California

As an actively practicing hand surgeon for the last 30 years, I have had an opportunity to see the improvement in hand function when hand therapists become involved at an early stage in the management of hand and upper extremity fractures. When I first began practice, the dogma was to immobilize for 6 weeks and then allow the hand therapist to start working on the patient after bones had healed, putting the hand therapist in a very difficult situation. Joints were very stiff, and tendons were often adherent to the fracture site. As we began working more closely with hand therapists, we asked them to become involved earlier in mobilizing fingers and joints. Our hope was to prevent tendon adhesion and joint contractures. At the same time, we had to walk the fine line between adequate mobilization and avoiding nonunion at the fracture site. Our results have improved with earlier intervention, and the rate of nonunion has not worsened. Patients have had earlier and better functional outcomes with earlier intervention by qualified hand therapists.

FAQ

When fabricating an orthosis for fracture management of the hand, how do you decide what joints and which fingers to immobilize in the orthosis design?

In most situations, the joint proximal and the joint distal to the fracture should be immobilized to minimize any stress or movement to the fracture site. In the case of children, it may be prudent to be more restrictive and include additional joints. For example, in the case of a proximal phalanx fracture in a 5-year-old, a forearm-based orthosis may prevent migration of the orthosis and improve fracture protection by preventing movements of adjacent finger during ADL. Additional joints may be added into the orthosis design in cases of unstable fractures or if profusion is a concern in complex fractures. As noted in this chapter, there may be times that the orthosis can be less restrictive such as in the case of stable, nondisplaced ulna fractures or stable metacarpal fractures where fracture bracing may be appropriate allowing or movement of proximal and/or distal joints.

---

[a]This chapter is based on the first-edition chapter written by Kristina E. Manniello, MS, OTR/L, CHT, and the second edition written by these authors.

When deciding which fingers to include in an orthosis, often, at least initially, the adjacent finger is immobilized for comfort and to minimize stress on the healing fracture site. This technique can make the hand less functional, promoting relative rest, further decreasing stress on the healing fracture. Typically, the index and middle fingers are immobilized together and the ring and the little fingers.

How do you know how long to immobilize a fracture in the hand?

Removing the support of an orthosis from a healing fracture is a matter of critical thinking, combining knowledge of fracture healing times, clinical signs, and radiographic information. The typical immobilization time for simple fractures of the upper extremity is 3 to 6 weeks. This time frame may vary depending on factors such as the location (i.e., slower healing due to arterial flow to small-finger bones), the nature of the fracture (i.e., comminuted, intra-articular), the stability, and method of fixation used to address the fracture and the health and age of the individual. In addition, ongoing clinical assessments (i.e., persistent edema, tenderness at the fracture site) and periodic radiographs will best help in determining when motion may progress in the rehabilitation process. It is important for clinicians to educate patients who have had ORIF procedures that this allows for earlier joint motion to be performed safely, but precautions still need to be taken to protect the healing fracture from weight-bearing and force-loading activities.

INTRODUCTION

The use of an orthotic device can play an important role in the aftercare of an acute fracture by providing protection, proper positioning to prevent deformities, and patient comfort during the healing process. The increased use of open reduction and internal fixation (ORIF) techniques to address upper extremity fractures has changed the timing and duration of orthotic application, but the aforementioned goals remain the same. The proper application of an orthosis during the initial fracture healing phase protects the fracture while allowing at least partial mobility of adjacent structures. Typical conservative practice for fractures is to immobilize the joints proximal and distal to the involved bone. In some situations, a fracture brace may replace traditional cast immobilization. The materials used in custom and prefabricated upper extremity orthoses are usually lighter in weight than those used with casting, promoting patient comfort. Additionally, the low-temperature thermoplastic materials used for custom devices can conform around small areas of the upper extremity, such as the metacarpals (MCs), and be easily modified to maintain proper fit as edema resolves or healing progresses, requiring less restriction in motion.

This chapter reviews the use of orthoses in the intervention of acute upper extremity fractures sequentially, from the shoulder complex through to the distal phalanx. Tables present a quick reference of recommended styles of orthoses for the types of fractures discussed. The devices, joint positioning, and timeline recommendations outlined in this chapter are meant as general guidelines only. Each fracture is unique, and therapeutic intervention must be individualized according to the clinical presentation and healing of each patient. However, a given fracture is described or classified by the physician; when it comes to the therapist's orthotic intervention and rehabilitation strategies, the most important elements to ascertain from the treating physician are the following:

1. Is the fracture extra-articular or intra-articular?
2. Is the fracture stable or unstable?
3. Are the surrounding joints stable or unstable?
4. After reduction or surgical intervention, was the anatomy restored?
5. Are there other injuries or conditions that may influence bone healing?

FRACTURE DESCRIPTION AND TREATMENT

Fractures are generally described by the anatomical location (base, neck, or shaft) and the direction of the break line (longitudinal, transverse, or spiral) (Fig. 16–1). They are further categorized by whether they are linear (two fragments) or comminuted (several fragments) (Fig. 16–2) and open (tissue disrupted; fragment exposed to environment) or closed (soft tissue intact) (Harkess & Ramsey, 1991). Table 16–1 highlights definitions of other frequently used fracture terms.

The treatment of fractures includes a closed, immobilization approach, which involves manipulation of the bone fragments to reduce the fracture, followed by casting, traction, or use of an orthosis to hold the bones in the corrected position. Traditional methods immobilize the joints proximal and distal to the fracture site. Functional fracture bracing immobilizes the fracture site only (Latta, Peng, Sarmiento, & Tarr, 1980). The physician directs the type of immobilization method to be used. Operative treatment is performed when closed reduction efforts are unsuccessful or may be the primary method of treatment for some types of fractures based on outcome evidence in the medical literature. Surgical techniques for fracture management include external fixation, percutaneous pinning, tension bands, and plate and screw fixation (Schutz & Ruedi, 2010).

| Longitudinal fracture | Transverse fracture | Spiral fracture |

FIGURE 16–1 Fractures can be classified by the direction of the fracture.

| Linear fracture | Comminuted fracture |

FIGURE 16–2 Linear fractures produce two fragments; comminuted fractures produce more than two fragments.

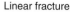

TABLE 16–1	**Common Upper Extremity Fracture Definitions**
Fracture	**Definition**
Avulsion	Occurs when a tendon or ligament attachment tears away from the bone with a fragment attached
Comminuted	More than two bone fragments result
Complicated/complex	May involve injury to nerves, arteries, viscera, or other soft tissues
Compound	Associated with an open wound; susceptible to infection if not properly treated
Extra-articular	Occurring outside of the joint
Greenstick	Impacted or buckling from bony cortex; associated with the pediatric population
Intra-articular	Involving the articular surface of a joint
Osteochondral	Involves the articular cartilage of the bone
Pathologic	An underlying health condition that weakens the bone (i.e., cancer, osteoporosis, or other metabolic disease) contributes to the fracture
Stress	Results from repetitive forces stressing the bone

SCAPULA FRACTURES

Scapula fractures occur infrequently, accounting for only 1% of fractures (Lapner, Uhthoff, & Papp, 2008). This is likely due to the fact that the scapula is well protected because it is enveloped by muscles and is in close proximity to the rib cage (Fig. 16–3). The scapula body is fractured mainly in cases of direct, high-energy trauma such as with motor vehicle accidents and falls from elevation. Acromion and coracoid fractures are usually isolated injuries caused by a direct blow to the area (Fig. 16–4). Often, scapula fractures can be managed nonoperatively and heal without complication (Jeong & Zuckerman,

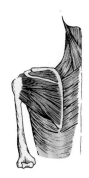

FIGURE 16–3 Scapula fractures are rare, owing to the large number of muscles that surround the bone.

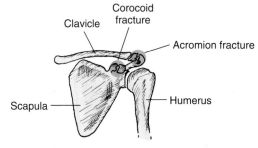

FIGURE 16–4 Fractures of the acromion and coracoid process.

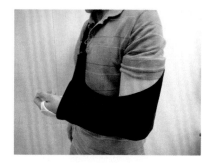

FIGURE 16–5 An arm sling can be used for many diagnoses, including injuries to the scapula, clavicle, humerus, and elbow.

2005). A systematic review by Zlowodzki, Bhandari, Zelle, Kregor, and Cole (2006) concluded that 99% of isolated scapula body fractures were treated nonoperatively with 106 of 123 achieving good to excellent results. Surgical intervention is indicated for displaced glenoid, neck, and body fractures (Jeong & Zuckerman, 2005).

Standard nonoperative management of scapula fractures includes ice and immobilization of the shoulder for 2 to 4 weeks with a sling or sling and swathe (Fig. 16–5) (Baronicek, 2015). The patient should be instructed in donning the sling, positioning the strap across the lateral aspect of the contralateral clavicle to avoid undue stress across the neck. The involved shoulder girdle should rest as close to anatomical position as tolerated to limit scapular protraction. Padding may be placed in the axilla to reduce pain and to position the arm properly. Education regarding edema control, activity limitations, and range-of-motion (ROM) exercises for the uninvolved distal joints to prevent contracture is indicated initially post injury. As pain subsides, pendulum exercises, passive ROM (PROM) for the shoulder, and pulley exercises are introduced as tolerated. Strengthening exercises are deferred until the fracture is healed at approximately 6 weeks post injury (Barei, Taitsman, & Nork, 2006). Postoperative care may include a sling for patient comfort in between PROM exercises and/or use of a continuous passive motion (CPM) device begun 1 to 2 days post surgery. AROM exercises may begin 3 to 4 weeks post surgery depending on the surgical fixation (Gross & Walcott, 2017).

FRACTURES OF THE CLAVICLE

The clavicle serves as a strut between the shoulder girdle and the axial skeleton, provides attachment for several muscles of the shoulder girdle, and protects the brachial plexus and subclavian vessels as they enter the upper extremity. The ends of the clavicle are held firmly in place to the adjacent sternum and acromion by the sternoclavicular and the acromioclavicular ligaments, respectively. The sternoclavicular joint is further reinforced by the interclavicular and costoclavicular ligaments, whereas the acromioclavicular joint obtains further stability from the coracoclavicular ligament.

Fractures of the clavicle typically occur from a direct fall or blow to the shoulder but may also occur indirectly from a fall onto an outstretched hand (Kubiak, Koval, & Zuckerman, 2005). The bending and torsional forces transmitted through the clavicle are highest in the midportion of the diaphysis, making this region the most susceptible to injury (Fig. 16–6) (Preston & Egol, 2009). Displacement is also common in midclavicle fractures due to the unopposed pull of the sternocleidomastoid muscle, which draws the medial fragment superiorly while the weight of the arm displaces the lateral fragment inferiorly. A prominence and/or skin tenting may result.

Historically, clavicular fractures have been described by the classification system introduced by Allman in 1967 and

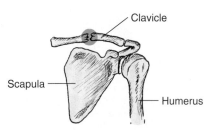

FIGURE 16–6 The middle third of the clavicle is the most common area of the clavicle to be injured.

expanded upon by Neer in 1968. Allman system divided fractures into three groups:

- *Group 1*: midshaft fractures
- *Group 2*: lateral third fractures
- *Group 3*: medial third fractures

In 1968, Neer further classified group 2 fractures into stable or nondisplaced fractures (type 1) and displaced fractures (type 2). Type 2 fractures were subdivided according to the coracoclavicular ligaments being (1) intact or (2) disrupted (Allman, 1967; Neer, 1968).

The "Edinburgh system" appeared in the literature in 1998 and has been used in outcome studies (Robinson, 1998). This system serves to describe clavicular fractures by four characteristics: anatomical location, whether there is articular involvement, whether there is displacement, and whether there is comminution. This classification system defines the following types:

- *Type 1*: the medial fifth of the clavicle
- *Type 2*: the middle three-fifths
- *Type 3*: the lateral fifth of the clavicle

Each type has further subdivisions according to the other characteristics noted earlier. Note how the numerical designations in this system differ from Allman.

Most clavicle fractures continue to be managed nonoperatively with immobilization of the upper extremity. ORIF may be indicated in situations of neurovascular compromise or to restore anatomy with significantly displaced, comminuted, or angulated bone fragments (Preston & Egol, 2009).

Immobilization options for patients with a clavicle fracture are a sling, a sling and swathe, or a figure-8 strap (Figs. 16–5 and 16–7). The figure-8 strap, sometimes recommended for midshaft fractures, requires patient education in properly positioning and adjusting the strap tension as edema resolves. If the straps are too tight, discomfort and compression of the neurovascular structures in the axilla

or skin irritation may result. The broad arm sling is appropriate for all types of clavicle fractures when used alone or in conjunction with a figure-8 strap. Andersen, Jensen, and Lauritzen (1987) compared the use of the figure-8 bandage versus a sling and concluded the sling was more comfortable with fewer clinical complications. A 2009 literature review study concluded that there is insufficient evidence to determine which conservative method is most effective (Lenza, Belloti, Andriolo, Gomes Dos Santos, & Faloppa, 2009).

Immobilization is typically recommended for 2 to 3 weeks and then weaned as pain subsides. ROM of the uninvolved joints is begun immediately with gentle active and passive shoulder motion beginning as pain allows, 7 to 14 days post injury. Isometric exercises for the rotator cuff, biceps, and triceps muscles may be introduced as tolerated. In postsurgical care of clavicular fractures, shoulder flexion and abduction should be limited to 90° initially to minimize rotation of the clavicle, which may stress fixation of the healing fracture site (Kubiak et al., 2005; Basamania & Rockwood, 2017).

HUMERAL FRACTURES

The humerus is a long bone that articulates with the glenoid fossa of the scapula proximally and the trochlear notch of the ulna and radial head of the radius distally, connecting the shoulder girdle with the forearm. **Humeral fractures** are caused by various insults including, but not limited to, falls, motor vehicle accidents, gunshot wounds, or other direct trauma to the humerus (Biangini, 1991; Tejwani & Metha, 2007). Commonly fractured sites of the humerus are the surgical neck, greater and lesser tuberosities, anatomical neck, humeral shaft, and distal humerus about the condyles (Fig. 16–8) (Beredjiklian, 2011; Brown, 1983).

Proximal fractures—involving the surgical neck, humeral head, or greater or lesser tuberosities—that are stable may be managed with a sling, sling and swathe, or collar and cuff immobilizer (Fig. 16–5) (McKoy, Bensen, & Hartsock, 2000). Humeral shaft fractures may be successfully managed conservatively using a functional humeral fracture orthosis or brace (Fig. 16–9A,B) (Sarmiento, Horowitch, Aboulafia, & Vangsness, 1990; Sarmiento, Zagorski, Zych, Latta, & Capps, 2000). As a singular long bone, enveloped by soft tissue, the humeral shaft is ideal for fracture bracing. The functional brace design is a circumferential orthosis that works by soft-tissue compression of the fracture while restricting movement of the bony fragments, even when the muscles are actively contracting. The pressure from the orthosis stabilizes the fracture, and the gravity-assisted weight of the arm can help reduce minor angulation deformities (Sarmiento et al., 2000; Sarmiento & Latte, 1999, 2006). Fracture braces are available commercially or can be custom

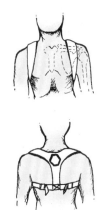

FIGURE 16–7 The figure-8 strap places the shoulder in a retracted and upright position, supporting the clavicle.

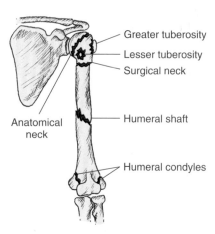

FIGURE 16–8 Areas of the humerus susceptible to fracture.

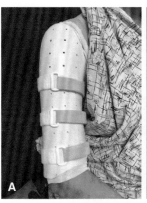
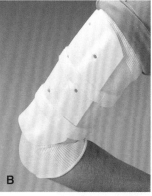

FIGURE 16–9 A, A custom-molded functional humeral brace (nonarticular humeral orthosis) that allows partial shoulder and elbow ROM. Notice the use of D-rings to allow adjustments to the amount of compression. **B,** The circumferential Rolyan® Preformed Humerus Brace allows elbow and forearm motion while providing good immobilization and support to the healing fracture. (Photo courtesy of Performance Health; Rolyan is a registered Trademark of Performance Health.)

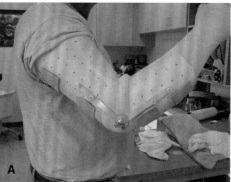
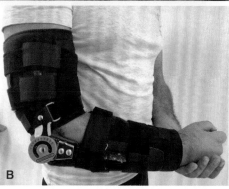

FIGURE 16–10 A, An elbow restriction orthosis using the Phoenix elbow hinge that permits protected elbow ROM. Note that the hinge is set to restrict elbow extension while allowing full flexion. **B,** A prefabricated elbow restriction hinge orthosis allowing for a selected arc of motion while restricting varus and valgus forces during fracture healing.

fabricated by the therapist. The primary benefit of this nonarticular orthotic intervention is the freedom of motion afforded to the adjacent joints, whereas slings or casts usually immobilize the joints proximal and distal to the fracture site (Beredjiklian, 2011; Sarmiento, Kinman, Galvin, Schmitt, & Phillips, 1977). Patients should be instructed in proper donning of the fracture brace for skin care and hygiene. Leaning on the elbow is discouraged during healing because this may contribute to fracture angulation (Sarmiento et al., 2000). The orthosis may require adjusting as edema resolves to maintain a proper conforming fit to stabilize the fracture. Shoulder pendulum exercises and ROM for elbow, forearm, wrist, and hand are initiated as early as safely possible to maximize motion without compromising the stability of the fracture.

Patients with humeral shaft fractures may have an associated radial nerve injury because the nerve wraps around the humerus in the spiral groove at this level. In cases where the radial nerve has been lacerated or tractioned, additional orthotic intervention should be provided to support the wrist and digits (refer to Chapter 20, for further details). This provides improved patient comfort, positions the hand for light activities of daily living (ADLs), and prevents elongation of the extensors and shortening of the flexors. Depending on the needs of the patient, a wrist immobilization orthosis may be adequate initially and progressed to a tenodesis or a forearm-based dynamic digit extension orthosis.

Functional fracture bracing has also been found to be effective for distal humerus fractures. Sarmiento et al. (1990); Sarmiento & Latta (2006) demonstrated a 96% union rate in a study performed on 85 patients with extra-articular comminuted fractures. For these fractures, the humeral cuff may be extended distally and molded around the lateral and medial condyles for additional support. In some cases, the addition of a circumferential forearm cuff attached with a hinge device may be desired to reduce varus and valgus forces at the elbow (Fig. 16–10A) (Beredjiklian, 2011; Colditz, 2011). Careful attention must be paid to align the hinge with elbow axis of rotation.

Orthotic intervention for humeral head and shaft fractures managed surgically may include the use of a sling, a cuff and collar sling, or functional fracture bracing. Distal humeral fractures managed surgically may be supported and protected by use of a sling, a posterior elbow immobilization orthosis (Fig. 16–11), a humeral fracture brace with or without a hinge (Fig. 16–10A), or a prefabricated hinged elbow orthoses (Fig. 16–10B). Table 16–2 summarizes management of fractures in the shoulder region.

EXPERT PEARL 16–1

Hinged Elbow Orthosis
CHANTAL ETCHEVERRY, OT
France

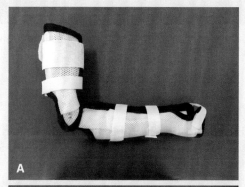
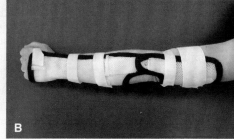

This articulated elbow orthosis is indicated for stable arm traumas (for example, a radial head fracture) allowing flexion and extension of the elbow without wrist movement or pro/supination. The two parts are molded separately and attached together with a rivet placed at the joint center.

Custom Sling
JANINE THOMAS, OTR/L, CHT, COMT
Virginia

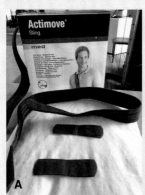
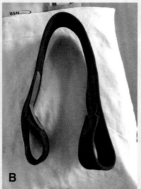
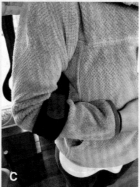
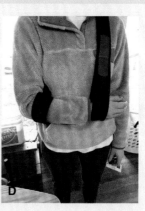

Creating a "sling" can be helpful for patients who have difficulty with positioning of arm or have issues with an elbow brace migrating. Actimove® (Essity) is a comfortable padded strapping system with Y-Tab closure to secure the upper extremity. Therapists can also create a "homemade" version with soft strapping material.

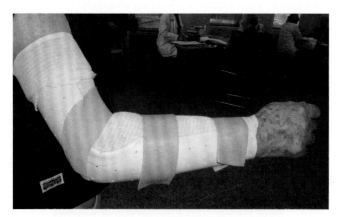

FIGURE 16–11 A posterior elbow immobilization orthosis; notice the rolling away of material about the lateral epicondyle region.

ELBOW FRACTURES

The elbow joint is inherently stable due to its bony anatomy and design. The articulations of the humeroulnar, humeroradial, and proximal radioulnar joints provide stability with additional support from the joint capsule, annular, and collateral ligaments. One of the complexities in rehabilitation of the elbow is that all three of these articulations are within a single joint capsule. Early motion following elbow fractures is always a goal because prolonged immobilization can result in fibrosis and limit ROM in any or all of these articulations (Davila, 2011). When freely mobile, the combined actions of these joints allow for effective placement of the hand for function with elbow flexion and extension and forearm pronation and supination without movement of the shoulder.

A fall on an outstretched hand (FOOSH) with the elbow partially flexed and pronated can result in a **radial head fracture** because the radial head absorbs as much as 60% of the axial load transmitted through the elbow (Ring & Jupiter, 1998a). These injuries account for 33% of all elbow fractures (Beredjiklian, 2011; Tejwani & Metha, 2007; Van Riet, Van

Glabbeck, & Morrey, 2009). Radial head fractures are divided into three types:

- *Type 1*: small fragment that does not interfere with ROM (Fig. 16–12)
- *Type 2*: fragment with greater than 2 mm of displacement that may result in limitations of movement
- *Type 3*: severely comminuted radial head or neck fractures (Adams & Steinmann, 2009; Ring & Jupiter, 1998a, 1998b)

Type 1 fractures can be managed conservatively with reduction under anesthesia and protected by use of a sling (Fig. 16–5), hinged elbow orthosis (Fig. 16–10), or posterior elbow immobilization orthosis (Fig. 16–11). Early ROM should be initiated (Bano & Kahlon, 2006). Type 2 and 3 fractures require surgical fixation to achieve articular congruity and stability to the joint.

Radial head fractures may be further complicated by a concurrent coronoid fracture and dislocation of the humeroulnar joint, known as the "**terrible triad**" (Seijas et al., 2009). Following surgical reduction, fixation, and stabilization, a posterior elbow and wrist immobilization orthosis with the elbow in 80° to 90° flexion and the wrist in neutral is applied (Fig. 16–13A,B). The position of the forearm will be according to the reconstruction performed at the elbow: pronation when the lateral collateral ligament (LCL) is repaired, supination when the medial collateral ligament (MCL) is repaired, and neutral rotation if both ligaments are repaired (Pipicelli, Chinchalkar, Grewal, & Athwal, 2011). Carefully supervised early ROM exercises may be performed, maintaining the appropriate forearm positioning.

Olecranon fractures account for 10% of elbow fractures and often occur from a direct impact to the posterior elbow, from direct high-energy loading of the joint from a fall, or from forceful hyperextension of the elbow (Tashjian, 2018; Adams & Steinmann, 2009). Although not as common, a fall on a partially flexed elbow may avulse the triceps tendon from the olecranon with a bony fragment (Fig. 16–14A), affecting the dynamic stability of the elbow (Adams & Steinmann, 2009; Ring & Jupiter, 1998b). When applying an orthosis to the elbow after an olecranon avulsion fracture, the therapist must appreciate the degree

TABLE 16–2	**Management of Shoulder Girdle, Clavicle, and Humeral Fractures**[a]	
Fracture	**Orthosis Options**	**Time Frame**
Shoulder girdle		
Scapula	• Arm sling, sling and swathe	2–4 wk, wean as pain resolves
Clavicle		
Midshaft	• Figure-8 strap, arm sling, sling and swathe	2 wk full time, wean as pain resolves until healed at 6–8 wk
Lateral	• Arm sling, sling and swathe	2–6 wk, wean as pain resolves until healed
Humerus		
Surgical neck or greater tuberosity	• Sling, humeral fracture brace with proximal extension	Variable depending on healing
Shaft	• Humeral fracture brace with or without sling	6+ wk until healed
Distal	• Humeral fracture brace with or without elbow hinge, arm sling, posterior elbow and wrist immobilization orthosis, hinged elbow orthosis	4–6+ wk depending on healing

[a]*Note that the orthosis options and time frames depend on the individual patient. Obtain clear orders from the referring physician before providing the patient with any therapy intervention.*

of elbow flexion in relation to the tension on the triceps repair. Positioning the elbow in a semiextended position places less tension on the healing structures (Fig. 16–14B).

Although literature presents limited information on orthotic intervention for fractures of the elbow, goals are the same as for other fractures: to protect healing structures, to maintain stability, and to encourage protected mobility for optimal healing with minimal residual stiffness or contractures (Davila, 2011). Initially, a sling or orthosis is applied to protect the elbow, whether managed conservatively or surgically. Slings may be applied for type 1 radial head injuries with early gentle ROM initiated in 2 to 3 days, with physician approval (Fig. 16–5). A posterior elbow immobilization orthosis may be fabricated for immobilization and protection of a stable reduced fracture or after surgical repair (Figs. 16–11 and 16–13). When early mobility is indicated, orthoses allowing for controlled elbow flexion

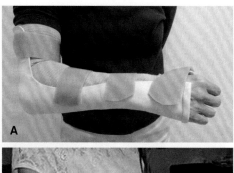
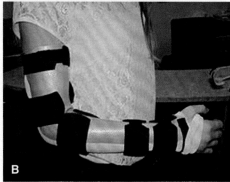

FIGURE 16–13 A, A posterior elbow/wrist immobilization orthosis is often used after radial head injuries and repairs. The wrist is included to restrict forearm rotation. **B,** An anterior approach was used with this patient making fabrication easier since gravity is assisting. The key is to make sure the straps are wide and conforming as shown here.

and extension and restricted supination and pronation such as a Muenster (Fig. 16–15A–D), sugar tong (Fig. 16–16A,B), or prefabricated hinged elbow brace (Fig. 16–10B) may be used. Therapists should be aware that neither the sugar tong nor the Muenster-style orthoses fully restrict forearm rotation. A study by Slaughter, Miles, Fleming, and McPhail (2010) suggests that if the patient is cued to respect sensory feedback provided by the orthosis, then an arc of approximately 31° rotation is available. However, if the patient is not compliant and forces to the limits of the orthosis, significantly more rotation can be achieved: 71° for the sugar tong and 92° for the Muenster-style orthoses. Ultimately, selecting the best orthosis and timing of ROM to minimize joint contractures following complex elbow fractures requires consideration of the joint stability, the structures injured, and the intrinsic healing factors of the patient. Collaboration between the surgeon and the therapist is recommended. Table 16–3 summarizes orthotic management of fractures in the elbow region.

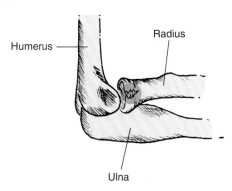

FIGURE 16–12 Type 1 radial head fracture.

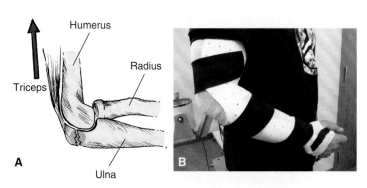

FIGURE 16–14 A, With an olecranon avulsion fracture, the triceps tendon pulls proximally with a fragment of bone. **B,** Inclusion of the wrist in an elbow orthosis may be needed to restrict forearm rotation and for the comfort of the patient. Notice the anterior/posterior design in this orthosis to unload pressure at the fracture site.

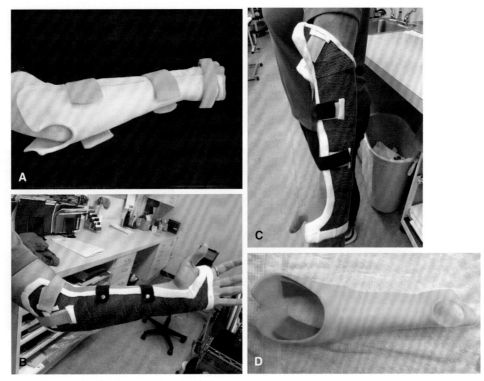

FIGURE 16–15 A, A Muenster-style orthosis supports the wrist and forearm and extends around the medial and lateral epicondyles of the humerus, allowing for elbow flexion and extension but limiting forearm rotation. **B and C,** Orthosis fabricated using Delta-Cast®—with proximal straps loosened, the patient is able to work on elbow ROM with forearm restricted in neutral. **D,** Thumb-hole, radial-based Muenster-style design—notice padding over medial and lateral epicondyles proximally.

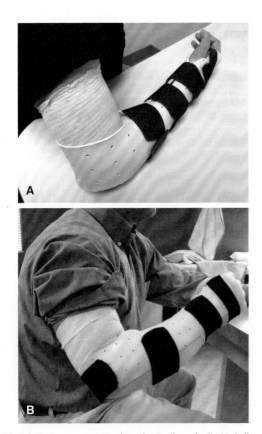

FIGURE 16–16 A, A sugar tong–style orthosis allows for limited elbow flexion and extension while restricting forearm rotation. **B,** This design allows for fluctuation in forearm edema. Notice the use of elasticized stockinette beneath for edema management.

FOREARM FRACTURES

Fractures in the forearm include isolated and concurrent fractures of the radius and ulna and more complex injuries with associated dislocations of the proximal or distal radioulnar joints (DRUJs). Singular ulna shaft fractures usually result from a direct blow to the forearm, for example, when the arm is raised to protect one's head or face from an attack or falling object. In cases where displacement is less than 50% of the width of the bone and angulation is less than 10°, cast immobilization or functional forearm fracture bracing is indicated (Fig. 16–17) (Chow & Leung, 2010; Osterman, Ekkernkamp, Henry, & Muhr, 1994). This concept is similar to functional humeral fracture bracing previously described. A circumferential custom or prefabricated orthosis is fit over the fracture site, placing pressure along the interosseous membrane to provide soft-tissue compression between the radius and ulna. This will effectively limit end-range supination and pronation but allow free forearm rotation through the midrange and early motion of the uninvolved joints. The brace is used full time until fracture healing is noted on x-ray at approximately 8 to 10 weeks. Research suggests functional fracture bracing provides greater patient satisfaction, earlier return to work, and improved ROM over immobilization in a long arm cast for these injuries (Gebuhr et al., 1992; Latta et al., 1980; Sarmiento & Latta, 2006; Sarmiento, Latta, Zych, McKeever, & Zagorski, 1998).

Fractures of both bones often result from a motor vehicle accident, direct blow, gunshot wound, or other high-energy traumatic event (Streubel & Peantez, 2015; Geissler, Valdes, & Kaiser, 2010).

TABLE 16–3	Management of Radius and Ulna Fractures[a]		
Fracture	**Orthosis Options**	**Position**	**Time Frame**
Elbow			
Radial head	• Sling • Posterior elbow immobilization orthosis • Hinged elbow orthosis	Elbow: 90°; forearm: neutral Variable	2 wk (removed for exercise)
"Terrible triad" LCL repair MCL repair LCL and MCL repair	• Posterior elbow/wrist immobilization orthosis potentially progressing to a hinged elbow orthosis	Elbow: 80°–90°; wrist: neutral Forearm: Pronated Supinated Neutral	Depending on healing and joint stability
Olecranon	• Posterior elbow (wrist) immobilization orthosis • Hinged elbow orthosis	Elbow: 45°–70°; forearm: neutral Wrist: neutral if needed	3–4+ wk depending on bone healing
With triceps avulsion	• Posterior elbow (wrist) immobilization orthosis • Hinged elbow orthosis	Elbow: 40°; forearm: neutral Wrist: neutral if needed	4+ wk depending on bone healing
Coronoid	• Posterior elbow immobilization orthosis • Hinged elbow orthosis for nonoperative intervention	Variable depending on associate injuries	2–3 wk depending on bone healing
Forearm			
Ulna, midshaft	• Posterior elbow immobilization orthosis • Forearm fracture brace	Elbow: 90°; forearm: neutral Forearm: neutral	Variable
Radius, midshaft	• Posterior elbow immobilization orthosis (after surgical repair) • Forearm fracture brace (after surgical repair)	Elbow: 90°; forearm: neutral	Variable
Galeazzi	• Sugar tong orthosis • Posterior elbow/wrist immobilization orthosis or cast • Muenster	Forearm: neutral Elbow: 90°; forearm: supinated Forearm: neutral	4–6 wk
Monteggia	• Posterior elbow/wrist immobilization orthosis or cast	Elbow: 70°–100°; forearm: neutral	4–6 wk
Essex-Lopresti	• Posterior elbow/wrist immobilization orthosis	Elbow: 70°–90° Forearm: supinated Wrist: neutral	3–4 wk
Distal radius			
Colles, Smith, or Barton	• Wrist immobilization orthosis	Variable depending on radiograph Wrist: in slight extension unless specified by MD	2–4 wk after cast removal 3–6 wk (ORIF)

[a]Note that the orthosis options and time frames depend on the individual patient. Obtain clear orders from the referring physician before providing the patient with any therapy intervention.

ORIF is the current standard of care. Depending on the alignment achieved and the integrity of the fixation, a cast or orthosis may or may not be required.

Examples of more complex conditions of the forearm that include fractures with associated soft-tissue trauma and joint dislocation include Galeazzi, Monteggia, and Essex-Lopresti injuries. A **Galeazzi fracture** (Fig. 16–18) is a fracture of the lower third of the radial shaft, resulting in DRUJ disruption, often caused by a FOOSH with forearm pronation (Ring, 2006). These fractures usually require ORIF to restore forearm and DRUJ stability. An elbow and wrist immobilization orthosis with the forearm in supination (Fig. 16–19) is indicated when DRUJ instability persists postoperatively for 4 to 6 weeks (Giannoulis & Sotereanos, 2007; Ring, 2006). Galeazzi fractures may also be managed with a Muenster (Fig. 16–15) or sugar tong (Fig.

16–16A,B) orthosis to restrict DRUJ motion but allow early elbow flexion and extension when the DRUJ is pinned and/or stable postoperatively.

A **Monteggia fracture** (Fig. 16–20) involves the proximal third of the ulna with radial head dislocation caused by high-energy injuries (Earhiraju, Mudgal, & Jupiter, 2007). Dislocation of the radial head may cause traction to the posterior interosseous nerve (PIN), resulting in a concurrent PIN palsy (Chow & Leung, 2010). Monteggia fractures are classified into four types (Bado, 1967; Streubel & Peantez, 2015; Earhiraju et al., 2007):

- *Type 1*: anterior dislocation of the radial head with anterior angulation of the fracture of the ulna diaphysis
- *Type 2*: posterior or posterolateral dislocation of the radial head with posterior angulation of the fracture of the ulna diaphysis

- *Type 3*: lateral or anterolateral dislocation of the radial head with fracture of the ulna metaphysis
- *Type 4*: anterior dislocation of the radial head with fracture of the proximal third of the radius and ulna

These complex fracture dislocations are managed surgically with the goal of restoring anatomy and forearm stability for immediate motion. Postoperatively, a removable posterior elbow immobilization orthosis is appropriate for protection between ROM exercise sessions (Fig. 16–11).

Essex-Lopresti injuries involve concurrent fractures of the radial head with soft-tissue disruption of the interosseous membrane and the DRUJ. Due to the injury to the interosseous membrane and possible forearm instability, they are often clustered with forearm fractures. These high-velocity complex injuries are typically treated surgically and stabilized postoperatively in a long arm cast or posterior elbow and wrist immobilization orthosis in elbow flexion with supination for 3 to 4 weeks (Fig. 16–19) (Chow & Leung, 2010; Dodds, Yen, & Slade, 2008).

EXPERT PEARL 16-3

Custom Wrist Wrap
NANCY BEAMAN, OTR/L, CHT
Massachusetts

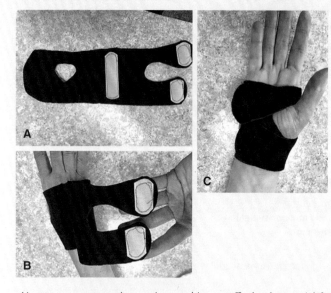

Neoprene support using sewing machine to affix hook material for closure. Helpful to use as a transition out thermoplastic or cast immobilization. Commonly used on patients who have a hard time weaning from more protective device or for those who have chronic wrist pain and require a light support during functional use.

EXPERT PEARL 16-4

Chip Bags for Edema
BETH PERKO, OTR/L, CHT
Virginia

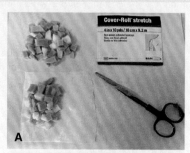
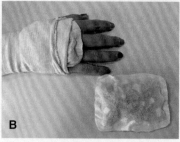

These are fabricated from small pieces of foam (various densities) encased in a custom-sized pouch (Cover-Roll stretch adhesive bandage). Their purpose is to provide constant gentle pressure, light traction on the skin, facilitate lymphatic flow, and to promote warmth. The increased body heat under the chip bag and the light pressure exerted by the foam can help soften thickened or fibrotic tissue, leading to decreased edema. They are placed directly against the skin under a compression sleeve/edema glove or positioned strategically inside orthosis to target area to maximize edema control and decrease scar adherence.

DISTAL RADIUS FRACTURES

There is a plethora of published classification systems for **distal radius fractures** documented and used in the literature, including those of Frykman, Melone, the Mayo Clinic, and the Association for Study of Internal Fixation (AO), just to name a few (Fernandez & Wolfe, 2005; Laseter & Carter, 1996; Medoff, 2011). Most of these systems define and group fractures at the distal radius as either extra-articular or intra-articular, and the AO classification system adds a third category of complex articular fractures. Within these categories are additional subsets of the fracture types. The Fernandez classification system classifies injuries according to the mechanism of injury: bending, shearing, compression, avulsion, or combined high-energy injuries (Ilyas &

Jupiter, 2010). These classification systems are well described in the medical literature.

In spite of efforts to scientifically classify all fracture patterns of the distal radius, physicians still may opt to note eponyms on prescriptions; thus, it is important for the therapist to be familiar with these common terms. A **Colles fracture** is a distal radius fracture with dorsal angulation and displacement and radial shortening (Fig. 16–21A). This type of distal radius fracture is frequently sustained by a FOOSH (Fernandez & Wolfe, 2005; Laseter & Carter, 1996; Michlovitz & Festa, 2011; Medoff, 2011).

A **Smith fracture**, also known as a reverse Colles fracture, is a fracture of the distal radius with volar displacement of the distal fragment and usually results from a fall on the dorsum of the hand

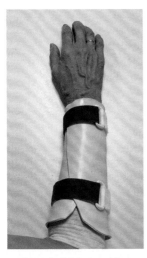

FIGURE 16–17 A custom-fabricated, functional forearm fracture brace indicated for stable, nondisplaced ulna fractures or for additional support ORIF.

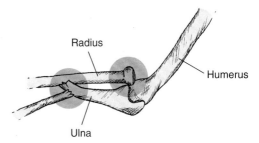

FIGURE 16–20 Monteggia fractures affect the proximal third of the ulna, resulting in radial head dislocation. These fractures often require ORIF.

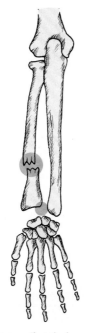

FIGURE 16–18 Galeazzi fractures affect the lower third of the radial shaft, resulting in distal radioulnar disruption.

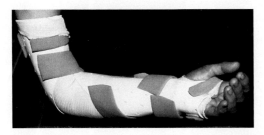

FIGURE 16–19 An elbow/wrist immobilization orthosis made from thermoplastic material to maintain fracture reduction. Note the unique spiral design to facilitate supination positioning. This positioning may be indicated to promote distal radioulnar joint (DRUJ) stability in Galeazzi and Essex-Lopresti lesions.

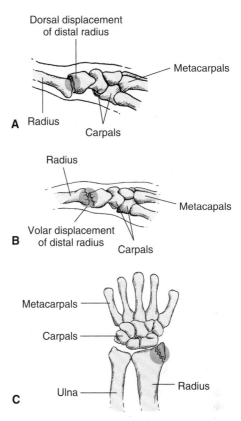

FIGURE 16–21 **Common fractures of the distal radius. A,** Colles fracture with dorsal displacement. **B,** Smith fracture with volar displacement. **C,** Barton fracture is a displaced, unstable articular fracture.

A short arm cast (below-elbow) for extra-articular fractures may be applied initially allowing for early mobility of the elbow and minimizing stiffness (Caruso et al., 2019). With more complex fractures, a sugar tong or long arm cast may be applied for a 2- to 3-week period initially and then replaced with a short arm circumferential cast for an additional 2 to 4 weeks. Colles fractures may be placed in slight wrist flexion and pronation initially to promote reduction of the dorsally angulated fragments, whereas Smith fractures may be positioned in mild wrist extension and supination (Jiuliano & Jupiter, 2006). In cases where the fracture is determined to be unstable, the duration of a long arm cast may be extended or the patient may require a more invasive intervention for fracture stabilization with percutaneous pinning, placement of an external fixator, or ORIF.

Once the cast is removed, a custom or prefabricated forearm-based wrist immobilization orthosis is appropriate intermittently for 2 to 4 weeks to provide comfort and support with easy donning and doffing as wrist motion and upper extremity function is restored (Fig. 16–22A–F). The device should allow for full metacarpophalangeal (MCP) motion of the fingers. To enhance wrist stabilization, a dorsal piece can be added to a volar-based orthosis (clamshell), or a circumferential design may be implemented (Fig. 16–22G,H).

(Fig. 16–21B). A **Barton fracture** is an unstable, displaced intra-articular fracture of the distal radius resulting in subluxation of the carpus, typically sustained from a fall on an extended and pronated wrist (Fig. 16–21C). A **Chauffeur fracture** is an intra-articular fracture of the radial styloid that may result in displacement of the carpus (Fernandez & Wolfe, 2005).

Conservative treatment via closed reduction and cast immobilization remains a widely accepted option for distal radius fractures.

Over the past decade, with the improvement in designs of volar plating systems, the use of ORIF has become more common in the management of distal radius fractures (Michlovitz & Festa, 2011). The benefits to this procedure include better restoration of the original bone and joint anatomy and earlier implementation of ROM to the wrist joint postoperatively (Brehmer & Husband, 2014; Ruch & McQueen, 2010). Use of a removable custom or prefabricated wrist immobilization orthosis postoperatively allows for early wound care, edema control, ROM exercise, and proper hand hygiene. The orthosis is weaned gradually over 3 to 6 weeks following surgery depending on the patient's pain complaints, clinical presentation, and visible callus formation on x-ray (Fig. 16–22A–C,F).

In more complex fractures with bone loss or injury with associated soft tissue requiring reconstruction, an external fixator or an option of a spanning bridge plate (internal fixation) may be used (Lauder & Hanel, 2017). When applied, the fixator is drilled into the radial shaft and the second MC spanning the wrist joint. Tension across the device results in traction across the fracture and ligamentotaxis (distracting tension on ligaments), keeping the fracture fragments in alignment and preserving the length of the radius. Spanning bridging plates are internally placed, allowing for early motion of the hand and left in place for the duration of bone healing before removal. With external fixators, adjustments can be made to the device during the healing process to correct angulation and/or reduction of the bony fragments. A bulky dressing is typically applied postoperatively and an ulnar-based wrist orthosis is provided for support, protection, and patient comfort as needed (Fig. 16–23). Some complications associated with the use of external fixators include index-finger (IF) MCP joint stiffness, first web space contractures, superficial radial nerve irritation or injury, chronic regional pain syndrome, and pin tract infections (Ruch & McQueen, 2010).

CARPAL FRACTURES

The wrist is an intricately balanced structure, consisting of eight small bones tightly articulated and bound by multiple ligaments that allow the motions of wrist flexion, extension, ulnar and radial deviation, and intercarpal rotation. Fracturing one of these bones can disrupt wrist kinematics and result in an alteration of wrist stability or mobility impairing hand and upper extremity function (Christie & Michelotti, 2019).

The most frequently fractured carpal bone is the scaphoid, accounting for approximately 70% of all carpal fractures and 11% of all hand fractures (Fig. 16–24) (Hove, 1999; Suh, Benson, Faber, MacDermid, & Grewal, 2010). A FOOSH or a high-velocity impact into forced wrist extension with radial or ulnar deviation is common mechanism of injury (Mayfield, 1980; Weber & Chao, 1978). Most **scaphoid fractures** occur through the waist of the bone (75%), followed by the proximal pole (20%) and the tubercle (5%) (Christie & Michelotti, 2019). Due to the vascular anatomy, the blood supply

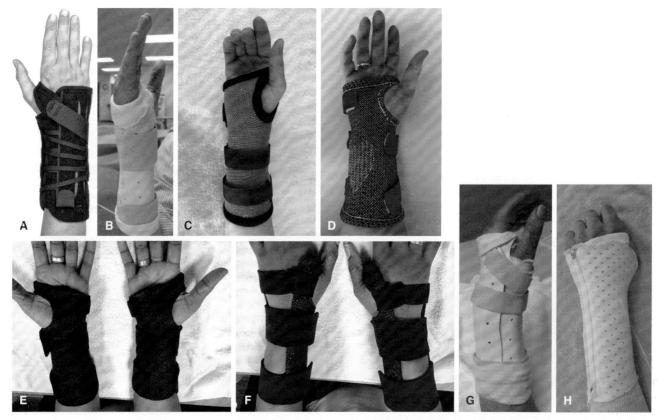

FIGURE 16–22 A, The Titan Wrist™ Lacing Wrist Orthosis allows for adjustability in fit and rigidity making it customizable to fit each patient. (Photo courtesy of Hely & Weber®.) **B,** A wrist immobilization orthosis including two-thirds of the length of the forearm for maximal comfort. **C,** *Wrist orthosis fabricated using Delta-Cast®—flexibility of material allows for modification of fit by tightening/loosening straps to accommodate for edema fluctuations often seen acutely.* **D,** X-Lite® PLUS used for this wrist orthosis providing breathability. **E and F,** 3-inch Orficast® More material makes a simple and easy-to-fabricate alternative for stable wrist immobilization. Notice unique distal strapping technique—making a slit in material and weaving strap thru itself—to avoid need for adhesive hook on such a small region of orthosis. (Images courtesy of Barbara Gaunt MHS, OTR, CHT Milford, DE.) **G,** A dorsal clamshell piece added to a wrist immobilization orthosis provides stability at the fracture site. The dorsal 1/2″ overlapping piece of thermoplastic material is applied after the volar piece has been fabricated and is fully set. Manual pressure along the edges creates an interlocking groove. **H,** A circumferential design of a wrist immobilization orthosis. This precut zipper design can be effective in promoting compliance with pediatric patients by using a zip tie to "lock" the zipper (shown is the Rolyan® AquaForm™ Zippered Wrist Splint available through Performance Health, Warrenville, IL).

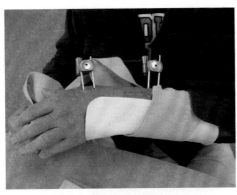

FIGURE 16–23 An ulnar-based immobilization orthosis may be used for comfort and support following placement of an external fixator. The orthosis may be held in place with soft strapping or an elasticized wrap.

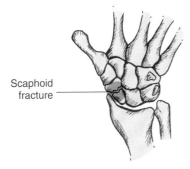

Scaphoid
fracture

FIGURE 16–24 Scaphoid fractures are the most common carpal fracture and often occur from a fall on an outstretched hand (FOOSH).

to the proximal pole is more tenuous, resulting in slower healing, requiring longer immobilization when treated conservatively (Adams & Steinmann, 2010). Nonoperative management requires immobilization with a long or short arm thumb spica cast until osseous healing is confirmed, which may take as long as 3 to 6 months. A review of the literature suggests there is insufficient evidence to support which immobilization technique is most effective (Yin, Zhang, Kan, & Wang, 2007). However, more recent research suggests that immobilization of the thumb may not be necessary with nondisplaced or minimally displaced scaphoid fractures (Buijze et al., 2014).

Indications for surgical intervention include displaced, comminuted, and proximal pole fractures or when diagnosis of the scaphoid fracture has been delayed (Knoll & Trumble, 2006). Operative treatment options for scaphoid fractures are well represented in the literature; however, it remains unclear which approach is most effective (Suh et al., 2010). When referred for treatment after surgery, a forearm-based wrist and thumb immobilization orthosis may be fabricated for continued protection during healing and remobilization of the wrist and hand (Fig. 16–25A–C). If included initially, the interphalangeal (IP) and MCP joints may later be freed for thumb mobility to decrease joint stiffness. A dorsal clamshell piece can be added to a volar orthosis or a circumferential design may be used to provide further stabilization of the wrist.

The therapist's involvement in managing other carpal bone fractures typically occurs following cast immobilization when remobilization of the wrist is indicated. Most carpal fractures can be managed with a wrist or a wrist and thumb immobilization orthosis for 4 to 6 weeks (Christie & Michelotti, 2019). Then, therapy is directed at controlling residual edema, addressing joint stiffness to increase ROM, and progressing upper extremity strength to restore ADL function. Knowing mechanisms of injuries and concurrent injuries associated with fractures of the other carpal bones can be helpful in designing rehabilitation programs.

Lunate fractures can occur acutely from a FOOSH but are more frequently associated with pathologic changes in the bone from avascular necrosis of the lunate known as Kienböck disease (Dell, Dell, & Griggs, 2011). Cast immobilization is recommended for 4 to 6 weeks for minimally displaced stable fractures, but immobilization may be prolonged if healing is delayed (Papp, 2010). Surgery may be performed if the fracture is unstable or if restoration of the joint congruity is needed. In cases of avascular necrosis, procedures to unload forces transmitted through the lunate such as a radial shortening osteotomy or salvage procedures such as a proximal row carpectomy or wrist arthrodesis may be performed (Dell et al., 2011).

Fractures of the triquetrum may occur from a hyperflexion injury avulsing the dorsal intercarpal or radiocarpal ligament or from a shearing mechanism with wrist flexion and ulnar deviation impingement of the triquetrum between the hamate and distal ulna. These fractures affecting the dorsal ridge are typically stable and can be addressed with wrist immobilization for 4 to 6 weeks (Dell et al., 2011). Triquetral body fractures are rare but, when seen, tend to occur with other significant injuries to the carpus such as perilunate dislocations.

Pisiform fractures can result from direct trauma or from forceful avulsion of the flexor carpi ulnaris (FCU). They may be addressed with wrist immobilization for 2 to 4 weeks or with excision of the bone (Dell et al., 2011). Following surgical excision, an orthosis lined with silicone gel may offer protection and support to the hypothenar eminence area.

Trapezium fractures can result from a blow to the abducted thumb or trauma, resulting a forceful wrist extension and radial deviation (Christie & Michelotti, 2019; Prosser & Herbert, 1996). Stable and minimally displaced fractures can be conservatively addressed with wrist and thumb cast immobilization for 4 to 6 weeks, whereas ORIF is recommended if the fracture is displaced greater than 2 mm to restore the intra-articular anatomy of the first carpometacarpal (CMC) joint (Papp, 2010).

Fractures of the trapezoid bone are rare, resulting from high-velocity trauma that forces the second MC into the trapezoid. Frequently, there is an associated fracture and/or dislocation of the second MC (Brach & Goitz, 2003; Christie & Michelotti, 2019). Cast immobilization for 4 to 6 weeks is the standard of care if nondisplaced. Displaced fractures may require ORIF using Kirschner wire (K-wire) fixation or a screw.

Fractures of the capitate are caused by an impact to the second and third MCs, with the wrist flexed and radially deviated (Papp, 2010). The therapist should be aware of other associated injuries such as scaphoid fractures, lunotriquetral ligament injuries, or other perilunate dislocations (Seng & Blazar, 2006). Proximal pole fractures are sometimes associated with late-onset avascular necrosis. Depending on the nature of the fracture, it may be treated with 4 to 6 weeks of cast immobilization, however, closed reduction and pinning, or ORIF may be needed to stabilize the capitate and reestablish carpal height (Christie & Michelotti, 2019).

Hook of the hamate fractures is often associated with sports that use a club, bat, or racquet. Injury can occur either from a direct blow, for example, when the club is inadvertently driven into the ground, or indirectly from strong muscle contraction while grasping the racquet or bat with wrist in extension and ulnar deviation as the ball makes contact resulting in an avulsion injury. Hamate body fractures may present with concurrent MC base fractures of the ring and little fingers (Dell et al., 2011). Minimally displaced fractures of the hamate (hook or body) can be immobilized with a cast for 4 to 6 weeks, whereas displaced fractures may be addressed with fixation or excision. A wrist immobilization orthosis may be used during the remobilization phase (Fig. 16–22A). In addition to

ROM, intervention for scar management and hypersensitivity may be indicated post surgery. Table 16–4 summarizes orthotic management for carpal fractures.

EXPERT PEARL 16-5

"Donut" Padding
LISA RAY, OTR/L, CHT
Virginia

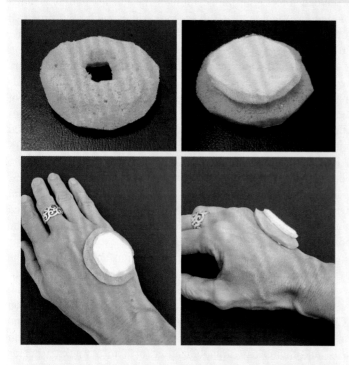

Useful for prepadding when molding over pins or bony prominences. Shown using Rolyan Temper Foam padding (Performance Health) 3/8″ with adhesive backing, edges beveled so orthosis material drapes over better. Top with thinner padding, stick directly on the patient's skin or leave paper partially on if skin is fragile. Apply prior to molding thermoplastic to create a conformable space in orthosis to accommodate these regions.

EXPERT PEARL 16-6

Sport Specific Fit
MELISSA CEPEDA, OTR/L
Colorado

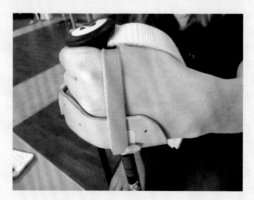

Hand-based orthosis to protect healing SF metacarpal fracture. Orthosis was custom molded to fit a ski pole to protect healing injury and allow patient to return to light skiing.

EXPERT PEARL 16-7

Fabrication Over Exposed K-wires
TRISH GRIFFITHS, OT
South Africa

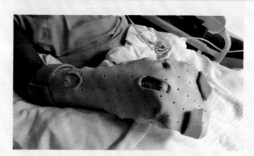

If the MD prefers to keep K-wires exposed for visualization/cleansing, a precise pattern is helpful in getting the "window" in the right spot.

EXPERT PEARL 16-8

Functional Fracture Orthosis
VERUSCHKA MOREIRA COÊLHO SAVOLDELI, OT
Brazil

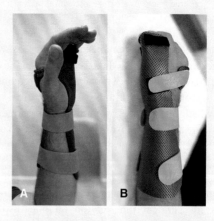

Orthosis for wrist immobilization and MCPs of ring and small fingers after fifth metacarpal fracture. Provides a functional position of the hand with active mobility of the thumb, index, and middle fingers along with PIP/DIP of ring and small fingers. Notice how distal borders of orthosis clear creases in hand that relate to allowing unrestricted motion—thenar, distal palmar crease (DPC) radially, and PIP ulnarly.

METACARPAL FRACTURES

Finger Metacarpal Fractures

Proximally, the MC bones are anchored into the carpal arch by interosseous ligaments with more stability in the index and middle CMC joints and more joint mobility in the ring, small, and thumb CMC joints. MC fractures account for 40% of hand fractures and are classified according to their anatomical location: base, shaft, neck, or head (Wong & Higgins, 2019). Metacarpal base fractures may be associated with carpal fractures and occur from direct axial loading. These fractures can be either

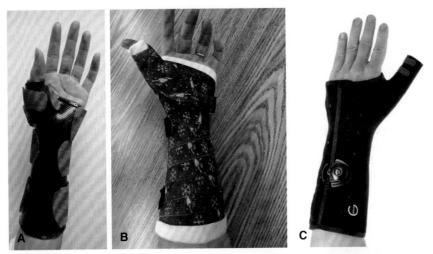

FIGURE 16–25 A, A wrist/thumb immobilization orthosis with the IP joint free is a management option for scaphoid, trapezium, and Bennett fractures. **B,** *Delta-Cast®* utilized to fabricate this wrist/thumb immobilization orthosis with extra strips of material placed radially prior to fabrication to provide reinforcement over the fracture site. **C,** The Long Thumb Spica Fracture Brace from EXOS® (distributed by DJO® Global) provides an alternative to casting or a circumferential orthosis. (Photo courtesy of DJO® Global.)

intra-articular or extra-articular but tend to be stable. Base extra-articular fractures are frequently managed with closed reduction and acute MC fracture bracing. Intra-articular fractures, like a reversed Bennett fracture with dislocation at the fifth MC and hamate joint, may require surgical repair due to forces of the FCU and extensor carpi ulnaris (ECU) tendon on the ulnar portion of the small-finger MC (Gallagher & Blackmore, 2011; Wong & Higgins, 2019).

Metacarpal shaft fractures appear as transverse, oblique, or spiral and occur with axial loading through the MC or by direct blows onto the dorsum of the hand. Transverse fractures may result in dorsal angulations at the fracture apex due to forces from the volar interosseous muscles. This angulation may leave an aesthetically unpleasing "bump" but is rarely functionally disabling (Jones, 1996). Oblique and spiral fractures may be affected by rotational torsion forces on the MC leading to rotational deformities with overlap or scissoring of digits with finger flexion. These may require closed reduction with pinning or ORIF (McNemar, Howell, & Chang, 2003).

The neck is the area of transition between the shaft and head of the MC. When excessive forces from the hand impacting an object or person transfer to the metacarpal neck, this may result in fracturing the ring or small MCs. This is known as a **boxer fracture** (Fig. 16–26). Interventions range from no treatment for nondisplaced fractures to surgical repair. Metacarpal head fractures are less common and occur from direct impact with a clenched fist (McNemar et al., 2003).

TABLE 16–4	**Carpal Fracture Management**[a]		
Fracture	**Orthosis Options**	**Position**	**Time Frame**
Scaphoid	• Long or short arm cast • Wrist/thumb immobilization orthosis	Wrist: extension Thumb: midpalmar/radial abduction	6+ wk depending on radiograph 6+ wk depending on radiograph
Trapezium	• Wrist/thumb immobilization orthosis or cast	Wrist: extension Thumb: midpalmar/radial abduction	4–6 wk
Trapezoid	• Wrist immobilization orthosis or cast	Wrist: extension	4–6 wk
Capitate	• Wrist immobilization orthosis or cast	Wrist: extension	4–6+ wk may be prolonged depending on radiograph
Hamate			
Hook excision	• Soft orthosis (after excision, if needed)		
Body/hook conservative	• Wrist immobilization orthosis or cast	Wrist: extension	4–6+ wk depending on radiograph
Triquetrum	• Wrist immobilization orthosis or cast	Wrist: extension	4–6 wk
Pisiform	• Wrist immobilization orthosis	Wrist: neutral	2–4 wk
Excision	• Soft orthosis as needed		
Lunate	• Wrist immobilization orthosis or cast		4–6+ wk may be prolonged depending on radiograph

[a]*Note that the orthosis options and time frames depend on the individual patient. Obtain clear orders from the referring physician before providing the patient with any therapy intervention.*

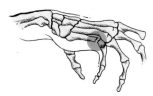

FIGURE 16–26 A boxer fracture of the fifth metacarpal (MC) neck often presents with apex dorsal angulation.

EXPERT PEARL 16–9

Why I Dislike Ulnar/Radial Gutter Splints?
HandLab: Clinical Pearls

JUDY C. COLDITZ, OT/L, CHT, FAOTA
North Carolina

Perhaps it is the name "gutter" I dislike. But long ago, I quit making splints that encase only the radial or ulnar aspect of the wrist and hand.

The indication for such a splint/orthosis is likely a metacarpal fracture. Although such a design (Fig. 1) provides the necessary stability to the healing fracture, it is challenging to make it comfortable for the patient. The edge of the splint always rests at the midline of the wrist dorsally and volarly, providing uncomfortable pressure points.

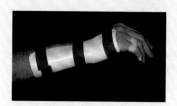

FIGURE 1 Typical ulnar gutter splint with straps.

If one of the goals of the splint is to stabilize the wrist, respecting the basic principle of three points of well-distributed pressure (Fig. 2) will increase comfort. This can only be accomplished by eliminating the edge of the splint at the wrist level which can be easily done by simply extending the splinting material further across the dorsum of the wrist as well as extending the palmar splinting material further across. With flexible thermoplastic splinting materials, this extended design still allows application and removal of the splint as needed, while greatly increasing the patient's comfort.

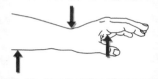

FIGURE 2 Splint should cover the three points of pressure comfortably.

Another reason the ulnar or radial gutter splint is uncomfortable may be its ability to shift on the patient's arm because the straps do not stabilize it. Either wrapping the gutter splint in place with an elastic wrap or making wide but self-contouring straps (neoprene or leather) can also potentially increase comfort. The final question is always "Could you comfortably wear the splint you have made?"

Clinical Pearls reprinted with permission from Clinician's Classroom at BraceLab.com written by Judy Colditz, OT/L CHT FAOTA, copyright HandLab/BraceLab, Raleigh NC. April 2011, No. 13.

MC fractures can be protected using functional MC fracture bracing or more traditional immobilization methods such as a forearm-based, hand-based radial- or ulnar-based orthosis (Figs. 16–27A–C and 16–28A–F). The following recommendations may be used as a guideline to select the appropriate orthosis for surgical and nonsurgical patients. Base and shaft fractures usually include the wrist for proper immobilization. Traditional management of the index-, middle-, ring-, and small-finger MC fractures involves an immobilization orthosis using an ulnar- or radial-based design with the MCP joints at 60° to 70° of flexion. The proximal interphalangeal (PIP) and distal interphalangeal (DIP) joints may be immobilized for comfort or to prevent movement of the fracture, or if stable, they may be left free to prevent stiffness of unaffected joints. It is important to hold these digits in the described position to prevent MCP joint extension contractures and maintain fracture stability (Freiberg, Pollard, MacDonald, & Duncan, 2006). Similar positioning and immobilization are required after surgical treatment depending on the type and placement of percutaneous K-wire fixations (Wong & Higgins, 2019). Inclusion of wrist may be dependent on patient compliance and MD preference.

In more progressive nonoperative treatment, Colditz (2011) recommends that MC shaft fractures be immobilized in a hand-based orthosis (ulnar or radial design) with buddy taping of the injured finger to the adjacent fingers. If additional protection from external forces is needed for shaft or neck fractures, the proximal phalanx can be included in the orthosis with the MCP joints in flexion and the IP joints free. This allows for functional ROM and can help prevent extensor tendon adherence to the fracture site. Table 16–5 summarizes orthotic intervention for MC fractures of the fingers.

EXPERT PEARL 16–10

External Fixation Protection
TRISH GRIFFITHS, OT
South Africa

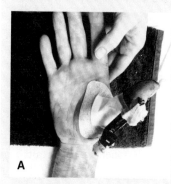
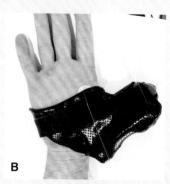

Utilize a thermoplastic material with a lot of drape to mold over the top. Ensure that the splint is easy to don and doff and does not catch on the fixation. Cover the hardware with gauze prior to molding to prevent stickage during the molding process.

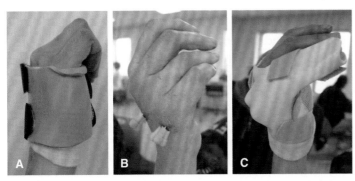

FIGURE 16–27 **A,** A nonarticular metacarpal (MC) orthosis (fracture brace) can be used to support stable MC shaft fractures and allow for early unrestricted motion of the digits and wrist. **B and C,** Ulnar-based MCPIP immobilization orthosis; notice dorsal pins are protected by forming a protective "bubble" around this region.

Thumb Metacarpal Fractures

Thumb MC fractures also occur at the base, shaft, and head. A **Bennett fracture**, occurring at the base, results from an axial blow with dislocation of the first MC and CMC joint. This may also be associated with avulsion of the palmar oblique ligament or displacement by the pull of the abductor pollicis longus (APL) tendon dorsal and radially (Fig. 16–29). A greater axial load may result in a **Rolando fracture**, a comminuted intra-articular fracture with fragments in "Y" or "T" configuration. Management of

these thumb base fractures with surgery is preferred due to the inherent instability of the CMC joint and risk of first web space narrowing (Wong & Higgins, 2019). Extra-articular fractures may be transverse or oblique. With stable reduction, transverse fractures may only require immobilization; however, oblique fractures are usually repaired via percutaneous pinning (McNemar et al., 2003). Forearm-based wrist/thumb immobilization orthoses are usually chosen to manage this level of thumb injury (Fig. 16–25A–C).

Shaft fractures of the thumb are rare as the mobility of the thumb allows forces to dissipate proximally. More common are first MC **head** fractures with bony avulsion of the ulnar collateral ligament (UCL) from the MC head, referred to as a **gamekeeper** or **skier thumb** injury (Freeland, 2000). This injury may be managed conservatively or surgically depending on the severity of the ligament disruption. A hand-based design including the ulnar side of the hand is necessary to prevent any deviation stress on the healing UCL (Fig. 16–30A–C).

Thumb MC fractures require the wrist and thumb to be immobilized (except in the case of a UCL injury as noted earlier). The thumb is positioned in midpalmar and radial abduction to preserve the first web space. The IP may be immobilized initially or free if the MC fracture is stable. However, once there is evidence of bone healing, the IP joint should be freed to minimize joint stiffness (Fig. 16–25A). Table 16–6 summarizes orthotic management of thumb fractures.

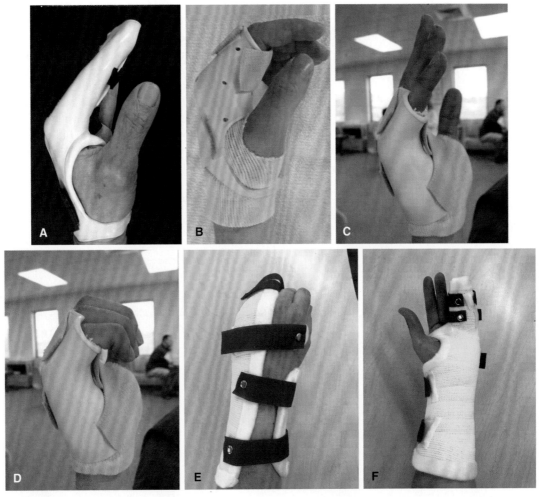

FIGURE 16–28 **A,** A hand-based radial orthosis ("gutter") for a second MC fracture with the IP joints included. **B,** A radial MCP immobilization orthosis for an index MC neck fracture. **C and D,** An ulnar-based orthosis for a fifth metacarpal neck fracture; note clearance for IP flexion. **E and F,** Delta-Cast® utilized to fabricate this forearm-based immobilization orthosis including IP joints.

TABLE 16–5	Metacarpal Fracture Management[a]		
Fracture	Orthosis Options	Position	Time Frame
Base	• Wrist immobilization orthosis	Wrist: neutral MCP: free	3–4 wk
Shaft	• Radial/ulnar forearm-based wrist/digit immobilization orthosis • MC fracture brace	Wrist extension MCP: 60°–70°, PIP: 0° or free; with or without buddy taping	3–4 wk
Neck	• Radial/ulnar hand-based digit immobilization orthosis	MCP: 60°–70°, PIP/DIP: 0° or free	3–4 wk
Head	• Radial/ulnar hand-based digit immobilization orthosis	MCP: 60°–70°, PIP/DIP: 0°; immobilize involved finger or with adjacent finger; include adjacent MC for stability	3–4 wk

[a]Note that the orthosis options and time frames depend on the individual patient. Obtain clear orders from the referring physician before providing the patient with any therapy intervention.

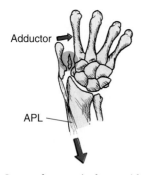

FIGURE 16–29 With a Bennett fracture, the fractured fragment separates from the MC shaft, which is further displaced by the pull of the APL tendon dorsally and radially.

PHALANGEAL FRACTURES

Proximal, Middle, and Distal Phalanx Fractures

The therapist frequently fabricates orthoses for finger fractures acutely. Goals for intervention include maintaining fracture stability, preventing joint stiffness, and minimizing adhesions of tendons during the healing process. **Proximal** and middle phalanx fractures mainly involve the neck and the shaft. Shaft fractures may be transverse, spiral, oblique, or comminuted. Simple fractures may be treated with reduction, with or without fixation. However, due to the anatomical relationship of the soft tissue surrounding these bones, injury and treatment may become more complex. Unstable proximal phalanx fractures often produce an apex volar angulation, owing to the pull of the interossei muscles on the base of the proximal phalanx (Fig. 16–31). Unstable middle phalanx fractures also present with volar angulation of the neck caused by the strong pull of the flexor digitorum superficialis (FDS) tendon on the proximal side of the fracture. If the base of the middle phalanx is fractured, a dorsal angulation will likely occur (Fig. 16–32) (Henry, 2010). Surgical interventions may include ORIF with placement of K-wires, mini screws, or plates (Lögters, Lee, Gehrmann, Windolf, & Kaufmann, 2018). Orthoses are used after surgical intervention to protect the fracture repairs and allow for safe mobility of tendons and joints (Freeland, Hardy, & Singletary, 2003; Gutow et al., 2003). Management of these injuries can be difficult as K-wire fixation delays joint motion until the pins are removed, 4 to 6 weeks following the procedure. Even when plates or screws are used, these injuries are highly susceptible to developing tendon adhesions of the extensor mechanism to the fracture site resulting in decreased extensor glide (Lögters et al., 2018; Chen & Kalainov, 2017). These patients may be candidates for a surgical tenolysis to release tendon adhesions after the initial stages of bone healing are complete.

For proximal **phalanx fractures**, hand-based digit immobilization orthoses are often used with the MCP joints generally positioned at 60° to 70° of flexion to keep the collateral ligaments at length, preventing MCP joint extension contractures. The PIP and DIP joints may be placed in near to full extension to prevent potential flexion contractures (Fig. 16–33A–C). Some therapists include the wrist positioned in 30° of extension with the MCP joints flexed and the IP joints at 0° for additional protection or for patient comfort. Nonarticular functional fracture bracing may also be used for

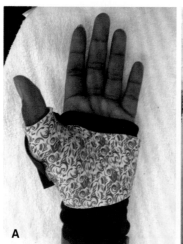

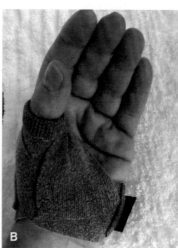

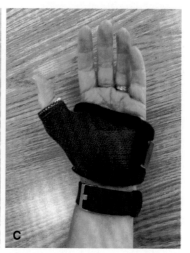

FIGURE 16–30 **A,** This thumb MCP immobilization orthosis is appropriate for an adult. It may be modified to include the thumb IP joint and or the wrist when further protection is needed for proper healing of the UCL. Similar orthoses fabricated from Orficast® **(B)** and *Delta-Cast®* **(C)**.

TABLE 16–6	Thumb Fracture Management[a]		
Fracture	Orthosis Options	Position	Time Frame
Metacarpal	• Wrist/thumb immobilization orthosis or cast	Wrist: neutral Thumb CMC: midpalmar and radial abduction	4–6+ wk depending on healing
Proximal phalanx	• Thumb immobilization orthosis	MCP: slight flexion MCP: 10°–20° flexion; IP: 0°; CMC: midpalmar and radial abduction	4–6+ wk
Distal phalanx	• Thumb immobilization orthosis	IP: 0°–5° hyperextension	3+ wk

[a]*Note that the orthosis options and time frames depend on the individual patient. Obtain clear orders from the referring physician before providing the patient with any therapy intervention.*

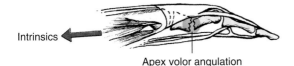

FIGURE 16–31 A proximal phalanx fracture with apex volar angulation. Note pull of intrinsic muscles.

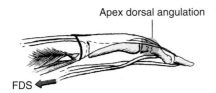

FIGURE 16–32 A middle phalanx fracture can produce apex dorsal angulation. Note the pull of the FDS tendon which can influence the position of the distal bone fragment.

stable proximal phalanx fractures because it provides the immobilization necessary for the healing fracture yet allows tendon gliding and motion of uninvolved joints (Gutow et al., 2003; Oxford & Hidreth, 1996). Fabrication of this orthosis needs to be well contoured providing stability across the fracture site. Remolding or refabricating may be required to maintain proper fit as edema decreases.

Middle phalangeal fractures can be successfully managed with a digit-based orthosis (Fig. 16–34A). However, a hand-based design may be fabricated to provide additional support, protection, and rest as in the pediatric population, postoperatively, or when other structures and/or multiple digits are involved (Fig. 16–34B,C).

Distal phalangeal fractures commonly result from a crush injury and generally can heal without complicated treatment (Kaplan, 1940). These injuries occur frequently with a finger becoming caught between two objects such as a door and a door jam. According to Kaplan (1940), distal phalanx fractures are described as tuft, shaft, or base fractures. Tuft fractures do not necessarily require immobilization; however, concurrent nail bed injuries may require an orthosis for protection and comfort. A clamshell design can be used to provide further protection for a hypersensitive fingertip (Fig. 16–35A,B). Distal phalanx shaft or base fractures may require surgical repair, usually with K-wire fixation. When

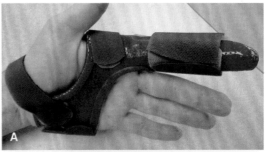
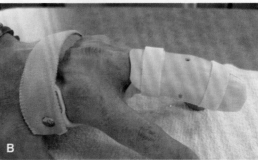
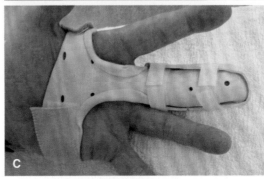

FIGURE 16–33 **A,** A hand-based volar digit immobilization orthosis for a proximal phalanx fracture. **B and C,** Hand-based design with protective dorsal "clamshell" segment to offer additional protection.

providing a protective orthosis, the PIP joint may be incorporated to improve stability and prevent the device from migrating distally off the finger (Fig. 16–36). This can be modified later to free the PIP joint as healing progresses.

PHALANGEAL FRACTURE/DISLOCATIONS

Proximal Interphalangeal Joint

PIP joint fractures or dislocations occur more commonly because they are more vulnerable to injury during normal functional, occupational, and athletic activities. Because they are often diagnosed as sprains, proper and timely intervention may be delayed (Lögters et al., 2018; Chen & Kalainov, 2017). According to Kiefhaber (1996), there are three categories of these injuries. Dorsal lip fracture dislocations are hyperflexion injuries with volar dislocation of the PIP joint causing an avulsion-type fracture of the central tendon. If nondisplaced, the PIP joint can be immobilized in extension for 6 weeks with a clamshell or circumferential orthosis with the DIP joint left free for active ROM (AROM) (Fig. 16–37A–D). Displaced fractures most often require ORIF and may be immobilized with MCP in flexion, PIP extended, and DIP free (Fig. 16–37C,E) (Chinchalkar & Gan, 2003; Freiberg et al., 2006).

Volar lip fracture dislocations involve hyperextension injuries with dorsal forces dislocating the PIP joint, resulting in volar plate avulsion and injury to collateral ligaments. They may be classified based on stability with stress testing: type 1 (stable), type 2 (tenuous), and type 3 (unstable) fractures (Kiefhaber & Stern, 1998).

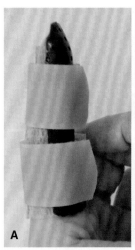
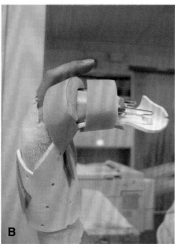
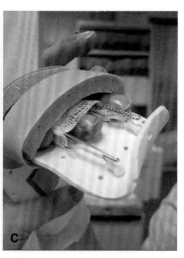

FIGURE 16–34 **A,** A digit immobilization orthosis for a middle phalanx fracture. **B and C,** This hand-based digit immobilization orthosis extends distally to provide protection for extruding pins. Notice the foam overlying the PIP joints to encourage extension.

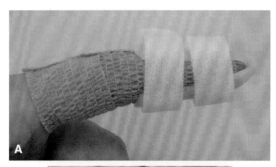

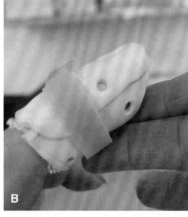

FIGURE 16–35 **A,** A volar-/dorsal-style DIP joint immobilization orthosis may be used to manage distal phalanx fractures and mallet finger injuries. **B,** This clamshell design can assist in protecting associated nail bed injuries.

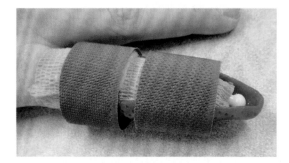

FIGURE 16–36 A digit immobilization orthosis may be applied for a distal phalanx fracture repaired with K-wire fixation.

Type 1 and 2 fractures may be protected with a PIP extension restriction orthosis or with buddy taping of the affected finger to adjacent fingers (Fig. 16–38A,B). Early movement is highly encouraged for these injuries to minimize joint stiffness and tendon adhesions. Type 3 fractures require surgical intervention and a postoperative hand-based orthosis to protect repairs.

Pilon fractures result from high-energy axial force with the finger in full extension. This causes a severe, centrally impacted comminuted fracture of the middle phalanx and collapse of soft tissue surrounding the PIP joint. Often, these difficult intra-articular fractures are treated with dynamic traction orthoses (Fig. 16–39) to regain length of tissue surrounding the joint (ligamentotaxis) and to provide early passive motion (Gallagher & Blackmore, 2011; Schenck, 1994). In some cases, the traction assists in stabilizing the fracture, and passive motion would not be used immediately.

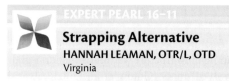

EXPERT PEARL 16–11

Strapping Alternative
HANNAH LEAMAN, OTR/L, OTD
Virginia

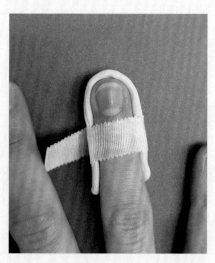

Adhesive tape can be used instead of traditional strapping to secure a finger orthosis that has a difficult time staying on. Replace tape often to prevent skin irritation.

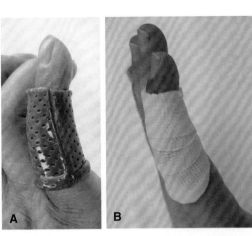
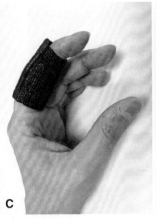
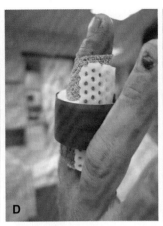
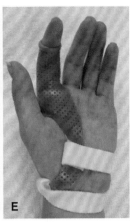

FIGURE 16–37 A, Finger-based circumferential PIP immobilization orthosis for nondisplaced PIP joint fracture dislocation injuries, allowing for DIP ROM exercises. As edema and pain resolve, the orthosis can be serially remolded to increase extension at the PIP joint. QuickCast 2 **(B)** and Orficast® **(C)** materials circumferentially applied to maximally distribute pressure and immobilize the PIP joint, allowing MCP and DIP motion. **D,** If a circumferential design is not appropriate due to fluctuating edema, a volar PIP immobilization orthosis with elasticized wrap beneath may be indicated. **E,** A hand-based PIP joint immobilization orthosis to protect a repaired dorsal lip fracture/dislocation of PIP joint, leaving DIP joint free for motion.

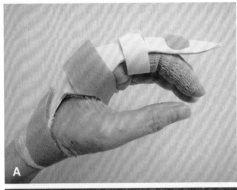
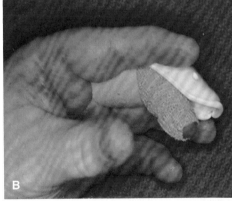

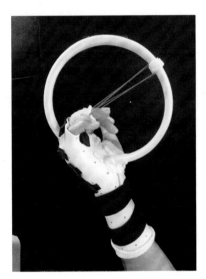

FIGURE 16–39 A dynamic traction orthosis maintains ligamentotaxis throughout a specific ROM.

FIGURE 16–38 A, A hand-based dorsal proximal interphalangeal (PIP) extension restriction orthosis used for a PIP joint volar lip fracture dislocation to allow early protected flexion but to restrict end-range extension. **B,** Finger-based design may allow for greater function of unaffected digits.

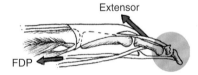

FIGURE 16–40 Distal phalanx avulsion fracture. Note the pull of the flexor and extensor tendon attachments and the resulting deformity.

Distal Interphalangeal Joint

Tension and compression forces can produce DIP joint fracture and dislocations. For example, sudden forced flexion of the DIP joint while the finger is actively extended may result in avulsion of the terminal tendon with a bone fragment of distal phalanx. This is known as a bony mallet finger injury (Fig. 16–40). Conservative management for these injuries includes wearing a protective DIP immobilization orthosis positioned in extension continuously for 6 to 8 weeks until the bone appears healed (Fig. 16–41A–D) (Cannon, 2003). If surgical repair is performed, an orthosis is made to protect the fixation (Fig. 16–41E). Refer to Chapter 18, for details.

Injuries to the DIP joint also may appear as a volar margin fracture with flexor digitorum profundus (FDP) rupture, a palmar plate avulsion fracture (hyperextension force with dorsal DIP joint dislocation), or impaction shear fractures (when fingertip is slightly flexed with force) (Kiefhaber, 1996). In the case of a fracture involving the FDP tendon, a dorsal blocking orthosis is made to include the wrist, and treatment would be initiated as per postflexor tendon repair guidelines. Refer to Chapter 19 for details.

Options for orthotic management to address phalangeal fractures vary greatly owing to differing physician preferences. The therapist

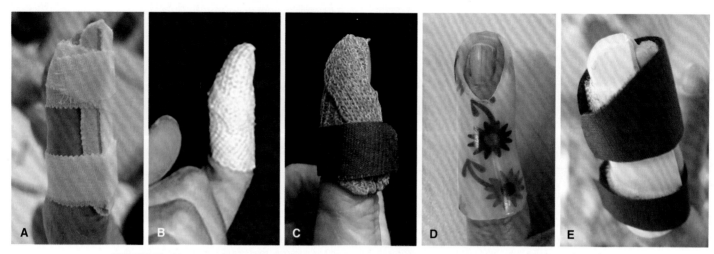

FIGURE 16-41 A, Dorsally applied AlumaFoam® positioning the DIP joint in slight hyperextension. **B,** QuickCast 2 applied circumferentially maximally distributes the pressure, minimizing incidence of irritation dorsally at DIP joint. **C,** Orficast® used to immobilize the DIP while allowing PIP motion. **D,** Thermoplastic option with nail free to ease donning. **E,** Finger-based DIP immobilization orthosis extended distally to protect pins.

may need to modify the orthosis repeatedly as the fracture heals to maintain support as edema decreases, to modify joint positioning as motion improves, or to free joints from the orthosis as healing progresses. A material that can withstand being repeatedly reheated is the material of choice for managing these injuries. Therefore, an elastic or rubber material is preferable for convenience as well as cost-effectiveness. Table 16-7 summarizes orthotic management of hand fractures.

TABLE 16-7	**Phalangeal Fracture Management**[a]		
Fracture	**Orthosis Options**	**Position**	**Time Frame**
Phalangeal			
Proximal	• Volar hand-based digit immobilization orthosis	MCP: 60°–70°; PIP: 0°–15°; DIP: 0°–10°	2–4 wk
Middle	• Digit immobilization orthosis	MCP: free, PIP: 0°; DIP: 0°	3+ wk
Distal	• Stax splint • DIP immobilization orthosis	Prefabricated DIP: 0°	4–6 wk 4–6 wk
Fracture or dislocation of PIP joint			
Dorsal lip			
Nondisplaced	• Digit immobilization orthosis	PIP: 0° as tolerated DIP: 0° or free	6 wk
Displaced	• Hand-based digit immobilization orthosis after surgical repair	MCP: 60°–70° PIP: 0°; DIP free	6 wk
Volar lip			
Type 1 and 2	• PIP extension restriction orthosis (hand based or finger based) • Buddy taping	PIP flexed per physician recommendation (increase extension by10° each week until full extension achieved) To adjacent digit	6 wk
Type 3	• Digit- or hand-based immobilization orthosis • Traction orthosis	MCP: 60°–70°; PIP: 0° Per physician: wrist extension MCP: 60°–70°; PIP: per physician	Variable 6+ wk
Pilon	• Digit- or hand-based immobilization orthosis • Traction orthosis	MCP: 60°–70°; PIP: 0° Per physician: wrist extension MCP: 60°–70°; PIP: per physician	Variable
Fracture or dislocation of the DIP joint			
Volar margin with FDP rupture	• Wrist/hand extension restriction orthosis (dorsal blocking orthosis)	Wrist: 0°–45° depending per physician flexion; MCP: 45°–60° flexion; PIP/DIP: 0°	4–6 wk based on healing
Volar plate avulsion	• Digit immobilization orthosis	PIP/DIP: 0°	4 wk
Bony mallet finger	• Digit immobilization orthosis	DIP: 0°	6–8 wk

[a]Note that the orthosis options and time frames depend on the individual patient. Obtain clear orders from the referring physician before providing the patient with any therapy intervention.

CONCLUSION

This chapter reviewed orthotic intervention for common upper extremity fractures. The appropriate selection and judicious use of orthoses can aid in managing fractures early while maximizing functional use of uninjured structures. Orthoses applied immediately post injury or post surgery can offer excellent conformability for secure fracture stabilization while allowing joint mobility and gliding of surrounding soft-tissue structures. Orthoses used during the remobilization phase of rehabilitation provide continued protection and help guard against reinjury during the patient's return to activity. Close communication with the physician regarding fracture stability and proper joint positioning within the orthosis is essential to prevent secondary problems such as joint or soft-tissue contracture, tendon adherence, or chronic instability.

FIELD NOTE

Michelle Coil, MOT, OTR, CHT, PYT, CEAS I
Texas

I first learned how to make functional casts in 2009 and was immediately drawn to the colorful end product that was more appealing than the traditional white or beige thermoplastic splint. Patients also enjoy the choice of colors and patterns and are pleasantly surprised with the washable, lightweight cast.

The use of functional casts in fracture management is an ideal solution due to the localized rigidity and protection of the fracture site while reducing the chance of preventable stiffness of adjacent digits or proximal joints. Fractures and soft-tissue injuries are stabilized with minimal muscle atrophy, while maximizing early return to function. Due to the circumferential application and improved functionality, a reduction of digital edema is noted fairly quickly. Often, the patient's confidence is quickly restored with the rigid support while maintaining comfort and compliance.

Delta-Cast provides this strong, yet lightweight alternative for patients in need of protection for their injury. The polyester casting material is silicone free, fiberglass free, and latex free which makes it a very appealing option for patients and therapists with skin sensitivities. The multidirectional polyester fabric allows for easy application around the delicate contours of the upper extremity. With no heat required or patterns needed, the Delta-Cast tape has a 3- to 5-minute setup time and is fully weight-bearing in 20 minutes. This makes it an optimal choice for busy therapists looking for time-efficient splinting methods.

The Delta-Cast padding is water resistant which contributes to reduced complications from skin maceration and maintains its bulk around bony prominences. There is no need for multiple splints to be fabricated since it is made circumferentially. You can fabricate one opening for the patient to don/doff or bivalve the cast to allow for a clamshell-type support.

The breathable stockinette makes its moisture wicking properties an optimal choice to reduce skin maceration. The multipurpose fleece liner not only makes for a comfortable edge but also holds padding in place, secures velcro to the cast, and prevents strap fraying. Finally, there are no worries about whether your patient is going to come back with a warped splint from keeping it in their hot car since the material will not deform under high temperatures.

Prior to fabrication, it is important to have a clear understanding of your patient's fracture diagnosis so you know where to add reinforcement, apply padding, and place the cut strip for the cast opening. Preparing your work station with your casting materials is necessary due to the quick setup time. This can also help you reduce the chance of forgetting the cut strip, which is likely to happen at least once. To apply the tape, simply tear open the package and submerge the tape in water. Since the casting tape is one long roll, your first cut will be the reinforcement piece to apply over the fracture site. Then begin application with slight tension to the tape, making sure to only allow two layers of overlap. Making the cast too thick will make it extremely difficult to cut.

Due to its conformable nature, the casting tape is easily applied around joints and bony prominences such as the olecranon, metacarpal heads, or through the thumb web space. This type of fracture bracing allows for the reinforcement piece to be placed where additional fracture stability is needed. I have fabricated Sarmiento functional casts for stable proximal and distal humerus fractures by overlapping the cast tape where fracture support is needed. However, its important to keep the remainder of the cast flexible enough for distal extremity mobility, which greatly reduces excessive edema commonly associated with these diagnoses. This also makes it easier for the patient to remove independently. As postfracture edema decreases, the cast opening will likely overlap, therefore access can be cut and relined with fleece edging.

Long arm functional casts are one of my favorites to make with this material. The fabrication process is faster and less painful for the patient. Olecranon, distal humeral, supracondylar, and radial head fractures are protected with the application of a long posterior reinforcement piece. From my experience, overlapping the casting material over the olecranon will allow for added protection while reducing the chance of making the cast too thick to cut at the elbow crease. Patient comfort is improved with the soft cushion padding applied to accommodate tenderness commonly associated with the ulnar head, olecranon, medial, and lateral epicondyles. The completed long arm orthosis is lightweight, therefore reducing proximal shoulder pain commonly seen with bulky casts and heavy braces. Less strapping is needed by keeping the cast material through the thumb web space when wrist immobilization is required. Delta-Cast is also an optimal rigid solution to prevent excessive forearm rotation as needed in Muenster or sugar tong orthoses. Our current splinting options make these long orthoses difficult to fabricate due to the large piece of thermoplastic material needed.

Thumb functional casts provide optimal stability to the thumb with radial reinforcement that extends down to the wrist or you can cut a small piece for a short opponens. From experience of getting a few thumb IPs stuck in the cast, I quickly learned to apply coban to the thumb IP prior to fabrication. This allows comfortable donning and doffing of the thumb orthosis. There are no seams to bond together or overlapping of thermoplastic material which can cause pinching of the patient's skin. The Delta-Cast thumb stockinette can be rolled down past the thumb IP prior to application to ensure clearing the thumb IP crease to avoid unnecessary stiffness. However, if needed, the stockinette is long enough to immobilize the thumb IP such as with a thumb proximal phalanx fracture.

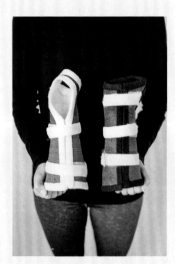

FIELD NOTE FIGURE 16–1

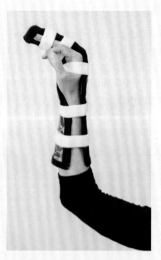

FIELD NOTE FIGURE 16–2

To enhance wrist immobilization, functional casts can be fabricated with the option to provide palmar, dorsal, or both palmar and dorsal reinforcement (Field Note Fig. 16–1). The cast opening can be dorsally placed making it easy for the patient to don and doff. Additional cast can be easily cut to allow for a larger opening for the patient to get in and out of, while continuing to provide circumferential stability. The Delta-Cast padding provides additional comfort for sensitive volar plate distal radius fractures and tender ulnar styloid fractures. Making a small cut in the cast tape as you roll through the web space will reduce blocking the metacarpals unnecessarily.

Radial gutters and ulnar gutters are easily fabricated using the Delta-Cast and a preferred choice for patients with metacarpal fractures and proximal phalanx fractures due to the palmar and dorsal protection of the fractured digit (Field Note Fig. 16–2). Unstable proximal phalanx fractures requiring x-ray do not require cast removal since the cast tape is translucent in nature. Metacarpal fractures and proximal phalanx fractures with pins can be safely protected in many different ways without the need to heat thermoplastic material. Normally, I bulk the pin site prior to casting application to make a roof for the pins. I have also applied the casting material around the pins leaving a window to allow for pin care, then making a removable cover with leftover material. Adjustments to functional gutter casts due to edema reduction can be made by adding padding, cutting excess cast off, or simply cinching the straps tighter.

Luckily, many patients of all ages can continue to work and play in their functional casts. Athletes and school-aged children can safely return to sport or play without fear of reinjury. Parents like it because it can be easily removed for bath or shower time. In fact, I prefer to make the functional cast thicker at the opening so young children are unable to remove the cast on their own. Luckily, you have the ability to reinforce a cast for our older patients that may need to use a cane or walker, yet create a flexible opening that will promote independence in donning and doffing. Once you use Delta-Cast, you more than likely will love this material choice for your fractures and utilize it for many more diagnoses.

Case Study Section

The case studies presented here are meant as a teaching guideline only. Treatment and orthosis protocols vary greatly from surgeon to surgeon and from therapist to therapist. The therapist should check with the referring physicians and colleagues to define the preferred treatment and appropriate orthotic intervention.

Case Study 1: Small-Finger Metacarpal Head Fracture

AM is a 27-year-old man who fell onto a clenched fist while trying to catch a football and sustained a right small-finger MC head fracture. ORIF with placement of two screws through the MC head was performed. AM was followed by the medical doctor (MD); however, referral for outpatient hand therapy was delayed until 4 weeks post surgery. Upon evaluation, AM's wound was healed, but he was noted to have thick scarring and joint stiffness with severe limitation in ROM throughout the small finger. He was unable to grip or lift using his left hand.

Initially, a hand-based, ulnar-based orthosis was fabricated to protect the small finger and adjacent ring finger at night and with daily activity to limit stress on the healing MC head fracture for an additional 2 weeks per MD orders (Fig. 16–42). The MCP joints were placed in end-range flexion as tolerated with the IP joints in extension. AM was instructed to wear this orthosis at night and for

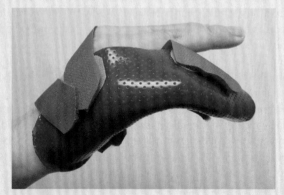

FIGURE 16–42 An ulnar-based digit immobilization orthosis for MC head fracture of the small finger.

heavier ADLs during the day. On follow-up visit, an ulnar-based MCP protective orthosis was made for only the small finger, allowing AM to better incorporate his right hand for grasping light objects and full use of unaffected fingers for ADLs.

Passive/active/active assistive ROM (PROM/AROM/AAROM) exercises were initiated including tendon gliding exercises and blocking exercises for isolated movements of PIP and DIP joints. He was instructed in methods to increase scar mobility and to decrease edema around the small finger. At 6 weeks postoperative, AM was weaned from the daytime MCP protection orthosis and instructed in use of buddy straps, allowing full use of his right hand for ADLs. Passive intrinsic plus and minus stretching as well as grip and pinch strengthening exercises was introduced.

Despite his diligence in following his home program, AM had developed scar adhesions of the small finger, limiting full active MCP extension (−25°). A night extension orthosis was made to rest the small finger in full extension at night, and active MCP extension exercises with skin mobilization were emphasized. He continued to have limited passive MCP flexion of 40°. A dynamic MCP flexion orthosis was fabricated, and he was instructed to wear it intermittently during day (four–six times per day, beginning with 15 minutes and increasing as tolerated to 30 minutes). The tension on the dynamic orthosis was checked and adjusted. As his ROM progress slowed, the dynamic component of the orthosis was changed to a static progressive force (Fig. 16–43).

At 8 weeks post surgery, AM had returned back to most light to moderate ADLs using his right-dominant hand and, after follow-up with MD, was cleared for full weight bearing and lifting as tolerated. His grip strength was 60% of his left nondominant hand and with near tight grip. PROM of his small-finger MCP extension/flexion was 0/70° with AROM of −10/65° and with full ROM of PIP and DIP joints. By 10 weeks post surgery, AM's right grip strength had improved to 75% of the left, and his MCP joint PROM was 0/80°; AROM was 0/75°. He had returned to performing most ADLs including workout activities and was discharged from therapy with a home exercise program of ROM, stretching, and strengthening exercises.

Case Study 2: Intra-articular Proximal Interphalangeal Joint Fracture

DG is a 49-year-old male who sustained an intra-articular fracture dislocation of the IF PIP joint from falling onto his hand with his finger in a hyperextended position. He was initially seen at the emergency room of a community hospital, where closed reduction was attempted. Upon returning home 2 days later, DG consulted his orthopedist, who scheduled surgery for fracture reduction/fixation. On the same day, he saw the surgeon; DG was referred to therapy for preoperative fabrication of an intra-articular PIP traction mobilization orthosis (Fig. 16–39). The orthosis was to be applied in the operating room, and gentle therapy was to begin in the recovery room.

A radial-based wrist and MCP immobilization orthosis (with wrist extended and MCPs flexed) was fabricated with a hoop-shaped outrigger attachment for the application of dynamic tension. The hoop allows equal rubber band tension from the middle phalanx to the hoop throughout PIP joint ROM. To achieve this tension, the surgeon placed a wire through the middle phalanx, leaving a small loop on each side of the protruding wire from which the rubber bands were attached and directed to the hoop. A variety of rubber bands were chosen to estimate the appropriate tension necessary to maintain fracture reduction. The rubber bands were given to the surgeon to attach to the orthosis in the operating room after reduction. An AlumaFoam® duchess cap was fabricated for attachment of the rubber bands against the hoop (Fig. 16–44). The orthosis was fabricated from a plastic material with moderate drapability. The hoop was made out of a 1/4″ AquaTube® for ease of fabrication.

The tension applied to the PIP joint was set at 300 g force as measured by a Haldex gauge to allow proper alignment of the joint as well as to preserve the joint space (Oxford & Hidreth, 1996). Alignment was confirmed by x-ray postoperatively.

DG wore the orthosis continuously, except for hygiene and skin inspection. For exercises, he was instructed to move the duchess cap with the rubber band traction, allowing excursion of his finger from extension to flexion or flexion to extension, alternating every 10 minutes during the day. This provided safe movement of the joint while maintaining reduction of the fracture and joint stiffness. When sleeping, the finger was positioned midway between full extension and flexion (Kearney & Brown, 1994).

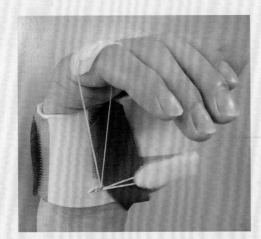

FIGURE 16−43 Static progressive MCP mobilization orthosis to improve MCP joint flexion of the small finger.

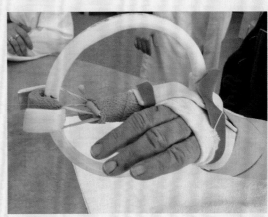

FIGURE 16−44 Intra-articular PIP traction mobilization orthosis.

At 5½ weeks post surgery, the orthosis was removed; a protective hand-based digit immobilization orthosis was fabricated with the IF MCP flexed to 60° and the PIP/DIP joints gently flexed. This was worn for continued protection and was gradually weaned as DG regained ROM and strength. A mild PIP flexion contracture developed and was managed with gentle serial static PIP extension casting (Fig. 16–45). The cast was changed weekly, and within 4 months of surgery, the patient had obtained functional PIP joint ROM and strength.

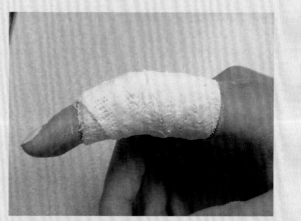

FIGURE 16–45 Serial static casting using plaster of paris into end-range extension is an effective way to address a flexion contracture of the PIP joint.

CHAPTER REVIEW QUESTIONS

1. Name three common hand fractures that a hand therapist would treat and manage with an orthosis.
2. What is the importance of properly positioning joints acutely?
3. Describe a minimum of two design choices for orthotic management of a distal radius fracture.
4. What position should the thumb MCP be placed in after a skier injury? Why is this position so important?
5. Describe the three common locations a metacarpal bone tends to fracture and the proper orthotic management and position for each fracture location.

17 Arthritis[a]

MaryLynn A. Jacobs, MBA, MS, OTR/L, CHT
Kristen MacDonald, MScOT, CHT, OT Reg. (Ont)
Shrikant Chinchalkar, M.Th.O, BSc.OT, OTR, CHT
Joey Pipicelli, MScOT, CHT, OT Reg. (Ont)

CHAPTER OBJECTIVES

After study of this chapter, the reader should be able to:
- Understand the disease process and general characteristics of osteoarthritis and rheumatoid arthritis of the elbow, wrist, and all joints of the hand.
- Explain the general goals and precautions for the use of orthoses in various arthritic conditions that affect the upper extremity.
- Understand the rationale and evidence-based information for orthotic management of the nonsurgical and postsurgical osteoarthritic or rheumatoid elbow, wrist, and hand.
- Explain the specific differences in immobilization, mobilization, restriction, or prefabricated orthoses for use with this patient population.

KEY TERMS

Arthritis	Grind test	Swan-neck deformity
Arthrodesis	Heberden nodes	Synovectomy
Arthroplasty	Interposition arthroplasty	Synovial fluid
Arthroscopic debridement	Juvenile rheumatoid arthritis	Synovial membrane
Articular cartilage	Low-load prolonged stress	Synovitis
Basal joint complex	Mannerfelt syndrome	Systemic lupus erythematosus
Bouchard nodes	Mucus cysts	Systemic sclerosis
Boutonniere deformity	Osteoarthritis	Tenolysis
Caput ulnae syndrome	Osteophytes	Tenosynovectomy
Crepitation	Pannus	Tenosynovitis
DeQuervain tenosynovitis	Psoriatic arthritis	Trapeziometacarpal joint
Dorsal Chamay repair	Rheumatoid arthritis	Vaughan-Jackson syndrome
First carpometacarpal joint	Scleroderma	Zigzag deformity
	Stenosing tenosynovitis	

MD NOTE

Janet Pope, MD
Canada

Osteoarthritis (OA) is the most common form of arthritis, and the pharmacological treatment has not changed much over the years. This includes acetaminophen and nonsteroidal anti-inflammatory drugs (NSAIDs) either topically or orally and sometimes intra-articular steroid injections. There have been trials of medications to potentially decrease joint damage including cartilage loss, but none are yet approved. Heberden and Bouchard nodes at the distal interphalangeal (DIP) and proximal interphalangeal (PIP) joints, respectively, are common in hand OA as is first carpometacarpal (CMC) OA (at the base of the thumb). Orthosis intervention is helpful for the CMC joint (such as a thumb immobilization orthosis). Several other designs of orthoses can rest joints that are malaligned.

Rheumatoid arthritis (RA) occurs in approximately 1% of the population. Despite many advances in treatment such as treating to a target with combination disease-modifying anti-rheumatic drugs (DMARDs) and biologics (tumor necrosis factor [TNF] inhibitors, IL6 inhibitors, costimulatory molecule inhibitor, and CD20 B cell depletion) and JAK inhibitors, two out of three patients are not in sustained remission. Intra-articular injections and NSAIDs are an adjunctive treatment. Some will develop deformities where orthosis intervention is very helpful. In addition, actively swollen joints of the hands such as wrists may be helped by rest including wrist or wrist and hand immobilization orthoses, and, if there is damage, some people are helped with working wrist orthoses. Custom-fabricated orthoses around the PIP joints can be made that appear to be jewelry and help to reduce swan-neck or boutonniere deformities. Rheumatoid deformities have decreased over the last 15 years but still occur in some patients and could also benefit from orthosis intervention. Other aids and therapy intervention may be helpful in OA and RA such as home exercise programs, assistive devices, walking aids, taping techniques, and other interventions that allow for pain relief, resting of a joint, and/or improvement of function.

Dr. Janet Pope

[a]This chapter is based on the first-edition chapter written by MaryLynn Jacobs, MBA, MS OTR/L CHT.

355

What type of material is best for the patient with osteoarthritis or rheumatoid arthritis?

Thermoplastic materials for the patient with OA should be carefully chosen. The selection ranges from heavyweight to lightweight materials, and the choice of which depends on the purpose of the orthosis, the patient's skin tolerance and joint integrity. An orthosis intended to provide gentle pressure for adequate joint stabilization may require greater rigidity than one used to position an inflamed joint. Materials should easily contour about bony prominences such as the ulnar styloid and the dorsal metacarpal heads. As changes in bony prominences and joint widths may occur over time with OA, consideration should be given to a material that can be reheated and reshaped repeatedly such as an elastic-based material. Neoprene material is an excellent choice to be considered. It provides light support when used alone and more rigid support when a thermoplastic material is adhered to it.

How is the diagnosis of CMC joint arthritis first made?

The diagnosis of first CMC joint OA is made primarily through a comprehensive physical examination followed by radiographic confirmation. Patients may complain of pain, pinch weakness, and/or crepitus at the first CMC joint.

Typically, patients note pain during functional activities, such as opening jars, brushing teeth, and turning a doorknob. Pain is generalized to the thenar eminence but may also be noted proximal and distal to the involved joint. Palpation may reveal tenderness over the volar aspect of the first CMC joint; in approximately half the population, concurrent pain is appreciated at the STT joint. The patient may have a positive grind test—pain elicited when the examiner imparts axial compression and rotation of the base of the first metacarpal into the trapezium. In the earlier stages of the disease, gross appearance may be normal. Progression of the disease often results in subluxation of the metacarpal dorsoradially over the trapezium; this positive "shoulder sign" may be seen at the base of the first CMC.

How important is the straps and strap placement when fabricating an orthosis on this patient population?

The strapping design of the orthosis should allow for easy independent donning and doffing. Straps should be wide, soft, and conforming as patients with any type of arthritis often have thin, fragile skin owing to their age, medications, or the disease process itself. Straps can be fabricated to allow extra length or loops on the end of the strap for easy application and removal.

Soft strapping material can also be used as digit dividers on wrist/hand immobilization orthoses. These dividers can aid in alignment and prevent maceration between the digits. Care should be taken to place straps advantageously. They can be used as an aid in gently redirecting joints into an antideformity position, straps can successfully provide light joint positioning.

INTRODUCTION

The word **arthritis** is derived from the Greek word *arthros* (joint) and *itis* (inflammation). Arthritis encompasses approximately 100 rheumatic diseases, all of which have joint disease as a prominent manifestation. In addition to joint involvement, the adjacent bones, ligaments, tendons, and muscles can also be involved. The two most common rheumatic diseases are **osteoarthritis (OA)** and **rheumatoid arthritis (RA)**. Less commonly, but often encountered by the hand therapist, are **juvenile rheumatoid arthritis (JRA)** also known as juvenile idiopathic arthritis, **systemic lupus erythematosus (SLE)**, **psoriatic arthritis (PA)**, and **scleroderma**, also known as **systemic sclerosis (SS)** (Beasley, 2011). For most forms of arthritis, there is as yet no cure; therefore, the main goals for treating these diseases are to minimize pain, control the inflammatory process, preserve joint structures, minimize progression of deformities, and maintain as much functional independence as possible.

The patient with arthritis of the upper extremity is best served by a supportive team approach including the primary care physician; rheumatologist; either hand, orthopedic, or plastic surgeon; physical therapist; occupational therapist; the patient themselves; and family members. The therapist is uniquely qualified to educate the patient regarding joint protection, energy conservation, exercise programs, and orthotic management (Beasley, 2011; Bernstein et al., 2010; Crepeau & Schell, 2009; Estes, Bochenek, & Fasler, 2000; Henry & Kramer, 2009; Kelley & Ramsey, 2000; Kozin, 1999; Kozin & Michlovitz, 2000; Poole & Pellegrini, 2000).

This chapter reviews joint disease, patient assessment, general characteristics of OA and RA, common surgical procedures, and the value of orthoses for these conditions. Threaded throughout this chapter are evidence-based highlights related to historically applied orthoses for the management of common arthritic conditions. Specific rehabilitation techniques, therapeutic modalities, medical management, related inflammatory diseases, and detailed surgical procedures are not reviewed; see "Suggested Readings" section of this chapter for further study.

GOALS FOR THE USE OF ORTHOSES

Initial conservative management of OA and RA may include an orthosis, often in combination with patient education, anti-inflammatory medication, and/or a local steroid injection. Although most physicians would agree with initial conservative management of arthritis involving the implementation of orthoses, including the American College of Rheumatology, there exists controversy within the literature regarding the efficacy of orthotic interventions. However, there is agreement among experts in the field that there is clinical evidence to support that orthoses can play a role in protecting the joints, potentially slowing joint and soft-tissue degeneration, providing pain relief, managing edema, and enhancing functional performance (Barron, Glickel, & Eaton, 2000; Beasley, 2011; Fess, Gettle, Philips, & Janson, 2005; Kozin, & Michlovitz, 2000; Melvin, 1982; Philips, 1995; Seeger & Furst, 1987; Stern et al., 1997; Swigart, Eaton, Glickel, & Johnson, 1999; Valdes, 2012; Weiss, LaStayo, Mills, & Bramlet, 2000). Immobilization orthoses can be custom molded with a variety of thermoplastic material or other materials such as neoprene. The reader is referred to Chapter 14 for information. Alternatively, many prefabricated orthoses are widely available, and some of these prefabricated designs can be custom-fit to a patient.

The use of orthoses also plays a key role in the postoperative management of surgical interventions for these patients. The type of postsurgical orthosis is determined by many factors, including the procedure performed, the integrity of the patient's tissue, and goals of the procedure. Typically, orthotic intervention is introduced following the removal of postoperative dressings or casting (Bernstein et al., 2010; Fess et al., 2005; Kozin, & Michlovitz, 2000; Melvin, 1982; Philips, 1995; Seeger & Furst, 1987; Stern et al., 1997; Swigart et al., 1999; Tomaino, 2011; Weiss et al., 2000). General management of orthoses for each joint of the wrist and hand, as well as the elbow, will be discussed in this chapter.

GOALS FOR THE USE OF ORTHOSES IN PATIENTS WITH ARTHRITIS

Use of orthoses in patients with arthritis includes the following (Fess et al., 2005; Jacobs, 2003; Melvin, 1982; Philips, 1995; Weiss et al., 2000):

- Reduce pain and inflammation of the involved joints
- Rest and support the weakened structures
- Position the involved joints as close to proper alignment as possible and address or prevent secondary deformity
- Help prevent, minimize, and/or slow joint deformity
- Provide external support (increase stability) to improve functional use of the hand
- Position healing structures appropriately after postoperative procedures

JOINT ASSESSMENT

COMPONENTS OF A NORMAL JOINT

Before discussing the diseased joint, normal joint anatomy must be understood. A joint is comprised of many components, each of which has a definite role and function (Fig. 17–1). Altogether, in a carefully orchestrated balance, they provide smooth, fluid, complete, and pain-free joint motion. The main components and functions of a joint are described in the following text.

Bone

Bone is living tissue with both blood and nerve supply that provide the framework of the body. This hard, porous material is composed of osteocytes which secrete a dense fibrous ground substance. This ground substance then calcifies into a strong and stiff matrix. Aside from aspects of teeth, bone is considered the hardest structure in the body. Bone is dynamic, constantly being remodeled in reaction to physical and metabolic stresses.

Articular Cartilage

Articular cartilage is a tough connective tissue that covers the articulating surfaces of bones with a synovial joint and functions as a shock absorber by lessening transmitted forces. Cartilage goes through adaptive changes in response to joint loading and possesses the ability to deform and reform many times. Cartilage has traditionally been thought to be incapable of regrowth, although recent research may prove that cartilage has some regenerative capacity (Medvedeva et al., 2018).

Fibrous Joint Capsule

The fibrous joint capsule is comprised of two layers: the stratum fibrosum and the stratum synovium. The stratum fibrosum is a relatively dense outer layer of tissue that envelops the joint and

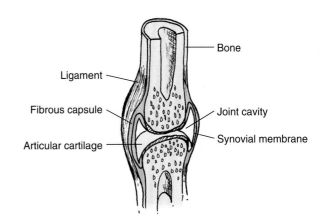

FIGURE 17-1 Normal joint anatomy and surrounding structures.

maintains the integrity of the joint structure. This layer is comprised of both collagen, which provides stability and strength, and elastin, which gives the capsule its ability to stretch and return to its previous state. This elastic capability plays a significant role in joint mobility. This layer is poorly vascularized but is highly innervated with joint receptors, giving continuous feedback to the central nervous system.

The stratum synovium is the inner layer beneath the joint capsule; it is highly vascularized and contains a **synovial membrane.** This membrane produces **synovial fluid**, which is responsible for nourishing and lubricating the joint. This layer also provides the mechanism by which fluid is removed from the joint. With the rheumatoid patient, this is the primary site of inflammation; as the synovium is attacked by immune cells, the synovium thickens into a rough and uneven tissue (pannus) which invades the joint space and leads to increased fluid production containing destructive enzymes.

Ligaments

Ligaments are strong fibrous bands that connect bone to bone, reinforcing joint position and providing static stability. Ligaments are composed of dense longitudinal connective tissue bundles with little ground substance. They are somewhat elastic; however, this can vary from person to person and can be affected by disease processes, thus impacting joint stability.

Muscles

Muscle is the contractile tissue which brings about joint motion. The attachment into the skeletal structure is via cordlike tendons which translate force produced via muscle contraction into joint motion. Tendons have a high tensile strength; their ability to lengthen is variable and is affected by its cellular makeup and length. However, tendon overall is much stiffer than muscle. This "team" is often referred to as the muscle-tendon or musculotendinous unit. Muscles also provide dynamic stability to joints.

JOINT DISEASE AND INFLAMMATION

The disruption of any healthy and intact component of a joint, either through injury or disease processes, can affect the quality of joint motion. This includes the range of motion available and the stability with movement or loading; both of which can be painful. This change in motion may significantly limit a person's ability to perform even the simplest of daily tasks. OA is a noninflammatory joint disease of the articular cartilage which typically occurs with advancing age, as well as post joint trauma, for example, an intra-articular fracture. The cartilage deteriorates over time as bony osteophytes simultaneously proliferate at the borders of the involved joint(s) (Bernstein et al., 2010; Melvin, 1982; Poole, & Pellengrini, 2000; Swanson, 1995a). Conversely, RA is an inflammatory joint disease localized to the synovial lining. As the disease progresses, the synovial membrane thickens, fluid accumulates within the joint, leading to the stretching and herniation of the fibrous joint capsule, causing damage to both the capsule as well as supporting structures (Fig. 17–2A–D) (Bernstein et al., 2010; Melvin, 1982; Swanson, 1995a).

Clinicians working with clients with arthritis should apply their fundamental knowledge of normal joint anatomy as well as the pathology and potential sequela of soft-tissue involvement of these joint diseases in order to develop an effective therapeutic regime.

OSTEOARTHRITIS

CHARACTERISTICS

Osteoarthritis is referred to as degenerative joint disease (DJD). It affects approximately 27 million people in the United States, usually between 40 and 50 years of age. Generally, women are more often affected than men. There are usually no systemic features; it occurs as a chronic, noninflammatory disease, leading to cartilage destruction and reactive changes about the periphery of joints and subchondral bone. The cause of the disease is chronic or repetitive biomechanical stress and mechanical loading and can be influenced by genetic factors, trauma (via work or sports), mechanical problems, metabolic issues, and/or age.

The most common sites of OA are the weight-bearing joints (e.g., hips, knees, feet, and spine); it may affect only one side or one aspect of the body such as *only* the hands or one thumb. The joints of the hand and wrist which tend to be the most involved are the DIP joints; the PIP joints; the metacarpophalangeal (MCP) joints; the basal joint of the thumb, specifically, the **first carpometacarpal joint**, also known as the **trapeziometacarpal (TM) joint**; and the **scaphotrapeziotrapezoid** (STT) joint (Fig. 17–3) (Kennedy, Manske, & Huang, 2016; Barron et al., 2000; Bernstein et al., 2010; Melvin, 1982; Poole, & Pellegrini, 2000; Swanson, 1995a; Tomaino, 2011). To increase clarity and consistency for the reader of this chapter, the authors will use the term *first CMC* throughout this chapter. It is important to note that the term *TM joint* is widely used in clinical practice and in the literature.

GENERAL SIGNS AND SYMPTOMS

Initially, patients may present with one or more of the following clinical symptoms: pain, stiffness, crepitation, osteophytes, and mucus cysts discussed in further detail in the following text. Over time, radiographs may reveal asymmetric joint space narrowing and actual joint damage; however, the degree of radiologic involvement may not always correspond with the patient's presentation and concerns (Nwawka, &Weinstock-Zlotnick, 2019; Bernstein et al., 2010).

Pain

One of the early symptoms is joint pain with motion which subsides with rest. Patients often complain of aching joints in cold, damp weather. As the disease progresses, pain tends to be noted during both motion and rest and, sometimes, may be accompanied by muscle spasm.

Stiffness

Stiffness of the involved joints may occur, especially after an extended rest period or immobilization. This may, in turn, influence active range of motion (AROM) and gross functional use of the involved joint becoming limited and painful. As the disease progresses, strength may also diminish due to pain or disuse.

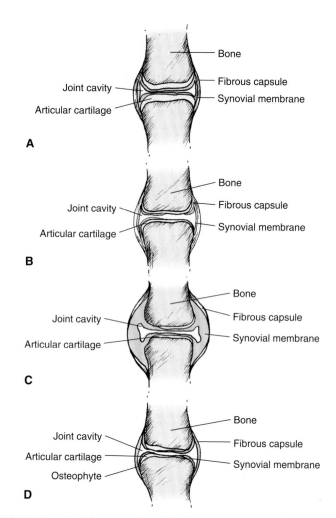

FIGURE 17-2 Healthy joint surfaces (**A**). Changes owing to OA and RA: early inflammation (**B**), advanced inflammation with herniation of synovial fluid and bone and cartilage destruction (**C**), and noninflammatory disease with cartilage breakdown and osteophyte formation (**D**).

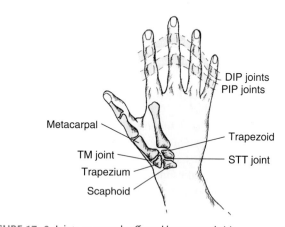

FIGURE 17-3 Joints commonly affected by osteoarthritis.

Crepitation

Crepitation may be noted within the joint or within the tendon sheath with motion. This is indicated by a crunching sensation or sound.

Osteophytes

Bone spurs, or **osteophytes**, are common in the OA disease process, forming at the borders of the joint between the bone and cartilage boundary (Buckland-Wright, Macfarland, & Lynch, 1991; Swanson, 1995a) (Fig. 17–2D). These bony enlargements can appear gradually over time or have a rapid onset. The degree of discomfort resulting from bone spurs is variable. Some patients describe a functional hindrance (e.g., putting on rings), whereas others describe episodes of pain (Buckland-Wright et al., 1991; Burkholder, 2000; Estes et

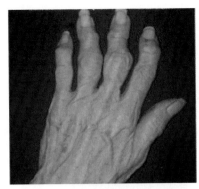

FIGURE 17–4 Note the Heberden and Bouchard nodules at the PIP and DIP joints, respectively.

al., 2000; Melvin, 1982). Osteophytes at the DIP joint are termed **Heberden nodes**; at the level of the PIP joint, they are referred to as **Bouchard nodes** (Fig. 17–4) (Burkholder, 2000; Melvin, 1982).

Mucus Cysts

Mucus cysts tend to appear in the fifth to seventh decade of life. They are firm, nontender, painless cysts in the vicinity of the dorsum of the DIP joint and are often indicative of DIP joint OA (Cassidy & Green, 2011). The first symptoms may be a subtle variety of nail deformities (grooving, splitting). If left untreated, some may progress to cyst rupture (Bernstein et al., 2010).

ORTHOTIC MANAGEMENT

Most health practitioners agree on conservative management being the first line of treatment for OA. Early referral to therapy is paramount. Conservative management for patients with OA may consist of orthoses for support, joint protection, and prevention of further harm or secondary deformity; anti-inflammatory medications; thermal agents for pain control; topical ointments; exercise programs; as well as instruction on joint protection and activity modification. Patient education is imperative with respect to compensatory techniques in all activities of daily living (ADLs) as well as vocational and recreational pursuits in order to moderate mechanical stresses and loading of the joints. If this is not addressed, continued joint stress may contribute to further deformity and/or pain (Estes et al., 2000; Kelley & Ramsey, 2000; Kozin, 1999; Poole, & Pellegrini, 2000). Education on adaptive equipment and/or custom-fabricated adaptations for ADLs may be extremely helpful in maintaining functional use of the hand as well as decreasing pain associated with use (e.g., increasing the size of grips on utensils, changing a round door knobs for a lever handle, adapting a steering wheel, modifying a grip on a golf club, use of large pens for writing).

Orthoses made with thermoplastic materials may not always be well tolerated by some patients due to the following factors:

- Pressure felt at bony prominences
- Fragility of the patient's skin
- The weight/heaviness of the orthosis is to great or cumbersome
- Restrictive nature of the orthosis limits necessary use
- Bilateral involvement may limit strength and/or dexterity required to apply the device

Some patients may prefer a softer, more conforming orthosis for immobilization or restriction of movement. Chapter 14 describes many examples of custom neoprene orthoses for this patient population. Whether custom or prefabricated, when applied early in the DJD process, an orthosis can assist in stabilizing the involved joint(s) during at-risk activities (activities or postures that stress the involved joint), minimize further joint damage, and decrease pain during activity (Barron et al., 2000; Colditz, 2000; Jacobs, 2003; Weiss et al., 2000).

MATERIAL SELECTION

THERMOPLASTICS

Thermoplastic materials for the patient with OA should be carefully chosen. The selection ranges from heavyweight to lightweight materials, and the choice of which depends on the purpose of the orthosis, the patient's skin tolerance, and joint integrity. An orthosis intended to provide gentle pressure for adequate joint stabilization may require greater rigidity than one used to position an inflamed joint (Austin, 2003; Colditz, 2000). Materials should easily contour about bony prominences such as the ulnar styloid and the dorsal metacarpal heads. As changes in bony prominences and joint widths may occur over time with OA, consideration should be given to a material that can be reheated and reshaped repeatedly such as an elastic-based material (see Chapter 5).

Another consideration is material flexibility. Materials that are thin (1/16″) and/or highly perforated tend to be more flexible than traditional (1/8″) solid materials (see Chapter 5 for further details) (Austin, 2003). However, a highly perforated material may irritate the fragile skin, owing to the friction of the perforations on the skin's surface. Cotton stockinette worn under the orthosis can minimize this irritation. Meticulous placement of straps with properly placed foam padding over or around bony prominences can minimize mobility within the orthosis, which in turn will additionally aid in decreasing friction on the skin's surface (Fig. 17–5A–F).

Materials may need to be "popped" apart to allow the orthosis to pass over an enlarged area and/or joint. This can be done by using coated thermoplastic (nonsticky) or by placing a wet paper towel or hand lotion between overlapping pieces of thermoplastic material. This is often referred to the patient as making them a "trap door" to allow for fluctuations in edema and ease of donning and doffing. Not only does this provide a way for the patient to slip in and out of the orthosis, but it also provides a sense of security for the patient who may be worried about not being able to remove the orthosis. An excellent example involves an orthosis of the thumb MP joint. In some patients, the interphalangeal (IP) joint can be significantly wider than the proximal phalanx, making removal of a thumb orthosis difficult unless it includes this design feature that allows it to be popped open (Fig. 17–5A).

STRAPPING

When securing straps onto the orthosis, consideration should be given to where the straps are going to traverse. Is the skin under the strap fragile? Are there bony prominences? Are Bouchard or Heberden nodes and/or mucous cysts present? If so, are they tender and will straps irritate them? Strapping considerations for the extremity with arthritis should include soft, conforming, and flexible material (Fig. 17–5F). Straps can be lined with foam to soften the contact points around bony areas. Larger widths of strapping can properly spread pressure across a greater area and help to minimize compression. Consider soft foam straps for night use and less bulky elasticized straps for day use (such as thin neoprene material). Both soft and elasticized strapping systems are comfortable, durable, and, when applied correctly, contribute to minimizing shear, distribute pressure evenly, and decrease compression stress on tissue (see Chapter 4 for details) (Fig. 17–6).

PREFABRICATED ORTHOSES

Prefabricated orthoses can be used for many patients with OA. Soft prefabricated wrist and thumb orthoses are a popular choice with physicians (Fig. 17–7) (Boozer, 1993; Murphy, 1996; Pagnotta, Baron, & Korner-Bitensky, 1998; Stern, Ytterberg, Krug, & Mahowald, 1996). Most patients initially do well with these orthoses. However,

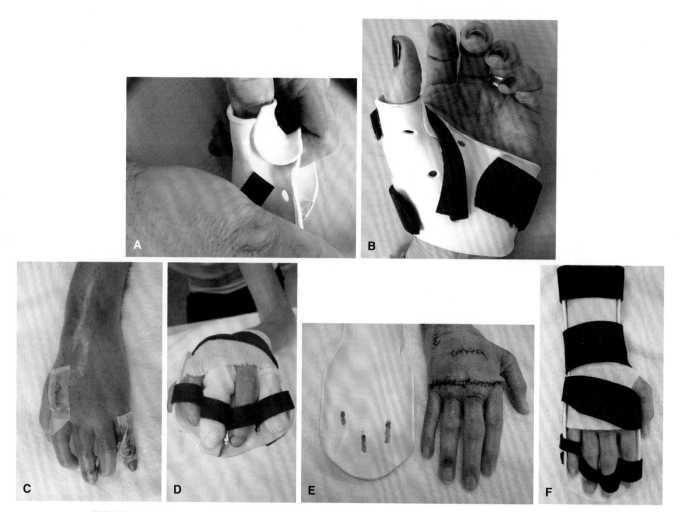

FIGURE 17–5 Enlargement of the IP joint of the thumb with OA can make removal of an orthosis difficult. **A and B,** By lightly and carefully overlapping the material during molding, a "trap door" can be made as shown here. This type of design provides for an expansion during application and removal and may also provide a sense of security to the patient that may feel "trapped" in the device. **C,** A patient with scleroderma who underwent IF PIP fusion, MF DIP fusion, and RF MCP arthroplasty. **D,** A hand-based orthosis was created to support procedures, properly align , and, yet, allow for some light wrist motion. **E,** IF-SF MCP arthroplasty post surgery. **F,** A resting orthosis fabricated to align digits and support procedure. Note the holes in the thermoplastic base that were incorporated (with a traditional hole punch) which allowed a way to maintain the digit in proper position.

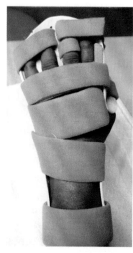

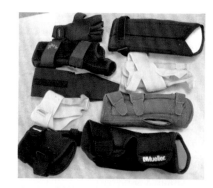

FIGURE 17–7 Various prefabricated orthoses are available and widely used to manage the early intermittent symptoms of arthritis. These are all orthoses that one patient purchased while trying to seek relief from first CMC OA.

FIGURE 17–6 Soft strapping should be considered when applying an orthosis to this patient population, who often have thin fragile skin. Note the cushion on the IF radial border to assist in alignment and the cushions under the soft strapping.

many of these prefabricated designs are meant to fit the population at large and may not provide the exacting support the patient or referring professional is seeking. For instance, a prefabricated thumb first CMC stabilization orthosis does not fully immobilize this joint nor can it reposition the joint and provide proper alignment of the metacarpal (Grenier, Mendonca, & Dalley, 2016). Prefabricated orthoses have a role when fit by a skilled clinician. If an appropriate fit is not achieved, insufficient support is provided, and/or joint/bony changes begin to alter the shape of the wrist and/or thumb, a more customized design may be necessary. In the clinical experience of the authors of this chapter, with end-stage disease, patients tend to do better with soft neoprene options as the primary management option.

PIP AND DIP JOINTS WITH OSTEOARTHRITIS

Osteoarthritis of the PIP and DIP joints can result in pain, edema, decreased digital AROM, and difficulty in tasks requiring gripping and pinching. The alterations in physical appearance that osteophytes can cause may be disturbing to some patients as they see their fingers as becoming deformed (Estes et al., 2000; Melvin, 1982). Bony changes and swelling can also have functional or meaningful implications with simple tasks such as donning rings. Although osteophytes and cysts are not always painful, they can be episodically tender (Burkholder, 2000; Cassidy & Green, 2011; Estes et al., 2000). Pain is reported as localized to the involved joints during functional activities. The intensity of the pain does not necessarily correlate to the amount of joint destruction or deformity as appreciated radiographically (Nwawka & Weinstock-Zlotnick, 2019; Estes et al., 2000).

NONSURGICAL ORTHOTIC MANAGEMENT GUIDELINES

Fitting an orthosis is usually reserved for the acutely painful PIP or DIP joint. Lightweight volar immobilization orthoses can be supportive and prevent lateral stress to the PIP and DIP joints (Fig. 17–8A,B) (Cassidy & Green, 2011). The orthoses support the joints in a comfortably extended position and are worn generally at night. Gel-lined products (such as the Silopos® Mesh Gel Tubing or various silicone-lined thermoplastic materials) may provide an absorbent cushion and layer of warmth to a painful joint (Fig. 17–9A). A piece of silicone gel can be incorporated into an orthosis for added protection and cushioning (Austin, 2003). An alternate option for the painful DIP or thumb IP joint is the use of a figure-of-eight splint worn to better align the joint (Fig. 17–9B,C). This allows the fingertip or thumb tip to be free and be less intrusive to functional pinching or picking up objects. Conversely, Dycem® can be affixed to the volar aspect of the tip of a finger-based orthosis to allow better grip and support greater functional use.

EXPERT PEARL 17–1

Neoprene Buddy Stalls
NATALIE ALFARO, OT, CHT
Australia

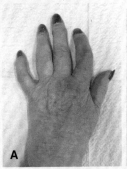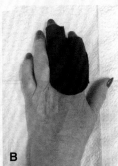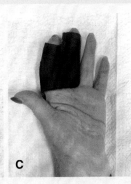

Fabricated from thin neoprene (1.6 mm) to support collateral ligaments while allowing movement after PIP joint replacement. Adjust the size of the dart between the fingers to either provide more ulnar or radial support.

EXPERT PEARL 17–2

Neoprene Orthosis
ANGELA FRIGERIO, OT, CHT
Australia

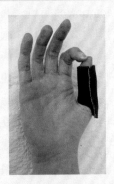

Thick (2.4 mm) neoprene used to prevent IP joint flexion in trigger thumb allows thumb pulp free for light function.

EXPERT PEARL 17–3

Neoprene DIP Sleeve
MELISSA CEPEDA, OTR/L
Colorado

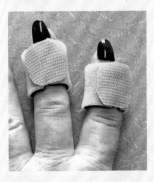

Fabricated from neoprene with nonadhesive hook for closure. These sleeves provide ability for patient to vary tension to accommodate for edema or joint enlargement. Utilized post DIP fusion in this patient to protect sensitive incisions and healing joints after initial immobilization period. The thickness of the neoprene prevents DIP motion but allows proximal motion and functional use.

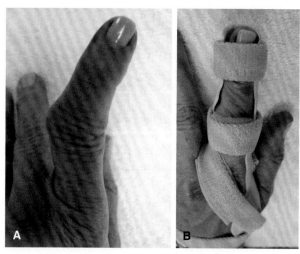

FIGURE 17–8 A, A volar RF digit immobilization orthosis that extends proximally to include the MCP joint. This extension provides a longer lever arm for increased stability and comfort, especially for patients with small hands or digits. **B,** This patient had significant radial deviation at the PIP joint, and the use of the longer orthosis combined with the precise strapping placed this joint back into anatomical alignment.

POSTSURGICAL ORTHOTIC MANAGEMENT GUIDELINES

DIP Joint Arthrodesis

There are few surgical options for the patient with DIP joint osteoarthritis, with the exception of arthrodesis (fusion); for this small but important joint, stability takes priority over mobility (Bernstein et al., 2010; Cassidy & Green, 2011; Estes et al., 2000; Melvin, 1982; Pelligrini & Burton, 1990). Along with providing stability, the purpose of the arthrodesis is to also decrease intractable pain and can enhance cosmetic appearance (Bernstein et al., 2010; Cassidy & Green, 2011; Pelligrini & Burton, 1990).

The DIP joint is immobilized after **arthrodesis** for 6 to 8 weeks, until sufficient osseous healing has occurred as evaluated radiographically (Cassidy & Green, 2011; Pelligrini & Burton, 1990). Postsurgically, the patient can be fabricated a protective distal interphalangeal joint (DIPJ) immobilization orthosis until the DIPJ has fused. The distal portion of the fingertip should be protected in the presence of an external K-wire, to protect a sensitive fingertip, or a compression screw (Fig. 17–10A–C). For added length and support, the orthosis can be hand based or finger based including the proximal interphalangeal joint (PIPJ) as well, which may make the orthosis more secure particularly in cases with significant dressings (Fig. 17–10D–G). Orthoses can later be modified to include only the DIP joint allowing for full range of motion and use of the PIP joint (Cassidy & Green, 2011; Rizio, & Belsky, 1995).

PIP Joint Arthrodesis

PIP joint arthrodesis is considered for patients who use their hand for activities that require a forceful grip, such as a butcher or construction worker. Surgical fusion has been recommended for the index finger (IF) where ulnarly directed force is exerted by the thumb with pinching (Bernstein et al., 2010). Other factors when considering candidacy for PIP arthrodesis include to provide increased functional use of the hand when the soft tissues in the joint cannot support an arthroplasty, when stability is more important than mobility (as in the index finger), and to provide a pain-free joint. The postoperative orthosis should protect the PIP joint in the fused position for 6 to 8 weeks or until the arthrodesis has sufficiently fused, as evaluated radiographically. Initially, the orthosis should include both the PIP and DIP joints for pain control and, as mentioned for DIP arthrodesis, should envelop any exposed hardware as shown in Figure 17–10F,G. In the

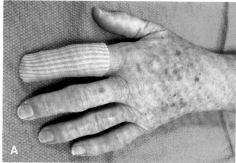

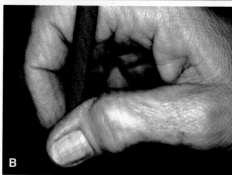

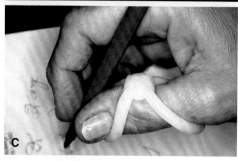

FIGURE 17–9 A, A mesh digital silicone-lined cap used to provide warmth and pain relief to a patient with OA of the IF DIP joint. **B,** Thumb IP during writing, an option is **C,** a custom-made IP ulnar deviation orthosis. As noted, with the small orthosis in place, this patient is able to write with a stable thumb.

latter weeks, the DIP joint may be cut free, or a second orthosis could be fabricated leaving the DIP joint free, permitting flexor digitorum profundus (FDP) tendon gliding to prevent tendon adherence and DIP stiffness (Estes et al., 2000; Rizio & Belsky, 1995). Lightweight thermoplastics or casting materials can be used.

The position of fusion for the PIP or DIP joint is based on which digit is involved and the functional demands of that particular joint as determined by preoperative discussion with the patient (Cassidy & Green, 2011; Estes et al., 2000). In normal hand function, the IF and middle finger (MF) are used mostly for prehension and do not require as much flexion as the ring-finger (RF) and small-finger (SF) PIP joints. The RF and SF require greater flexion, especially at the DIP joints, as they contribute the most to grip strength (Estes et al., 2000; Rizio & Belsky, 1995).

PIP Joint Arthroplasty

PIP joint arthroplasty can be considered to restore motion, alleviate pain, and enhance PIP joint stability. An arc of motion of 0° to 70° can be anticipated (Bernstein et al., 2010; Goldfarb, 2011; Kozin, 1999; Pelligrini & Burton, 1990; Rizio & Belsky, 1995; Swanson, Swanson, & Leonard, 1995). Exercise protocols vary and depend on the surgical approach and procedure, implant, and intraoperative joint stability (Feldscher, 2010). Therefore, postoperative rehabilitation and orthosis application depend on close communication between the surgeon and therapist. Common surgical approaches to PIP joint arthroplasties include the central slip sparing technique, palmar approach, lateral approach, and **dorsal Chamay repair.** All approaches typically permit immediate early active flexion and extension of the affected digit

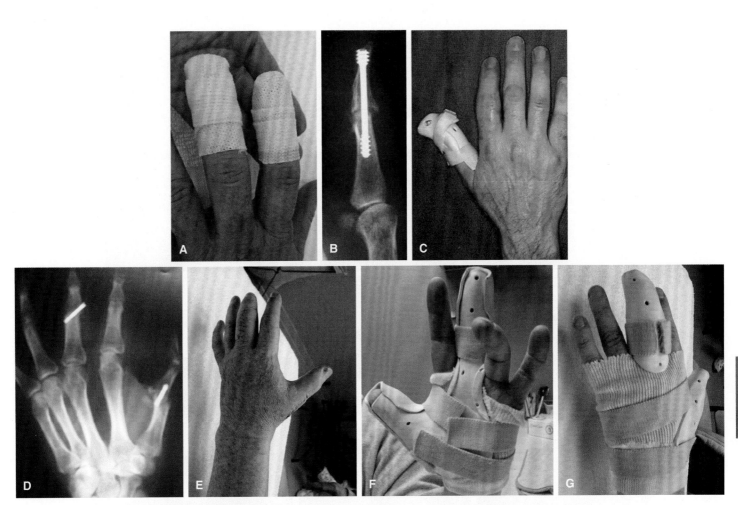

FIGURE 17–10 **A,** QuickCast 2 used to fabricate DIP immobilization orthoses for protecting recent DIP joint fusions. **B,** Radiograph of a thumb IP fusion. **C,** A thumb-based orthosis for postoperative thumb immobilization. **D,** Radiograph of a thumb MP and MF PIP arthrodesis. **E,** Postoperative day 2. **F and G,** Hand-based "clamshell" designed postoperative orthosis.

and should include DIP joint flexion and extension exercises with the PIP joint blocked in neutral. They do not require the application of a mobilization orthosis (dynamic) for movement (Bechenbaugh & Linscheid, 1993; Chamay, 1988; Feldscher, 2010; Lipscomb, 1967; Schneider, 1991). With dorsal and lateral approaches, it is important to consider retention of the PIP joint extension. An extension lag at the PIP joint along with DIP hyperextension may lead to a secondary pseudoboutonniere. It is critical that the PIP joint be positioned in neutral. A silastic implant has a greater tendency to develop an extension lag. Whereas with a volar approach, it is critical that the PIP be positioned on 10° to 15° of flexion to prevent a secondary swan-neck posture (Ceruso, Planner, & Caulli, 2017) (Fig. 17–11A–E). Another common surgical approach is the central slip splitting technique, which often delays mobilization for 2 to 4 weeks with the use of an extension mobilization orthosis (dynamic) during the day to allow active PIP joint flexion with a gentle, "dynamic," passive assist into extension (Swanson, Maupin, Gajjar, & Swanson, 1985) (Fig. 17–11F). Postoperative management may be affected by the type of implant used, including a silicone spacer or pyrolytic carbon/ceramic resurfacing implant, as well as surgeon preference; however, postoperative management and orthosis positioning are guided primarily by surgical approach and may be altered during the rehabilitation process as necessary to prevent development of secondary complications.

Therapeutic management should take into account other surgical procedures that may have been performed in tandem, such as tenolysis, extensor tendon reconstruction, or volar plate release. In general, AROM exercises are initiated between 2 and 7 days postoperatively (Fig. 17–11C,E). A recommended exercise schedule is 5- to 10-minute sessions, four to six times a day.

Typically following a PIP joint arthroplasty, a hand-based IP extension immobilization orthosis is fabricated and worn at all times for 4 to 6 weeks; it is removed only for hygiene, wound care, and exercise sessions, although the orthosis can be created to allow for just distal strap removal for exercise sessions (Fig. 17–11A–E). The MCP joint is usually included, at least initially, for improved purchase and comfort. If the patient had a swan-neck deformity (PIP hyperextension, DIP flexion) prior to surgery, consider positioning the involved joints in some degree of MCP and PIP flexion (approximately 10°–30°) within the orthosis (Fig. 17–11B). This may help prevent the tendency for the PIP joint to rebound into hyperextension given likely the dorsal orientation of lateral bands and deficient volar plate. Extension mobilization orthoses are an alternative postoperative management option (Fig. 17–11F). These orthoses are fabricated to position the PIP gently in extension yet allow gentle active flexion against rubber band traction.

Regardless of whether immobilization, restriction, or mobilization orthoses are implemented postoperatively, the orthoses should protect the joint from lateral stress and facilitate the encapsulation process (Estes et al., 2000). Immobilization and restriction orthoses should have sufficient depth for lateral protection and allow the patient to easily perform the home exercise program prescribed (Fig. 17–11C,E). Mobilization orthoses should maintain the line of pull centrally over the middle phalanx and avoid any undesired rotation or lateral deviation stresses (Fig. 17–12). It is important to recognize any tendon adherence, extension lag, and prolonged inflammation. The orthosis fit and effectiveness should be monitored often (at least at each therapy visit) because the tissue will undergo changes due to its wear. Adjustments to the orthosis should be based on these factors.

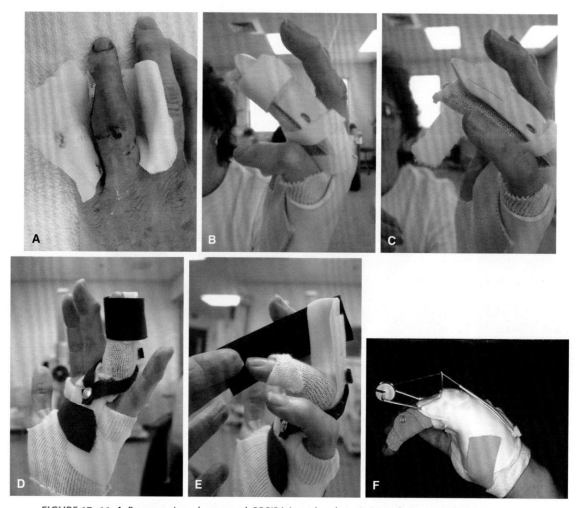

FIGURE 17–11 A, Postoperative volar approach RF PIP joint arthroplasty. **B,** PIP orthoses used after arthroplasty, note the gentle MCP and PIP flexion positioning. **C,** Strategically placed straps allow for ease of exercise execution. **D and E,** This volar-/dorsal-designed orthosis positions the MCP joint in extension and allows for PIP immobilization in slight flexion and also permits strap removal for AROM. **F,** A PIP extension mobilization orthosis (using a Phoenix Outrigger, Performance Health) may be indicated to allow frequent motion of PIP joint.

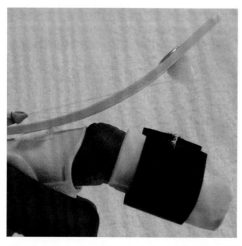

FIGURE 17–12 PIP extension mobilization orthosis: Note the 90° line of pull and the placement directly aligned over the middle phalanx (Digitec Outrigger system, Performance Health).

THUMB WITH OSTEOARTHRITIS

The thumb has a large, unique, and vital arc of motion allowing opposition to all the digits. Through the aging process, the first CMC joint can be subjected to a significant amount of stress. The cumulative impact of these stresses may exceed the load tolerance of the tissues including the articular cartilage, joint capsule, and ligaments. It is believed that ligamentous laxity and instability, either through the aging process or the demands placed on the joint, are the initiators of OA at the first CMC joint (Grenier et al., 2016; Kennedy et al., 2016; Barron et al., 2000; Boozer, 1993; Estes et al., 2000; Freedman, Eaton, & Glickel, 2000; Kelley & Ramsey, 2000; Pelligrini & Burton, 1990; Poole & Pellegrini, 2000). Additional predisposing factors to first CMC joint OA (Katarincic, 2001; Pellegrini & Burton, 1990) include the following:

- Subtle joint anatomical abnormalities, which lead to an increase in contact stress on the articular structures
- Periarticular soft-tissue trauma
- Base fractures of the first metacarpal
- Thinning of the articular cartilage combined with incongruency of the joint
- Excessive capsular laxity associated with hormonal changes (primarily postmenopausal women)

CLINICAL EXAMINATION

The diagnosis of first CMC joint OA is made primarily through a comprehensive physical examination followed by radiographic confirmation. Generally, patients complain of pain, pinch weakness, and/or crepitus at the first CMC joint (Kennedy et al., 2016). In an exploratory study by Valdes and Quegulin (2019), the researchers revealed that patients with CMC OA also demonstrated a decrease in joint position sense when compared to their healthy counterparts (Valdes, & Quegulin, 2019).

Typically, patients note pain during functional activities, such as opening jars, brushing teeth, and turning a doorknob. Pain is generalized to the thenar eminence but may also be noted proximal and

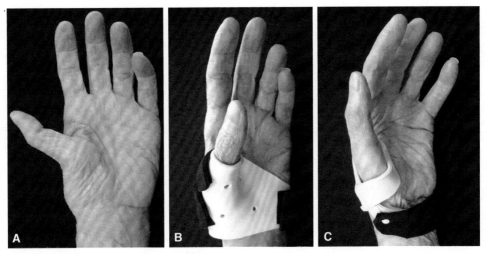

FIGURE 17–13 A, Note the subluxation of the TM joint, first metacarpal adduction, and MP joint hyperextension in this patient with advancing first CMC OA. **B and C,** These are two types of orthoses intervention that worked for this patient to reduce her subluxation.

distal to the involved joint. Palpation may reveal tenderness over the volar aspect of the first CMC joint; in approximately half the population, concurrent pain is appreciated at the STT joint (Kennedy et al., 2016; Glickel, Kornstein, & Eaton, 1992; Kozin, 1999; Poole & Pellegrini, 2000). The patient may have a positive **grind test**—pain elicited when the examiner imparts axial compression and rotation of the base of the first metacarpal into the trapezium (Bernstein et al., 2010; Estes et al., 2000). In the earlier stages of the disease, gross appearance may be normal. Progression of the disease often results in subluxation of the metacarpal dorsoradially over the trapezium; this positive "shoulder sign" may be seen at the base of the first CMC (Fig. 17–13A–C). As the disease progresses, motion at the first CMC joint diminishes. Patients often develop an adduction contracture, a loss of radial abduction, and exaggerated IP flexion. Compensatory thumb MCP joint hyperextension may develop leading to a "Z" or swan-neck deformity of the thumb. This classic deformity is the hallmark of advanced-stage first CMC joint arthritis (Kennedy et al., 2016) (Fig. 17–14).

Radiographic examination will confirm as well as determine the stage of osteoarthritic change present at the first CMC joint (Fig. 17–15). The severity of first CMC OA based on radiographic findings may be graded according to the well-accepted staging system applied by many surgeons. Refer to Table 17–1.

PATHOMECHANICS OF FIRST CARPOMETACARPAL OSTEOARTHRITIS

The first CMC joint is the key articulation responsible for imparting mobility to the thumb. The trapezium also articulates with the scaphoid, trapezoid, and the index metacarpal. This complex of articulations is also commonly referred to as the **basal joint complex**. Osteoarthritis of the CMC joint is due to a transfer of exponentially greater load on the trapezium by the first metacarpal during grasp and pinch. The trapezium is inherently unstable due to its anatomical location and relatively poor ligamentous stability. Because of these two factors, it is believed that the first CMC joint over time develops excessive axial and cantilever bending forces during thumb use. Adaptively, the trapezium begins to tilt radially, causing the base of the metacarpal to slide in a dorsoradial direction. Consequently, the adductor pollicis pulls the metacarpal medially, increasing the tension on the abductor pollicis longus (APL) tendon, contributing to the zigzag collapse of the TM joint. This in turn results in attenuation or failure of the anterior oblique ligament (AOL) which is the primary stabilizer of the first CMC in preventing dorsal translation; as the metacarpal translates, this can progress cartilage degeneration (Katarincic, 2001). Also considered part of the basal thumb complex and often involved in later stages of first CMC OA are the scaphotrapezial, scaphotrapezoid, and trapeziotrapezoid joints (Bernstein et al., 2010).

 EXPERT PEARL 17–4

"Swan-Neck" Thumb in RA
MAGDALENA KOLASIŃSKA, PT
Poland

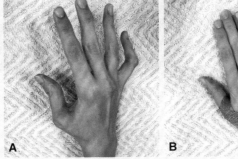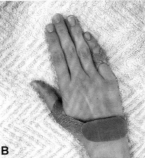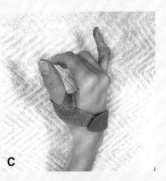

Restricting MP flexion corrects the IP extension. Orficast More utilized, start application from the dorsal side of the wrist toward the thumb, cross dorsal MP joint to then palm side to join. Be mindful to maintain correcting position of the MP while material sets. (Notice Figure-8 design utilized on SF to address boutonniere deformity.)

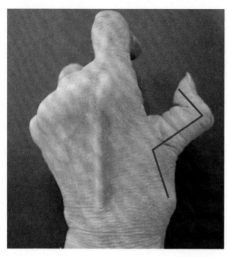

FIGURE 17–14 Advanced first CMC disease with significant thumb IP flexion. Thumb mechanics are greatly altered.

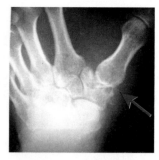

FIGURE 17–15 Stage IV radiograph of the basal joint of the thumb with significant sclerosis and joint destruction (arrow).

NONSURGICAL ORTHOTIC MANAGEMENT GUIDELINES

Orthosis application is the mainstay of conservative (nonsurgical) management of first CMC joint OA. However, other common methods of conservative treatment include pain control, principles of joint protection teaching including the use of adaptive devices, exercise, dynamic stability training (as described by O'Brien, & Giveans, 2013) thermal modalities, nonsteroidal anti-inflammatory medications, and corticosteroid injections (Medvedeva et al., 2018). The overall objectives of an orthosis are to stabilize the first CMC joint, provide pain control, and prevent adduction contracture (Grenier et al., 2016; Barron et al., 2000; Colditz, 1995; 2000; Jacobs, 2003; O'Brien & Giveans, 2013; Poole & Pellegrini, 2000; Weiss et al., 2000).

The designs of orthoses can vary, and many options are available (Fig. 17–16A–E). Common to most of these designs is the maintenance of a wide first web space because as the disease process advances, adduction and subluxation of the first metacarpal may occur, causing a contracture and/or narrowing of the first web space (Bernstein et al., 2010; Colditz, 2000; Diaz, 1994; Melvin, 1982, 1995; Poole & Pellegrini, 2000; Swigart et al., 1999; Tomaino, 2011; Wajon, 2000; Weiss et al., 2000). Ideal orthotic management for first CMC joint arthritis involves positioning the thumb in palmar abduction and approximately 30° of MP flexion (Grenier et al., 2016; Bernstein et al., 2010; Colditz, 1995; Jacobs, 2003; O'Brien & Giveans, 2013; Poole & Pellegrini, 2000; Weiss et al., 2000). The orthosis can be custom made from thermoplastic material or neoprene material (see Chapter 14), or a clinician may choose a prefabricated design. There are many prefabricated designs, discussed in Chapter 9, which may work very well for this population. As noted above, there is no superior orthosis design as indicated by the body of literature; however, the choice is dependent on clinician preference, stage of disease process, and most importantly should always be in partnership with the patient. Proper fit is a key factor for any orthoses chosen for a patient.

Recommendations differ with respect to the orthosis design, wearing schedule, and accompanying education and exercise regimens. A systematic review by Bertozzi et al. explored conservative therapeutic interventions regarding the first CMC joint. Results indicated that there was overall low quality of evidence exploring the use of therapeutic methods and the treatment of first CMC OA. However, there was moderate quality of evidence to support that orthoses can improve hand function long term (Grenier et al., 2016; Bertozzi et al., 2015). Bernhard et al. in their systematic review, indicated a positive effect on pain and hand function regardless of orthosis design with the use of a thumb immobilization (Spica design) orthosis for the management of CMC OA (Bernhard, Simone, & Taeymans, 2016). Another study compared thermoplastic and neoprene orthoses with this patient population. They found that despite a statistically significant improvement in pain relief with the use of the orthoses with a thermoplastic component, patients indicated a preference for the prefabricated neoprene thumb orthosis (Grenier et al., 2016; Sillem, Backman, Miller, & Li, 2011). It has been suggested that conservative management of first CMC joint OA, regardless of the stage of progression, should begin with a trial of a 6-week course of orthosis wear and hand therapy including strengthening exercises. Tshie et al. indicated that patients with the greatest pain and dysfunction initially benefitted the most from this intervention, and that outcomes at 6 weeks versus 3 months had no statistically significant difference (Tsehaie et al., 2019).

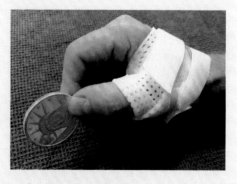

EXPERT PEARL 17-6

MP Hyperextension Restriction Orthosis
KATHY VILLACRES, OTR/L, CHT
Ohio

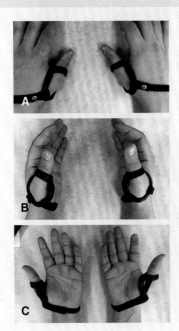

Fabricated from 1/16" elastic-based material; strap is riveted on one side and has a fold over loop tab on the other side.

EXPERT PEARL 17-7

Thumb MP Orthosis: Low-Profile Design
NIAMH MASTERSON, OT
Australia

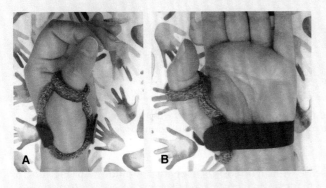

Fold a long narrow piece of wet-heated orfitcast at desired length and cut along the open edge to seal the material. Double layer provides strength, and edges can be smoothed using the heat gun. Ensure the hook material remain on the outer aspect to reduce risk of irritating skin.

CLINICAL PEARL 17-1

Postsurgical Orthotic Management Guidelines

In the authors practice, it is important to consider the stage of disease progression both clinically and radiographically, including subluxation of the metacarpal over the trapezium, as well as hyperextension of the MP joint when recommending orthoses in treatment of first CMC OA. We like to use the analogy of shoes: you have different shoes for different activities,

TABLE 17-1	Stages of Carpometacarpal Joint Osteoarthritis
Stage I	Appears normal on radiographic examination; there may be no degenerative joint changes to minimal changes or widened joint space secondary to synovitis.
Stage II	May present with a reduction of joint space and possible appearance of sclerosis and osteophytes less than 2 mm in diameter; STT joint is normal.
Stage III	More dramatic joint space narrowing and notable subchondral sclerosis as well as sclerosis and/or osteophytes measuring more than 2 mm in diameter.
Stage IV	Characterized by advanced degenerative changes involving the first CMC and the ST joint and could involve neighboring joints as well (Fig. 17-15).

From Barron, O. A., & Eaton, R. G. (1998). Save the trapezium: Double interposition arthroplasty for the treatment of stage IV disease of the basal joint. The Journal of Hand Surgery, 23, 196–204; Barron, O. A., Glickel, S. Z., & Eaton, R. G. (2000). Basal joint arthritis of the thumb. Journal of American Academy of Orthopaedic Surgery, 8, 314–323; and Tomaino, M. M. (2011). Thumb carpometacarpal joint resection arthroplasty. In T. R. Hunt (Ed.), Operative techniques in hand, wrist and forearm surgery (pp. 684–691). Philadelphia, PA: Lippincott Williams & Wilkins.

running shoes, heels, and so on, then having various orthoses may be beneficial for different tasks and activity demands, for example, gardening versus folding laundry. It is the author's preference to suggest to patients the use of both a neoprene soft wrap as well as a custom-fabricated hand-based immobilization orthosis. A custom design should be considered particularly in the presence of subluxation of the metacarpal at the first CMC and with MP joint hyperextension. The authors fabricate a hand-based design in which the CMC is positioned in extension and abduction (tip pinch with index) and the MP rests in slight flexion (30°) to correct the classic Z deformity (Fig. 17–51A,B). At times, a prefabricated neoprene soft wrap with a thermoplastic insert can be considered (Fig. 17–17A–D).

For a custom design, it may help to extend the orthosis border proximally on the radial aspect just beyond the STT joint to secure the thumb column. A conforming, lightweight material (e.g., 3/32" Aquaplast, Polyform light, Polyflex light, or TailorSplint) is an excellent choice for fabricating this orthosis (Austin, 2003). The material's thinness can make fabrication challenging to a novice fabricator, and it may not offer the strength necessary to stabilize the first metacarpal (Fig. 17–16A) (Austin, 2003; Colditz, 2000). These orthoses are used during daily activities to promote pain-free function. The selection of thermoplastic material (thickness and perforations) should take into consideration the activity level and functional demands of the patient wearing the orthosis. The dosage for precise wearing time of an orthosis has yet to be established. In these authors' experience, orthoses are most likely to be beneficial in patients who suffer from stages I to III of first CMC joint OA. Refer to Table 17–1 for reference. In general, a 6-week period of orthosis use is suggested in combination with patient education, range-of-motion exercises, and exercises to strengthening stabilizing muscles of the first CMC when initiating conservative treatment. Studies were able to determine a significant difference in participant's pain and dysfunction by 6 weeks of orthosis use.

It is generally accepted that people with severe stage IV degenerative stages will be less likely to respond to conservative management and should be referred for surgical consultation. Some physicians request that the daytime orthoses be complemented with a more substantial resting orthoses for night use (Jacobs, 2003; Weiss et al., 2000).

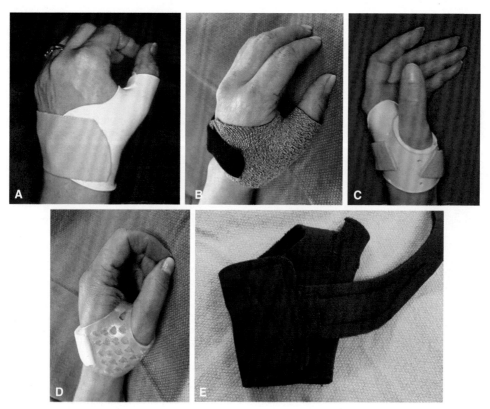

FIGURE 17–16 A, Hand-based first CMC immobilization orthosis to limit motion at the thumb first metacarpal and to place the thumb column in a position of function. Note the intimate contouring of the material about the proximal orthosis border. **B,** Similar in design to A, however, in a fabric material: Orficast. **C,** This orthosis (described by (Colditz, 2000) places an extension force to the volar/ulnar aspect of the distal metacarpal with counterpressure to the dorsal/radial portion of the metacarpal base. **D,** Similar in design to C, however, from a 3D-printed plastic. **E,** A prefabricated neoprene wrap support may be appropriate when nonrigid support is recommended. (Shown Comfort Cool orthosis, North Coast Medical, Morgan Hill, CA.)

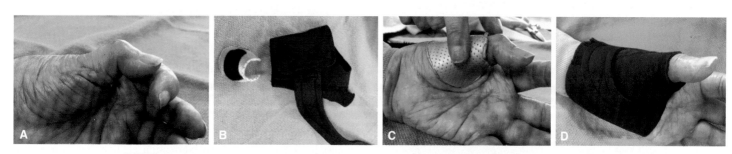

FIGURE 17–17 A, MP hyperextension deformity. **B and C,** A custom-molded thermoplastic insert is used in combination with a prefabricated neoprene wrap. **D,** Note support to correct MP joint hyperextension. (Shown Comfort Cool orthosis, North Coast Medical, Morgan Hill, CA.)

Forearm-based night orthoses can be fabricated to immobilize a wider and/or longer surface area, incorporating proximal and distal structures to achieve a greater degree of immobilization (Austin, 2003; Colditz, 2000; Fess et al., 2005; Jacobs, 2003; Leonard, 1995; Simmons, Nutting, & Bernstein, 1996; Weiss et al., 2000). Therapists may find that patients become concerned about wearing an orthosis too much, possibly leading to joint stiffness and/or weakness. In some cases, stiffness may be the desired outcome as a decrease in joint motion may also produce a decrease in pain. If pain persists without relief from orthotic intervention (use a trial period of 4–6 weeks), other modalities such as injection or surgical consult should be considered (Barron et al., 2000; Estes et al., 2000; Kozin, &Michlovitz, 2000). Refer to additional information on orthoses for thumb OA in Box 17–1.

POSTSURGICAL ORTHOTIC MANAGEMENT GUIDELINES

Surgical intervention may be an option for patients with painful, progressive OA of the thumb. In these advanced cases, there typically has been first CMC subluxation and/or dislocation. Managing this disease with an orthosis is likely to be of little help (Fig. 17–18A,B) (Ataker, Gudemes, Ece, Canbulat, & Gulgonen, 2012; Bernstein et al., 2010; Colditz, 1995). Several surgical procedures (and variations of these procedures) for ligament reconstruction of the first CMC joint have been described (Ataker et al, 2012; Bernstein et al., 2010; Estes et al., 2000; Freedman et al., 2000; Kozin, 1999; Poole & Pellegrini, 2000; Rozental & Bora, 2000; Tomaino & King, 2000; Tucker et al., 1994; Trumble et al., 2000; Varitimidis, Fox, King, Taras, & Soreranes, 2000). All have the primary goals of pain relief and reestablishing the thumb/IF web space to provide a stable post for digits to pinch against and preventing further joint destruction. One such procedure uses a tendon interposition graft with a slip of the flexor carpi radialis (FCR) tendon as a spacer with excision of the trapezium (Poole & Pellegrini, 2000; Tomaino, Pellegrini, & Burton, 1995; Tomaino, 2011). The successful outcome of ligament reconstruction of the thumb requires stabilization of the base of the thumb metacarpal and simultaneous adjustment of distal deformity (Ataker et al, 2012; Colditz, 1995; Estes et al., 2000; Poole & Pellegrini, 2000; Tomaino et al., 1995; Tomaino, 2011).

BOX 17–1   EVIDENCE-INFORMED ORTHOTIC MANAGEMENT: THUMB OSTEOARTHRITIS

Therapeutic interventions for persons with osteoarthritis commonly involve the use of orthoses. To date, there have been few systematic reviews on the effectiveness of orthotic application in the patient with osteoarthritis. Orthotic management in persons suffering from OA has been most studied when applied to the thumb. Positioning with an orthosis is the mainstay of conservative management of the osteoarthritic thumb. The success of an orthosis positioning program is determined by the reduction in pain and improved hand function along with dynamic thumb-stability training/strengthening (O'Brien, & Giveans, 2013). A review of the literature has shown only limited evidence on the effectiveness of static orthosis positioning for persons with varying stages of CMC joint OA of the thumb (Grenier et al., 2016; Kennedy et al., 2016; Beasley, 2011; Buurke, & Baten, 1999; Sillem et al., 2011; Swigart et al., 1999; Weiss et al., 2000, 2004).

Three types of orthoses are commonly used in the treatment of first CMC joint OA. They are the following:

1. Wrist/thumb immobilization orthosis (Fig. 17–19A,B)

2. Hand-based thumb immobilization orthosis (Figs. 17–13 and 17–16A–D)

3. Custom or prefabricated soft/neoprene orthosis (Figs. 17–7, 17–16E, and 17–17D)

There is no evidence that one type of orthotic design is more effective than another (Egan et al., 2003; Grenier et al., 2016; Kennedy et al., 2016; Valdes & Marik, 2010). There is evidence that rigid custom orthoses provide better pain reduction compared to soft prefabricated neoprene orthoses; however, patients may prefer the neoprene designs (Sillem et al., 2011) (Weiss, LaStayo, Mills, & Bramlet, 2004). These findings suggest that therapists should be patient centered when providing orthoses to meet the individual needs of patients.

To the knowledge of the authors of this chapter, orthosis application to digits with osteoarthritis in either the PIP or DIP joints to date have not been studied in the literature. Furthermore, orthosis application following an operative procedure to the osteoarthritic hand or wrist has not been studied in the literature. Managing osteoarthritis with an orthosis, in these instances, is based on expert opinion and the clinical experience of the authors of this chapter.

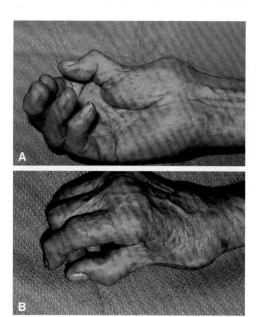

FIGURE 17–18 A and B, This patient presents with end stages of CMC OA, note the adducted posture and shoulder sign as well as thumb MP hyperextension. CMC, carpometacarpal; OA, osteoarthritis.

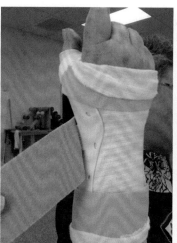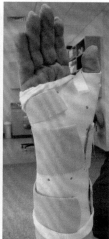

FIGURE 17–19 A wrist/thumb immobilization orthosis is often used after first CMC joint arthroplasty. Note the additional support that wraps around the radial dorsal thumb base. CMC, carpometacarpal.

Ligament reconstruction procedures of the first CMC joint normally require a short period of cast immobilization, followed by transitioning into an orthosis during the first 2 to 4 weeks post surgery; however, protocols vary from surgeon to surgeon (Fig. 17–19) (Ataker et al, 2012; Bernstein et al., 2010; Colditz, 1995; Kozin, 1999; Poole & Pellegrini, 2000; Tomaino, 2011; Tomaino et al., 1995; Tomaino, 2011; Weiss et al., 2000). Post cast removal, typically a forearm-based wrist/thumb immobilization orthosis is fabricated that allows the IP joint to move freely. The orthosis is typically worn full time during the first 6 weeks postoperatively and is gradually weaned as tolerated by the patient. Some surgeons prefer to shorten the orthosis after 6 to 8 weeks to allow wrist motion. After approximately 12 weeks, the orthosis can be discontinued or worn only at night, if necessary (Jacobs, 2003; Poole & Pellegrini, 2000). The therapist must appreciate that depending on the type of ligament reconstruction used and the preference of the surgeon's

postoperative rehabilitation protocol, the type and duration of orthosis wear may be influenced. Some patients may prefer to use a soft custom or prefabricated orthosis for added comfort and stability during the first 3 to 6 months postoperatively (see Chapters 9, 18, and 19).

WRIST WITH OSTEOARTHRITIS

Osteoarthritis of the wrist presents most often at the STT joint. Confusion can exist between clinical presentation of STT arthritis and first CMC joint arthritis; the literature has clearly outlined clinical distinctions of each (Kozin, & Michlovitz, 2000; Poole & Pellegrini, 2000).

STT JOINT VERSUS FIRST CMC JOINT OSTEOARTHRITIS: WHAT IS THE DIFFERENCE?

Patients with *STT joint arthritis* may exhibit pain with radial deviation of the wrist (e.g., using scissors, pulling up socks), a decrease in active radial deviation, tenderness with palpation over the STT area, a positive grind test, joint space narrowing with radiographic examination, pain with the scaphoid shift test, and, only occasionally, first CMC joint changes.

Patients with *first CMC joint arthritis* may demonstrate difficulty with fine motor tasks (using clothespins, writing, doing needlepoint, turning a car key), a positive grind test, and subluxation of the first CMC joint with possible MP hyperextension. Approximately half of patients with first CMC joint OA show STT joint space narrowing with possible osteophyte formation on radiographs (Bernstein et al., 2010; Kozin, 1999; Kozin, & Michlovitz, 2000; Poole & Pellegrini, 2000; Weiss et al., 2000).

NONSURGICAL ORTHOTIC MANAGEMENT GUIDELINES

Patients with STT arthritis may find some temporary relief from such interventions as cortisone injection, pain-modulating modalities, activity modification, and orthosis use (Kozin & Michlovitz, 2000). A recommended orthosis design is a wrist/thumb immobilization orthosis with the thumb IP free (Fig. 17–18A,B). Wrist immobilization orthoses may also be successful in controlling pain and permitting limited hand use. Circumferential wrist orthoses (such as the Rolyan® AquaForm™ Zippered Wrist orthosis) may be more appropriate for heavy labor workers, whereas a lightweight volar wrist immobilization orthosis will likely suffice for a person with lighter functional demands. There are several prefabricated orthosis designs that can work well for this population that are well described in Chapter 9 (Boozer, 1993; Stern et al., 1997; Stern, Ytterberg, Krug, & Mahowald, 1996; Trumble et al., 2000).

EXPERT PEARL 17–8

Tips for using OhioF
LAURA CONWAY, OTR, CHT, COMT UE
Florida

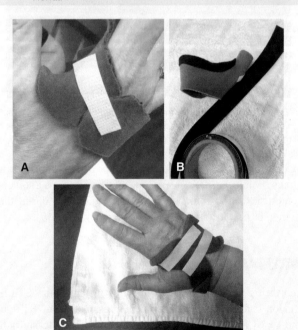

A. Use small tabs of hook to secure Ohio F during the molding to free hands and attend to contours and assuring a good fit.
B. Felt edging tape (Essity) can soften the perforated edges making orthosis very comfortable on delicate skin.
C. Due to the flexible and soft nature of Ohio F, it is ideal for orthosis where weight-bearing is needed such as when using a cane.

POSTSURGICAL ORTHOTIC MANAGEMENT GUIDELINES

Several procedures have been described for managing OA of the wrist, including scaphoid excision with four-corner fusion, proximal row carpectomy, wrist arthrodesis, arthrodesis of the distal radioulnar joint, arthrodesis of the STT joint, and distal ulna resection (Beer & Turner, 1997; Bernstein et al., 2010; Cross & Baratz, 2011; Feinberg, 1999; Kozin, 1999; Michlovitz, 1999; Shapiro, 1996; Swanson, 1995b; Tijhuis, Vliet Vlieland, Zwinderman, & Hazes, 1998; van Vugt, van Jaarsveld, Hofman, Helders, & Bijlsma, 1999; Watson & Ballet, 1984; Watson, Weinzweig, Guidera, Zeppieri, & Ashmead, 1999; Wilson & Fredick, 1994). Common to these surgical procedures is the judicious postoperative orthosis intervention. Orthoses are used after bulky dressing removal to further stabilize and protect the surgical site. Position of the wrist and the length of time the orthosis is worn may depend on the procedure performed. A wrist/thumb immobilization orthosis with the IP joint free may be used 6 to 8 weeks after STT fusion (Fig. 17–19). Once satisfactory radiographic union is observed, gentle motion of the wrist is often initiated (Cross, & Baratz, 2011; Kozin, 1999).

EXPERT PEARL 17–9

Neoprene Orthosis
SABRINA CASSELLA, M.ED, OTR/L, CHT
Massachusetts

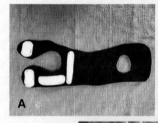
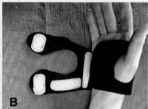
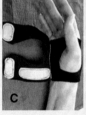
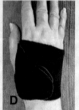

A custom neoprene orthosis with sewn hook closures—ideally fabricated using sewing machine or can be hand-sewn as well.

ELBOW WITH OSTEOARTHRITIS

Primary OA of the elbow is a relatively rare condition that comprises only 1% to 2% of patients with elbow arthritis (Morrey, 1992). It almost exclusively affects males and has a strong association with strenuous use of the arm in activities ranging from operating heavy machinery, throwing athletes, to aggressive weight training. The pattern of pain in patients suffering from primary elbow OA is very different than that of patients suffering from the rheumatoid elbow. Patients with elbow OA classically complain of impingement pain at the extremes of motion. Unlike OA of other joints, elbow OA is characterized by the relative preservation of articular cartilage and the maintenance of joint space but with hypertrophic osteophyte formation and capsular contracture. Osteophytes may be present in the olecranon fossa and on the olecranon, which may cause pain in maximal extension. Osteophyte formation may also occur in the coronoid process or the trochlea, which may cause impingement pain in full flexion. As the disease progresses, patients may complain of pain throughout the arc of ulnohumeral motion. This is most often present typically in advanced stage disease. Classically, patients will complain of pain while carrying heavy objects at the side of the body with the elbow in extension. They often complain of painful catching or locking, which may represent the presence of a loose body or a synovialized osteocartilaginous fragment, which can be found in approximately 50% of patients (Antuna, Morrey, Adams, & O'Driscoll, 2002; Forster, Clark, & Lunn, 2001; Morrey, 1992; Oka, 2000). The extension/flexion arc of ulnohumeral joint motion is often limited and patients may have up to a 30° flexion contracture (Antuna et al., 2002; Oka, Ohta, & Saitoh, 1998; Wada, Isogai, Ishii, & Yamashita, 2004).

NONSURGICAL ORTHOTIC MANAGEMENT GUIDELINES

Conservative management for the painful elbow with OA consists of rest, anti-inflammatory medication, long-term activity modification, referral to physical/occupational therapy, and orthotic management. A soft neoprene orthosis that provides soft-tissue compression, warmth, and protection can provide patients with symptom improvement during aggravating activities. These can be custom made or purchased commercially (Fig. 17–20A,B) (McAuliffe & Miller, 2000). A hinged elbow orthosis that limits full extension and flexion may be trialed to prevent anterior and posterior ulnohumeral impingement (Fig. 17–21). These can be custom made as shown or alternatively prefabricated. Prefabricated, commercially available orthoses are further described in Chapter 9.

POSTSURGICAL ORTHOTIC MANAGEMENT GUIDELINES

Current surgical treatment options for elbow OA include **arthroscopic debridement**, open debridement with ulnohumeral arthroplasty, distraction **interposition arthroplasty**, and total elbow arthroplasty (Cheung, Adams, & Morrey, 2008). Orthosis application will vary based on the surgical procedure and physician preference.

An arthroscopic debridement involves decompression of the impinging osteophytes, capsular release, and joint debridement with the removal of any loose bodies within the joint. Advantages of this approach include less postoperative pain and decreased intraoperative bleeding, which allows for early gains in range of motion (ROM) (O'Driscoll, 1995). Following such procedures, patients are often placed simply in a "collar and cuff" or some type of sling during the day to assist with pain control (Fig. 17–22). In addition, patients are instructed in frequent ROM exercises to prevent stiffness. A night static progressive extension orthosis is often applied to maintain any extension achievements made during the operative procedure. This is preferably applied the same day as the operative procedure and can be progressively remolded as edema decreases and extension improves. This orthosis can be either custom fabricated or obtained through commercial sources. If custom fabricated, the orthosis can be either applied anteriorly or posteriorly. The authors' preference is a custom-fit anterior design with the forearm positioned in supination or neutral (Fig. 17–23). The distal portion of the orthosis must be flared to prevent irritation to the dorsal sensory branch of the radial nerve or any bony prominences at the level of the wrist.

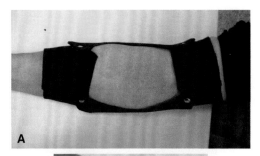
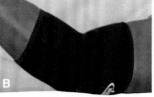

FIGURE 17–20 A and B, Soft, conforming custom or prefabricated neoprene-type orthoses are available in many sizes and lengths.

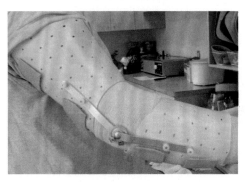

FIGURE 17–21 A custom-fabricated extension restriction orthosis can be fabricated to allow movement in one direction while limiting movement in another (Phoenix Elbow Outrigger; Performance Health).

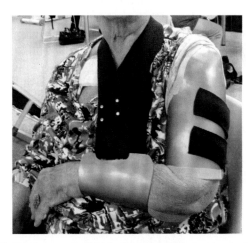

FIGURE 17–22 Custom-modified, "collar and cuff" designed orthosis for a patient who underwent an elbow debridement and, a few days later, sustained a nondisplaced humerus fracture.

If more extensive procedures are performed, then patients should be placed in an elbow immobilization orthosis or restriction orthosis similar to those used following rheumatoid elbow procedures, such as a posterior resting splint at 90°. The patient must be instructed in edema management and a carefully guided exercise program to prevent stiffness. The precise exercise regime will be dependent on the surgical procedure performed, patient and tissue factors, and surgeon preference, all of which require close communication between the patient, therapist, and surgeon.

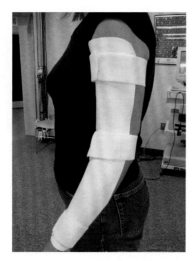

FIGURE 17–23 Custom anterior design with forearm in neutral.

RHEUMATOID ARTHRITIS

CHARACTERISTICS

RA is an unpredictable, systemic, autoimmune, chronic, and potentially debilitating disease affecting the synovial tissue of joints. It affects roughly 2.1 million people in the United States, touching the lives of women more than men in a 3:1 ratio. The disease process is inflammatory and may be characterized by exacerbations and remissions that occur over the course of time. If the inflammation remains unchecked, the disease process may eventually cause severe joint destruction, attenuation or rupture of tendons, ligament laxity, joint deformity, and a generalized decrease in function (Bernstein et al., 2010; Fess et al., 2005; Kozin, 1999; Massarotti, 1996; Melvin, 1982; Poole & Pellegrini, 2000; Swanson, 1995a, 1995b). Advancements in anti-inflammatory medications and disease-modifying drugs (biologics) have greatly influenced the goals of reducing pain, inflammation, and slowing joint damage and have influenced the severity of deformities experienced by patients and presenting to hand therapists as in years past.

Early onset is often seen in the shoulders, wrists, and knees but later on may then involve other joints of the upper and lower extremities including the MCP and PIP joints of the hand (Fig. 17–24). RA is a systemic disease, and patients may also complain of intermittent fevers, weight loss, fatigue, muscle atrophy, and prolonged morning stiffness (Swanson, 1995a, 1995b).

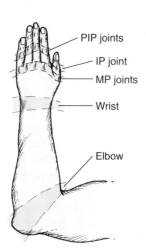

PIP joints

IP joint

MP joints

Wrist

Elbow

FIGURE 17–24 Upper extremity joints commonly affected by RA.

In the early stages of the disease, orthotic management and medical management may be all that is required. As the disease progresses, surgical intervention such as joint replacement and tendon transfer may be considered, depending on the degree of functional impairment and tissue involvement (Poole & Pellegrini, 2000; Shapiro, 1996). A generally accepted operative sequence usually involves initially stabilizing the affected proximal structures (Wilson & Fredick, 1994). For example, procedures would first address to the wrist (arthrodesis) followed by the MCP joints (arthroplasty). Some procedures can be performed simultaneously, such as a wrist and thumb metacarpophalangeal (MP) fusion or a first CMC arthroplasty, carpal tunnel release, and thumb MP arthrodesis (Fig. 17–25A–D) (Wilson & Fredick, 1994). When surgical intervention is planned, the hand dominance and ambulatory status of the patient must also be considered. If the patient is presently using a cane or crutches, he or she should be instructed in the use of platform crutches before surgery to allow ambulation without placing undue stress on the surgically repaired structures (Wolf, Patel, Zusstone, & Wolfe, 2019).

GENERAL SIGNS AND SYMPTOMS

RA is characterized by joint redness, inflammation, and tenderness over involved areas on gentle palpation (Fess et al., 2005; Massarotti, 1996; Melvin, 1982; Swanson, 1995b). The involved joint(s) may be warm and swollen, with a decrease in joint ROM. Unlike the normal healing process in which the inflammation subsides and the patient progresses through the stages of healing, patients with RA often remain in an extended inflammatory phase, which results in damage and deformity to the joints, pain, and impaired function (Swanson, 1995a; Terrono, Feldon, & Kimball, 2011).

Pain

Joint pain can occur during rest and may indicate acute inflammation (Melvin, 1982). Gentle pressure at the lateral aspects of an inflamed joint can cause some degree of pain, depending on the severity of the inflammation and joint damage. The joint(s) involved are generally described as sore with a notable decrease in AROM and functional use.

Stiffness and Decreased Function

Fluctuations in AROM can be related to joint pain and the extent of joint damage. Most patients with RA describe an increase in joint stiffness in the morning, after prolonged inactivity, and during periods of exacerbation when pain limits functional use (Fess et al., 2005; Melvin, 1982).

Synovitis

Synovitis, inflammation of the joint lining (synovium), occurs slowly in the patient with RA. There are biochemical and autoimmune responses that cause changes in the synovium (Swanson, 1995a). Inflammatory cells and enzymes attack the synovial lining of the joints, and the synovial tissues can eventually become fibrotic and form a scar tissue–like substance (pannus), which may invade tendons and ligaments (Fig. 17–2B). This process is progressive; continued swelling causes greater thickening of the synovium, capsular stretching, pain, and eventually destruction of the cartilage and bone (Fig. 17–2C) (Blank & Cassidy, 1996).

The synovitis associated with RA may be divided into three phases: acute, subacute, and chronic active (Melvin, 1982). Each phase has the same symptoms of pain, tenderness, warmth, and limited ROM. The disease is most active in the acute phase, which leads to joint destruction. The symptoms begin to subside as the subacute phase is entered. The disease may be considered to be in the chronic

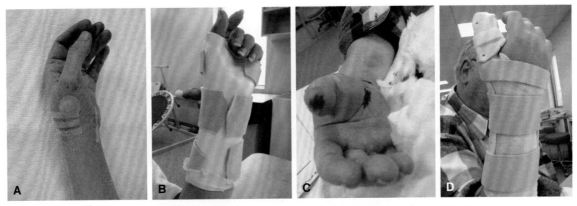

FIGURE 17–25 A, A first CMC joint arthroplasty with MP joint fusion. **B,** Thumb/wrist immobilization orthosis. **C and D,** A patient that underwent a thumb IP fusion and CTR. Postoperatively, the patient was placed in a thumb/wrist mobilization orthosis with a "clamshell" dorsal component.

active phase if the symptoms persist over a long period of time. The course of the disease varies and is unique to each patient; not all progress through these phases (Melvin, 1982; Swanson, 1995a).

Tenosynovitis

Tenosynovitis is an inflammation of the synovial lining of the tendon sheaths. In patients with RA, tenosynovitis usually occurs at the level of the flexor tendons, as they traverse at the level of the wrist (under the flexor retinaculum), and at the dorsum of the wrist, deep to the extensor retinaculum, the only site of extensor synovial lining (Leslie, 1999; Wilson & Fredick, 1994). These tunnels are lined with the same synovial fluid that surrounds the joints. If left untreated, the lining becomes thickened, and plaques and nodules may form, disrupting normal tendon excursion (Alter, Feldon, & Terrono, 2011; Leslie, 1999).

Tenosynovitis in a *digit* usually appears as a sausage-type swelling in which the entire digit may be enlarged and tender to palpation. Digital flexion can be significantly impaired by even a small amount of tenosynovitis (Leslie, 1999). Pain, mild triggering, and/or crepitation may be noted with attempted ROM (Ferlic, 1996; Melvin, 1982; Valdes, 2012).

Tenosynovitis in the *volar wrist* can present with median nerve irritation or carpal tunnel syndrome. The group of thickened, enlarged flexor tendons within the carpal canal secondarily place pressure on the median nerve as it passes through the shared carpal tunnel (Ferlic, 1996; Leslie, 1999).

Tenosynovitis in the *dorsal wrist* is quite evident by swelling, which can occur in one or all six dorsal compartments. Dorsal tenosynovitis can be distinguished from dorsal wrist synovitis by observing movement of the distended tenosynovium with active digital flexion and extension (Leslie, 1999; Wilson & Fredick, 1994).

DeQuervain Tenosynovitis

DeQuervain tenosynovitis is inflammation of the extensor pollicis brevis (EPB) and the APL tendons within the first dorsal wrist compartment. Tenderness, thickening, and crepitation are often present over the radial styloid. Pain may radiate proximally and dorsally with active wrist radial/ulnar deviation (Kirkpatrick, & Lisser, 1995).

Stenosing Tenosynovitis

Stenosing tenosynovitis, also known as *trigger finger*, commonly occurs at the RF and/or MF but can also occur in the thumb and small finger. Stenosing tenosynovitis is the result of swelling and

thickening of the flexor tendon proximal to the A1 pulley, as well as is linked to a potential changes of the histology of the pulley itself (thick, inelastic) (Teo, Ng, & Wong, 2019; Ferlic, 1996; Kirkpatrick & Lisser, 1995; Valdes, 2012). As the tendon attempts to traverse through the pulley, it catches, holding the digit in a flexed position that has to be manually released or forcefully extended by the patient. Attempted movement and direct palpation over the A1 pulley can be painful. Oftentimes, the patient will complain of simultaneous dorsal PIP joint pain. This is at least in part due to the extensor mechanism working to overcome the resistance from the "stuck" flexor tendon. Custom orthosis intervention (MCP or PIP based) has been shown effective in the early management of stenosing tenosynovitis (<6 months), with reports of the subjective reduction of pain and objective increase in functional use (Teo et al., 2019; Valdes, 2012).

Tendon Ruptures and Repairs

Tendon ruptures can occur when tendons are invaded by inflamed synovium or when tendons rub on a rough edge of a bone, an attritional rupture (Alter et al., 2011; Leslie, 1999). These rough edges or bony spurs are most likely the result of joint inflammation that has led to joint damage (Fig. 17–26A–E) (Ferlic, 1996; Shapiro, 1996; Swanson, 1995b; Wilson & Fredick, 1994). Tendon ruptures in the hand occur most commonly at prominent bony sites, such as the scaphoid waist, the distal ulna, and Lister tubercle on the dorsal radius. As a result, most common ruptures are of the flexor pollicis longus (FPL), index FDP, the extensor digiti quinti (EDQ), and the extensor pollicis longus (EPL) tendons (Ferlic, 1996; Katz & Moore, 2000; Leslie, 1999; Shapiro, 1996; Swanson, 1995b; Wilson & Fredick, 1994). Extensor tendon ruptures are more common with RA.

PATHOMECHANICS OF DEFORMITIES IN RHEUMATOID ARTHRITIS

As mentioned earlier, RA is the most common connective tissue disorder. It is a systemic disease that produces a joint inflammation. This is as a result of immunologic response occurring from the synovial tissue. The pathogenesis in RA causes synovitis and the synovium produces a **pannus**; the growth of abnormal tissue within and between joints; infiltrates cartilage, tendon, and ligaments. This pannus eventually produces significant stress on the joint capsule causing it to attenuate and the cartilage and subchondral bone to erode. Subsequently, there is often ligamentous disruption that affects both tendon(s) gliding and eventually joint motion.

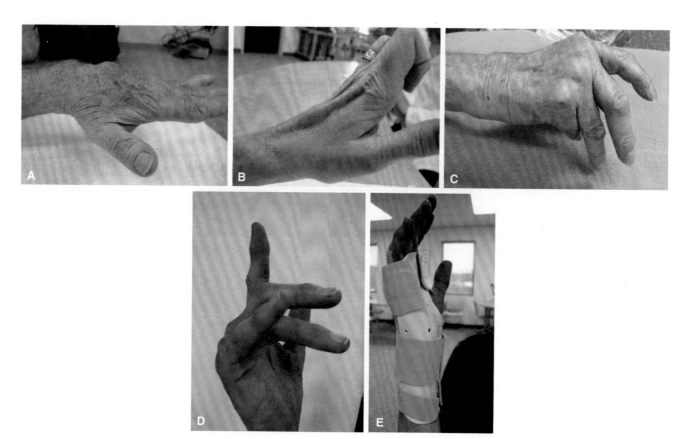

FIGURE 17–26 A, Dorsal synovitis. **B,** IF extensor digitorum communis (EDC) tenosynovitis. **C,** Rupture of the EDQ and EDC tendons of the RF and SF in a patient with RA. **D and E,** Rupture of MF and RF EDC tendons and orthosis management post surgery. Elastic therapeutic tape is used in conjunction with the orthosis to assist in maintaining MCP extension while allowing some active flexion.

Over time, with use of the hand and/or wrist, abnormal stressors continue to produce a significant load on tendons and other tendon-supporting structures. Because of instability and derangement of the joint-tendon relationship, patients often have pain. Alteration of joint motion, along with the abnormal tendinous pull, often produces crepitus associated with swelling and pain. The hand pathomechanics in RA is progressive in nature. Pathogenesis of deformities of the wrist and hand is divided into four stages; see Table 17–2 for the typical characteristics of each of the stages.

The entire upper extremity is a kinematic chain supported and/or stabilized by various ligaments and joint capsules and is controlled by the musculotendinous units. The degree and amplitude of joint motion are dependent on the precise functioning of the neuromuscular structures. The articulation of various joints may depend on the skeletal configuration and is either classified as stable or inherently unstable. Once the ligamentous and capsular stability is lost, along with tenosynovitis due to the disease process, sequential disturbance in the affected joint(s) follows. The distal joint position is a consequence of the altered musculotendinous vectors, causing progression of the deformities (Fig. 17–27A,B). In addition, an abnormal compressive load placed on the joints, due to the aforementioned factors, also contributes to joint degenerative changes. For instance, looking at the various stages of pathogenesis of RA deformities, derangement occurring at the radioulnar joint subsequently will produce changes at the wrist followed by changes at the digital levels. Imbalance occurring at the digital level thus will produce changes at the proximal joints.

Therefore, it is critical to assess *both* the rheumatoid wrist and hand together when applying an orthosis because altered mechanics at the proximal level will affect the distal levels and vice versa.

NONSURGICAL ORTHOTIC MANAGEMENT GUIDELINES

A combination of rest (with an immobilization orthosis) and medical management can aid in reducing the symptoms of RA (Fig. 17–28A,B). The therapist should teach the patient adaptations to ADLs and other techniques for joint protection and energy conservation as this can aid the patient with coping with arthritis on a daily basis (Colditz, 2000; Fess et al., 2005; Massarotti, 1996; Poole & Pellegrini, 2000; Simmons et al., 1996; Terrono, Nalebuff, & Philips, 1995).

Physicians should be encouraged to refer patients early for therapeutic interventions including patient education, joint protection, orthoses, pain management techniques, and an exercise regime. Although orthosis application is a treatment component, it is rarely used alone. Other interventions should be integrated into the treatment plan. Thermal agents can be useful adjuncts in preparing the joints for exercise and reducing pain (e.g., paraffin, hot packs, and ultrasound) (Katz & Moore, 2000). A well-instructed home exercise program can aid in maintaining joint flexibility and daily function. When implemented early after diagnosis, orthoses can provide support to weak structures around a joint, reduce stress to the joint capsule, decrease pain during use, and perhaps slow soft-tissue damage (Blank & Cassidy, 1996; Jacobs, 2003).

Material Selection

Thermoplastics

The need for and type of orthosis may change as the disease process evolves. The therapist must use his or her knowledge of the disease process, biomechanics, hands-on skills, and experience to create

TABLE 17-2	**Stages of Rheumatoid Arthritis**
Stage I	Synovitis of the joints and tendons, pain and swelling, impaired tendon gliding associated with crepitus, and no obvious deformity.
Stage II	Synovitis of the joint and tendon continues; with use, the wrist and hand joints may demonstrate a tendency for subluxation and/or dislocation because of joint laxity. The deformity is apparent at the joints; however, it is passively correctable.
Stage III	Deformities become fixed. The joints may demonstrate minimal or no joint destruction.
Stage IV	Evidence of joint destruction and presence of soft-tissue disturbance associated with multiple wrist and hand deformities.

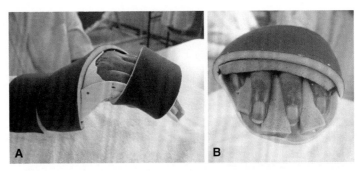

FIGURE 17–28 **A,** Soft straps aid in proper anatomical positioning of the digits into the orthosis. **B,** Digit dividers are added by using high-density foam wedges to align and separate digits.

the most appropriate orthosis and orthosis regime. For example, a wrist/hand immobilization orthosis (resting hand orthosis) may be ordered for a patient, but lifestyle and daily demands may require at least some use of the hand and may not be feasible for the patient to use. An option may be to fabricate a wrist immobilization orthosis for day use (digits and thumb free) and a wrist/hand immobilization orthosis for night use (Simmons et al., 1996). Before fabrication, consideration must be given to the acuteness of the disease, material choice for skin type, wearing schedules, patient's lifestyle, and ability to don and doff the orthosis independently.

The choice of orthotic material should take into account conformability and weight. Orthoses should be lightweight and allow for fluctuating edema and synovitis whenever possible. Materials that are highly conforming (minimal resistance to stretch, such as plastic-based material) may not be the best choice if joint swelling fluctuates or if frequent adjustments are anticipated to accommodate joint and soft-tissue changes. Materials that are more rigid (high resistance to stretch, such as a rubber-based material) tend not

to fit as intimately to the contours of the body part and may be a better choice for this patient population (Austin, 2003). These materials provide joint support, are more forgiving than highly conforming materials, and may better accommodate fluctuations in edema.

During the orthotic planning process, a clinician must take into account the likelihood of the patient having variability of edema/synovitis and then account for this as they are fabricating the orthosis. Several options include (1) layering cotton stockinette, (2) using elastic wrap over the intended body segment, (3) choosing a material with flexibility such as a 3/32″ highly perforated material, and/or (4) incorporating a softer material into the design such as a neoprene and thermoplastic combination (Fig. 17–29A,B).

The therapist must also keep in mind that an orthosis worn for a specific problem may aggravate a proximal or distal condition. For example, a wrist immobilization orthosis may work well to stabilize the wrist, but during functional use, altered patterns of movement or potential transfer of forces proximally to the elbow may irritate existing elbow inflammation or distally increasing forces to the MCP joints.

Strapping

The strapping design of the orthosis should allow for easy independent donning and doffing. Straps should be wide, soft, and conforming as patients with RA often have thin, fragile skin owing to their age, medications, or the disease process itself. Straps can be fabricated to allow extra length or loops on the end of the strap for easy application and removal (Fig. 17–30A,B).

Soft strapping material can also be used as digit dividers on wrist/hand immobilization orthoses. These dividers can aid in alignment

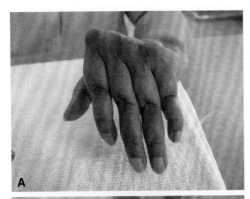

FIGURE 17–27 **A and B,** A patient with severe RA of the wrist and digits; note the ulnar deviation, MCP subluxation, and swan-neck deformities.

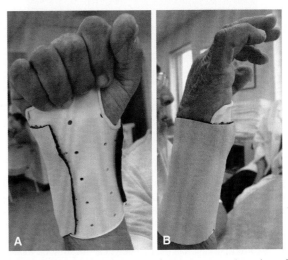

FIGURE 17–29 **A and B,** A custom-cut wide neoprene strap/wrap is used to compliment this wrist orthosis. This wide 1/8″ thick neoprene material provides an even dorsal pressure distribution as well as warmth to the underlying tissue.

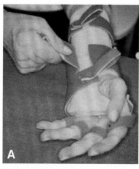
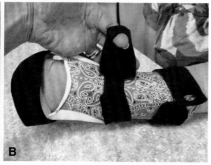

FIGURE 17–30 **A,** A patient with severe RA of the wrist and digits uses a custom-made strapping system to don and doff this orthosis by combining soft strap closures with loop attachments. **B,** A small hole is made in this neoprene strap to ease application for this patient. The neoprene material will not fray and will hold up to repeated stress.

and prevent maceration between the digits (Fig. 17–31A). Care should be taken to place straps advantageously. They can be used as an aid in gently redirecting joints into an antideformity position (Fig. 17–31B), straps can successfully provide light joint positioning (Fig. 17–32A–C).

Prefabricated Orthoses

As previously mentioned in this chapter, commercially purchased neoprene orthoses can often work well to provide intermittent light

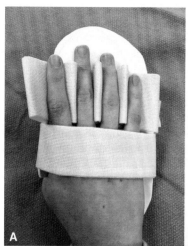
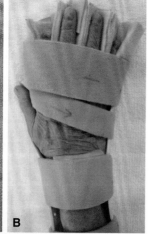
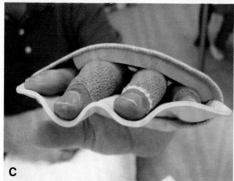

FIGURE 17–31 **A,** Soft straps are used for "finger separator" liner as well as light and comfortable support to this orthosis. The soft strapping used here has adhesive backed hook between the layers to keep the finger separators in place. **B,** Adhesive-backed foam padding is placed judiciously between digits. This technique can be extremely effective in gently directing individual joints to a more anatomically correct position, and this can prevent undue stress on vulnerable joints. **C,** The thermoplastic material was molded to incorporate "gulley's" for the digits to rest in. Incorporating digits troughs while the thermoplastic material is setting can be challenging but well worth the results.

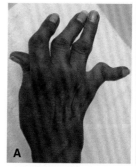
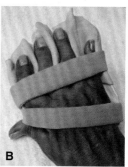

FIGURE 17–32 **A,** A patient with psoriatic arthritis. **B,** A night-resting orthosis with soft straps strategically placed to help improve joint alignment and prevent joint contracture.

support to joints during times of symptom exacerbation (Fig. 17–7). For some patients, these orthoses are easy to apply and care for. Chapter 9 reviews these options in more detail.

Surgical Orthotic Management Guideline

Postsurgical management with the use of orthotics follows similar indications as reviewed above with the OA population. Postsurgical patients should be instructed in digital motion to decrease the chance of adhesions and maximize motion. Gentle, early ROM, and blocking exercises aid in optimizing tendon excursion and reducing intrinsic tightness. The therapist needs to have an understanding of the pathomechanics of the disease in being able to effectively treat postoperative cases and with preventing potentially secondary complications given preoperative tissue imbalances.

ELBOW WITH RHEUMATOID ARTHRITIS

RA in the elbow can manifest itself similarly as it does in other joints (Bernstein et al., 2010). Elbow involvement in the patient with RA can be noted as joint synovitis and, occasionally, the presence of subcutaneous nodules at the posterior aspect of the elbow joint (Fig. 17–33). Chronic synovitis can lead to elbow flexion and extension contractures as well as limitations in forearm rotation. These contractures tend to result from reduced motion secondary to joint pain and patient guarding. Ulnar nerve irritation may occur owing to tension on the nerve resulting from local trauma, static posturing, joint inflammation, osteophyte formation, or pressure from a subcutaneous nodule (McAuliffe & Miller, 2000). As with other joints in RA, disease-modifying medications have made a substantial change in managing the disease and its progression.

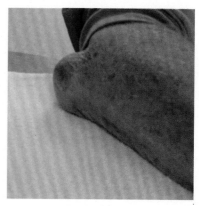

FIGURE 17–33 Subcutaneous rheumatoid nodules are often seen about the posterior elbow of a patient with RA.

Should pain and joint destruction continue, surgical options such as **synovectomy** and **arthroplasty** are recommended with this population (Stanley, 2011).

NONSURGICAL ORTHOTIC MANAGEMENT GUIDELINES OF THE ELBOW

Conservative management of the painful rheumatoid elbow typically consists of anti-inflammatory or disease-modifying antirheumatoid medications, referral to physical/occupational therapy, activity modifications, and orthotic management (Bernstein et al., 2010; McAuliffe, & Miller, 2000; Nirschl & Morrey, 1993). Orthoses at the elbow joint should be used cautiously due to the high risk of joint contracture (Morrey, 2000b). Soft devices can be used as an option in the early stages of the disease to provide protection and support to the painful elbow. Commercially available or custom-fabricated elbow sleeves or protectors can limit full range of elbow flexion and extension and protect tender nodules or skin ulcerations (Fig. 17–34). A custom-made donut design fabricated from foam padding, silicone gel sheeting, neoprene, or a combination of these can absorb shock, protect a painful nodule/bursa, cushion the ulnar nerve, or decrease pressure about painful tissue (Fig. 17–35A–C). Neoprene orthoses produce gentle soft-tissue compression and have the added benefit of neutral warmth and insulation (see Chapter 14) (McAuliffe, & Miller, 2000).

When greater support is needed, an anterior or posterior orthosis can be applied. An anterior elbow immobilization orthosis is recommended if nodules are present on the posterior elbow; it can be used at night as it allows the arm to relax on the bed or pillow rather than against hard material (Figs. 17–23 and 17–36) (McAuliffe, & Miller, 2000). The anterior design may be less complicated to fit as there are fewer bony prominences and less potential for developing pressure areas. Figure 17–36C shows an anterior design with the wrist included, and Figure 17–36E shows a posterior design with the same desired effect, both to reduce distal migration. The anterior approach also allows for gravity-assisted application with precise conformability.

When posterior orthoses are used, the wrist should be considered in the design. Patients with elbow arthritis may be more comfortable with the wrist included in the orthosis to control forearm rotation and excess motion. Posterior orthoses should be cautiously molded and, if necessary, well-padded about the condyles, ulnar styloid, and the olecranon process (Austin, 2003).

Contractures of the elbow can cause devastating limitations in all ADLs, leisure, and vocational pursuits. The development of an elbow flexion contracture is a common sequela following elbow trauma as well as postsurgically. With early intervention, contractures can be managed with gentle serial static or static progressive mobilization via an orthosis in the desired direction of correction.

POSTSURGICAL ORTHOTIC MANAGEMENT GUIDELINES OF THE ELBOW

An elbow joint synovectomy can be performed to alleviate pain and increase functional joint ROM in the early stages of the disease, with or without a radial head resection (Varitimidis, Plakseychuk, & Sotereanos, 1999). Orthosis application following synovectomy is based on surgeon preference and is used with caution. If the surgery was relatively simple and less invasive due to mild synovitis, the patient can use a sling and remove frequently for active ROM. If more extensive dissection is undertaken, the forearm is often positioned in neutral rotation with the elbow comfortably positioned at approximately 90° of flexion within an orthosis. The orthosis is typically worn for 2 to 4 weeks postoperatively, removing frequently for ROM.

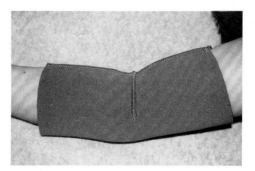

FIGURE 17–34 Custom-made or prefabricated protection about the elbow.

Elbow joint arthroplasty is reserved for the severely involved joint. Pain, joint instability, ulnar nerve involvement, and the inability to perform simple ADLs may lead a patient to this decision. Several procedures have been described (Bryan & Morrey, 1982; Ferlic, 1999; Gill & Morrey, 1998; Morrey, 2000a; Wright, Froimson, & Stewart, 1993). Regardless of the procedure, early orthosis application and postoperative therapy play significant roles in achieving maximal results (Ferlic, 1999; Gill & Morrey, 1998; Melvin, 1982; Morrey, 2000b; Nirschl & Morrey, 1993; Wolf, 2000). Following the arthroplasty, elbow immobilization or restriction orthoses are used cautiously and in combination with a carefully guided exercise and edema management regime (Brach, 1999; Edmond, 1993; Wolf, 2000). The position of the elbow is dependent upon the procedure(s) performed. The capsule of the elbow is at its greatest capacity at approximately 80° of flexion (Johansson, 1962).

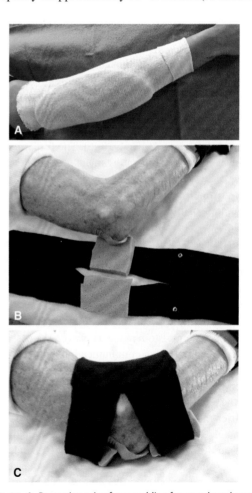

FIGURE 17–35 **A,** Protection using foam padding for a tender subcutaneous nodule is secured with an elasticized sleeve. **B and C,** This patient with a right elbow ulceration from advanced scleroderma receives comfort with this custom-made orthosis from neoprene and Tee foam padding. The orthosis allows her to rest her elbow without direct pressure on tender, sore tissues.

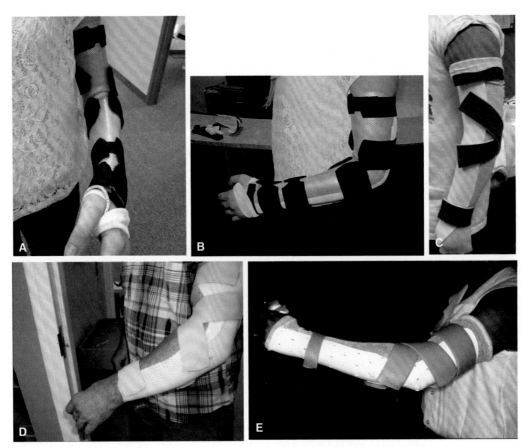

FIGURE 17–36 A, An anterior elbow extension immobilization orthosis. **B,** A wide or a crisscross designed strap at the anterior elbow crease may help enhance fit of this posterior elbow immobilization orthosis. **C,** Anterior elbow design with the wrist included. **D,** Posterior elbow orthosis with 2″ wide straps aid in securing the orthosis within the elbow. **E,** Posterior elbow design with the wrist included.

Therefore, positioning the elbow in approximately 80° to 90° of flexion reduces pressure within the joint, making this position quite comfortable for the patient. The position of the forearm within the orthoses will depend on whether or not ligamentous reconstruction was performed (Szekeres, & King, 2006). The forearm is placed in supination if the medial collateral ligament was repaired, pronation if the lateral collateral ligamentous complex was repaired, and in neutral if both were repaired in surgery (Szekeres, & King, 2006). Furthermore, the position of the elbow will depend on the status of the triceps tendon. For example, if the surgical approach involved the triceps being detached and repaired, the elbow may be positioned in some degree of extension, the angle of which is based on the tension of the repair assessed intraoperatively, strength of repair, and surgeon preference (Fig. 17–37).

The anterior or posterior elbow resting orthosis should be removed four to eight times a day for ROM exercises. The orthosis can be prefabricated or custom made. However, the precise exercise regime is dependent on close communication between the surgeon and therapist, type of arthroplasty, surgical procedure, condition of the ulnar nerve, triceps status, collateral ligament status, and overall stability of the elbow joint. The prolonged use of an immobilization orthosis carries the risk of joint contractures, as previously emphasized (Edmond, 1993; Wolf, 2000). Circumferentially wrapping the orthosis on the arm (e.g., using an elasticized bandage) instead of using straps may aid in postoperative edema management and prevent orthosis migration as the edema subsides. Orthotic fabrication over the olecranon, medial and lateral epicondyles, and the bony grooves of the cubital tunnel require particular care as these bony prominences are prone to irritation from direct pressure (Fig. 17–38). A hinged orthosis (mobilization or restriction) may

be prescribed versus an immobilization orthosis following elbow arthroplasty. This will allow for a precise controlled arc of motion in flexion and extension and can facilitate joint and tendon glide, increase blood flow and nutrition to the repair site, and aid in preventing joint stiffness while healing (Fig. 17–39). However, hinge orthoses at the elbow can be difficult to fit comfortably. There are few contours about the elbow that contribute to a congruent fit. Obtaining a secure mechanical hold of the orthosis in the proper position (axis of the elbow hinge lined up with the elbow's joint axis) may warrant fabrication of some type of shoulder harness to prevent migration as the forearm moves.

Orthotic interventions that apply a mobilization force in the latter healing stages can elongate soft tissue in the event that a joint flexion or extension contracture has developed (Fig. 17–40). These orthoses can be custom fabricated or purchased/rented commercially. This form of orthotic intervention is not used until at least 6 to 8 weeks postoperatively and is only used if the patient is not making adequate gains in ROM with his or her prescribed exercise program (Szekeres, & King, 2006). The rationale behind this form of orthotic intervention is based on **low-load prolonged stress (LLPS)** to mobilize a stiff joint (Flowers & LaStayo, 2012; Hepburn, 1987; Light, Nuzik, Personius, & Barstrom, 1984) (refer to Chapter 15, for further details). These mobilization orthoses are used to apply LLPS to the stiff elbow through the mobilization device maintaining the joint at the end of available ROM for a long period resulting in the tissue adaptively changing to the stress applied. It is critical to ensure that minimal lateral force is being applied in order to protect the collateral ligaments of the elbow joint and are generally applied with the forearm in a neutral rotation (McAuliffe, & Miller, 2000; Morrey, 2000a, 2000b).

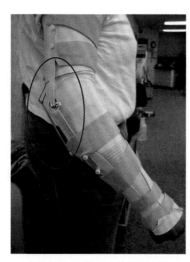

FIGURE 17–37 This patient had a custom elbow flexion restriction orthosis (Phoenix elbow hinge, Performance Health) with the forearm in neutral. Note the "dynamic" extension assists to aid in triceps extension and the flexion block positioned on the center of the hinge. As the surgeon's protocol allows, the flexion arc can be increased by moving the block counterclockwise.

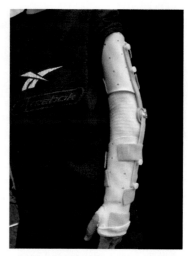

FIGURE 17–39 This Phoenix elbow-hinged orthosis (Performance Health) is used after elbow reconstruction on this young boy with juvenile RA. The orthosis restricts elbow AROM and prevents lateral stress.

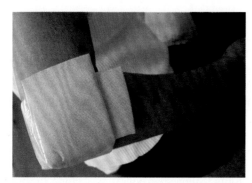

FIGURE 17–38 Prepadding the condyles and/or posterior elbow may aid in decreasing direct pressure over bony prominences while custom molding.

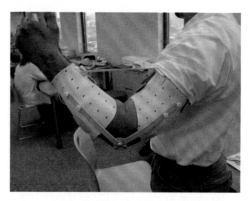

FIGURE 17–40 At 12 weeks after elbow arthroplasty, this patient was unable to gain functional elbow flexion. Thus, a "dynamic" elbow flexion mobilization orthosis with a Phoenix elbow hinge (Performance Health) was prescribed. Note the D-rings proximally that are used to secure the rubber band traction and the home-made distal hook for the terminal attachment. Including the wrist in this design could be an option to assist with forearm rotation.

WRIST WITH RHEUMATOID ARTHRITIS

Wrist and hand deformities caused by RA are often the first joints affected within the upper extremity (Colville, Nicholson, & Belcher, 1999; Melvin, 1982; Swanson, 1995a, 1995b; Vamos, White, & Caughey, 1990; Wilson & Fredick, 1994). Deformity results from a combination of ligamentous laxity and the location of the synovitis.

The patient with acute RA presents with diffusely swollen and red appearance of the involved joints (Fess et al., 2005). Any attempt to move the wrist or fingers may be exquisitely painful. On palpation, the wrist and hand may be warm, owing to a combination of joint and tendon inflammation. Rest (orthosis) is one of the first treatment choices that may be prescribed (Blank & Cassidy, 1996; Fess et al., 2005; Kozin, 1999; Melvin, 1982; Stirrat, 1996).

The wrist is a complex joint with multiple ligamentous connections on both the volar and dorsal surfaces. Many combinations of deformities may occur, depending on the location of the inflammation and the ligaments affected. The three most common patterns of deformity are subluxation of the distal radioulnar joint, volar subluxation/supination of the carpus at the radiocarpal joint, and radial deviation of the wrist (Feinberg, 1999; Michlovitz, 1999; Rizio, & Belsky, 1995; Shapiro, 1996; Swanson, 1995b; Talesnick, 1989; van Vugt et al., 1999; Wilson, 1986; Wilson & Fredick, 1994).

The triangular fibrocartilage complex (TFCC) stabilizes the distal radioulnar joint. If synovitis invades the TFCC, it can weaken and damage the supportive ligaments. As a result, the radius subluxates volarly, making the ulnar head appear more prominent dorsally. This is typically termed **caput ulnae syndrome** (Shapiro, 1996; Swanson, 1995b). This deformity may be appreciated radiographically or on clinical examination with palpation and observation of the prominent distal ulna, particularly with the forearm in pronation. The patient is likely to present with pain during active forearm rotation and wrist range of motion.

Synovitis in the radiocarpal joint also weakens its surrounding ligamentous structures. There is often attenuation and laxity of the radioscapholunate and radiocapitate ligaments volarly, as well as radiocarpal and intercarpal ligaments dorsally. This laxity, in combination with the natural volar inclination of the radius, may facilitate volar carpal subluxation. The moment arm of the extensor carpi ulnaris (ECU) tendon shifts from extension to flexion. Volar subluxation can contribute to carpal supination, ulnar translocation of the carpus, and ulnar deviation of the metacarpals; all of these changes can decrease support to wrist extension and decrease effectiveness of the digital extensor tendons (Fig. 17–41) (Shapiro, 1996; Swanson, 1995b; Wilson & Fredick, 1994).

Disturbance of radioulnar alignment subsequently produces instability of the radiocarpal joint and progressively the proximal carpal row and midcarpal instability. This instability occurring at

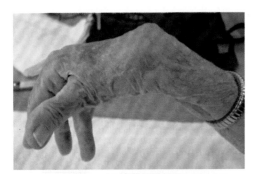

FIGURE 17–41 Synovitis in the radiocarpal joint weakens the surrounding ligamentous structures.

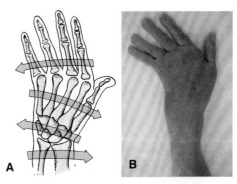

FIGURE 17–43 A and B, Typical deforming forces: The wrist deviates radially, the carpal bones deviate ulnarly, the metacarpals deviate radially, and the proximal phalanges deviate ulnarly and often sublux volarly as well.

the wrist joint eventually leads to the deforming forces produced by the digital flexors and extensors affecting both the MCP and IP joints. Altered orientation of the flexors and extensor tendons at the level of the wrist as well as at the MCP joints causes failure of the sagittal bands dorsally and the fibro-osseous sheath volarly, further contributing to the ulnarly directed forces at the MCP joints (Fig. 17–42). The extensor tendons fall in the ulnar valley between the MCP joints when the weaker radial sagittal bands fail, causing an extensor lag at the MCP joints. This contributes to various secondary deformities at the distal joints, including a secondary swan-neck deformity. An alteration in radioulnar, radiocarpal, and midcarpal kinematics increases the gliding resistance (friction) to the extensor tendons in conjunction with bony degeneration and leads to potential tendon ruptures.

Radial deviation of the wrist is mainly caused by an ulnar translocation of the carpus with ulnar shift of the metacarpals. This shifting of the carpal bones can contribute secondarily to ulnar deviation of the digits, commonly referred to as **zigzag deformity**. In the normal resting hand, the wrist is positioned in about 10° of ulnar deviation, causing the radius to align with the IF (Leslie, 1999; Swanson, 1995b). In the zigzag deformity, the body seems to attempt to recreate this balance (Fig. 17–43A–B).

NONSURGICAL ORTHOTIC MANAGEMENT GUIDELINES FOR THE WRIST

Orthosis options for RA of the wrist are similar even when the pathology is different. A wrist immobilization orthosis is often the treatment of choice for the patient with wrist inflammation (Blank,

& Cassidy, 1996; Fess et al., 2005; Kozin, 1999; Melvin, 1982; Stirrat, 1996). A lightweight, rubber-based material may be a good option for these immobilization orthoses. To avoid increased pressure on the median nerve, the suggested wrist position is neutral to 10° of extension if the deformity allows (Fig. 17–44A,B) (Melvin, 1982).

Rigid orthoses that immobilize the wrist and hand may be initially recommended for night use as full-time wear can greatly limit any function of the hand(s) (Leonard, 1995). It is important to incorporate volar support within the orthosis at the distal ulna and MCP joints (Philips, 1995). This support helps protect against carpal and MCP joint subluxation and MCP joint ulnar deviation. A wrist/hand/thumb immobilization (resting hand) orthosis can provide this position for night use (Fig. 17–45). This design is selected as it positions the thumb comfortably between midpalmar and radial abduction while supporting the wrist and digits. Suggested positions include the wrist at neutral to 10° extension, MCP joints at 25° to 30° of flexion, and IP joints in slight, relaxed flexion (Fess et al., 2005; Melvin,

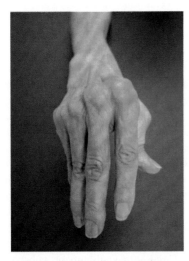

FIGURE 17–42 Note the ulnarly oriented extensor digitorum communis (EDC) of the MF and RF over the MCP joints. This in turn will influence ulnar migration of the digits and volar subluxation of the proximal phalanges.

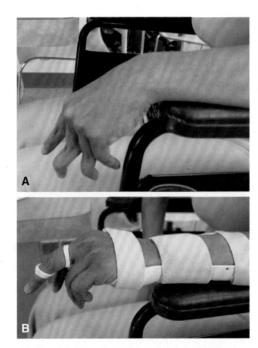

FIGURE 17–44 A and B, Note the position of the distal digits once an orthosis has been applied to stabilize the wrist. The middle digit had a long-standing swan-neck deformity that was not corrected with wrist positioning; therefore, a simple, functional PIP extension restriction orthosis was fabricated.

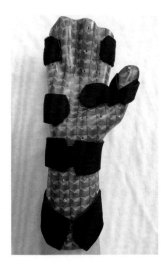

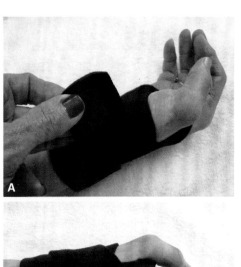

FIGURE 17–45 A (mitten design) wrist/hand/thumb immobilization orthosis is generally worn at night to provide volar support to the wrist and MCP joints to properly align inflamed structures. Note the use of a plastic-based thermoplastic material that has excellent comfortability about the volar aspect of the digits.

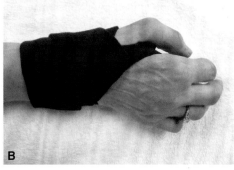

FIGURE 17–46 A and B, Custom neoprene orthoses, such as this wrist wrap design, can be considered as an alternative to hard thermoplastic materials.

1982). The MCP joints should be in no more than 30° of flexion as any greater flexion could force the joints into a position of deformity: volar subluxation of the MCP joints and strained IP joint extension (Philips, 1995; Shapiro, 1996; Wilson & Fredick, 1994). Positioning the IP joints in full extension with the MCP joints flexed may contribute to intrinsic muscle spasm, tightness, and IP stiffness, which is difficult to overcome and can contribute to further deformity.

RA is often bilateral and symmetrical, requiring the patient to wear immobilization orthoses for both hands. Without assistance at home, it can be challenging to don or doff bilateral orthoses. Consider alternating the use of right and left orthosis each night. Wearing schedules depend on the presenting condition. If only wrist synovitis is present, the wrist orthosis may be worn as necessary. However, patients often present with coexisting MCP joint synovitis, therefore immobilizing the wrist alone could place increased stress on the MCP joints with functional use of the hand (Melvin, 1982; Philips, 1995). If MCP pain and/or swelling become an issue, consideration should be given to alternating the orthosis regime (wrist orthosis for functional day use, wrist/hand orthosis for night).

Prefabricated wrist orthoses with a removable metal stay can be an option for daytime activities that contribute to wrist pain (Leonard, 1995; Murphy, 1996; Pagnotta et al., 1998; Stern et al., 1997; Stern et al., 1996b; Tijhuis et al., 1998; Veehof, Taal, Heijnsdijk-Rouwenhorst, & Van de Laar, 2008). The metal stay can be removed, allowing a small amount of wrist motion when necessary, which may decrease the forces placed on the MCP joints. Neoprene wrist orthoses may also help provide a light support while allowing some degree of motion. Neoprene may provide some pain relief owing to its neutral warmth properties. Careful fitting of soft prefabricated orthoses is paramount. Not all of these orthoses designs fit well given the often encountered alteration in bony anatomy and size of the forearm in relationship to the wrist (Leonard, 1995). A neoprene orthosis can be custom fabricated to accommodate bony changes (Fig. 17–46A,B). Thermoplastic materials can be added to neoprene as a hybrid to provide additional reinforcement and support (see Chapter 14). Refer to additional information on orthoses for wrist RA in Box 17–2

 EXPERT PEARL 17–10

Night Resting Orthosis
NANCY BEAMAN, OTR/L, CHT
Massachusetts

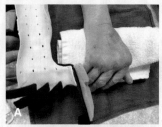

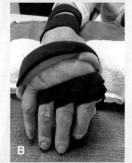

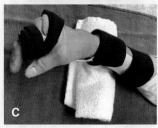

Custom strapping to reduce ulnar deviation—notice strategically placed slits in volar orthosis for optimal angle of pull. Foam beneath distal strap helps to position MCPs in extension, IP joints free for motion.

BOX 17–2 EVIDENCE-INFORMED ORTHOTIC MANAGEMENT: RHEUMATOID WRIST

Wrist orthoses are mainly prescribed for pain reduction in persons who suffer from RA. Prefabricated, off-the-shelf–type wrist orthoses have been found to be effective in reducing wrist pain (Kjeken, Møller, & Kvien, 1995; Nordenskiold, 1990; Pagnotta et al., 1998; Pagnotta, Mazer, Baron, & Wood-Dauphinee, 2005; Veehof et al., 2008). With regard to improvement in grip strength, the literature is conflicting because some studies found an improvement, whereas others found no effect or a reduction in grip strength (Anderson & Maas, 1987; Kjeken et al., 1995; Nordenskiold, 1990; Stern et al., 1996). These findings suggest that off-the-shelf orthoses may provide a positive reduction in pain relief, which may enhance overall function with their use. Precise dosage or wearing regimes have not been determined.

Wrist/hand immobilization orthoses are one of the most widely used orthosis applications in persons who suffer from RA. These orthoses are generally worn at night to provide volar support to the wrist and MCP joints and aid in proper aligning of inflamed structures. These are prescribed to both newly diagnosed as well as for persons who suffer chronic RA. To date, studies indicate that hand immobilization orthoses provide no beneficial effect in improving hand function in patients with early RA. Thus, current evidence to support immobilization orthoses is lacking (Adams, Burridge, Mullee, Hammond, & Cooper, 2008; Egan et al., 2003; Steultjens et al., 2004; Steultjens, Dekker, Bouter, Leemrijse, & van den Ende, 2005). Clinicians have been providing these orthoses for decades based on expert opinion. RA is a chronic, systemic, autoimmune disorder that orthosis application likely has some effect on in delaying the progression of hand deformity, pain, and dysfunction. However, orthoses in conjunction with patient education and pharmacologic management may assist with short-term pain relief, especially in the event of a flare. This is based on expert opinion; orthosis application remains a rational biomechanical form of treatment that likely has a positive effect on the mechanics of joint motion and musculoskeletal function.

POSTSURGICAL ORTHOTIC MANAGEMENT GUIDELINES FOR THE WRIST

There are numerous surgical procedures that have been described for managing pain, increasing stability, improving functional use, and minimizing deformity of the wrist with RA (Wolf et al., 2019; Blank & Cassidy, 1996; Colville et al., 1999; Linscheid, 2000; Nalebuff, 1990; Shapiro, 1996; Stirrat, 1996; Talesnick, 1989; Terrono et al., 2011; van Vugt et al., 1999; Watson & Ballet, 1984; Watson et al., 1999; Wilson, 1986). Relevant surgical procedures include synovectomy, tenosynovectomy, tendon repair or transfer, arthroplasty, and arthrodesis (Shapiro, 1996).

Synovectomy or Tenosynovectomy

Wrist synovectomy (surgical removal of damaged synovium) or **tenosynovectomy** (surgical excision of the tendon sheath) is designed to decrease pain, increase function, prevent tendon rupture, and improve appearance. Synovectomy is not usually performed when there is advanced bony erosion, subluxation of the carpus, ruptured tendons, or flexion contractures (Wilson & Fredick, 1994). Orthoses are used to position the wrist joint after the postoperative dressing is removed. If tenosynovectomy has been performed in combination with wrist synovectomy, the orthotic protocol should protect the tendons as well (Fig. 17–47A,B). Carefully instructed exercise sessions are essential for preventing tendon adherence postoperatively. The following are suggested positioning guidelines; however, the referring surgeon should recommend the positions of the involved joints (Fess et al., 2005; Leonard, 1995; Melvin, 1982; Philips, 1995).

- Wrist synovectomy: wrist positioned in neutral.
- Dorsal wrist tenosynovectomy: wrist positioned in some extension with the MCP joints in 35° to 40° of flexion.
- Volar wrist tenosynovectomy: wrist positioned in neutral to 25° extension.
- Digital flexor tenosynovectomy: If wrist is included, wrist positioned in approximately 20° of extension, and MCPs in 30° flexion. For a hand-based orthosis, MCPs blocked at approximately 30° of flexion.

EXPERT PEARL 17–11

Strap Customization
SABRINA CASSELLA, M.ED, OTR/L, CHT
Massachusetts

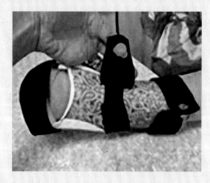

Finger loop slit for ease of don/doff of orthosis for patients with limited hand mobility. Be mindful to orient straps to make patient's angle of pull optimal.

Tendon Ruptures and Tendon Repairs

The cause of **tendon rupture** in patients with RA is relatively common in the hand and wrist. Tendon ruptures are typically attritional, as the tendon becomes abraded by roughened bone or osteophyte as the tendon crosses over and rubs during active motion and normal daily use (Ferlic, 1996; Leslie, 1999; Michlovitz, 1999; Shapiro, 1996; Wilson & Fredick, 1994). Furthermore, the destructive effects of chronic tenosynovitis may weaken the tendon, leading to eventual rupture. The common sites for tendon ruptures include the following:

- The tendons of the fourth, fifth, and occasionally sixth dorsal extensor compartment: extensor digitorum communis (EDC) and extensor digiti minimi (EDM). This is often referred to as **caput ulnae** or **Vaughan-Jackson syndrome** (Vaughan-Jackson, 1948).

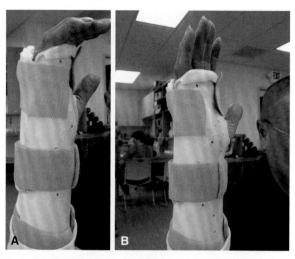

FIGURE 17–47 A and B, This orthosis supports the wrist and MCP joints in comfortable extension post extensor tenosynovectomy. It also places the tendons that were involved in the synovectomy in a stress-free, protected position. The patient can gently glide tendons per MD protocol.

- The FPL and FDP to the index and long fingers may be abraded by a spur formed at the level of the scaphotrapezial joint. This is often referred to as **Mannerfelt syndrome** (Mannerfelt & Norman, 1969).

Refer to additional information on orthoses for tendon ruptures and tendon repairs in Box 17–2.

Tendon ruptures in patients with RA are rarely repaired primarily. Surgical reconstruction is typically through tendon transfers or grafts. Prior to undergoing tendon reconstruction, the status of the MCP joints and wrist must be assessed thoroughly via physical and radiographic examination. Any reconstructive wrist procedures should be carried out simultaneously with tendon reconstruction. Orthotic management guidelines for tendon repairs and tendon transfers are similar to those described in detail in Chapters 18, 19, and 21; however, due to the slower healing rates with this population, the postoperative rehabilitation program will likely need to be adjusted. The therapist must keep in mind the extent of surgical intervention and whether other procedures were done simultaneously, such as tenosynovectomy or arthroplasty (Fig. 17–48). Management of the tendon-repaired hand greatly depends on the extent of disease and surgical procedure; close communication with the referring surgeon is essential. Some physicians prefer complete cast immobilization for several weeks, whereas others prefer restrictive mobilization through a carefully guided orthosis program and therapy regime.

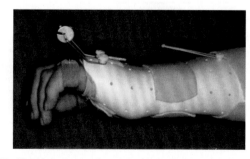

FIGURE 17–48 This patient underwent an SF MCP joint implant arthroplasty and carpal tunnel release (CTR). The MCP extension mobilization orthosis (Phoenix Single Finger Outrigger; Performance Health) positions the wrist appropriately for the CTR and supports the MCP joint arthroplasty, allowing gentle ROM via rubber band traction.

Arthroplasty

There are several indications for partial or total wrist arthroplasty: significant articular cartilage degeneration, pain, increasing difficulty with simple ADL tasks, and wrist deformity. The main goal is to preserve some painless wrist motion. After the postoperative dressing is removed, a wrist immobilization orthosis can be applied, including the MCP joints depending on physician protocol (Fig. 17–47). This orthosis can be removed for carefully guided exercises. AROM is generally initiated within 1 to 6 weeks postoperatively, depending on soft-tissue integrity, prosthetic fit and stability, and surgical preference (Anderson & Adams, 2005; Kozin, 1999; Michlovitz, 1999). The therapist's goal for total arc of motion in flexion and extension should be approximately 60° (Feinberg, 1999; Michlovitz, 1999).

Arthrodesis

A limited or total wrist arthrodesis sacrifices motion for stability, however, provides maximal function of the distal and proximal joints for the severely arthritic wrist (Hayden, & Jebson, 2005; Kozin, & Michlovitz, 2000). This procedure is typically reserved for patients with exquisite wrist pain, tendon rupture, poor bone stock, and significant wrist deformity (Hayden, & Jebson, 2005; Shapiro, 1996; Watson et al., 1999). It is often performed after other options have failed. A circumferential orthosis is sometimes used preoperatively to simulate the outcome of a wrist arthrodesis. Often, this same orthosis can be reheated and adjusted in the postoperative phase (Fig. 17–49A–C). Whether the arthrodesis is partial or total, postoperative orthotic management is essentially the same. In general, the cast is removed 1 to 2 weeks after arthrodesis, and the patient is placed in a wrist immobilization orthosis. Digital tendon gliding exercises are performed to prevent tendon adherence over the fusion site. The orthosis is generally worn until the fusion site is considered well healed, which is evaluated radiographically or by CT scan (6–8 weeks postoperatively) (Feinberg, 1999).

THUMB WITH RHEUMATOID ARTHRITIS

As with any chronic synovitis, the thumb may develop many different deformity patterns as described in the literature (Nalebuff, 1968; Stein & Terrono, 1996). In 1968, a classification system for thumb

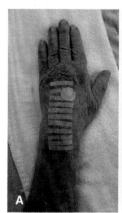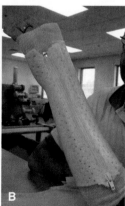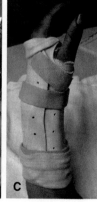

FIGURE 17–49 A, A patient 2 weeks after undergoing a wrist arthrodesis. **B,** An option to consider for this patient is a Rolyan® Aquaform™ Zippered Wrist orthosis. This elastic-based material allows for easy remolding and refitting, and the circumferential design ensures secure immobilization. **C,** Another option to consider is a "clamshell" orthosis design as shown here. This was fabricated for a woman who underwent a wrist synovectomy and limited arthrodesis; she was exquisitely tender over the surgical site and slow to heal. The design allows the patient to remove the dorsal piece easily for wound care and dressing changes.

deformities in RA was devised by Nalebuff. Any or all of the thumb joints may be involved to some degree. Management of the thumb with RA is based on the pattern of deformity and the functional needs of the patient. Orthosis application, used early in the disease process, can enhance function and reduce pain of the thumb by stabilizing the joint(s) involved during hand use and support joints in an antideformity position. Orthosis application is used as a conservative measure but can also be used during the management of postoperative thumb procedures.

The **boutonniere deformity** of the thumb is commonly seen in RA and is characterized by MP flexion and IP hyperextension (Fig. 17–50A–C) (Gellman, Statson, Brumfield, Costigan, & Kuschner, 1997; Rizio, & Belsky, 1995; Tomaino et al., 1995). Prolonged synovitis at the MP joint causes attenuation of the extensor mechanism including EPB and EPL tendons. This results in EPL tendon subluxation volarly and ulnarly. In turn, the proximal phalanx assumes a flexed position and often subluxates volarly. Early on, the patient may maintain passive MP joint extension but may not be able to extend the joint actively. As a compensatory mechanism, the patient radially abducts the first metacarpal and hyperextends the IP joint. Accentuation of this hyperextension occurs when pinch forces are applied. With progression of the disease, this deformity often becomes fixed and can no longer be corrected passively.

Swan-neck deformity of the thumb is also frequently seen in the RA population (Stein & Terrono, 1996). This deformity is characterized by metacarpal adduction, MP joint hyperextension, and IP joint flexion (Fig. 17–14). The deformity is initiated by synovitis of the first CMC joint, which results in attenuation of the joint capsule and leads to radial subluxation of the base of the first metacarpal. This imbalance of forces progresses to the development of an adduction contracture of the first CMC joint. As the deformity progresses, the volar plate of the MP joint becomes lax, allowing the joint to hyperextend. Dorsal and radial subluxation of the first metacarpal progresses which further contributes to the imbalance of the extensor forces. This leads to CMC adduction with MP joint hyperextension and IP joint flexion (Stein & Terrono, 1996; Swanson, 1995b).

Deformity of the thumb MP joint can occur without first CMC involvement (Stein & Terrono, 1996). Synovitis at the MP joint can result in attenuation of the ulnar collateral ligament (UCL) and volar plate. UCL attenuation allows the proximal phalanx to deviate radially. This in turn may cause the first dorsal interossei and the adductor muscles to tighten and the web space to contract. With volar plate involvement, the MP joint hyperextends and the IP joint secondarily flexes with increased pull from FPL. The pattern of thumb deformity is varied and may occur in different patterns and combinations. The goal of both conservative and operative treatment is restoration of pain-free balance and stability (Glickel et al., 1992; Stein & Terrono, 1996).

NONSURGICAL ORTHOTIC MANAGEMENT GUIDELINES

Orthoses can be used conservatively to protect the passively correctable joints from increased damage and to slow the progression of a fixed contracture (Stein & Terrono, 1996). In thumb boutonniere and swan-neck deformities, the goal is stabilization of the thumb in gentle abduction to prevent adduction contracture of the first web space, to provide pain relief, and to protect during rest and activity. A hand-based orthosis can allow for functional use, permitting full wrist mobility while performing ADLs (Figs. 17–50C and 17–51A,B). For advanced thumb boutonniere deformity—in which the IP joint significantly hyperextends—an orthosis that stabilizes the MP in slight flexion and provides a dorsal block to IP hyperextension may be of value for light functional use (Fig. 17–52), alternatively with the swan-neck

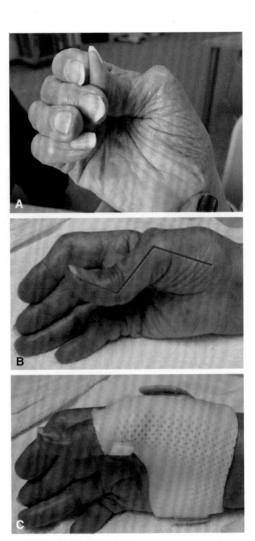

FIGURE 17–50 A, A patient with advanced rheumatoid disease. The boutonniere deformity of the thumb is exacerbated by tasks requiring pinch. **B and C,** This patient had psoriatic arthritis and was able to function well with the use of a thumb immobilization orthosis supporting the MP joint, preventing further collapse.

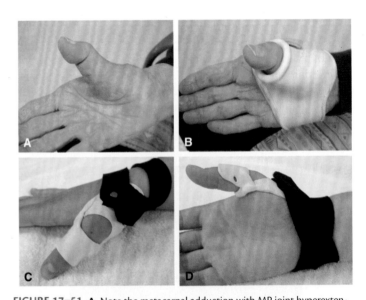

FIGURE 17–51 A, Note the metacarpal adduction with MP joint hyperextension and IP flexion in this patient with a swan-neck deformity of the thumb. The initial stage of this deformity is CMC subluxation. **B,** This hand-based orthosis applies gentle three-point pressure to correct the CMC subluxation passively, which in turn aids in realignment of the MP and IP joints. The device design allows the patient to perform light ADLs. **C and D,** Offer an alternative orthosis design for an MP hyperextension deformity that does not include CMC subluxation.

deformity the MP joint should be positioned in flexion to correct its hyperextension tendency. A forearm-based wrist/thumb immobilization orthosis is recommended for all other times to reduce pain and properly stabilize the CMC joint (Fig. 17–19) (Colditz, 1995; Terrono et al., 1995). Patients should be encouraged to wear this orthosis at night.

To address isolated thumb MP joint deformity, the joint should be positioned as close to full extension as possible and the web space maintained, even if there is no pain (Colditz, 1995). The orthosis supplies the external stability to maintain the MP in extension and allows IP flexion; little motion is necessary at the MP joint for good thumb function. Various orthotic designs can be used, depending on the preference of the surgeon or therapist (Figs. 17–5B and 17–16A). Thinner materials (3/32″) are recommended for fabrication if the deformity is easily passively correctable. If there are tight volar structures, a more rigid material should be considered to provide adequate support to maintain desired positioning (1/8″).

Protection with an orthosis can also be provided to the thumb IP joint if instability occurs (Philips, 1995; Terrono et al., 1995). A small dorsal thermoplastic orthosis can be fabricated or commercially available orthotics (e.g., Silver Ring™ orthoses from Silver Ring™ Company, Charlottesville, VA) can be ordered to provide lateral support, prevent hyperextension, and provide stability for functional use or while awaiting surgical intervention (Fig. 17–53). An option to increase functional use with gripping onto options with a thermoplastic orthosis is to use dycem at the volar aspect at the fingertip.

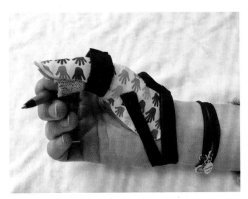

FIGURE 17–52 A dorsally applied orthosis holds the MP in slight flexion and prevents IP hyperextension.

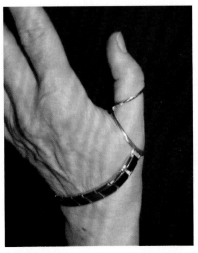

FIGURE 17–53 A thumb orthosis for MP joint hyperextension. This Silver Ring orthosis provides MP joint positioning and lateral joint stability. This orthosis is measured by the therapist and custom made by the company. It is a durable, attractive, and low-profile design for long-term wear.

EXPERT PEARL 17–12

"Butterfly" Pattern
LAURA CARTER, OT
Australia

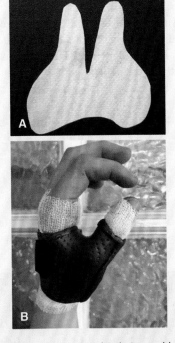

Hand-based thumb orthosis option—this design enables good immobilization of the CMC, metacarpal, and proximal phalanx to adequately stabilize the MP joint. Cutting the material along the dorsum of the thumb while the thermoplastic is still warm on the client creates a contoured fit and smooth seal that sits flush with the skin. This area can then be reinforced if needed by dry heating a strip of thermoplastic and applying over the seal.

POSTSURGICAL ORTHOTIC MANAGEMENT GUIDELINES FOR THE THUMB

The goals of surgery for the patient with RA of the thumb depend on which joints are involved and extent of disease progression. The stability of each joint depends on the extent and direction of forces applied to it during use as well as the direction and counterforce of the muscle-tendon units acting on it (Stein & Terrono, 1996).

Thumb Interphalangeal Joint

Surgical intervention at the IP joint may consist of extrinsic tendon reconstruction, if tendon integrity allows. Thumb extensor tendon repairs should be positioned in an orthosis for at least 5 weeks in wrist extension, thumb radial abduction and extension, and MP/IP extension (Stein & Terrono, 1996). After thumb flexor tendon repair, the patient is positioned in a safe degree of wrist flexion, thumb midpalmar/radial abduction, and slight MP/IP flexion (see Chapter 19 for details).

IP arthrodesis is reserved for the unstable, painful joint, providing there is minimal involvement of the first CMC, STT, and MP joints (Nalebuff, 1968). This procedure provides a stable joint for the digits to pinch against. A small thermoplastic orthosis can be applied to protect the IP joint until fusion is solid.

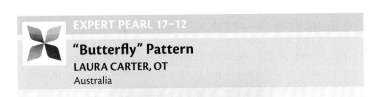

Thumb Metacarpophalangeal Joint

Surgical intervention for the thumb MP joint may include synovectomy, arthrodesis, relocation of EPL, capsulodesis, and arthroplasty (Chung, Kowalski, Myra, & Kazmers, 2000; Rizio, & Belsky, 1995; Terrono et al., 1995). **Synovectomy** is reserved for patients who have had chronic synovitis for 6 months or more (Chung et al., 2000). Orthotic positioning in extension is typically the postoperative position to prevent MP flexion contracture (Fig. 17–54A,B).

For severe instability and articular damage of the thumb MP, surgical options include MP joint arthrodesis or arthroplasty. The decision is influenced by vocational and avocational demands, the integrity of the MP joint, the condition of the bordering first CMC and IP joints, and the anticipated future activity level (Chung et al., 2000; Colditz, 1995; Rizio, & Belsky, 1995). Some protocols limit the use of implant arthroplasty at the MP level to only those with flexion deformity (Chung et al., 2000; Terrono et al., 1995).

Thumb MP joint arthroplasty is done when the joint is painful, unstable, or demonstrates articular destruction. If the thumb IP joint necessitates fusion, attempts may be made to preserve some motion of the MP joint through arthroplasty. The goal of the procedure is to gain stability with some motion, that is 10° to 35° of flexion (Chung et al., 2000; Swanson et al., 1995). Patients are positioned in an orthosis close to full extension for 4 to 5 weeks at which time AROM is begun (Chung et al., 2000).

The goal of thumb MP joint arthrodesis is to provide thumb stability. The postoperative orthotic intervention program is based on the surgeon's protocol. In general, after the initial postoperative immobilization phase, the patient is placed in either a hand-based or forearm-based protective orthosis that maintains the fused position and protects it from injury. Initially, a forearm-based orthosis may be preferred to intentionally limit the use of the hand. A hand-based orthosis can be an alternative with a compliant patient and when the pins may be less exposed. Hand-based orthoses with this patient population can allow more functional use of the wrist and the nonimmobilized digits as shown in Figures 17–16A, 17–50C, and 17–51B. In both designs, the importance is placed on early IP joint motion to decrease the risk of extensor tendon adherence over the surgical site.

DIGIT MCP JOINTS WITH RHEUMATOID ARTHRITIS

The MCP joints of the digits of hand are frequently involved in patients with RA. Chronic inflammation with aggressive synovial proliferation may damage the surrounding structures (Flatt, 1996; Gellman et al., 1997; Nalebuff, 1968; Rothwell, Cragg, & O'Neil, 1997; Stirrat, 1996; Terrono et al., 2011). An orthosis should be applied to the MCPJs for the following reasons: to rest the acutely inflamed hand, minimize deformity, and provide pain relief. Orthoses are also applied following operative procedures to the MCP joints such as arthroplasty or joint fusion (Boozer, 1993; Murphy, 1996; Rennie, 1996; Theisen, 1993).

The two major deformities that occur to the digital MCP joints are ulnar drift and volar subluxation/dislocation of the proximal phalanx (Fig. 17–55). These deformities may result from several factors (Rizio & Belsky, 1995; Shapiro, 1996; Stirrat, 1996; Swanson, 1995b; Swanson et al., 1995; Wilson & Fredick, 1994):

- The flexor tendons approach the MCP joints ulnarly and, therefore, exert a stronger ulnar pull with muscular contraction.

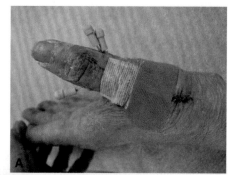
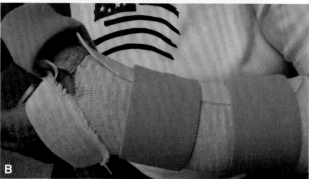

FIGURE 17–54 **A,** Thumb MP joint fusion increases stability and improves the ability to pinch. **B,** Used after the postoperative immobilization period, this MP immobilization orthosis protects the MP joint fusion. Note the incorporation of the thermoplastic "bump-outs" for the pins.

- Most functional activities involving MCP function (prehension) increase ulnar and palmar displacement of the flexor tendons across the MCP joint.
- The shape of the metacarpal heads influences ulnar drift; the ulnar side of the metacarpal is shorter than the radial side, influencing the proximal phalanx to favor an ulnar-oriented position during flexion. Any ligamentous laxity allows the joint to slip ulnarly.
- Chronic synovitis weakens the soft tissues surrounding the MCP joint. As a result of the weakening of these structures, distention of the capsule, laxity of the radial and UCLs, as well as laxity of the radial sagittal band, the tendinous line of pull becomes more ulnarly directed.
- Wrist involvement can ultimately influence ulnar deviation of the digits. Often seen in early RA, the wrist radially deviates, and consequently affects the ulnar position of the digits (Figs. 17–43 and 17–56).

NONSURGICAL ORTHOTIC MANAGEMENT GUIDELINES

During periods of exacerbation, the wrist should be included when applying an orthosis to the MCP joints to prevent or minimize any

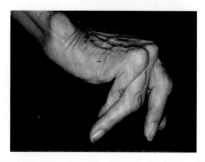

FIGURE 17–55 Volar MCP subluxation and ulnar deviation of the proximal phalanxes.

zigzag deformity (Stirrat, 1996). The optimal position of the orthosis includes wrist in 10° to 15° of extension and 10° of ulnar deviation and MCP joints in full extension and central alignment (Stirrat, 1996). The MCP joints should be positioned in extension to support weakened structures, prevent volar subluxation, minimize reflex intrinsic muscle contracture, and correct for ulnar drift (Boozer, 1993; Fess et al., 2005; Melvin, 1982; Murphy, 1996; Rennie, 1996). The orthosis is generally worn at night (Fig. 17–57A and 17–5F). Carefully positioned straps can be the key to guiding the wrist and MCPs gently into an antideformity position (Fig. 17–57B). A strap attaching to the inside of the orthosis (just beneath the second metacarpal head) and traversing obliquely toward the fifth metacarpal can aid in gently directing the wrist and digits into the antideformity position (Boozer, 1993; Flatt, 1996; Melvin, 1982; Philips, 1995).

Daytime functional orthosis application for ulnar drift can be challenging to fabricate, especially for a novice therapist. This is due in part to the necessity of molding the material between each digital web space, while simultaneously accounting for adequate digital flexion/extension. It is also important to consider how easily the MCPJs passively extend. This will indicate the degree of resistance and/or friction the digits will encounter against the thermoplastic material. For these few reasons alone, one can appreciate the skill needed to make this type of orthosis comfortable, effective, and cosmetically acceptable to the wearer (Fig. 17–58A–D). Various forms of prefabricated orthoses can be tried to aid in support and central alignment of the MCPJs (Fig. 17–59A,B) (Flatt, 1996; Rennie, 1996).

EXPERT PEARL 17–14

MCP Deviation Orthosis
HOANG TRAN, OT/L, CHT
Florida

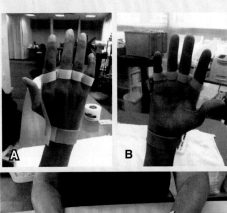

Fabricated using soft, thin strapping sewn together to decrease ulnar drift at MCP joints often seen with RA. Digits pulled radially and secured to loop around wrist. Another option using leather finger loops: trim to size, sew together, and attach to a strap on IF radial side to wrist loop.

EXPERT PEARL 17–13

MCP Joint Alignment
ANNA OVSYANNIKOVA, MD, HAND THERAPY
Russia

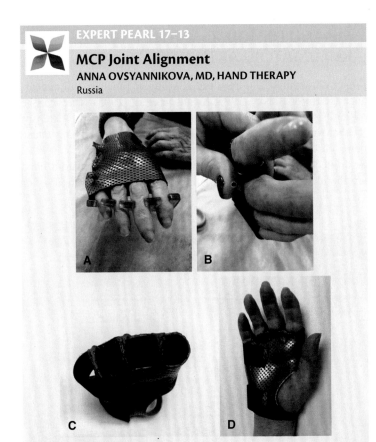

Orthosis for blocking and/or improving alignment of MCP joints. Use small pieces of thermoplastic to separate fingers and make the orthosis more stable. Utilize a "toe separator" at the level of the middle phalanges when forming to maintain web spaces.

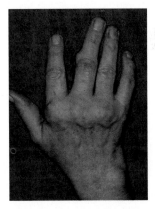

FIGURE 17–56 Zigzag deformity with radial deviation at the wrist and ulnar deviation at the MCP joints. Note the tenosynovitis over the dorsal MCP joints.

POSTSURGICAL ORTHOTIC MANAGEMENT GUIDELINES

A common surgical option for advanced MCP joint arthritis is an **MCP joint implant** arthroplasty (Fig. 17–60A). Indications for this procedure include ulnar drift not amenable to soft-tissue repair alone, pain, subluxation, or dislocation that severely limits function, and displeasing appearance (Flatt, 1996; Gellman et al., 1997; Melvin, 1982; Nalebuff, 1968; Rennie, 1996;Rizio, & Belsky, 1995; Rothwell et al., 1997; Terrono et al., 2011; Theisen, 1993; Wilson &

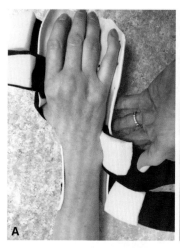
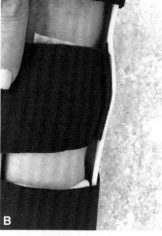

FIGURE 17–57 **A,** A night wrist/hand immobilization orthosis that uses straps to enhance the antideformity position of the wrist and digits. **B,** Note the orientation of the strap from the ulnar border which imparts a gently radially directed force. The radial MCP IF strap imparts an ulnarly directed force.

Carlblom, 1989). MCP arthroplasty involves resection of inflamed soft tissue, the metacarpal head, and the base of the proximal phalanx. A silastic implant is typically used as a spacer between these bones. During the healing process, a capsule typically forms about the new joint; this is referred to as encapsulation (Philips, 1995; Stirrat, 1996; Swanson, 1995a; Tomaino et al., 1995).

The therapist's role is critical in the postoperative management of these patients (Swanson et al., 1995; Terrono et al., 2011). A typical protocol would include the use of a daytime forearm-based MCP extension mobilization orthosis, allowing controlled and limited active MCP flexion to facilitate the encapsulation process (Fig. 17–60B–D) (Melvin, 1982; Stirrat, 1996; Theisen, 1993; Wilson & Carlblom, 1989). If there has been reconstruction of the radial collateral ligament of the IF MCP joint, a radial outrigger is used to prevent pronation and support the MCP in slight radial deviation (overcorrection). The MCP of the SF should be allowed unrestricted flexion, which may require removal from the extension component (sling) to that finger during exercise sessions (Stirrat, 1996). SF MCP flexion can be inadequate because of the significant instability preoperatively or owing to weakness resulting from surgical release of the ulnar-sided intrinsic muscles (Rizio & Belsky,

1995). If not carefully fit, the sling may actually position the SF in MCP hyperextension. The clinician may consider casting the SF PIP and DIP joints into extension, then applying the sling over the cast to better target the forces of active flexion at the MCP joint (Terrono et al., 2011). The mobilization orthosis is normally worn during the day for a period of 4 to 6 weeks. The expected outcome for arc of flexion at the MCP joints is approximately 40° to 60° (Kozin, 1999; Rizio, & Belsky, 1995; Stirrat, 1996; Terrono et al., 2011). This dynamic mobilization orthosis is often prescribed in combination with a night wrist/hand immobilization orthosis (Fig. 17–61) (Michlovitz, 1999; Stirrat, 1996; Theisen, 1993; Terrono et al., 2011). The immobilization orthosis maintains the wrist in slight extension, while the MCPs are slightly flexed to approximately 10° in central alignment, with the IPs gently extended. The immobilization orthosis is worn for 3 or more months postoperatively to maintain good MCP alignment (Terrono et al., 1995; Terrono, Nalebuff, & Philips, 2011).

A hand-based orthosis can be fabricated from thermoplastic material 4 to 6 weeks postoperatively for intermittent light activity (Flatt, 1996; Kozin, 1999; Rennie, 1996; Rizio, & Belsky, 1995; Stirrat, 1996). This small orthosis can provide external support for continued MCP extension, preventing ulnar deviation, especially with attempted pinch with the thumb against the IF. Care must be taken to decrease bulk and rough edges between the fingers, which can lead to discomfort and impaired function (Fig. 17–58). Soft neoprene orthoses can also be used postoperatively to provide some volar MCP support, guidance against ulnar deviation, and increased digital function (Fig. 17–59). Refer to additional information on orthoses for digit arthroplasties in Box 17–3.

PIP AND DIP JOINTS WITH RHEUMATOID ARTHRITIS

Finger deformities as a result of RA impair function and appearance (Rizio & Belsky, 1995; Swanson et al., 1995). They can be difficult to treat due to the critical involvement of the extensor mechanism at this level. Synovitis of these small joints may cause pain, chronic edema, and stiffness (Wilson & Fredick, 1994). Swan-neck and boutonniere deformities of the rheumatoid hand are the most common finger pathologies. Implant arthroplasty or

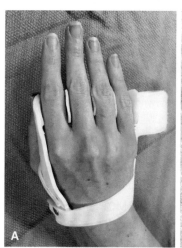
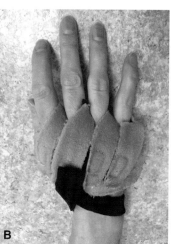
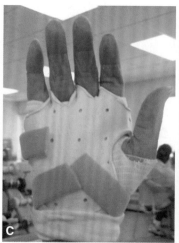
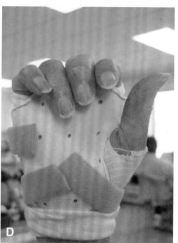

FIGURE 17–58 **A,** At 4 to 6 weeks after MCP joint arthroplasty, a small, hand-based orthosis can be used for light functional tasks. **B,** A prefabricated orthosis can be an option; this one has been slightly customized (strap at wrist) to allow for better fit. **C and D,** Volar view of another orthosis design to allow IP extension/flexion while maintaining MCP support.

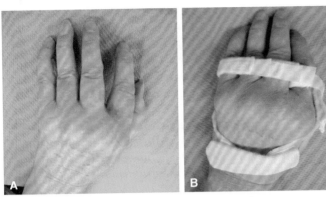

FIGURE 17–59 A, Ulnar drift at the MCP joint. **B,** This orthosis is a less rigid support with soft strapping and a thermoplastic base, providing centralization of the MCP joints, while allowing functional use of the hand.

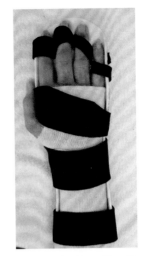

FIGURE 17–61 Volar forearm-based wrist and hand immobilization orthosis used postoperatively for an IF-SF MCP implant arthroplasty. Such orthoses are used to maintain MCP extension alignment. Note the soft neoprene straps forming comfortable troughs for the digits to rest in.

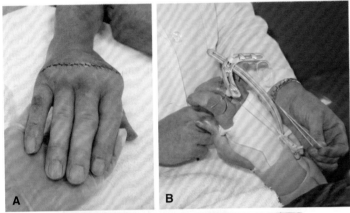

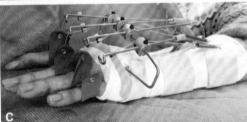

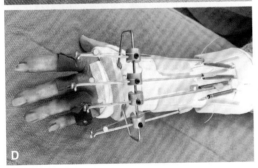

FIGURE 17–60 A, Postoperative view of an IF-SF MCP joint arthroplasty with reconstruction of all radial collateral ligaments of the MCP joints. **B,** Dynamic MCP extension mobilization orthosis applied 5 days postoperatively using Digitec Outrigger system (Performance Health). Note the slight radial pull at the proximal phalanges to protect the reconstructed MCP joint radial collateral ligaments. Active MCP flexion can be performed within this orthosis, therefore care must be taken not to place excessive tension through the rubber bands; use just enough to hold the MCPs in extension while allowing gentle gliding in flexion. **C and D,** This is another choice for dynamic mobilization using the Rolyan system and spring coils (Rolyan® Adjustable Outrigger Kit; Performance Health).

arthrodesis can be considered for the rheumatoid PIP or DIP joint. They are managed in the same way as discussed for OA earlier in this chapter. Orthotic intervention in the early stages of the disease process can be used as an external support to place joints in a mechanically advantageous position to enhance their function. Orthoses can also be used as a postoperative tool to support and protect surgical procedures.

SWAN-NECK DEFORMITY

Swan-neck deformity in the digit presents as PIP joint hyperextension and DIP flexion, as noted in Figure 17–44A. An anatomical classification of swan-neck deformity of the fingers was first introduced by Zancolli (1979), whereas clinical classification was expanded by Nalebuff (1989). Refer to Table 17–3.

The first two stages of the Nalebuff classification are responsive to orthotic management, and the latter two should be considered for surgical intervention. The intrinsic/extrinsic muscle imbalance in the rheumatoid hand may occur from synovitis about the wrist, MCP, PIP, or DIP joint(s) or along the flexor tendon sheath (Eckhaus, 1993; Rizio & Belsky, 1995; Swanson, 1995b; Wilson & Fredick, 1994). The most common cause is synovitis at the level of the MCP joint, which can lead to extensor tendon subluxation (ulnarly) as a result of radial-sided sagittal band attenuation. This subluxation eventually produces an extensor lag leading to MCP joint subluxation and accentuating the swan-neck deformity (Chinchalkar & Pitts, 2006). Chronic synovitis appears to cause a reflexive intrinsic muscle contracture. This contracture increases the extension pull at the PIPJ, leading to volar plate laxity, PIP hyperextension, attenuation of the transverse fibers of the retinacular ligaments, dorsal subluxation of the lateral bands, and attenuation of the oblique retinacular ligament (ORL) distally (Swanson, 1995b). The DIP tends to flex secondarily to the proximal pathology (Melvin, 1982; Swanson, 1995b).

Swelling of the DIP joint may cause attenuation or a rupture in the terminal extensor tendon with resultant DIP flexion. The harmony of the entire extensor mechanism is disrupted, producing hyperextension at the PIP joint, a secondary swan neck. Synovitis of the PIP joint itself may lead to stretching of the volar ligaments with a resultant dorsal migration of the lateral bands (Fig. 17–62).

BOX 17–3   EVIDENCE-INFORMED ORTHOTIC MANAGEMENT: POSTOPERATIVE MCP AND PIP JOINT ARTHROPLASTY

Application of an orthosis following MCP and PIP joint arthroplasty is an important component of postoperative management. The purpose of the dynamic or mobilization orthosis is to allow for ROM while controlling the position and alignment of the reconstructed joint(s). However, many papers fail to discuss this orthosis application process within the rehabilitation program in any detail (Burr, Pratt, & Smith, 2002; Hansraj, Ashworth, & Ebramzadeh, 1997; Jensen, Boeckstyns, & Kristiansen, 1986; Mannerfelt & Andersson, 1975; Massy-Westropp, Johnston, & Hill, 2008; Nicolle & Gilbert,

1979; Pereira & Belcher, 2001; Wilson, Sykes, & Niranjan, 1993). It is difficult to compare outcome studies for the application of an extension mobilization orthosis (which allows controlled active flexion and dynamically assisted extension) compared to an immobilization orthosis, which is removed by the patient to perform *active* flexion and extension. Therefore, immobilization (static) versus mobilization (dynamic) orthosis application following MCP and PIP joint arthroplasty should be based on physician preference and expert opinion.

TABLE 17–3	**Swan-Neck Deformity**
Stage I	Joints are supple and mobile. Preventing hyperextension at the PIP joint corrects the flexion of the DIP joint.
Stage II	Presence of mild interosseous contracture is often seen.
Stage III	Retraction of tendons, dorsal joint capsule, and interosseous contracture is profound. Surgical management should be considered.
Stage IV	Deformity is more profound with articular destruction.

From Nalebuff, E. A. (1989). The rheumatoid swan-neck deformity. Hand Clinics, 5, 203–214.

Early management may consist of joint injections and corrective "anti–swan-neck" orthoses (Figs. 17–44B and 17–63A–C) (Rizio, & Belsky, 1995). A swan-neck deformity can result from multiple pathologies: the arthritic hand, including, but not limited to, intrinsic tightness, volar plate attenuation, and sagittal band rupture. Refer to additional information on orthoses for swan-neck deformities in Box 17–4.

NONSURGICAL ORTHOTIC MANAGEMENT GUIDELINES

The primary goal of fitting an orthosis for swan-neck deformity is to reduce and/or minimize the progression of the deforming stages. The goal of the orthosis application to a passively

correctable swan-neck deformity is to allow near to full flexion of the PIP joint while preventing PIP joint hyperextension (Eckhaus, 1993). A supple swan-neck deformity can be managed with an extension restriction orthosis (Fig. 17–63B,C). These small, ring-type orthoses can be beneficial for short-term solutions. More permanent orthoses can be purchased from various companies and/or catalogs that may be less bulky and work well for some patients. These tend to be more durable, fit well, and are more cosmetically pleasing (Fig. 17–53).

EXPERT PEARL 17–15

Long Figure-8 Orthosis
ANA CANDICE COELHO, PT
Brazil

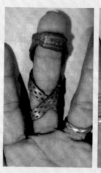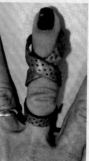

Utilized for finger with swan-neck deformity with significant DIP flexion. Folding the thermoplastic to double to thickness makes the orthosis stronger.

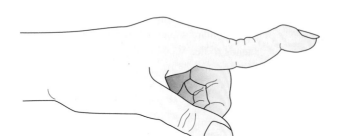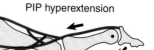

FIGURE 17–62 Swan-neck deformity. (Adapted with permission from American Society for Surgery of the Hand. (1990). *The hand: Examination and diagnosis* (3rd ed.). New York, NY: Churchill Livingstone.)

PIP hyperextension

DIP flexion with extensor lag

EXPERT PEARL 17-16

PIP Extension Restriction
DEBBIE FISHER, MS, OTR, CHT
Texas

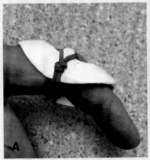
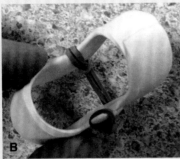

Utilize a rubber band to secure an orthosis to target a swan-neck deformity for a patient with a large PIP joint. This will make adjusting tension and donning/doffing much easier because of the stretchy nature of a rubber band. This is also much more comfortable on the volar surface as there is no thermoplastic bulk to interfere with flexion.

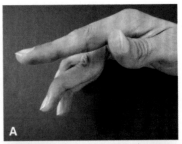
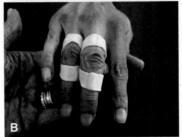
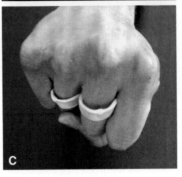

FIGURE 17-63 A, Swan-neck deformity with hyperextension at PIP and flexion at DIP joint. **B and C,** This deformity be managed with an extension restriction orthosis (Figure-8 design) that allows near full digital flexion, yet limits PIP joint hyperextension.

POSTSURGICAL ORTHOTIC MANAGEMENT GUIDELINES

Surgical restoration of the hyperextended PIP joint may involve the use of a tendon transfer, such as a superficialis tendon. In some situations, DIP joint pin fixation in 0° is warranted. Postoperative orthosis application depends on individual physician preferences; however, most include early fabrication of an orthosis, which positions the wrist in neutral to slight extension, slight MCP flexion, PIP flexion of 20° to 30°, and the DIP in neutral. If the PIP joint is pinned in flexion, the orthosis should support this position. This orthosis is generally worn for 2 to 3 weeks. The patient can then be transferred to the use of a hand- or finger-based extension restriction orthosis. At approximately 6 weeks, the degree of extension allowed is gently and gradually increased at the PIP joint. The orthosis should carefully accommodate these gradual changes based on healing timelines (Fig. 17–64A–E).

BOUTONNIERE DEFORMITY

Boutonniere deformities of the digits are characterized by PIP flexion and DIP hyperextension (Fig. 17–65A–C). Similar to the swan-neck classification, boutonniere deformity is also classified based on clinical stages (Tubiana, 1981). Refer to Table 17–4.

In the first three stages of boutonniere deformity, MCP joint hyperextension during digital motion is observed, whereas in stage IV, fixed hyperextension of the MCP joint may be a contributing factor. The most common cause of this deformity in the rheumatoid hand is chronic PIP joint synovitis (Eddington-Valdata, 1993; Nalebuff & Millender, 1975; Rizio & Belsky, 1995; Swanson et al., 1985; Wilson & Fredick, 1994). The synovitis migrates dorsally between the lateral bands, displacing them laterally and volarly (Swanson, 1995b). This, in turn, creates lengthening of the central tendon. The lateral bands eventually orient themselves below the axis of the PIP joint, becoming PIP joint flexors. This places a secondary pull on the DIP joint into extension. Left untreated, the ORL shortens, causing the DIP joint to become tight in extension (Fig. 17–66). A true boutonniere is pathology specific to the central slip

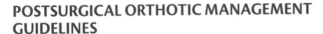

BOX 17-4   EVIDENCE-INFORMED ORTHOTIC MANAGEMENT: SWAN-NECK DEFORMITY

The swan-neck deformity is a common finger deformity associated with RA, and orthoses are often prescribed for newly diagnosed patients as well as for patients who suffer from chronic RA. Studies indicate that Silver Ring™ orthoses or similar, prefabricated orthoses, and custom-made orthoses can improve dexterity and reduce pain (Schegget & Knipping, 2000; Zijlstra, Heijnsdijk-Rouwenhorst, & Rasker, 2004). All of these orthoses have been found beneficial. Some studies have reported that patients prefer Silver Ring™ orthoses versus custom-made orthoses due to the small thin ring design and attractive appearance (Schegget & Knipping, 2000).

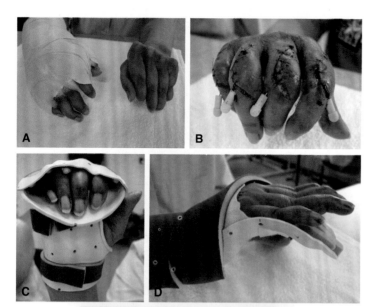

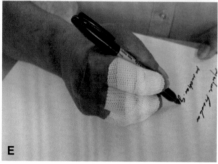

FIGURE 17–64 **A and B,** MCP deformity and swan-neck deformities in this 26-year-old college graduate student. Postoperative dressing removed and an orthosis was fabricated **(B)**. Note the similar deformity of her left hand. **C,** A hand-based protective orthosis. **D,** The "dorsal thermoplastic hood" could be removed for pin care and gentle AROM on the noninvolved structures. Note the swan-neck deformities of her digits. **E,** Small digits casts were used at 6 weeks to simulate PIP fusions. The patient went onto require IF-SF PIP joint fusions.

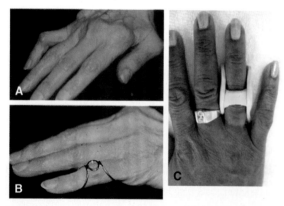

FIGURE 17–65 **A,** Boutonniere deformity with flexion at the PIP joint. This deformity may be managed with a PIP extension orthosis on a long-term basis. Many patients find a ring-type orthosis **(B)** to be more cosmetically appealing than a thermoplastic PIP extension restriction orthosis **(C)** (SIRIS Boutonniere Splint shown). (Photo courtesy of Silver Ring™ Splint Company.)

TABLE 17–4	**Boutonniere Deformity**
Stage I	Minimal deficiency of less than 30° of extension is noted.
Stage II	Mild flexion contracture of the PIP joint along with volar subluxation of the lateral bands; hyperextension of DIP joint and a negative retinacular test are also present.
Stage III	Presentation of contracture of the retinacular ligaments; enabling passive extension of the PIP joint with associated positive retinacular test
Stage IV	Deformity exhibits a fixed contracture of the PIP and DIP joints.

From Tubiana, R. (1981). The hand. Philadelphia, PA: Saunders.

at the level of the PIP joint; however, a pseudoboutonniere may arise from various causes including PIP joint contracture, triangular ligament laxity, and others.

NONSURGICAL ORTHOTIC MANAGEMENT GUIDELINES

Applying an orthosis for a passively correctable boutonniere deformity is best achieved with a twofold process. The patient should have a digit immobilization orthosis for night use, which positions the PIP joint in full extension (Fig. 17–67A) (Glickel et al., 1992). An effective option for daytime orthotic application includes the use of a custom-made PIP extension immobilization orthosis which allows full MCP and if desired, DIP motion. If the deformity is the result of an attritional rupture of the central tendon, uninterrupted PIP extension immobilization must be maintained for approximately 6 weeks before motion is gradually initiated (Eddington-Valdata, 1993). In these authors' opinion, the best way to achieve uninterrupted motion is to apply a circumferential nonremovable orthosis (Fig. 17–67B). Gentle isolated DIP active and passive motion or joint-blocking exercises can help maintain the length of the extensor mechanism, ORL, and dorsal mobility of the lateral bands (Poole & Pellegrini, 2000; Wilson & Fredick, 1994).

If the patient presents with a fixed flexion contracture of the PIP joint, a gentle serial static extension mobilization approach may be implemented until full PIP extension is achieved (Eddington-Valdata, 1993). Full PIP extension is critical to achieve before the patient is considered for surgical intervention, such as a flexible implant arthroplasty (Nalebuff & Millender, 1975). Once fully extended, the PIP is held in extension for an additional 4 to 6 weeks (Eddington-Valdata, 1993). If, at that time, the patient cannot maintain extension, surgical intervention should be considered. Refer to additional information on orthoses for boutonniere deformities OA in Box 17–5.

POSTSURGICAL ORTHOTIC MANAGEMENT GUIDELINES

Surgical intervention may be considered to reestablish PIP extension if conservative management has failed. Postoperative management varies depending on the exact procedure or combination of procedures performed, such as pinning, **tenolysis**, and/or volar plate release (Eddington-Valdata, 1993; Nalebuff & Millender,

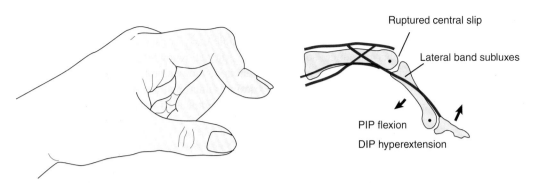

FIGURE 17–66 Boutonniere deformity. (Adapted with permission from American Society for Surgery of the Hand. (1990). *The hand: Examination and diagnosis* (3rd ed.). New York, NY: Churchill Livingstone.)

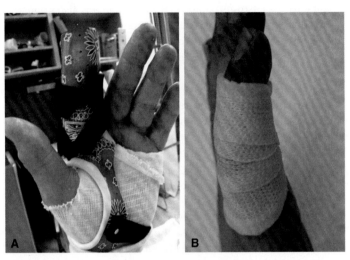

FIGURE 17–67 **A,** Orthosis fabrication for night extension is important for reducing the possibility of a PIP flexion contracture. This hand-based design incorporates the thumb which aides in securing the orthosis fit—a good option for night wear. **B,** A circumferential cast is used for uninterrupted PIP immobilization to allow for better compliance and assured healing. Note the lining of paraffin that was applied to the proximal and distal borders.

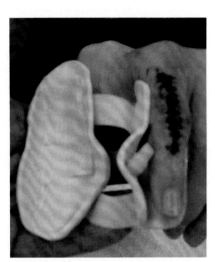

FIGURE 17–68 A protective orthosis used after PIP joint reconstruction. Note how the pin was incorporated into this small "clamshell-type" design. This design protects the repair yet allows for easy removal for wound care and gentle, guarded DIP exercises as dictated by the surgeon.

1975; Rizio & Belsky, 1995) (Fig. 17–68). The PIP joint is most often positioned in extension for approximately 4 weeks, after which, gentle active exercises are introduced. A mobilization device can be used as seen in Figure 17–12. This allows for gentle flexion while the extensor mechanism is assisted back into extension. Active DIP joint flexion exercises should begin as soon as possible postoperatively to aid in advancing the extensor mechanism, allowing for lateral band dorsal migration and preventing tendon adhesions (the PIP joint should be held in extension during this exercise) (Eddington-Valdata, 1993; Nalebuff & Millender, 1975; Wilson & Fredick, 1994).

BOX 17–5   EVIDENCE-INFORMED ORTHOTIC MANAGEMENT: BOUTONNIERE DEFORMITY

To date, there have been no randomized control trials on the effectiveness of orthosis application to correct this deformity. Studies are needed to determine the clinical effectiveness. In the authors' expert opinion, orthosis application can be of benefit with passively correctable deformities in the compliant patient who follows the prescribed orthosis regime carefully.

CONCLUSION

Although medical options, particularly pharmaceutical developments, and surgical advancements have greatly influenced the prevention and further progression of joint deformity in the patient with rheumatic disease, the use of orthoses remains both a valuable early conservative treatment and an important postoperative adjunct. Knowledge of the disease process, joint anatomy and function, biomechanics of secondary deformity, and the patient's desired functional goals is crucial to providing effective and appropriate therapeutic interventions.

FIELD NOTE: WHAT IS *DYNAMIC STABILITY* OF THE THUMB ALL ABOUT?

By Virginia H. O'Brien, OTD, OR/L, CHT
Minnesota

The thumb appears to be at risk. Why does it seem there is only a 35-year warranty on the first CMC joint? Thumb use contributes up to 60% to 70% of the function of the hand. It is inherently unstable due to its anatomy and wide range of motion. It is the joint of the hand that is most affected by osteoarthritis (OA), has the highest report of pain and disability, and is the joint most commonly operated on in the hand. So, if this is such an important joint of the hand, what can be done to reduce its pain? I suggest that part of that answer is dynamic stability.

Evidence for conservative care shows positive effects of exercise, orthoses, and joint protection education (JPE) for CMC OA to reduce pain and improve function. However, evidence is not conclusive for which orthosis or which exercises are best? Also, little is known about dosage of exercise for the small muscles of the hand[1].

Dynamic stability rehabilitation strategies are used for injuries and OA at other joints in the body, such as the knee and the shoulder.[2–3] What is *dynamic stability*, and why is it used? Dynamic stability is a term to signify the restoration of functional motion, the reeducation of specific muscles to improve the strength, and the reduction of pain and disability. It also includes the promotion of self-management of pain during function. It is only recently that evidence for this approach is available for the intervention of the thumb.

The first dorsal interosseous (FDI) and the opponens (OP) are *emerging* as key muscles for thumb stability. Multiple studies show radiographically the FDI and OP can act to help center the metacarpal on the trapezium. Interestingly, one study showed concomitant activation of the FDI and OP reduced subluxation significantly, and when more force was applied, a greater radiographic reduction was noted.[4–7] This may be our first understanding of dosage. More research is required for force, frequency, and repetitions and when this should be applied in rehabilitation or prevention of thumb pain.

There are three important points for a stable thumb: release the adductor to widen the thumb web space and keep it supple; use *appropriate* thumb motors to stabilize and centralize the first metacarpal on the trapezium, with an emphasis on the combined motions of the FDI and opponens; and educate the person to care for their own thumbs for a lifetime.

Since there is no consensus for one specific orthosis to provide thumb stability, this predisposes the need for the custom fitting of the "best orthosis" for each person individually; be it custom or off the shelf, hand or forearm based. Jan Albrecht, the author of "Caring for the Painful Thumb"[8] would often say, "No two thumbs are alike." She would often even refer to the difference of even the thumbs of a person's own two hands.

It is the author's opinion that the conservative intervention of every thumb includes an individualized program of dynamic stability, with a customized orthosis as needed. It is also important to include the wear schedule to wear as pain and stability dictate with a plan to wean out of the orthosis. It is imperative to educate on joint protection and adaptive techniques and tools as well.

Another area of emerging evidence surrounds the proprioceptive end organs in the stout CMC dorsoradial ligament structure and its influence on thumb motors. A most interesting finding is proprioception of OA CMC ligaments responds differently than those of non-OA ligaments. Joint instability ALONE may not be the primary etiological factor in development of OA of CMC. Dynamic proprioceptive function of the joint is subject of exciting continuing studies and more to come.[9–11]

As regards to orthotic intervention, knowing that evidence has not demonstrated the optimum orthosis for the CMC joint of the thumb, the answer may be found in the clinical decision between the person and the therapist. It is in the essential and complete evaluation of that person and their thumb that will reveal the needful orthosis or orthoses. Of course, this may also be based on the medical information from the physician. It may be the choice is an orthosis for rest or for daily use or both. However, an uncomfortable orthosis is useless. Even more useless is one that does not provide the appropriate support where needed.

A thumb-based orthosis may be sufficient if it provides adequate support at the CMC. However, if the person has hyperextension of the MP thumb joint, this person may require support to prevent this. Others may need an orthosis to provide a wider thumb web space, allowing MCP joint motion or the traditional thumb spica orthosis. This may be thumb or hand based or forearm based.

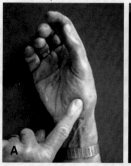
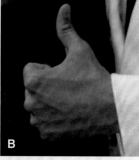

FIGURE 1 The usual point of pain: the thumb CMC joint. Even normal thumbs can have a typical deformity: a boutonniere thumb.

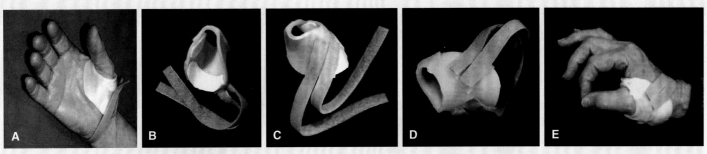

FIGURE 2 Thumb-based CMC stability orthosis, designed by Jan Albrecht, OTR, CHT (2001–2015).

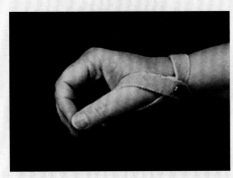

FIGURE 3 Another alternative orthosis designed by Julie Liebelt, PT, CHT, may also provide thumb abduction with CMC support for use in situations where force may overwhelm the person's ability to maintain a stable position of the thumb.

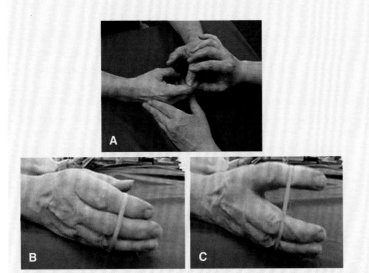

FIGURE 4 The first dorsal interosseous may be strengthened using AROM, progressing to isometric and then isotonic strengthening. The use of a rubber band as the exercise band may be a good tool for retraining this muscle.

References

1. American College of Sports Medicine. (2011). Position stand. Quantity and quality of exercise for developing and maintaining cardiorespiratory, musculoskeletal, and neuromotor fitness in apparently healthy adults: guidance for prescribing exercise. *Medical Science of Sports Exercise, 43,* 1334–1359.
2. Wilk, K. E., Macrina, L. C., & Reinold, M. M. (2006). Invited clinical commentary: Non-operative rehabilitation for traumatic and atraumatic glenohumeral instability. North American Journal Sports Physical Therapy, 1, 1–10.
3. Chmieleweski, T. L., Hurd, W. J., Rudolph, K. S., Axe, M. J., & Snyder-Mackler, L. (2005). Perturbation training improves knee kinematics and reduces muscle co-contraction after complete unilateral anterior cruciate ligament rupture. Physical Therapy, 85, 740–749.
4. Adams, J. E., O'Brien, V. H., Magnusson, E., Rosenstein, B., & Nuckley, D. J. (2018). Radiographic analysis of simulated first dorsal interosseous and opponens pollicis loading upon thumb CMC joint subluxation: A cadaver study. Hand, 13(1), 40–44. doi:https://doi.org/10.1177/1558944717691132
5. O'Brien, V. H., & Giveans, M. R. (2013). Effects of a dynamic stability approach in conservative intervention of the carpometacarpal joint of the thumb: A retrospective study. Journal of Hand Therapy, 26, 44–52.
6. McGee, C., O'Brien, V. H., Van Nortwick, S., Adams, J., & Van Heest, A. (2015). First dorsal interosseous muscle contraction results in radiographic reduction of healthy thumb carpometacarpal joint. Journal of Hand Therapy, 28, 375–381.
7. Mobargha, N., Esplugas, M., Garcia-Elias, M., Lluch, A., Megerle, K., & Hagert, E. (2015). The effect of individual isometric muscle loading on the alignment of the base of the thumb metacarpal: A cadaveric study. Journal of Hand Surgery (European Volume), 41(4), 1–6
8. Albrecht, J. (2015). *Caring for the painful thumb* (3rd. ed.). Mankato, MN: Author.
9. Hagert, E., Lee, J., & Ladd, A. L. (2012). Innervation patterns of thumb trapeziometacarpal joint ligaments. *Journal of Hand Surgery, 37A,* 706–714.e1.
10. Halilaj, E., Rainbow, M. J., Moore, D. C., Laidlaw, D. H., Weiss, A-P. C., Ladd, A.L., & Crisco, J. J. (2015). In vivo recruitment patterns in the anterior oblique and dorsoradial ligaments of the first carpometacarpal joint. *Journal of Biomechanics.* doi:10.1016/j.jbiomec.2015.04.028.
11. Mobargha, N. (2015) *The proprioception and neuromuscular stability of the basal thumb joint* (Unpublished doctoral dissertation). Karolinska Institutet, Stockholm, Sweden.

CHAPTER 17

Case Study Section

The case studies presented here are meant as a teaching guideline only. Treatment and orthosis protocols vary greatly from surgeon to surgeon and from therapist to therapist. The therapist should check with the referring physicians and colleagues to define the preferred treatment and appropriate orthotic intervention.

Case Study 1: Osteoarthritis: Thumb Carpometacarpal Joint

LS, a 45-year-old physically active and fit right-handed woman was diagnosed with bilateral first CMC joint OA. She was referred to therapy for evaluation and treatment. She presented with bilateral thumb pain that was localized to the thenar eminences and reported pain with all functional activities involving grasp and pinch.

Clinical examination revealed bilateral tenderness on palpation and thickening at the first CMC joints. No acute swelling was noted. She had a positive grind test bilaterally. AROM was equal in both hands, with thumb opposition to the SF MCP joint. Grip strength was bilaterally equal. Pinch strengths (lateral, tip, and three-point) were decreased and associated with pain.

LS was referred to therapy with a prescription for bilateral hand- and forearm-based thumb immobilization orthoses. The hand-based orthoses were to be used for days, and the forearm-based orthoses were to provide further joint rest, support, and protection while sleeping. The day orthoses were fabricated from 1/16″ Aquaplast (Fig. 17–16A). This elastic-based thermoplastic material provided the right amount of stretch and conformability to fit the first web space intimately and stabilize the first CMC joint. The night orthoses were made out of a perforated 1/8″ plastic-based material (Fig. 17–19).

LS wore the orthoses with some pain relief at home and work. However, the intensity of her thumb pain increased to the point that even with these devices, she had consistent, unrelenting pain day and night. After 5 years of conservative management, LS opted for surgical intervention of her nondominant hand first. Her surgeon performed a ligament reconstruction with a tendon interposition graft (LRTI).

The postsurgical wrist/thumb immobilization cast was worn for 4 weeks. At the time of cast removal, a wrist/thumb immobilization orthosis was applied and gentle wrist/thumb AROM was begun. The orthosis was the same night orthosis she had worn with adjustments made for postsurgical edema and dressings (Fig. 17–19). This orthosis was worn at all times except for hygiene and exercise sessions. The same device was cut down to a hand-based design at 6 weeks, and a gradual decrease in the wearing schedule was begun (Fig. 17–5B). At 8 weeks, therapy focused on grip and light thenar/pinch strengthening with orthosis use for only at-risk activities.

LS was instructed in joint protection principles and activity modifications to provide ways to decrease external stress on the thumb with ADLs. She was made a custom neoprene orthosis, which allowed her to comfortably transition from guarded use of her hand to having a light external support to aid in protection. She used this device when she engaged in activities that required repetitive wrist and thumb use. This orthosis worked well for returning to work and recreational activities (Fig. 17–69). When last seen, 12 weeks after surgery, LS was able to do her normal activities with little discomfort and was scheduling this same surgery for her dominant hand.

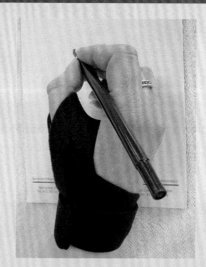

FIGURE 17–69 A custom-fabricated neoprene orthosis is used for ongoing support for ADL and vocational and recreational activities. See Chapter 14 for more information and orthotic designs with neoprene materials.

Case Study 2: Rheumatoid Arthritis: Metacarpophalangeal Joint Arthroplasty

PF is a 62-year-old right hand–dominant male who works during the day as a computer programmer and nights and weekends as an amateur musician (drummer and guitarist). He had an 8-year history of RA and was referred for fabrication of day orthoses to address ulnar drift at the MCP joints to enhance functional use. PF had limited digital ROM secondary to volar subluxation and ulnar drift of the proximal phalanges. This deformity was passively correctable at that time (Fig. 17–55). Slight radial deviation was also noted at both wrist joints.

A hand-based MCP extension and radial deviation immobilization orthosis was fabricated (Fig. 17–58C). The orthosis redirected the MCPs into extension and neutral deviation (antideformity position). Although full MCP flexion was not possible with this small design, the IP joints were free to fully flex and oppose the thumb for light functional use. Using this orthosis, PF was able to continue to use the computer keyboard. Thin thermoplastic material (3/32″) was an excellent choice for this orthosis to avoid bulk between the digits. A forearm-based wrist/hand immobilization orthosis was also fabricated for night use to complement the day device (Fig. 17–6). A carefully molded orthosis that incorporated troughs for each digit, along with a meticulous strapping technique, aided in minimizing the common zigzag deformity. This conservative treatment was satisfactory for 1 year until he began having difficulty with fine motor skills and was finding it nearly impossible to perform the simplest of work and ADL tasks. Because this decrease in function affected all aspects of his life, he sought surgical intervention.

An IF-SF MCP joint arthroplasty was performed with reconstruction of all the radial collateral ligaments (Fig. 17–60A). The patient was seen 5 days postoperatively and was placed in a daytime MCP extension mobilization orthosis and a night wrist/hand immobilization orthosis (Figs. 17–60B and 17–61). At approximately 8 days, individual PIP/DIP extension casts were placed on the fingers so that the patient could gently direct flexion forces to the MCP joints (Fig. 17–67B). These casts were used three times a day for short periods of exercise. At 2 weeks, SF MCP joint was excluded from the day orthosis because of difficulty achieving MCP flexion. At approximately 4 weeks post surgery, PF was given an IF-SF IP extension orthosis to aid in achieving MCP flexion (Fig. 17–70A,B). This exercise orthosis is effective in blocking IP flexion, directing flexion force to the MCP joint. At approximately 6.5 weeks, the patient was placed into a neoprene hand-based orthosis that supported the MCPs in extension and aided in resisting ulnar deviation forces, similar to Figure 17–59B. He wore this for light activity. PF continued to wear the forearm-based night immobilization orthosis. At 8 weeks post surgery, he had functional MCP motion. The patient and his surgeon were delighted by the improvement in his hand function and appearance.

Case Study 3: Osteoarthritis: Elbow

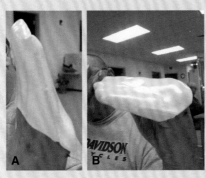

FIGURE 17–70 **A and B,** An IP extension orthosis is being used as an exercise tool to gently redirect the forces of flexion to the MCP joints.

RM is a 47-year-old right hand–dominant firefighter of 21 years. He enjoys playing various sports, including hockey and basketball, and is an avid weight lifter. He notes a gradual onset of right-sided elbow pain, stiffness, and intermittent locking of his elbow during simple ADLs and weight lifting. These symptoms first began approximately 1 year ago. RM was referred to therapy for evaluation and treatment of right elbow OA.

On his initial visit to therapy, a thorough examination of the entire upper quadrant was performed. ROM of the shoulder, wrist, and hand was within normal limits bilaterally. However, his right elbow active extension and flexion arc of motion was −25° to 120° compared to +10 (hyperextension) to 135° of elbow flexion on the contralateral elbow. Passive overpressure to both right elbow flexion and extension produced pain with minimal improvement in ROM. Both extension and flexion joint end feels were hard. Pronation and supination ROM were normal. Grip strength was 52 kg bilaterally and did not produce any pain.

RM was instructed in a home exercise program consisting of active-assisted and active elbow ROM. Furthermore, he was instructed to modify his weight lifting routine to prevent further overload to his right elbow. He was especially advised to discontinue specific elbow flexor and extensor strengthening exercises because this may cause a significant increase in joint compressive forces likely contributing to pain. He was permitted to continue strength training, monitoring the frequency, and duration

of which exercises produce the most pain. He was also instructed in proper application of heat and cold at home to assist with pain control. RM was given a soft neoprene elbow sleeve to wear during aggravating activities or when the elbow is painful (Fig. 17–20).

RMs symptoms of right elbow pain persisted, and he was extremely frustrated and opted for surgical intervention. RM underwent an arthroscopic debridement to his right elbow with removal of osteophytes and loose bodies. Also, an ulnar nerve decompression was performed at the time of surgery. Intraoperative elbow extension and flexion was −10° to 135°. He was seen in therapy on postoperative day 1. RM referral stated active-assisted, active, and passive ROM as tolerated, edema control, and an elbow extension immobilization orthosis was fabricated (Fig. 17–71). The orthosis positioned the elbow in approximately −25° of flexion and the forearm in neutral rotation. RM elbow extension and flexion ROM were −20° and 120°, respectively. He demonstrated moderate anterior elbow edema.

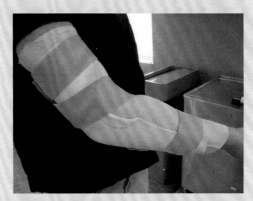

FIGURE 17–71 This orthosis was designed using a posterior approach; however, an anterior approach, similar to Fig. 17–36C, can also be considered. The choice of orthotic design is dependent on several factors including surgical incisions and dressings, the ability to position the patient for comfortable fabrication, and the material and strapping systems that are available.

RM was instructed in hourly active-assisted, active, and passive ROM exercises and edema control techniques consisting of elevation, compression, and icing. RM was instructed to wear the orthosis at night and three 20-minute periods during the day, increasing time spent in the orthosis as tolerated. RM was seen weekly in therapy to monitor his ROM improvements and for serial orthosis adjustments. After 3 weeks of therapy, his elbow ROM was −15° to 130°. Therapy for RM consisted of superficial heating via hot packs to his elbow in extension, followed by gentle passive extension ROM. Elbow extension gradually increased to −10°. Thus, his extension orthosis was remolded to accommodate this improvement in ROM. He was instructed to continue orthosis wear day and at night. At 6 weeks, his elbow ROM was −10° to 130°, and light strengthening, with an emphasis on triceps, was added to his program.

At 12 weeks after surgery, his surgeon advised him he could resume normal activities but cautioned him on returning to avid weight lifting. He recommended swimming as a resistive exercise as well as to take on more cardiovascular activities. RM final elbow ROM was −10° to 135° with little discomfort and no intermittent locking. He was able to return to firefighting with no concerns.

CHAPTER REVIEW QUESTIONS

1. Describe the general difference between osteoarthritis (OA) and rheumatoid arthritis (RA), including all joints that are commonly affected.

2. What are the general indications for use of immobilization and mobilization orthoses in both populations? Give an example of each.

3. What are the considerations for material choice in this patient population and why is it so important?

4. What is the conservative orthotic management of first CMC OA? What are the choices described in this chapter?

5. What is the difference between a swan-neck deformity and a boutonniere deformity, and how does the orthotic management differ? What material choices would one consider?

18 Extensor Tendon Injuries

Alexandra MacKenzie, OTR/L, CHT

CHAPTER OBJECTIVES

After study of this chapter, the reader should be able to:

- Identify the extensor tendon anatomy.
- Describe the three phases of wound healing and how they impact the healing tendon.
- Determine the appropriate therapeutic management and orthotic intervention for each zone of tendon injury.
- Have an understanding of the various extensor tendon protocols and indications for use.
- Appreciate the important role of communication between the patient, therapist, and surgeon.

KEY TERMS

Boutonniere
Central slip
Dorsal hood
Early active mobilization (EAM)
Early passive mobilization (EPM)
Extrinsics

Immediate active tension
Immediate controlled active motion (ICAM)
Intrinsics
Juncturae tendinum
Lateral bands
Oblique retinacular ligament
Relative motion orthosis

Sagittal bands
Short arc of motion (SAM) protocol
Swan neck
Tendon adhesion
Tendon gap
Terminal tendon

 ## MD NOTE

Steve K. Lee, MD
New York

Collaboration between the hand therapist and upper extremity surgeon is paramount to getting the best result for the patient with an extensor tendon injury. When a tendon in the hand is injured, the balance of the digits and hand is altered. After repair of the extensor tendon, there is delicate timing between adequate postoperative immobilization and postoperative movement and exercise. Clear communication between a therapist and surgeon is necessary. I prefer a combination of a detailed prescription and verbal communication. A copy of the operative note is also helpful to send to the therapist. In verbal communication, nuances can be discussed such as severity of injury and strength and confidence of the tendon repair. The prescription should have detailed instructions of splint type, exact joint positions, and precise directions of what exercises to perform and when. Continued communication is performed throughout the healing process if conditions change after surgery. Also helpful in this process if attendance at conferences where lectures and case discussions are held with therapists and surgeons. For a patient to have the best result possible, it takes teamwork of a dedicated hand therapist and surgeon.

 ## FAQ

Which thermoplastic materials work best for relative motion orthoses?
A smoother material like Polyform or TailorSplint tends to be tolerated better by the patient because so much of the plastic is laying on skin between fingers (which tends to be more sensitive). If your material is perforated, those perforations can irritate the skin (if the material is cut along the perforations), so when you are cutting the material, cut between the perforations to create a smooth surface.

What is your favorite orthosis design and treatment approach for mallet fingers?

It is preferable to check the skin and orthosis fit every 2 weeks, with the patient leaving it on full time. Sometimes it is not always possible for the patient to return (for example, if the patient lives far away from the clinic or if there are insurance constraints). If the patient is unable to return to the clinic, it is important to make sure that the patient is able to independently don/doff the orthosis while supporting the DIP in full extension on a tabletop while letting the skin air out periodically. Orthosis design depends on so many variables, but a circumferential design usually works well. For an orthosis that the patient will not be removing independently, QuickCast works well in being lightweight, fairly breathable, and easily tolerated. However, if the patient has an enlarged DIP joint or edema, a design that is open on the side seams and is taped shut may work better. This makes it easier to accommodate changes in edema.

It has been 8 weeks and it is time for the patient to come out of the mallet orthosis but after the patient left it off all day, there is a lag—what should I do?

It is important that the patient weans out of the orthosis slowly. They can wear it on and off during the day (such as wearing it with heavier hand use or when out and about). It should still be worn at night for another 4 weeks. Taping the finger in extension with either paper tape or Kinesio Tape can be helpful in gently encouraging DIP extension. If the extensor lag is particularly profound, the patient may need to resume full-time mallet orthosis use. It is important to maintain good communication with the referring physician to make sure that everyone is communicating the same information and expectations to the patient.

INTRODUCTION

Extensor tendon injuries can be disruptive to the function of the hand and can be daunting to treat. These injuries are common; however, there is more literature about flexor tendon injuries. The tendon anatomy is complicated, and scar tissue can wreak havoc with the intricate motions required of the hand. Therapeutic intervention plays a critical role in the recovery process. Tendon repair, rehabilitation techniques, and orthoses have evolved through the years, allowing for earlier motion and better outcomes. The issues for extensor tendon injuries are similar to flexor tendon injuries: risk of tendon adhesions, **tendon gapping**, risk of rupture, and loss of motion in both flexion and extension. Multiple studies have demonstrated the benefit of controlled stress to the healing tendon (Evans, 2011) and treatment techniques have evolved to incorporate these concepts.

The goal of this chapter is to give the reader a thorough understanding of extensor tendon anatomy, the healing process, common protocols, the type and timing of orthotic intervention, and how to integrate this knowledge for the most appropriate clinical decision-making in this patient population. The goals for therapy are to protect the tendon repair while providing controlled stress to the healing structures and prevention of complications.

EXTENSOR TENDONS: ANATOMY AND FUNCTION

The extensor tendon system is not designed for power, but rather to balance the power of the flexors as well as providing hand balance and coordination. The flexor system is muscle to tendon to bone, where each muscle acts primarily on one joint (secondarily contributing to flexion at each joint it crosses). Much of the extensor system is not so straightforward: there is no one single muscle/tendon unit to achieve digit extension. Contributions from both extrinsic and intrinsic muscles work together to extend the fingers, and the muscles are smaller in mass than the flexors. Fibrous bands arising from the tendons contribute greatly to finger extension. The extensor tendons balance out the power of the flexor tendons and play a large role in fine motor control.

There are nine extrinsic extensors: three each for the wrist, fingers, and thumb (extensor carpi radialis longus [ECRL], brevis and ulnaris, extensor digitorum communis [EDC], extensor indicis proprius, extensor digiti minimi [EDM], extensor pollicis longus [EPL], extensor pollicis brevis [EPB], and abductor pollicis longus [APL]). Similar to the extrinsic flexors, these muscles all originate in the forearm and insert distal to the wrist to elicit motion at the designated joint(s) (Fig. 18–1). At the level of the wrist, the tendons traverse the extensor retinaculum: a fibro-osseous tunnel system that is partitioned into six dorsal compartments (A–F) (Fig. 18–2). Compartment one contains APL and EPB, compartment two contains extensor carpi radialis brevis (ECRB) and ECRL, compartment three contains EPL, compartment four contains EDC, compartment five contains EDM, and compartment six contains extensor carpi ulnaris (ECU). In addition to acting as a source of nutrition, the extensor retinaculum acts as a pulley to give biomechanical advantage and prevent bowstringing of the extensor tendons. There is great potential for scar and adhesions to develop within the peritendinous fascia and within the synovial retinaculum with injury to the extensor tendons (Rosenthal & Elhassan, 2011). Where the digital extensors are round as they enter the retinaculum, distal to the wrist, they fan out into broad and flat tendons (Dy, Rosenblatt, & Lee, 2013). They receive nutrition from vascular mesotendon fibers (similar to vinculae in flexor tendons), from the peritendinous fascia that surrounds the tendons, and via synovial diffusion from the extensor retinaculum at the wrist.

MCP JOINT EXTENSION

The extrinsic digital extensors are the EDC, the extensor indicis proprius (EIP), and the EDM. The musculotendinous junction for EDC is approximately 4 cm proximal to the wrist, while the EIP musculotendinous junction is more distal, located at the level of the wrist joint (Dy et al., 2013). These three muscles extend the metacarpophalangeal (MCP) joints, while the EIP and the EDM allow for independent extension of the index and small fingers. The EIP and EDM tendons lie ulnar to the EDC. The EDC has tendons to the index, middle, and ring fingers, but not everyone has an EDC to the small finger. In addition, people can maintain independent function of the index finger even without an EIP because of an independent EDC muscle belly to the index finger (Moore, Weiland, & Valdata, 1987).

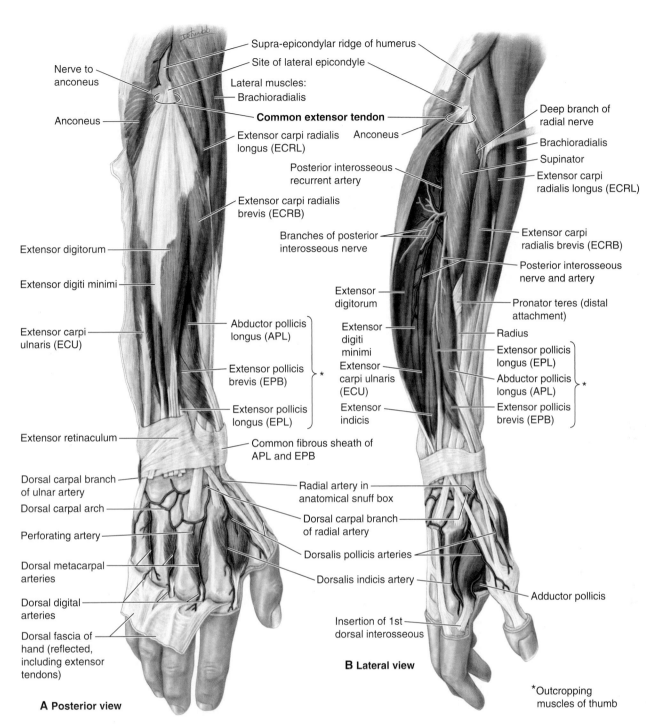

FIGURE 18-1 Muscles and neurovascular structures of the posterior compartment of forearm and hand. A, Superficial dissection. B, Deep dissection. (Reprinted with permission from Moore, K. L., Agur, A. M., & Dalley, A. F.II (2019). *Moore's Essential clinical anatomy* (6th ed.). Philadelphia, PA: Wolters Kluwer.)

The EDC does not insert on the base of the proximal phalanx; instead, MCP extension occurs as muscle contraction of EDC leads to tensioning of the fibers of the **sagittal bands**, causing MCP extension (Van Sint Jan, Rooze, Van Auderkerke, & Vico, 1996) as well as tensioning of the fibers of the **juncturae tendinum** (intertendinous connections) on the dorsum of the hand (Fig. 18–3). The **dorsal hood** is a broad fibrous structure at the MCP joint, which is composed of fibers from the EDC, the juncturae tendinum, and the sagittal bands, which work together to provide stability to the MCP joints. Injury to one structure will place excessive forces on the other (Chinchalkar, Barker, & Owsley, 2015).

The sagittal bands are ligamentous structures at the MCP joints. Their vertical fibers surround the MCP joint to insert on the volar plate and intermetacarpal ligaments. They serve two functions: (1)

to centralize the EDC over the MCP joints and (2) to transmit forces from the EDC to provide MCP extension. While the EDC does not insert directly onto the proximal phalanx, it still extends the MCP joint due to the function and anatomy of the sagittal bands. When the finger is fully flexed, the sagittal band is distal to the MCP joint. As the EDC contracts, tension on sagittal bands pulls them proximally toward the MCP, and this circumferential design helps pull the MCPs into extension. Injury to the sagittal bands (either through rupture or laceration) will result in subluxation of the EDC off the MCP joint, and this will usually occur in an ulnar direction as radial sagittal bands are not as robust as ulnar sagittal bands (Fig. 18–4).

The juncturae tendinum are bands arising from the ring-finger EDC, which branch out to the EDC of the small, middle, and

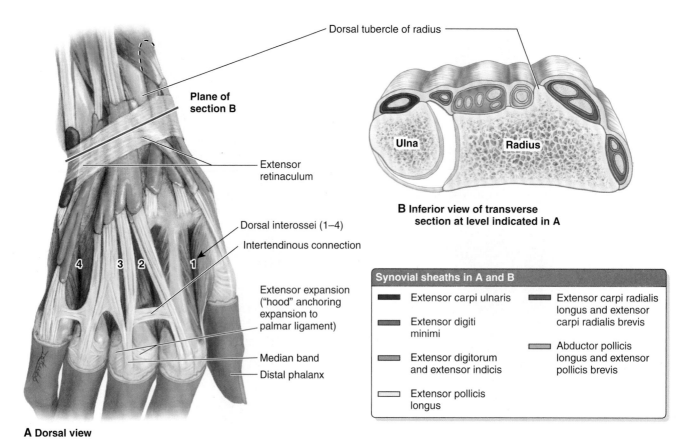

FIGURE 18–2 Synovial sheaths of extensors tendons on distal forearm and dorsum of hand. A, Illustration with color-coded synovial sheaths. B, Transverse section through distal end of radius and ulna to show extensor tendons in their synovial sheaths. (Reprinted with permission from Moore, K. L., Agur, A. M., & Dalley, A. F.II (2019). *Moore's Essential clinical anatomy* (6th ed.). Philadelphia, PA: Wolters Kluwer.)

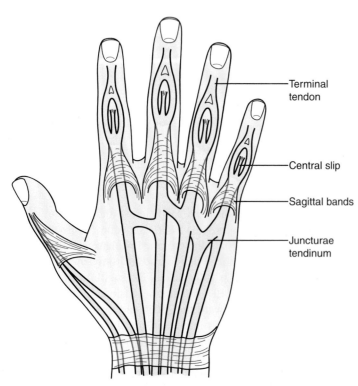

FIGURE 18–3 Juncturae tendinum function to coordinate forces between extensor tendons, while sagittal bands help centralize EDC over metacarpal heads.

occasionally the index finger as well as to the EDM. They also send fibers to the sagittal bands. The juncturae tendinum between the middle and index fingers is a smaller, thinner fibrous band (Dy et al., 2013). As the fingers flex, the juncturae become more transverse and help in stabilizing the EDC tendons. The juncturae help provide uniform extension of the fingers. If a tendon is lacerated proximal to the juncturae, tension through this structure can provide extension to the injured finger (thereby masking whether the tendon is actually lacerated). If a tendon is lacerated distal to the juncturae, those fibers help prevent proximal migration of the tendon.

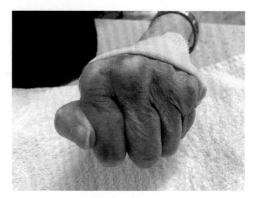

FIGURE 18–4 Subluxation of middle-finger EDC. Note how, with a full fist, the extensor tendon slides in ulnar direction in relation to metacarpal head.

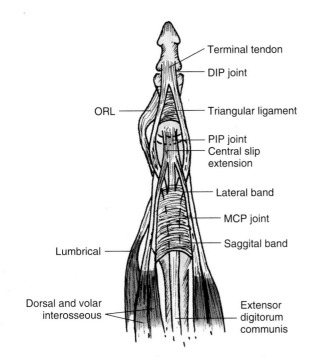

FIGURE 18-5 The intricate extensor apparatus.

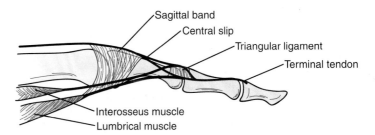

FIGURE 18-6 Lateral view of extensor mechanism to digit.

The fibers on the dorsal hood at the MCP joint continue on to the proximal phalanx and combine with fibers from the intrinsic hand muscles to form the dorsal apparatus (Fig. 18–5). These fibers contribute to both flexion and extension of the MCP joint. The more proximal vertical fibers contribute to MCP flexion, whereas the more oblique distal fibers contribute to IP extension.

IP JOINTS

If the MCP joints are not hyperextended, the EDC can also secondarily assist with IP extension, however, the prime muscles acting on IP extension are the intrinsic muscles. The fibers from EDC divide into three parts: central fibers go on to become the **central slip** (inserting at the base of the middle phalanx), while the lateral fibers combine with fibers from the intrinsic muscles to form the conjoined **lateral bands** (Dy et al., 2013).

The lumbricals are the primary IP extensors, whereas the dorsal and palmar interossei act secondarily as extensors. The lumbrical muscles originate on the flexor digitorum profundus (FDP) tendons and insert radially onto the fibers of the dorsal hood (Fig. 18–5). The lumbricals act secondarily as MCP flexors. If the FDP is contracted, the lumbricals are on slack and the IPs will not extend (the opposite is also true: if the lumbricals are contracted, the FDP relaxes). The interossei muscles originate along the metacarpals and send fibers to insert on the bases of the proximal phalanges (for finger abduction and adduction and MCP flexion), but they also send fibers to the dorsal apparatus to secondarily contribute to IP extension (if the MCP joints are extended).

The lateral fibers from the extrinsic EDC tendon combine with fibers from the intrinsic tendons to form the **lateral bands** (Fig. 18–6A–D). The lateral bands lay dorsal to the axis of proximal interphalangeal (PIP) joint motion during extension and migrate volarly during PIP flexion. The PIP joint has fibers in similar orientation as the sagittal bands. These fibers arise from the flexor tendon sheath and encircle the joint to help stabilize the lateral bands. Dorsal to the lateral bands, these fibers are called the triangular ligament and help centralize the lateral bands over the middle phalanx. The triangular ligament prevents palmar subluxation of the lateral

bands as the PIP flexes. The fibers below the lateral bands form the transverse retinacular ligament, which prevents dorsal subluxation of the lateral bands as the PIP extends. Too much volar or dorsal migration of the lateral bands can lead to deformity (**boutonniere** or **swan neck**).

The lateral bands come together over the middle phalanx to form the **terminal tendon**, which inserts on the base of the distal phalanx (Fig. 18–5). The **oblique retinacular ligament** (ORL; also known as Landsmeer's ligament) arises volarly from the flexor sheath and crosses obliquely over the middle phalanx to blend with fibers from the terminal tendon. The ORL likely does not contribute to active distal interphalangeal (DIP) extension; however, tightness of this ligament can contribute to decreased DIP flexion, particularly if the PIP joint is extended (Shrewsbury, 1977). In the normally functioning hand, extension of the PIP and DIP joints occurs together; the joints cannot extend independently (Fig. 18–7).

EXTENSOR TENDONS: THUMB

There are three extrinsic tendons for the thumb: the extensor pollicis brevis, abductor pollicis longus, and the extensor pollicis longus. In the thumb, there is one muscle per joint for extension (Figs. 18–1 and 18–2).

EXTENSOR TENDON EXCURSION

To promote tendon healing and to prevent the formation of scar adhesions, it is widely accepted that a range of 3 to 5 mm of tendon excursion is necessary, based on the work of Duran and Houser (1975) in flexor tendon models. We can apply this knowledge to how we choose a treatment option for extensor tendons. There is greater excursion of extensor tendons in proximal zones compared to distal zones, and these excursion requirements should be taken into consideration when contemplating treatment protocols. In zones I and II, there is normally only 1 to 2 mm tendon excursion, so immobilization is the treatment of choice. To prevent tendon adhesions after repair, 4 mm of glide is required in zone III and IV and in zones V to VII, 5 mm of glide is required (Howell & Peck, 2013; Evans, 2012). Flexion of the MCP joints to 30° will result in 5 mm of tendon glide in zones V to VII, while 21° of wrist extension will result in little tension on a repaired EDC in zones V to VI with active finger flexion (Chinchalkar & Pipicelli, 2009).

WOUND HEALING

In treating tendon injuries, it is important to be aware of the basic concepts of tissue/wound healing. Review of Chapter 3 and further reading in this area is recommended. Having an understanding of the concepts of healing will help guide the therapist

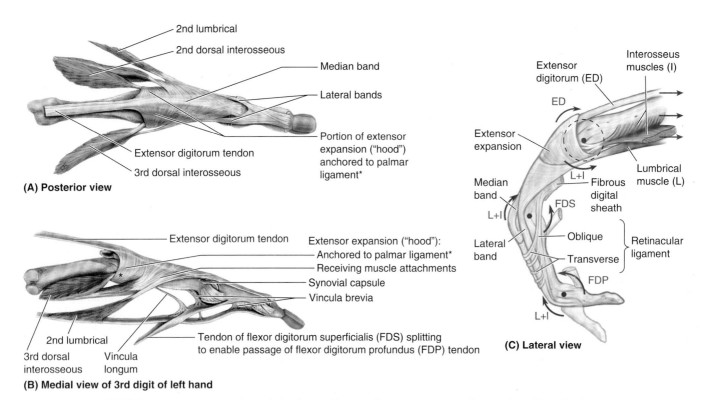

FIGURE 18–7 Extensor expansion and vincula. A and B, Parts of extensor expansion. The vincula are fibrous bands that convey small vessels to the tendons. C, Retinacular ligaments. (Reprinted with permission from Moore, K. L., Agur, A. M., & Dalley, A. F.II (2019). *Moore's Essential clinical anatomy* (6th ed.). Philadelphia, PA: Wolters Kluwer.)

in the clinical decision-making process. Not only is the tendon undergoing healing but also all of the surrounding tissues. There are three phases that all overlap as the body moves from one phase to the next.

INFLAMMATORY PHASE

The first phase is the inflammatory phase; this is the body's immediate response to a traumatic event (surgery can also be considered a traumatic event) (Fig. 18–8A). This phase can last anywhere from 3 to 7 days postoperatively.

FIBROBLASTIC PHASE

The second phase is called the fibroblastic or proliferative phase. In this phase, fibroblasts start the production of collagen fibers (Fig. 18–8B). Early collagen fibers are weak, disorganized, and have little tensile strength, but they begin to lay the foundation for stronger collagen fibers that will be produced in the later phase. The fibroblastic phase lasts from around day 5 to day 21.

REMODELING/MATURATION PHASE

The third and longest phase is the remodeling or maturation phase. Early collagen fibers begin to become more differentiated and more linear, and the tendon gains tensile strength (Fig. 18–8C). The early collagen fibers are broken down (lysis) and newer, stronger, more mature fibers are produced. In the earlier phases of scar production, collagen fibers are dense and disorganized, but over time, the collagen fibers lie in a more parallel orientation (e.g., cooked spaghetti in a pot vs. dry spaghetti in the box). Collagen fibers that are more parallel take up less room and do a better job of gliding through surrounding tissue. This phase can last anywhere from 3 weeks postoperatively to well over a year. Externally, we can watch the scar and determine how well it will

respond to therapeutic techniques. A pink-red scar is metabolically active and is still undergoing the remodeling phase, whereas a scar that has faded to a color paler than the surrounding skin is no longer active and is less likely to respond to efforts aimed at changing scar tissue properties.

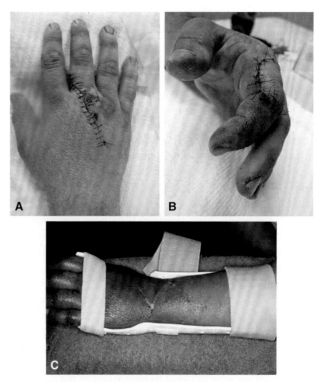

FIGURE 18–8 Stages of wound healing. **A,** Inflammatory stage shown after saw injury 2 days postoperatively. **B,** Attempts at active flexion during proliferative stage during the height of collagen synthesis. **C,** Scar maturation phase noted by fading of scar and dense adhesion formation during active digital extension.

EXTENSOR TENDON SURGICAL REPAIR

Much has been written about surgical technique and tendon healing principles for flexor tendons, however, there is much less in the literature about this same information for extensor tendons despite how common extensor tendon injuries are. Surgical techniques and postoperative protocols are based on what is known about extensor tendon anatomy as well as on flexor tendon research. Ultimately, the goal is a repair that will not attenuate or rupture and will glide smoothly, resulting in functional range of motion (ROM). Studies have shown that **early protected mobilization** has beneficial effects on healing tendon, leading to increased tensile strength and increased ability for tendon gliding to occur (Buckwalter & Grodzinsky, 1999; Fong et al., 2005; Gelberman, Woo, Lothringer, Akeson, & Amiel, 1982). In order for the tendon to withstand the forces required of it during early protected mobilization, the repair itself must be strong but not so bulky as to be unable to glide through the surrounding tissue. The information gleaned from flexor tendon research can be applied to healing extensor tendons.

Most of the excursion occurring in the extensor tendon system is proximal to the wrist: there is very little excursion occurring after the wrist. Therefore, it is crucial to try to restore the normal length of the tendons so as not to disrupt the delicate balance. An extensor tendon which heals too long (on stretch) will lead to an extensor lag, while a tendon that is too short will lead to difficulty fully flexing the digit.

Extensor tendons distal to the extensor retinaculum are thinner and flatter than flexor tendons, making it more challenging to perform a repair that is strong enough to tolerate early motion as there is simply not enough tendon to perform core sutures, as is done in flexor tendons. A running horizontal mattress suture has been found to be biomechanically strong enough to handle early motion for extensor tendon injuries in zones II to V (Dy et al., 2013).

It is important to watch for signs of infection during the postoperative course of recovery. Infection may interfere with the stages of wound healing and prolong the healing process as well as create more scar tissue.

POSTOPERATIVE TREATMENT

THERAPY EVALUATION

Treatment of tendon injuries requires a team approach: a skilled surgeon, an experienced hand therapist, and a patient who can follow through with the home exercise program (HEP). If an early mobilization program is going to be used, therapy should begin 3 to 5 days postoperatively in order to prevent adhesions, limit joint stiffness, and promote tendon glide. Communication with the referring surgeon is essential. All measurements (e.g., PROM, edema, sensation) that are safe to document should be taken at the initial visit and at regular intervals throughout the course of therapy. Box 18–1 outlines important questions to consider asking the referring doctor.

IMPORTANT INFORMATION TO GATHER

Choosing the right treatment approach will depend on several factors; a thorough history must be taken at the initial visit. Information gathered should include the following (Tan et al., 2010; van Adrichem, Hovius, van Strik, & van der Meulen, 1992):

- Mechanism of injury
- Past medical history (conditions such as diabetes and arthritis may have a negative impact on healing potential)
- Medications: NSAIDs have been shown to inhibit production of tendon cells and increase the production of collagen, both potentially leading to more scar tissue (Su & O'Connor, 2013). However, Tan et al. in 2010 demonstrated that NSAIDs appear to reduce flexor tendon adhesions. Use of NSAIDs should always be discussed with the physician as there are differing thoughts on the benefits versus the risks.
- Social habits such as smoking or drinking (van Adrichem et al. in 1992 demonstrated that cigarette smoke negatively impacts microcirculation after surgery)
- Any preexisting injuries to the affected hand that would lead to a decrease in ROM
- Concomitant injuries may prevent early mobilization; these can include fracture, nerve or vascular repair, skin grafts, and a tenuous repair that is unable to withstand the forces necessary that occur during mobilization
- Age plays a factor in clinical decision-making. The patient must be cognizant and able to understand the precautions and exercise program. Patients who are too young may not be able to participate in an early mobilization postoperative program. Older patients may have a decreased capacity for healing

FACTORS THAT MAY HINDER ATTENDANCE TO THERAPY

There are other significant factors that may hinder the patient coming to therapy for the prescribed frequency or being able to come at all. These may include,

- Lack of or limited insurance coverage or high co-pays, co-insurance, and/or deductibles
- Being able to get to and from therapy because of distance or transportation issues
- Having a clear understanding of the importance and value of therapeutic intervention with this serious injury
- Family and work commitments

BOX 18–1   PHYSICIAN QUESTIONS

Note: These are only a few of the many questions a clinician should discuss with the referring surgeon.

- What was the condition of the tendon?
- Were there any other structures involved? Nerves, arteries, bones?

- Was the tendon repaired and what is the strength of the repair?
- Will the patient be able to tolerate an early AROM program?
- What joints should be included or left free in the orthosis?

For these reasons and more, education is paramount. An overeager patient may exercise too much, potentially leading to increased swelling, scar tissue, gapping, and/or rupture. A patient who does not understand the importance of or comply with the home program may be overly fearful and more likely to develop stiffness and motion-limiting adhesions.

A smooth and freely gliding tendon that is able to produce a functional ROM is always the goal. As the tendon passes through the soft-tissue structures of the hand, a certain amount of normal "drag" is encountered. However, in an injured hand, drag may be heightened by postinjury and postoperative edema, sutures, scar tissue, and/or a dressing that is bulky or too tight. Edema, adhesions, and other injured tissues can create biologic resistance. Tendon rupture, gapping, or attenuation at the repair site are consequences that could occur if the tendon is moved too forcefully. It is difficult to assess if gapping has occurred, but it can lead to problems such as increased scar formation, a weaker tendon, and an extensor tendon lag.

FACTORS INFLUENCING PROGNOSIS

Other factors that may have an impact on prognosis and tendon healing include the following:

- Level of injury (zone)
- Type of injury
- Other structures involved (bone, nerve, ligaments)
- Clean laceration versus a crush injury: the more trauma there is to the tissue at time of injury, the greater the potential for scar tissue (Pettengill & Van Strien, 2011)
- Surgical technique (careful handling of the tendon will minimize scar tissue and risk for adhesions)
- Suture strength
- Timing of repair (after 2 weeks, the ends tend to scar down to surrounding tissue)

CLINICAL DECISION-MAKING

The therapist will need to evaluate when the patient can be advanced through the next stages of therapy or when the patient needs to be held back. Some people tend to produce more scar than others; therefore, it is necessary to individually tailor each therapy program. A patient may need to be progressed a little sooner if they are particularly stiff or held back a little longer if the patient is moving too well.

SCAR REMODELING

Scar management techniques can begin once the wound is closed. Silicone gel sheeting (sold by various manufacturers) may assist in preventing the formation of excessive scar tissue. The mechanisms by how silicone gel sheeting works are not fully understood, however, there are a few hypotheses. First, the silicone is able to keep the scar at a balanced level of hydration, and this balance signals to the body to not produce excessive amounts of collagen. Secondly, the silicone gel sheet absorbs the tension from the wound edges, preventing hypertrophic scar formation. Thirdly, silicone dressings inhibit excessive circulation leading to less collagen formation at the scar area. By reducing collagen at the targeted area, the scar becomes paler and less visible, without the red and purple skin tone that scars can often become (Bleasdale et al., 2015) (Fig. 18–9A–C). Scar remodeling materials can be incorporated into techniques

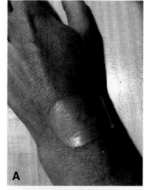
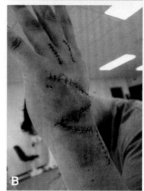
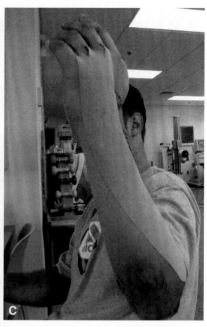

FIGURE 18–9 A, Silicone gel sheeting is an effective tool in scar management and conforms well around joints and curved surfaces. **B and C,** Zone IV–VI extensor tendon injury; the use of elastic therapeutic tape applied early postoperative can assist to mobilize edema and give light tension on the skin for adhesion intervention.

for edema reduction to create gentle compression to the scar during resting hours. The compression properties contribute to desensitizing a hypersensitive scar and assists in remodeling dense, thick, hypertrophic scars. Elastic therapeutic tape may also be helpful for dorsal hand scars which have a propensity to becoming adherent (Fig. 18–10A–E).

EXTENSOR TENDON PROTOCOLS: USING CLINICAL JUDGMENT

To mobilize or not to mobilize a repaired extensor tendon is something that needs to be considered when determining the postoperative course of treatment. The treatment of choice will primarily depend on the zone of injury. Extensor tendon injuries can be treated with either immobilization, early passive mobilization (EPM), or early active mobilization (EAM). Extensor tendon injuries tolerate early motion well in all zones except for zone I. The risks of rupture or tendon attenuation from an early mobilization program do not seem to be as great with extensor tendons as with flexor tendons (Evans, 2012; Newport & Tucker, 2005; Griffin, Hindocha, Jordan, Saleh, & Khan, 2012). Ruptures that occur may be caused by the powerful force of flexion rather than via forced extension as the extensors are not as powerful as the flexors.

There are multiple benefits to mobilizing a tendon early, such as decreased potential for joint contractures, tendon adhesion, decreased time in therapy, and earlier return to function. It has been demonstrated in multiple studies that early loading of healing tissue helps strengthen material properties of the tissue (Buckwalter & Grodzinsky, 1999; Fong et al., 2005; Gelberman et al., 1982; Kubota, Manske, Mitsuhiro, Pruitt, & Larson, 1996). The rationale

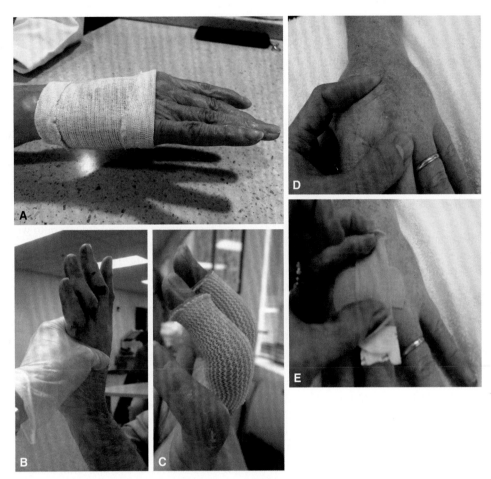

FIGURE 18–10 A, Otoform˜ is an effective silicone mold for scar management and can be held in place on the hand with an elasticized stockinette; **B and C,** Silipos® sleeves used to manage these zone III for digital scars and provides circumferential management of edema; **D and E,** Elastic therapeutic tape applied in a crisscross fashion over an adherent zone V scar. The direction of the tape assists in scar mobilization.

is that early stress to the tendons promotes healing both intrinsically and extrinsically. Most research on properties of tendon healing has been on flexor tendons within a synovial sheath or on animal models. Knowledge of flexor tendon healing properties can be applied to extensor tendon healing, as the principles and timelines of wound healing should be similar. Please refer to Chapter 3 for further information on tendon healing.

Another consideration with any tendon injury is that there may be concomitant injuries (fractures, neurovascular repairs, etc.), and those injures may dictate the postoperative course of treatment. The greater the bony and/or soft-tissue damage, the greater the likelihood for the formation of adhesions. Tendon adhesions can cause loss of motion in both flexion and extension. Loss of flexion and decreased grip strength both have a greater impact on function than an extensor lag. However, lags are more difficult to correct than soft-tissue tightness, and, therefore, a repaired extensor tendon should be positioned in slack postoperatively.

Hall, Lee, Page, Rosenwax, and Lee (2010) compared all three treatment options: immobilization, EPM, and EAM. These studies showed no long-term differences between the treatment protocols, although it was found that patients who were immobilized were more likely to have extensor lags and decreased flexion than other treatment groups and that patients using EAM saw the earliest gains in motion and return to function.

IMMOBILIZATION

Immobilization is the only treatment option for injuries occurring in zone I. For injuries occurring in more proximal zones, there is evidence that the tendons tolerate immobilization as well, although the recovery process will take longer than if an early mobilization protocol is used. Multiple studies have looked at injuries in zones V to VIII and compared early mobilization (either active or controlled dynamic passive motion) with immobilization. They have shown that although patients performing an early mobilization protocol have more motion at week 4, in the long term, there are no functional differences between the protocols (Bulstrode, Burr, Pratt, & Brobbelaar, 2005; Talsma, de Haart, Beelen, & Nollet, 2008). One study found that by 6 months, there were no significant differences in grip strength between the immobilized and mobilized groups (Mowlavi, Burns, & Brown, 2005). Purcell, Eadie, Murugan, O'Donnell, and Lawless (2000) found 95% good or excellent results with the use of an immobilization orthosis at 4 months postoperatively.

With early mobilization, patients may return to previous level of function sooner than if immobilized; however, not every patient may be appropriate for an early mobilization protocol. Patients who are very young or who are unable to be compliant with an early mobilization exercise program may be appropriate for an immobilization protocol.

EARLY MOBILIZATION PROTOCOLS

There are differing opinions on when to initiate early motion. Several studies (Halikis, Manske, Kubota, & Aoki, 1997; Zhao et al., 2004) found that the tendon encounters the least amount of work when motion is initiated anywhere from 3 to 7 days postoperatively (compared to initiating motion days 0–2 postoperatively). The first few days after surgery, the tendon is presented with a lot of resistance (due to newly traumatized tissue), and more force is required of the tendon to achieve motion. Waiting a few days allows the tissue to rest and inflammation to go down.

Early Passive Mobilization

Early passive mobilization protocols for injuries in zones V to VII were developed in the 1980s in an effort to promote intrinsic tendon healing. In the early passive mobilization protocol for injuries in zones V to VIII, the orthosis positions the wrist in 45° of extension, and the MCPs are positioned in full extension via dynamic rubber band tension. The MCPs are allowed to actively flex to 40°, and they are passively extended back to neutral via rubber band tension. In order to get a correct line of pull, there is a dorsal outrigger for the rubber bands to pass over.

There are few studies which compare early active with early controlled dynamic mobilization, and there is no evidence to show that EPM is superior to EAM (Chester, Beale, Beveridge, Nancarrow, & Titley, 2002; Khandwala, Webb, Harris, Foster, & Elliot, 2000; Hall et al., 2010). Eissens, Schut, and van der Sluis (2007) recommend adding protected wrist motion to the dynamic orthosis for zones V to VII, although there is no evidence to show this as being more effective than other early mobilization protocols. Newport and Shukla (1992) found that in a dynamic orthosis, it is unlikely that the extension is truly passive and that some degree of active extension is occurring.

With EPM, the orthosis is time-consuming and can be costly to fabricate. The exercise regime is more complicated and the orthosis, if dynamic, is more cumbersome for daily life, both of which may reduce overall compliance. If feasible, EAM should be the treatment of choice for treatment of extensor tendon injuries in zones V to VII.

Early Active Mobilization

Early active mobilization protocols were developed to encourage tendon movement while preventing buckling of the tendon (Hall et al., 2010). With EPM protocols, the tendon achieves some glide, but the tendon is more likely to be compressed or "bunched up" rather than actually gliding through soft tissue. True gliding has better potential to help prevent adhesions.

Early controlled active range of motion (AROM) protocols require orthoses that are simpler and less expensive to fabricate than an early passive mobilization orthosis; they are also less cumbersome for the patient to wear, which is likely to maximize compliance. There are various early controlled active mobilization protocols that allow for AROM within the limitations of the orthosis (Khandwala et al., 2000; Merritt, Howell, Tune, Saunders, & Hardy, 2000; Sylaidis, Youatt, & Logan, 1997).

Multiple studies have shown favorable outcomes with early mobilization, with earlier return of total arc of motion and without an increase in rate of complications (Chow, Dovelle, Thomes, Ho, & Saldana, 1989; Howell, Merritt, & Robinson, 2005; Ip & Chow, 1997; Russell, Jones, & Grobbelaar, 2003; Sameem, Wood, Ignacy, Thoma, & Strumas, 2011; Sylaidis et al., 1997; Wong et al., 2017). There is evidence that patients using an EAM protocol can return

to work earlier: as soon as 18 days with a relative motion extension orthosis (RMO), 6 weeks with the Norwich regime protocol, and 10 weeks with dynamic extension mobilization (Canham & Hammert, 2013).

The nomenclature for EAM in the literature varies. **Controlled active motion (CAM)** can refer to any early protected active motion, and **relative motion extension** refers to a protocol where the injured digit is placed approximately 20° more extension than the neighboring digits and is reserved for tendon injuries in zones V to VI. Relative motion orthoses are discussed in greater detail in Chapter 7.

A recent systematic review comparing different EAM protocols found that RME studies tend to be newer compared to CAM studies and that patients were able to return to work earlier with the RME protocol although ROM and grip strength outcomes were similar with both protocols. There were fewer reports of ruptures in the RME groups compared to CAM (Collocott, Kelly, & Ellis, 2018).

Hirth, Howell, and O'Brien (2016) did a literature search and found that treatment using RME for zones IV to VII had either similar or superior results compared to other treatments including early controlled mobilization, early passive mobilization using a dynamic orthosis, or immobilization. They also found variability of inclusion of a wrist orthosis, with later studies being less likely to include a wrist orthosis as well as overall shorter duration of orthosis wear. Few complications with this protocol have been reported after EDC repair zones IV to VII, with earlier return-to-work times (Hirth et al., 2016). A systemic review (Ng et al., 2012) found similar results. As EAM and EPM outcomes are similar, the simpler EAM protocol is favored due to overall lower cost, shorter time investment, and increased patient comfort.

Collocott, Kelly, & Foster, (2020) compared CAM to RME and found superior results with RME. They did not use a wrist orthosis with the RME orthosis; however, they did have patients wear a wrist, hand, and finger immobilization orthosis (WHFO) at night. The CAM protocol used a static orthosis with MCP joints positioned in 30° of flexion and the wrist in 40° of extension and the interphalangeal joints (IPs) free, with an additional extension orthosis to hold the IPs straight at night. There were no ruptures in either group and patients in the RME group had earlier return to work, earlier total active motion (TAM), and improved satisfaction with orthosis design.

With any early AROM protocol, it is the *quality* of motion achieved that is important: The exercises should be performed correctly in order to achieve the most glide with the lowest load on injured structures. Increasing the exercise frequency will not have an impact on adhesion formation if the tendon is not gliding. In addition, over-exercising may incite an inflammatory response, which may lead to more adhesions. However, frequency of exercise has been associated with improved tensile strength of the tendon (Evans, 2011).

ZONES OF INJURY AND TREATMENT BY ZONE

The extensor tendons are separated into eight zones. Treatment of extensor tendon injuries varies greatly depending on the zone of injury. All of the odd-numbered zones are over joints. Zone I is over the DIP joint, zone III is over the PIP joint, zone V is over the MCP joint, and zone VII is over the wrist. The zones are numbered distal to proximal (as in the flexor tendon zones) (Fig. 18–11) (Table 18–1).

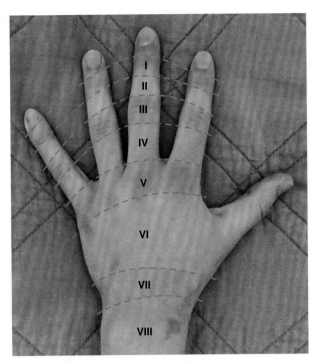

FIGURE 18–11 Extensor tendon zones of injury.

TABLE 18–1	Extensor Tendon Zones of Injury
Zone I	Over the DIP joint. This zone includes the terminal tendon.
Zone II	Over the middle phalanx.
Zone III	Over the PIP joint. This zone contains the central slip and the lateral bands.
Zone IV	Over the proximal phalanx. There is a large amount of contact between the tendon and bone in this zone, which can lead to significant adherence to the bone.
Zone V	Over the MCP joint. This zone contains the sagittal bands.
Zone VI	Over the dorsum of the hand. This zone contains the juncturae tendinum, where the tendons are broad and flat.
Zone VII	Over the wrist. This zone contains the extensor retinaculum, which is synovial and may lead to increased scarring in this zone. Without the retinaculum, the tendons will have a tendency to bowstring, which will decrease excursion and strength.
Zone VIII	Dorsal forearm just proximal to the extensor retinaculum. Includes the musculotendinous junctions of the digital and wrist extensors.
Zone TI	At the thumb IP joint. This is where the EPL inserts.
Zone TII	Over the proximal phalanx.
Zone TIII	Over the thumb MCP joint. In addition to the EPL passing through here, this is where the EPB inserts.
Zone TIV	At the level of the first metacarpal.
Zone TV	At the level of the wrist. This includes the extensor retinaculum, which is synovial and may lead to increased scar tissue formation in this zone.

Note: Zones are described distal to proximal. All of the odd-numbered zones are over joints.

ZONES I AND II

Zone I lies over the DIP joint and, when injured, is commonly referred to as a mallet finger. The structure of importance in this zone is the terminal tendon. Injury can occur through tendon rupture, laceration, avulsion fracture of the bone where the tendon inserts, or through crush injury (Fig. 18–12A,B). Mucous cysts from osteoarthritis at the DIP joint can also secondarily lead to a mallet finger. Even if the terminal tendon is completely lacerated, the DIP joint will not assume a fully flexed position; rather, it will rest in approximately 45° of flexion. This is because of the action of the collateral ligaments and the ORL.

Zone II lies over the middle phalanx. Injuries here are usually the result of laceration or crush injury. After the tendon is repaired, treatment is the same as it is for zone I injuries.

Mallet injuries are usually the result of forceful flexion of an extended finger and the mechanism can often seem relatively benign (making a bed, cleaning a carpet, tucking in a shirt). An avulsion of the terminal tendon off the bone or a fracture at the site of tendinous insertion will both result in a mallet finger. Regardless of the mechanism of injury, the mallet finger is treated by immobilizing the DIP joint in extension and maintaining that position for 6 to 8 weeks, followed by 2 to 4 weeks of night immobilization and with strenuous activity to prevent an extension lag (Fig. 18–13A–H) (Griffin et al., 2012; Lamaris & Matthew, 2017; Dy et al., 2013). If the DIP joint is allowed to flex at any point in the initial 6 to 8 weeks, the integrity of the healing process is interrupted, and the immobilization regimen must start again. A gap of just .5 mm will lead to a 10° extensor lag (Howell & Peck, 2013). Tendon repair is not a surgical option at this level of injury, although placement of a K-wire through the DIP joint is an option for some patients (in patients with chronic mallet, complex open injuries or patients who may be less compliant with an orthosis regimen). K-wire placement is also recommended if there is a fracture with disruption of the joint surface which is greater than 1/3 or if there is subluxation of the DIP joint (Lamaris & Matthew, 2017; Dy et al., 2013; Lin & Samora, 2018).

For most mallet finger injuries, the treatment of choice is immobilization with an orthosis. The PIP joint is left free in the orthosis. The mallet orthosis can be challenging to fabricate. An orthosis which provides rigid stability both volarly and dorsally (as in a circumferential orthosis) is preferred to maintain DIP hyperextension. Volarly, the orthosis must be long enough to provide sufficient support for DIP extension, but it must not be so long that it blocks PIP flexion or causes the orthosis to migrate distally as the PIP flexes. The small finger is the most difficult finger to achieve this balance because of the shortened lever arms (see Chapter 4, for detailed instructions and helpful hints). Prior to orthosis fabrication, it may be helpful to place paper tape or elastic therapeutic tape to hold the DIP in extension. This can give added security in the orthosis (Fig. 18–14A–D). A pilot study by Devan (2014) advocated the use of elastic therapeutic tape. Custom orthoses have been shown to have more favorable outcomes and decreased skin complications when compared to prefabricated or aluminum foam–type orthoses (O'Brien & Bailey, 2011; Witherow & Peiris, 2015).

An untreated mallet finger may lead to a swan-neck deformity over time as the fibers from the ORL are stretched for a prolonged period of time (Chinchalkar et al., 2010; Griffin et al., 2012). A combination of a flexed DIP joint and a hypermobile PIP joint may lead to dorsal migration of the lateral bands as the triangular ligament tightens and the transverse retinacular ligaments stretch. This can eventually lead to difficulty flexing the PIP. If the patient has a hypermobile PIP, it

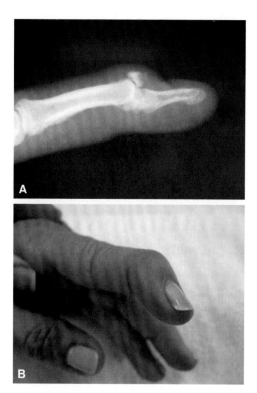

FIGURE 18–12 A, Zone I extensor tendon injury (mallet finger) with bony avulsion; **B,** mallet injury posture.

is recommended that a separate PIP extension restriction orthosis be made, which allows PIP flexion but not hyperextension, with the aim of preventing a swan-neck deformity (Fig. 18–15A–C).

Extensor lags are a complication with mallet finger injuries, and weaning out of the orthosis slowly is recommended, with nighttime extension recommended up until 12 weeks post initiation of treatment. Lutz, Pipicelli, and Grewal (2015) recommend gradually allowing DIP flexion over time: 20° to 30° for the first 2 weeks, 40 to 50 over the next 2 weeks, and then unrestricted DIP motion after that. An exercise template can be used to prevent overstretching of injured structures (Fig. 18–16A,B). Saito and Kihara (2016) found that patients had improved DIP extension outcomes when a two-step orthosis program was used: the PIP joint is held in slight flexion and the DIP in slight hyperextension for the first 2 to 3 weeks of immobilization (Fig. 18–17). After the initial treatment period, the PIP is freed up and only the DIP is held in slight hyperextension for the remainder of the 6-week treatment course.

EXPERT PEARL 18–1

Mallet Orthosis Fabrication Tip
KIM ROSINSKI OTR/L, CSCS, CHT
Pennsylvania

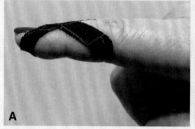

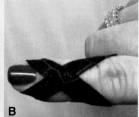

Kinesio Tape used to extend DIP during mallet orthosis fabrication or apply it when the orthosis is discontinued and extensor lag persists. Rip middle of the tape, pull in opposite directions, apply the middle onto the fingertip. Apply pull to keep the DIP extended. Crisscross the ends over the dorsal DIP.

EXPERT PEARL 18–2

Alternative Mallet Orthosis
KERRY A. RAYMOND, MS, OTR, CHT, CFCE
New Hampshire

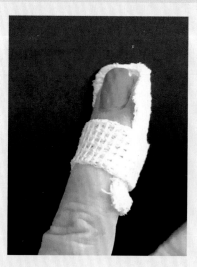

QuickCast material can be easily and quickly used to fabricate a low-profile Mallet orthosis. Several layers of material are used to improve stability for the volar segment. The dorsal piece can be fashioned by folding the 1″ width in half and wrapping around the DIP to secure.

EXPERT PEARL 18–3

Thin Edging Material
JANINE THOMAS, OTR/L, CHT, COMT
Virginia

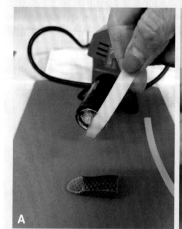

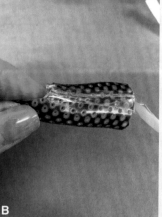

Use of Rolyan® Aquaplast® Ultra thin edging material on Mallet and Boutonniere orthoses. Cut the width in 2, activate with heat gun and use this to seal the seam. This material can also be used to line the rough edges when perforated materials are used.

ZONES III AND IV

Zone III lies over the PIP joint and contains the central slip as well as the lateral bands and transverse retinacular ligaments. Zone IV lies over the proximal phalanx. Injuries in either zone are treated the same and can be either closed or open.

The central slip is the portion of the tendon that can initiate PIP extension from a flexed position. The lateral bands can maintain extension once the joint is extended and if they lie dorsal to the axis of joint motion (Rosenthal & Elhassan, 2011).

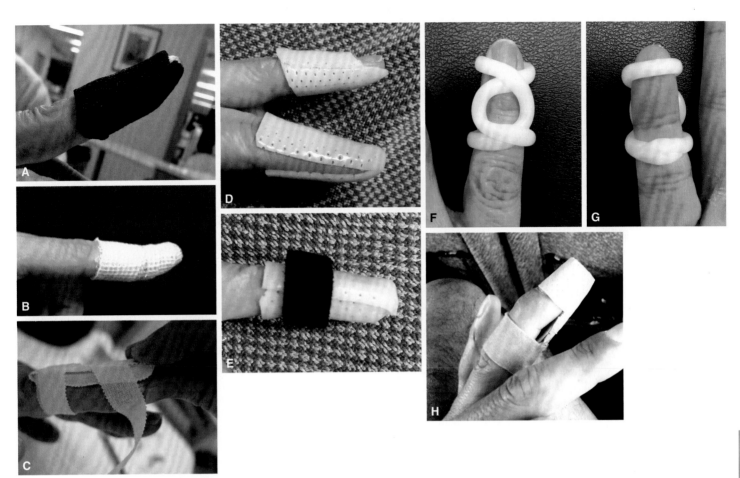

FIGURE 18–13 Various styles of orthoses for mallet finger, where the DIP is positioned in slight hyperextension and the PIP is left free: **A,** Mallet-finger orthosis made with Orficast® (Orfit Industries); **B,** Orthosis fabricated using QuickCast 2 (Patterson Medical). **C,** AlumaFoam® applied dorsally—note placement of tape at an angle to contour at tip. **D and E,** Options fabricated from 1/16″ 11% perforated thermoplastic **(F and G)** figure-8 design using Aquatube. **H,** Ineffective mallet-finger orthosis—notice how DIP is positioned in flexion.

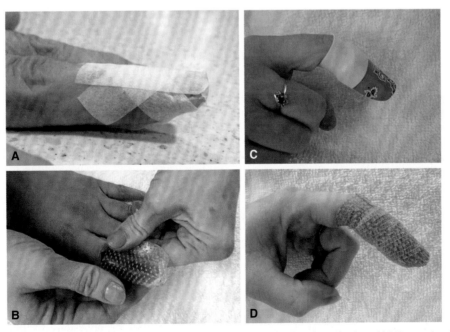

FIGURE 18–14 A, Paper tape placed in a figure-8 fashion can be used within the orthosis to aid DIP extension; **B,** elastic therapeutic tape is used to assist the DIP into extension and the orthosis is fabricated over this. **C,** Microfoam™ surgical tape (3M) is a soft flexible tape that can be used to assist in securing the orthosis on the distal phalanx and preventing distal migration; **D,** elasticized wrap can also be used to ensure immobilization. Note that in both **(C and D)** the wraps encompass both the proximal end of the orthosis as well as the proximal "skin."

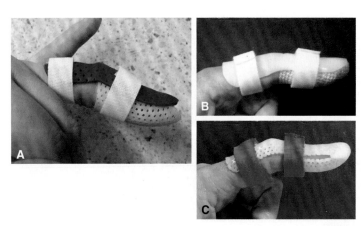

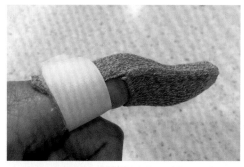

FIGURE 18-17 Two-step "mallet-finger" orthosis, where the PIP is held in flexion for the first 2-3 weeks of immobilization before transitioning to a traditional mallet finger orthosis. Orficast® material shown here.

FIGURE 18-15 Mallet-finger orthosis options with dorsal PIP extension restriction chosen with hypermobile PIP causing finger to assume swan-neck deformity (PIP hyperextension/DIP flexion). **A,** Orficast® used for PIP dorsal block and **(B)** QuickCast 2 used for DIP orthosis. The dorsal gutter can be removed for PIP flexion exercises. **(C)** Alternate method of using a single orthosis to position DIP in extension and PIP in flexion—this one is more challenging to fabricate due to positioning of joints.

Boutonniere Injury

A boutonniere deformity will result from injury to three structures: the central slip, the triangular ligament, and dorsal hood fibers from the interossei. In this scenario, the PIP joint assumes a flexed posture after "button-holing" through damaged structures and the DIP is hyperextended. The lateral bands, untethered from the triangular ligament, are allowed to migrate volarly. This shortens the connection to the terminal tendon, pulling the DIP into hyperextension, while paradoxically flexing the PIP. The flexor digitorum superficialis (FDS), which is now unopposed, further pulls the PIP into flexion, accentuating the deformity. The lateral bands also act as flexors of the PIP joint when they are volar to the axis of motion (Fig 18–18A–C). Over time, tissues shorten and the deformity becomes fixed. If this is the case, then the flexion contracture must be treated before the tendon injury. Even partial injury to any of the extensor structures at the PIP joint can lead to decreased PIP extension, without it being a true boutonniere. However, even with partial injury to central slip, there is increased tension on intact structures (triangular ligament) which may lead to a latent or chronic boutonniere deformity (Grau et al., 2018).

The Elson test can be a helpful diagnostic tool if injury to the central slip is suspected. In this test, the PIP joint is flexed to 90° over the edge of a table. The patient is asked to extend the finger with resistance placed over the middle phalanx (Fig 18–19A). If the central slip is intact, resistance will be felt and the DIP will be unable to extend fully. If there is disruption to the central slip, the forces of extension will instead be directed to the lateral bands and the DIP will extend (Amirtharajah & Lattanza, 2015; Lutz et al., 2015).

The Boyes test is another test which can be used in chronic boutonniere deformities when trying to rule out whether a PIP flexion contracture is due to volar plate or flexor tendon pulley injury (aka a "pseudo-boutonniere") or if there is extensor tendon involvement. The DIP joint is passively flexed with the PIP in extension and then again with PIP flexion. If the DIP is more difficult to passively flex with the PIP in extension than flexion, then it is more likely to be a boutonniere deformity due to lateral band involvement (Fig 18–19B) (Merritt, 2014).

Closed Injuries

A closed boutonniere is treated conservatively: the PIP joint is immobilized at 0° for 6 weeks (Figs. 18–18B and 18–20). Flexion exercises are introduced gradually, with the focus on maintaining active extension. The orthosis is worn between exercise sessions for another 2 to 4 weeks. A circumferential orthosis is commonly the best immobilization option; the pressure aids in reducing swelling, and the circumferential nature of the design maximizes the pressure distribution making the orthosis comfortable for the patient (Fig. 18–18B). A volar- or dorsal-based orthosis often is unable to maintain the PIP joint in full extension and pressure problems or inadequate positioning may arise. The orthosis can be made out of thin thermoplastic strips such as QuickCast 2, Orficast® Tapes, or plaster of paris. The DIP is left free, and the patient is instructed in active DIP exercises. This allows the lateral bands to advance and the ORL to stretch, which will further prevent the boutonniere deformity. Frequently, a patient, coach/trainer, or family member may assume this injury is a "finger sprain" and will wait to see if it heals on its own before seeking medical attention.

Commonly, the PIP will develop a flexion contracture (Fig. 18–18C) caused by adhesions forming in the volar plate with a swollen, inflamed PIP joint that is allowed to rest in a flexed position. The contracture must be treated first (via a serial static extension mobilization orthosis). Once the PIP reaches full passive extension, the 6-week immobilization regimen is initiated.

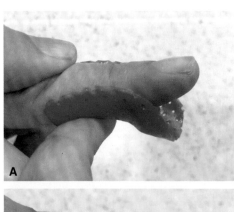

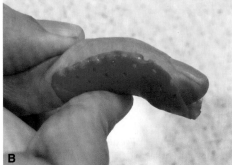

FIGURE 18-16 **A and B,** Exercise template for DIP flexion in the early mobilization phase preventing unrestricted DIP flexion.

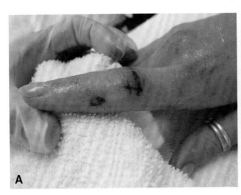
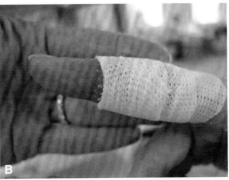
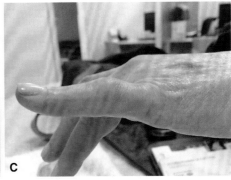

FIGURE 18-18 A, Open boutonniere injury due to laceration; **B,** immobilization with a circumferential cast; **C,** closed boutonniere injury due to a "jammed" finger.

However, once the deformity is fixed, then the prognosis for a good outcome is reduced. These patients should be monitored weekly while they are in the orthosis to check the skin as well as to assess for any changes in swelling. If swelling decreases, the orthosis may become too loose, requiring adjustment. After the 6-week period, PIP flexion is gradually introduced with extension immobilization continued between exercise sessions for another 2 to 4 weeks. The immobilized tendon is fragile and lacks the normal tissue properties (tensile strength, hydration, and collagen cross-linking); therefore, care must be taken to not be overly aggressive when initiating flexion. Most importantly, watch for increases in swelling and any developing extension lag. Because of the unique anatomy in zones III and IV, there is a high risk for scarring and adhesions to occur.

In zone IV, there is a high surface area ratio of tendon to bone and this fact, combined with poor tendon excursion in this zone, leads to a large area for the tendon to adhere to the bone. When the tendon is immobilized for 6 weeks, it is relying on extrinsic healing to occur (i.e., healing via scar tissue). As PIP joint motion is initiated, if the tendon is adhered in zone IV, attenuation can occur over the PIP joint, which leads to an active extension lag. Therefore, progression of motion must begin slowly.

Evans (2011) advocates treating closed boutonniere injuries with a short arc motion (SAM) protocol (discussed later in this chapter), while multiple authors (Merritt, 2014; Hirth, Howell, & O'Brien, 2017; Merritt, Wong, & Lalonde, 2020) advocate treating boutonniere injures with an RMF orthosis which places the MCP joint in 15 to 20° of relative flexion in relation to adjacent digits (Fig. 18–21A,B). This takes the tension off of the FDP while increasing the tension on the dorsal hood, bringing the lateral bands more dorsally which thereby encourages PIP extension. This technique is effective if the joints are supple and the patient is able to achieve full active PIP extension when the MCP joint of the injured digit is placed in relative flexion. If the patient is unable to actively fully extend, then the injury is treated in the same way as a chronic boutonniere. For chronic boutonnieres with fixed contractures, it is recommended that the PIP is initially serially casted to achieve a minimum of −20° extension. The DIP should also be able to achieve flexion. If the DIP remains in a hyperextended position, it will be difficult to achieve PIP extension. If this is the case, the DIP can be held in a neutral position with an orthosis (Merritt et al., 2020). This is also a nice treatment technique if the patient has an extensor lag due to adhesions after proximal phalanx fracture. As the published data for either of these protocols for closed boutonniere injuries is limited, it is recommended that different treatment options are discussed with the referring physician to determine the best fit for the patient.

EXPERT PEARL 18-4

Modification of a Relative Motion Flexion Orthosis
CLYDE JOHNSON PT, CHT
Washington

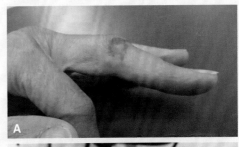
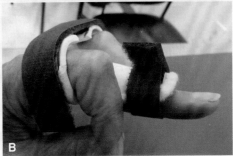
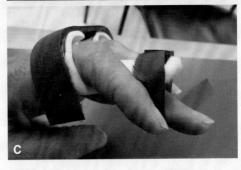

Involved digit is placed in relative flexion, with addition of dorsal expansion or "hood" that extends to DIP joint. The distal strap is pulled tight to keep the PIP joint in full extension when at rest and loosened several time per day to allow a prescribed amount of flexion at the PIP joint. Initially 30° then increasing 10° per week as long as no lag develops. The cut length of the distal strap determines how far the patient is allowed to flex the PIP. This is used as a single orthosis throughout the protected phase of boutonniere rehabilitation.

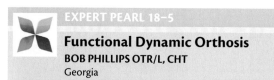

EXPERT PEARL 18–5

Functional Dynamic Orthosis

BOB PHILLIPS OTR/L, CHT
Georgia

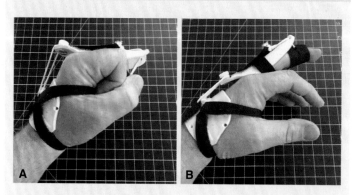

Design allows for functional use of hand while addressing minor flexion contractures of the PIP joint that respond well during treatment. Note: this particular orthosis is not advised for a hard-end feel.

Short Arc Motion Protocol

For this protocol, the patient is immobilized in full extension, and two exercise orthoses are fabricated for the patient (Fig. 18–22A–D). The first exercise orthosis is for PIP flexion, and it allows the PIP to flex to 30°. The patient actively flexes to the orthosis block then actively extends the PIP fully. The second exercise orthosis is for DIP flexion. If the lateral bands are not repaired, then the DIP is allowed to flex fully during exercise sessions while the PIP is held at zero. If the lateral bands are repaired as well as the central slip, the template is fabricated with the PIP held at zero and the DIP allowed to flex to 30°. During exercise sessions, the patient positions the wrist in slight flexion, which decreases the viscoelastic tension on the tendons. After the second postoperative week, if no extensor tendon lag has developed, then the patient is allowed to flex to 40°. Approximately 10° of flexion are added each week as long as no active lag has developed. Full composite flexion is allowed by week 5 and gentle strengthening exercises by week 6 (at which point the extension orthosis is discontinued). The rationale for this protocol, as outlined by Evans (2011), is to allow for tendon excursion in a protected range as well as to promote tendon healing (applied from the principles gleaned from flexor tendon research).

EXPERT PEARL 18–6

Exercise Orthosis

ANDREA MOSER, OT, HAND THERAPIST
Austria

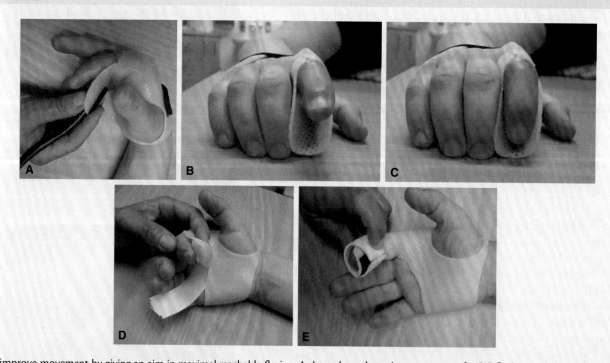

Used to improve movement by giving an aim in maximal reachable flexion. A shows how therapist overcorrects for PIP flexion position with help of a scar tool during the molding process. B/C: Active movement exercise. D: Make it more challenging by pressing down into a piece of putty. E: Between exercises, the finger can be immobilized with loop strapping to provide prolonged stretch.

Open Injuries

Open injuries are less common. Depending on the amount of soft-tissue loss, the patient can begin a **short arc of motion (SAM) protocol** after surgical repair, as outlined by Evans (2011).

Functional impairments for the untreated boutonniere can include difficulty with fine motor coordination because of lack of DIP flexion as well as lack of ability to extend the finger when reaching into a small space (pockets, gloves, etc.). While the lack of

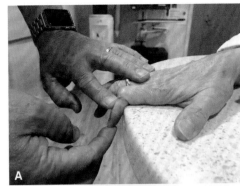

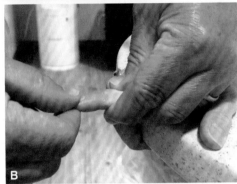

FIGURE 18–19 **A,** Elson test for injury to central slip; **B,** Boyes test for injury to central slip.

PIP extension may be cosmetically unappealing for the patient, it is the inability to flex the DIP which creates a greater functional loss for fine motor coordination. It is important to restore this balance in order to improve function.

ZONES V TO VII

Zone V lies over the MCP joint and contains the sagittal bands and the EDC tendon. Zone VI spans the length of the metacarpals and involves the EDC tendons just distal to the wrist.

Treatment Options

Rupture of the sagittal bands can lead to subluxation of the extensor tendon off of the MCP joint. Usually, it is rupture of the radial bands, which are weaker than the ulnar bands. The long finger is the most commonly involved finger with this type of injury (Young & Rayan, 2000). This can happen both from trauma (usually in younger patients) or from nontraumatic chronic attenuation (in older patients) (Peelman, Markiewitz, Kiefhaber, & Stern, 2015). Treatment of the closed injury can be done conservatively with immobilization (Slater & Bynum, 1997) (Fig. 18–23A–D) or with RMO (even if more than one digit is involved). Operative treatment may be indicated in cases of complete radial sagittal band disruption or in instances of failed conservative treatment.

Immediate Controlled Active Motion (Relative Motion)

This protocol, also referred to as "relative motion splinting," was first described by Merritt et al. in 2000 and again by Howell et al. in 2005, although they had been doing some form of immediate CAM since the 1980s. In this text, Chapter 7, Relative Motion, goes into great detail on this form of controlled motion. This protocol was developed based on the anatomy of the EDC: four tendons arising from a single muscle. By placing the affected digit in 15° to 20° extension in relation to adjacent digits, tension on

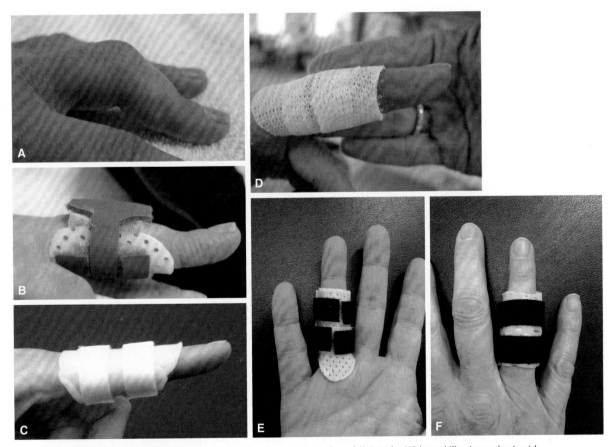

FIGURE 18–20 **A,** Closed boutonniere deformity sustained after a fall. **B,** Volar PIP immobilization orthosis with dorsal padding to secure extension position. **C,** Circumferential clamshell design using thermoplastic material. **D,** QuickCast 2 used offering maximal pressure distribution making this a comfortable option. **E and F,** Adjustable circumferential boutonniere orthosis with DIP free—notice extension volarly into palm to maximal mechanical advantage.

the injured tendon is offloaded and the injured tendon ends can approximate. The excursion of an injured/repaired tendon can occur in a protected environment and early motion can progress without placing stress on the repair as long as this relative motion is maintained (Fig 18–24A–C) (Howell et al., 2005; Merritt, 2014). Biomechanical studies support this theory (Sharma, Liang, Owen, Wayne, & Isaacs, 2006). Intraoperative observation has shown that by placing the repaired tendon in relative extension, that tendon's excursion decreases from 12 to 6 mm, thereby preventing tension on repaired structures while still allowing for sufficient gliding of the tendon to prevent adhesions (Merritt et al., 2020). This regime can be used with both simple and complex repairs as long as there is one intact extensor tendon.

Relative Motion Orthosis
TRISH GRIFFITHS, OT HAND THERAPIST
South Africa

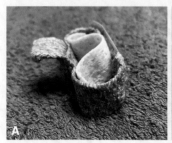 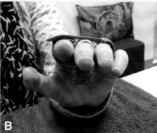

Woodcast (not currently available in the United States) used to fabricate this RM orthosis chosen because it adheres to itself and is strong. Notice volar block to limit PIP flexion which may be used with some short arc protocols to manage Zone III extensor tendon injuries over the PIP joint.

The relative motion concept has evolved over the years in regard to the degree of relative extension, whether or not to include the wrist and for how long. There have also been several names to describe the same orthosis: the Wyndall Merritt orthosis, the immediate controlled active motion (ICAM) orthosis, a yoke orthosis, or a bridge orthosis. It has been suggested to streamline the nomenclature and name the orthosis based on whether the injured digit is positioned in extension or flexion in relation to the neighboring digits (i.e., RMO or RMF orthosis). This orthosis has gained popularity and been used to treat a variety of conditions beyond extensor tendon injuries and can be used not only as a protective orthosis, but in some scenarios, it can also be used as an exercise orthosis and an adaptive orthosis (Hirth et al., 2016).

This protocol as originally written requires two orthoses. A wrist immobilization orthosis is fabricated placing the wrist in 20° of extension. The distal palmar crease is cleared to allow for full MCP ROM. Then a separate **relative motion extension orthosis** is fabricated that places the involved digit in 15° to 20° of extension relative to the adjacent digits (Fig. 18–25A,B) (Howell et al., 2005). If the index finger is lacerated, then the RMO also places the small finger in extension to create balance (and vice versa if it is the small finger that is lacerated).

Identifying and Lessening the Dreaded EDC Lag
HandLab: Clinical Pearls
JUDY C. COLDITZ, OT/L, CHT, FAOTA
North Carolina

How does one identify the cause of this posture when finger extension is attempted? Either adherence or weakness of the extrinsic finger extensors or the presence of severe interosseous muscle tightness can create this posture.

In the case of severe interosseous muscle tightness, both MCP joint extension and interphalangeal (IP) joint flexion are limited.

Determining the cause of extensor lag is more complex. The lag can result from weakened muscles which are most often seen when muscle innervation is returning following a nerve injury. In the injured hand, the active lag is usually caused by adherence of the extrinsic extensor tendons somewhere along their path.

Consider the extrinsic extensors (herein referred to as EDC) in an uninjured hand. Since IP joint extension is accomplished primarily by the intrinsic finger muscles, testing the EDC focuses on MCP joint extension. Since the EDC also crosses the wrist, the ability of the EDC to extend the MCP joints is made more difficult with greater wrist extension because simultaneous wrist and MCP joint extension require maximum muscle contraction to produce maximal proximal tendon glide. Conversely, wrist flexion creates passive tension on the EDC, thereby passively extending the MCP joints without requiring active EDC muscle contraction. When the wrist is positioned close to neutral, the EDC excursion (and muscle contraction) required to accomplish MCP joint extension is less than when the wrist is in extension.

To test the maximum proximal excursion of the EDC, the patient must actively hold both the wrist and the MCP joints in extension simultaneously, without IP joint extension. In this photo of a patient without a nerve injury, one sees that with the wrist extended about 30°, there is a 45° extension lag at the MCP joints. In this case, the first question is whether the MCP extension lag changes when the wrist position changes. If MCP joint extension decreases as the wrist moves into extension and increases as the wrist moves to neutral, the adherence is proximal to the wrist. If, however, the MCP extension lag does not change when the wrist position is changed, the adherence is distal to the wrist; (over the metacarpals) assuming passive MCP joint motion is present.

To reduce EDC lag/adherence regardless of the location of the adherence, start by determining the wrist position where the patient demonstrates the best MCP joint extension, even though less than full. If the adherence is over the metacarpals, less wrist extension may not alter the MCP joint extension at all, but a wrist position closer to neutral maximizes the EDC pull across the metacarpals because the muscle does not have to work so hard.

The patient repeats active MCP joint extension with the wrist in the chosen position and the IP joints in relaxed flexion until almost full MCP joint extension is regained. When MCP joint extension is gained in the initial position, the wrist is then serially repositioned in greater extension until the patient is able to simultaneously maximally extend both the wrist and the MCP joints. Only then is it appropriate to ask the patient to add active IP joint extension as part of the exercise.

One should keep in mind that an injured stiff hand may have both interosseous muscle tightness as well as an extensor lag from adherence, requiring more than one exercise to remediate the problems.

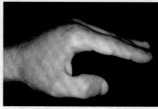

(Clinical Pearl reprinted with permission from Clinician's Classroom at BraceLab.com written by Judy Colditz OT/L CHT FAOTA, copyright HandLab/BraceLab, Raleigh NC. July 2016, No. 41.)

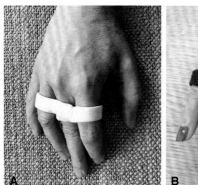
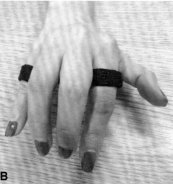

FIGURE 18–21 Relative motion flexion orthosis, **A,** for middle finger; **B,** for index finger.

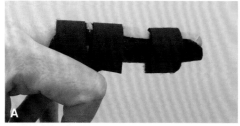
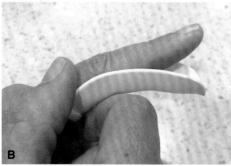
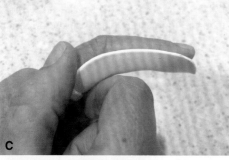
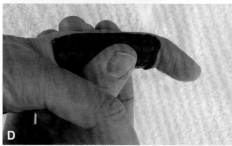

FIGURE 18–22 Short arc motion protocol: **A,** Finger orthosis immobilizing IP joints are worn between exercise sessions; **B,** full active extension in exercise template orthosis; **C,** exercise orthosis limits active flexion to 30°; **D,** second exercise orthosis holds PIP in extension and allows for full distal DIP flexion to encourage advancement of lateral bands distal to the repair site.

Phase of RMO Protocol

The following describes the phases of this protocol:

- **Phase 1 (days 0–21):** The patient is allowed full AROM within the confines of the orthoses (which are not to be removed by the patient).
- **Phase 2 (days 22–35):** The wrist orthosis is removed for wrist AROM and light activities, but the RMO stays on at all times.
- **Phase 3 (days 36–49):** The wrist orthosis is discontinued, and the patient can remove the relative motion orthosis for AROM exercises but continues to wear the RMO with ADLs.

This protocol cannot be used if more than three digits are involved. Canham and Hammert (2013) advocate using the Norwich regime in those cases (described in this chapter). For injuries distal to the juncturae tendinum, it has been shown that a wrist support is not needed and patients can have good results; however, injuries proximal to the juncturae tendinum should include a wrist orthosis for the first 3 to 4 weeks (Svens, Ames, Burford & Caplash, 2015).

In treating sagittal band injuries, Peelman et al. (2015) demonstrated that RME positioning was effective in 94% of patients presenting with acute subluxation (either traumatic or nontraumatic) and 90% of subacute presentations. Sagittal band injuries that were addressed in more chronic stages still had a success rate of 62%. Patients wore a RMO (but no wrist orthosis) full time for 6 weeks and then weaned over the next 2 to 4 weeks. Catalano et al. (2006) also demonstrated good results in treating sagittal band injuries with a relative motion orthosis. Timelines varied for duration of treatment with orthosis wear anywhere from 4 to 8 weeks of full-time wear after injury, with 2 to 4 additional weeks of wear with heavy tasks. Complications include persistent symptoms in three patients.

EXPERT PEARL 18–9

Relative Motion Orthosis Fabrication Tip
JEANINE BEASLEY, EDD, OTR, CHT, FAOTA
Michigan

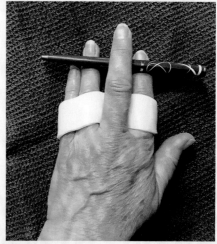

When fabricating a relative motion orthosis for a zone 5 extensor tendon repair, the digit often relaxes to be in line with the other digits. Placement of a pencil distally can assure that the necessary 15° to 20° greater extension of lateral digits is maintained as the material cools.

Controlled Active Motion: The Norwich Regime

This protocol came out of the United Kingdom as a way to mobilize extensor tendons early without the bulk of a dynamic orthosis (Sylaidis et al., 1997). The orthosis includes the wrist placed in 45° of extension, the MCP joints flexed to 50°, and the IP joints in full extension.

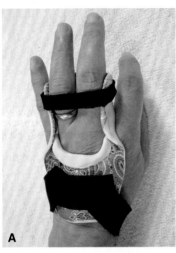
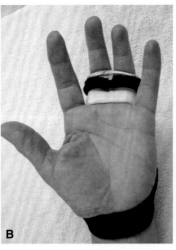
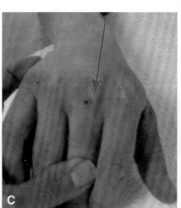
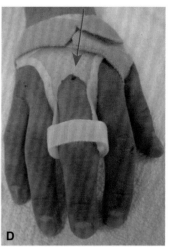

FIGURE 18–23 Closed extensor tendon zone V injury. **A and B,** Two digits involved and **(C and D)** middle finger only included in this volar/dorsal MCP joint immobilization orthosis. Note the radial orientation of the extensor tendon over the third MCP indicated by the arrow.

During the first 4 weeks, the patient performs two exercises within the orthosis: full MCP/IP extension and full MCP extension with IP flexion. At 4 weeks, if there is no extension lag, the orthosis is discontinued, and progressive flexion exercises are allowed. If there is a lag, then the orthosis is continued another 2 weeks. In this study, 92% of patients had good/excellent results (Sylaidis et al., 1997).

Khandwala et al. (2000) took the EAM premise of the Norwich regime and modified the orthosis to allow for synchronous motion at the MCP, PIP, and DIP joints. The orthosis includes the wrist in 30° of extension, the MCP joints at 45° of flexion, and the IP joints left free (Fig. 18–26A–C). During the first 3 weeks, the patient is allowed full AROM within the orthosis (extension to neutral only). At week 3, the MCP joints are flexed to 70° in the orthosis. The exercise regimen remains the same with full active extension, with the addition of a hook fist within the orthosis. The orthosis is discontinued by week 5. In this study, 93% of patients had good/excellent results, which were comparable to results experienced with patients in a dynamic orthosis group (Khandwala et al., 2000).

Tendons in zones V and VI that are repaired may be treated with immobilization. This may be appropriate if the patient cannot be compliant with a more complicated early mobilization protocol or if there are other structures that need to be immobilized. It is important to keep in mind that the more traumatic the injury, the greater the likelihood of scar tissue and adhesion formation.

If only the EIP or EDM is lacerated, then only the involved digit needs to be immobilized. However, if the EDC is lacerated, then all digits need to be included in the orthosis because of the action of the juncturae (Fig. 18–27A). The orthosis positions the wrist in 30° of extension and the MCP joints in full extension for 4 to 6 weeks, with buddy taping to provide protection for another 2 weeks (Griffin et al., 2012). The IP joints are left free in the orthosis, but there must be enough thermoplastic volarly on the proximal phalanx to support the MCP joint, yet not so long as to prevent IP flexion. It is

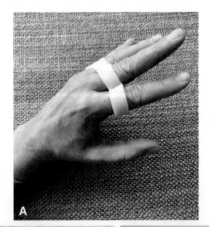

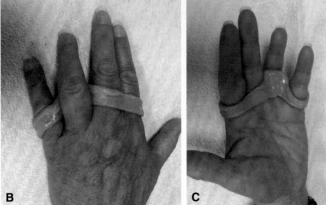

FIGURE 18–24 **A,** Relative motion extension orthosis (middle finger). **B and C,** Relative motion extension orthosis (ring finger).

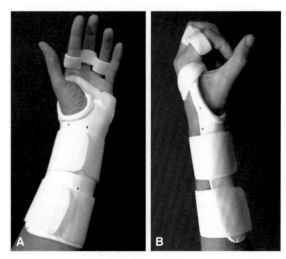

FIGURE 18–25 **A and B,** Two orthoses used in ICAM protocol: relative motion orthosis which positions the injured finger in slight extension relative to the adjacent digits, and a wrist orthosis which clears the distal palmar crease to allow for MCP flexion.

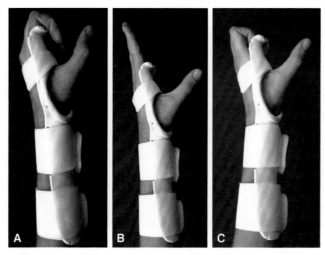

FIGURE 18–26 Early active motion, Khandwala protocol. **A,** MCP joints are placed in 45° of flexion; IPs are left free. **B,** Full AROM is allowed within the orthosis, and patient can actively extend MCP joints to neutral. **C,** At week 3, hook fist within the orthosis is added and the orthosis is modified to allow for 70° of MCP flexion.

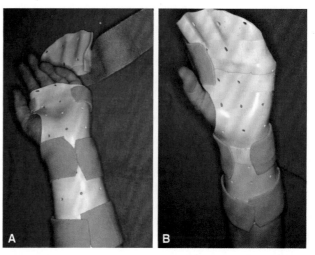

FIGURE 18–27 **A,** Wrist and MCP extension orthosis, allowing for PIP flexion during the day; **B,** Extension pan attachment to be worn at night to prevent IP flexion contractures.

important to monitor the patient and make sure that he or she is not developing PIP flexion contractures. If there seems to be a potential for this, the patient can wear a night orthosis that positions the entire hand in full extension (Fig. 18–27B).

Gentle active motion is initiated at week 3, with the initial focus on isolated MCP joint motion. Using the principles of tenodesis decreases the tension from the surrounding soft tissue: MCP flexion with the wrist in slight extension and MCP extension with the wrist in slight flexion. Composite flexion is begun at postoperative week 4 or 5 if there is no extension lag, and the orthosis is discontinued at week 6.

Early Passive Mobilization

The use of dynamic orthoses for zone V and proximal is considered a passive mobilization protocol (although it is likely that there is some active extension occurring in the dynamic orthosis). The orthosis itself is time-consuming and expensive to fabricate. It is heavier than orthoses used in other protocols and can be cumbersome, making dressing and sleeping difficult. A less bulky extension immobilization orthosis for sleeping can be made, although insurance may not cover both orthoses (Fig. 18–28A,B).

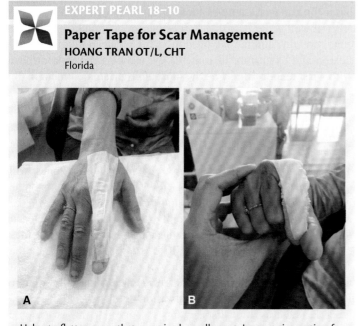

EXPERT PEARL 18–10

Paper Tape for Scar Management
HOANG TRAN OT/L, CHT
Florida

Helps to flatten scars that are raised or adherent. Inexpensive option for home program. Place tape on the scar at least a few inches above and below; apply in two layers that overlap at least 50% to give it better pressure. May wear for 1 to 2 hours when most active, with motion the tape will gently pull on the skin/scar and provide "massage" while the pressure from the motion and tape will help flatten the scar. Remove by gently pulling the tape off or wash under soap and water to remove easier.

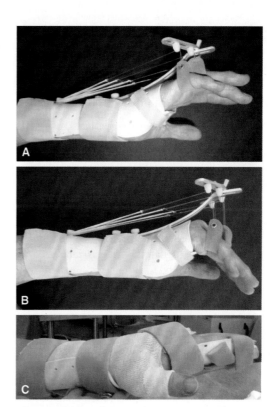

FIGURE 18–28 **A and B,** A dynamic MCP extension mobilization orthosis used for an EPM program for zones V to VII extensor tendon repair (Digitec Outrigger System shown, Performance Health). The amount of flexion can be restricted by adding a volar orthosis block or by applying small beads on each monofilament line to prevent further excursion through the line guide. **C,** A wrist/hand extension immobilization orthosis is worn at night or during rest periods to complement an EPM program for zones V to VII extensor tendon repair.

In addition, there are no studies which demonstrate the superiority of an early passive motion protocol over an early active motion protocol.

In this protocol, the orthosis is molded dorsally with the wrist in 40° of extension. The outrigger (custom made with copper wire or via a commercially available kit) is attached dorsally, allowing for finger sling placement holding the MCP joints at neutral. The slings are attached to the outrigger with rubber bands or elastic thread. The MCP joints are allowed to flex to 30° (a mechanical block can be placed on the outrigger to prevent further flexion). The elastic tension of the rubber bands then passively extends the MCP joints back to neutral. The IP joints can flex with the MCP joints held in neutral via the sling. After 3 weeks, progressively more MCP flexion is allowed with full composite fist and the orthosis is discontinued by week 6.

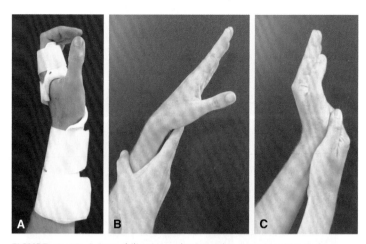

FIGURE 18–29 **A,** Immobilization orthosis used in zones V to VIII. Early-phase exercise regimen performed with therapist: **B,** Active place/hold MCP extension with the wrist in 20° of flexion. Patient can also flex MCP joints to 30° and actively extend to neutral from this position. **C,** Wrist extension with MCP flexion to 40°.

EXPERT PEARL 18–11

Blocking Mechanism
JEANINE BEASLEY, EDD, OTR, CHT, FAOTA
Michigan

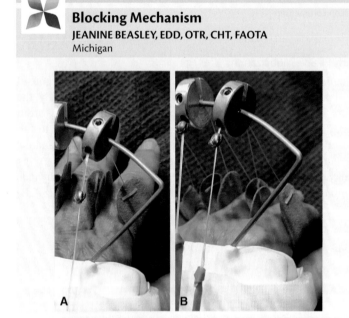

When utilizing a dynamic approach to rehabilitate a zone V extensor tendon repair—allowing 30° of flexion after is simplified by placing a fishing line sinker or bead on the line. The fishing sinker is too large to go through the outrigger allowing only the desired motion.

Immediate Active Tension

The immediate active tension protocol as outlined by Evans (2011) includes a mobilization (dynamic) orthosis fabricated as described earlier. Gentle passive tenodesis exercises are performed (but not allowing more than 40° of MCP flexion with the wrist in full extension and not allowing the wrist to flex more than 20°). This is followed by active place and hold exercises: performed with the wrist in 20° of flexion and MCP joints at neutral. Then, with the wrist still in 20° of flexion, the MCP joints are actively extended from 30° of flexion to neutral. These exercises are done under the supervision of the therapist in the clinic while the patient performs the PROM protocol (mentioned earlier) while at home. Progression of exercises is the same as in the dynamic EPM protocol. Evans (2011) advocates using a dynamic orthosis with this protocol; however, this same tenodesis exercise progression can also be performed using a less cumbersome static orthosis between exercise sessions: The wrist is positioned in 30° to 45° of extension, MCP joints flexed to 20°, and the IP joints free. Active place and hold tenodesis exercises are performed in a protected range as mentioned earlier (Fig. 18–29A–C) (Gallagher, 2006).

ZONES VII AND VIII

Zone VII is over the wrist and contains the extensor reticulum—the broad fibrous structure divided into six compartments for the tendons to pass through. The retinaculum is synovial, which provides nutrition to the tendons, yet there is increased risk for scar formation in this region. Loss of extensor retinaculum may lead to bowstringing of the tendons and result in an extension lag at the MCP joint(s). Zone VIII is the area of the dorsal forearm just proximal to the extensor retinaculum and includes the musculotendinous junctions of the digit and wrist extensors. The orthosis and the exercise regimen are essentially equal to the treatment for zones V and VI, with a slight modification: The wrist is placed within the orthosis at no more than 20° of wrist extension to prevent buckling of the tendons within the retinaculum. This is based on cadaveric studies looking at tendon excursion in zone VII (Howell & Peck, 2013). Adhesions are a complication in this zone, creating limitations in motion for wrist and digits in both flexion and extension. In some cases, use of a dynamic orthosis with wrist tenodesis may be the most appropriate treatment in this zone (Lutz et al., 2015).

THUMB EXTENSOR TENDONS

The extensor tendons in the thumb are divided into five zones (with odd numbers over the joints) (Fig. 18–30). The EPL inserts on the base of the distal phalanx of the thumb and is the only tendon that can *hyper*extend the IP joint. IP joint extension to neutral can occur through contributions to the dorsal hood from the intrinsic muscles but not hyperextension. The EPL is also the only tendon that can perform retropulsion (the ability of the thumb to extend off of the table). Injury can occur either through laceration or rupture. Rupture can occur at the distal insertion or at the level of Lister's tubercle (such as after distal radius fracture). If this is the case, the patient will likely need a tendon transfer (e.g., EIP to EPL) because the ruptured tendon ends are often not in suitable condition for direct repair. After direct repair or tendon transfer, the thumb and wrist are positioned in extension to put slack on the repair. The EPB inserts on the base of the proximal phalanx and passes through the first dorsal compartment at the extensor retinaculum (along with the APL).

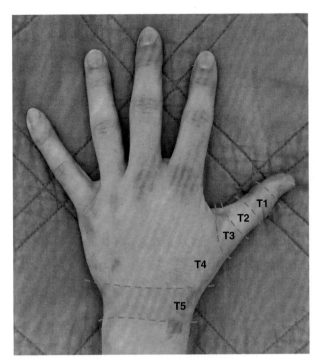

FIGURE 18-30 Extensor tendon zones of injury in the thumb.

ZONE TI

This is a mallet type of injury to the EPL and is treated the same as zone I digit extensor tendon injuries. The IP joint of the thumb is held continuously in slight hyperextension for 6 to 8 weeks if there is no surgical repair. Unlike zone I injuries in the digits, the EPL is large enough to be able to be sutured in this zone (Howell & Peck, 2013). If the tendon was repaired, then active flexion can begin earlier, at week 5 or 6. In either situation, motion is initiated gradually, with the orthosis worn between exercises for an additional 2 weeks (Fig. 18–31A–C).

ZONE TII

Zone TII lies over the proximal phalanx and also involves the EPL tendon. The orthosis is hand based, with the MCP and IP joints in extension and the thumb in radial abduction (Fig. 18–32A,B). A short arc active mobilization protocol can be initiated at week 3 and gradually progressed weekly. The orthosis is discontinued by week 6 as long as there is no active extension lag.

ZONES TIII AND TIV

Zones TIII and TIV reside over the MCP joint and thumb metacarpal, respectively. The orthosis used is forearm based, with the wrist in 30° of extension and the thumb in radial abduction and MCP/IP extended (Fig. 18–33A–C). There is little published

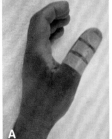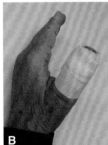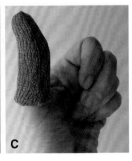

FIGURE 18-31 **A,** Zone TI injury **(B and C)** circumferential mallet thumb orthoses using QuickCast 2 **(B)** and Orficast® **(C)** thermoplastic tapes.

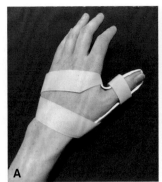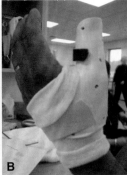

FIGURE 18-32 **A,** a volar hand-based orthosis for extensor tendon injury in zone TII, immobilizing the MP and IP joints. **B,** a dorsal design can also be applied.

information on rehabilitation in this zone. Injuries here can be treated with immobilization, early AROM, or with dynamic passive mobilization. As mentioned earlier, knowledge of flexor tendon healing and early mobilization can be applied to the thumb. Khandwala, Blairm, Harris, Foster, and Elliot (2004) and Elliot and Southgate (2005) found that EPL tendons treated with a dynamic passive mobilization orthosis had good to excellent results (Fig. 18–34). However, both authors point out the promising results seen with early AROM in the finger extensors and advocate a move toward an early AROM protocol for the EPL (as opposed to passive mobilization via dynamic orthosis), which will require a less bulky orthosis. Howell and Peck (2013) advocate using a hand-based orthosis which allows the IP to flex to 30° to 40°. Active flexion and place and hold extension exercises are performed throughout the day. The IP joint can be held in full extension at night to prevent an extensor lag. Full IP flexion is allowed by week 3%, and 50% MCP flexion with IP in extension is initiated at this time.

ZONE TV

Injuries in this zone involve the extensor retinaculum, which is synovial. This poses an increased threat to adhesion formation. If there is limited ability for the tendon to glide, changes in wrist position can affect the position of the thumb (Chinchalkar, Pipicelli, Laxamana, & von Dehn, 2010). Because of this increased risk, early AROM or PROM is recommended. It has been found that the EPL achieves the greatest amount of glide at the wrist when the wrist is positioned in 30° of extension when compared to other wrist positions (Chen, Tsubota, Aoki, Echigo, & Han, 2009).

The orthosis recommended places the wrist in 30° of extension, the MCP at neutral, and the IP dynamically held in extension (allowing for up to 60° of active IP flexion) (Fig. 18–34). In therapy, the orthosis is removed for passive tenodesis exercises (no more than 20° of wrist flexion) and place/hold exercises with the wrist in 20° of flexion and the thumb in radial abduction and MCP/IP joints in extension. Consideration can be given to the application of elastic therapeutic tape that is worn under the orthosis to (1) assist with extension and (2) place gentle tension on the incision area to prevent adherence (Fig. 18–35A–C). Graded increases in individual joint motion are initiated at weeks 3 to 4, and composite flexion is initiated at week 5. The orthosis is discontinued by week 6.

SPECIAL CONSIDERATIONS

Extensor tendon adhesions of the EDC due to tendon repair zones V-VII or metacarpal fractures can lead to the phenomenon of

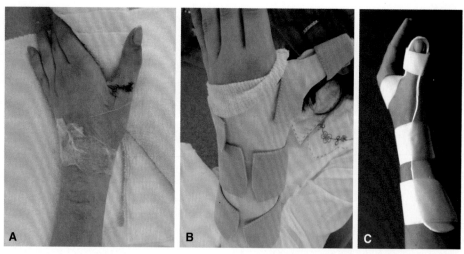

FIGURE 18–33 A, Zone TIII injury postoperative dressing removed. **B,** Dorsal immobilization orthosis applied; **C,** alternative design—a volar immobilization orthosis. These two types of orthoses can be used to manage zones TIII-V.

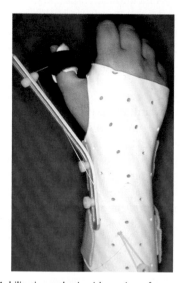

FIGURE 18–34 Mobilization orthosis with outrigger for extensor tendon laceration in zones TIII-V. (Digitec Outrigger System shown, Performance Health.)

quadriga. Tendon adhesions form a pseudo-insertion at the site of the adhesion, creating an extensor lag distally. The fourth and fifth digits are more prone to contributing to extensor lag due to the increased mobility at the fourth and fifth carpometacarpal (CMC) joints: if there is an adhesion, EDC forces will be directed toward hyperextending fourth and fifth CMC, which will subsequently decrease the tension on adjacent digits. This can have a cascade effect, leading to intrinsic tightness as well as decreased tendon excursion of adjacent tendons. Intrinsic tightness can lead to extension forces being directed at the PIP joint. Treatment should be directed at preventing PIP hyperextension as well as preventing intrinsic tightness and increasing EDC glide (Chinchalkar, Gan, McFarlane, King, & Roth, 2004).

Extensor tendon lags in more distal zones are more difficult to treat due to the low excursion these tendons have in these zones, which is why it is important to recognize and address issues early. Motion loss is most likely to occur at the joint just distal to the tendon adhesion (Graham et al., 2019).

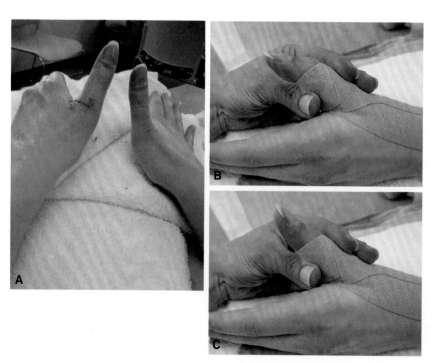

FIGURE 18–35 A, Zone TIII laceration. **B and C,** Use of elastic therapeutic tape applied to assist with EAM protocol and protect repair; this can be used in combination with orthosis use.

CONCLUSION

Rehabilitation to extensor tendon injuries has come a long way in the past 30 years. Research and experience have shown that early mobilization tends to result in better functional outcomes for the patient. However, tendon adhesions, extensor lags, and joint stiffness continue to be issues faced by physicians and therapists. Further research in this area is recommended, particularly in concern to rehabilitation of the tendons of the thumb where research is scant. The general trend has been toward early ROM, either passive or active, and toward orthoses that are less bulky and less complicated, which not only saves time and money but also increases patient compliance with the postoperative protocol. Tendons can be interesting and exciting to treat; however, choosing an appropriate treatment protocol and accompanying orthosis require sound clinical judgment skills and good communication among the treating team.

FIELD NOTE: RELATIVE MOTION ORTHOSES

Julianne Wright Howell, PT, MS, CHT
Michigan
Melissa Jayne Hirth, B (OT), MSc (OT-Hand & Upper Limb Rehab)
Australia

"All things relative motion" is a phrase we hear a lot since hand therapists and hand surgeons have discovered a 40-year-old concept; Relative Motion. Chapter 7 reviews the use of relative motion extension (RME) as applied in the EAM of zones IV to VII extensor tendon repairs of the fingers. We have also included evidence by zone of repair to substantiate RME-*only* orthoses without the wrist orthosis for certain zones. This chapter will also introduce you to a variety of ways in which RME orthoses are being used, including postoperative and nonsurgical intervention of sagittal band injuries.

We are elated that an international survey of hand therapists reported RME to be the most commonly used early active motion approach following zone V to VI extensor tendon repairs of the fingers.[1] Equally impressive was that 85% of the therapist respondents who were not using the RME approach said they wanted to switch to RME so their patients could more quickly recover motion, resume hand function, and return to work.[1] Surprising to us, 70% of those wanting to switch to RME reported surgeon preference as the #1 barrier to implementation![1] Our intent in Chapter 7 is to furnish sufficient rationale, supportive evidence and practical tips from which therapists can structure their conversations with hesitant hand surgeons, if any still exist.

Relative motion flexion (RMF) orthoses are being increasingly used for nonsurgical management of acute/chronic boutonniere deformity, zone III central slip repairs, and boutonniere deformity reconstruction. In Chapter 7, you will find the rationale for the concept of RMF, which is supported by a few clinical cases incorporating RMF orthoses.

Because relative motion has so many applications, there are now three categories of classification, "protective," "exercise," and "adaptive." Soon, we predict the addition of a fourth category, "assessment," which will include the RME/RMF "Pencil Test" and more.

We invite you to view Chapter 7 so that you too may share in our enthusiasm for "all things, Relative Motion"!

Julianne Howell and Melissa Hirth

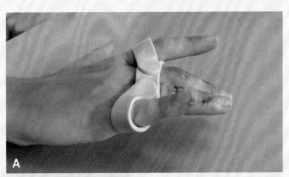

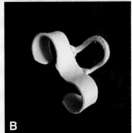 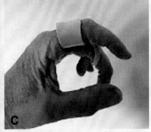

RMF orthosis for early CAM after central slip repairs of the long and ring fingers. (Courtesy Melissa Hirth 2019.)

A uniquely designed RMF orthosis for the long finger that combines short arc motion for management of boutonniere deformity or central slip repairs (Orthosis design, courtesy of Gwendolyn van Strien MSc, PT © 2019).

Reference

1. Hirth M. J., Howell J. W., Feehan L., et al: International Extensor Tendon Survey. Project registration identification # 13,583 Monash University, Melbourne Australia June 06, 2018.

Case Study Section

The case studies presented here are meant as a teaching guideline only. Treatment and orthosis protocols vary greatly from surgeon to surgeon and from therapist to therapist. The therapist should check with the referring physicians and colleagues to define the preferred treatment and appropriate orthotic intervention.

Case Study 1

A 51-year-old male was trying to catch a falling glass jar when it shattered and lacerated his right small and ring fingers. His ring finger sustained a laceration to his central slip and ulnar collateral ligament to his PIP joint. The lateral bands were intact. His small finger sustained a laceration to the extensor tendon in zone II. He underwent repair to lacerated structures in both digits. A few days postoperatively, he developed an infection to his ring finger and was started on a course of antibiotics. His ring finger was placed in a finger immobilization orthosis, and his small finger was placed in a DIP immobilization orthosis (Figs. 18–13 and 18–18B). Due to his infection, the decision was made by his physician to delay early motion to his ring finger. At 3 weeks postoperatively, he was started on a SAM protocol for his ring finger PIP joint (Fig. 18–22B–D), while his small finger DIP remained immobilized.

At 7 weeks postoperatively, all protective orthoses were discharged. His ROM was as follows:

	PIP	DIP
Ring	−15/60	30
Small	0/55	30

A circumferential static progressive orthosis, to increase ring finger PIP extension, was fabricated for him to wear at night; however, as he began to use his hand more with daily activities, his extensor lag increased to −30. At that point, an RMF orthosis for his ring finger was fabricated for him to wear during the day while he continued to wear the extension orthosis at night. Therapy focused on scar management and exercises to increase ROM and functional use of his hand. His range of motion at discharge (4 months postop) was as follows:

	PIP	DIP
Ring	0/95	0/55
Small	0/90	0/60

Case Study 2: Zone V: Sagittal Band Rupture

AK is a 44-year-old jeweler who ruptured his right middle finger sagittal band in a martial arts class. The original prescription from the physician asked for a forearm-based orthosis blocking the middle and ring MCP joints in extension with the IP joints free. The patient reported that he would most likely not wear the orthosis because it would interfere too much with the fine motor requirements of his job, so after discussion with the physician, it was decided to go with an early ICAM protocol.

An orthosis placing the wrist in 30° of extension was fabricated. A relative motion orthosis (RMO) placing the middle finger in 20° of extension relative to the ring and index fingers was also fabricated (Fig. 18–25A,B). The patient was instructed in AROM exercises within the orthosis. He was seen 1 week later to adjust the RMO because of a decrease in swelling. He reported that he was compliant with the orthosis program, and he was much happier with this option.

The wrist orthosis was discontinued at 3 weeks post injury, and wrist ROM exercises were initiated. The RMO was used until he was 7 weeks post injury. He maintained excellent ROM throughout the program and was able to work in a limited fashion.

CHAPTER REVIEW QUESTIONS

1. Describe the structures that are within each zone of injury in relation to extensor tendons.
2. What are the series of events leading to a chronic boutonniere deformity? What diagnostic tests can be performed if injury to the central slip is suspected?
3. What is the function of the juncturae tendinum?
4. What are the theories behind early passive mobilization (EPM) and EAM in extensor tendon repair management?
5. Describe the various orthoses that may be used to address a mallet finger or injury in zone I.
6. Describe at least two appropriate diagnoses for the use of a relative motion orthosis.

19 Flexor Tendon Injuries

Rebecca Neiduski, PhD, OTR/L, CHT

CHAPTER OBJECTIVES

After study of this chapter, the reader should be able to:
- Describe the anatomy of the flexor tendon system and zones
- Identify key aspects of tendon repair, healing, and nutrition that inform rehabilitative choices
- Relate fundamental flexor tendon concepts to assessment and intervention
- Design a strategy for the initiation of therapy, including assessment, intervention, and education
- Contrast and categorize rehabilitation regimens
- Evaluate outcomes and subsequently progress therapeutic interventions
- Summarize complications and potential causes

KEY TERMS

Annular pulleys
Camper chiasm
Cruciform pulleys
Dorsal blocking orthosis
Early passive flexion
Force

Indiana protocol
Kleinert
Manchester short splint/orthosis
Modified duran
Place and hold
Pyramid of progressive force
Saint John protocol

Strickland percentage
Synergistic motion
Synovial sheaths
Tendon excursion
True active motion
Vincula system
Work of flexion

MD NOTE

Don Lalonde, MD
Canada

It was not easy to create the ideal situation in Saint John where hand therapists and surgeons work together before, during, and after flexor tendon repair with our patients as partners of the team. This came about after countless hours of lobbying many people about the importance of therapists and surgeons working together to see patients. It is worth the concerted effort required by hospitals, surgery centers, surgeons, and therapists to make this happen.

In my view, the six most important new things in flexor tendon repairs in the last 15 years are the following improvements in surgery and therapy: (1) At least four strands in a bulky (10%–30%) very solid repair with 1 cm bites; (2) judicious venting of up to 1.5 to 2 cm of pulley length, including either the A2 or A4 pulleys when required; (3) intraoperative full fist flexion and extension testing in the awake patient to reveal/repair gaps and perform adequate pulley venting; (4) intraoperative patient education by the surgeon and therapist in the awake patient; (5) up to half a fist of true active movement starting at 3–5 days postoperation; (6) relative motion orthoses to improve flexor and extensor lag beginning at 4 to 6 weeks after surgery. A "must read" reference for all surgeons and therapists is the following paper by Professor Jin Bo Tang, which is as important as Kleinert's 1967 paper which dispelled the "No Man's Land" myth (*Tang JB, Zhou X, Pan ZJ, Qing J, Gong KT, Chen J. (2017)*. Strong digital flexor tendon repair, extension-flexion test, and early active flexion: Experience in 300 tendons. *Hand Clinics, 33(3), 455–463.*

This chapter is based on the first-edition chapter written by Lisa Cyr OTR/L, CHT, and second-edition chapter by Alexandra MacKenzie OTR/L, CHT.

What is one of the "tricks" to get the wrist and the MCP joints in the proper position when molding the thermoplastic material?
As shown in Figure 19–10A,B, this homemade thermoplastic "hand stand" allows the therapist to gently position the angle of the wrist and the MCP joints *prior* to application of the material. By allowing the patient to "rest" on this hand stand, the therapist is not juggling with constant repositioning of the wrist and redirecting the patient.
This stand can be made from scrap thermoplastic material. The key in making one of these is to

a. make sure the vertical bars are tall enough to clear the digit tips as they drape over the stand.
b. the horizontal bar that lays across the palmar aspect of the hand should follow an oblique angle from the index finger to the small finger (following the contour of the proximal palmar crease). This will allow the clinician to incorporate this angle within the orthosis. If not, this may risk the fourth and fifth MCP joints to be held in unwanted extension compared to second and third MCP joints, which in turn may lead to collateral ligament tightness.

What is the best material to use when making a forearm-based wrist/hand extension restriction orthosis for a flexor tendon injury?
Rubber-like materials (low conformability/high resistance to stretch) give the therapist a long working time which can be helpful when multiple joint levels are involved. If the patient presents with significant edema or bulky dressings—using a material in this category might be helpful since it can be reheated multiple times and a more general fit is achieved which can be altered with remolding.

For the skilled clinician, a plastic-based material can be a great choice for this patient population. There is a high degree of conformability with these materials which makes defining the dorsal MCP joints and the creases between the digital web spaces easy to achieve (due to the assistance of gravity). These materials also stretch effortlessly about and around joint angles. Therefore, in fabricating a flexor tendon orthosis, the therapist with appropriate skill can blend the wrist and the MCP joints easily into this orthosis design (Fig. 19–18).

For therapists who prefer a conformed fit with some control during the molding process, a blend material—combination of rubber and plastic qualities—may be the best choice. These combination materials offer moderate conformability and stretch. With some guidance of the material, it can conform nicely to the wrist and MCP joint angles as well as the dorsum of the digits (Fig. 19–9A). (Refer Chapter 5 for specific material choices.)

What are the best types of blocking exercise orthoses to isolate specific tendon gliding?
Blocking orthoses that are circumferential in design and hold the proximal joint(s) as "quiet" as possible may be the best choice. As shown in Figure 19–23C, the proximal joint (PIP) is held in full extension so that all the forces of flexion are directed to the DIP joint allowing the FDP to flex the DIP joint. Application of a DIP orthosis and manually holding the adjacent digits in extension will isolate FDS glide. In Figure 19–23A,B, all the MCPs are held in extension in order to facilitate differential FDP/FDS tendon gliding.

INTRODUCTION

Tendon injuries pose a significant risk to the function of the hand and can be daunting to treat. The anatomy of the flexor tendon system is complicated, and scar tissue can wreak havoc on the intricate sequence of motions that facilitate efficient and functional use of the hand. Therapy plays a critical role in the recovery process and is optimally initiated early in the postoperative phase.

The history of flexor tendon repair and rehabilitation has gone through many incarnations, slowly progressing toward acceptance of early motion as safe and effective in helping patients regain full function of their hands. Early conservatism led surgeons to immobilize patients after tendon repair, founded in the concept that extrinsic processes were necessary for tendon healing prior to initiation of tendon gliding (Mason & Allen, 1941; Potenza, 1963; Peacock, 1965). Some surgeons questioned whether tendons could be successfully repaired without having to use tendon grafts (Riboh & Leversedge, 2011; Seiler, 2011). Landmark studies in the 1970s and 1980s provided evidence to support intrinsic healing (Lundborg & Rank, 1978, 1980); the myriad benefits of applying modulated stress to the healing tendon (Gelberman, Vande Berg, Lundborg, & Akeson, 1980, 1981, 1982, 1986; Gelberman, & Woo, 1989); and the negative effects of immobilization relative to loss of strength in the healing tendon (Hitchcock et al., 1987).

Parallel to surgical advances, rehabilitation regimens and the architecture of orthoses have also evolved over time. The application of postoperative orthoses began with simple casts and dorsal blocks with an emphasis toward flexion; transitioned to intricate designs with rubber bands and springs intended to replicate the flexor tendon system; and has more recently returned to more basic dorsal blocks with a greater focus on wrist positioning and motion.

The goal of this chapter is to give the reader a thorough understanding of tendon anatomy; the healing process; historic and progressive regimens; and the type and timing of orthotic intervention. Integration of these concepts will afford an effective and evidence-based approach to flexor tendon rehabilitation.

ANATOMY OF THE FLEXOR TENDON SYSTEM

EXTRINSIC TENDONS

The extrinsic flexor tendons originate in the forearm and insert within the hand. There are nine extrinsic digital flexor tendons (Fig. 19–1): the flexor pollicis longus (FPL), flexor digitorum superficialis (FDS) to digits two to five, and flexor digitorum profundus (FDP) to digits two to five. Approximately 20% of the population does not have FDS to the fifth digit (Austin, Leslie, & Ruby, 1989). The FDS is innervated by the median nerve, the FPL and FDP to index and middle fingers are innervated by the anterior interosseous branch of the median nerve, and the FDP to the ring and small fingers are innervated by the ulnar nerve. There are two extrinsic wrist flexors: flexor carpi radialis (FCR) and flexor carpi ulnaris (FCU). The palmaris longus is not considered in this discussion because of its relative insignificance in flexor tendon rehabilitation.

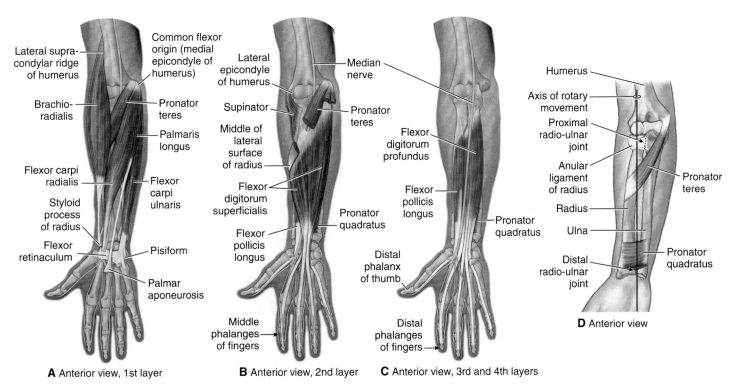

FIGURE 19–1 Muscles of the anterior compartment of forearm and hand. A, First layer. **B,** Second layer. **C,** Third layer. **D,** Fourth layer. (Reprinted with permission from Moore, K. L., Agur, A. M., & Dalley, A. F.II. (2019). *Moore's Essential clinical anatomy* (6th ed.). Philadelphia, PA: Wolters Kluwer.)

The FDP and FPL form the deep muscle layer in the flexor compartment of the forearm just superficial to the pronator teres (Fig. 19–1C,D). The FDP originates on the anterior surface of the shaft of the mid-ulna, the interosseous membrane, and occasionally the proximal radius. Typically, the muscle belly of the FDP separates into a radial and ulnar bundle in the mid-forearm. The radial bundle becomes the tendon to the index finger, and the ulnar bundle forms the tendons to the long finger, ring finger, and small finger. The muscle bellies transition to tendons in the distal forearm. These four tendons traverse the carpal tunnel, occupying its floor, and then diverge to their respective digits in the palm. The FDP tendons enter the particular flexor sheaths at the level of the metacarpophalangeal (MCP) joints and insert on the palmar base of the distal phalanx of each finger. The primary function of the FDP is to flex the dorsal interphalangeal (DIP) joints of the digits. Each FDP tendon acts as a point of origin for an associated lumbrical muscle; an intrinsic that serves to flex the MP and extends the proximal interphalangeal (PIP) and DIP joints of each digit via attachment to the extensor mechanism. The relationship between the FDP and lumbricals has important anatomic implications in cases of severe adhesion and will be further discussed later in this chapter. The FPL originates from the proximal radius and the interosseous membrane. The tendon also lies on the floor of the carpal tunnel, enters the flexor sheath of the thumb, and inserts on the proximal volar surface of the distal phalanx. Its primary function is to flex the interphalangeal (IP) joint of the thumb.

The FDS occupies the intermediate layer of the flexor compartment superficial to the FDP and FPL (Fig. 19–1B). Proximally, two separate heads originate from the elbow region. The humeroulnar head arises from the medial epicondyle of the humerus and the coronoid process of the ulna; the radial head originates from the proximal shaft of the radius. The FDS evolves into four distinct muscle bellies as it traverses distally in the mid-forearm and becomes four individual tendons in the distal forearm. The tendons travel through

the carpal tunnel with the tendons to the long and ring fingers, superficial and central to those of the index and small fingers. The FDS enters the flexor sheath at the level of the MP joint with the FDP tendon. At the level of the mid-proximal phalanx, the FDS tendon bifurcates, and the radial and ulnar slips insert into the proximal aspect of the middle phalanx (Fig. 19–2). This bifurcation, referred to as **Camper chiasm**, allows the FDP tendon to pass through on its course to the distal phalanx. When the digit is flexed, the bifurcation migrates proximally, making the FDP extremely vulnerable to injury in this position (Kleinert, Schepel, & Gill, 1981). The primary function of the FDS is to flex the PIP joints of the fingers while the FDP primarily flexes the DIP joints.

The FCR and FCU are parts of the superficial layer of the flexor surface (Fig. 19–1A). The FCR inserts proximally with the common flexor tendon at the medial epicondyle. Distally, the tendon passes through the flexor retinaculum to insert on the base of the second metacarpal. The FCU has two sites of origin: the humeral head arises from the common flexor tendon, and the ulnar head originates from the medial border of the olecranon and the upper two-thirds of the posterior ulna border. Distally, it inserts on the pisiform, the hook of the hamate, and the base of the fifth metacarpal. The FCR and FCU are the primary wrist flexors.

SYNOVIAL SHEATHS

The **synovial sheaths** in the hand are fibro-osseous tunnels that serve several functions: to provide a better gliding system, to supply nutrition to the tendons, and to contribute to biomechanical efficiency of the tendons during flexion (Fig. 19–2). The sheaths to the index, long, and ring fingers originate at the level of the volar MP joint, whereas the sheaths to the thumb and small fingers extend into the carpal tunnel, becoming the radial and ulnar bursae (Doyle, 1988). The digital tendon sheath has two layers. The outer, parietal layer attaches to the fibrous part of the sheath and pulley system, whereas the inner, visceral layer is attached to the tendon.

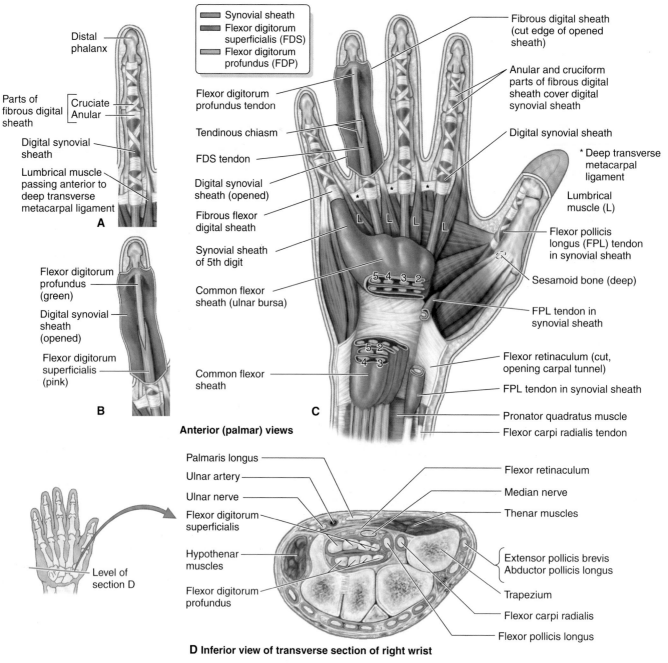

Anterior (palmar) views

D Inferior view of transverse section of right wrist

FIGURE 19-2 **Synovial and fibrous sheaths of long flexor tendons of hand. A,** Parts of fibrous digital sheath. **B,** Digital synovial sheath opened. **C,** Dissection of common flexor sheath and synovial sheaths of digits 1 to 5 (purple). **D,** Transverse section of wrist showing carpal tunnel and its contents. (Reprinted with permission from Moore, K. L., Agur, A. M., & Dalley, A. F.II. (2019). *Moore's Essential clinical anatomy* (6th ed.). Philadelphia, PA: Wolters Kluwer.)

PULLEY SYSTEM

The flexor tendon pulley system is a complex arrangement of connective tissues. There are **annular pulleys**, which are thicker and whose fibers lay perpendicular to the tendon fibers, as well as thinner, more flexible **cruciform pulleys**, which form an "X" over the tendons. From a biomechanical standpoint, the pulleys hold the tendon close to the surface of the bone as the finger flexes. Without an intricate pulley system, the tendon would bowstring, compromising both strength and motion. If the tendon takes the shortest path possible, the muscle fibers may reach a state of full contraction before the tendon can pull the finger through its full range of motion (ROM). The A1, A3, and A5 pulleys originate from the volar plates of the MP, PIP, and DIP joints. The pulleys are numbered proximal to distal, with odd numbers over the joints. The A2 and A4 pulleys originate from the bases of the proximal phalanx and middle phalanx (Fig. 19–3) (Seiler, 2011). These are

the two most structurally important pulleys. The surgeon may elect to repair these pulleys if they were also injured, and a pulley ring may be incorporated in an attempt to further protect the repair (Fig. 19–4).

There are three pulleys over the FPL (Fig. 19–3). The A1 pulley arises from the volar plate of the MP joint, and the A2 pulley arises from the volar plate of the IP joint. The most important pulley in the thumb, the oblique pulley, lies diagonally in between the A1 and A2 pulleys, originating from the fibers of the adductor pollicis.

FLEXOR TENDON ZONES

The flexor tendons are divided into zones, used to identify the location of injury (Fig. 19–5) (Table 19–1). There are different anatomical considerations in each zone. An injury in one zone may require different therapeutic approaches than an injury to the same tendon in another zone.

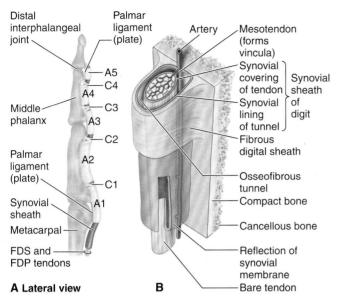

FIGURE 19–3 Fibrous digital sheaths of digits. A, Annular and cruciate parts ("pulleys"). **B,** Structure of osseofibrous tunnel of finger. (Reprinted with permission from Moore, K. L., Agur, A. M., & Dalley, A. F.II. (2019). *Moore's Essential clinical anatomy* (6th ed.). Philadelphia, PA: Wolters Kluwer.)

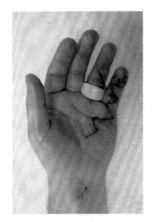

FIGURE 19–4 Nonarticular proximal phalanx orthosis (pulley ring) fabricated to protect pulley repair in zone II injury.

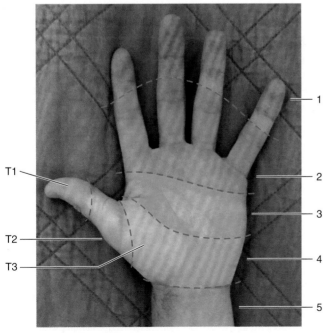

FIGURE 19–5 The flexor tendon zones.

TABLE 19–1	**Flexor Tendon Zones of Injury**
Zone I	Distal tips of digits to just proximal to the DIP joint crease. This zone contains the insertion of the FDP.
Zone II	Starts from middle of middle phalanx and goes to distal palmar crease. This zone contains the insertion of FDS on the base of the middle phalanx. Most rehabilitation protocols are based on injuries within this zone.
Zone III	Distal palmar crease to flexor retinaculum (carpal tunnel).
Zone IV	Flexor retinaculum. As the nine tendons enter the carpal tunnel, they are oriented in the following way: the FDS of middle and ring fingers is the most superficial, with the FDS of index and small fingers just underneath. The four FDP tendons and the FPL are in the deepest layer.
Zone V	Proximal to volar wrist crease to the musculotendinous junction.
Zone TI	Distal phalanx of thumb.
Zone TII	Proximal phalanx of thumb.
Zone TIII	Thenar muscles.

Note: Zones are described distal to proximal.

Zone I

Zone I originates immediately proximal to the DIP crease and extends to the tip of each digit. Injuries in this zone impact the FDP tendon only, resulting in loss of DIP flexion. Based on available tendon stump left for repair, the surgeon may elect to either use a bone anchor or to place suture material through the bone and attach a button on the fingernail to hold the suture in place (Fig. 19–6).

"Jersey finger" is an injury that occurs in zone I with FDP avulsion off the bone. It is so named due to observed incidence in football players when the tip of a finger gets caught in the jersey of another player. Sometimes, the avulsion may even take a part of the bone, which prevents the FDP from retracting too far proximally. The ring and long fingers are the most commonly involved. Oftentimes, this injury may go undiagnosed or be misdiagnosed as a "finger sprain."

Zone II

Zone II traverses from the distal palmar crease to the mid-middle phalanx, corresponding with the A1 pulley and the insertion of the FDS, respectively. Camper chiasm is found in this zone; the location where FDS bifurcates into two slips, which rotate 180° around and under the FDP, inserting on the base of the middle phalanx. Care must be taken to avoid injury to the pulley system during repair, particularly the A2 and A4 pulleys. Sometimes, the surgeon may elect to only repair one slip of the FDS tendon if repairing

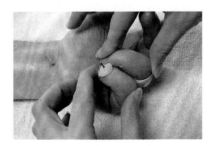

FIGURE 19–6 Button (pull-out suture) in place during the initial stages of healing to keep distal repair secure.

both will make the tendon too bulky to smoothly glide through the pulley system. Historically, this area was referred to as "no man's land" because injuries in this zone were perceived to have poorer prognoses. This nomenclature has unfortunately perpetuated a hesitance to consider progressive approaches to flexor tendon repair and rehabilitation.

Zone III

Zone III spans the volar aspect of the hand from the flexor retinaculum to the distal palmar crease. Injuries in this zone are not within the fibro-osseous tendon sheath, and scar tissue may not be as functionally limiting as injuries in zones II and IV.

Zone IV

Zone IV is located beneath the flexor retinaculum, including all extrinsic flexors of the digits and thumb as well as the median nerve (see Table 19–1). Injuries in this zone are within the carpal tunnel and not as frequent. During tendon repairs in this zone, the transverse carpal ligament is not always repaired. Similar to a standard carpal tunnel release, the wrist should be positioned in neutral in the orthosis to prevent bowstringing of the tendons. Tendon adhesions must be monitored closely in this zone as the tendons lie in close proximity within the synovial sheath.

Zone V

Zone V is located in the distal, volar forearm, spanning from the wrist crease to the musculotendinous junction. Injuries in this zone may include other structures in addition to the finger flexors, such as nerves, vessels, and wrist flexors. Prognoses tend to be better for injuries in this zone. Tendon adherence can occur in this zone but generally does not lead to functional loss as the overlying tissue is loose and mobile.

Zones TI Through TIII

The flexor tendon zones of the thumb include TI, TII, and TIII, corresponding with the distal phalanx, proximal phalanx, and thenar eminence, respectively. The FPL tendon lies alone in its sheath and only crosses one IP joint. However, this tendon is more likely to retract proximally because there is only one vinculum and no lumbrical muscle attached. This may lead to increased tendon adhesions with injuries to this tendon.

TENDON REPAIR, HEALING, AND NUTRITION

SURGICAL REPAIR

Injury to the intricate anatomy of the flexor tendon system requires prompt surgical attention and meticulous repair techniques. Advances in these techniques over the past few decades have led to improvements in postoperative functional outcomes. Ultimately, the goal is a repair that is strong enough to allow early motion and smooth enough to glide easily through the synovial sheaths and within the pulley system.

From a surgical perspective, there have been changes in suture material and suture technique. While therapists can choose to pursue an understanding of the technical details such as named suture techniques and where knots and loops are placed, it is imperative to know how many strands cross the repair site. A two-strand core suture creates a repair that does not gain strength until 3 weeks postoperatively (Hatanaka, Zhang, & Manske, 2000). The very common, four-strand tendon repair involves a single suture crossing the repair site four times with a cross in the middle (Fig. 19–7). Six- and eight-strand repairs have been shown to be even stronger; however, surgical skill is necessary to minimize tendon bulk and adhesions (Winters et al., 1998). Increased strength of the tendon repair is achieved if the epitenon is repaired, also decreasing propensity for gapping at the repair site (Dy, Hernandez-Soria, Ma, Roberts, & Daluiski, 2012; Mashadi & Amis, 1992).

The timeframe between injury and surgery is critical to final outcomes. Ideally, it is best to repair the tendon shortly after injury. Delaying repair may lead to increased scar tissue and contracted muscles. If the tendon has retracted into the palm, which may occur if the finger was flexed at time of injury, there is additional trauma to the tendon due to the greater chance of vincula disruption as well as increased handling of peritendinous structures during tendon retrieval. The surgical incision is typically completed in a zigzag pattern, known as a Bruner incision, which allows for maximal exposure of the tendon. Alternately, a surgeon may elect to place the incision on the lateral border of the digit in an attempt to decrease external scar and increase ROM. This approach is technically more difficult as care must be taken to avoid the digital nerve branches and the vascular supply to the digit.

TENDON HEALING

Tendon healing was originally postulated to occur only through extrinsic processes, including scar tissue and adhesions (Mason & Allen, 1941; Potenza, 1963; Peacock, 1965). This antiquated notion was based on the idea of adhesions being the sole source of blood supply and fibroblasts needed for collagen production and healing. Until the late 1970s, surgeons favored immobilization to allow tendons to heal during the early postoperative phase, deferring tendon glide and accrual of strength until the later stages of wound healing.

The deleterious effects of immobilization cannot be understated and were finally disrupted through a set of groundbreaking studies by Lundborg and Rank (1978, 1980), who demonstrated that flexor tendons are completely capable of intrinsic healing without associated external scar adhesions. During a similar timeframe, Dr. Richard Gelberman and his colleagues published a series of impactful studies showing that the application of stress through early passive motion leads to more rapid recovery of tensile strength, fewer adhesions, improved excursion, and better nutrition (Gelberman et al., 1980, 1981, 1982, 1986; Gelberman & Woo, 1989). The concept of tendon softening in the early postoperative phase was also refuted through studies that supported early mobilization as a means to enhance tensile strength while limiting adhesions (Hitchcock et al., 1987; Strickland & Glogovac, 1980). The work of these authors and many since reinforces the notion

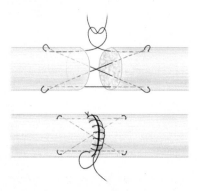

FIGURE 19–7 Four-strand cruciate repair with epitenon stitch. (Reprinted with permission from Hunt, T. R. (2011). *Operative techniques.* In *Hand, wrist and forearm surgery* (pp. 466). Baltimore, MD: Lippincott Williams & Wilkins.)

that the practice of immobilization following flexor tendon repair, unfortunately not obsolete, should be replaced by early mobilization in the vast majority of situations.

TENDON NUTRITION

Tendon nutrition is integral to tendon healing. Tendons, especially in zone II, lack robust vascular supply, primarily receiving their nutrition through vascular and synovial diffusion. The tendon receives blood supply from the bone at the site of tendon insertion. There is also a **vincula system**, vascular "highways" leading directly from the bone to the dorsal surface of the tendon. Each FDS and FDP tendon has a brevis and profundus vincula.

The pulley system plays an important role in the nutrition of the tendons; the mechanical action of the pulleys "pumps" nutrition via diffusion into the volar surface of the tendons. In addition to nutritional benefits, this action aids in creating a better environment for the gliding of the tendon. Active flexion of the digit creates a high-pressure system within the pulleys to push the nutrients into the tendon. This may be part of why patients performing early motion tend to have better results and is something to consider when choosing a rehabilitation protocol (Amadio, Jaeger, & Hunter, 1990).

WOUND HEALING

In treating tendon injuries, it is important to be aware of the basic concepts of tissue/wound healing to help guide clinical decision-making. Review of Chapter 3 and further reading in this area is recommended. As the tendon is healing, the surrounding tissues are also healing in three overlapping phases. The first phase is the inflammatory phase, the body's immediate response to a traumatic event. It is important to consider surgery as traumatic event, resulting in an inflammatory response (Fig. 19–8A). This phase can last anywhere from 3 to 7 days postoperatively.

The second phase is called the fibroblastic or proliferative phase. In this phase, fibroblasts initiate the production of collagen fibers (Fig. 19–8B). Early collagen fibers are weak, disorganized, and have little tensile strength, but they begin to lay the foundation for stronger collagen fibers that will be produced in the later phase. The fibroblastic phase typically lasts from day 5 to day 21. Important work by Urbaniak, Cahill, and Mortenson (1975) demonstrated that the tensile strength of tendon repairs may decrease in this phase, specifically between days 7 and 21. Consideration of this evidence affords therapists an opportunity to modulate exercise carefully during this phase.

The third and longest phase is the remodeling or maturation phase. Early collagen fibers begin to become more differentiated and more linear, and the tendon gains tensile strength (Fig. 19–8C). The early collagen fibers are broken down through a process called lysis and newer, stronger, more mature fibers are produced. In the earlier phases of scar production, collagen fibers are dense and disorganized, but over time, the collagen fibers lie in a more parallel orientation. A simple visual that reinforces this concept is cooked spaghetti in a pot compared with spaghetti in the box. Collagen fibers that are more parallel require less space and glide more effectively through surrounding tissue. This phase can last anywhere from 3 weeks postoperatively to well over a year.

Scars can be observed externally to determine response to therapeutic techniques. A pink-red scar is metabolically active and is still undergoing the remodeling phase, whereas a scar that has faded to a color paler than the surrounding skin is no longer active and is less likely to respond to efforts aimed at changing scar tissue properties. It

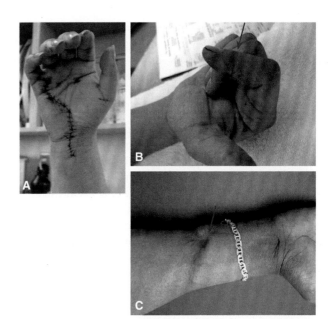

FIGURE 19–8 Stages of wound healing. A, Inflammatory stage shown after saw injury 2 days postoperatively. **B,** Attempts at active flexion during proliferative stage during the height of collagen synthesis. **C,** Scar maturation phase noted by fading of scar and dense adhesion formation during active digital extension.

is imperative to recognize that scar modulation techniques employed to disrupt external scar, such as massage and vibration, have little impact on internal adhesions that have formed between the tendon and sheath. There is also no evidence to support ultrasound as an effective technique for internal scar tissue. Early and consistent evaluations of tendon glide, paired with safe and progressive exercise, are the primary means by which to avoid internal adhesions.

It is important to watch for signs of infection during the postoperative course of recovery. Infection may interfere with the stages of wound healing, prolong the healing process, and potentially create more scar tissue.

FUNDAMENTAL CONCEPTS

A smooth and freely gliding tendon that is able to produce ROM and return to function is the ultimate goal of flexor tendon repair and rehabilitation. In addition to understanding flexor tendon anatomy, surgical repair, and healing, therapists who can apply the fundamental concepts of tendon gliding, force, synergistic motion, and work of flexion to their rehabilitative strategies will advance therapy beyond the standard protocols.

EXCURSION AND FORCE

The smooth movement of the tendon within the synovial sheath is typically referred to as **tendon excursion** or tendon gliding. Tendon glide is measured as the amount of differential motion that occurs between the tendon and surrounding structures, including other tendons, the tendon sheath, the pulley system, and the local bony architecture. Mathematical calculation of tendon glide affords the knowledge that a normal FDP tendon with 270 of combined, active motion at the MP, PIP, and DIP will demonstrate 3.6 cm (36 mm) of tendon excursion as it moves from full extension to full flexion (Brand, 1985). More specifically, the FDP tendon is calculated to glide 1.3 mm during every 10 of PIP motion and 0.9 mm during every 10 of DIP motion. Creating at least 3–5 mm of tendon gliding in the early postoperative phase has been suggested as a baseline to avoid tendon adhesions (Duran & Houser, 1975; Gelberman, Botte, Spiegelman, & Akeson, 1986). Promising bench research has been published about the addition of surface lubricants, applied to the tendon at time of repair, to improve tendon glide (Kim et al., 2010).

FORCE

According to Zhao et al. (2002), "the ideal postoperative therapy would use the smallest **force** to achieve the largest tendon excursion." As muscles activate, forces are transmitted across the musculotendinous junction and through tendons to create joint motion. Passive and active exercises submit forces through the healing tendon, and wrist position can be utilized to carefully modulate those forces. As stated previously, it is imperative that therapists know the number of strands crossing the repair site. This information provides essential guidance regarding the amount of force a healing tendon can safely accept. Urbaniak et al. (1975) suggested that two-strand repairs can withstand 1250 g of force between 1 and 3 weeks post repair, while four-strand repairs safely allow up to 2150 g. Table 19–2 outlines the evidence-based force and excursion parameters paired with standard therapeutic exercises. Knowing both the number of strands and the forces created by exercises helps therapists create safe progression after tendon repair.

SYNERGISTIC MOTION

Synergistic motion is the active, agonist-synergist balance that negates active insufficiency in the digital flexors. Wrist extensors act as synergists during digital flexion, facilitating the length-tension relationship and offsetting passive tension created by the long extensors. The opposite occurs during digital extension when wrist flexors take over the synergist role. Multiple studies have established the importance of synergistic motion after flexor tendon repair to decrease passive tension and increase tendon excursion (Savage, 1988; Cooney, Lin, & An, 1989; Evans & Thompson, 1993; Lieber, Amiel, Kaufman, Whitney, & Gelberman, 1996, Lieber, Silva, Amiel, & Gelberman, 1999; Zhao et al., 2002). Asking the patient to perform active digit flexion with the wrist positioned in flexion, an unfortunately common practice in the postoperative phase, increases force on the healing flexor tendon and should be avoided.

WORK OF FLEXION

Work of flexion is the work necessary to create active flexion, influenced by both intrinsic and extrinsic factors including surface friction, bulk of the repaired tendon, tendon adhesions, edema, joint stiffness, and resistance of the antagonistic musculature (Tanaka et al., 2003; Zhao et al., 2004, 2005). Multiple studies have suggested day 4 or 5 after surgery as the timeframe when work of flexion is minimized and therapy should be initiated (Tanaka et al., 2003; Zhao et al., 2004, 2005; Cao & Tang, 2005, 2006; Cao et al., 2008). Therapists often delay therapy when edema is observed; however, a series of studies by Cao & Tang, (2005), Cao et al. (2008), and Cao and Tang (2006) demonstrated that gentle motion actually reduced gliding resistance and work of flexion. As therapists, this conclusion affords the opportunity to modulate the range, frequency, and speed of exercise when edema is present. Having the patient create a short arc range, slowly and with fewer repetitions, is safe, effective, and preferable to delaying treatment. Conversely, a common wound care and edema strategy that markedly increases work of flexion is a self-adherent wrap. A study by Buonocore et al. (2012) noted that digits with self-adherent wrap in place during ROM experienced significant increases in work of flexion. While exercise can be performed carefully in the presence of edema, self-adherent wrapped must be removed to protect the healing tendon.

TABLE 19–2	Force and Excursion Parameters	
Exercise	**Excursion**	**Force**
Passive protected extension	3–8 mm distal (Duran & Houser, 1975)	200–300g (Urbaniak et al., 1975)
Place and hold digital flexion during wrist extension (synergistic motion)	FDS 26 mm FDP 33 mm proximal (Wehbe & Hunter, 1985a, 1985b)	900g (Lieber et al., 1999)
Active straight fist	Wrist neutral FDS 28 mm FDP 27 mm Max FDS proximal (Wehbe & Hunter, 1985a, 1985b)	1100g (Greenwald et al., 1994)
Active hook fist	Wrist neutral FDS 13 mm FDP 24 mm Maximum differential proximal (Wehbe & Hunter, 1985a, 1985b)	1300g (Greenwald et al., 1994)
Active composite fist	Wrist neutral to extended FDS 24–26 mm FDP 32–33 mm Maximum FDP proximal (Wehbe & Hunter, 1985a, 1985b)	400–4000g (Schuind et al., 1992)
Active, isolated PIP flexion	~13 mm (calculated) FDP proximal	900g (Schuind et al., 1992)
Active, isolated DIP flexion	~6.5 mm (calculated) FDP proximal	1900g (Schuind et al., 1992)

INITIATION OF THERAPY

Treatment of flexor tendon injuries requires a team approach: a skilled surgeon, an experienced hand therapist, and a patient who can participate in the rehabilitative process. Ideally, the patient should be seen for therapy within the first week postoperatively, with 4 to 5 days being the optimal timeframe. The longer it takes to initiate therapy, the more likely limiting adhesions will form along with joint stiffness. Communication with the referring surgeon is essential. Refer to Box 19–1 for the essential questions that will guide flexor tendon rehabilitation.

INITIAL EVALUATION

Choosing the right treatment approach will depend on several factors; a thorough history must be taken at the initial visit. Information gathered should include the following (Tan et al., 2010; van Adrichem, Hovius, van Strik, & van der Meulen, 1992):

- Mechanism of injury.
- Past medical history. Conditions such as diabetes and arthritis may have a negative impact on healing potential.
- Medications. A recent study by Tan et al. (2010) demonstrated that NSAIDs appear to reduce flexor tendon adhesions.
- Social habits such as smoking or drinking. van Adrichem et al. (1992) demonstrated that cigarette smoke negatively impacts microcirculation after surgery.
- Any preexisting injuries to the affected hand that would lead to a decrease in ROM.
- Concomitant injuries that will impact tendon gliding and therapy progression, such as fractures and nerve repairs. Yu et al. (2004)

BOX 19–1   ESSENTIAL QUESTIONS

Note: These are only a few of the many questions a clinician should discuss with the referring surgeon.

- Mechanism of injury? Condition of tendon?
- Issues around potential patient compliance?

- Zone of injury?
- Number of strands crossing the repair site? Epitendinous suture?
- Integrity of repair?
- Other structures involved? Nerves, arteries, pulleys?

demonstrated that limited, protected motion does not impact the results of digital nerve repairs.

- Surgical procedures that create precautions such as vascular repairs and skin grafts.
- Age plays a factor in clinical decision-making. The patient must be able to understand the precautions and exercise program. Patients who are too young may not be able to participate in an early mobilization postoperative program. Older patients may have a decreased capacity for healing.

Financial factors may hinder therapy, such as uninsured patients, those with limited insurance, and those with high co-pays or deductibles. Some patients may need to travel from far away to attend therapy. For these reasons and more, education is paramount. An overeager patient may exercise too much, potentially leading to increased swelling, gapping, and/or rupture. A patient who does not understand the importance of or adhere to the home program may be overly fearful and more likely to develop stiffness and limiting adhesions.

Baseline measurements that are safe to document are an essential part of the initial visit and every visit thereafter. Passive ROM, with the exception of MP extension and composite digital extension, provides a baseline of joint mobility and provides the therapist with a comparative data point to assess tendon glide. A gentle place and hold flexion measurement with the wrist in a neutral position will allow the therapist a first look at flexor tendon function. This practice is invaluable for future assessment but indicated only when the surgeon has verified integrity of the repair and/or has requested a **place and hold** or **true active motion** protocol. A tendon with normal glide and function will be recognized when active motion is equal to passive motion; tendon adhesions are present when passive flexion is greater than active flexion.

In addition to goniometric measurement, assessment of pain, edema, and sensation are vital evaluative measures. The use of a self-report outcome measure at baseline, such as the Disabilities of the Arm, Shoulder, and Hand (DASH), will help the therapist and patient incorporate essential conversations about activities of daily living and adaptation during the healing phase (Powell & von der Heyde, 2014).

Other factors that may have an impact on prognosis and tendon healing include the following:

- Level of injury (zone).
- Type of injury.
- Other structures involved.
- Clean laceration versus a crush injury. Greater trauma to the tissue at time of injury creates a greater potential for scar tissue (Pettengill & Van Strien, 2011).
- Tendon sheath integrity.
- Surgical technique. Careful handling of the tendon will minimize scar tissue and risk for adhesions.
- Suture strength created by number of core strands crossing the repair site and a circumferential, epitendinous suture.
- Timeframes between injury and surgery, surgery and initiation of therapy. Greater timeframes are correlated with higher incidences of tendon adhesions and worse outcomes.

POSTOPERATIVE ORTHOSIS

The historical **dorsal blocking orthosis** restricts composite extension and maintains the flexor tendons in a shortened position. Positioning of this orthosis traditionally held the wrist at 10° to 30° of flexion, MP joints at 40° to 60° of flexion, and IP joints in full extension (Fig. 19–9A–C). A greater understanding of synergistic motion and work of flexion has modified the traditional wrist and MP positions, with multiple authors suggesting alternative approaches. Coats, Echevarria-Ore, and Mass (2005) and Clancy and Mass (2013) suggest moving the wrist to 20° to 30° extension with the MPs in 60° to 75° flexion, while Peck et al. (2014) and Higgins and Lalonde (2016) allow up to 45° of wrist extension while limiting MP flexion to 30° (Fig. 19–9D). For those therapists and surgeons who are not yet ready to move the wrist into extension, positioning the wrist in neutral is a reasonable compromise that will provide both protection to the healing tendons and safely allow place and hold and true active motion within the orthosis (Fig. 19–9E–G).

Several issues must be taken into consideration when fabricating an extension restriction orthosis. It may be helpful to position the patient's arm on a foam ramp or on a homemade hand rest, preferably with a towel roll under the arm and the digits draped over the edge (Fig. 19–10A,B). Padding placed over the ulnar styloid prior to orthosis fabrication will increase comfort and prevent skin breakdown (Fig. 19–11A,B).

Full MP flexion may not be comfortable for the patient, especially if the wound extends into the palm. Too little MP flexion, however, may not be sufficient enough to put slack on the repair. To maintain position of the orthosis, it should conform to the MP joints with attention to potential areas of pressure. The palmar strap should securely maintain the dorsum of the hand to the hood of the orthosis (Fig. 19–12A). The orthosis itself can be contoured adequately, but if the strap across the palm is not sufficient, the patient can unknowingly rest in too much MP extension, potentially putting the tendon repair at risk (Fig. 19–12B).

During fabrication, it is important that the roof of the orthosis is made to allow for full IP joint extension, even if the IP joints have not yet achieved full extension. It is challenging, yet crucial, to ensure that the MP joints are flexed to the intended angle while keeping the IP joints straight. Not only does full IP extension in the orthosis help prevent PIP flexion contractures but also it allows the tendon to glide distally when actively extending to the orthosis, helping to prevent adhesions (Fig. 19–13A–C). Though refuted in current literature (Yu et al., 2004), some surgeons continue to request restriction of extension at the PIP joint following a concomitant, digital nerve repair. Adding a small foam wedge dorsally at the middle phalanx will allow for this restriction of motion and can be altered as the weeks progress to provide greater available extension. This open-packed positioning of the PIP can quickly lead to a flexion contracture and should be monitored carefully.

EXPERT PEARL 19-1

Volar digit orthosis within flexor tendon orthosis

THERESA BELL-NAGLE, OTR/L, CHT
Massachusetts

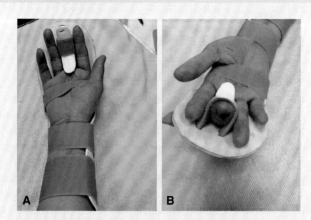

Addition of digit orthosis within larger protective orthosis to gently hold PIP/DIP joints in extension to prevent flexion contracture. The hook strap is being pulled through on the dorsal side through slits in the material.

REHABILITATION REGIMENS

Rehabilitation regimens, often referred to as protocols, have been developed to provide timelines for progression of therapy. As previously stated, seminal research has shown that early mobilization leads to improved ability for the tendon to glide as well as increased strength of the repair (Lundborg & Rank, 1978, 1980; Gelberman et al., 1980, 1981, 1982, 1986; Gelberman & Woo, 1989; Hitchcock et al., 1987). In current practice, regimens are categorized by type of exercise, including immobilization, **early passive flexion**, place and hold flexion, and true active flexion.

IMMOBILIZATION

Despite advances in knowledge of tendon healing and tendon repair, there may be situations where postoperative immobilization is the best choice. A patient who is too young, cognitively unable, or unwilling to participate in therapy is best suited for this protocol. When a tendon is immobilized, it loses strength after initial repair due to softening of the tendon ends. This loss of strength lasts until the second week postoperatively and must be taken into consideration during the rehabilitation process.

0 to 3–4 weeks: The patient is allowed to move any joint not protected by the orthosis including the elbow and shoulder.

3 to 4 weeks: The wrist is brought to neutral in the orthosis and the patient can initiate an exercise program: PROM to each joint, followed by active tendon gliding exercises. The orthosis can be removed for bathing and exercise but otherwise should be worn throughout the day and night.

4 to 6 weeks: The dorsal blocking orthosis is discontinued. Exercises are progressed to include joint blocking. At this time, if flexion contractures have developed or extrinsic flexor tightness is present, an orthosis that creates gentle mobilization toward extension may be initiated at night.

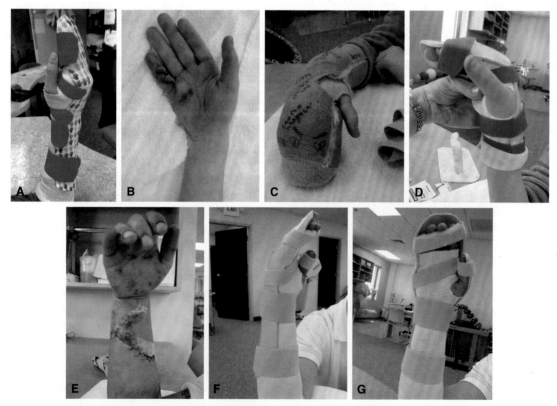

FIGURE 19-9 A, Wrist and hand extension restriction orthosis for flexor tendon repair with the wrist in 30° flexion and the MP joints in approximately 60° of flexion. **B–D,** A 9-year-old boy is casted per the immobilization protocol then the cast is removed, incision site cleansed, and a custom wrist extension restriction orthosis is applied. **E–G,** A zone V injury shown, wrist is in neutral with the MP joints in 30° of flexion. The amount of wrist and MP flexion depends on the protocol used, severity of injury, type and extent of repair, and/or the MD preference. Note the use of wide elasticized 2-inch strapping. This allows for even pressure distribution and comfort.

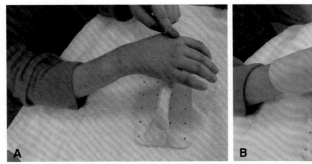
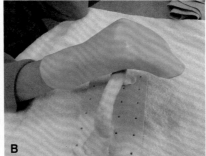

FIGURE 19–10 A and B, Homemade thermoplastic hand stand used to prevent flattening of forearm musculature during the molding process as seen when using foam supports. This also allows for easy adjustments of wrist and MP joint angles.

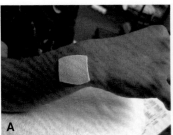
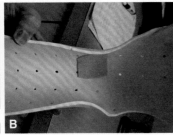

FIGURE 19–11 A, Prepad the distal ulna and **(B)** invert the foam into the orthosis for a permanent solution to prevent bony irritation.

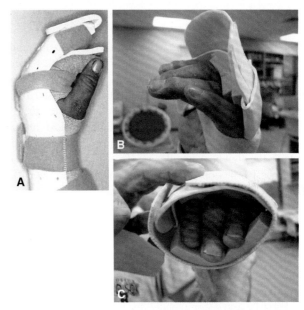

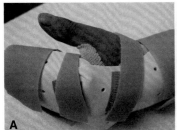
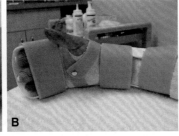

FIGURE 19–12 A, When molding about the MP joints, use a strategy such as this cut/overlap technique to obtain contour about this bony area (dorsal second MP). **B,** Riveting a strap that contours around the thumb carpometacarpal (CMC) joint secures the orthosis on the arm, preventing migration.

FIGURE 19–13 A, An AlumaFoam® insert positions the index MP joint in flexion, facilitating active proximal interphalangeal (PIP) extension with exercise and allowing the PIP to be safely strapped into extension to prevent PIP flexion contracture. **B and C,** Applying foam dorsally over the proximal phalanges and volarly on the distal strap can be another way to achieve greater PIP extension within the orthosis.

EARLY PASSIVE FLEXION

Early passive flexion protocols came into use in the 1970s. These protocols are rarely used in isolation, but it is important to understand the history behind their development. They are based on the work of Kleinert, Kutz, Ashbell, and Martinez (1967) and Duran and Houser (1975), who demonstrated that early mobilization increased tendon gliding and produced better outcomes. Passive motion affords minimal tendon glide without the forces created by active motion. Each protocol has specific timeframes and exercises, but in practice, most therapists using early passive flexion protocols use a combination of approaches. Early passive flexion protocols are a safe and potentially effective option in situations where the surgeon was only able to do a two-strand repair or if the number of strands crossing the repair site is unknown.

Duran and Houser

Duran and Houser (1975) observed that 3 to 5 mm of glide was sufficient to prevent adhesions. According to the original protocol,

the patient is positioned in a wrist and hand extension restriction orthosis with the wrist in 20° of flexion, MP joints in relaxed flexion, and IP joints held in flexion with dynamic traction, such as rubber bands. Isolated PIP and DIP PROM is performed with wrist and MP joints held in flexion, six to eight repetitions, two times per day. After 4.5 weeks, the orthosis is discontinued and a wristlet is placed with a rubber band attached from the wrist strap to the fingernail to allow for finger flexion/extension to occur with tenodesis (Fig. 19–14A, B). Resisted flexion does not begin until 8 weeks.

The **modified Duran** protocol discontinued the use of rubber band traction, positioning the IP joints in extension against the orthosis between exercise sessions. Passive flexion and extension exercises are performed as previously stated. The patient is also allowed to actively extend IP joints to the extension block of the orthosis, which is the component that makes this the "modified" Duran protocol (Fig. 19–15A,B).

Kleinert

The original **Kleinert** protocol placed the wrist in 45° of flexion and the MP joints in 10° to 20° of flexion. However, the original protocol

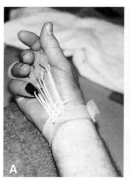
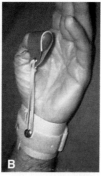

FIGURE 19–14 **A wristlet is worn during the intermediate phase of treatment with the modified Duran protocol. A,** The force can be secured distal to the proximal phalanx directly to the nail of the small finger or applied via a sling on the proximal phalanges of the index, long, or ring. **B,** Flexor pollicis longus repairs can be managed in a similar fashion with a passive thumb IP flexion cuff.

is rarely, if ever, used and this wrist and MP joint positioning is no longer recommended. Kleinert's research showed that extension against resistance actually quieted the activity of the flexors based on electromyography (EMG) findings. Using the rubber band traction as described in the Duran protocol, the patient is asked to create active extension of the IP joints toward the hood of the orthosis and against the resistance of the rubber bands. The tension of the rubber band passively pulls the digit back into flexion. This sequence of active extension and passive flexion is completed 10 times every waking hour. Gentle active flexion is initiated at 3 to 6 weeks and resistance at 6 to 8 weeks.

Washington

The Washington Regimen, also referred to as the Brooke Army Hospital modification, combines the passive flexion recommended by Duran and Houser with the controlled active extension/passive rubber band flexion recommended by Kleinert, adding a pulley in the palm for increased DIP flexion (Fig. 19–16). Active flexion is

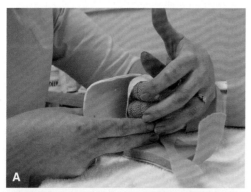

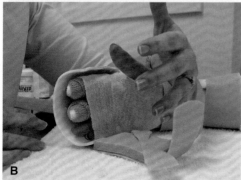

FIGURE 19–15 Modified Duran protocol: passive digit flexion performed in clinic under supervision **(A)** with active digit extension to the confines of the orthosis **(B)**.

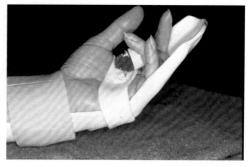

FIGURE 19–16 Rubber band traction is used for gentle digital flexion in an early passive flexion program; modified orthosis with palmar pulley shown here.

not begun until week 4, the wrist position in the orthosis is brought to neutral at week 5, and the orthosis is generally discontinued at week 6 (Dovelle & Heeter, 1989).

PLACE AND HOLD

With early passive flexion protocols, the tendon achieves some glide, but the tendency is for the tendon to be compressed or "bunched up" rather than actually gliding through the sheath. True tendon excursion has better potential to help prevent adhesions. Place and hold regimens are based on the concept of synergistic motion, optimizing agonist-synergist balance, decreasing passive tension, and increasing tendon excursion (Savage, 1988; Cooney et al., 1989; Evans & Thompson, 1993; Lieber et al., 1996, 1999; Zhao et al., 2002). Place and hold regimens mobilize all four digits simultaneously, a practice that has been suggested to maximize tendon glide (Korstanje et al., 2012; Silfverskiold, May, & Oden, 1993). A landmark, experimental study offering the highest level of evidence to date for flexor tendon rehabilitation was published by Trumble and colleagues (Trumble et al., 2010; Neiduski & Powell, 2019). The authors observed that patients have better outcomes, including increased active flexion and decreased flexion contractures, with a place and hold protocol than with early passive flexion (Trumble et al., 2010).

Indiana

A commonly used place and hold protocol proposed by Strickland (1993) and Cannon (1993), the **Indiana Protocol**, includes a synergistic exercise sequence where the wrist is placed in flexion, the fingers are placed in flexion, the wrist is moved toward extension, and the patient gently and actively holds the digits in flexion. This exercise can be practiced using the contralateral hand until the sequence feels natural and can be demonstrated with smooth movements.

Two orthoses are used in the original Indiana protocol. When not exercising, the patient is in a wrist and hand extension restriction orthosis that holds the wrist at 20° of flexion, the MP joints at 50° of flexion, and the IPs in full extension against the hood of the orthosis. The exercise orthosis is hinged at the wrist and blocks wrist extension at 30°, allowing the place and hold exercise to occur safely within the orthosis (Fig. 19–17A–C). In the interest of saving time and resources, the exercise orthosis can be fabricated with a removable block placing the wrist in 20° of flexion to be worn between exercise sessions. In this protocol, modified Duran exercises followed by place and hold exercises are performed hourly. At 4 weeks, the patient is allowed to initiate active flexion in a synergistic fashion outside of the orthosis: active digital flexion with wrist extension followed by active wrist flexion with digit extension. At 7 to 8 weeks, the extension restriction orthosis is discontinued, and resistive exercises are initiated.

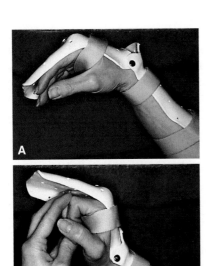

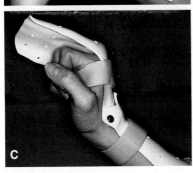

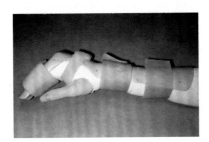

FIGURE 19–17 This tenodesis orthosis allows full flexion of the wrist but blocks extension at 30°. **A,** Wrist flexion with digit extension. **B,** Passive digit flexion with wrist extension. **C,** Active digit flexion hold. The orthosis shown is one of many design options for this protocol.

TRUE ACTIVE FLEXION

True active flexion regimens include those in which the patient is asked to produce a determined range of volitional, active digital flexion. Gaining momentum over the past decade, the majority of these regimens include a static, dorsal blocking orthosis that positions the wrist in extension rather than flexion (Coats et al., 2005; Clancy & Mass, 2013; Higgins & Lalonde, 2016; Fig. 19–18). Based on the seminal work by Evans and Thompson (1993), positioning the wrist in up to 45° extension helps create minimal active muscle tendon tension in the healing flexor tendon. This wrist extension is paired with partial ranges of true active flexion, including first third (Peck et al., 2014), midrange (Higgins & Lalonde, 2016), and available range (Coats et al., 2005; Clancy & Mass, 2013).

Manchester Short Orthosis

Published by Fiona Peck in 2014, the **Manchester Short Orthosis** regimen includes an innovative, hand-based orthosis that allows

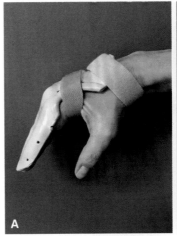
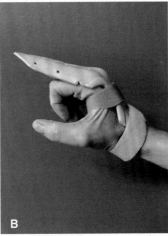

FIGURE 19–19 **A,** The Manchester Short Splint, a hand-based dorsal blocking orthosis. **B,** Allows up to 45° of wrist extension.

up to 45° of wrist extension, holding the MPs at 30° flexion and the IPs in full extension against the dorsal hood of the orthosis (Fig. 19–19A,B). Peck et al. (2014) suggested that placing the MP joint in too much flexion after repair biases motion toward the PIP joint and increases forces on the FDP tendon during attempts to produce DIP flexion. True active flexion is initiated at the DIP joint to optimize differential glide, is limited to the first third of the total available range, and is completed synchronously with active wrist extension.

In a comparative study, Peck et al. (2014) demonstrated that patients who were rehabilitated using the Manchester Short Orthosis had significantly less flexion contractures at the PIP joint at 6 and 12 weeks, had significantly greater arcs of DIP flexion, and were more likely to have good or excellent results.

Saint John Protocol

Drawing on Peck's innovation, the **Saint John Protocol** begins with a dorsal blocking orthosis that includes the wrist and transitions to the Manchester Short Orthosis between 2 and 4 weeks after surgery (Higgins & Lalonde, 2016). Using the same joint positioning, this regimen also incorporates true active flexion to the first third or half of the available range, initiated at the DIP. Both protocols call for a passive ROM warm-up to prepare the joints and tendons for active exercise.

FLEXOR POLLICIS LONGUS REHABILITATION

Rehabilitation and orthosis management for FPL repair is more complicated as there are limited studies to guide practice. Most protocols are based on research to FDS and FDP tendons. Brown and McGrouther (1984) noted that more FPL glide occurs when the thumb MP is held in extension while the IP is passively flexed as compared to passive composite flexion. The FPL tendon is more prone to scar formation as it is more likely to retract after laceration. Muscle shortening makes tendon retrieval challenging and IP flexion contractures are common.

There is no formal FPL protocol. Therefore, the clinician must apply knowledge about tendon rehabilitation for FDS and FDP laceration/repair and apply it to the FPL tendon. Four-strand repairs have been shown to better tolerate early motion with lower rupture rates (Elliot, Moiemen, Flemming, Harris, & Foster, 1994).

In general, the orthosis for FPL injuries should position the wrist in slight flexion and the thumb in palmar abduction with the IP extended (Fig. 19–20). The fingers are left free; however, the patient should be cautioned against gripping or attempting to use the hand

FIGURE 19–18 Static, dorsal blocking orthosis with wrist positioned in extension.

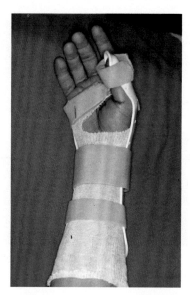

FIGURE 19–20 Extension restriction orthosis for flexor pollicis longus repair. The thumb should be positioned between palmar and radial abduction.

functionally due to possible intertendinous connections between the FDP of the index finger and the FPL, known as Lindberg anomaly. This orthosis can be used with early passive flexion protocols but should be modified to wrist neutral or extended to initiate place and hold or true active flexion of the thumb.

THERAPY PROGRESSION AND OUTCOMES

With any flexor tendon protocol, it is the quality of motion achieved that is important; exercises should be performed correctly in order to achieve the most glide with the lowest load. Increasing the frequency will not have an impact on adhesion formation if the tendon is not gliding. In addition, overexercising may incite an inflammatory response, which may lead to more adhesions.

The therapist will need to evaluate when the patient can be advanced through the next stages of therapy or when the patient needs to be held back. Some people tend to produce more scar than others; therefore, it is necessary to individually tailor each therapy program. Based on consistent goniometric measurement and comparison of passive to active motion, tendon glide should be assessed at each therapy visit. Patients who are demonstrating consistent increases in tendon glide are treated more conservatively; there is no need to add force or additional exercise if the tendon is responding favorably to the current exercise regimen. Conversely, patients who demonstrated worsening or plateaued tendon glide are treated with progressive exercises that increase force and excursion. **Strickland percentage** and the **pyramid of progressive force** are two tools that therapists can use to help guide therapeutic progression after tendon repair.

STRICKLAND PERCENTAGE

Published by Strickland and Glogovac, 1980, the formula commonly known as Strickland percentage affords therapists and surgeons a percentage comparison to normal tendon glide. Based on the combined normative value of 175°, the patient's PIP and DIP flexion are added together, any extensor lags are subtracted, and the final number is divided by 175. Multiplication by 100 provides a percentage of normal PIP and DIP motion (Box 19–2). This percentage can be tracked along with ROM at each visit to determine whether tendon glide is increasing over time.

PYRAMID OF PROGRESSIVE FORCE

In 2004, Groth proposed a theoretical guideline to help therapists and surgeons decide how to progress the rehabilitation of the injured flexor tendon. Traditional flexor tendon protocols as outlined within this chapter are based on chronologic timelines and the wound healing process. Time-based regimens do not accommodate individual healing differences from patient to patient. The pyramid of progressive force (Groth, 2004) is used to support clinical decision-making as opposed to serving as a precise protocol (Fig. 19–21). As such, it can be used in conjunction with other regimens to determine exercise prescription and progression.

The pyramid of progressive force was developed based on knowledge of tendon excursion and amount of force encountered during motion. Exercises creating the least force are located at the bottom of the pyramid, while those requiring more force are found at the top. The use of a pyramidal shape indicates that most patients will participate in the exercises on the bottom, while fewer will need to be progressed through those at the top. The goal of the pyramid is to allow the therapist to progress exercises based on how the tendon is performing. It is vital to remember that if the tendon is responding well to treatment, the therapist should stay the course and not add additional exercises.

- Base level: The first level of the pyramid is protected passive finger extension, based on Duran, Houser, and Kleinert protocols. This exercise is an excellent warm-up and affords distal glide of the healing flexor tendon.
- Second level: The second level includes place and hold with a loose fist and wrist extension, also known as synergistic motion.
- Third level: The third level includes advancing to an active, composite fist. Groth (2004) advocated for the wrist to be protected in 20° of flexion; however, current literature encourages moving the wrist toward a neutral or extended position and decreasing the range between the first third up to midrange (Coats et al., 2005; Clancy & Mass, 2013; Higgins & Lalonde, 2016).
- Fourth level: The fourth level includes active straight and hook fist. The wrist is held at neutral to provide even stress to the tendon. It is important to note that a tendon with a two-strand repair is not strong enough to withstand an active hook fist until 21 days after surgery (Urbaniak et al., 1975; Greenwald, Shumway, Allen, & Mass, 1994).
- Fifth level: Groth (2004) identified discontinuation of the protective orthosis as an important milestone that would inherently increase forces on the healing tendon due to increased functional use. No new exercises are added while the patient adjusts to the new stresses of being orthosis-free. The patient can be weaned from the orthosis gradually over the course of 1 to 2 weeks.

BOX 19–2 STRICKLAND PERCENTAGE

$$\frac{\left(\text{Active PIP} + \text{DIP flexion}\right) - \left(\text{PIP} + \text{DIP extensor lags}\right)}{175} \times 100 = \% \text{ of normal PIP and DIP motion}$$

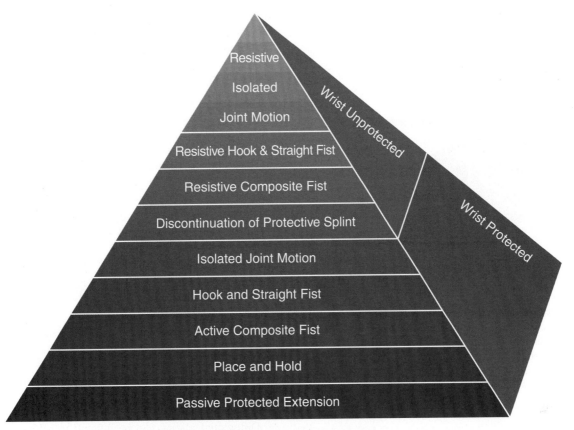

Pyramid of progressive force application

FIGURE 19–21 Pyramid of progressive force exercises to the injured flexor tendon. (Reprinted with permission from Groth, G. N. (2004). Pyramid of progressive force exercises to the injured flexor tendon. *Journal of Hand Therapy*, 17, 31–42.)

TABLE 19-3	**Tendon Adhesion Grading System**

- **Absent:** Greater than or equal to 5° discrepancy between digital active and passive flexion
- **Responsive:** Greater than or equal to 10% resolution of active lag between therapy sessions
- **Unresponsive:** Less than 10% resolution of active lag between therapy sessions

- Final levels: The final levels include progression through resistive exercises and should only be used if the tendon is adhered to the surrounding tissues.

A tendon adhesion grading system helps to guide the progression of exercise. This grading system allows the therapist to assess the difference between active and passive motion and evaluate the responsiveness of the tendon to the exercise program. A tendon that is adherent not only prevents full flexion of the joint but can also limit extension when the tendon is tethered down to adjacent tissue (Table 19–3).

COMPLICATIONS

A newly repaired tendon is only as strong as the sutures that bind it. The tendon cannot withstand the forces required to actively pull the finger into flexion. Gapping and rupture are consequences that could occur if the tendon is moved too forcefully. Conversely, a lack of tendon gliding in the early phase can lead to adhesions, while poor positioning over time can create flexion contractures.

GAPPING AND RUPTURE

It is difficult to assess if gapping has occurred, but it can lead to problems such as increased scar formation, a weaker tendon, and an insufficient excursion of the digit. A tendon that is too long creates an inability to produce composite flexion. Triggering of the digit in the early postoperative phase may be an indication of a gapped tendon that is subsequently catching on the annular pulley and is at risk of rupture. All exercises must be halted if triggering occurs and the patient should be sent back to the referring surgeon for evaluation.

In the unfortunate case of a rupture, the patient typically reports experiencing a popping sensation followed by an inability to create active motion in the affected digit. Rupture can occur due to functional use of the hand or due to exercise that is progressed too rapidly. Education and careful progression are essential to safe and effective outcomes after flexor tendon repair.

ADHESIONS

The most common problem following flexor tendon repair is the formation of limiting adhesions. As previously stated, adhesions are typically present when passive ROM is greater than active ROM. In a study by Duran, Houser, Coleman, and Postlewaite (1976), it was noted that adhesions could be minimized if the tendon was allowed 3 mm of excursion. With the exception of immobilization, all regimens described in this chapter afford the exercise necessary to create tendon excursion and help decrease adhesion formation. The concepts offered in the pyramid of progressive force help the therapist modulate treatment and add exercise when the tendon is unresponsive.

"Finger treadmill" board
LISA RAY, OTR/L, CHT
Virginia

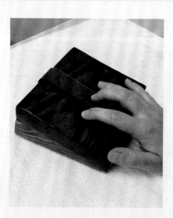

Helpful for isolating a single digit to work on both flexion and extension, similar to a towel crawl—but with the ability to adjust the resistance. Vary strap tension to vary resistance—tighter will create more tension and be harder and vice versa. Consider having several straps on one board in varying resistances. Works best if underside covered with Dycem to prevent slippage during use.

Active grasp guide
JULIANNE LESSARD, OTR/L, CHT
Massachusetts

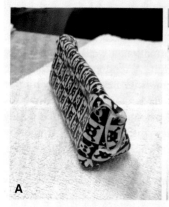 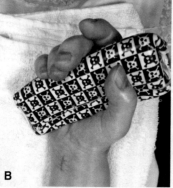

A   **B**

With a triangular shape and one side dented in, it provides opportunities for grasp to a guide, start wide and work to the narrow side blocking MCP or encouraging PIP/DIP flexion. Can be adjusted or can create a series of these to progress active grasp patterns.

FLEXION CONTRACTURES

Flexion contractures are a common complication in zone II injuries. Scar tissue tends to contract the PIP joint, and the extensor tendons are not strong enough to overcome the power of the contractile force of scar tissue. This can also occur from too much time spent in dynamic traction or from the hood of the orthosis not molded in a fully extended position combined with the swollen PIP joint preferring a position of slight flexion at rest. Early in the course of therapy, a digit extension orthosis can be fabricated for the patient

to wear inside the forearm-based orthosis. Once the long orthosis is discontinued, an extension mobilization orthosis can be fabricated to promote finger extension (Fig. 19–22A–F).

QUADRIGA

Quadriga is a syndrome that occurs when the FDP tendon is repaired too tightly, often noted after the tendon is advanced greater than 1 cm during the repair process. This shortening of the FDP can lead to flexion contractures of the affected digit. Because the FDP to the middle, ring, and small fingers share the same muscle belly, the tendons to these three digits need to be tensioned equally to ensure full flexion. If one is shorter, muscle contraction will bend that finger first and the other unaffected digits will be unable to flex completely. The FDP does not have a lot of glide in this zone, which means that there is not a lot of room to shorten the repair without secondary consequences.

ORTHOSES TO ADDRESS POSTOPERATIVE COMPLICATIONS

Early in the postoperative course, the orthosis is a protective mechanism. Over time, as the patient progresses and no longer needs the same level of protection, motion deficits may become apparent. A new orthosis can be fabricated to help gain motion and facilitate exercises or the existing orthosis can be reconfigured into a new design to save money.

Differential gliding can be difficult to achieve because of tendinous adhesions. For up to 6 weeks, the patient has been held in a position of intrinsic plus. Because the lumbricals originate on the FDP tendons, DIP joint flexion is compromised. The normal cascade of motion is affected: when the patient attempts to initiate DIP joint flexion, they may initiate with the lumbricals instead of initiating at the DIP joint. To promote DIP flexion and differential tendon glide, the lumbricals need to be deactivated. An MP joint blocking orthosis holds the MP joints in full extension while the IP joints are left free (Fig. 19–23A,B). This helps to guide the hook fist while preventing the lumbricals from taking over. A PIP joint blocking orthosis, a cylinder holding the PIP joint in extension with the DIP joint free, helps to encourage DIP flexion. If the dorsal portion of the orthosis extends to the fingertip, a rubber band can be added to give resistance to the FDP when the patient has reached a safe timeframe (Fig. 19–23B,C).

Dynamic DIP extension orthosis
KIMBERLY GOLDIE STAINES, OTR, CHT
Texas

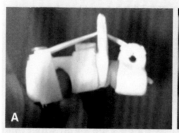 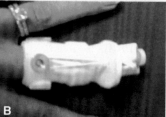

A   **B**

Can be utilized for isolated FDP finger strengthening (once resistance permitted) or to address active DIP flexion lag to promote flexor glide. Also helpful for boutonniere deformity to increase active ORL stretching.

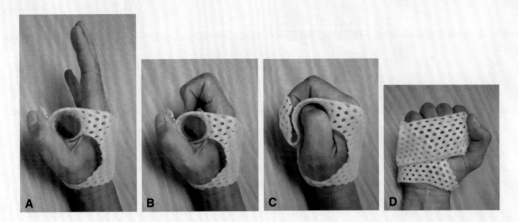

A,B: Exercise orthosis works by giving an aim for movement. To reach the end position in full fist you have to bend the IPs joints first—effective for improving flexor tendon gliding. The thermoplastic material is rolled over a pipe—vary dimension to form the optimal fist position.

C,D: The orthosis can also immobilize the digits into fist position to provide prolonged stretch into flexion.

SCAR REMODELING

Silicone gel dressings applied under an orthosis may assist in preventing the formation of excessive scar tissue. Silicone sheeting, as sold by various manufacturers, is thought to prevent moisture from entering the scar area. If moisture at the scar area is lessened, blood flow in turn is reduced, leading to less collagen formation at the scar area. By reducing collagen at the targeted area, the scar becomes paler and less visible, without the red and purple skin tone that scars often become (Fig. 19–24A). Scar remodeling materials can be incorporated into the orthosis for gentle compression to the scar

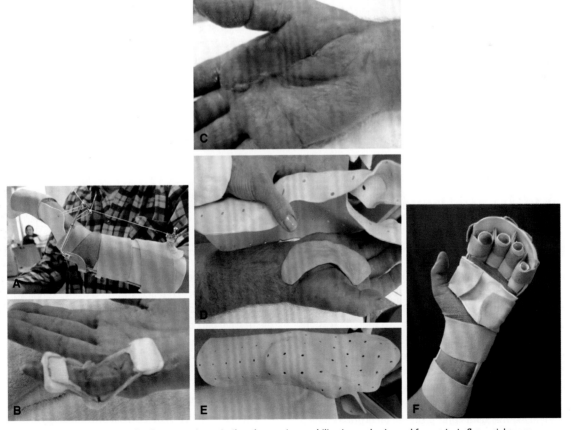

FIGURE 19–22 A, A Static progressive wrist/hand extension mobilization orthosis used for extrinsic flexor tightness. Tension is adjusted as the tissues gently elongate. **B,** Digit proximal interphalangeal extension mobilization orthosis used to stretch contracted volar structures (LMB Spring Finger Extension Assist Splint, DeRoyal, Powell, TN). *Note: the therapist should consult with the physician prior to using any mobilization orthosis that may place stress on a healing tendon.* **C–E,** Note the residual adhesions post tendon injury and repair. Elastomer is applied over the area and held on with a night wrist/hand/thumb serial static extension mobilization orthosis. **F,** A Dorsal approach can be used to gently elongate flexor tendons while controlling the wrist position.

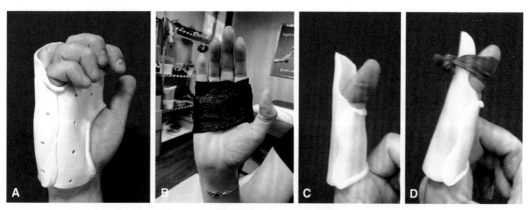

FIGURE 19–23 **Exercise orthoses. A,** MP blocking orthosis: This is worn for exercise sessions to encourage IP joint motion and differential tendon glide. **B,** MP blocking shown fabricated with 3-inch Orficast® material. **C,** Proximal interphalangeal blocking orthosis to encourage flexor digitorum profundus (FDP) glide. **D,** The addition of an exercise band adds resistance to the exercise once the patient is cleared for heavier activities. This puts a lot of stress on the FDP and should be used cautiously. (B, Image compliments of Courtney Garbade, OTR/L CHT, Greenville, SC).

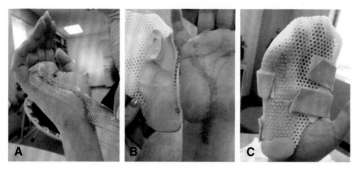

FIGURE 19–24 **A,** Silicone gel applied to a healing incision and **(B and C)** elastomer mold incorporated into a night orthosis.

during resting hours. The compression properties that are applied by using these materials under an orthosis contribute to desensitizing a hypersensitive scar and assist in remodeling dense, thick, ropelike scars (Fig. 19–24B,C).

CONCLUSION

The repair and rehabilitation of an injured flexor tendon requires meticulous surgical technique; careful and consistent communication between surgeon and therapist; thorough understanding of anatomy, fundamental concepts, and rehabilitative regimens; and a strong therapist-patient relationship built on education and mutual trust. The literature pertaining to this complex and exciting diagnosis continues to progress, offering therapists the opportunity to play an important role in careful and consistent assessment with subsequent progression of intervention. Current evidence challenges the notion of traditional orthoses protecting the wrist in flexion, moving instead toward wrist extension between and during exercise. Choosing the appropriate regimen and accompanying orthosis requires sound clinical reasoning and excellent communication and leads to optimal, functional outcomes following flexor tendon repair.

FIELD NOTE: ZONE I AND ZONE II FLEXOR TENDON REPAIR REHABILITATION PROGRAM: THE SAINT JOHN PROTOCOL

By Amanda Higgins, BScOT, OT Reg (NB)
Canada

In 2008, we recognized that we needed to make changes to the way we were managing flexor tendon repairs in zones I and II. These changes were primarily patient-driven. Despite being taught place and hold exercises, patients were coming back to therapy sessions performing early active tuck and fist exercises, and they were getting really good results with their ROM. Those patients who were still following our instructions were getting stuck in scar. A literature search on early active ROM programs for flexor tendon repair management led us to the programs Dr. Jin Bo Tang published in 2007 and Dr. Fiona Peck in 2014. The Saint John protocol incorporates ideas from both of these leaders in flexor tendon management. Through this learning adventure we realize now that the most resistance to

glide of a repaired tendon is during the final one-third of active flexion. We do not teach place and hold exercises early in the program as we know this causes the tendon to bunch at the repair site during the passive part of the movement and then during the active phase, when the resistance is at the highest, the flexor tendon is roughly jerked at the repair site. We are able to witness this movement pattern with the use of WALANT.

First 4 days post surgery

- The hand is placed in a dorsal block orthosis with IP joints of all fingers in full extension, MCP joints in 30° of flexion,[1] and wrist in slight comfortable extension.

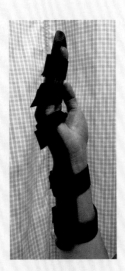

Four days post surgery to 14 days

- The patient is taught passive composite flexion exercises to all fingers within the orthosis. The patient is then taught to let go of the finger and to actively extend the fingers within the dorsal block limits. Keeping the MCP joint in a flexed position will help to encourage PIP joint extension. If this is taught early enough, PIP joint flexion contractures can be avoided during the rehabilitation phase of tendon repair.

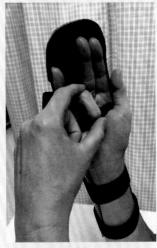

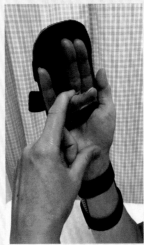

- Patients perform active tendon glide of all the fingers within the dorsal block orthosis. They try to actively flex at least a quarter to a half fist position[2]. This movement should be gentle without forceful pulling or strenuous force on the repaired tendon. Encourage the patient to lead with the DIP joint; a modified tuck movement with MCP joint in 30° of flexion to achieve differential tendon glide between FDP and FDS.

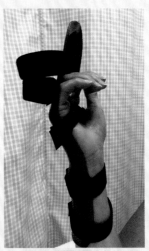

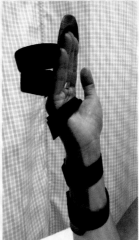

- The dorsal block orthosis is changed to the Manchester Short Splint by the 2 weeks post surgery[3] point in recovery. This splint allows the wrist to fully flex but limits wrist extension to 40° to 45°. Fingers are still kept in the same position as described above.

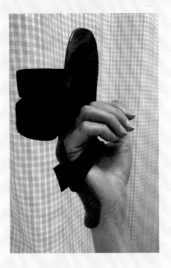

14 to 28 days

- The patient continues to work on full passive composite flexion of all fingers and active extension of each finger in the orthosis.

(Continued)

- The patient continues to work on gentle active tendon glide trying to achieve a 3/4 or near full fist position.[4]
- With Manchester Short Splint on, patients are taught to flex wrist while extending fingers, hold for 5 second count, and then extend wrist (up until the block) while curling fingers into a tuck position. This helps to promote differential glide of the FDS and FDP tendons.[3]

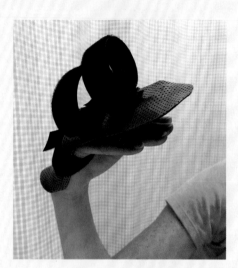

29 to 42 days

- The patient continues to work on full passive composite flexion of all fingers within the orthosis and active extension of each finger in the splint.
- To really work on PIP joint extension, the Manchester Short Splint can be replaced with a Relative Motion Flexion orthosis.

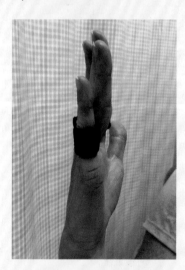

- The patient is shown activities that are more in line with typical daily activities but help to achieve active tendon glide. Patients can wear a Relative Motion Flexion orthosis or remove the splint

completely to bend fingers around cell phone, try to turn a water glass or wine glass on a table surface, try to drag fingers through cream on a table top surface, try to scrunch tissue or towel, and extend fingers.

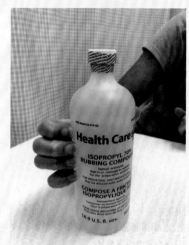

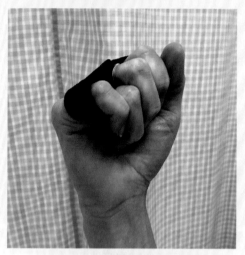

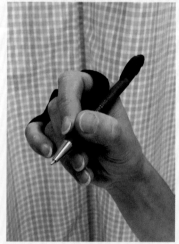

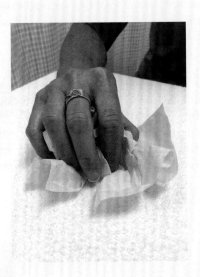

43 to 56 days

- Manchester Short Splint or Relative Motion Flexion orthosis is discontinued.

- The patient can start to incorporate the hand into regular activity.
- A night extension orthosis or Relative Motion Flexion orthosis can be used to treat PIP joint flexion contractures.

Do not lose patience! Sometimes it can take 6 to 8 months for a patient to achieve full hand function status! But it will come!

References

1. Wong, J. K., Peck, F. (2014).Improving results of flexor tendon repair and rehabilitation. *Plastic and Reconstructive Surgery*, 134, 913e–925e.
2. Tang, J. B. (2007). Indications, methods, postoperative motion and outcome evaluations of primary flexor tendon repairs in zone 2. *Journal of Hand Surgery*, 32E(2), 118–129.
3. Peck, F. H., Roe, A. E., Ng, C. Y., Duff, C., McGrouther, D. A., Lees, V. C. (2014). The Manchester short splint: A change to splinting practice in the rehabilitation of zone II flexor tendon repairs. *Hand Therapy*, 19(2), 47–53.
4. Tang, J. B., Zhou, X., Pan, Z. J., Qing, J., Gong, K. T., & Chen, J. (2017). Strong Digital Flexor Tendon Repair, Extension Flexion Test, and Early Active Flexion: Experience in 300 Tendons. *Hand Clinics*, 33, 455–463.

Case Study Section

The case studies presented here are meant as a teaching guideline only. Treatment and orthosis protocols vary greatly from surgeon to surgeon and from therapist to therapist. The therapist should check with the referring physicians and colleagues to define the preferred treatment and appropriate orthotic intervention.

Case Study 1: Flexor Digitorum Profundus Avulsion

JF is a 56-year-old lawyer who ruptured his left long finger FDP tendon when his hand caught in someone else's shirt while dancing at a wedding. He was seen preoperatively for orthosis fabrication and education about what to expect postoperatively. He had a high level of anxiety regarding his injury and the surgeon wanted him placed in a protected position to prevent retraction of the tendon. A wrist and hand extension restriction orthosis was fabricated for him with his wrist in 10° of flexion, his MP joints in 70° of flexion, and his IP joints straight. He wore this until surgery. During surgery, his FDP was reattached to the distal phalanx with a pull-through suture to a button on his nail. He also suffered a middle phalanx fracture that was treated with screw fixation. He brought his orthosis with him to his first postoperative visit at day 3, when his dressing was removed. The physician felt that the fracture was stable enough and the tendon repair strong enough to participate in place and hold regimen. He was started on an exercise program of passive digital flexion and active extension to the roof of the orthosis. Gentle passive tenodesis was also performed in the clinic. Due to his level of anxiety, coupled with notable stiffness and edema, synergistic place and hold exercises were deferred until visit two.

At his next visit (postoperative day 5), his home program was reviewed. He demonstrated almost full passive flexion, and synergistic place and hold exercises were added to his home program (10 repetitions, 5 times per day). He was followed three times per week for edema control, wound care/scar management, and upgrade of home program. At 2 weeks postoperatively, place/hold hook fist was initiated to increase glide of the FDP tendon and place/hold straight fist to maximize FDS glide. He also was developing a PIP flexion contracture, so at 2.5 weeks, a finger immobilization orthosis was fabricated for him to wear at night within his dorsal block orthosis.

JF continued to make nice progress and was able to maintain the place/hold composite, hook, and straight fists. It was decided to continue him on his current home program until 4 weeks postoperatively when active tendon glide exercises were introduced as well as active synergistic motion. His PIP flexion at that point was 90° and DIP flexion was 3°. At 5 weeks, his DIP flexion remained the same, so gentle blocking exercises were introduced.

At 6 weeks, his button was removed, and the dorsal block orthosis was discontinued except when in crowds (on the subway, while out jogging, etc.). Light functional tasks were introduced in the clinic. Because he still had a slight PIP flexion contracture, his finger immobilization orthosis was continued at night. It was felt that the PIP contracture was likely caused by soft tissue tightness around the PIP joint and not caused by extrinsic flexor tightness. He continued to make gains in PIP/DIP flexion, so resistive exercises were not begun until 8 weeks postoperatively. JF continued in therapy until 12 weeks postoperatively. Final ROM measurements taken are the following: PIP, 10/100; DIP, 0/50. At that point, he was discharged from therapy.

Additional case studies can be found on the companion website on the Point.

CHAPTER REVIEW QUESTIONS

1. Why is early motion beneficial to the healing tendon?
2. Define tendon excursion and force. What exercises provide low levels of force and high levels of excursion to the healing tendon? Which exercise effectively creates distal glide and is safe for all tendon repairs in the early postoperative phase?
3. Describe the activity of the wrist and digit muscles during synergistic motion. Why should patients complete digital flexion with the wrist in extension rather than flexion?
4. What does the literature regarding work of flexion suggest regarding initiation of rehabilitation and exercise in cases of edema?
5. How is tendon glide measured?
6. Identify five key current concepts about dorsal blocking orthoses.
7. Describe the common regimens for early passive flexion, place and hold, and true active flexion following flexor tendon repair.
8. What are the benefits of incorporating Strickland percentage and/or the pyramid of progressive force into assessment strategies?
9. Identify two strategies for avoiding tendon adhesions.

20 Peripheral Nerve Injuries

MaryLynn A. Jacobs, MBA, MS, OTR/L, CHT
Danielle Wojtkiewicz, MSOT, OTR/L, CHT

CHAPTER OBJECTIVES

After study of this chapter, the reader should be able to:
- Appreciate the motor, sensory, and vasomotor pathways as well as the healing and regeneration principles of a peripheral nerve.
- Identify the deficiencies of the three main peripheral nerves to the hand: **radial**, **ulnar**, and **median nerves.**
- Appreciate the various degrees of injury associated with traumatic and compressive nerve insults.
- Determine the appropriate therapeutic and orthotic intervention for each nerve injury.
- Understand the popular surgical techniques and the various types of peripheral nerve repairs.
- Appreciate and describe the role of **nerve grafts**, conduits, and allografts in this patient population.

KEY TERMS

Anterior interosseous nerve syndrome	Froment sign	Pronator syndrome
Ape hand deformity	Guyon canal	Radial nerve
Axonotmesis	Jeanne sign	Radial tunnel syndrome
Carpal tunnel syndrome	Median nerve	Resistant tennis elbow
Claw hand deformity	Multiple-crush syndrome	Saturday night palsy
Cubital tunnel syndrome	Nerve grafts	Second-degree injury
Double-crush syndrome	Nerve laceration	Sixth-degree injury
Elbow flexion test	Nerve transfers	Third-degree injuries
End-to-end repairs	Neurapraxia	Tinel sign
Epineurial repair	Neurotmesis	Ulnar nerve
Fifth-degree injuries	Peace sign deformity	Wallerian degeneration
First-degree injury	Peripheral nerve injury	Wartenberg sign
Fourth-degree injury	Phalen test	Wartenberg syndrome
	Posterior interosseous nerve syndrome	Wrist drop

The need for corrective splintage in peripheral nerve injuries has been recognized for a long time, but only recently has it been appreciated that a good splint should do more than merely prevent deformity, it should also encourage function.

Wynn Parry, 1981

MD NOTE

Mitchell A. Pet, MD
Missouri

While communication and collaboration between the surgeon and therapist is always important, there is perhaps no time when this is a more critical issue than in the treatment of a nerve injured patient. The root of this truth is that the care of the nerve injured patient occurs over an enormously long timescale. Because of this, a one-time discussion or "order" is never sufficient to offer optimized care. Over the years that it takes to reconstruct and rehabilitate a severe nerve injury, these patients undergo constant change. These changes may be positive (return of motor or sensory function, improved range of motion, increased strength), or negative (contracture, noncompliance, increased pain/anxiety/depression). These changes can be difficult to detect, but with each change, the surgeon and therapist each need to weigh in and the plan must be adjusted. On the therapy side, orthoses may need to be remolded or refabricated, and objectives may need to be modified. On the surgical side, medications may need to be adjusted, or return to the operative room may even be indicated.

Making this more difficult is the fact that peripheral nerve injuries are so varied and manifest so differently in patients of different age, background, and demand. Especially for the surgeon and therapist who may not see a high volume of these patients, this means that each patient's "protocol" must be individually developed and actively managed. This communication is in fact a very difficult task to keep up with, and surgeons rely heavily on therapists to detect the slow and incremental changes that characterize recovery from a peripheral nerve injury or reconstruction. For these reasons, therapists should feel empowered to communicate frequently, and surgeons should be appreciative of the therapist who can collaborate on this difficult task!

INTRODUCTION

Orthotic intervention for **peripheral nerve injury (PNI)** is challenging, thought provoking, and always specific to the individual. This chapter describes orthotic management for deficiencies of the three main peripheral nerves: median, ulnar, and radial—**nerve lacerations**, common mixed lesions, compression neuropathies, and lesions associated with other injuries. Tendon and nerve transfers will not be addressed in great detail as Chapter 21 is dedicated to this topic. A table is provided to aid the therapist in nerve injury identification and appropriate selection of orthoses.

Assessment of the nerve-injured hand requires sound knowledge of nerve healing, functional anatomy, physiology, and kinesiology as well as a thorough understanding of motor, sensory, and vasomotor pathways. With this information, the therapist can recognize abnormalities and determine the appropriate therapeutic and orthotic intervention. The therapist must appreciate (1) the type and degree of motor and sensory loss, (2) the importance of cortical reintegration, (3) the impact of pain on function and recovery, (4) protection of the healing nerve, (5) prevention of deformity, (6) education of adaptive techniques, (7) the role of exercise, and (8) continual reassessment of nerve return to achieve the best functional results for the patient (Fig. 20–1).

Advances in nerve repair have allowed surgeons to employ the peripheral nerve's regenerative capabilities and apply these to creative techniques for nerve reconstruction. This has opened the door for the therapist to participate in pioneering complimentary orthotic management and rehabilitation protocols.

DEFINITION

PNIs commonly seen by a therapist are either traumatic in nature or as a result of an entrapment or a compression neuropathy. Most traumatic injuries occur in association with other injuries, such as fractures or tendon lacerations. Compression neuropathies usually occur in specific anatomic areas where the nerve is vulnerable as it passes through a soft-tissue restraint, such as the median nerve as it traverses beneath the transverse carpal ligament in carpal tunnel syndrome (American Society for Surgery of the Hand [ASSH], 1995; Diao, 2011; Eaton, 1992; Mackinnon, 1992; Thomas, Yakin, Parry, & Lubahn, 2000). Compression neuropathies are typically chronic in nature because they are a result of prolonged compression to the nerve. Acute compression neuropathies are associated with traumatic events, such as in compartment syndrome or with a direct hit or blow to the nerve (Elfar et al., 2010). A nerve can also be entrapped at more than one site along the nerve's pathway, resulting in a **double-crush** or **multiple-crush syndrome** and/or phenomenon (Bindra & Johnson, 2011; Jacoby, Eichenbaum, & Osterman, 2011; Mackinnon, 1992). Nerves are vulnerable to injury as they slide, glide, pass, and/or rub over or between soft tissue structures and bony prominences (e.g., ulnar nerve at the cubital tunnel, radial nerve as it traverses through the soft tissue structures of the forearm) (Topp & Boyd, 2012). Neuropathies can occur secondary to repetitive use/cumulative trauma, endocrine disorders (e.g., diabetes or hypothyroidism), renal failure, hormonal changes (e.g., pregnancy or menopause), electrical injury, traction,

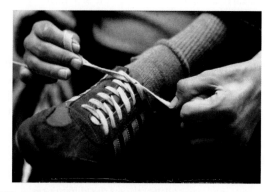

FIGURE 20–1 Although nerve injuries are devastating, many patients can learn adaptive methods for functioning independently. Note the ulnar nerve atrophy of the left thumb dorsal web space.

ischemia, rheumatoid arthritis, Guillain-Barré syndrome, myasthenia gravis, amyotrophic lateral sclerosis, sarcoidosis, or tumors/soft tissue masses (Cameron & Klein, 2010; Dellon, 1992; Diao, 2011; Smith, 1995, 2011).

A nerve injury produces changes within the nerve itself and in the tissues that it innervates. Symptoms of nerve injury include weakness or paralysis of the muscles innervated by the motor branches of that particular nerve and sensory loss to areas innervated by the sensory branches of the injured nerve. Early symptoms of compression neuropathy may be vague but usually include some combination of pain, tingling, numbness, and weakness. Pain may be sharp and burning with accompanying paresthesias over the corresponding dermatome or sensory distribution. These signs may occur proximal and/or distal to the site(s) of compression (Bell-Krotoski, 2004; Mackinnon, 1992; Slutsky, 2005a; 2011; Smith, 1995). Applying an orthosis that positions the limb in such a way that tension or compression stress is decreased on the nerve may relieve some, or all, of the nerve symptoms (Topp & Boyd, 2012; Walsh, 2012).

The reader should keep the following points in mind while progressing through this chapter:

- Atrophy begins immediately.
- The more proximal the diagnosis, the worse the prognosis.
- The more severe the injury, the worse the prognosis.
- A more favorable prognosis is associated with early repair.
- Sensation can return up to 3 years postinjury.
- Peripheral nerves have excellent regeneration potential.
- Complete functional recovery is rarely attained in an adult.
- Nerve transfer should be undertaken as soon as it is determined that spontaneous recovery, primary repair, or grafting will be of little benefit (refer to Chapter 21).

NERVE ANATOMY

The nervous system is made up of two parts: the peripheral nervous system (PNS) and the central nervous system (CNS). The PNS consists of the spinal and cranial nerves, and the CNS incorporates the brain and spinal cord (Carpenter, 1978). The PNS serves as the mediator (or transporter) of neural impulses traveling between the sensory receptors, muscles, and CNS. A bundle of axons (nerve fibers) in the PNS is called a nerve, and a network of nerves is referred to as a nerve plexus. A collection of nerves outside the cell bodies is a ganglion. Peripheral nerve fibers are made of an axon, myelin sheath, and neurolemma or sheath of Schwann cells. After a nerve has been injured, the changes that happen to the nerve are collectively termed Wallerian degeneration (Bindra & Johnson, 2011; Boscheinen-Morrin, Davey, & Conolly, 1985; Carpenter, 1978; Elfar et al., 2010; Mackinnon, 1994; Parry, 1981; Smith, 1995, 2011; Walsh, 2012).

Figure 20–2 shows the anatomy of a nerve cell and its pathway to the target organ. A peripheral nerve is surrounded by three layers of connective tissue that offer strength and protection to the nerve itself (Elfar et al., 2010). The layers are the epineurium, a sheath that encompasses the entire nerve; the perineurium, which encloses a small bundle (fasciculus) of nerve fibers and forms a more fragile connective tissue sheath than the epineurium; and the endoneurium, a thin connective tissue sheath that surrounds the individual nerve fibers (Bindra & Johnson, 2011; Boscheinen-Morrin et al., 1985).

Figure 20–3 illustrates nerve injury and regeneration (Boscheinen-Morrin et al., 1985). After any significant neural insult, degeneration of the axon and myelin sheath occurs distal to the injury site. Degeneration also occurs proximal to the injury and to the previous node of Ranvier (constrictions of the myelin sheath). During this process of **Wallerian degeneration**, the axon atrophies, but the connective tissue sheath remains open to accept regenerating axonal fibers. In general, axons grow approximately 1 to 2 mm/d or, in an adult, 1 inch per month. If there is no axonal activity soon after injury or if axons never make contact with a motor end organ, muscle atrophy will occur with irreversible loss by 18 months (Slutsky, 2011). This may account for poor motor outcomes in above elbow injuries, especially in the adult (Slutsky, 2005a, 2011; Terzis, 1991). In contrast to motor end plates, the sensory end organs remain preserved after denervation (Elfar et al., 2010). The potential for reinnervation of a sensory nerve is therefore more optimistic by comparison, providing protective sensation even several years after insult (Elfar et al., 2010; Slutsky, 2011).

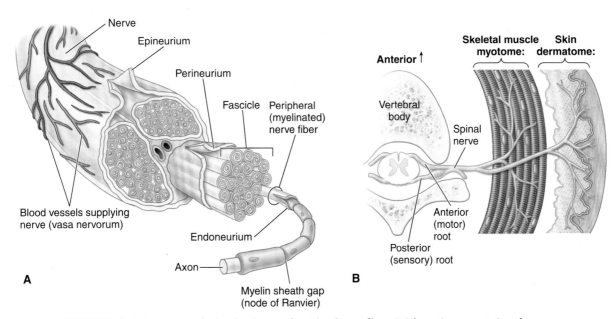

FIGURE 20–2 A, Arrangement and ensheathment of peripheral nerve fibers. **B,** Schematic representation of a dermatome (the unilateral area of skin) and myotome (the unilateral portion of skeletal muscle) receiving innervation from a single spinal nerve. (Reprinted with permission from Moore, K. L., Agur, A. M., & Dalley, A. F.II.(2019). *Moore's Essential clinical anatomy* (6th ed.). Philadelphia, PA: Wolters Kluwer.)

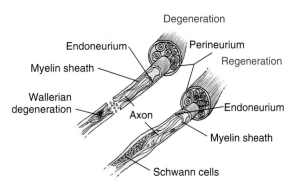

FIGURE 20–3 Nerve degeneration and regeneration.

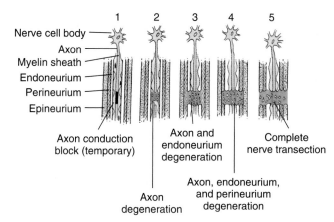

FIGURE 20–4 Sunderland's five degrees of nerve injury: (1) conduction block; (2) axonal degeneration; (3) axonal and endoneurial degeneration; (4) axonal, endoneurial, and perineurial degeneration; and (5) complete nerve transection.

Different types of nerve lesions result in different prognoses; therefore, it is important to appreciate the effect and extent that each type of nerve injury may have on its respective nerve cell, axon, and target organ. This information is also important for assessing nerve regeneration, applying appropriate orthoses and therapy intervention, and timely orthotic modifications. The more proximal the injury, the worse the prognosis, because there is a greater distance from the site of insult to the target organ (Lundborg, 1988; Lundborg & Rosen, 2004; Moore & Agur, 1995). By the time the regenerated axon reaches the end organ, significant end plate degeneration may have occurred. Regenerated axons may not always find their end organs (Bathen & Gupta, 2011; Smith, 2011). For example, a sensory axon may reach a motor plate or vice versa. Age can be a significant factor in potential nerve recovery. In general, young children have a better functional result than adults. This may be due to the shorter distances axons have to grow (smaller, shorter limbs) to reach their target organ and for the great capacity young brains have to integrate centrally and reorganize incoming information (Bindra & Johnson, 2011; Elfar et al., 2010; Parry, 1981). Cortical plasticity and its importance to nerve recovery gained increased attention, particularly with sensory relearning techniques (Anastakis, Chen, Davis, & Mikulis, 2005, 2008; Duff, 2005; Novak, 2011; Walsh, 2012). Proximal injury in adults may require that functional or antideformity orthoses be worn for extended periods of time.

A crush or compression injury may cause damage to the axon but can leave the connective tissue layers of the nerve intact, maintaining a conduit to guide the growing axons to their ultimate destinations. However, when a nerve is severed, the part distal to the injury degenerates, and only careful surgical anastomosis will provide a chance of functional recovery (Elfar et al., 2010; Lundborg, 1988; Mackinnon, 1994; Mackinnon & Nakao, 1997; Moore & Agur, 1995). Some of these surgical options are reviewed later in this chapter.

NERVE INJURY CLASSIFICATION

Seddon (1943) was the first to classify nerve injuries (Smith, 1995), using the terms **neurapraxia**, **axonotmesis**, and **neurotmesis**. In 1951, Sunderland (1952) expanded this classification to five more precise degrees of injury (Fig. 20–4) (Horn & Crumley, 1984; Smith, 1995). Mackinnon (1994) identified a sixth lesion, a mixed injury that includes normal fascicles with some or all of Sunderland's five degrees (Bathen & Gupta, 2011). Regardless of which classification the reader chooses to reference, the most important part of these classifications is the prognosis. Table 20–1 summarizes and compares the Seddon and Sunderland classifications.

TABLE 20–1	**Comparison of Classification of Nerve Injuries**	
Degree of Injury	**Descriptive Term**	**Nature of Injury/Neuropathology**
I	Neurapraxia	Demyelinating injury with a temporary conduction block
II	Axonotmesis	Distal degeneration of the injured axon but with almost always complete regeneration due to intact endoneurium
III		Axon and endoneurial loss of continuity, perineurium intact
IV	Neuroma in continuity	Axon, endoneurium, and perineurium are disrupted with extensive scarring that blocks axonal regeneration and often results in a neuroma in continuity
V	Neurotmesis	Complete disruption of nerve without possibility of spontaneous regeneration
VI	Mixed injury (I-V)	Injury where some fascicles may be injured, and others show varying degrees of recovery

From Ray, W. Z., Mackinnon, S. E. (2010). Management of nerve gaps: Autografts, allografts, nerve transfers, and end-to-side neurorrhaphy. Experimental Neurology, 223, *77–85.*

FIRST-DEGREE INJURY (NEURAPRAXIA)

First-degree injury involves a localized area of conduction block, which is reversible. Recovery is quick, usually complete motor and sensory function within 12 to 16 weeks. The mechanism of injury is commonly acute compression and local ischemia (Elfar et al., 2010). Wallerian degeneration does not occur in neurapraxic lesions because the perineurium is left intact.

SECOND-DEGREE INJURY (AXONOTMESIS)

In the **second-degree injury**, damage to the axon occurs, and regeneration of the nerve proceeds at the standard rate of approximately 1 mm/d or 1 inch per month. An advancing **Tinel sign** is present. The

Tinel sign is a common technique used to assess nerve regeneration; a gentle tapping is performed along the nerve's pathway, distal to proximal (although many therapists perform this proximal to distal), which, when performed carefully, should elicit paresthesias into innervated tissue (Allan & Vanderhooft, 2005; Bell-Krotoski, 2004; Diao, 2011; Lundborg, 1988; Mackinnon, 1994; Parry, 1981). The recovery rate for second-degree injuries is slow; yet, complete return of function can be expected. If the injury occurs proximal to the distal target, the time required to reach the end organ makes the recovery pattern slower than normal (Lundborg, 1988; Mackinnon & Nakao, 1997).

THIRD-DEGREE INJURY (AXONOTMESIS OR NEUROTMESIS)

Third-degree injuries have the most unpredictable degree of recovery, which ranges from almost normal to no recovery at all. With this type of injury, there is some scarring within the endoneurium, making it difficult for the axon to reach the appropriate receptor. These injuries recover slowly, and patients eventually achieve some, but usually not all, function.

FOURTH-DEGREE INJURY (NEUROTMESIS)

In a **fourth-degree injury**, a segment of the nerve is completely blocked by scar. This can also be referred to as a neuroma in continuity (Ray & Mackinnon, 2010). The nerve is in continuity but only because of the fibrous bond. The internal structure of the nerve is severely damaged. There is no function or nerve conduction through the fibrous block of scar. Surgical repair or grafting is most often recommended.

FIFTH-DEGREE INJURY (NEUROTMESIS)

In **fifth-degree injuries**, the nerve is completely severed. The patient must undergo surgical intervention, which may include direct repair or a nerve graft, depending on the size of the deficit. Functional recovery depends on factors such as the time since injury and/or repair, wound status, patient's age, surgeon's skill, and the degree of tension on the repair.

SIXTH-DEGREE INJURY (MIXED INJURY)

The **sixth-degree injury** is a mixed lesion that includes some normal fascicles in combination with all or any of Sunderland's five degrees of injury (Bathen & Gupta, 2011; Mackinnon, 1994). This lesion includes several patterns of injury from fascicle to fascicle. The variation in injury can also be seen along the length of the nerve. Complicated upper extremity lesions are often the result of devastating injuries such as gunshot wounds, traumatic crushing, and traction injuries, or they can occur from a combination of the previously stated mechanisms. Surgical intervention may include a combination of procedures such as neurolysis, nerve graft, and/or direct repair. Mixed lesions are challenging injuries for the surgeon to treat and the therapist to rehabilitate, owing to the variability of injury, repair, and recovery.

NERVE REPAIRS AND RECONSTRUCTION

Prior to treating a nerve-repaired structure, the clinician must have knowledge of the exact procedure performed. Questions presented in Box 20–1 are only *some* of the questions that a

| BOX 20–1 | QUESTIONS THE CLINICIAN SHOULD ASK THE SURGEON |

1. What type of repair/reconstruction was done (epineurial, perineurial, end-to-end, end-to-side)?
2. Was there tension on the nerve repair? What was the situation?
3. How much and which portion of the nerve was injured and/or repaired?
4. Was the injury/repair to a motor, sensory, or combined nerve?
5. Was the repair primary or via nerve graft, conduit, or transfer?
6. If a donor nerve was used, what is the expected deficit from the donor site (sensory, motor)?
7. When orthotic protection/positioning is prescribed, what are the exact joint positions desired?
8. What are the parameters for immobilization, mobilization, and/or restriction of the repaired structure?
9. What future surgery is planned or is the patient eligible for?

clinician should consider when referred a patient with a postoperative nerve repair. Close communication with the surgeon is paramount.

INTRODUCTION OF NERVE RECONSTRUCTION

It is not the intent of this chapter to discuss the vast options and advances in surgical procedures, because there are many resources available that delve into this topic in great detail. Rather, this chapter is meant to provide the clinician with a basic foundation and familiarity with terms related to PNI and surgery in order to fully appreciate the selection and application of appropriate orthotic intervention. The clinician will find short descriptors of the most common procedures for quick reference and are encouraged to seek further study in this exploding area of nerve repair and reconstruction. The definitions listed in the following text highlight common definitions the therapist will encounter in the realm of peripheral nerve surgery.

DEFINITIONS RELATED TO PERIPHERAL NERVE REPAIR

- Primary repair is typically done within 48 hours (Smith, 2011) and does not involve the use of grafting or other supplemental techniques.
- Early secondary repairs are performed within the first 6 weeks.
- Late secondary repairs are done after 3 months (Smith, 2011).
- **Epineurial repair** is a quick, simple, and most common technique used to repair a completely transected nerve. The outer epineurium is debrided proximal and distal from the nerve stumps until all signs of damage are removed. The nerve stumps are then realigned, and sutures are placed in the epineurium to secure closure (Smith, 2011). The goal is to establish continuity of the nerve with minimal tension (Elfar et al., 2010) (Fig. 20–5A–C).
- **Perineurial repair** (group fascicular repair) is the second most common peripheral nerve repair technique. In this repair, the outer and inner epineurium are dissected away from the nerve stumps. The fascicles are then matched and aligned using the

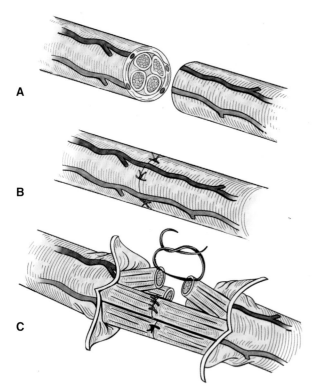

FIGURE 20–5 **A,** Schematic representation of a traumatic nerve laceration. **B,** A traditional epineurial repair done to establish proper alignment while minimizing tension. **C,** A group fascicular repair is often advantageous over epineurial repair if the sensory and motor group fascicles are in near alignment to their corresponding sensory and motor group fascicles in the distal stump. (Borrowed with permission from Elfar, J., Petrungaro, J. M., Braun, R. M., Cheng, C. J., Gupta, R., LaBore, A., & Wong, J. E. (2010). Nerve. In Hammert W. C., Calfee R. P., Bozentka D. J., & Boyer M. I. (Eds.), *ASSH manual of hand surgery* (pp. 332). Baltimore, MD: Lippincott Williams & Wilkins.)

least amount of suture to close. An advantage of this repair is the matching of similar fascicles (motor and sensory), but the disadvantage can be the risk of intraneural fibrosis secondary to the increased use of suture and the overall surgical handling (Elfar et al., 2010; Smith, 2011).

- **End-to-end repairs** are direct clean nerve ends sutured together.
- **End-to-side transfers** have been described mainly for sensory recovery. The distal stump of the injured nerve is sutured to the side of an uninjured donor nerve. This is performed when the proximal injured stump is inaccessible or not available for repair.
- Reverse (supercharge) end-to-side transfer is a procedure in which the donor nerve is completely transected. The epineurium and perineurium of the recipient nerve are opened. The transected end of the donor nerve (distal) is coapted to the side of the recipient denervated nerve (Mackinnon, 2016).
- **Fibrin glue** can be used with epineurial repairs in order to reduce suture materials and adequately seal the repair site. The role of fibrin glue in peripheral nerve repair is becoming more popular due to the ease of application versus microsuture (Sameem, Wood, & Bain, 2011).
- Neurotization is the implantation of a nerve into a paralyzed muscle.
- **Neurorrhaphy** is the suturing of a divided nerve.
- Nerve grafting is used to bridge a deficit in a nerve using a donor graft. A nerve graft can be nonvascularized (a conventional graft) or vascularized. A vascularized graft is either pedicled or free flaps (Slutsky, 2005a; Terzis & Kostopoulos, 2005).

- **Nerve conduits** are also used to bridge nerve gaps. The conduits can be of biologic or nonbiologic origin (Herman, Diaz, & Strauch, 2005).
- **Neurosensory flaps** are innervated flaps that provide sensory feedback. These flaps can be either pedicled or free flaps (Slutsky, 2005b).

NERVE HEALING

After insult, a peripheral nerve can regenerate spontaneously, but this requires both axon regrowth and remyelination by Schwann cells. Without surgical intervention, healing naturally may lead to poor results such as (1) a mismatch when the end organ is attempting to innervate a receptor, (2) the axon may lose its continuity, and (3) the end organ may have too long a distance to travel, therefore becoming degenerated by the time it reaches the end target (Bathen & Gupta, 2011). Other factors that influence healing are patient's age, the length of time since injury, level of injury, the quality of surrounding tissues, and the amount of scar formation about the injured area (Smith, 2011).

NERVE GRAFTING

A nerve graft (Fig. 20–6A) provides a regenerating axon with a protective pathway to the distal stump (Slutsky, 2005b). The nonvascularized nerve graft is considered to be the treatment of choice in reconstructing nerve gaps. The grafting procedure may take place approximately 3 weeks after injury using a suitable, accessible donor (Elfar et al., 2010). This timeline is variable, however, and is dependent on when the zone of injury is more clearly defined. The patient should be accepting of the choice of donor nerve. Some of the more commonly used nerves are the

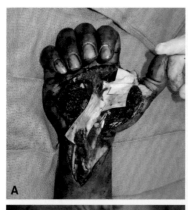
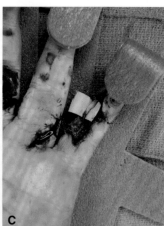

FIGURE 20-6 **A,** Nerve repair using a cable nerve graft. **B,** Digital nerve repair utilizing a nerve conduit. **C,** Digital nerve repair utilizing nerve allograft. (Photos courtesy of Mitchell Pet, MD, St. Louis, MO.)

anterior and posterior interosseous nerve (PIN), the medial and lateral antebrachial cutaneous nerves, and the sural nerve from the lower extremity (Elfar et al., 2010; Slutsky, 2005a). The length of the donor nerve needs to be long enough to allow a tension-free repair. This is a critical question the clinician must ask when applying an orthosis to these patients.

NERVE CONDUITS

A nerve conduit (Fig. 20–6B) can act as a guide, connecting the neural gap in order to contain, align, and direct the regenerating axons (Taras, Nanavati, & Steelman, 2005). A nerve conduit is made of either an autogenous material (i.e., vein) or a synthetic material (i.e., collagen) that is placed between the nerve ends, incorporating the end stumps into the conduit. Soon after the nerve ends are placed into the conduit, a serous fluid begins the process of creating a platform for regeneration (Elfar et al., 2010). Tension on the repair site is not a factor in regard to initiation of early rehabilitation; therefore, early active motion can commence soon after repair, incorporating appropriate orthotic management; protective, guarded motion; and motor and/sensory reeducation principles (Slutsky, 2011). Orthosis positioning should include a degree of flexion if the nerve repair is volar and extension if the repair is dorsal (Taras et al., 2005). Extension restriction and flexion restriction orthoses are excellent choices for this patient population. Restriction orthoses do not completely block motion; instead, they allow a protected arc of motion that will assist in prevention of adhesion formation and facilitate gentle nerve and tendon glide. A digital nerve repair that is tensionless will most often not require orthosis management (Taras et al., 2005). Most orthotic intervention is discontinued between 4 and 6 weeks

NERVE ALLOGRAFT

The use of a nerve allograft (Fig. 20–6C) provides increased treatment options for devastating or segmental nerve injuries. Nerve allografts are cadaveric nerve tissue that has been decellularized while preserving the endoneurial structure (Safa & Buncke, 2016). Allograft benefits include the microenvironment inherent to nerve tissue, avoiding donor site morbidity, utility with larger gap lengths, and they are readily accessible (Ray & Mackinnon, 2010; Safa & Buncke, 2016). It is important to note that allograft recipients require temporary immunosuppression of approximately 24 months, or until the Tinel sign has crossed the distal graft site (Ray & Mackinnon, 2010). Rehabilitation focus is on early protected range of motion followed by sensory and motor re-education. Orthotic positioning during the period of time the muscles are denervated, will help facilitate recovery once reinnervation occurs by keeping the muscles at a normal resting length (Mackinnon, 2016).

NERVE TRANSFERS

Nerve transfers are briefly mentioned below as the reader will need to appreciate their role in this patient population. Much greater detail is available in the Chapter 21. Recent developments in peripheral nerve reconstruction introduced nerve transfer to the upper extremity. In injuries where primary nerve reconstruction or grafting is not possible or where the outcome is expected to be poor, the surgeon may consider nerve transfer. Nerve transfers can restore at least some degree of motor or sensory function (Slutsky, 2011). A donor nerve is required;

therefore, thoughtful discussion with the patient is important to consider how the loss of the donor would impact function. The patient must clearly understand the deficit left by the harvesting of the donor, the purpose of the transfer, and the intended outcome. The therapist is well versed in functional (motor and sensory) anatomy and can be of great help to the patient and family through this decision-making process.

A therapist may see such transfers in patients with a brachial plexus lesion, a high ulnar nerve injury, or traumatic injury to several of the peripheral nerves of the same extremity such as seen in a gunshot wound (Elfar, 2010). Protective orthotic intervention, motor reeducation, sensory retraining, and ongoing patient education are a large part of postoperative management.

Motor Transfers

The best donor for a motor transfer is a pure motor nerve. This muscle should be of adequate strength (grade 4) being able to work against gravity, ideally with light resistance (Elfar, 2010). Orthotic management is based on close communication with the surgeon because the surgeon has firsthand knowledge of the quality of the tissue transferred and the amount of tension desired for that transfer. Orthotic management may consist of weekly adjustments as the tissue heals and motor innervation commences.

Examples of common motor donors that a clinician may see (Elfar, 2010) are as follows:

- Elbow flexion
  - Intercostal nerve or partial ulnar nerve transfer to biceps branch of musculocutaneous nerve
- Shoulder abduction/flexion
  - Spinal accessory nerve transfer to suprascapular nerve
- Hand intrinsic function
  - Anterior interosseous nerve (AIN) to motor branch of ulnar nerve or recurrent branch of median nerve

Sensory Nerve Transfers

Most devastating to functional use of the hand, besides loss of motor innervation, is sensory loss. When there is sensory loss to the volar aspect of the hand, radial border of the index finger (IF), ulnar border of the thumb, and ulnar border of the hand, sensory nerve transfer should be considered (Elfar et al., 2010; Slutsky, 2011). These can restore, at best, protective sensation (Elfar et al., 2010). The sensory nerve end organs remain viable for longer periods of time than do those of a motor nerve, making sensory nerve transfer less common than a motor nerve transfer. In a patient that has sustained a severe nerve injury, the therapist may commonly see a sensory nerve transfer performed at the same time as a motor transfer. An example would be a patient with a high ulnar nerve injury losing intrinsic function and sensation to the ulnar innervated digits as seen in Figure 20–1. Orthotic management is similar to that described for a motor transfer.

Examples of common sensory nerve donors that a clinician may see (Elfar, 2010) are as follows:

- Radial sensory nerve transfer to ulnar aspect of the thumb and/or radial aspect of IF.
- Ulnar digital nerve of IF to the radial aspect of IF.
- Ulnar digital nerve of middle finger (MF) to ulnar aspect of small finger (SF).

NERVE INNERVATIONS AND PATHOLOGY

The extent of functional loss from a nerve injury depends on where along the nerve's pathway it has been injured. In this chapter, the author will discuss injuries that affect the forearm, wrist, and hand.

Lesions and/or lacerations are generally referred to as high (injury proximal to the elbow) or low (injury near or distal to the elbow joint). Figures throughout this chapter detail the specific muscles an individual nerve innervates and at what level/order the innervation generally occurs. There can be variations in nerve innervations that can be functionally significant. Clinicians should be aware of these possible connections and how they may complicate the clinical presentation (Bas & Klienert, 1999). The two most common examples are the links between the median and ulnar nerves in the proximal forearm and the hand (Figs. 20–7 and 20–8).

- **Martin-Gruber Connection.** This association is seen when a portion of the median nerve communicates with the ulnar nerve in the proximal one-third of the forearm. There are many variants of Martin-Gruber connections that have been identified. Several are noted in Figures 20–7 and 20–8 (Elfar et al., 2010). These connections are generally proximal to the AIN branch or distal

within the flexor digitorum profundus (FDP) muscle occurring in approximately 10% to 25% of the population (Gellman & Owens, 2011; Leversedge, Goldfarb, & Boyer, 2010a; Toby & Ritter, 2011). This connection may contain a mix of fibers from the median nerve or AIN or just motor fibers or just sensory fibers. When this anastomosis is present, a complete lesion of the median nerve may not cause paralysis or sensory loss in all the median nerve–innervated muscles because some of the muscles may be receiving innervation from the ulnar nerve. This puzzling presentation, which can exist at various levels, may make the therapist question whether the nerve has been completely severed (Leversedge et al., 2010a; Matloub & Yousif, 1992; Moore & Agur, 1995).

- **Riche-Cannieu Connection** (refer to Figs. 20–7 and 20–8). This is a connection between the recurrent branch of the median nerve and the deep branch of the ulnar nerve in the volar hand, offering ulnar nerve innervation to the intrinsic thenar muscles (Elfar et al., 2010). This occurs in approximately 50% to 77% of the population (Gellman & Owens, 2011; Leversedge et al., 2010a). Variations in this anastomosis have been observed, but the most common effect seen by a clinician would be ulnar innervation to intrinsic thenar muscles such as the body of the flexor pollicis brevis (FPB). Other variations include the thenar common digital nerve connecting to the deep ulnar nerve and connections appearing deep within the abductor pollicis brevis or in the first

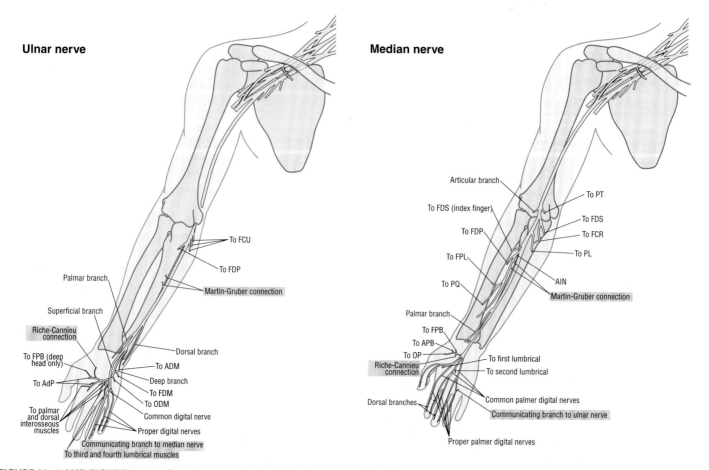

FIGURE 20–7 AND FIGURE 20–8 Schematic representation of the ulnar nerve and median nerves with their common connections to each other. Of these variant connections, the most common are those between either the median and ulnar nerve, or the anterior interosseous nerve and ulnar nerve. When these variant connections are present, a complete lesion of the involved nerve (median or ulnar) may not cause full motor or sensory loss because of the "additional" communication from the neighboring nerve.

lumbricals (Elfar et al., 2010). When this anomalous interconnection is present, clinicians will note that full or near-full thumb motion will be preserved.

PERIPHERAL NERVE PATHOLOGY

The following section will describe the pathology associated with each of these peripheral nerves, further divided into sections for high lacerations, low lacerations, and compressive neuropathies.

MEDIAN NERVE INJURIES

Laceration to the Median Nerve

HIGH LACERATION

High median nerve injury is often associated with traumatic injury of the upper extremity, which may include several neurovascular structures (Fig. 20–9, Box 20–2). Clinical signs of isolated high median nerve injury are a loss of the following:

- Forearm pronation
- Wrist radial flexion
- Independent proximal interphalangeal (PIP) joint flexion from the IF through the SF
- IF and middle finger (MF) distal interphalangeal (DIP) and metacarpophalangeal (MCP) joint flexion
- Thumb interphalangeal (IP) flexion, opposition, and palmar abduction
- Thumb MP flexion weakness caused by the partial innervation of the FPB radial head
- Sensation to the volar radial aspect of the hand

The hand will posture in a **peace sign deformity**–like position (Fig. 20–10). This devastating injury robs the hand of normal function. Rehabilitation should involve preservation of joint

BOX 20–2	ORDER OF INNERVATION FOR MEDIAN NERVE

1. Pronator teres
2. Flexor carpi radialis
3. Palmaris longus
4. Flexor digitorum superficialis
5. Radial half of flexor digitorum profundus
6. Flexor pollicis longus
7. Pronator quadratus
8. First lumbrical
9. Second lumbrical
10. Abductor pollicis brevis
11. Flexor pollicis brevis
12. Opponens pollicis

range of motion (ROM), education on sensory precautions, and careful orthtic intervention to maximize function and prevent deformity.

LOW LACERATION

Low median nerve injury, at the level of the wrist, may be associated with flexor tendon injury. Motor, sensory, and sometimes vascular innervation to all structures distal to the injury site may be affected. In this laceration, there may be loss of the following:

- IF and MF MCP flexion (lumbricals IF and MF)
- Thumb opposition and palmar abduction
- Thumb MP flexion (weakness caused by partial innervation of the FPB radial head)
- Sensation to the volar radial aspect of the hand

The sensory loss is extremely disabling because there is no sensory input to most of the volar surface of the radial digits. The clinical presentation of this injury is often referred to as **ape hand deformity** because of the loss of stabilizing thenar musculature to the volar radial aspect of the hand with inability to position the thumb out of the palm (Fig. 20–11A–C). Simple activities such as writing and holding a utensil can be greatly impaired not only due to the motor loss but also to the inability to feel the object with the radial digits and thumb.

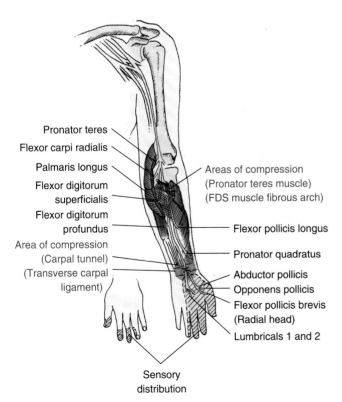

Pronator teres
Flexor carpi radialis
Palmaris longus
Flexor digitorum superficialis
Flexor digitorum profundus
Area of compression (Carpal tunnel) (Transverse carpal ligament)

Areas of compression (Pronator teres muscle) (FDS muscle fibrous arch)
Flexor pollicis longus
Pronator quadratus
Abductor pollicis
Opponens pollicis
Flexor pollicis brevis (Radial head)
Lumbricals 1 and 2

Sensory distribution

FIGURE 20–9 The motor portion of the median nerve innervates most of the wrist and digital flexors. The sensory distribution of the median nerve plays an integral role in providing sensation to the volar radial aspect of the hand.

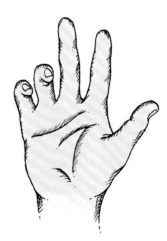

FIGURE 20–10 A high median nerve laceration causes a peace sign posturing of the hand, owing to the loss of the FDP, FDS, and intrinsics of the IF and MF.

If wrist, thumb, or digital flexor tendons are involved, treatment includes a wrist/hand flexion immobilization or restriction orthosis (also referred to as a dorsal blocking orthosis) to decrease tension on the nerve repair and associated soft tissue structures (Fig. 20–12). If the median nerve was repaired in isolation, an orthosis that positions the wrist in flexion (allowing MCP and IP motion) with the thumb in opposition and palmar abduction is often acceptable (Fig. 20–13). When healing allows (at 4–6 weeks), a small opposition strap can be used to enhance

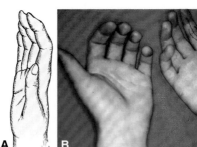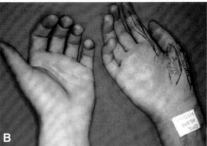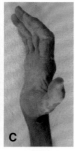

FIGURE 20–11 **A and B,** A low median nerve laceration leaves an apelike hand. Note left hand thumb adduction secondary to the loss of thumb abductor and opponens pollicis. Posture further influenced by the innervated thumb adductor and first dorsal interossei. **C,** In this radial view, the devastating loss of the hand's arches and muscular tone is appreciated.

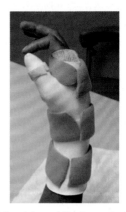

FIGURE 20–12 A wrist/thumb immobilization orthosis (dorsal blocking) is used to protect a repaired median nerve, thumb flexor tendon, and other soft-tissue structures.

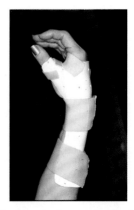

FIGURE 20–13 An option for orthosis management of a median nerve repair is incorporating gentle wrist flexion, thumb opposition/palmar abduction, with the metacarpophalangeals (MCPs) free. If the thumb web is not supported in opposition and abduction, the unopposed ulnar-innervated intrinsics will pull the thumb web into adduction, eventually leading to contracture.

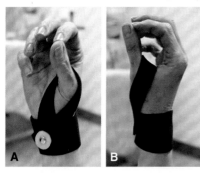

FIGURE 20–14 **A and B,** A simple strap can be used to allow functional opposition. This neoprene strap allowed an OB/GYN surgeon to resume limited work activities by giving assistance to weak reinnervating median nerve musculature.

and facilitate functional pinch (Fig. 20–14A,B). Orthotic fabrication is used in combination with the referring physician's postoperative protocol, which may include such techniques as pain management, wound care, edema reduction, and guarded active or passive ROM.

Compression Neuropathies of the Median Nerve

PROXIMAL MEDIAN NERVE NEUROPATHY (PRONATOR SYNDROME)

Compression in the proximal forearm is commonly referred to as **pronator syndrome**; however, proximal median nerve compression is not localized solely to the pronator teres muscle. The most common site of proximal neuropathy is in the region of the fascial bands and muscular anomalies of the pronator teres muscle and the fibrous arcade of the flexor digitorum superficialis. Other less common potential sources of compression are the ligament of Struthers, lacertus fibrosis, an accessory bicipital aponeurosis, an anomalous muscle, a space-occupying lesion, or scarring from trauma (Eversmann, 1992; Hartz, Linscheild, Gramse, & Daube, 1981; Moore, Dalley, & Agur, 2010; Toby & Ritter, 2011). Symptoms may include intermittent or consistent pain and paresthesias in the volar forearm and hand, which increases with active use or provocative positioning. The thenar muscles may feel weak and fatigued with only an occasional loss of sensation in the median nerve distribution of the hand. There is often a positive Tinel sign in the volar forearm, weak or negative **Phalen** and reverse Phalen tests (positioning in extreme wrist flexion/extension, creating paresthesias in the median nerve distribution), pain with resistive pronation, and pain in the forearm with resistance to the flexor digitorum superficialis (FDS) of the MF and ring finger (RF).

Proximal median nerve neuropathy or pronator syndrome is often seen in patients who do heavy manual labor; those whose jobs require resistive, repetitive forearm rotation; and quite often in musicians who maintain awkward postures or bear the weight of their instruments on their hands for long periods of time (Charness, 1992; Eversmann, 1992; Mackinnon & Novak, 1997). Care must be taken to examine and rule out carpal tunnel syndrome and cervical radiculopathy. Orthosis management is usually in combination with rest, activity modification, appropriate therapeutic modalities, gentle nerve-gliding exercises, and anti-inflammatory medication. Suggested orthosis positioning includes elbow flexion, forearm pronation, and wrist neutral.

ANTERIOR INTEROSSEOUS NERVE SYNDROME

The AIN is a motor branch of the median nerve, originating 5 to 8 cm distal to the level of the lateral epicondyle (Lundborg,

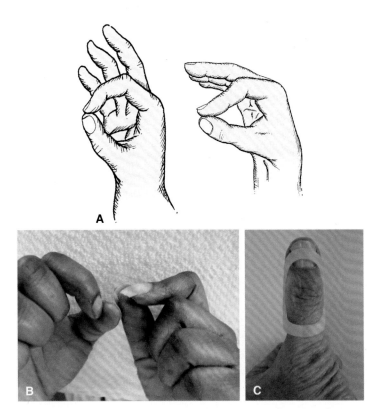

FIGURE 20-15 **A and B,** With an AIN injury, loss of thumb IP and IF DIP flexion results in the inability to perform the okay sign as seen in this patient's right hand. **C,** This Oval-8° Finger Splint (3-Point Products, Stevensville, MD) applied to the thumb IP joint helps maintain a small degree of flexion for an improved pinch.

1988). **Anterior interosseous nerve syndrome** is purely a motor lesion and may occur secondary to trauma (fracture, puncture, and compression), vascular insult, or compression under tendinous bands. Symptoms can include weakness or paralysis of the flexor pollicis longus (FPL), FDP of the IF and MF, and pronator quadratus muscle. Injury to the AIN results in the inability to perform tip and three-point pinch properly (Eversmann, 1992). If the patient is unable to make the "OK" sign, it is likely there is AIN loss (Fig. 20–15A,B).

Orthosis intervention is not common but may be considered to prevent thumb IP (Fig. 20–15C), IF DIP, and sometimes MF DIP extension contractures if applicable. The clinician must impart the importance of maintaining passive motion of these distal joints as the patient is awaiting nerve return. If nerve regeneration is not noted after a reasonable amount of time, other treatment options for complete loss of this branch may be considered, including surgical decompression, nerve, or tendon transfer.

CARPAL TUNNEL SYNDROME

Carpal tunnel syndrome (CTS) may be recognized as one of the most common compression neuropathies of the upper extremity. The carpal tunnel is a narrow space in which the median nerve and nine digital flexor tendons traverse. The tunnel is bordered on three sides by carpal bones and on the volar aspect by the thick, dense transverse carpal ligament (Lundborg, 1988). This narrow space is just wide enough for the structures within it to pass (Fig. 20–16). Any additional pressure, inflammation, or obstacle—such as an osteophyte or scar tissue—within this space may cause compression of the nerve. Compression of the median nerve at this level may occur owing to a multitude of factors, including inflammatory conditions, metabolic disorders, status post fracture or dislocation of the distal radioulnar joint, and tenosynovitis of the digits and wrist flexors caused by arthritis or repetitive stress motions (Lundborg, 1988).

The median nerve is a mixed nerve with both motor and sensory fibers; and because of this, the symptoms can be varied. Some complain of only numbness, whereas others may complain of shooting volar forearm pain and weakness. Most commonly, however, the patient experiences nocturnal burning pain and paresthesias, clumsiness with routine tasks (e.g., drying hair, taking dishes out of the dishwasher), or radiating pain along the volar forearm. Continued compression and irritation to the nerve may result in weakness of thumb abduction, opposition, and the median nerve–innervated intrinsics (Fig. 20–17A). The patient may have difficulty with fine motor manipulation (Fig. 20–17B) because of the described weak musculature and the sensory disturbance to the volar thumb, IF, MF, and radial half of the RF (Boscheinen-Morrin et al., 1985). The patient may have a positive Tinel sign with tapping over the carpal tunnel and a positive Phalen test. Conservative treatment consists of rest; activity modification; a volar wrist immobilization orthosis, with the wrist in neutral for night use; nerve-gliding exercises; and anti-inflammatory medication and/or injection (Fig. 20–18A,B) (Sailor, 1996). Surgical intervention is an option if symptoms persist.

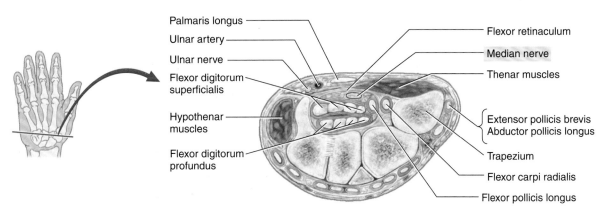

FIGURE 20-16 Cross section of the carpal tunnel through the wrist. Note how the median nerve is surrounded by nine tendons within a small space. (Reprinted with permission from Moore, K. L., Agur, A. M., & Dalley, A. F.II. (2019). *Moore's Essential clinical anatomy* (6th ed.). Philadelphia, PA: Wolters Kluwer.)

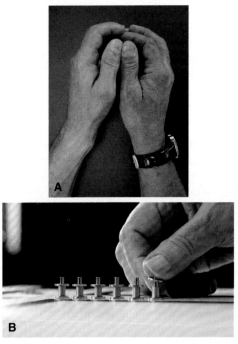

FIGURE 20–17 A, Note the thenar atrophy on the left thumb of this man as compared with his right. **B,** Fine motor manipulation is often challenging and training should be part of the rehabilitation regime.

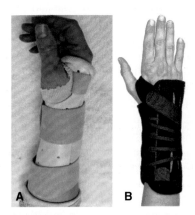

FIGURE 20–18 When the median nerve is compressed at the level of the wrist, an orthosis that positions the wrist in neutral can decrease symptoms since the nerve is in a relaxed, tension free position. **A,** Custom fabricated or **(B)** prefabricated option. The Titan Wrist™ Lacing Wrist Orthosis shown here allows for adjustability in fit and rigidity making it customizable to fit each patient. (Photo courtesy of Hely & Weber™.)

ULNAR NERVE INJURIES

Lacerations to the Ulnar Nerve

HIGH LACERATION

Lacerations of the ulnar nerve at or above the elbow result in loss of the following (Fig. 20–19) (Box 20–3):

- Ulnar wrist flexion
- DIP and MCP flexion of RF and SF
- Abduction and adduction of all digits
- Adduction of thumb
- Thumb MP flexion (weakness owing to partial innervation of the FPB ulnar head)
- Sensory loss of the dorsoulnar aspect of the hand, radiating along the ulnar side of the forearm
- Significant loss of grip and pinch strength

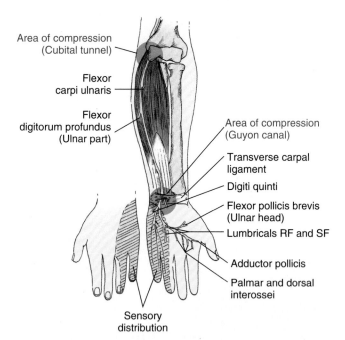

FIGURE 20–19 The ulnar nerve provides innervation to the ulnar aspect of the wrist and hand. The sensory branches innervate the dorsal ulnar and the volar aspect of the SF and the ulnar half of the RF.

BOX 20–3	ORDER OF INNERVATION FOR ULNAR NERVE

1. Flexor carpi ulnaris
2. Ulnar half of flexor digitorum profundus
3. Abductor digiti minimi
4. Flexor digiti minimi
5. Opponens digiti minimi
6. Fourth web space interossei
7. Third web space interossei
8. Second web space interossei
9. Fourth lumbrical
10. Third lumbrical
11. Adductor pollicis
12. First web space interossei

Clinical signs of chronic high-level ulnar nerve injury may include a mild **claw hand deformity** of the hand (hyperextension of the RF and SF MCP joints secondary to loss of the stabilizing intrinsics, weakened or stretched MCP joint volar plates, and overpull of the intact extensor tendons) with a loss of the hypothenar and interosseous muscles (Fig. 20–20). The patient may be unable to adduct the SF secondary to paralysis of the third volar interossei (**Wartenberg sign**) and abduct the IF owing to paralysis of the first dorsal interossei (Lundborg, 1988) (Fig. 20–21A). The patient may also exhibit the inability to contract the adductor pollicis, and when combined with the loss of the first dorsal interossei (Fig. 20–21B), attempted lateral pinch is significantly impaired. Lateral pinch is compensated for by the median nerve–innervated FPL, causing extreme flexion of the thumb IP joint during attempted pinch (**Froment sign**) (Fig. 20–22), and with chronic loss of innervation, this clinical picture may eventually include hyperextension of the thumb MP joint known as **Jeanne sign** (Fig. 20–23A) (Doyle, 2006; Lundborg, 1988; Parry, 1981).

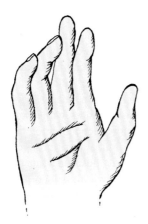

FIGURE 20-20 A high ulnar nerve laceration does not cause the pronounced RF and SF PIP DIP flexion posturing that is seen with a lower ulnar nerve lesion secondary to the paralysis of the associated FDP tendons.

Treatment may consist of education regarding sensory precautions, preservation of ROM, and orthotic intervention to maximize functional use and prevent joint contractures while waiting for nerve regeneration (Fig. 20–23B).

LOW LACERATION

Low ulnar nerve injury at the wrist is often seen in combination with flexor tendon, median nerve, and vascular injury.

Injury of the ulnar nerve at this level results in loss of the following:

- MCP flexion of RF and SF
- Abduction and adduction of all digits
- Adduction of thumb
- Sensory loss of the ulnar aspect of the hand; dorsoulnar sensation remains intact
- Thumb MP flexion (weakness caused by partial innervation of the FPB ulnar head)
- Significant loss of grip and pinch strength

A clawing deformity of the RF and SF is more prominent than with a high lesion secondary to the intact profundus tendon to these digits (Fig. 20–24A,B). In chronic conditions, the patient may progress to the point that the Wartenberg, Froment, and Jeanne signs are present. The use of an orthosis that places the MCPs in flexion can prevent overstretching of the supporting volar soft tissues and can facilitate functional use while waiting for nerve return (Fig. 20–24C,D).

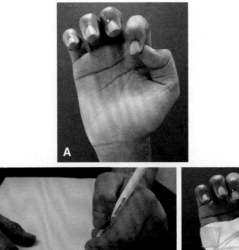
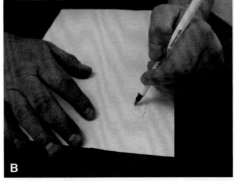
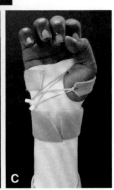

FIGURE 20-22 **A,** Froment sign: with ulnar nerve injury, the patient loses the ability to contract the adductor pollicis; and when combined with the loss of the first dorsal interossei, attempted lateral pinch is significantly impaired. **B,** Lateral pinch is compensated for by the median nerve–innervated FPL, resulting in flexion of the thumb IP as shown here. **C,** A thumb abduction mobilization orthosis can assist in functional use and prevent structures from overstretching. This is an option for day use.

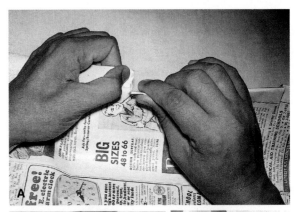
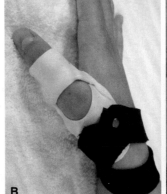
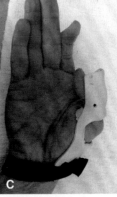

FIGURE 20-23 **A,** Jeanne sign: with ongoing chronic loss of the ulnar nerve, the patient displays all that is described with the Froment sign. In addition, over time, the volar structures of the thumb MP become lax, eventually causing pronounced thumb MP hyperextension . **B and C,** A thumb MP extension restriction orthosis can be used to position the thumb MP in slight flexion (better mechanical advantage), which supports a functional position for pinch and prevents further stretching of the volar MP structures. (A, Borrowed from Doyle, J. R. (2006). *Hand and wrist* (pp. 219). Philadelphia, PA: Lippincott Williams & Wilkins.)

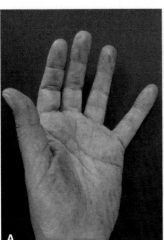
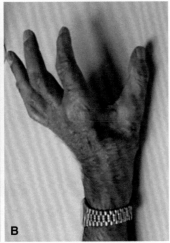

FIGURE 20-21 **A,** Wartenberg sign: demonstrating the inability of the small digit to actively adduct secondary to intrinsic weakness. **B,** Wasting of the first dorsal interosseous following ulnar nerve lesion.

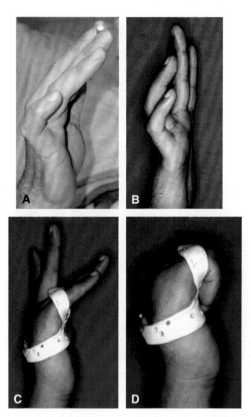

FIGURE 20–24 A low ulnar nerve laceration leads to partial claw deformity. A, Low lesion; note the DIP flexion here caused by the innervation of the FDP SF. **B,** High lesion; there is an increase in MCP volar laxity and a loss of distal innervation to the DIP. A RF/SF MCP extension restriction orthosis allows RF and SF digit extension **(C)**, and flexion **(D)**.

Combined Ulnar and Median Nerve Injury

A combined median and ulnar nerve injury can result in a claw hand deformity. In a low lesion, clawing of all the digits occurs secondary to complete loss of intrinsic control and a functioning profundus

tendon (Fig. 20–25A,B). If the injury is high, clawing still occurs but is significantly less pronounced.

Intervention (for high and low combined lesions) includes patient education regarding sensory precautions as well as fabrication of a daytime functional orthosis that includes all the MCPs in flexion (and thumb abduction/opposition if necessary) to prevent MCP joint extension/PIP flexion contractures while providing a position for functional use. Furthermore, depending on the deforming forces, a variety of nighttime immobilization orthoses can be used to place the structures in an antideformity position while waiting for nerve return (Fig. 20–25C–G). The elbow joint is incorporated into the orthosis (positioned at 90° flexion) if at least one of the involved muscle-tendon unit's origin is at or above the humeral condyles (Fig. 20–25F) (Doyle, 2006).

Compression Neuropathies of the Ulnar Nerve

CUBITAL TUNNEL SYNDROME

The cubital tunnel is formed by a tendinous arch joining the ulnar and humeral attachments of the flexor carpi ulnaris (FCU) tendon. The boundaries of the cubital tunnel are the medial epicondyle, the ulnohumeral ligament, and the fibrous arch formed by the two heads of the FCU tendon (Rayan, 1992). Many factors can cause or contribute to **cubital tunnel syndrome**, a common compression neuropathy, including direct trauma; fracture or fracture and dislocation of the medial or lateral epicondyles; arthritis; a subluxing ulnar nerve; or postural stress caused by sleeping positions, vocational demands, or recreational activities.

The clinical symptoms of cubital tunnel syndrome are paresthesias and numbness in the ulnar portion of the hand and forearm; vague, ulnar-sided arm pain that is sometimes described as a sharp, radiating pain that may worsen with an increase in activity level; and reported weakness of grip and pinch strength. Novak, Lee, Mackinnon, and Lay (1994) found that the cubital tunnel can be quickly screened by performing an **elbow flexion test** (prolonged

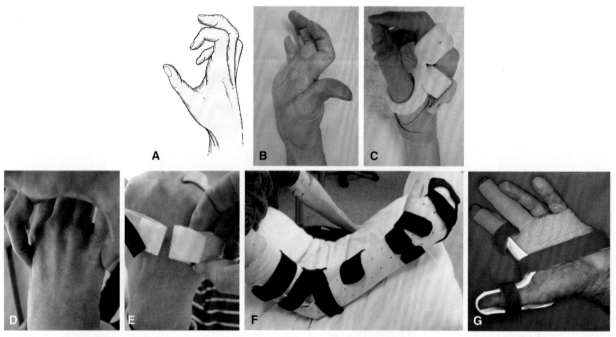

FIGURE 20–25 A–E, Atrophy of the hypothenar and the first dorsal interossei muscles may cause muscle atrophy/ indenting along the lateral borders of the hand, making application and removal of an orthosis quite difficult. A trap door (using hook loop closure) helps with orthosis application and removal. **F,** The elbow is incorporated after surgical repair of a high ulnar laceration and complex flexor tendon injury. Note the soft crossed neoprene strapping in the anterior elbow fossa. **G,** When necessary and especially with combined ulnar and median nerve lesions, attention should be given to maintaining a wide webspace with appropriate midpalmar and radial abduction.

elbow flexion positioning resulting in paresthesias along the ulnar nerve distribution) combined with pressure on the ulnar nerve. A positive Tinel sign over the ulnar nerve at the elbow, sensory changes in the ulnar nerve distribution, decreased grip and pinch strength, and atrophy of the intrinsic muscles of the hand are also common indicators (Novak et al., 1994). Performing the scratch collapse test may also be a quick screen for cubital tunnel. It has been shown to have a significantly higher sensitivity than the other existing clinical tests (Cheng, Mackinnon-Patterson, Beck, & Mackinnon, 2008). In some cases, chronic compression of the nerve may lead to positive Wartenberg, Froment, and Jeanne signs. The differential diagnosis should rule out thoracic outlet syndrome, C8/T1 nerve root compression, and compression of the ulnar nerve distally at the Guyon canal.

Conservative management usually involves rest and avoidance of provocative activities (e.g., prolonged elbow flexion, repetitive elbow flexion/extension, and weight bearing on the medial elbow), gentle nerve-gliding exercises, anti-inflammatory medication if appropriate, and some type of night elbow immobilization orthosis (slight elbow flexion, neutral forearm to slight pronation, and wrist neutral with slight ulnar deviation) (Fig. 20–26A–C) (Harper, 1990; Sailor, 1996; Tetro & Pichora, 1996; Warwick & Seradge, 1995).

If the patient cannot tolerate a thermoplastic orthosis for nighttime use (or insurance will not cover it), other options can be considered. A piece of foam or a small pillow can be placed on the anterior aspect of the elbow crease to prevent elbow flexion. The foam should extend proximally to the middle upper arm and distally to the mid-forearm; it can be held in place with a stockinette or a light circumferential wrap. Another option is to wind a towel around the elbow, securing it with a circumferential wrap (Fig. 20–27A–C). These methods are intended to restrict full elbow flexion and may be tolerated better than a rigid orthosis. During the day, soft padding (foam or silicone) about the posterior and medial elbow (cubital tunnel region) may protect the nerve from further trauma and provide a sense of security for the patient (Fig. 20–28A,B). If symptoms continue, surgical decompression or transposition of the nerve may be warranted.

ULNAR TUNNEL (GUYON CANAL) SYNDROME

The ulnar tunnel, also referred to as **Guyon canal**, is formed by the volar carpal ligament, hook of the hamate, and the pisiform bones. This space is small and somewhat superficial, making the nerve vulnerable to injury. Just proximal to the wrist, the nerve divides into a dorsal superficial sensory branch and a volar deep motor branch. Compression of the sensory branch, motor branch, or both branches may occur depending on the level of impingement. If only the motor branch is involved, the intrinsic muscles are affected, but sensation is left intact. An isolated lesion to the deep motor branch may be seen in people who use tools intensively, such as a screwdriver or pruning shears. They do not usually complain of pain, just weakness and atrophy (Boscheinen-Morrin et al., 1985; Matloub & Yousif, 1992).

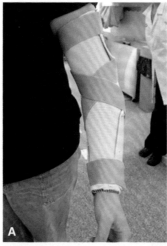

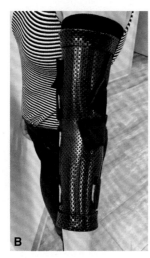

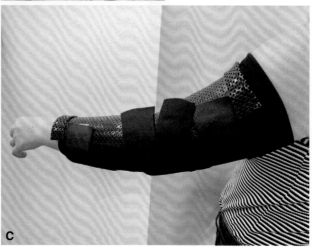

FIGURE 20–26 A, A night resting elbow immobilization orthosis—posterior design—minimizes compression on the nerve as it passes through the cubital tunnel. Restriction of elbow flexion during sleep may decrease irritation in this area. **B and C,** An anterior elbow immobilization orthosis is an alternate option to preventing elbow flexion to reduce ulnar nerve irritation at the cubital tunnel.

The compression of the ulnar nerve at this level can be caused by repetitive trauma (cycling, hammering, use of vibrating tools), fracture of the hook of the hamate or pisiform bones, arthritis in the pisohamate joint, ganglion, anomalous muscle or ligament, or possibly an ulnar artery aneurysm or thrombosis (Lundborg, 1988; Moore & Dalley, 1999; Moore et al., 2010). Symptoms include vague pain, paresthesias or numbness of the SF and ulnar half of the RF, and weakness of the intrinsic muscles. In some cases, the patient may demonstrate positive Wartenberg, Froment, and Jeanne signs owing to the weakness of the ulnar innervated muscles. When the sensory branch is involved, examination may reveal a positive Phalen test and Tinel sign over the ulnar tunnel.

Treatment of these low lesions focuses on rest, immobilization, avoidance of symptomatic activities, and anti-inflammatory medication. If symptoms persist, surgical intervention may be necessary. Orthoses may be used initially to immobilize the wrist and ulnar aspect of the hand for symptom relief. Once symptoms subside, orthoses can be fabricated to protect the ulnar tunnel during vocational or recreational activities. Padding the ulnar wrist over the ulnar tunnel area with gel or high-density foam may aid in absorbing vibration and compression stress to this vulnerable area. An orthosis can then be formed directly over this padded area (Fig. 20–29A–C).

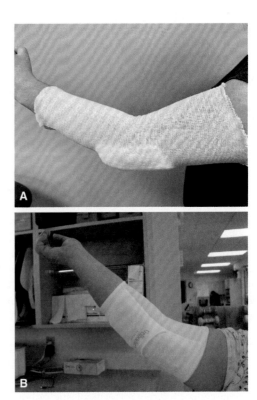

FIGURE 20–28 **A and B,** Soft padding or use of silicone gel sheets (or similar products) over the cubital tunnel area may help protect and absorb vibration/forces to a hypersensitive or regenerating ulnar nerve.

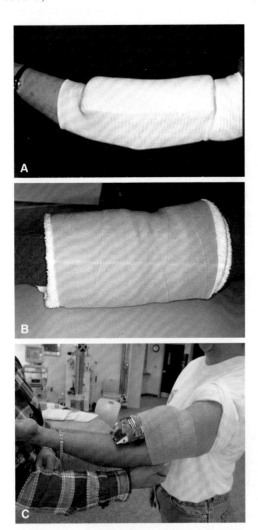

FIGURE 20–27 **A,** A foam pad applied to the anterior aspect of the elbow can provide some light resistance to full elbow flexion. **B,** A towel wrapped about the elbow can also prevent full elbow flexion while sleeping, allowing a less restraining option to rigid immobilization. **C,** A small pillow or rolled up towel can be secured with an elasticized bandage as yet another option.

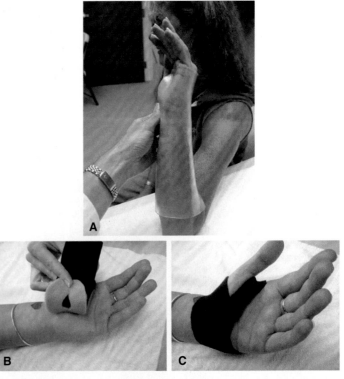

FIGURE 20–29 **A,** An ulnar wrist immobilization orthosis can be fabricated by incorporating silicone gel or high-density foam over the volar ulnar aspect of the wrist to protect the ulnar nerve in this region. **B and C,** A donut of foam rests over Guyon canal and is incorporated into this small custom-fabricated neoprene orthosis.

RADIAL NERVE INJURIES

Lacerations of the Radial Nerve

The radial nerve innervates the triceps muscle, which provides elbow extension, and innervates all of the wrist, digit, and thumb extensors as well as the supinator muscle (Fig. 20–30) (Box 20–4). Sensory loss of the radial nerve is much less functionally significant than that of the ulnar or median nerve. Despite this, pain can be functionally limiting and should be addressed.

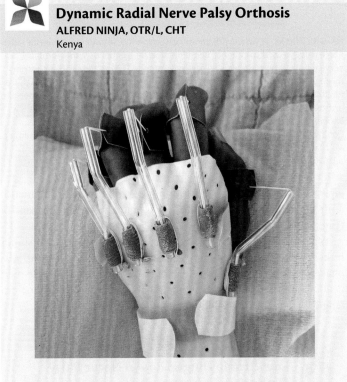

EXPERT PEARL 20–1

Dynamic Radial Nerve Palsy Orthosis
ALFRED NINJA, OTR/L, CHT
Kenya

Use segment of Orficast to attach Orfitubes to orthosis—dry heat then wrap around the Orfitube, also dry heat the spot on the orthosis to make it stick firmly.

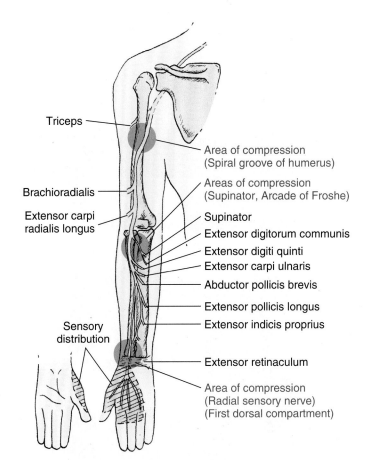

FIGURE 20–30 Injury to the motor portion of the radial nerve is functionally disabling.

Triceps

Area of compression (Spiral groove of humerus)

Brachioradialis

Areas of compression (Supinator, Arcade of Froshe)

Extensor carpi radialis longus

Supinator

Extensor digitorum communis

Extensor digiti quinti

Extensor carpi ulnaris

Abductor pollicis brevis

Extensor pollicis longus

Extensor indicis proprius

Sensory distribution

Extensor retinaculum

Area of compression (Radial sensory nerve) (First dorsal compartment)

BOX 20–4   ORDER OF INNERVATION FOR RADIAL NERVE

1. Brachioradialis
2. Extensor carpi radialis longus
3. Supinator
4. Extensor carpi radialis brevis
5. Extensor digitorum communis
6. Extensor carpi ulnaris
7. Extensor digiti minimi
8. Abductor pollicis longus
9. Extensor pollicis longus
10. Extensor pollicis brevis
11. Extensor indicis proprius

HIGH LACERATION

Laceration to the radial nerve in the upper arm is often associated with a midshaft humerus fracture or traumatic injury to the nerve from a gunshot or stabbing injury. The radial nerve travels in close proximity to the humerus and is extremely vulnerable to injury if the humerus is involved. If lacerated at this level, the patient experiences loss of the following:

- Wrist extension
- Forearm supinator (weak)
- Thumb and digital extension
- Independent IF and SF digital extension
- Sensation over the dorsal radial aspect of the forearm and hand

This clinical presentation is often referred to as **wrist drop** (Fig. 20–31). The radial nerve cannot innervate its distal musculature, making wrist and digital extension impossible. Orthosis intervention can be used to place the wrist and digits in a more neutral/functional position to prevent overstretching of the involved extensor muscle-tendon units, prevent joint contractures, and provide a mechanical advantage for the flexor tendons while waiting return of radial nerve function (Fig. 20–32) (Colditz, 1987; Duff, 2005). There are several options of orthoses available to the therapist, including both custom and prefabricated designs (Fig. 20–33A–H). These are mentioned in Table 20–2.

EXPERT PEARL 20-2

Radial Palsy Orthosis

ANNE WAJON, PT, CHT
CERI PULHAM, OT, CHT
Australia

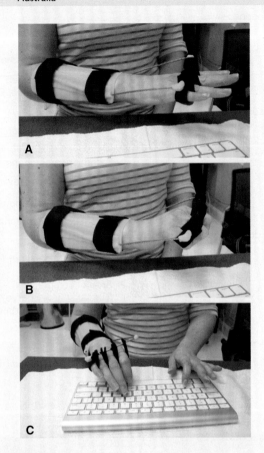

Fabricated with double-sided Velcro loop (to create finger loops). Ensure correct length of loops relative to each finger before finalizing the orthosis with thermoplastic stoppers.

A wrist extension immobilization orthosis can also be used for day functional use; however, the therapist should caution the patient on potential MCP flexion and IP extension contractures due to loss of active extension. Nighttime immobilization may consist of a simple wrist/hand/thumb immobilization orthosis. Figure 20–34A,B shows a simple wrist extension immobilization orthosis that is worn for day use; then for night, an extension attachment was added to prevent flexion contractures of the digits and of the first web space. The use of elastic therapeutic tape such as Balance Tex™ or Kinesio®

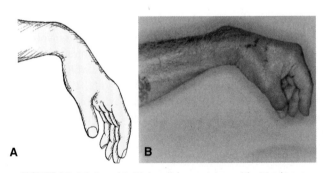

FIGURE 20–31 **A and B,** High radial nerve injury with wrist drop.

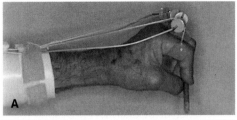

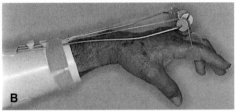

FIGURE 20–32 A wrist/MCP/thumb extension mobilization orthosis (for radial nerve palsy) is used to enhance hand function for a patient waiting for radial nerve reinnervation. The wrist is passively extended **(A)** as the digits actively flex through this mobilization device, and when the wrist actively flexes (through the functioning flexor tendons), the digits passively extend **(B)**. The proximal dorsal orthosis was fabricated out of 3/32″ material; the mobilization component is a Phoenix Extended Outrigger Kit. (Design of this orthosis modified from Colditz, J. C. (1995). Splinting the hand with a peripheral nerve injury. In Hunter J. M., Mackin E. J., & Callahan A. D. (Eds.), *Rehabilitation of the hand* (4th ed., pp. 679–692). St. Louis, MO: Mosby Year Book.)

tapes as well as neoprene strapping can be used in conjunction with an orthosis to assist the digits and thumb into extension (Fig. 20–35A–D).

When surgical tendon transfer or repair is warranted, similar orthosis intervention is appropriate after the initial postoperative phase. Postoperative orthoses can be used to facilitate muscle reeducation and functional use, maintain balance of muscle-tendon unit length(s), and prevent joint contractures.

EXPERT PEARL 20-3

Low-Profile Hinged Radial Nerve Palsy Orthosis

BOB PHILLIPS, OTR/L, CHT
Georgia

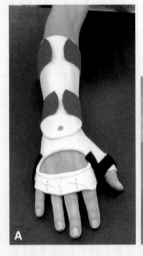

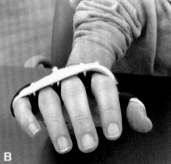

Dycem or other nonskid materials may be used to help prevent distal migration. Elastic Thread and/or Elastic Cord 600 g utilized to hold stretch loop 5/8″ material at digit level. Notice how pattern was cut with MCP joints free dorsally to prevent pressure points. Pay close attention to the thumb making sure it is midway between thumb radial and palmar abduction to allow for function. Adjust tension on elastic loop to allow desired MCP flexion specific for functional activity. Hinge allows for radial/ulnar deviation of wrist during use.

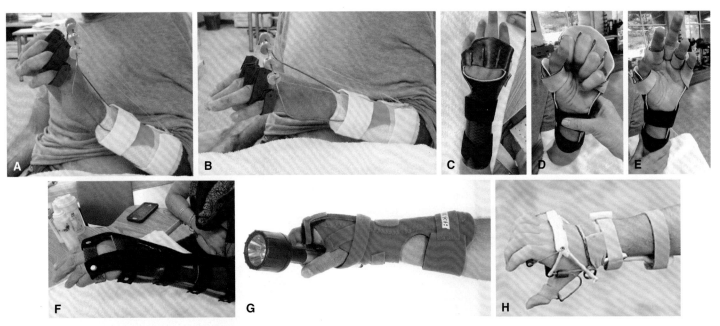

FIGURE 20–33 **A and B,** Custom-bent aluminum wire and soft neoprene slings can be an alternative when not all kit components are available, affordable, or appropriate for the patient. Note the dorsal orthosis "cuff" with elasticized strap closures. **C–E,** Custom option utilizing neoprene strapping for dynamic MCP extension assist with zip ties securing dorsally. Notice cut out over MCP joints to prevent irritation and ability to adjust tension of neoprene depending on functional activity. **F,** Custom design using elasticized loop attached to distal proximal phalanx circumferential segment which provides extension of MCP joints—adjustable tension to be able to vary allowable range of motion. **G,** The Tunnel Forearm Splint. (Photo courtesy of Benik Corp, Silverdale, WA.) **H,** LMB⁻ Radial Nerve Splint Wrist Extension with MCP Extension Assist and Adjustable Thumb Extension Assist. (Photo courtesy of DeRoyal Industries, Powell, TN.)

LOW LACERATION

Distal and anterior to the lateral epicondyle (at 8–10 cm), the radial nerve divides into a sensory and a motor branch. The sensory branch provides innervation to the dorsoradial forearm while the motor branch (PIN) continues distally to innervate the digit and thumb extensors. The radial wrist extensors—the extensor carpi radialis

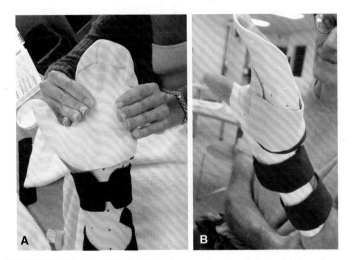

FIGURE 20–34 **A,** A night digit/thumb extension piece is being fabricated over the day wrist extension orthosis to prevent IP flexion contractures and shortening of the flexor tendons, which can occur as a consequence of this injury. **B,** A simple volar piece was added to this day orthosis in order to keep digits extended, the thumb IP is free, yet the orthosis incorporated the first web to provide for a wide first web space minimizing contracture.

longus (ECRL) and extensor carpi radialis brevis (ECRB)—are innervated proximal to this bifurcation. Therefore, with low injury to the PIN, wrist extension is normal with only the loss of digit and thumb extension. The intrinsics attempt to extend the PIP and DIP joints, but the MCPs cannot be extended by the inactive extrinsic extensor tendons. Orthosis management is essentially the same as for a high lesion. The inclusion of the wrist is optional and not recommended if there is adequate wrist extension strength (Fig. 20–36A–H). The reader is referred to Chapter 9 for alternatives to custom designs.

Compression Neuropathies of the Radial Nerve

HIGH COMPRESSION

The radial nerve courses about the humerus at the level of the spiral groove. Injury may occur owing to local compression of the radial nerve against the humerus for an extended period of time, also known as **Saturday night palsy** (i.e., falling asleep with arm against a hard object, a forceful squeeze). There may be tenderness directly over the compression site with little other pain noted. This area of compression block may cause a neurapraxia, resulting in impairment of the muscles innervated below this level. With time, this weakness or paralysis may resolve with little or no functional deficit (Eaton & Lister, 1992; Lundborg, 1988; Moore & Dalley, 1999; Moore et al., 2010; Parry, 1981). The goals of orthosis intervention consist of prevention of joint contractures, protection against overstretching of the involved extensor muscle-tendon units, and maximizing functional use of the hand and wrist while waiting for nerve return.

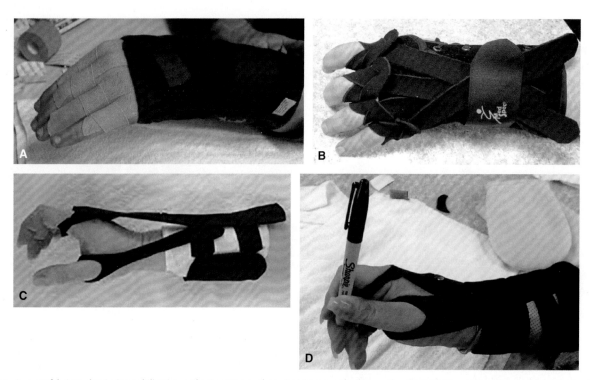

FIGURE 20–35 A, A prefabricated wrist immobilization orthosis supports the wrist into neutral, whereas the elastic therapeutic tape is applied to assist the digits into extension. **B,** Neoprene can also be considered for MCP extension assist. **C and D,** A low-profile wrist/MCP extension orthosis can be an alternative design for a radial nerve palsy orthosis. These orthoses utilize the elastic qualities of the neoprene material to support the wrist, digits, and thumb in extension. More can be found on the use of neoprene in Chapter 14.

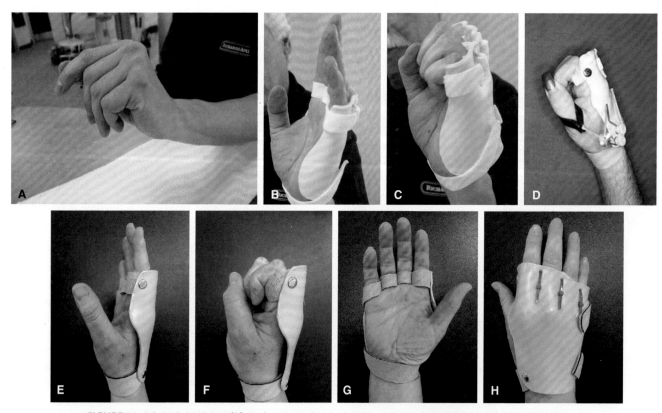

FIGURE 20–36 A–C, PIN injury **(A)** can be managed with a hand-based MCP/thumb MP extension mobilization orthosis. This orthosis maintains passive MCP/thumb MP extension **(B)** while allowing **(C)** active digital flexion. A lightweight material is used to contour about the dorsum of the hand. **D,** A thumb extension outrigger is not always necessary and may be cumbersome to some patients; however, here it helped the patient carry out work responsibilities. Prepadding the dorsal MCPs may assist in decreasing migration, shear stress, and increasing comfort. **E–H,** Low-profile custom design utilizing neoprene as dynamic MCP assist—notice adjustability on ulnar side and zip ties for creating digit loops. This design can easily be modified to include the thumb if required or the wrist for higher radial nerve lesions.

Dynamic Tenodesis Orthosis
LARISSA PÓVOA ALVES BARRADAS, OT
Brazil

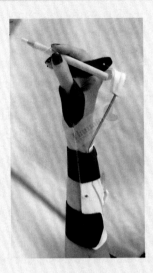

Designed to assist manual function after radial nerve injury. Elastic components provide extension of the MCPs and stability of the wrist. Function of the hand using the tenodesis effect is made possible. Notice hole in plastic on radial side for thumb line attachment.

Radial Palsy Orthosis
GRÉGORY MESPLIÉ, PHYSIOTHERAPIST
CHANTAL ETCHEVERRY, OT
BAPTISTE ARRATE, OT
France

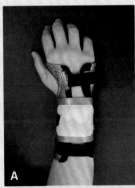

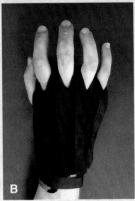

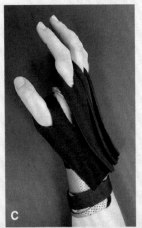

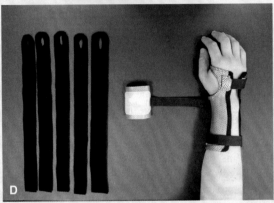

The Neoprene straps compensate for loss of extension at the wrist/fingers and abduction of the thumb. Neoprene strips are not only used for comfort but also to reduce the size of the orthosis. They facilitate daily tasks and can be cleaned/changed easily.

RADIAL TUNNEL SYNDROME

The PIN passes deep to the origin of the ECRB and the arcade of Frohse (proximal margin of the supinator) and then passes between the two heads of the supinator to supply the supinator (Lundborg, 1988; Moore & Dalley, 1999; Moore et al., 2010). Compression can occur at any one of the sites through which the nerve passes; however, the arcade of Frohse is by far the most likely anatomic structure to compress the PIN (Lundborg, 1988; Moore & Dalley, 1999; Moore et al., 2010). **Radial tunnel syndrome**, also known as **resistant tennis elbow**, is often characterized by pain with repetitive rotational movement of the forearm (Roles & Manudsley, 1972; Simmons & Wyman, 1992). Pain is described as aching and radiating toward the dorsal part of the wrist. There is profound tenderness on palpation directly over the extensor muscle group and supinator, 3 to 4 cm distal (over the arcade of Frohse) to the lateral epicondyle (Lundborg, 1988; Rayan, 1992). Resistance to supination, wrist extension, and MF extension usually reproduces the pain. Pain can occur during the day with forearm rotation activities; however, it is usually most evident at night. Radial tunnel can be misdiagnosed as lateral epicondylitis (tennis elbow). A careful differential diagnosis should be done. In lateral epicondylitis, pain is directly over the lateral epicondyle, wrist extension may be weak and painful, and pain is most often during and/or after work or recreational activity (Eaton & Lister, 1992; Lundborg, 1988; Newcomer, Martinez-Silvestrini, Schaefer, Gay, & Arendt, 2005).

Management should include rest, avoidance of provocative positions, activity modification, anti-inflammatory medication or modalities, nerve-gliding exercises, and orthosis application with the elbow gently flexed (optional) and forearm supinated with wrist extension.

Posterior Interosseous Nerve Syndrome

The same pathology and therapeutic intervention as described for the low radial nerve laceration applies to **posterior interosseous nerve syndrome**. Although not common, the PIN can be damaged, compressed, or lacerated at this level (Thomas et al., 2000). Injury may occur from a mass pressing on the nerve (e.g., ganglion, lipoma, or fibroma), from a traumatic incident (e.g., an injection, plate or pin fixation while repairing a proximal radius or ulna fracture), rheumatoid arthritis of the elbow, or a forearm compression injury (Dell & Guzewicz, 1992). Symptoms usually include some degree of pain and weakness. Physical examination reveals no sensory deficit and a temporary partial or complete paralysis of the extrinsic digit and thumb extensors.

Superficial Radial Sensory Nerve Syndrome (Wartenberg Syndrome)

The sensory branch of the radial nerve is vulnerable to injury as it approaches the radial styloid of the wrist. Therapists and surgeons often see injury and/or irritation at this level. In **Wartenberg syndrome**, the nerve becomes entrapped at the site of the brachioradialis in the distal third of the forearm. This compression site is about 9 cm proximal to the radial styloid (Fig. 20–37A,B). Additionally, in **superficial radial sensory nerve syndrome** the nerve can become entrapped in scar from a laceration or from a surgical incision, as occasionally seen with a deQuervain release. Irritation to this branch can also be caused by friction from pin placement, jagged orthosis edges, sharp or compressive orthosis straps, or excessive edema (Colditz, 1995). Sensory alterations (paresthesias and numbness) occur in the dorsoradial aspect of the hand

(Lundborg, 1988). Intervention focuses on orthosis management, with a silicone gel cushion or pad placed directly over the radial styloid (Fig. 20–37C). For an acute, painful injury, a doughnut may be used over this area to avoid direct contact. An orthosis can offer protection and decreased tension on the nerve. Other therapeutic modalities may be used as warranted. Surgical decompression is considered when all conservative management fails.

DIGITAL NERVE LACERATIONS

Digital nerves can be lacerated in isolation but most often are seen in combination with tendon injury in zones II to IV. If seen in isolation, the involved digit is placed into a hand-based immobilization or restriction orthosis (depending on the physician's protocol). The position of the digit is in a gently flexed posture to minimize stress on the surgical anastomosis. Protective orthotic management is used for 4 to 6 weeks; the patient is put into progressively greater extension per physician's orders (Fig. 20–38A–D).

During the initial weeks, a guarded ROM program is begun, which usually involves unrestricted flexion and some degree of restricted extension. If tendons are involved, the wrist and/or thumb must be incorporated into the orthosis, following the physician's preferred tendon protocol. Patient education regarding sensory precautions, wound care, edema control, and protected ROM must be reviewed.

BRACHIAL PLEXUS INJURY

Injuries to the brachial plexus are extremely varied, ranging from simple compression and irritation injuries to complex traumatic avulsions. The brachial plexus supplies the principal motor and sensory innervations to every muscle of the upper extremity with the exception of the levator scapulae and trapezius muscle (Leversedge et al., 2010; Moore et al., 2010). Trauma (i.e., gunshot wounds, avulsions), disease, stretching, and compression (Erb

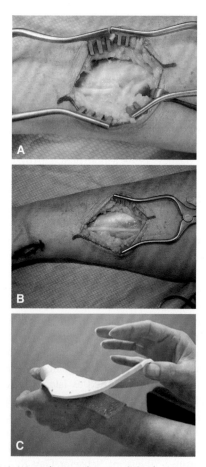

FIGURE 20–37 A, Wartenberg syndrome, radial nerve compression by brachioradialis. **B,** Following decompression of radial nerve. **C,** Place a silicone gel cushion or pad directly over or around the radial styloid process and under the orthosis for protection of the nerve absorption of vibration and distribution of pressure. (A, Photos courtesy of Mitchell Pet, MD (St. Louis, MO).)

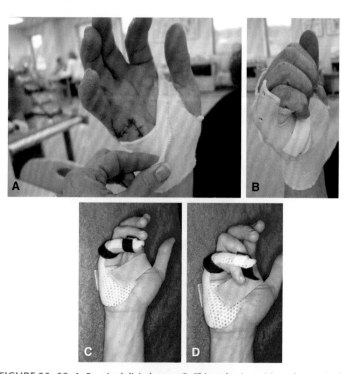

FIGURE 20–38 A, Repaired digital nerve. **B,** This orthosis positions the repaired digital nerve in a shortened position while allowing gliding of the flexor tendons through the incision area, minimizing the risk of adhesion formation. **C,** This design further protects the length of the nerve when increased precaution is necessary. **D,** Removal of the straps allows periodic gentle ROM within the orthosis confines.

palsy, Saturday night palsy) in the axilla or lateral cervical triangle of the neck may produce a brachial plexus injury (Moore et al., 2010). The type of distal pathology the clinician will see depends where the plexus was injured. The location of injury and the anticipated pathology can be appreciated in Figure 20–39A. Although a review of this nerve complex is beyond the scope of this chapter, it is important to value the complex path (root → trunk → division → cord → branch) the peripheral nerve takes to end in its terminal branch. It is also relevant to mention that orthotic intervention is based on the predicted distal pathology and potential deformity (Hunter & Whitenack, 1995; Jacobs, 2003; Lowe & O'Toole, 1995) (Fig. 20–39A). Pain is often a consequence of these injuries and can play a major role in the therapist's ability to manage the patient. The therapist should recognize that the peripheral nerves,

nerve plexuses, spinal nerves, and nerve roots may all become a source of pain and thus may limit the plan of care (Barbis & Wallace, 1995; Elvey, 1997).

PSYCHOSOCIAL IMPACT OF PERIPHERAL NERVE INJURIES

It is well established that upper extremity disorders affecting the peripheral nervous system have lasting implications on function (Novak, Anastakis, Beaton, Mackinnon, & Katz, 2010). In addition to biomedical measures of function, social and emotional well-being and function are negatively impacted and less frequently considered and addressed throughout the course of treatment and recovery. Pain associated with nerve injuries can often be severe and is associated with higher

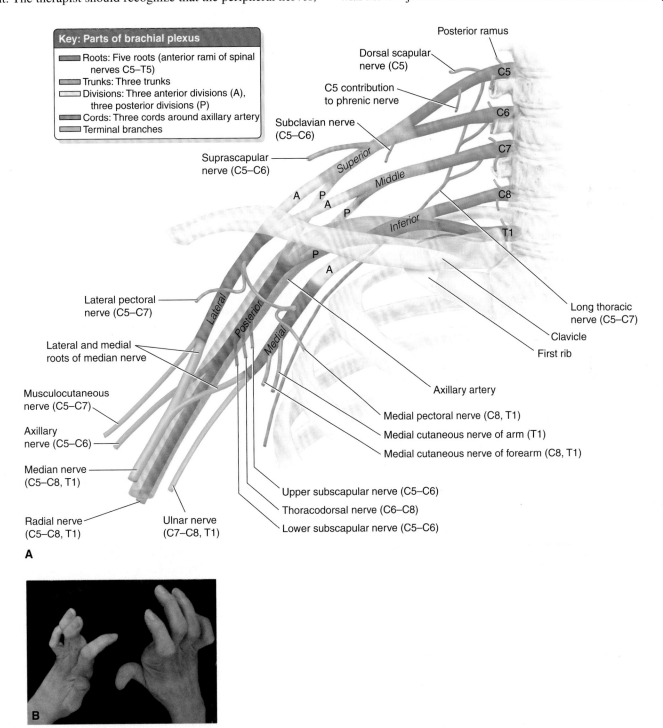

FIGURE 20–39 A, Brachial plexus. **B,** The clinician can appreciate the complex origin of each terminal branch and how this correlates with hand anatomy and function. (A, Reprinted with permission from Moore, K. L., Agur, A. M., & Dalley, A. F.II (2019). *Moore's Essential clinical anatomy* (6th ed.). Philadelphia, PA: Wolters Kluwer: Figure 3.27.)

disability using patient-rated outcome measures (Cocito et al., 2006; Novak, Anastakis, Beaton, & Katz, 2009). Patients with peripheral nerve injuries also experience a moderate to large negative impact on quality of life, regardless of the nerve-related diagnosis (Wojtkiewicz et al., 2015). Going forward, there remains a need for increased screening and assessment of factors that reach beyond the traditional biomedical model of treatment employed in most orthopedic clinics.

The same general orthosis management principles, considerations, and precautions discussed in this chapter apply to brachial plexus injuries as well. Orthosis intervention to preserve functional motion and minimize overstretching of the denervated muscles is most important especially with an extended recovery (Colditz, 1987).

The level at which the brachial plexus is injured determines the most appropriate orthotic intervention for preventing deformity and maximizing function (Hunter & Whitenack, 1995; Lowe & O'Toole, 1995). Often, there is not a clear-cut pattern of deformity, especially with untreated lacerations and long-standing compression injuries. In addition, the patient may have developed joint contractures and/or compensatory patterns, which may lead to deforming forces acting on the distal hand (Fig. 20–39B).

For example, a patient with an injured **medial cord** of the brachial plexus has involvement of the ulnar nerve as well contributions to the median nerve. This type of injury results in remarkable loss of the ulnarly innervated intrinsic hand muscles and causes some median nerve deficits as well. The patient essentially presents with a claw hand deformity as noted in Figure 20–39. Applying an IF through SF MCP flexion restriction orthosis may preserve function while the patient waits for nerve return. For those patients who will not fully regain normal function, these orthoses become a crucial component of everyday existence. The patient may need to depend on these orthoses in order to perform even the simplest of tasks (Fig. 20–40A–D).

Injury to the **posterior cord** of the brachial plexus results in damage to all of the extensors of the forearm, wrist, thumb, and fingers and to the deltoid, which abducts the shoulder at the glenohumeral

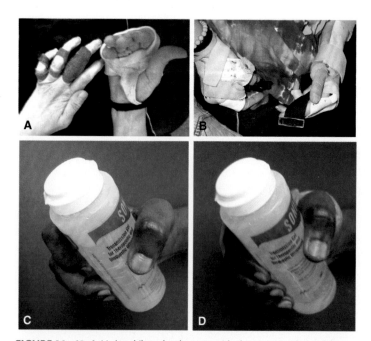

FIGURE 20–40 **A,** Various bilateral orthoses provide this patient with the ability to function somewhat independently. **B,** Bilateral orthoses are used to attach the seat belt and proceed to drive a car with a modified steering wheel. **C,** Note the gross grasp this patient displays without an orthosis and **(D)** the position of digits and thumb while wearing an metacarpophalangeal (MCP) extension restriction orthosis with the thumb included. The orthosis placed the MCPs in flexion and the thumb in opposition allowing a better mechanical advantage for the work of the flexor tendons.

joint. The patient presents with a wrist drop deformity that can be managed with an immobilization orthosis, a mobilization orthosis, or a combination of both as shown in Figures 20–31 and 20–32. The mobilization orthosis allows for a light functional grasp using the natural tenodesis of the hand. The therapist should teach the patient sensory precautions, passive ROM exercises, carefully guided nerve-gliding exercises, the use of adaptive techniques, and postural awareness (Barbis & Wallace, 1995; Lowe & O'Toole, 1995; Topp & Boyd, 2012; Walsh, 2012).

GENERAL PRINCIPLES OF ORTHOTIC INTERVENTION FOR PERIPHERAL NERVE INJURIES

Table 20–2 summarizes PNI management focusing on orthosis considerations. This table is not intended to include all the options of therapeutic procedures or orthotic interventions available to treat the nerve-injured hand.

GOALS IN MANAGING THE UPPER EXTREMITY PERIPHERAL NERVE INJURY

When caring for a patient with a PNI, the therapist should have the following goals in mind:

- Reduce pain and edema.
- Provide a balance among the innervated and denervated muscle-tendon structures while waiting for motor return.
- Keep denervated muscles from remaining in a lengthened position.
- Appreciate cortical plasticity while applying sensory relearning techniques.
- Promoting sensorimotor/sensory reeducation strategies.
- Prevent joint stiffness and joint/soft tissue contractures.
- Prevent development of abnormal substitution patterns.
- Position the hand and wrist in the best biomechanically prudent position to maximize functional use and substitute for loss of motor function.
- Decrease pain and paresthesias associated with nerve compression injuries.
- Protect the surgically repaired or injured nerve and associated injuries.
- Protect and teach the patient/caregiver how to protect insensate areas.
- Keep abreast on current findings on neural regeneration and cortical reorganization.

CONSIDERATIONS AND PRECAUTIONS FOR ORTHOTIC INTERVENTION

The therapist should keep the following considerations and precautions in mind when fabricating an orthosis for this patient population:

- Sensory and motor return should be monitored and orthoses modified accordingly.
- Watch for deformities that may not initially be clinically or functionally evident. As reinnervation occurs, the deformity may become increasingly more apparent; therefore, corrective orthotic intervention is mandatory (e.g., in a returning high ulnar nerve lesion, the FDP eventually becomes innervated and the distal claw deformity becomes more prominent) (Dell & Guzewicz, 1992).

TABLE 20–2	Peripheral Nerve Injury: Orthosis Management and Considerations		
Diagnosis	**Therapy Goals**	**Orthosis Guidelines and Recommendations**	**Considerations**
Median Nerve			
High and low lacerations	• Prevent adduction contractures of the thumb • Prevent overstretching of the thenar muscles • Prevent IF MCP joint contractures • Prevent tension on the surgical repair	• Week 1 (postsurgery): elbow flexed (high lesion only), wrist flexed, thumb midpalmar/radial abduction immobilization orthosis • Week 3: increase wrist extension of orthosis to tolerance • Weeks 4–5: discontinue elbow for high lesions • Weeks 5–6: discontinue wrist, continue protective orthosis for night and at-risk situations only; children and tenuous repairs 1 wk longer; thumb abduction/opposition mobilization strap for day; maintain thumb abduction at night • Week 8: begin gentle mobilization orthosis, if necessary	• Maintain IF passive ROM: extend distal borders of thumb abduction portion of the orthosis (for comfort) • Apply soft material under web portion of orthosis to provide intimate fit (elastomer or silicone gel) • Weeks 5–6: attempt thumb opposition to MF with day orthosis to allow functional pinch through the common origin of the FDP
Pronator syndrome	• Relieve pain and paresthesias • Rest inflamed structures • Prevent provocative motions of the wrist and forearm	• Day: forearm pronation, wrist neutral to slight flexion, immobilization orthosis • Night: for severe symptoms, include elbow in slight flexion	• Fabricate with patient in supine for gravity assist • Careful placement of straps to prevent direct pressure over tender area • The orthosis should be worn until symptoms have subsided and should be only part of a comprehensive rehabilitation program
Anterior interosseous nerve syndrome	• Simulate pinch while waiting for nerve return • Prevent thumb IP and IF DIP extension contracture	• IF DIP/thumb IP flexion immobilization orthosis (or casts); optional	• Consider orthosis in this position if thumb IP and IF DIP function is required for vocational functional tasks • Thin thermoplastic materials or thin casting materials such as QuickCast or Orficast™ can be used, leaving volar pads free for sensory input
Carpal tunnel syndrome	• Decrease pain and paresthesias • Avoid repetitive and/or provocative motions • Rest inflamed structures	• Mild symptoms: day use is optional or depends on physician's preference; wrist immobilized in neutral • Severe symptoms: consider night wrist/hand orthosis to immobilize entire muscle-tendon length	• Allow unimpeded MCP flexion and thumb mobility • The orthosis should be worn until symptoms have subsided and should be only part of a comprehensive rehabilitation program
Ulnar Nerve			
High and low lacerations	• Prevent RF/SF MCP extension, PIP flexion contractures • Prevent overstretching of intrinsic muscles • Prevent RF/SF MCP collateral ligament shortening • Protect and decrease the tension on surgical repair	• Week 1 (postsurgery): elbow flexed (high lesion only), wrist flexed, immobilization orthosis • Week 3: increase wrist extension in orthosis to tolerance • Weeks 4–5: discontinue elbow for high lesions • Weeks 5–6: discontinue wrist; continue MCP flexion protective orthosis for night and at-risk situations only; children and tenuous repairs 1 wk longer; use RF/SF MCP extension restriction orthosis for day • Week 8: begin gentle mobilization orthosis, if necessary	• Allow for full RF/SF MCP flexion • The dorsal component should be well molded to distribute pressure • Prevent RF/SF collateral ligament shortening • Atrophy of the hypothenar muscles may make the day orthosis difficult to don and doff; incorporate an opening (on dorsal aspect) to ease application
Cubital tunnel syndrome	• Prevent repetitive and prolonged elbow flexion • Decrease shearing stress on the nerve as it travels through the cubital tunnel • Position the nerve in a resting state	• Day: posterior medial elbow pad; buddy tape SF to RF (if needed) • Night: elbow at 30°–40°; wrist neutral with slight ulnar deviation immobilization orthosis • Alternative: elbow flexion restriction orthosis to allow a protected, limited ROM, avoiding full elbow flexion • Alternative: foam on anterior elbow or towel wrap around elbow to prevent elbow flexion at night	• Severe symptoms may require orthosis use during day • Avoid pressure over epicondyles • Posterior orthosis designs should be well padded over cubital tunnel • Restriction orthosis may be used for intermittent symptoms and does not allow elbow flexion beyond 90° • Avoid straps directly over tender or inflamed areas • The orthosis should be worn until symptoms have subsided and should be only part of a comprehensive rehabilitation program

(Continued)

CHAPTER 20

TABLE 20–2	Peripheral Nerve Injury: Orthosis Management and Considerations (Continued)		
Diagnosis	**Therapy Goals**	**Orthosis Guidelines and Recommendations**	**Considerations**
Ulnar tunnel/Guyon canal syndrome	• Decrease stress on the ulnar nerve as it passes through the ulnar tunnel • Protect from direct forces over the pisiform • Avoid provocative activities	• Day and night: immobilization orthosis with wrist 0° to slight flexion; consider padding ulnar/volar wrist area • Alternative: soft neoprene orthosis for work and leisure activities	• Consider applying a silicone gel patch directly over the sensitive area before orthosis fabrication, or use a foam doughnut • The orthosis should be worn until symptoms have subsided and should be only part of a comprehensive rehabilitation program
Combined Median and Ulnar Nerves			
High and low lacerations	• Same goals as listed for each nerve • Maintain three-point pinch	• Week 1 (postsurgery): elbow flexed (high lesion only), wrist flexed, thumb midpalmar and radial abduction immobilization orthosis • Week 3: increase wrist extension in orthosis to tolerance • Weeks 4–5: discontinue elbow for high lesions • Weeks 5–6: discontinue wrist, continue with IF-SF MCP flexion/thumb abduction orthosis for night and at-risk situations only; children and tenuous repairs 1 wk longer; use IF-SF MCP extension restriction orthosis for day, with or without thumb • Week 8: begin gentle mobilization orthosis, if necessary	• Orthosis may be difficult; some patients may benefit from an orthosis that recruits power from the radial nerve • These injuries most often occur in combination with tendon and vascular injury; check with physician for specific protocol • Paramount to maintain PROM of all involved joints
Radial Nerve			
High laceration or compression injury	• Recreate tenodesis action while waiting for nerve return • Prevent overstretching of the wrist, thumb, and digital extensors • Prevent joint contractures (wrist, MCP, and PIP flexion)	• Week 1 (postsurgery): if repair is proximal to the elbow, consider orthosis or casting as follows—elbow flexion/wrist extension/digit and thumb extension immobilization • Weeks 2–3: nonsurgical or compressive injury; use wrist/MCP/thumb extension immobilization orthosis (IPs are free) for day; use wrist extension/MCP flexion/IPs and thumb extension immobilization for night • Alternative: tenodesis orthosis (wrist flex/MCP extension; MCP flex/wrist extension) • Alternative: consider fabricating a wrist immobilization orthosis for work if the tenodesis orthosis is too cumbersome or not appropriate • Alternative: Robinson forearm-based radial nerve glove with wrist (AliMed®) • Alternative: Forearm-based Tunnel Splint* (Benik Corporation) • Alternative: Neoprene custom made (see Chapter 14) • Alternative: LMB™ radial nerve splint with MCP extension	• Avoid pressure over ulnar styloid; consider prepadding • Take care when fitting all the proximal phalanx slings • Check for appropriate tension when fabricating tenodesis orthosis • The orthosis should be worn until symptoms have subsided and should be only part of a comprehensive rehabilitation program • Prolonged orthosis use may contribute to weakened extensors.
Low laceration and posterior interosseous nerve injury	• Recreate tenodesis action while waiting for nerve return • Prevent overstretching of the wrist, thumb, and digital extensors • Prevent joint contractures	• Day: wrist flexion/MCP extension; MCP flexion/wrist extension mobilization orthosis (tenodesis orthosis) • Night: wrist/thumb/digit extension immobilization orthosis • Alternative: hand-based MCP extension mobilization orthosis, with or without thumb extension outrigger • Alternative: Robinson radial nerve glove (AliMed®) • Alternative: Hand-based Tunnel Splint* (Benik Corporation) • Alternative: use of elastic therapeutic taping to assist in digit/thumb extension; can be worn alone or under an orthosis • Alternative: Neoprene custom made (see Chapter 14)	• Take care when fitting all the slings • Avoid pressure over the ulnar styloid; consider prepadding • Check for appropriate tension when fabricating tenodesis orthosis • For hand-based orthosis, avoid MCP irritation • Correct thumb position

TABLE 20–2	Peripheral Nerve Injury: Orthosis Management and Considerations (Continued)		
Diagnosis	**Therapy Goals**	**Orthosis Guidelines and Recommendations**	**Considerations**
Radial tunnel syndrome	• Prevent repetitive resisted supination • Avoid provocative positions • Position the nerve in a resting state	• Day and night: wrist extension (30°–40°), forearm neutral rotation immobilization orthosis	• When in combination with lateral epicondylitis, orthosis the elbow in 60°–90° flexion and the forearm in supination • Avoid strap compression over tender area • The orthosis should be worn until symptoms have subsided and should be only part of a comprehensive rehabilitation program
Superficial radial nerve syndrome, Wartenberg syndrome	• Eliminate irritation of the cutaneous branch of the radial nerve about the radial styloid • Protect the area from direct trauma while healing	• Day and night: radial wrist immobilization orthosis that positions the wrist and thumb column to minimize tension on the radial sensory nerve	• Take care when molding; avoid direct pressure over the radial styloid • For severe irritation, consider lifting the material up by making a doughnut to relieve pressure on the entrapped nerve • Alternative: apply silicone gel or padding over this area before applying the orthosis
Digital Nerves			
Lacerations	• Protect and decrease tension on the surgical repair • Prevent joint MCP, PIP, or DIP contractures • Sensory precautions	• Day and night: hand-based MCP/PIP/DIP extension restriction orthosis (MCP: 45°, PIP: 30°; DIP slight flexion)	• Orthosis position depends greatly on level of digital nerve injury and involvement of other structures (e.g., neurovascular, tendon, ligament). • When orthosis, pay extra attention to the orthosis' borders, making sure they do not dig into insensate areas

The guidelines and recommendations outlined in this chart are not meant to be inclusive of every possible product or management technique; rather, the guidelines are to stimulate thought and provide a foundation to build a treatment plan.
This table is meant as only a guideline for injury management. Keep in mind that other nerve innervations may be present, and the pattern of nerve return is never predictable. This table does not include all possible mixed lesions. Remember that orthosis modifications occur frequently to accommodate motor return. Evaluate for sensory loss and teach patients careful skin inspection.
Data from Colditz, J. C. (1995). Splinting the hand with a peripheral nerve injury. In Hunter J. M., Mackin E. J., & Callahan A. D. (Eds.), Rehabilitation of the hand (4th ed., pp. 679–692). St. Louis, MO: Mosby Year Book; Data from Matloub, H. S., & Yousif, N. J. (1992). Peripheral nerve anatomy and innervation patterns. Hand Clinics, 8, 203–214; Bindra, R. R., & Brininger, T. L. (2010). Advanced concepts in hand pathology and surgery: Application to hand therapy practice (pp. 145–179). Rosemount, IL: ASSH and Elfar, J., Petrungaro, J. M., Braun, R. M., Cheng, C. J., Gupta, R., LaBore, A., & Wong, J. E. (2010). Nerve. In Hammert W. C., Calfee R. P., Bozentka D. J., & Boyer M. I. (Eds.), ASSH manual of hand surgery (pp. 294–342). Philadelphia, PA: Lippincott Williams & Wilkins.

- If patients with nerve injuries must wear an orthosis for function, keep the design simple and low profile. An orthosis that is cumbersome and bulky may interfere with the function of uninvolved joints. Patients are less likely to comply with an orthosis-wearing schedule when the orthosis is big and cumbersome.
- Be aware of the most common distributions of the sensory branches of the three major peripheral nerves in order to appreciate strap placement and orthoses borders and avoid compression of these structures.
- Educate patients regarding their sensory deficits, teaching careful skin examination after fabrication. This will prevent the possibility of excess pressure/friction caused by extended wear of the orthosis (Blackmore & Hotchkiss, 1995; Jacobs, 2003). Meticulous skin inspection after wear is crucial, especially with sensory loss.

prevent skin irritation and maximize the orthosis strength, comfort, and cosmesis. The perforated nature of some materials, although lighter in weight, can be problematic. The holes in the material may cause shear/friction stress against the skin as the patient attempts to move. *If* a perforated material is chosen, patient education regarding diligent and meticulous skin inspection is paramount (Austin, 2003).

Materials that tend to retain heat (during the molding process) may be uncomfortable and even painful for some patients with nerve involvement. Select a material that has a lower heating temperature but can still provide an intimate fit with minimal handling (refer to Chapters 5 and 6) (Austin, 2003). As mentioned throughout this chapter and detailed in Chapter 14, neoprene materials, either alone or in combination with thermoplastics, can provide an alternative for some patients.

MATERIAL SELECTION

Lightweight, contouring, and highly drapable materials may be the most appropriate choice for management of the nerve-injured hand. Many of these injuries have accompanying sensory loss, which limits the patient's ability to detect shear or compressive stress. Great care should be taken to ensure proper length, width, and weight distribution. Corners and borders should be rounded and flared to

COMPONENT SELECTION

The use of components, such as outriggers, slings, and line guides, should be minimized. Every additional component makes the orthosis more complicated to apply and wear. Finger and hand slings should be cautiously applied to the insensate hand. Close attention should be given to avoid creation of shear and/or compression stress under these slings (Austin, 2003). If components are necessary to maintain active function, the therapist must educate the patient, family, and/or caregiver in the correct application and wearing schedule as well as stress the precautions of orthosis wear. The selection of the components should be as low profile as possible. Carefully read instructions for applications and precautions. Commonly, mobilization orthoses are worn for functional day use, complemented by a night immobilization orthosis to prevent joint contractures.

STRAPPING SELECTION

Straps should be conforming and soft. They should be strategically placed to minimize migration and increase comfort. Neoprene and soft straps conform nicely around joints and through web spaces, minimizing skin irritation (Austin, 2003).

OTHER MANAGEMENT OPTIONS

Other options to manage PNIs may include simple taping techniques (see Chapter 13) or the creative use of neoprene (see Chapter 14). These other options can be performed either alone or in combination with thermoplastic material, casting material, or an orthosis that is either prefabricated or custom made as shown in Figures 20–35A,B. A simple "off-the-shelf" orthosis such as a wrist orthosis (sold by many manufacturers) can be a complement to a custom-fabricated program (worn only for certain events/activities), or in some cases can be used alone. For example, a patient may not be able to afford therapy sessions due to copayments/coinsurance/deductibles costs or the patient may object to wearing a custom orthosis; in this case, a cost-effective option to consider is a prefabricated device.

The Robinson InRigger soft leather glove (AliMed Corporation, Inc, Dedham, MA) or the Tunnel Splint® (Benik Corporation, Silverdale, WA) are just a few additional options for management of such nerve injuries. These are both prefabricated, low-profile, glove-like designs (they come with or without the wrist and/or with or without the thumb) that provide some degree of wrist and/or thumb and/or digit extension after active flexion. A few examples of such orthoses are shown in Figures 20–33C,D. These types

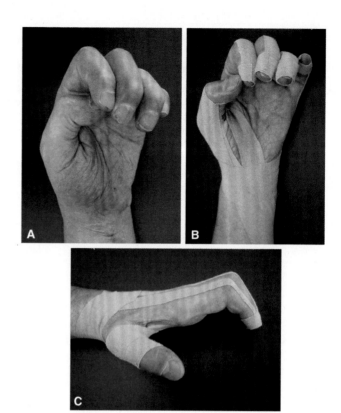

FIGURE 20–42 A, This patient had a traumatic laceration of his median and ulnar nerve as well as all his flexor tendons. Note that he is unable to formulate a productive pinch (thumb to digits) which greatly impairs functional performance. **B and C,** Elastic therapeutic taping is used to facilitate digit extension and thumb opposition. He was a late referral to therapy and had developed PIP flexion contractures. With this taping technique, he is able to laterally oppose his index finger. Note the hypothenar atrophy.

of gloves can be used to manage PIN injury, radial nerve injury, combined PNIs, distal pathology from a brachial plexus lesion, and distal nerve degeneration from a chronic neuromuscular disease. Reference to Chapter 9 is encouraged for a more thorough description of the available prefabricated options. Chapter 14 reviews the use of neoprene for the creative modification of prefabricated orthoses as well as using neoprene (and a combination of other materials) to fabricate "soft" low-profile options for this population.

Elastic therapeutic taping (such as Kinesio® Tape, Balance Tex™ tape, SpiderTech™ Tape, Dynamic Tape®) can be used to help position and increase the function of the hand. For example, the thumb can be taped in abduction and opposition after a median nerve injury. A figure-of-8 design around the proximal phalanx can enhance tip pinch during wrist extension (Figs. 20–41 and 20–42A–C). Chapter 13 provides additional information and techniques for the use of elastic therapeutic taping.

CONCLUSION

This chapter has focused on the role of the orthosis in various conditions of nerve injury and/or repair. With the information in this chapter, the reader should appreciate the importance of orthotic intervention in this patient population. Not only is the orthosis used to protect the body part after injury and/or surgical repair, but it also can play a critical role in granting functional independence. The future for the surgeon and clinician managing the nerve-injured hand is exciting. Early referral to a "nerve" specialist combined with developments in surgical techniques and procedures, innovative motor and sensory nerve grafting and transfers, and the skilled intervention of a hand therapist foster improved functional outcomes for this challenging patient population.

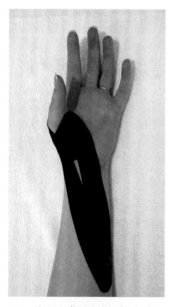

FIGURE 20–41 For a returning median nerve, elastic therapeutic tape is used to position the thumb gently in palmar abduction and opposition. As the wrist is extended, the thumb is carried farther into opposition and abduction, providing the capacity for light tip pinch. This taping technique can be used in conjunction with other orthosis interventions.

FIELD NOTE: LOW-PROFILE RADIAL NERVE ORTHOSIS

By Jeanine Beasley, EdD, OTR, CHT, FAOTA
Michigan

A radial nerve injury can limit the ability to complete active wrist, digit, and thumb extension as well as thumb radial abduction.[1,2,3] This injury can take months of recovery especially if a result of a mid-humeral fracture.[3] A radial nerve orthosis can be helpful in providing this extension while awaiting motor return.[5,6] A low-profile orthosis is often preferred by patients as they complete daily grasp and release activities.[5,7,8] Originally designed by Sally Fistler-DeSilva, OTR, CHT, and presented as a poster at the 1998 meeting of ASHT, the orthosis is economical and easy to fabricate.[4] This orthosis utilizes elastic Velcro and elastic thread instead of rubber bands to provide the extension to the digits. Two holes are punched in the orthosis between each digit. Elastic thread is inserted and tied into these holes to support the elastic Velcro making a dynamic sling supporting each digit. Elastic Velcro on the thumb provides the needed thumb extension. A dorsal cut out for the metacarpal heads allows a slight tenodesis grasp and release and avoids pressure at the metacarpal heads during digit flexion. The dorsal ulnar head is cut out to avoid any pressure to this area. Using a thumb spica precut for this orthosis reduces fabrication time. The precut is applied dorsally and the thumb post is trimmed to allow full thumb flexion. Antidotally observed in the clinic, this orthosis has had a high patient acceptance and utilization. Once fabricated, the patient reports immediate increase in use of the hand for daily activities.

References

Colditz, J. C. (1987). Splinting for Radial Nerve Palsy. *Journal of Hand Therapy*, 1, 18–23.

Colditz, J. C. (2002). Splinting the hand with a peripheral-nerve injury. In Mackin E. J., Callahan A. D., Skirven T. M., Schneider L. H., Osterman A. L., (Eds.), *Rehabilitation of the hand and upper extremity* (5th ed., Vol. 2, pp. 1875–1888). St. Louis, MO: Mosby, Inc.

Duff, S.V., Estilow, T. (2011). Therapist's management of peripheral nerve injury. In Skirven T. M., Osterman A. L., Fedorczyk J. M., Amadio P. C., (Eds.), *Rehabilitation of the hand and upper extremity* (6th ed., Vol. 1, pp. 619–633) Philadelphia, PA: Elsevier Mosby.

Fistler-DeSilva, S. (1998). *Dorsal Dynamic Radial Nerve Palsy Splint, ASHT Program 1998 Annual Meeting*, New Orleans Poster 205

Hannah, S. D., Hudak, P.L. (2001). Splinting and radial nerve palsy: a single-subject experiment. *Journal of Hand Therapy*, 14:195–201.

Ingari, J. V, Green, D. P. (2011). Radial nerve palsy. In Wolfe S. W., Hotchkiss R. N., Pederson W. C., Kozin S. H., (Eds.), *Green's operative hand surgery* (6th ed., pp. 1075–1092). Philadelphia, PA: Churchill Livingstone Elsevier.

McKee, P., Nguyen, C. (2007) Low-profile dorsal dynamic wrist-finger-thumb assistive-extension orthosis for high radial nerve injury – Fabrication instructions. *Journal of Hand Therapy*, 20(1), 70–72.

Peck, J., Ollason, J. (2015) Low profile radial nerve palsy orthosis with radial and ulnar deviation. *Journal of Hand Therapy*, 28(4), 421–424.

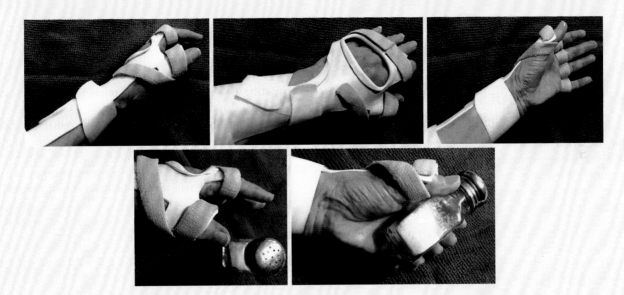

Case Study Section

The case studies presented here are meant as a teaching guideline only. Treatment and orthosis protocols vary greatly from surgeon to surgeon and from therapist to therapist. The therapist should check with the referring physicians and colleagues to define the preferred treatment and appropriate orthotic intervention.

Case Study 1: High-Level Radial Nerve Injury

GH is a 39-year-old, right-dominant female who sustained a right midhumeral fracture, right distal radius fracture, and radial nerve injury during a hit-and-run accident. In the emergency room, she was placed in a long arm cast with her elbow at 90°, forearm pronated, wrist in slight flexion, and digits left free. Because of the edema in her hand and digits and her inability to extend her digits, she was referred to hand therapy with a question of radial nerve injury.

Upon clinical examination, it was noted that she did indeed have symptoms consistent with radial nerve compression or injury. GH was unable to extend her digits or thumb actively within the cast. Therefore, an MCP extension mobilization orthosis was fabricated to fit directly over the cast. This allowed the patient to use her digits purposefully and prevent overstretching of the digit and thumb extensors.

The cast was removed 6 weeks later. Upon examination, GH demonstrated weak triceps function and no active wrist, digit, or thumb extension. She had impaired sensibility over the dorsoradial aspect of her forearm. She required continued orthosis intervention to substitute for loss of muscle function. A wrist flexion/MCP extension, wrist extension/MCP flexion orthosis was chosen (radial nerve orthosis). This design allowed the patient to take advantage of the natural tenodesis effect of the digits with wrist movement. When the wrist extends, the digits flex; when the wrist flexes, the digits extend (Fig. 20–33A,B). This orthosis design allows full use of the palmar surface of the hand and is light in weight. GH continued with the orthosis for approximately 6 weeks. At night, she wore a simple wrist/hand/thumb immobilization orthosis (Fig. 20–34A,B), which she found did not disrupt her sleep. In therapy, the patient worked on regaining wrist motion and strength.

When her wrist extensors were strong enough to support themselves against gravity, she was placed in a hand-based MCP/thumb extension mobilization orthosis (Fig. 20–36B,C) while waiting for the return of the distal motor branch of the PIN. GH wore the orthosis for activities of daily living (ADLs) and work-related tasks. Compliance with wearing the orthosis was not an issue because of its low-profile design. She was able to take it off with increased frequency while waiting return of nerve function, which took an additional 5 weeks. Eventually, she discarded all orthoses and worked on a general strengthening program.

Additional case studies can be found on the companion web site on thePoint.

Case Study 2: Median Nerve Compression (Carpal Tunnel Syndrome)

In her fifth month of pregnancy, NA began having numbness and tingling in the median nerve distribution of her hands bilaterally. She was experiencing nighttime symptoms that were so severe that she woke up several times during the night. She was experiencing pain and paresthesias during the day while driving, holding a book to read, pushing a grocery cart, and even putting on jewelry. She was referred by her primary care physician to therapy with a diagnosis of carpal tunnel syndrome.

Upon evaluation, NA had an acutely positive Phalen test and thenar weakness bilaterally. She was placed into bilateral wrist immobilization orthoses that held the wrists in neutral. In this position, compression of the median nerve is significantly decreased (Fig. 20–18). The orthoses also kept her from placing her wrists in provocative positions. She was instructed to wear the orthoses at all times initially, taking them off for hygiene purposes only. As her symptoms subsided, orthosis use was decreased to nighttime only.

The therapist taught NA about carpal tunnel syndrome and how to avoid activities and static postures that could irritate the nerve. The patient had great relief of symptoms with the use of the orthoses and nerve-gliding exercises and continued the nighttime regime throughout the remainder of her pregnancy.

CHAPTER REVIEW QUESTIONS

1. Name the three main peripheral nerves of the upper extremity, describing the motor and sensory function of each.
2. What are the general principles in managing a peripheral nerve injury? What are the unique roles of immobilization, mobilization, and restriction orthoses in this patient population?
3. Describe the conservative management for a compression injury of the median nerve.
4. Describe the injury associated with a high radial nerve laceration and what distal orthotic intervention(s) a therapist can provide to allow for some functional use.
5. Not initially prominent, in a high ulnar nerve injury, what must a therapist be concerned with? What interventions should a therapist consider?

21 Tendon and Nerve Transfers

Lorna Canavan Kahn, PT, CHT
Macy Miller Stonner, OTD, OTR/L
Anna VanVoorhis Miller, MS, OTR/L, CHT

CHAPTER OBJECTIVES

After study of this chapter, the reader should be able to:
- Identify common nerve and tendon transfers and their role in restoring upper extremity function.
- Describe the key principles that guide rehabilitation following nerve and tendon transfer surgeries.
- Understand the role of orthotic intervention following nerve and tendon transfers.
- Identify appropriate postoperative orthoses that correspond with specific peripheral nerve reconstruction.
- Define the timeframe of nerve recovery and how that influences the rehabilitation process.

KEY TERMS

Donor activation focused rehabilitation approach
Donor muscle

Free functional muscle transfers
Motor reeducation
Nerve transfers

Recipient muscle-tendon unit
Tendon transfers

MD NOTE

Susan E. Mackinnon, MD
Missouri

Speaking as a surgeon who has worked with skilled hand therapists for my entire career, it would be hard to overstate the importance of hand therapy in the realm of nerve and tendon transfers. Nerve and tendon transfers are complex procedures used among peripheral nerve and spinal cord injuries that require a team effort to maximize outcomes. I believe the hand therapist plays an important role in both pre- and postoperative phases. Their evaluation skills contribute valuable clinical information to the surgical decision-making process. I strongly rely on the hand therapist from their muscle testing skills to their perspective on functional adaption. Following nerve and tendon transfers, the therapist on my team manages the patients' recovery with respect to timing of orthotic needs, progression of motor reeducation, and preparation for return to work. Over the past few decades, I have learned that the functional outcomes following nerve reconstruction are dependent on the expertise of the therapist. Most certainly I have seen this with nerve transfers. Interdisciplinary collaboration has significantly augmented the results of such nerve transfer surgeries. Patients are experiencing earlier motor recovery as the therapists initiate comprehensive motor reeducation almost immediately following these transfers. Simply put, you cannot do nerve or tendon transfers without a skilled surgeon to perform the surgery, nor without a hand therapist to truly optimize results from that surgery.

FAQ

I have seen both one- and two-part orthosis designs used with tendon transfers for the hand that involve proximal donor muscles such as brachioradialis and pronator teres that cross the elbow joint. How do you decide which design is preferable?

The authors prefer the two-part orthosis; one part that immobilizes the hand and wrist and the other to immobilize the forearm and elbow. This design simplifies the fabrication of the orthosis that is often challenging as one must control and position the multiple involved joints.

In addition, the proximal donor muscles do not need to be immobilized the full 4 weeks. Making the orthosis in two parts enables the patient to independently remove the proximal component after 2 weeks. This limits elbow joint stiffness and eliminates the need for an additional hand therapy visit to cut back the proximal portion if it was fabricated as one unit (Mackinnon & Nakao, 1997).

If I am referred a patient with multiple nerve and tendon transfers, how do I prioritize positioning for their postoperative orthosis?

A nerve transfer should be considered a nerve repair, needing to be kept "quiet" for the first 2 to 3 weeks whereas a tendon transfer needs complete immobilization from movement of the involved tendons for 3 to 4 weeks. Develop your orthosis plan based on the need of the tendon transfer. You never want the tendon transfer to be put in a position that stretches the repair. If there are multiple tendon transfers you may need to be creative to achieve protection of all involved structures. Generally, this will involve limited movement of the limb, thus protecting the nerve transfer as well. Nerve transfers are performed with the nerve on slack making it easier to accommodate.

Following a tendon transfer how long should I encourage the patient to wear the orthosis during the exercise phase?

After the immobilization phase, the patient should be instructed in motor reeducation exercises and advised to remove the orthosis throughout the day for exercise. During this training phase, the patient may be weaned gradually from immobilization, but the timing for weaning is patient dependent. Some patients struggle to control the tendon transfer. In this situation, longer protection may be needed to avoid stretching out the transfer. For example, a patient with radial tendon transfers for wrist extension (PT to ECRB) may wear a prefabricated wrist immobilization orthosis while performing resisted forearm pronation exercises with a hammer to protect the repair and encourage greater response from the donor, pronator muscle. In between exercise sessions, he would return to his MCP and wrist extension orthosis until he is able to control extension against gravity.

INTRODUCTION

Peripheral nerve injuries (PNIs) in the upper extremity often lead to devastating functional loss. The initial goal of surgical intervention is to repair the nerve. Long considered the gold standard, direct repairs yield excellent results when conditions are ideal, but in reality, they are often impossible, too risky, or too far from the target end organ (muscle). These cases typically have a poor prognosis for functional recovery. Because of this, **tendon transfers** were developed to aid in the restoration of hand function in soldiers returning home from World War-I and -II (WWI and WWII) who had sustained PNIs. Many of these transfers are still performed today because they have been proven a reliable and effective form of reconstruction.

In the latter part of the 20th century, advancements in microsurgical techniques and a deeper understanding of the internal topography of peripheral nerves led to an interest in **nerve transfers** as a surgical reconstruction option for patients with PNI. Early nerve transfers offered promising results for the restoration of elbow flexion, which led to the development of nerve transfers in the forearm and hand to restore wrist and fine motor function. This chapter will address the role of orthoses in postoperative hand therapy for the more common tendon and nerve transfer surgeries.

TENDON TRANSFERS

Patients may undergo tendon transfers to regain motion of a weak or absent muscle in which peripheral nerve function has not been restored within a reasonable period of time (Bednar, Judson, & von der Hyde, 2010; Jones, 1994). The surgery involves rerouting a functional muscle-tendon unit to an injured or denervated muscle-tendon unit in order to restore balance to a joint or limb. The tendon of a functional muscle is detached distally at its insertion, mobilized, rerouted, and resutured to the tendon of a nonfunctional muscle or into a bony insertion (Bednar et al., 2010; Brand, 1995; Hammert et al., 2010; Jones, 1994).

This chapter focuses on common tendon transfers related to specific PNI of the median, ulnar, and radial nerves. Tendon transfers can be performed for similar deficits in patients with injuries such as spinal cord injury, stroke, traumatic brain injury, cerebral palsy, and brachial plexus lesions, in which the therapeutic and orthotic intervention may have a similar postoperative course. Refer to the

Suggested Reading list at the end of this chapter for a more in-depth review of such transfers and a detailed discussion of appropriate orthotic interventions that are outside the scope of this chapter.

Tendons are transferred and repaired with a distinct degree of tension, and the postoperative orthotic program should adequately protect the surgical reconstruction during the healing period (Barbis & Wallace, 1995; Blackmore & Hotchkiss, 1995; Brand, 1995; Chan, Jaglowski, & Kaplan, 1994; Colditz, 1995; Elvey, 1997; Hunter & Whitenack, 1995; Jones, 1994; Lowe & O'Toole, 1995; Smith, 1987). The postoperative orthosis should avoid tension on the surgically transferred muscle(s) by placing the joint that the transferred muscle-tendon unit crosses in a shortened position to allow rest (Bednar et al., 2010). It is also important that the orthosis positions the joint(s) in a manner that protects the proper direction of the transferred tendon's pull. For example, when an opponensplasty has been performed using a slip of the ring finger flexor digitorum superficialis (FDS) tendon guided through a flexor carpi ulnaris (FCU) pulley, the orthosis should hold the thumb in palmar abduction/opposition with the wrist in neutral to slight flexion and ulnar deviation. It is imperative that patients receive extensive education regarding the importance of compliance with full-time orthosis wear for the initial 4 weeks following tendon transfer surgery (Seiler, Desai, & Payne, 2013) to prevent stress to the repair site and avoid overstretching the tendon. Patients' understanding of the anatomy involved may increase compliance, avoid rupture, and improve functional outcome (Megerle, Przybilski, Sauerbier, Germann, & Giessler, 2008).

The therapist should review the exact reconstruction performed with the referring surgeon before treating the patient. With strong surgeon-therapist communication, a clear picture can be established regarding the muscle-tendon unit to be used, the function to be restored, and the appropriate orthosis design (e.g., dorsal vs. volar design, joint angle, etc). This information will guide the therapist in thorough patient education, proper orthosis fabrication, and optimal therapeutic intervention. The following orthosis recommendations are presented as general guidelines. Again, it is the therapist's responsibility to review the details of the tendon transfer prior to fabrication of the orthosis. Each patient must be evaluated and immobilized or mobilized according to his or her needs and in accordance with the surgeon's guidelines. Table 21–1 summarizes orthosis management for common tendon transfers.

TABLE 21–1 Common Tendon Transfers

RADIAL NERVE TENDON TRANSFERS

Functional Deficit	Common Tendon Transfer	Orthosis Description	Instructions and/or Image
Wrist extension (ECRB, ECRL, ECU)	PT to ECRB	Two-part orthosis: 1. Wrist in 35°–40° extension 2. Long arm posterior orthosis in 90° elbow flexion with forearm in full pronation molded over wrist orthosis	Discontinue long arm component after 2 wk of protection *
MCP joint extension of digits 2–5 (EDC)	FCR to EDC Other: • FCU to EDC • FDS (ring or middle) to EDC	MCP extension orthosis with wrist in slight extension, MCP joints in full extension, IP joints free	**
Thumb extension (EPL)	PL to EPL Other: • FDS (ring) to EPL	Thumb in radial abduction with MCP and IP joint in full extension	***

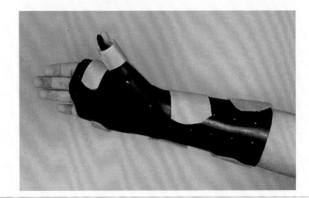

It is common for all three of the above procedures to be performed at the same time. The orthosis therefore reflects the elbow, wrist, finger, and thumb components together.
*If only wrist extension is restored, the thumb and finger components are not included.
**If only finger extension is restored, the thumb component is not included.
***If only thumb extension is restored, the finger component is not included.

(Continued)

TABLE 21–1	**Common Tendon Transfers** (Continued)		

ULNAR NERVE TENDON TRANSFERS

Functional Deficit	Common Tendon Transfer	Orthosis Description	Instructions and/or Image
High Ulnar Nerve Injury			
Ring and small finger DIP flexion (FDP)	Profundus tenodesis: side-to-side suturing of median FDP to ulnar FDP *Other:* • ECRL to FDP	Forearm-based extension restriction orthosis with wrist neutral, MCP joints in 50° flexion, and IP joints in slight flexion	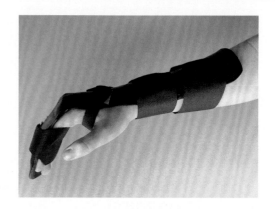
Low Ulnar Nerve Injury			
Ring and small finger MCP flexion and IP extension (lumbricals)	ECRL/B (with PL tendon graft) to lateral bands of ring and small *Other:* • FDS (middle) to lateral bands of ring and small • FDS (middle or index) to pulleys of ring and small	Forearm-based intrinsic plus with wrist slightly extended, MCP joints in 60°–70° flexion (or maximal available), and IP joints in extension Include a dorsal clamshell component to maintain MCP flexion and prevent clawing	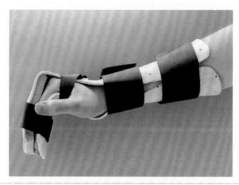
Power pinch Thumb adduction (adductor pollicis, AP) Index finger abduction (first dorsal interosseous)	ECRB to AP *Other:* • EIP to AP • FDS (ring) to AP • APL to first dorsal interosseous	Forearm-based orthosis with thumb in full adduction and wrist in 15°–30° extension	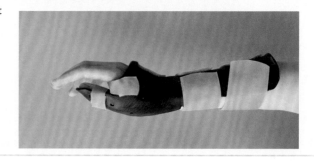

TABLE 21–1	**Common Tendon Transfers**	(Continued)	
MEDIAN NERVE TENDON TRANSFERS			
Functional Deficit	**Common Tendon Transfer**	**Orthosis Description**	**Instructions and/or Image**
High Median Nerve Injury			
Thumb IP joint flexion: FPL	BR to FPL *Other:* • ECRL to FPL • Split FPL to EPL	Two-part orthosis: 1. Forearm-based extension restriction orthosis with wrist in 15° flexion, thumb in palmar abduction, MCP and IP joints in 20° of flexion, fingers free 2. Long arm posterior orthosis in 90° elbow flexion with forearm in neutral rotation molded over dorsal block	Discontinue long arm component after 2 wk of protection. 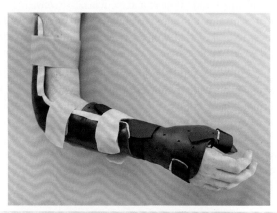
Index and middle finger flexion: FDS and FDP	Profundus tenodesis: side-to-side suturing of ulnar FDP to median FDP *Other:* • ECRL to FDP	Forearm-based extension restriction orthosis with wrist neutral, MCP joints in 50° flexion, and IP joints in slight flexion	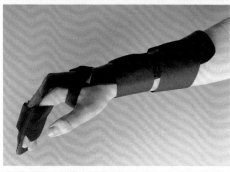
Low Median Nerve Injury			
Thumb opposition and palmar abduction: OP and APB	EIP to APB *Other:* • PL to APB • FDS ring to APB • ADM to APB • EDM to APB	Forearm-based extension restriction with wrist in 0°–30° flexion, thumb in full palmar abduction, slight CMC and MCP flexion, and fingers free Wrist position varies based on donor source (flexor or extensor)	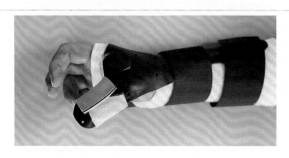

ADM, *abductor digiti minimi;* AIN, *anterior interosseous nerve;* AP, *adductor pollicis;* APB, *abductor pollicis brevis;* APL, *abductor pollicis longus;* BR, *brachioradialis;* ECRB, *extensor carpi radialis brevis;* ECU, *extensor carpi ulnaris;* EDC, *extensor digitorum communis;* EDM, *extensor digiti minimi;* EPB, *extensor pollicis brevis;* EPL, *extensor pollicis longus;* FCR, *flexor carpi radialis;* FDP, *flexor digitorum profundus;* FDS, *flexor digitorum superficialis;* FPL, *flexor pollicis longus;* OP, *opponens pollicis;* PIN, *posterior interosseous nerve;* PL, *palmaris longus;* PQ, *pronator quadratus;* PT, *pronator teres.*

SELECTION OF TENDON TRANSFERS

A team approach should guide the decision-making algorithm prior to tendon transfer surgery. The surgeon, patient, and therapist should collaborate when prioritizing the function to be restored and the adequacy of potential donor muscle(s). The selection process includes (1) analysis of the current and anticipated strength of a **donor muscle** after the transfer, (2) potential muscle-tendon excursion, (3) number of joints the transfer must cross, (4) direction of pull, and (5) effect of the transfer on the remaining muscle-tendon units in the extremity (Bednar et al., 2010; Brand, 1995; Colditz, 1995; Jones, 1994; Mackinnon, 1994; Smith, 1987).

PREOPERATIVE CONSIDERATIONS

In the upper extremity, the best functional results occur when (1) involved joints have full passive motion, (2) edema has subsided and scars have matured, and (3) ulnar and median nerve sensation is at least partially present, although some patients seem to do quite well despite sensory loss (Novak, 2011). Considering this, the following should be addressed with the patient/family prior to surgical intervention:

- Prevent or correct substitution patterns from developing or progressing while awaiting transfer by providing preoperative therapy and orthosis fabrication to encourage the natural use of the hand.
- Achieve and maintain full passive ROM of all involved joints (with or without the use of orthoses).
- Elongate the involved skin, soft tissue adhesions, and joint contractures when present (Brand, 1995; Colditz, 1995; Jones, 1994; Walsh, 2012).
- Strive to achieve maximal strength (4+) of the donor muscle(s) considered for transfer (Bednar et al., 2010; Brand, 1995; Elfar et al., 2010).
- Educate patient regarding therapy timeline, precautions, and the importance of orthosis compliance (Duff & Humpl, 2011).
- Set expectations for postoperative function.
- Consider patient ability (cognitive, psychosocial, financial, etc.) to participate in appropriate postoperative care.

POSTOPERATIVE CONSIDERATIONS

In order to ensure optimal outcomes following tendon transfer surgery, the following should guide the clinician's decision-making process during the **first** postoperative visit:

- Position the orthosis so that the joint angle(s) mimic the desired action of the **recipient muscle/tendon**.
- Consider patient age prior to immobilization. Children are more likely to be noncompliant with removable orthoses, which may jeopardize the surgical reconstruction. They tend to do well with the use of a cast for the required healing time.
- Consider cognitive and/or psychological deficits regarding immobilization options. Patients with impaired memory or inability to follow instructions may benefit from cast immobilization and/or a longer duration of immobilization (Duff & Humpl, 2011).
- Communicate with the corresponding surgeon to confirm the appropriate therapy plan regarding factors such as tendon quality, strength of transfer, and intraoperative findings.
- Inspect all orthoses for possible areas of compression. Sensation is often impaired, and it is the therapist's responsibility to teach the patient vigilant skin inspection.

ROLE OF ORTHOSES

There is no defined joint position described in the literature for each postoperative orthosis following tendon transfers. Guidelines are based on principles of tissue healing, which drive the treatment plan. The goal should be to protect the transferred tendon yet avoid secondary tissue restrictions. The custom orthosis must position the joint(s) properly by placing the recipient tendon in a shortened position to avoid tension at the coaptation site. Failing to position the orthosis in this manner may cause attenuation, rupture, or gap at the suture site. Conversely, an orthosis that places the transfer in an overly short position may cause excessive tightness, tissue contracture, edema, and/or nerve compression. For example, following tendon transfers to restore extensor carpi radialis brevis and longus (ECRB/L) function, the orthosis should be fabricated so that wrist extension does not exceed 45° (Neumann, 2013; Strickland & Kleinman, 1998).

The design of the orthosis should allow early motion of the uninvolved joints. Orthoses are generally worn for 3 to 4 weeks before active motion of the involved joint(s) is initiated. The postoperative exercise regimen is dependent on the surgeon's preference, strength of the transfer, and any other factors that may influence early motion. The use of a protective orthosis continues for an additional 3 to 6 weeks during at-risk activities and while sleeping. The extent of use should be based on the individual patient status. Patients who exhibit excessive tightness may need less time, and those who struggle to hold the expected position may need more time.

As the patient progresses, exercise orthoses are helpful to strengthen the transferred muscle. For example, exercising with a thumb interphalangeal (IP) immobilization orthosis after an opponensplasty can (1) block the strong extrinsic flexor pollicis longus (FPL) tendon from overpowering the weak, newly transferred tendon, (2) retrain the transferred muscle-tendon unit (cortical reorganization) to perform its new function, (3) minimize adhesion formation (Fig. 21–1). Orthoses used to augment motor reeducation can be fabricated out of lightweight material (including nonthermoplastic material) and used for a home program. For example, an anticlaw orthosis may prevent the extensor digitorum communis (EDC) from overpowering weak intrinsics following an ECRL to lateral bands tendon transfer (Fig. 21–2). Taping and strapping techniques may be used to facilitate appropriate movement, such as thumb palmar abduction and opposition (Walsh, 2012) (Fig. 21–3).

Daytime orthoses are generally discontinued at 6 weeks for flexor tendons and approximately 8 weeks for extensor tendons. Extensor tendons are generally weaker than flexor tendons and are therefore held in a protected position for a longer duration (Bednar et al., 2010; Smith, 1987; Stanley-Goodwyn, 1995). Night orthotic management may continue as long as necessary to address potential contractures and/or tension-related complications (Bednar et al., 2010).

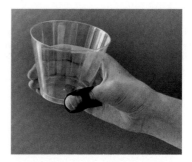

FIGURE 21–1 An interphalangeal (IP) immobilization orthosis may be used during tendon transfer training following an opponensplasty to discourage IP joint flexion (flexor pollicis longus [FPL] substitution).

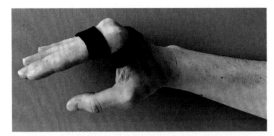

FIGURE 21-2 A four-digit metacarpophalangeal (MCP) extension restriction orthosis (also referred to as an anticlaw orthosis) may be used to limit extensor digitorum communis (EDC) substitution during training following extensor carpi radialis longus (ECRL) to lateral bands tendon transfer (or other anticlaw procedures).

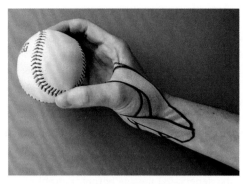

FIGURE 21-3 Taping the thumb into palmar abduction aids in functional reeducation to limit the faulty movement pattern of thumb carpometacarpal (CMC) extension following opponensplasty.

After 8 to 12 weeks, structures that have become excessively tight may require stretch or passive exercise. Uninvolved structures can be stretched early but stretching involved/transferred tendons should not be initiated until 12 weeks, if at all, and should be discussed with the referring surgeon. If tissue restrictions persist, mobilization orthoses may be used to gently stretch tight structures, such as tight intrinsic muscles after an extensor tendon transfer. However, with early intervention and careful progression, the implementation of mobilization orthoses to stretch transferred tendons should be limited.

 CLINICAL PEARL 21-1

Orthosis to Facilitate Movement

Individually designed exercise orthoses can be useful as the patient progresses in order to help strengthen a transferred muscle. Guarded active exercise should begin only under the supervision of a hand therapist. As shown in these images, a small thumb IP immobilization orthosis is fabricated specifically to isolate palmar adduction and opposition after an opponensplasty. The orthosis can be used alone and, as the patient progresses, used for active resistive exercises. The material shown here is QuickCast2, Performance Health.

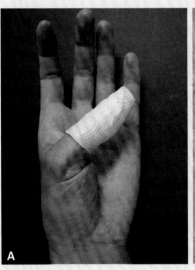 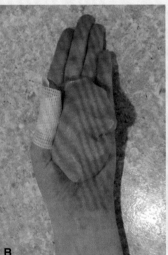 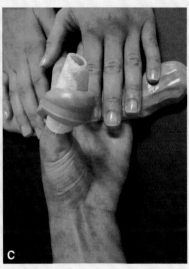

NERVE TRANSFERS

A nerve transfer is a surgical technique that is performed to reinnervate a denervated muscle where primary nerve repair is unachievable, inaccessible, or incomplete. Redundant motor nerve fascicles are cut distally from the donor muscle, rerouted, and attached to the recipient nerve. Once the nerve grows across the coaptation site and along the new pathway, the denervated muscle will ultimately become reinnervated by the donor nerve. Nerve transfers have demonstrated utility in restoration of function in many muscles in the upper extremity (Bertelli & Ghizoni, 2014; Garcia-Lopez, Martinez, & Rojas, 2014; Mackinnon, Novak, Myckatyn, & Tung, 2005; Ray, Chang, Hawasli, Wilson, & Yang, 2015).

ADVANTAGES OF NERVE TRANSFERS

Several of the potential advantages of nerve transfers include

- Avoidance of muscle or tendon repair, thus limiting the need for sustained protective postoperative immobilization
- Reinnervation of multiple muscles with a single transfer
- Restoration of both motor and sensory function
- Return of motor function in nerves in which the cell body has been injured (no available healthy proximal nerve)
- Restoration of isolated fine motor control and dexterity currently not achievable through tendon transfers

(Dy & Mackinnon, 2016; Ferrante & Wilbourn, 2015; Novak, 2015; Ray & Mackinnon, 2011; Weber & Davidge, 2015; Wood, Johnson, & Myckatyn, 2015)

CHALLENGES OF NERVE TRANSFERS

One of the great challenges to reconstructive surgery involving injured motor nerves is time. Long periods of denervation lead to atrophy of the affected muscle (Weng, Zhang, Yin, & Jiang, 2018). Following an axonometric nerve injury, a metaphorical clock starts "ticking" with respect to the longevity of muscle integrity (Ma et al., 2011). While the exact timeframe for irreversible atrophy in humans is unknown, it is generally believed that by 12 months the denervated muscle has little chance to recover function (Davidge & Fox, 2015; Weber & Davidge, 2015). The goal of a nerve transfer is to rescue the denervated muscle before it atrophies to the irreparable point of fatty infiltration. A surgical timeframe of 6 months or fewer following nerve injury is considered ideal (Coulet, Allieu, & Chammas, 2002).

The timeframe for functional recovery is much longer compared to tendon transfers because the transferred nerve will take several months to grow to the new target recipient muscle. Once reinnervation begins, the muscle will recover function gradually as it ascends the manual muscle testing (MMT) scale from trace (1/5) to active movement against gravity (>3/5). Functional strength outcomes will vary significantly for nerve transfers. The double fascicular nerve transfer for elbow flexion has been reported to recover *up to* 4+/5 MMT strength (Mackinnon et al., 2005). This variability in outcome depends on the quality of the donor and recipient nerves, timing of the transfer, and age of the patient.

DIFFERENCE BETWEEN TENDON AND NERVE TRANSFERS

When considering options for surgical reconstruction, the crucial differences between tendon and nerve transfers should be made clear. Tendon transfers may be performed at any point in time following injury and may recover motor function in 2 to 3 months. Nerve transfers, on the other hand, are limited by the time constraints of atrophying denervated muscle and must be performed within a year after injury. Among individuals with spinal cord injuries, the time constraints vary for nerve transfers. In this population, the cell body of the nerve is often intact with the injury occurring in the central nervous system (Davidge et al., 2014; Van Heest, 2005). When this is the case, nerve transfers maybe an option for years following injury with the primary limiting factor being the limited number of healthy, redundant donor muscles/nerves (Fox, 2016). While there is potential for greater functional recovery with the nerve transfer, it may take over a year to achieve.

SUCCESSFUL MOTOR REEDUCATION—NERVE TRANSFERS

Critical components to successful motor reeducation following nerve transfers include an understanding of the involved anatomy and an appreciation for the role of cortical plasticity and motor relearning strategies in the recovery process (Novak, 2008). The DAFRA (donor activation focused rehabilitation approach) model emphasizes the importance of the donor muscle's role in the relearning process. The key components include limb preparation, early patient education defining the donor and recipient muscles, instruction in donor muscle activation and combined donor and recipient muscle exercises, exercise instruction that is appropriate to the level of motor recovery, and setting realistic expectations for the patient (Kahn & Moore, 2016).

ROLE OF ORTHOSES

The role of orthoses in postoperative management of nerve transfers is relatively new. While protection of the repair site is standard, the use of orthoses beyond the initial postoperative period is developing conceptually as our understanding of nerve transfer recovery expands.

The objectives for orthosis use following nerve transfer are to (1) protect the repair site immediately following surgery, (2) limit substitution patterns during exercise (pre- and postoperatively), (3) protect the recipient muscle length, and (4) augment motor reeducation by supporting recipient recovery while challenging the donor muscle.

POSTOPERATIVE CONSIDERATIONS

Immediately following surgery there is an initial rest period similar to any nerve repair. About 2 to 3 weeks is common, although this may vary by surgeon preference. Once the protective phase is complete, the focus shifts to the maintenance of muscle length during the protracted motor recovery phase. As demonstrated in the length-tension curve, first described by Ramsey and Street in 1940, a muscle that is too long or too short has limited tension capabilities (Gordon, Huxley, & Julian, 1966; Ma et al., 2011). Supporting the denervated muscle in a functional position will enable it to develop greater contractile strength once it is reinnervated. We recommend supporting the muscle until it can resist antigravity positions and maintain the functional length independently. A classic example would be the patient with a posterior interosseous nerve (PIN) palsy. A common nerve transfer option is median (branch to flexor carpi radialis [FCR]) to radial/PIN. A trace contraction of the EDC muscle may be noted at 6 months, but active extension of the metacarpophalangeal (MCP) joints may not be regained until 12 months postoperatively. During this time, one should protect the length of the EDC and encourage functional use without substitution patterns by fitting the patient with a forearm- or hand-based MCP extension orthosis. An MCP immobilization orthosis may be used at night to maintain length, whereas a functional MCP extension orthosis is encouraged during the day (dynamic or low-profile neoprene) (refer to Chapter 14, Neoprene ideas on custom neoprene designs). These can be custom made, but many patients find the prefabricated option such as the Benik™ to be more comfortable and aesthetically pleasing. Refer to Table 21–2 which offers alternatives for orthosis intervention for common transfers.

Role of orthoses is to aid in motor reeducation. Motor reeducation relies heavily on early donor activation with repetitive combined motions of resisted donor with assisted recipient muscles. Cortical plasticity plays a large role in the rehabilitation process as the brain must relearn how to engage the donor muscle in order to activate the newly reinnervated recipient muscle. In the case of tendon transfers, the recipient muscle is able to move actively within 4 weeks of surgery. With nerve transfers, however, there will generally be no response in the recipient muscle for at least 4 to 6 months, depending on the transfer. Because of this protracted period of time, there is often an issue with motor memory loss. In these situations, an orthosis may augment motor reeducation by isolating recipient recovery while challenging the donor muscle. Ideally, such an exercise orthosis would provide assistance to the recovering denervated muscle while applying resistance to the donor muscle (refer to Table 21–2, second-to-last row).

TABLE 21–2	Common Nerve Transfers		
Functional Loss	**Common Nerve Transfer**	**Protective Phase Orthosis**	**Exercise Orthosis (optional)**	**Functional Orthosis (optional)**

ULNAR NERVE

Digit ab/adduction (interossei)	AIN (pronated quadratus branch) to deep motor branch of ulnar nerve	Wrist neutral orthosis Prefabricated orthosis is typically sufficient 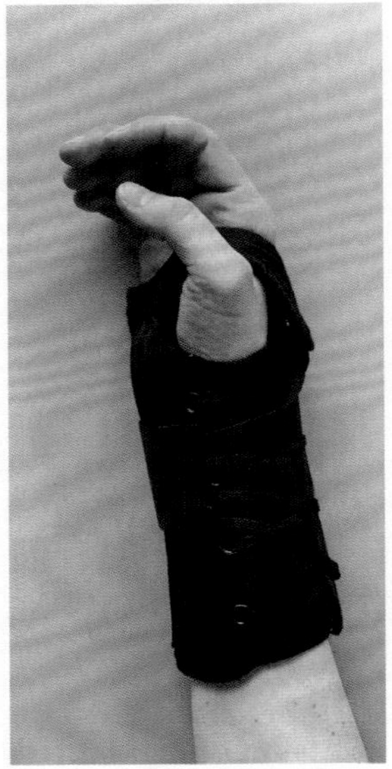	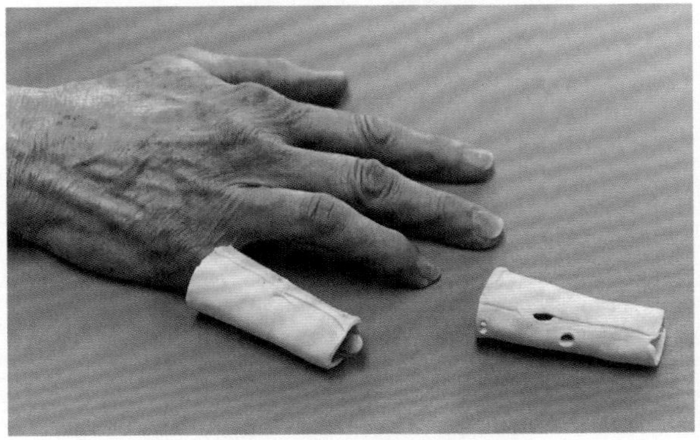 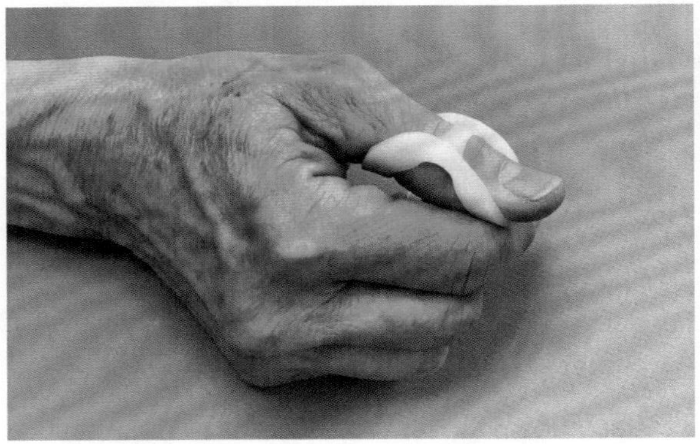 Finger tubes to prevent clawing during ab/adduction exercises	Extension restriction (anticlaw) orthosis to maintain muscular balance, prevent hyperextension at MCP joints, limit substitution patterns, and prevent PIP flexion contractures 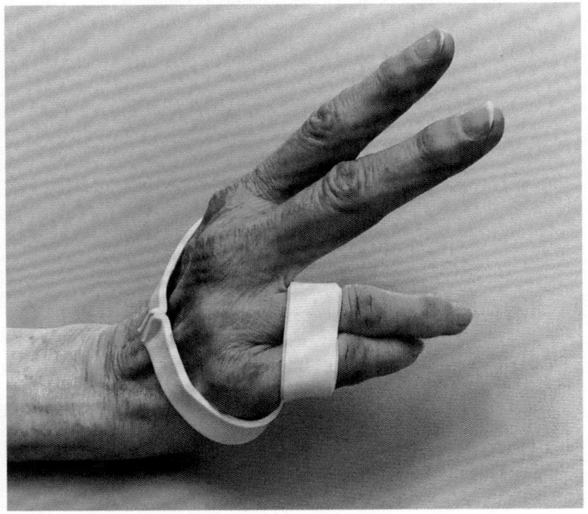
Lateral pinch (adductor pollicis)				
Clawing (lumbricals)			Figure-8 to prevent FPL substitution during pinch exercise	

(Continued)

TABLE 21–2 Common Nerve Transfers (Continued)				
Functional Loss	Common Nerve Transfer	Protective Phase Orthosis	Exercise Orthosis (optional)	Functional Orthosis (optional)
MEDIAN NERVE (AIN BRANCH)				
Index and middle DIP joint flexion (FDP)	ECRB to AIN	Wrist neutral orthosis Prefabricated orthosis is typically sufficient	Wrist wrap with Kleinert-style dynamic thumb attachment to enable synergistic thumb flexion with wrist extension; index may be included	Figure-8 orthosis to prevent hyperextension of thumb IP joint, index finger DIP joint, and to assist with stable pinch for prehension
Thumb IP joint flexion (FPL)				

MEDIAN NERVE (AIN BRANCH)

Index and middle finger flexion (FDP)	No orthosis is required, but a sling is recommended × 2–3 wk to limit elbow flexor activity and prevent seroma formation at the incision site in the medial arm	Buddy-style extension restriction orthosis to prevent hyperextension of index DIP while providing assisted flexion with the middle finger 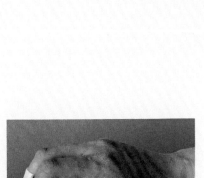
Thumb IP flexion (FPL)	Brachialis to AIN	Figure-8 orthosis to prevent hyperextension of thumb IP joint, index finger DIP joint, and to assist with stable pinch for prehension 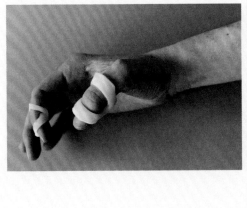

MEDIAN NERVE

Pronation (PT, PQ)	ECRB to pronator	Wrist neutral orthosis Prefabricated orthosis is typically sufficient 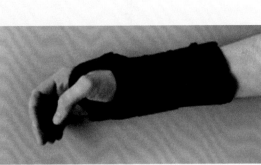
		No orthosis recommended unless passive pronation is limited or supination posture is persistent. In this case, either a static progressive pronation orthosis and/or night positioning orthosis may be beneficial No orthosis recommended

(Continued)

TABLE 21–2	Common Nerve Transfers	(Continued)		
Functional Loss	**Common Nerve Transfer**	**Protective Phase Orthosis**	**Exercise Orthosis (optional)**	**Functional Orthosis (optional)**
Opposition (OP) Palmar abduction (APB)	ADM to thenar motor branch of the median nerve	Forearm-based thumb immobilization orthosis 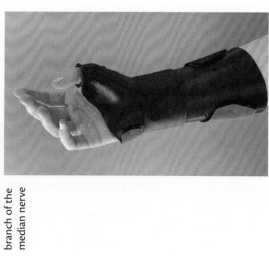	No orthosis recommended	Hand-based thumb immobilization orthosis in functional opposition 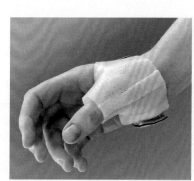

RADIAL NERVE

| Wrist extension (ECRB, ECRL, ECU) | FDS to ECRB | Wrist immobilization orthosis Prefabricated orthosis is typically sufficient | 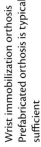 |

RADIAL NERVE (PIN BRANCH)

| MCP joint extension of digits 2–5 (EDC) | Supinator to PIN | MCP extension orthosis with thumb extension component to support digit and thumb extensors | 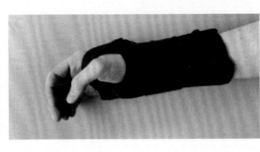 |
| Thumb extension (EPL) | | Low-profile forearm- or hand-based (dependent upon wrist extension strength) radial nerve palsy orthosis, such as a neoprene Benik™ moldable orthosis | 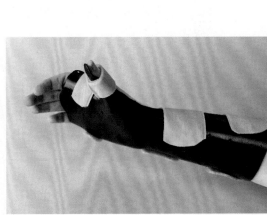 |

(Continued)

TABLE 21–2	Common Nerve Transfers (Continued)			
Functional Loss	**Common Nerve Transfer**	**Protective Phase Orthosis**	**Exercise Orthosis (optional)**	**Functional Orthosis (optional)**
MCP joint extension of digits 2–5 (EDC) Thumb extension (EPL)	FCR to PIN	MCP extension orthosis with thumb extension component to support digit and thumb extensors 	Dynamic orthosis to engage resisted wrist flexion with synergistic digit and thumb extension Static MCP extension orthosis to allow isometric self-resistance to FCR (patient is instructed to extend MCP from orthosis position) 	

FREE FUNCTIONAL MUSCLE TRANSFERS

Injuries to peripheral nerves often do not occur in isolation and may result in a complex array of motor and sensory deficits throughout multiple areas. Patients with brachial plexus injuries can have mixed motor and/or sensory loss in more than one nerve distribution, which does not follow a predictable pattern of axonal loss or recovery. These cases typically necessitate multiple nerve and tendon transfers that may be performed in a single surgery or a staged progression.

Severe injuries to the plexus such as complete avulsion injuries pose a challenge for restoration of distal function. Free functional muscle transfers (FFMTs) are a viable option to restore elbow and finger flexion in such cases where nerve transfers are not an option. FFMT combines principles from both nerve and tendon transfers to utilize a donor or "free functional" muscle, such as the gracilis, to power elbow and/or finger flexion (Seal & Stevanovic, 2011). Donor nerves, typically from the intercostals or rectus abdominis, are transferred to the donor muscle with a nerve graft and ultimately provide innervation for contraction of the grafted muscle (Krauss, Moore, & Tung, 2016).

ROLE OF ORTHOSES

Orthoses for these transfers must protect all the joints affected by the transfer including elbow, wrist, and digits. The required utilization timeframe is also much longer than with tendon or nerve transfers. The affected joint(s) are held in a protected position for 6 to 12 months to maintain muscle-length tension while awaiting reinnervation and to create a slight flexion contracture to augment function and force production. Regarding the more common gracilis muscle transfer to facilitate both elbow and finger flexion, the appropriate orthosis is two-part: (1) a forearm-based dorsal blocking orthosis with the MCP joints in 50° to 60° of flexion, with the proximal interphalangeal (PIP) and distal interphalangeal (DIP) joints in slight flexion, (2) a long arm posterior orthosis in 90° of elbow flexion and supination (molded over the dorsal blocking orthosis) as shown in Figure 21–4.

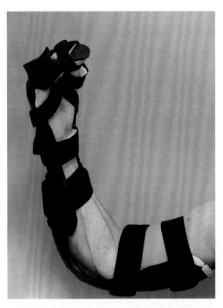

FIGURE 21–4 Following free functional muscle transfer (FFMT), a two-part orthosis positioned in elbow flexion, forearm supination, wrist neutral, and digital flexion is fabricated. Long-term orthosis use is required to protect muscle length while awaiting reinnervation.

CONCLUSION

Orthotic intervention can be an effective tool throughout the recovery of individuals undergoing nerve and tendon transfer surgery. Not only do orthoses protect and rest vital structures, but they also prevent faulty movement patterns, augment motor reeducation, and promote functional independence. Through the innovative techniques in surgery, a multidisciplinary approach to patient care, and the skilled intervention of the hand therapist, there are promising functional outcomes to improve the quality of life for individuals with PNIs.

The overview of orthotic intervention described in this chapter regarding nerve transfers is not all inclusive. Nerve transfer rehabilitation is in its infancy; this is a growing area of interest and expertise. Creative therapists will find many more examples of how to best utilize orthoses to maximize outcomes with their nerve transfer patients.

FIELD NOTE: CHOOSING A TENDON TRANSFER: CONSIDERATIONS

MaryLynn A. Jacobs, MBA, MS, OTR/L, CHT
Massachusetts

In an ideal situation, the therapist, patient, and surgeon decide on what is the best *functional* performance to be restored, followed by the choice as to what is *available* to use as a possible donor. The selection process includes the analysis of the anticipated strength of a donor muscle after the transfer, its potential excursion, how many joints it must cross, the direction it must pull in order to be effective, and the overall effect the transfer has on the balance of other muscle/tendon units in the extremity (Brand, 1995; Colditz, 1995; Jones, 1994; Mackinnon, 1994; Smith, 1987; Bednar et al., 2010). Before surgical intervention, the following therapy considerations should have been met:

- Prevent, correct, or minimize substitution patterns from developing or progressing while awaiting transfer by providing preoperative therapy and orthosis fabrication to encourage the natural use of the hand.

- Achieve and maintain full passive range of motion (ROM) of all involved joints.

- Maintain strength, if able and safe, of all noninvolved muscle tendon structures.

- Prevent or minimize the development of soft tissue contractures or adhesions.

- Maintain or gain tissue length of the involved skin and soft tissue adhesions and joint contractures (Brand, 1995; Colditz, 1995; Jones, 1994; Walsh, 2012).

- Strive to achieve maximal strength (4+) of the donor muscle(s) considered for transfer (Brand, 1995; Elfar et al., 2010; Bednar et al., 2010).

- Stress the importance to patient and caregivers, the understanding of the postoperative course of the therapy, and the significance of strict orthosis compliance.

Case Study Section

The case studies presented here are meant as a teaching guideline only. Treatment and orthosis protocols vary greatly from surgeon to surgeon and from therapist to therapist. The therapist should check with the referring physicians and colleagues to define the preferred treatment and appropriate orthotic intervention.

Case Study: Cubital Tunnel Syndrome With Ulnar Neuropathy

RK is a 55-year-old male who developed severe ulnar neuropathy 10 years following medial elbow trauma. By the time he was evaluated by a surgeon, he presented with both extrinsic and intrinsic ulnar motor deficits. His grip and pinch strength were less than 50% of the uninvolved side, and there is severe ulnar intrinsic wasting. He underwent an ulnar nerve transposition, release of the ulnar nerve at Guyon canal, and an end to side nerve transfer of the pronator quadratus branch of the anterior interosseous nerve to the deep motor branch of the ulnar nerve in the distal forearm.

At the first hand therapy visit, 3 days postoperatively, he was fitted with a prefabricated wrist orthosis with the wrist in neutral (0° extension). He was instructed to wear this full time for 3 weeks, removing only for hygiene, once or twice a day. He was given instructions to avoid full use of the arm and to keep it elevated, but he may gently move the extremity in a symptom-free range a few times per day. The patient follows up 3 weeks later and describes paresthesias and weakness in the involved hand. There is a mild claw deformity involving the ring and small digits. The patient is warned that this will likely increase in severity as the long (FDP) flexors recover strength in 3 months. Active ROM, ulnar nerve glides and scar management is initiated at this time. The patient is also instructed in nerve transfer motor reeducation with an emphasis on donor activation exercises with hourly forearm pronation. The wrist orthosis is no longer needed full time but may be used occasionally to protect the arm during travel or heavy activity.

Despite compliance to ROM instruction, a strong claw deformity is noted at the 3-month follow-up visit. A hand-based anticlaw orthosis is fabricated, blocking the MCP joints of the ring and small digits in slight flexion facilitating full active IP joint extension. Instruction is given to wear the orthosis during the day to improve function and prevent potential PIP joint contracture. Active assisted digital abduction/adduction exercises are reviewed, and due to the increased clawing, finger extension (tube) orthoses are fabricated to aid in isolation of the weak interossei during these exercises. A thumb-based oval-8 may also be fabricated to block FPL substitution during pinch activities. Refer to Table 21–2.

The patient is followed on a monthly basis, and 6 months later, resolution of the claw deformity is noted as intrinsic function improves. The anticlaw orthosis is no longer needed. The patient can now abduct/adduct the digits without clawing when the forearm is pronated. The exercises are advanced to include light resistance putty. The thumb orthosis continues to be used during resistive pinch strengthening in order to isolate and strengthen the adductor pollicis muscle. Once he can perform this without FPL substitution, this orthosis is also discarded, and the patient can advance his hand strengthening regimen.

CHAPTER REVIEW QUESTIONS

1. Why would a patient undergo a tendon transfer?
2. Why is patient orthotic education prior to tendon transfer critical?
3. What are some of the most important components of the decision-making algorithm in the selection of tendon transfer?
4. What are the main goals of the role of an orthosis in the tendon transfer patient?
5. What are three advantages of nerve transfers?
6. What is the difference between a tendon and a nerve transfer?

22 The Athlete[a]

Kimberly Goldie Staines, OTR, CHT

CHAPTER OBJECTIVES

After study of this chapter, the reader should be able to:
- Describe common sport-specific diagnoses of the upper extremity.
- Understand the clinical reasoning process for selecting the most appropriate orthosis for an athlete.
- Explain how management of the athlete differs from other patient populations when managing upper extremity diagnoses.
- Appreciate the unique sport-specific factors related to orthotic intervention.
- Identify various materials and application techniques used in the management of this unique population.

KEY TERMS

Bennett fracture
Biceps tendon rupture
Boutonniere deformity
Bowler's thumb
Carpal tunnel syndrome
Cubital tunnel syndrome
Cyclist palsy
DeQuervain tenosynovitis
Distal radius fractures

Distal ulna instability
Flexor digitorum profundus avulsion
Handlebar palsy
Intersection syndrome
Lateral epicondylitis
Mallet finger
Medial epicondylitis
Metacarpal fractures
Midcarpal instability
Olecranon bursitis

Phalangeal fractures
PIP joint dislocation
Playing orthosis
Pronator syndrome
Radial tunnel syndrome
Scaphoid fracture
Tendinosis
Thumb MP joint sprain
Triangular fibrocartilage complex

MD NOTE

David TJ Netscher, MD
Texas

Athletic upper extremity injuries are common. There is often pressure to return to high-level performance as rapidly as possible. These injuries include closed flexor and extensor tendon injuries, joint ligament destabilizing injuries, major muscle injuries, fractures that may be intra- or extra-articular as well as occasional nerve injuries. Some injuries can be so severe that they are career-ending, but still require optimal and meaningful rehabilitation. Most injuries are such that the athlete will be able to return to peak performance.

The hand therapist must understand not only the type of sport but also the position played on a team. These may or may not place constraints on the ability of the athlete to return to full activity. Being able to work with the athlete so that supportive orthoses can be worn within any required protective gear is important.

Orthoses in sports must be functional. It is equally important to understand which orthoses may potentially pose a danger to both the injured athlete and other players. Protective orthotic padding may be required. An orthosis that spans the finger MCP joints, for example, may load more distal skeletal structures in a fall, leading to additional potential injuries and even fractures.

In most injuries, there is acute management to reduce swelling and inflammation. Then there generally follows a period of immobilization (with or without surgery) and then protected mobilization and finally conditioning and strengthening. Often orthotic protection and cautious mobilization can occur simultaneously such as with a hinged orthosis that enables motion at a proximal interphalangeal (PIP) or elbow joint but protects collateral ligaments. Understanding the complex mechanisms of motion is important, especially with the wrist and distal radioulnar joints.

The eventual return to sporting activity involves coordinated teamwork with the assembled team being the injured athlete, coach, hand therapist, and hand surgeon. The birth of hand therapy as a specialty is relatively recent; hand surgery came into its own during the World War II years. A number of notable hand surgeons realized that specially trained hand therapists were required to help rehabilitate these patients. Independently both hand surgeons and hand therapists have evolved their own specialties. Collectively and collaboratively, surgeons and therapists bring their respective skills and together are indomitable. This unique collaboration is especially important in the treatment of the elite athlete. It is with great pleasure that I provide this introduction for the very comprehensive chapter authored by Kimberly Goldie Staines OTR, CHT, with whom I have had the pleasure of many years of collaboration in education, research, and high clinical standards.

---

[a]This chapter is based on the first-edition chapter written by Lisa Schulz Slowman, MS, OTR/L, CHT, with contributions in third edition from David TJ Netscher, MD.

FAQ

How does treating an athlete differ from a nonathlete?
The athlete is generally very motivated to return to a high level of activity—working out or sport-specific training. Education regarding the specifics of that fracture and healing timeframes is key. Close communication with the referring physician can allow for collaboration and returning the athlete to their desired activity safely as quickly as possible. Fabricating a protective orthosis in the early stages and progressing as aggressively as possible into less protective devices as healing allows, including a playing orthosis, can help facilitate a timely return to sport process.

What are the primary considerations in regard to material and strapping selection in this unique population?
Firstly, it is imperative to have a good understanding of the sport and demands on the injured body part. The sporting equipment must be on hand when fabricating an orthosis to be used during a sporting event. Choosing the thickness of material depends on the required rigidity. Opting for perforations is always wise due to perspiration. Consider taping or using a glove to hold the orthosis in place versus traditional often bulky hook/loop strapping. Taping offers a light support and may be all that is required in some cases to allow for safe return to sporting activity.

INTRODUCTION

Athletic competition in our current society has become paramount. The importance of athletics has allowed for a greater understanding of this specialty population and a greater evaluation for improved medical and sport-specific management of injuries. Common upper extremity injuries include bony and ligamentous injuries to the elbow, forearm, wrist, hand, thumb, and digits in addition to a variety of other soft tissue injuries. Despite improvements in protective equipment, upper extremity injuries continue to represent approximately 25% of all sport-related injuries that involve the hand or wrist (Avery, & Rodner, 2016; Bernadette, Brou, Fields, Erkenbeck, & Comstock, 2017; Hootman, 2007; Rettig, 2003; Rozenbaum, 2017). With 50% of sports injuries reported in the lower extremity, upper extremity injuries may not be as obvious or as well reported (Hootman, 2007). The rate of injuries in competition is higher than those in practice traditionally. The most common upper extremity injuries were fracture (45.0%), contusion (11.6%), and ligament sprains (9.0%) (Hootman, 2007). The purpose of this chapter is to highlight common sport-specific injuries and review options in orthotic management.

GENERAL ORTHOTIC CONSIDERATIONS

Protecting the injured athlete has consistently been a challenge to the hand therapy profession. With more aggressive approaches to medical care and treatment of the athlete, the challenge for the hand therapist is to determine a rehabilitation protocol that is safe and effective in protecting the injured tissue while not increasing the risk of re-injury or additional injury and that is acceptable to the athletes' league of play. Athletes with upper extremity injuries progress through the phases of rehabilitation which include no activity with formal rehabilitation (Phase One), limited/modified activity with supplemental rehabilitation (Phase Two), then to Phase Three including full activity with supplemental conditioning (Kibler & Sciascia, 2019).

PHASES OF REHABILITATION

In the early acute phases of rehabilitation, orthotic goals are generally to provide rest and protection to the injured structure(s) while allowing easy removal of the orthosis for initiation of a range of motion (ROM) program and management of soft tissue trauma. Other rehabilitation goals during this initial period are to decrease edema and pain. The clinician should recall that immobilization causes widespread morphological and biochemical changes to all of the involved tissues, injured and noninjured. At 4 weeks, the muscle tissue of injured animals demonstrates the wasting of mass and lower total content of myofibrillar proteins; this disuse atrophy occurs rapidly in immobilized muscle and may result in a longer recovery (Mobach et al, 2019; MacLennan et al., 2020).

As the athlete progresses, orthotic goals begin to focus on providing protection to the injured structure(s) while minimally interfering with the upper extremity function of the athlete. For example, a hockey player who sustains a metacarpal fracture initially requires a wrist and metacarpophalangeal (MCP) joint immobilization orthosis to protect the fracture; the player removes the orthosis to do protected ROM exercises. As the athlete advances to return to competition, he or she may be fitted with a similarly positioned hand-based orthosis that fits into the hockey glove; this facilitates early return to competition.

Phase One—No Activity With Formal Rehabilitation

In Phase one, rehabilitation focuses on the causative factors that may influence injury and also to re-establish proximal and distal kinetic chain activations that allow rehabilitation of the body to function as a unit. This is accomplished by working on posture and motion facilitation, as well as closed chain tasks when indicated, and working in multiple planes of motor recruitment while protecting the injured structure (Sciascia, Thigpen, Namdari, & Baldwin, 2012).

Any orthosis or protective device provided to an athlete should protect the injured structure(s) and prevent reinjury, should allow safe and effective participation in the sport, should not pose an injury threat to an opposing athlete, and should meet the demands of the governing bodies for the sport and the local game officials (Bertini et al., 2011) (Fig. 22–1A,B). Coppage and Carlson (2017) provide a detailed review of the specific rules regarding the use of orthoses, casts, and other types of protective equipment, dependent on the sport and the level of competition. Information regarding the rules and guidelines is readily available online. Refer Table 22–1 for contact information.

Phase Two—Limited Activity With Supplemental Rehabilitation

At this level, you will find the athlete presents comparable to the "no activity" level; however, their symptoms may be more general and may be secondary to Phase one restrictions versus injury-specific complaints. Secondary injuries that do not directly inhibit function may also be found in this phase. Return to some team

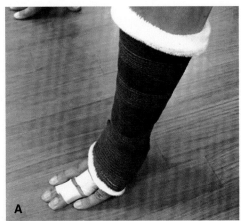

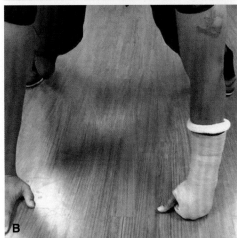

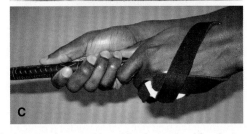

FIGURE 22-1 A, A wrist cast with padding is permitted for play in most professional leagues but care should be taken to protect other exposed joints. **B,** The use of buddy strapping protects the exposed digits from lateral stress but coaching to have a fisted hand placement in a weight bearing stance will limit to risk of an MCP or PIP hyperextension injury. **C,** The therapist must consider the injured athlete's sports equipment when fabricating or fitting an orthosis. This RF and SF digit immobilization orthosis is protecting a healing SF PIP joint injury in this golfer.

TABLE 22-1	**Sports Rules and Regulations**

National Collegiate Athletic Association (NCAA)
6201 College Blvd.
Overland Park, KS 66211-2422
913-339-1906
www.NCAA.org
College sports

National Federation of State High School Associations (NFHS)
P.O. Box 20626 (64195-0626)
11724 Northwest Plaza Circle
Kansas City, MO 64153
816-464-5400
www.NFHS.org
High school sports

American Alliance for Health, Physical Education, Recreation and Dance (AAHPERD)
1900 Association Dr.
Reston, VA 20191
703-476-3400
www.AAHPERD.org
High school sports

when any orthosis is fabricated. This allows the therapist to make any necessary modifications to permit continued effective use of the equipment while protecting the injury without creating pressure areas or impingement from the orthosis (Fig. 22–1C).

Phase Three—Full Activity With Supplemental Conditioning

Finally, basic supports and pre-exercise/post exercise regimes may be required for return to all aspects of the sport after injury. It is not uncommon for athletes returning to have underlying deficiencies ranging from soft tissue inflexibility to muscle weakness or imbalance that may result in post play soreness. Educating the athlete and team staff about the purpose of the orthosis is imperative. The athlete should understand why the orthosis is necessary, when and how it should be used and cared for, and the plan for duration of use and weaning from the orthosis. The better the athlete understands the purpose of the orthosis, the greater the chance for compliance and the lower the patient's risk for reinjury. It is also important that the athlete's coach, athletic trainer, team members, and family understand the purpose and importance of the orthosis to help reinforce its use.

Stretching, strengthening, and conditioning exercises are critical to the successful return to sport; they include eccentric and concentric loading as well as sport-specific drills. The clinician or athletic trainer should review proper technique, provide information for equipment modification, teach adequate warm-up and cool-down exercises specific to the injury, and, if appropriate, provide orthoses or taping for use during and/or after exercise. The athlete should initially monitor the intensity and duration of exercise and report any signs and symptoms of reoccurring symptoms.

Communication with the physician, athlete, coaching staff, and trainers ensures that the most appropriate orthosis options are being considered. Appropriate prefabricated orthoses or sport-specific equipment that may not be commonly used (skiing gloves with thumb MP support) may be available to meet the performance demands of the athlete (refer Chapter 9 on prefabricated orthoses for further information). The athletes, coaches, or trainers may be familiar with such equipment, and it is important for the therapist to investigate these options as well. If other management options are explored, the therapist must make sure that the equipment meets the medical needs of the athlete.

In some cases, taping may be an option for protection of the injured structures (Little & Jacoby, 2011). For example, after acute

activities may be allowed at this point of rehabilitation as well. Activity modification would likely be included during return to team practice such as limited frequency of throwing or participating in fielding activities versus more specific tasks. Close communication between the treating physicians, team athletic trainers, and/or coaches is crucial to provide safe return to play while limiting stress to the involved structures in order to limit the risk of reinjury (Singletary & Geissler, 2009). These team members provide valuable information regarding the injury and help the therapist gain an understanding of the sport-specific demands to help optimize the orthotic intervention. Specific demands include the level of competition, type of sport, and position played. It is also important to know the athlete's goals for continued participation in the sport. For example, a high school lacrosse player with the prospect of a collegiate sports scholarship may have a stronger desire to return to competition compared to a high school freshman playing lacrosse for the first time.

If the athlete uses gloves or other equipment (sticks, clubs, bats, braces, handlebars), it is important that the athlete brings them management of volar plate injuries, buddy taping adjacent fingers helps prevent undue stress to healing structures. Some of the goals that can be met with taping are restriction of ROM, managing edema, providing anatomical support, and protecting against reinjury. Athletes with a prior injury are four times more likely to sustain another injury; premature return to play may result in complications and potentially permanent sequelae that would otherwise be preventable (Coppage & Carlson, 2017). Taping of the wrist, thumb, and digits is common after injuries to these areas and can be used with or without custom thermoplastic supports (refer Chapter 13 on taping for further information) (Porette-Loehrke, 2016; Wegener, Brown, & O'Brien, 2016; Cai, Au, An, & Cheung, 2016).

Also, the hand therapist should stay abreast of any changes in the sport and make necessary modifications as the sport evolves. For example, the potential for decreased impact attenuation properties of artificial turf compared to natural turf may require increased padding and/or rigid support for hand and wrist injuries (Williams, Hume, & Kara, 2011).

MATERIAL SELECTION

There are various materials and strapping systems that may be good options for athletes. The choice of material depends on the objective for the orthosis. In the initial phases of rehabilitation, the goal for the orthosis may be to provide protection during daily activities and to allow removal for hygiene and ROM exercises. For protective purposes, a 1/8″ material is typically appropriate for orthotic fabrication. As the athlete returns to practice and competition, a **playing orthosis** may be appropriate. Thick external padding of a rigid orthosis works well as a transitional orthosis by providing impact absorption, while continuing to rigidly protect healing structures. If only soft support is necessary, a neoprene or soft canvas orthosis with or without a rigid support may be appropriate (Fig. 22–2A,B). Neoprene material is a synthetic, latex-free rubber that is available in various thickness, densities, elasticity, and perforations. It is able to provide flexible support and compression via prefabricated or custom-fabricated orthoses (see Chapter 14 on neoprene for further information).

The body part being fitted also influences the material selection. A thinner thermoplastic material with memory, 1/16″ or 3/32″, is an option to consider for digit-based immobilization orthoses used after a fracture (Fig. 22–3). This thinner material may not be appropriate for a wrist and thumb immobilization orthosis, for example, following a scaphoid fracture, a 1/8″ thermoplastic should be chosen for greater durability, rigidity, and protection (Fig. 22–4).

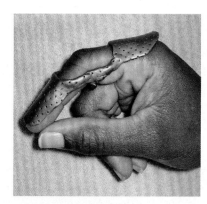

FIGURE 22–3 A PIP extension restriction orthosis for a volar plate avulsion fracture fabricated from 1/16″ material.

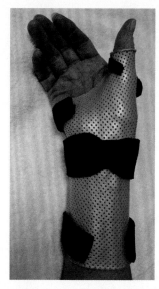

FIGURE 22–4 Wrist and thumb immobilization orthosis fabricated from 1/8″ material to provide a rigid support for a healing scaphoid fracture. Note full clearance of the IP joint.

When determining the best material to use for a protective orthosis for an athlete returning to competition, the therapist should consider the hardness (rigidity) of the material (must be strong enough to protect and stabilize the injured structures), the ability of the material to absorb an impact (flexibility), and the rules of the sport's governing body and local officials regarding playing with orthoses and/or casts (Coppage & Carlson, 2017). Consider that professional and collegiate athletes can usually return to competition with a hard cast or an orthosis provided that it is covered with soft padding, but this is generally not allowed in high school contact sports. The sports governing body may dictate the thickness and type of padding material, but generally closed-cell foam at least 3/4″ thick is appropriate to encompass the device. If the athlete requires padding only in competition, consider securing the padding in place with an elastic wrap so that it can be removed when the athlete is not competing (Fig. 22–5A,B).

Material options include low-temperature thermoplastics, room-temperature vulcanizing (RTV) silicone rubber, tape, fiberglass-based materials (Scotchcast™ and Plastazote®), Delta-Cast® Conformable Casting Tape (Essity, Charlotte, NC), and neoprene materials. Materials applied circumferentially, such as QuickCast 2 (Performance Health) and Orficast® (Orfit) have simplified many orthotic applications. A circumferential digit orthosis fabricated from these materials eliminates the need for strapping. If the orthosis is made from QuickCast 2 without a liner, the athlete does not have to remove the cast for hygiene because of the material's meshlike quality. In addition to the benefit of air exchange, this material is extremely durable (depending on number of layers), may allow the athlete to sweat, bathe, or swim with limited

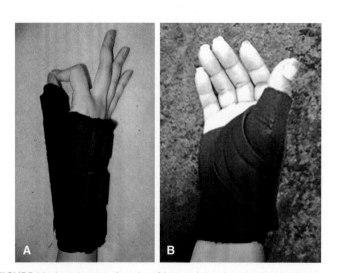

FIGURE 22–2 A, Forearm-based prefabricated thumb orthosis with hard stays. **B,** Neoprene brace offers support, warmth, and restriction of joint motion.

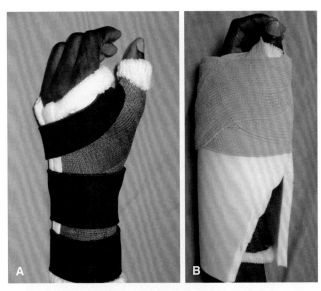

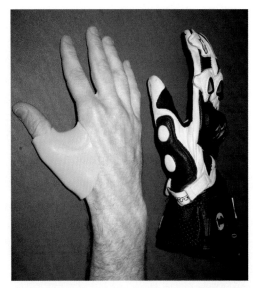

FIGURE 22–5 **A,** A Delta-Cast° conforming thumb and wrist orthosis for a scaphoid fracture; split and secured with elasticized loop to allow for edema and skin care. **B,** Cast covered with ½″ closed cell padding and secured with an elastic bandage for return to sport.

FIGURE 22–7 Thumb MP immobilization orthosis using thermoplastic material and that can be secured inside a motocross glove without additional strapping.

risk of maceration. This works especially well for acute boutonniere and mallet injuries; the ability to get the hand wet is appreciated along with the slim custom fit (Fig. 22–6A,B).

Additional considerations for orthotic material selection include the use of perforated materials to decrease perspiration and minimize skin irritation. The use of colored materials and strapping to coordinate with uniforms should also be considered, which may improve wear compliance. The therapist should be aware of the temperature and environment in which the athlete will be wearing the orthosis. A diver may require a perforated orthosis to limit skin irritation, and a rugby player in Texas may not tolerate thermoplastic material due to the heat exposure and humidity.

STRAPPING SELECTION

The strapping systems used for athletic orthoses are unique, especially for those used in conjunction with other equipment. For example, a thumb immobilization orthosis that is fabricated for a motorbike racer who is returning to competition may not require a strap. Rather, the orthosis may be held in place by the bike glove

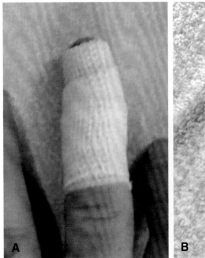

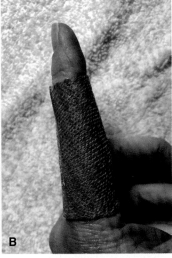

FIGURE 22–6 **A,** Circumferential digit immobilization orthosis fabricated from QuickCast 2 allows this patient with an acute central tendon injury to bathe with the orthosis on. **B,** PIP immobilization orthosis fabricated from Orficast° used to address acute boutonniere injury.

(Fig. 22–7). A strap in this case is unnecessary and could interfere with the cyclist's feel and grip of the handlebars in the palm. However, if strapping is to be used under equipment, consider soft strapping material (neoprene) or taping to minimize the risk of skin irritation from friction due to traditional loop material.

Sometimes, it is appropriate to use a circumferential elasticized wrap, such as an elastic bandage (Coban™ or Ace™ Wrap) to hold an orthosis in place. This secures the orthosis while distributing the pressure evenly on the body part. A padded wrist orthosis used during practice by a football blocker may best be secured with an elasticized bandage (Fig. 22–5B).

Another option for securing a return to sport orthoses is tape, see Chapter 13 on taping. There are a multitude of options that can be used to limit migration of the orthosis and bulk under equipment. You may use 1/2″ paper or silk tape for the application of a finger orthosis, whereas athletic tape or elastic therapeutic tape (Kinesiotape®, Dynamic Tape, or Theraband tape) may be used to secure a hand- or forearm-based orthosis. Be sure that the tape selected has enough adhesion to secure the orthosis with sweat, water, and friction from external sports equipment. When using high tack tapes, such as athletic tape, be sure to use roll gauze (Kerlix, Hypafix) or prewrap to allow for easy removal and reuse of the orthosis (Fig. 22–8A,B).

It is important that the strapping best suits the needs of the athlete. Whenever possible, the athlete should bring the sports equipment that will be used or worn while wearing the orthosis to the clinic. The athlete should simulate practice using the orthosis with the equipment prior to leaving the clinic so the therapist can make any reasonable alterations to the orthosis. The therapist must work with the athlete to customize the strapping system and allow maximal upper extremity use while maintaining the function of the orthosis and protecting the injury. Athletes should be given additional sets of strapping, especially those involved in aquatic activities such as rowing, kayaking, swimming, water polo, and diving so that dry straps are always available for securing the orthosis. This is necessary for maintaining good skin integrity under the straps.

ORTHOSIS OPTIONS

Orthotic fabrication includes articular and nonarticular, immobilization, and restriction orthoses involving the elbow (EO), wrist hand (WHO), hand (HO), hand finger (HFO), and finger (FO) that includes the thumb (Bash et al., 2011). Articular orthoses stabilize or restrict the motion across a joint. Examples of articular orthoses

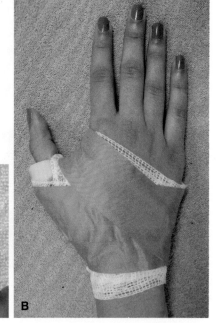

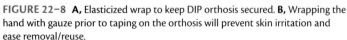

FIGURE 22–8 **A,** Elasticized wrap to keep DIP orthosis secured. **B,** Wrapping the hand with gauze prior to taping on the orthosis will prevent skin irritation and ease removal/reuse.

include a thumb MP immobilization orthosis (FO) used to protect a healing ulnar collateral ligament (UCL) on a cyclist (Fig. 22–7) and a PIP joint extension restriction orthosis (FO) used to prevent reinjury of the volar plate in a soccer player (Fig. 22–3). Nonarticular orthoses do not cross a joint but provide stability to soft tissue or bony structures to treat or prevent injury. Examples of nonarticular orthoses are a proximal phalanx orthosis (FO), also known as a pulley ring, for a rock climber to protect against flexor tendon sheath injury (Fig. 22–9A,B) and a proximal forearm orthosis (EO), also known as an epicondylitis strap, used to absorb and disperse forces of the forearm muscles as they approach the medial and/or lateral epicondyle(s) (Fig. 22–10A,B) (Warme & Brooks, 2000; Whaley & Baker, 2004).

SPORT-SPECIFIC INJURIES

Management of specific common upper extremity injuries such as fractures, fracture/dislocations, ligamentous injury, muscle/tendon ruptures, and nerve injury is discussed in detail elsewhere in this book (see Chapters 16, 18–20).

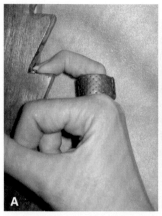

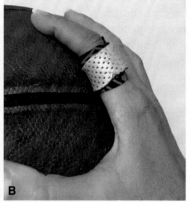

FIGURE 22–9 **A,** Nonarticular proximal phalanx orthosis (pulley ring) to limit bowstringing of flexors for return to sport after tendon injury. **B,** Note use of Dynamic Tape under the ring orthosis for added stability.

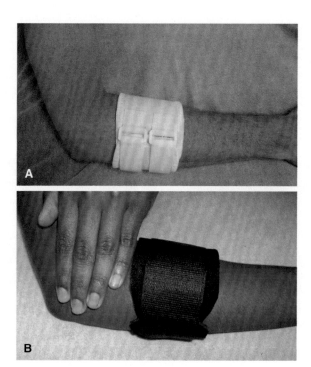

FIGURE 22–10 **A,** A proximal forearm orthosis (counterforce brace or epicondylitis strap) used to reduce stress at the proximal muscle insertion (shown: Count-R Force Strap, NorthCoast Medical). **B,** Custom-made counterforce strap—note that by placing the index finger on the epicondyle, the small finger will locate the correct placement of pressure.

The four main mechanisms for the most common sports injuries include twisting, weight bearing, throwing, and impact. The hand, wrist, and elbow are especially exposed areas for injury in many sports. As the incident of lower extremity injury limits the athlete's mobility, the upper extremity performs highly technical and demanding prehensile tasks and as such is often left unprotected. In addition, external pressure from family, parents, coaches, fans, teammates, school officials, team owners, sponsors, and managers can be strong considerations in competitive sporting and aggressive return to play. The sport-specific provider team should include the patient, family, physician, therapist, athletic trainer, and coach in order to determine the soundest recommendation for care and allow the athlete to choose the most effective intervention for their needs. An informed willingness of the athlete to take a reasonable risk of jeopardizing treatment and the future function of the body part may have to be honored, although the "worst possibility" must be thoroughly reviewed with the athlete (Strickland & Rettig, 1992). The obligation on the part of the sports medicine team must include detailed information that would allow the athlete and his sports training team to consider the potential consequences of returning to competition with a given injury. The therapist plays a crucial role in this discussion regarding the orthotic device and protection to allow a decided risk with protected return to play.

A brief description of common sport-related injuries is reviewed in the following text. Table 22–2 summarizes orthotic selection and fabrication for sport-specific injuries. Relying on basic science knowledge of connective tissue healing, protection, and immobilization is important in the first phase of healing (Kannus, Parkhari, Jarvinen, Jarvinen, & Jarvinen, 2003).

FRACTURES

In sports, upper limb fractures are much more common than lower limb and axial skeletal fractures, accounting for 76.7% of sports fractures seen (Aitken & Court-Brown, 2008). When treating an athlete with an acute fracture, the therapist must consider the stability of the injury as well as the patient's age, level of competition, position played, and desire to return to sport. Fractures sustained by athletes during competition due to low impact forces can be stable injuries treated with immobilization followed by a transition into a playing orthosis for early return to competition (Rettig, 1991). Fabrication of an orthosis for an unstable fracture requires the stabilization of the joint proximal and distal to the fracture. Unstable fractures may require surgical intervention, resulting in a more variable course of treatment. Refer Chapter 16 for more comprehensive information regarding orthotic management for fractures.

TABLE 22–2 Orthoses for Sports Injuries

Diagnosis	Orthosis Options	Return to Sport	Considerations	Return to Play
Distal radius and/or ulna fracture	After surgery or cast removal: • Wrist immobilization orthosis	• Circumferential wrist orthosis (primarily with contact sports) • Neoprene wrist orthosis	• Adapt playing orthosis to athlete's upper extremity demands • Well padded on outside for contact sports	• With confirmed healing, protective orthosis worn for 2–4 wk per physician recommendation and sport-specific position requirements
Scaphoid fracture	After surgery or cast removal: • Wrist and thumb MP immobilization orthosis	• Circumferentially padded wrist and thumb immobilization orthosis • Neoprene wrist/thumb orthosis • Wrist/thumb taping	• Adapt playing orthosis to athlete's upper extremity demands • Trim thumb portion of neoprene orthosis to allow necessary motion • Tape to limit full thumb motion, protecting against hyperextension and radial deviation forces	• Per physician recommendation and sport-specific position requirements • Use of playing orthosis depends on status of scaphoid healing and sport demands on the hand/wrist
Metacarpal fracture	After surgery or cast removal: • Wrist and MCP or hand-based MCP immobilization orthosis	Depends on fracture stability and sport-specific demands • Buddy taping • Wrist and MCP or hand-based MCP immobilization orthosis	• Make sure orthosis is adapted to equipment used by athlete (hockey stick and glove, bicycle handlebars, ski glove and pole) • Pad the exterior of return to play orthosis to prevent slipping on equipment	• Per physician recommendation and sport-specific position requirements • May return to play with sport orthosis depending on fracture healing and demands of sport
Phalangeal fracture	After surgery or cast removal: • Hand-based digit immobilization orthosis • Buddy taping	Depends on fracture stability and sport-specific demands • Digit or hand immobilization orthosis for injured digit(s) only • Digit or hand immobilization orthosis for injured and adjacent digits • Buddy taping to adjacent digits	• Orthosis should provide enough stability to protect fracture and be adapted to allow athlete to meet upper extremity demands • Adapt orthosis to equipment as necessary	• Per physician recommendation and sport-specific position requirements
PIP fracture and/or dislocation (volar plate injury)	Acute (nonoperative management): • Hand-based PIP extension restriction orthosis (extension allowed is increased weekly until full extension is attained)	• PIP extension restriction orthosis • Buddy taping to adjacent digit	• Orthosis should position PIP in appropriate degree of flexion determined by fracture reduction • Early motion program and edema management are important	• PIP extension restriction orthosis used for initial 2-4 wk • Buddy taping continues for 4-6 mo during competition
Central tendon rupture (acute boutonniere injury)	Acute (nonoperative management): • PIP or IP extension immobilization orthosis • Serial digital cast immobilizing PIP joint while allowing DIP flexion	• Digital cast with PIP and DIP extension to protect DIP from hyperextension injury • PIP or IP immobilization orthosis • Taping	• Watch for problems with skin maceration or breakdown at dorsal PIP joint • Changes in edema require frequent adjustments • Orthosis must maintain PIP in full extension when DIP is actively flexed with exercise	• Used 4-6 wk (day and night) • Used 4-8 wk between ROM exercises and at night • Used 8 or more weeks at night and as required during the day
Terminal tendon rupture (Mallet finger)	Acute (nonoperative management): • DIP extension immobilization orthosis • Digital cast immobilizing DIP joint while allowing PIP flexion	• DIP extension immobilization orthosis • Digital cast immobilizing DIP joint while allowing PIP flexion • Circumferential IP taping • Neoprene DIP orthosis	• Watch for problems with skin maceration or breakdown at dorsal DIP joint • Changes in edema require frequent adjustments • Watch for inadvertent removal of orthosis if used under glove	• Use 6 wk (day and night) • Use 6-8 wk ROM exercise and at night • Use 8 or more weeks at night and as needed during the day
FDP avulsion (jersey finger)	After surgical repair: • Wrist flexion/MCP flexion/IP extension immobilization orthosis	• Dorsal DIP immobilization orthosis with DIP slightly flexed • Circumferential DIP cast • Circumferential DIP taping	• With repaired tendon, follow protocol precautions • Generally, athlete will not return to competition for at least 12 wk	• Use 4-6 wk (day and night) • Use 6-8 wk for additional protection only

CHAPTER 22

(Continued)

TABLE 22–2	**Orthoses for Sports Injuries** (Continued)			
Diagnosis	**Orthosis Options**	**Return to Sport**	**Considerations**	**Return to Play**
Thumb UCL injury (skier's or gamekeeper's thumb)	After surgical repair (Stenar lesion): • Wrist/thumb MP immobilization orthosis After cast immobilization: • Thumb immobilization orthosis Return to sport: • Hand-based orthosis during sport for 1-2 mo Partial tear: • Hand-based thumb MP immobilization orthosis • Taping	• Hand-based thumb MP immobilization orthosis • Neoprene thumb orthosis • Thumb MP circumferential taping	• Adapt orthosis to equipment used by athlete	• After surgery: use for approximately 8 wk • After casting: use 6-8 wk • Partial tear: use 4-6 wk
Medial epicondylitis (golfer's elbow)	• Proximal forearm orthoses (counterforce brace: Epitrain, Nirschl Count'R Force brace) or custom-made nonarticular forearm orthosis • Taping (Chapter 13)	• Proximal forearm orthosis • Taping (Chapter 13)	• In addition to bracing, patient education, anti-inflammatory treatment, massage, ice, activity modification, and equipment modification (wider handle) may help	• Depends on symptoms
Lateral epicondylitis (tennis elbow)	• Proximal forearm orthoses—prefabricated or custom (counterforce brace: Epitrain, Nirschl Count'R Force brace) • Taping	• Proximal forearm orthosis • Taping	• In addition to orthotic management, patient education, anti-inflammatory treatment, massage, ice, activity modification, and equipment modification (wider handle, string tension) may help	• Depends on symptoms
Guyon canal syndrome (handlebar palsy)	Acute symptoms: • Wrist immobilization orthosis in neutral to slight flexion and ulnar deviation Return to sport: • Padded biking gloves	• Padded biking gloves • Custom strap with padding	• Padding may require modification (doughnut) to relieve pressure on the nerve	• Depends on symptoms
Dorsal impaction syndrome (gymnast's wrist)	Return to sport: • Wrist immobilization orthosis to decrease wrist hyperextension • Neoprene orthosis • Taping	• Neoprene orthosis	• Minimize palmar contact area in the hand with orthotic material and strapping • Patient education regarding changing hand position and periodic stretching • Consider prefabricated or neoprene orthosis to restrict hyperextension	• Continuous use for practice and competition • Not used for daily activities

Distal Radius Fractures

Distal radius fractures are common in sporting activities; the usual mechanism of injury is a fall on an outstretched hand (FOOSH). In the athlete, these injuries tend to be high-energy fractures and involve the articular surfaces, causing disruption of the distal radioulnar and distal radiocarpal joints (Rettig & Raskin, 2000). After cast removal, a wrist immobilization orthosis with a circumferential design may offer the most protection for the athlete while they begin to progress through the later stages of rehabilitation. A custom bivalved or zipper-type orthosis may be used for initial return to practice and conditioning as well as transition to return to play with padding (Fig. 22–11A,B). Returning to full sport participation depends on the sport-specific requirements and the demands placed on the healing extremity. For example, a soccer player (except the goalie) may be able to return to play before a football player because of the individual upper extremity demands of the sports.

Scaphoid

A scaphoid fracture in sports can occur with a fall on an outstretched arm with maximum wrist extension (football, soccer, biking). Stable nondisplaced fractures are often immobilized in either a long arm or a short arm thumb cast (Fig. 22–12), followed by orthosis application during the initial return to play (Fig. 22–4) (Rettig & Raskin, 2000). If bone healing is slow and both the physician and the athlete agree that return to a guarded level of performance may be of benefit, then a protective playing cast made from conforming cast material and external padding may be appropriate (Canelon & Karus, 1995; Rettig, 1991). In the collegiate or professional athlete, percutaneous fixation of nondisplaced scaphoid fractures may be done to facilitate early return to competition in a playing cast. Whether or not the athlete may return to play with a scaphoid fracture is controversial and depends on the sport, athlete, location of the fracture, stability of the fracture, and ability to safely participate in a cast/protective orthosis (Jaworski, Krause, & Brown, 2010).

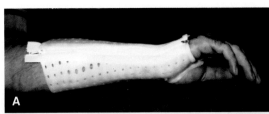

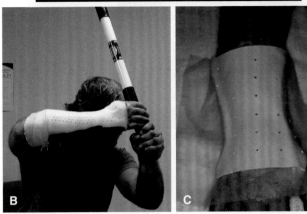

FIGURE 22–11 **A and B,** Circumferential wrist immobilization orthoses (Rolyan® AquaForm® Zippered Wrist Splint, Performance Health). **C,** Wrist immobilization orthosis—clamshell design with interlocking volar and dorsal pieces. Notice use of wet paper towel during fabrication to prevent adherence.

Thumb Metacarpal

Fracture of the base of the first metacarpal, a Bennett fracture, is often associated with a fall on a hyperextended thumb, as in a baseball player diving for a ball or sliding into a secured base. The fracture is accentuated by the strong pull of the abductor pollicis longus (APL) tendon as it inserts on the base of the first metacarpal. The athlete generally undergoes a period cast immobilization (Fig. 22–12), progressing to a return-to-sport wrist and thumb immobilization orthosis (Fig. 22–4). For unstable first metacarpal fractures in athletes, especially for the professional athlete, surgical fixation may be the treatment of choice because surgical fixation may facilitate an earlier return to play (Werner et al., 2014).

Digit Metacarpals

Fracture of the neck, shaft, or base of the metacarpal bone(s) can be sustained from blunt trauma (hit with a lacrosse stick, goalie block in soccer) and, more commonly, from punching-type sports (boxing, karate, blocking sports) (Shaftel & Capo,

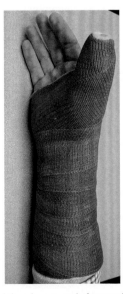

FIGURE 22–12 Wrist and thumb cast used after scaphoid fracture. IP joint may or may not be included depending on MD preference.

2014). Initially, metacarpal shaft fractures may be immobilized in a cast or orthosis including the wrist and digits (Fig. 22–13A,B). In some instances, stable metacarpal shaft fractures may be adequately treated with a simple nonarticular metacarpal immobilization orthosis (Fig. 22–13C), which traverses the involved metacarpal and adjacent structures. Often, this orthosis is supplemented with finger buddy taping to limit lateral and rotational forces across the fracture. When treating a young athlete, the therapist should consider adding the proximal phalanx within the orthosis (Fig. 22–13D,E). Including the MCP joint in the orthosis provides greater protection and stability against external forces across the proximal injury (Jaworski et al., 2010; Etier, Scillia, Tessier, & Aune, 2015).

A metacarpal neck fracture of the ring finger (RF) or small finger (SF) can be managed after cast removal with an orthosis that immobilizes the ulnar two metacarpals along with the middle finger (MF) metacarpal, positioning the MCP joints in flexion (Fig. 22–13D). Anchoring the RF and SF to the MF decreases the natural mobility in the ulnar side of the hand. Metacarpal base fractures are treated in the same manner; however, the wrist is included in the orthosis to provide optimal fracture alignment with or without the digits (Fig. 22–13B,F).

Phalangeal

Fractures of the proximal or middle phalanges are common in the athlete (Jaworski et al., 2010). Phalangeal fractures can occur in various sports, including tumbling events in gymnastics, wrestling maneuvers, football, and lacrosse. Fracture management using an orthosis depends on the location (articular vs. nonarticular), type of fracture, stability of the fracture, presence of dislocation/ligamentous injury, and need for surgical intervention. There are many options for orthotic intervention: fracture bracing (Fig. 22–14A,B), circumferential casting (Fig. 22–6A,B), restrictive orthoses (Figs. 22–3 and 22–14C,D), and buddy taping (Fig. 22–14E,F).

SPRAINS, LIGAMENTOUS INJURIES, DISLOCATIONS

Injury to ligamentous structures in the upper extremity is common in athletes. The degree of injury depends on the amount of force applied to the body part and the direction of that force on the joint. These two factors directly affect the recommended medical and orthotic intervention.

Elbow Ulnar Collateral Ligament Injuries

Medial-side elbow injuries are common in any sport requiring forceful overhead or side arm movements, for example, with baseball pitching (Fig. 22–15A). Owing to the combination of forces on the elbow during the final stages of cocking and initiation of the acceleration phase, the ulnar collateral ligament (UCL) and ulnar nerve can undergo significant microtrauma, resulting in both acute and chronic injuries, such as progressive degeneration of the UCL. Rest (immobilization in an orthosis to limit lateral stress to the elbow), followed by strengthening of the flexor pronator mass, stabilization of the proximal joints, and evaluation of throwing mechanics are the initial treatment recommendations. In chronic cases, reconstruction of the UCL may be indicated. Symptoms of ulnar neuropathy often occur simultaneously; therefore, an ulnar nerve release or transposition may be performed at the same time (Alley & Pappas, 1995). Postoperative management involves protection in a long arm orthosis immediately after surgery and initiation of gentle elbow flexion and extension 1 week later. Protection against lateral stresses is accomplished with an elbow restriction orthosis (hinged) that can allow for progressive increases in elbow mobility until the athlete achieves full ROM (Fig. 22–15B–E).

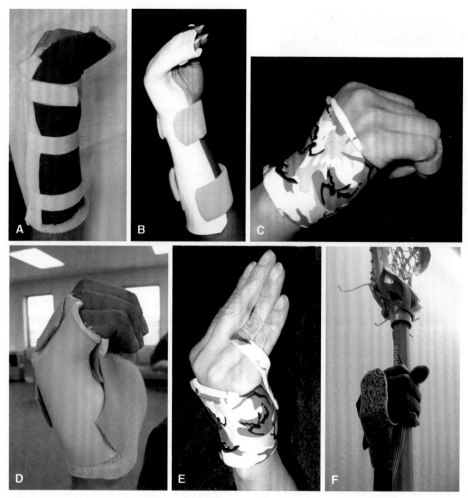

FIGURE 22–13 Various ways to immobilize a metacarpal fracture. **A,** Ulnar-based wrist and digit immobilization orthosis fabricated from Delta-Cast˚. **B,** Forearm-based design in the antideformity position. **C,** Nonarticular metacarpal orthosis with buddy taping RF/SF. **D and E,** Hand-based design with MCP joint included to further protect distal metacarpal fractures. **F,** Wrist in distal forearm-based design for lacrosse player.

Triangular Fibrocartilage Complex Tears

As the primary stabilizer of the radioulnar joint, injuries to the TFCC can result in significant disability for the athlete. Injury is often a result of a FOOSH, resulting in compression of the TFCC between the head of the ulna and the carpus or torqueing of the forearm while loaded (Rettig, 2003). This injury is seen in athletes who break a fall with the hand (gymnasts) or who undergo excessive rotational force (e.g., racket and throwing sports) (Howse, 1994). A nonsurgical or surgical approach may be taken with this population, depending on the severity of the disruption. Orthoses can be an important component of the rehabilitation plan and return to competition. Initial injury may require a rigid cast for complete immobilization. As rehabilitation progresses, a wrist immobilization orthosis can be used and weaned to a less rigid support, such as taping or neoprene orthosis. Soft supports may be appropriate to allow initiation of guarded activity with continued protection (Fig. 22–16A,B). Chapter 14 reviews the fabrication of a neoprene orthosis for this patient population and those with wrist instability.

Weight bearing forearm and wrist maneuvers seen in gymnastics and other impact sports can lead to ulnar impaction syndrome and triangular fibrocartilage ligament complex (TFCC) injuries. In ulnar impaction syndrome, typically there is swelling at the distal radioulnar joint or in the lunotriquetral joint. In TFCC injuries, the forces of impact with torsion can result in rupture of the ulnar collateral ligament or cartilage complex.

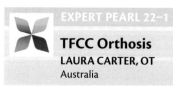

TFCC Orthosis
LAURA CARTER, OT
Australia

For TFCC injuries that are stubborn, a thermoplastic wrist cuff can be fabricated for wear under a Wrist Widget˚ (wristwidget.com). When molding, do not forget to trim the orthosis down to account for wrist flexion and extension. Using putty or padding over the ulna head and positioning in a neutral wrist position also stops aggravation over this prominence with forearm rotation.

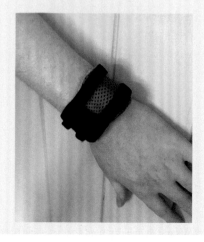

Wrist Strap for TFCC
LISA RAY, OTR/L, CHT
Virginia

Simply fabricate a homemade version of Wrist Widget* to test on patient prior to purchasing actual product. Soft foam padding and nonadhesive hook utilized and fit to wrist. This version is not as durable as product purchased through wristwidget.com but can be helpful in identifying patients that would benefit from the more permanent device.

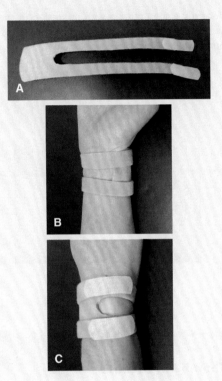

Distal Ulna Instability

Distal ulna instability can be acute or chronic in nature. Acute instability is often associated with a fracture of the ulna styloid and disruption of the TFCC. Treatment of this type of injury may be surgical or may require 6 weeks of cast immobilization. Millard, Budoff, Paravic, and Noble (2002) evaluated the effect of both prefabricated commercial braces and custom-made braces on joint stability and was documented by computed tomography. Both braces markedly reduced DRUJ translation in both full pronation and full supination and suggested that functional forearm bracing may be effective in reducing instability of the DRUJ without greatly restricting motion of the wrist, forearm, or elbow. Chronic instability often results from a late diagnosis after a "wrist sprain" (common with gymnasts and snowboarders). Treatment of these injuries is generally surgical and involves a period of immobilization after surgery. After using a wrist immobilization orthosis, a soft support such as therapeutic taping, neoprene, or custom nonarticular orthosis may be recommended to aid in the transition from practice to competition (Monasterio & Brou, 2007) (Fig. 22–17A,B). Of note, the Monasterio DRUJ Stability orthosis is a good support for contact impact sports as well as martial arts.

Wrist Instability

Carpal instability is associated with attenuation of the ligamentous support in the carpus and can often be seen with club sports (baseball, lacrosse, golf, polo) requiring wrist deviation along with rotation of the forearm. Midcarpal instability often presents with a trivial injury or no injury at all, clinically presenting with a painful wrist and spontaneous "clunk." The laxity of the extrinsic stabilizing ligament of the wrist can lead to a carpal instability (Lichtman & Wroten, 2006). Management includes the fabrication of a pisiform boost orthosis (Skirven & DeTullio, 2006), a carpal instability nondissociative orthosis (Staines, Konduris, & O'Brien, 2003; O'Brien, 2013), or ulnar wrist support (Chinchalkar & Yong, 2004) (Fig. 22–18A–D). These orthoses are designed to stabilize the extrinsic ligaments of the carpus and are used in conjunction with activity modification and strengthening exercises.

Scapholunate Instability

It has become clear that the stability of the scapholunate joint is not dependent wholly upon the scapholunate interosseous ligament but rather upon both primary and secondary stabilizers, which form a scapholunate ligament complex. Each diagnosis of scapholunate instability is unique and therefore should be treated with tissue-specific repairs, which may partly explain why a single procedure cannot successfully restore joint stability in every case. Not all lunotriquetral ligament tears are traumatic. The optimal treatment of symptomatic tears is still uncertain. Wrist arthroscopy has a pivotal role in both the assessment and treatment of these derangements.

In recent years, the use of a dart thrower's orthosis has come into favor during early phase one and two rehabilitation (Anderson & Hoy, 2016) (Fig. 22–19A,B). Orthotic intervention incorporating the dart thrower's motion has become a part of conservative management guidelines for treatment of scapholunate injury (Tang, Gu, Xu, & Gu, 2011; Bergner, Farrar, & Coronado, 2020). While this orthosis is functional for rehabilitation, it is not a return to play orthosis. The return to play will require either a cast with padding or a 1/8″ thermoplastic orthosis. Once the instability has been stabilized, taping or neoprene supports are beneficial during competition.

Darth Thrower's Motion Orthosis
JOANNA JOURDAN, OT
Germany

Allows radial extension and ulnar flexion in the wrist. This limits and minimizes movement of the proximal carpal bone row. May be used in early controlled motion after injuries to the proximal carpal row. Utilizes thumb nuts to create moveable hinge and uncoated thermoplastic to allow for easy bonding.

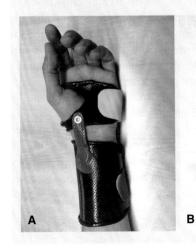

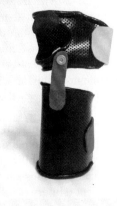

A   **B**

Wrist Hinge
KIMBERLY GOLDIE STAINES, OTR, CHT
Texas

When fabricating a wrist/thumb orthosis to allowing flexion/extension and restrict radial/ulnar deviation (DeQuervain or scaphoid fracture)—an Aquatube (Performance Health) can be heated in the center using a heat gun and crimped with needle nose pliers to make a simple, strong wrist hinge.

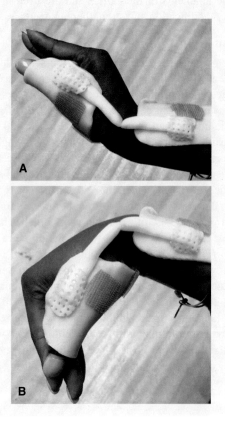

Thumb MP Joint Injury

Thumb MP joint sprain most often occurs from forceful thumb MP hyperextension, resulting in MP volar dislocation. In addition, lateral forces at the MP joint can disrupt the collateral ligaments, resulting in joint instability. A UCL sprain, also known as gamekeeper's or skier's thumb, occurs commonly in sports after a fall onto the hand with the thumb in abduction, such as when gripping a ski pole or racquet (Melone, Beldner, & Basuk, 2000) (Fig. 22–20A). Orthoses are commonly used to place the ligament in a stress-free, shortened position while healing occurs (Fig. 22–20B–D). As with other ligamentous injuries, a range of damage can occur, from a midsubstance tear to an avulsion fracture where the ligament inserts on the thumb proximal phalanx. In a pure ligamentous injury, a Stenar lesion can occur (the adductor is interposed between the UCL and its insertion). A rotated fracture or a Stenar lesion is generally an indication for surgery (Badia & Khanchandani, 2011; Baskies & Lee, 2009; Melone et al., 2000). Patients who require surgery usually undergo a period of postoperative immobilization in a thumb cast progressing to an immobilization orthosis that can be used for protection during sport to prevent reinjury (Little & Jacoby, 2011). Radial collateral

ligament (RCL) disruptions can also occur, but those injuries are much less common. Injury to the RCL is also managed with a thumb immobilization orthosis with weaning to taping or a neoprene restriction orthosis for return to competition.

Early Active Motion Orthosis
BOB PHILLIPS, OTR/L, CHT
Georgia

Designed for early guided motion with protection to the thumb MP joint after a UCL injury/repair. Provides support, preventing radial/ulnar directed motion while allowing flexion/extension.

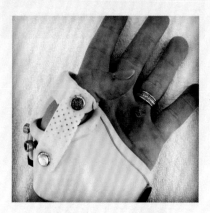

Thumb MP Orthosis
DIANE COKER, PT, DPT, CHT
California

When fabricating a thumb orthosis for an MP collateral injury or post surgery, it may be useful to add a side buttress to prevent stress to the healing ligament. Often the distal border of the thumb ends up a bit lower than what would offer MP joint stability, or there is commonly too much laxity in the thumb hole itself. Add a radial buttress for a UCL injury, or an ulnar buttress for an RCL injury.

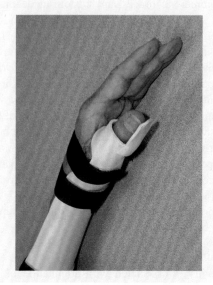

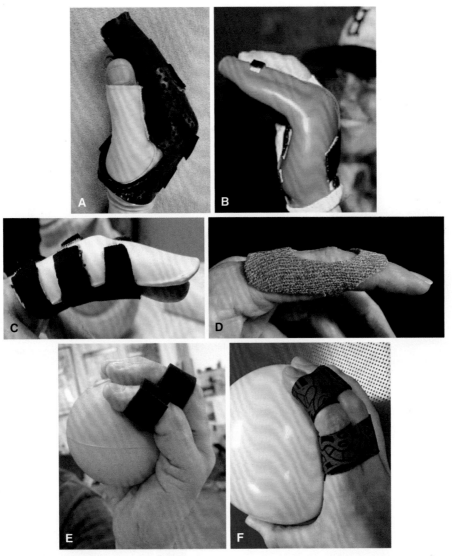

FIGURE 22–14 A, Hand-based index finger (IF) and MF orthosis for proximal phalanx fracture; notice edema glove used beneath. **B,** Hand-based SF orthosis for proximal phalanx fracture—RF included for increased stability and protection for this active athlete. **C,** PIP joint extension restriction orthosis for volar plate avulsion fracture—strapping can easily be removed for active flexion exercises if permitted. **D,** Alternative PIP extension restriction design for a volar plate avulsion fracture—Orficast® utilized to form this low-profile design. **E,** Buddy taping of RF and SF can be challenging because of the difference in the length of the digits. Custom straps to accommodate for this difference are necessary to allow unrestricted joint motion. **F,** Therapeutic taping can also offer a low profile, easy to don/doff option—Dynamic Tape shown here.

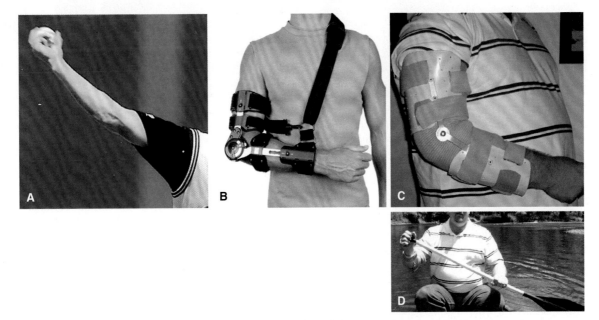

FIGURE 22–15 A, Pitching places tremendous stress on the medial structures about the elbow. Note the prominence of the ulnar nerve at the medial elbow. **B,** Innovator X® Post-Op Elbow has a user-friendly hinge allowing for easy adjustments of ROM restrictions. (Photo courtesy of Össur® Americas, Inc., Reykjavik, Iceland.) **C and D,** Custom orthosis utilizing Phoenix Elbow Hinge (Performance Health) preventing lateral stress during club sports such as rowing.

CHAPTER 22

Thumb Pad
KIMBERLY GOLDIE STAINES, OTR, CHT
Texas

This can be used with any grip irritation at the ulnar thumb, first web space, or index radial MP (the web side/ulnar side of pad is wider than the radial side). In sports, it is designed for batters during practice and can also be used in golf or gardening gloves. Simply tape or use cohesive bandage to secure to area. This device can be purchased premade at most sporting stores or handmade using 1/8″ neoprene. Patients may benefit from having more than one at their disposal due to sweating during activity.

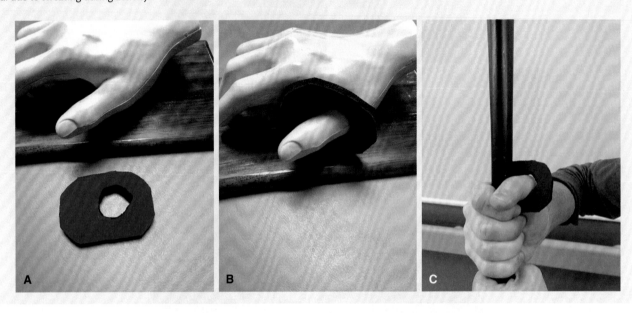

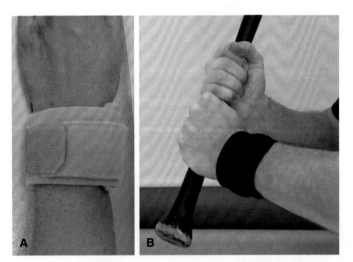

FIGURE 22–16 **A,** Custom nonarticular distal forearm orthosis (using hook, loop, and padding) to stabilize the distal radioulnar joint (DRUJ) for impact activities such as biking, cheerleading, and gymnastics. **B,** Prefabricated orthosis for stabilization of the TFCC while allowing wrist extension in this baseball player—shown is "Squeeze" Ulnar Compression Wrap from Hely & Weber.

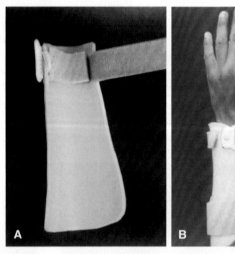

FIGURE 22–17 **A and B,** Modified Anti-Pronation DRUJ Instability Orthosis—custom design using strapping to stabilize ulnar head—allows for hand and elbow (Monasterio & Brou, 2007).

CMC Dislocation

Presenting in both chronic and acute settings, CMC dislocations, particularly of the index and middle fingers, are a common problem when the hand is used for combat sports. Surgical intervention is typically indicated with the use of percutaneous pinning and/or CMC arthrodesis. A wrist orthosis may be used immediately after surgery and a circumferentially designed hand-based CMC orthosis for return to training (Fig. 22–20B). Taping techniques are often helpful with return to competition.

Prevention of hand injuries in martial arts includes four main concepts: hand and wrist wraps/taping, modification to glove padding and design, proper striking technique/form, and proper global conditioning (Drury, Lehman, & Rayan, 2017).

Sagittal Band Injury

The term "Boxer's Knuckle" is used interchangeably to describe an injury to either the sagittal bands resulting in pain or instability of the extensor tendon as it traverses the MCP joint or dorsal MCP joint capsule (Drury et al., 2017). The injury more often impacts the middle finger MCP as this is the most common

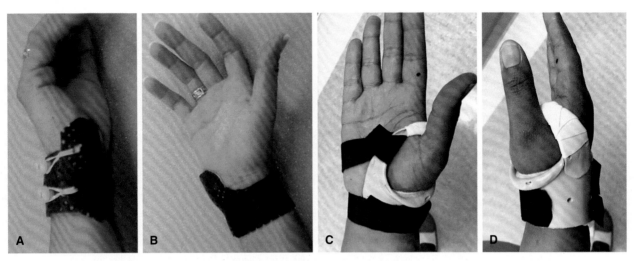

FIGURE 22–18 **A and B,** "Pisiform boost" and **C and D,** CIND (carpal instability nondissociative) orthoses for midcarpal instability will allow wrist extension while stabilizing the ulnar side of the carpus. Note the use of neoprene in C&D as the counterforce, anchoring the volar and dorsal segments.

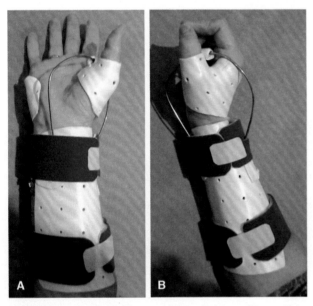

FIGURE 22-19 **A and B,** Dart Thrower Orthosis which is used for retraining after scapholunate ligament reconstruction and can be used to address chronic wrist instability as well.

point of impact and most prominent of the metacarpal heads. The injury often involves the radial side of the MCP; pain with or without extensor tendon instability. When mild, these injuries can be treated with rest through buddy taping or immobilization, but when severe surgery may be indicated (Fig. 22–14E,F). MCP dislocation is less common, they present with focal point of tenderness and often will require surgical intervention for stability. Often many patients with these injuries present months to years after the acute event making conservative treatment and prognosis poorer.

Proximal Interphalangeal Joint Injury

PIP joint dislocation can result from an axial load, lateral stress, or hyperextension force applied to the PIP joint in sports such as volleyball, basketball, soccer (primarily goalie), rock climbing, and gymnastics (Fig. 22–21A). The severity of this injury depends on the amount and direction of force applied as well as any concurrent injury such as fracture (Glickel & Barron, 2000; Little & Jacoby, 2011; Vitale, White, & Strauch, 2011). Injury can occur to a single collateral ligament, both collateral ligaments, and/or the volar plate.

If the volar plate is disrupted, then at least one of the collateral ligaments is usually involved. This injury can include an avulsion fracture of the middle phalanx associated with the volar plate (fracture dislocation of the PIP joint).

Orthosis selection is affected by the degree of injury and stability of the joint. Collateral ligament injuries may be managed with buddy taping to an adjacent digit (Fig. 22–14E,F) or a restrictive orthosis including hinge or figure-8 type (Fig. 22–21B–E); whereas volar plate involvement usually requires a dorsal-based PIP extension restriction orthosis (Fig. 22–14C). Orthotic fabrication after surgical intervention may also be necessary and should be customized to the surgical procedure (Little & Jacoby, 2011; Najarian & Lawton, 2011).

EXPERT PEARL 22–8

Figure-8 Orthosis
EMMA HIRST, OT
New Zealand

Orficast may be used for PIP joint volar plate injuries for a return to sports and eliminating hyperextension of an unstable PIP joint presurgery. After heating the material, fold in half lengthways and wrap the Orficast around the finger forming an 8. The patient should flex the PIP at this stage to approximately 20° and hold this position until the material has hardened.

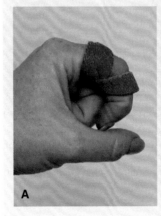

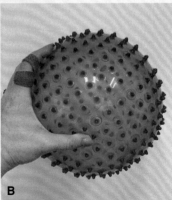

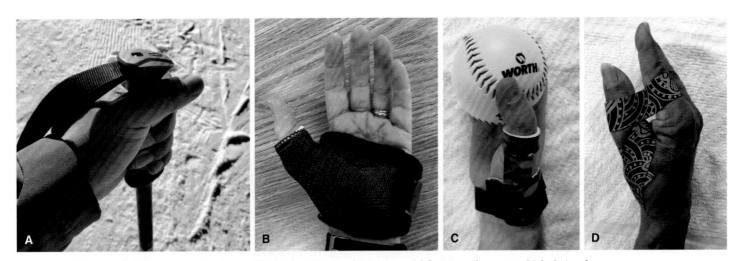

FIGURE 22-20 **A,** Holding a ski pole places the thumb MP joint at risk for injury. There are multiple designs for protection after UCL tear. For partial UCL tears, 4 weeks of full-time immobilization followed by 2 to 4 weeks of protective splint during play is recommended. **B,** Custom orthosis utilizing Delta-Cast'; **C,** dorsal thumb-based orthosis (Galindo & Lim, 2002). **D,** Taping while weaning from rigid support of the orthosis is encouraged for an additional 4 to 6 weeks (Dynamic Tape shown).

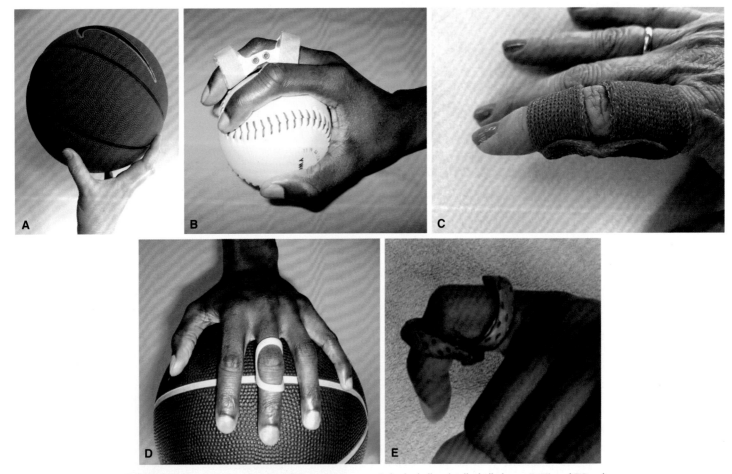

FIGURE 22–21 **A,** PIP hyperextension injuries are common in basketball and volleyball players. **B,** Hinged PIP orthosis prevents lateral stress to healing ligaments. **C,** Custom version utilizing Orficast' with rolled/crimped material to form hinges. **D,** PIP extension restriction orthosis prevents hyperextension stress while playing sports—Oval-8' Finger Splint shown (3-Point Products'). **E,** Custom orthosis utilizing 1/16″ elastic-based material to form more intimate fit also allowing for precise restriction of motion.

Distal Interphalangeal Joint Injury

A forceful blow to the distal finger is most often the cause of a distal interphalangeal (DIP) joint dislocation (Hritcko, 2006; Little & Jacoby, 2011). Sprain and/or dislocation of the DIP joint can occur in many sports, but these injuries are most often associated with ball-handling sports such as volleyball, basketball, and football. Thermoplastic materials, taping techniques, and silicone-lined products are a few options available for protecting an injured distal phalanx.

TENDON INJURIES

Tendon injuries can occur in any sport in which the tendon is placed in a vulnerable position (e.g., excessive force loading, forceful hyperextension, or flexion). Refer Chapters 18 and 19 for more comprehensive information regarding orthotic management for tendon injuries.

Distal Biceps Tendon Rupture

Distal biceps tendon rupture can occur after a fall on a hyperextended elbow or with a sudden eccentric load to the biceps brachii muscle during a sport such as snowboarding, rock climbing, wrestling, and bodybuilding (Bertini et al., 2011; Williams, Hang, & Bach, 1996). Athletes usually note a "pop" during the activity and present with a deformity of the upper arm (fullness in bicep area) with pain and difficulty supinating the forearm. Management of these patients can be surgical or nonsurgical. Surgical repair to preserve elbow flexion and supination strength is one option for the highly competitive athlete. Rehabilitation protocols after surgical repair of the ruptured biceps tendon depend on the method and stability of the repair. Newer protocols advocate early, restricted ROM in a hinged elbow restriction orthosis, whereas older protocols favor an extended period in an elbow immobilization orthosis. The elbow restriction orthosis allows for gradual increases in amount of allowed ROM (Fig. 22–15B). Returning to preinjury level of competition is dictated by the surgeon and may warrant several months of rehabilitation for regaining full strength for sports participation (Cohen, 2008; Morrey, 1993). More recently, postoperative care may only involve a few weeks of immobilization beginning protective active motion as early as 10 days to 2 weeks (Blackmore, 2011; Ivy & Spencer, 2011).

Bicep/Triceps Tendinosis

Tendon-specific inflammation in sports is generally characterized as acute (macrotrauma) or chronic (micro traumatic overuse, cumulative trauma, or overuse syndrome) (Bertini et al., 2011). Clinically, sport-induced soft tissue inflammation may resolve spontaneously; however, often this may become chronic and a major problem for the athlete. Excessive forces are applied to the tendon when propelling the body especially during vaulting, floor exercise, rings and weight lifting. Biceps tendinosis is seen primarily at the biceps proximal insertion and is often seen in a sport that requires repetitive overhead reaching (basketball, weight lifting) or in sports in which handheld equipment may come in contact with resistance (lacrosse, golf). Triceps tendinosis, also known as "jumper's knee" of the elbow, develops after the triceps tendon at the distal attachment to the olecranon gets irritated. This is specifically seen in sports requiring excessive forces to propel the body such as gymnastics, track and field, and snow sports (Vidal, Drakos, & Allen, 2004). The aging process contributes a tendency toward chronic soft tissue inflammation (Leadbetter, 1993). Medical management of these injuries often includes the use of nonsteroidal and steroidal anti-inflammatory treatments as well as altering the technique that causes inflammation of the specific structure. In addition, orthotics and bicep/triceps counterforce strapping can off-load the inflamed area to limit fraying and inflammation while allowing return to play, much as a Cho-Pat™ strap is used for patellar tendon inflammation (Fig. 22–22).

Epicondylosis

Injury to the muscles and tendon origins at both the medial and lateral elbow and are seen in a variety of athletes. Repetitive microtrauma to either the wrist extensor mass (lateral epicondylosis—"tennis elbow") or the flexor pronator mass (medial epicondylosis—"golfer's elbow") can result in injury, ranging from acute inflammation to chronic degeneration and fibroblastic changes (Ciccotti, Schwartz, & Ciccotti, 2004; Fedorczyk, 2011; Whaley & Baker, 2004) (Fig. 22–23A). In boating, fishing, water polo, and diving, these microtraumas can develop to a tendinosis and limit access to sport. Management of these injuries focuses on rest (refraining from the sport), nonsteroidal anti-inflammatory drugs (NSAIDs), and/or injection (corticosteroid, platelet-rich plasma or prolotherapy) (Sanchez, Anitua, Orive, Mujika, & Andia, 2009). Wrist orthosis use or therapeutic taping (Fig. 22–23B) to decrease activity of the involved muscle-tendon units may be beneficial, including the use of a nonarticular

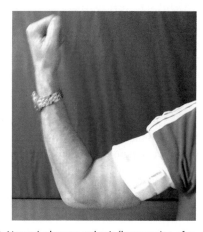

FIGURE 22–22 Nonarticular arm orthosis (large version of counterforce brace) used to off-load the bicep for management of tendinosis.

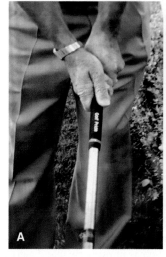
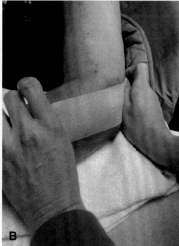

FIGURE 22–23 A, When treating a golfer or tennis player with elbow pain, the therapist should critique technique as well as equipment. **B,** Therapeutic taping is one intervention that can improve muscular symptoms and provide low-profile support.

forearm orthosis (counterforce strap) (Borkholder, Hill, & Fess, 2004; Meyer, Pennington, Haines, & Daley, 2002; Struijs et al., 2001) (Fig. 22–10A,B). At times a more elaborate hinged elbow support may need to be fabricated to limit the valgus stress to the arm and encouraged decreased stress on the involved tissues during practice and competition. It is important for the athlete and therapist to determine the factors that may be contributing to the development of the condition (grip size, equipment tension, and technique). Although the orthosis may decrease the advancement of the microtrauma and allow for tissue healing, appropriate activity changes should be made to deter recurrence.

Medial epicondylosis occurs when the club strikes the ground before the ball, which would propel the energy from the handle of the club into the elbow and hamate region. This can also cause a hook of hamate fracture as discussed previously. The differences between various racquet sports can cause dramatic differences in the tissues involved and the injury management. While tennis requires a stiff wrist with frequent overhead reach, sports such as squash and racquetball use a quick snapping motion and a smaller racquet (shorter lever arm) for impact. Olecranon impingement can also be seen with poor racquet or club mechanics. This can result in pain at the olecranon fossa of the humerus. Loose bodies may form that can cause pain, swelling, restrict motion and may cause locking of the elbow.

Extensor Carpi Ulnaris Tenosynovitis

The ECU tendon is a prime muscle providing wrist extension and ulnar deviation. ECU tenosynovitis can occur in athletes who participate in racket, stick, and rowing sports because of the repetitive ulnar deviation involved in these activities. Management consists of rest, evaluation of equipment, and technique modification. The wrist should be positioned in extension and slight ulnar deviation in order to off-load the ECU tendon (Fig. 22–24). The athlete should be transitioned from immobilization to a conditioning program once the inflammation and pain have been controlled.

Intersection Syndrome

Intersection syndrome is inflammation or tenosynovitis at the junction of the first and second dorsal compartments of the wrist (Servi, 1997). Intersection syndrome most often occurs from overuse of the radial wrist extensors, for example, in skiing when the pole is pulled from deep snow. It may also be seen in weight lifters, rowers, and indoor racket sport players (Servi, 1997). Signs and symptoms include tenderness, crepitus, and swelling over the dorsal radial aspect of the forearm. Crepitation, or squeaking, may be noted with active wrist extension or passive motion. Treatment is similar to that for DeQuervain tenosynovitis: orthoses, NSAIDs, and activity/equipment modification. Orthosis use should incorporate the wrist positioned in extension, usually with the thumb left free to move (Fig. 22–24). Care should be taken not to irritate the median nerve by positioning the wrist in extreme extension (>30°).

Radial Styloid Tenosynovitis

Radial styloid (DeQuervain) tenosynovitis involves the tendon and synovial sheath of two thumb muscles: the extensor pollicis brevis (EPB) and the APL. These tendons share a common tendon sheath (first dorsal compartment) and can become inflamed when there is too much friction within the sheath as a result of activities requiring grip with wrist deviation such as improperly using a golf club or racquetball racket (Fig. 22–23A). Radial styloid tenosynovitis is an overuse injury that can be caused by a tight grip on the club as well as radial and ulnar deviation of the wrist during

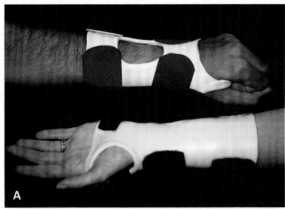
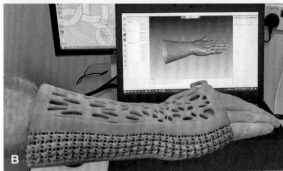

FIGURE 22–24 **A,** A wrist immobilization orthosis is commonly used to treat tendonitis about the wrist, forearm, and elbow regions. Note the position can be modified for the specific wrist condition. **B,** 3-D printed orthosis.

swing. A direct blow to this area can also result in an acute onset of radial styloid tenosynovitis. Pain occurs with ulnar deviation of the wrist with thumb flexion (Finkelstein test) and most often radiates proximally along the thumb column into the forearm. Management is similar to other tendinopathies, including rest (orthoses and activity modification), NSAIDs, anti-inflammatory injection, and activity/equipment modification. The appropriate orthosis for this condition is one that immobilizes the wrist and thumb such as a wrist and thumb immobilization orthosis (Fig. 22–2A, and 22–4). Taping and soft orthosis use can also be considered (Fig. 22–25).

Flexor Digitorum Profundus Avulsion

Flexor digitorum profundus (FDP) avulsion (jersey finger) usually occurs when a player grabs the jersey of another player and gets the fingertip caught in the uniform while the opposing player continues forward momentum, most commonly seen in the RF FDP tendon (Allan, 2011; Stamos & Leddy, 2000) (Fig. 22–26). This is a severe injury requiring surgical intervention to restore FDP function and should be managed according to the treating physician's flexor tendon protocol (see Chapter 19 for details). For professional athletes and promising collegiate athletes, the option to not repair the ruptured tendon may be considered. The athlete may require taping of the digits upon return to sport. Postseason or at the end of the athlete's career, secondary tendon repair options or a DIP fusion may be considered.

Extensor Tendonitis

This is also known as "abused karate hand," a chronic condition described as a hypertrophic infiltrative tendonitis of the long finger extensor tendon secondary to impact from various martial arts moves (Drury et al., 2017). Treated similar to a trigger finger with rest, tendon gliding and resting orthosis at night, with buddy taping during the day (Fig. 22–14E,F).

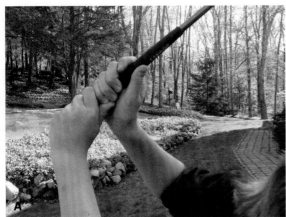

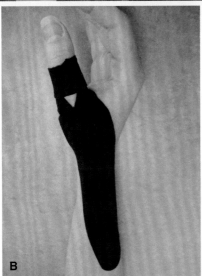

FIGURE 22-25 **A,** Assessment of golf swing in regard to wrist deviation is essential. **B,** Therapeutic taping is a low-profile way to address symptoms without the bulk of an orthosis.

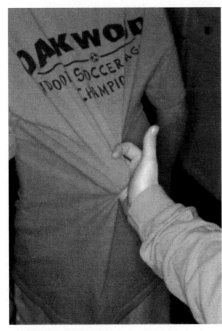

FIGURE 22-26 If a player has a finger stuck in an opponent's jersey, the DIP joint will be forced to flex strongly as the opponent continues to run, possibly resulting in an FDP rupture.

Acute Boutonniere Injury

Rupture of the extensor mechanism at the PIP joint can result in flexion posturing of the PIP, a boutonniere deformity, owing to rupture of the insertion of the central tendon and volar migration of the lateral bands (Scott, 2000) (Fig. 22–27A). These injuries can occur from a fall or from striking the hand against another player or athletic equipment. Immobilization of the PIP joint in extension for 6 to 8 weeks is necessary for conservative management of these injuries. Various orthoses can be used to achieve this goal. In most cases, the DIP joint is left free for ROM to encourage and facilitate gliding of the lateral bands dorsally. Orthosis use may be continued throughout the rest of the sport season as a precautionary measure (Marino & Lourie, 2012) (Fig. 22–27B–E).

Mallet Injury

Mallet finger injuries are common in ball sports such as baseball, basketball, and football (Yeh & Shin, 2012). It is usually a result of forced hyperflexion of an extended finger on a ball or direct contact with another player (Fig. 22–28A). The middle, ring, and small fingers are the most frequently involved digits. The athlete typically presents with a flexed posture at the DIP joint and impaired active extension (extension lag). Wehbe and Schneider have advocated nonsurgical management of closed mallet fractures with large fracture fragments, even with volar subluxation of the distal phalanx. The authors found that subluxated mallet fractures will heal and remodel the DIP joint articular surface with preservation of the joint space.

Immobilization of the DIP joint in full extension may prevent optimal play for athletes, and some may opt to delay treatment or for no treatment at all. Effective treatment for stable, closed mallet finger injuries involves full-time orthosis for at least 6 to 8 weeks followed by nighttime orthosis of a similar duration (Simpson et al., 2001). Athletes are expected to adhere strictly to the full treatment course and continue with immobilization during strenuous activity including return to training/play. Orthosis use during training and play runs the risk of maceration, loss of immobilization, and injury to other joints. During immobilization, consider including the adjacent joints in the orthosis, using a circumferential cast (QuickCast), and buddy taping to limit risk of injury to PIP and MCP joints. Also, the use of Dynamic Tape or Kinesiotape in conjunction with the orthosis or cast can dramatically decrease the risk of maceration (McMurtry & Isaacs, 2015; Hovgaard & Klareskov, 2005) (Fig. 22–11B–F).

If the player cannot tolerate the external orthosis or is unable to maintain the immobilization through the entire 8 weeks period due to the demands of his/her positions, an alternative is internal fixation by percutaneous pinning (contraindicated in play but acceptable for training with digit cast or orthosis) also for at least 6 weeks. However, there is a risk for another jamming injury that could break the pin in the joint or for pin migration. Following discontinuation of immobilization, players are permitted to return to play and to resume ball handling as tolerated. Athletes must be aware that even with strict compliance to orthotic wear, a residual 5- to 10-degree extensor lag and dorsal joint prominence may be present. Without treatment, permanent flexion deformity, swan-neck deformity, or DIP joint osteoarthritis can develop.

Chronic mallet deformities, categorized as more than 4 weeks from injury, may be successfully treated with an extension orthosis even several weeks after the injury (Chauhan et al., 2014). Swan-neck deformity is characterized by hyperextension of the PIP joint

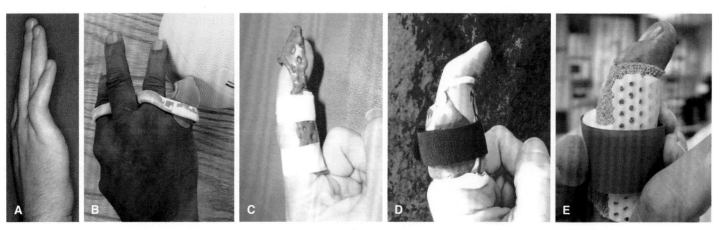

FIGURE 22–27 A, Posturing of digit with disruption of the central tendon overlying the PIP joint. **B,** Relative motion flexion orthosis and edema sleeve are used to address injury to small finger. **C,** PIP joint immobilization orthosis allowing DIP motion to mobilize the lateral bands. **D,** Digit immobilization orthosis ("drop out" design); note the DIP is in slight flexion while the PIP is held in extension for correction of deformity. **E,** Volar design with foam over PIP joint to assist with maintaining full PIP extension. Notice use of Coban wrap for edema.

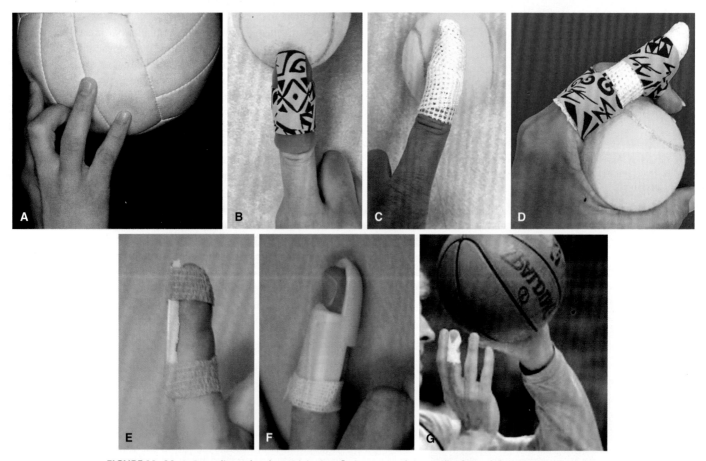

FIGURE 22–28 A, Force directed at the DIP joint into flexion can result in a mallet finger deformity. Various types of orthoses can be used for mallet finger management: **B,** Thin thermoplastic material; **C and D,** QuickCast 2 material (Performance Health); **E,** Prefabricated orthosis such as AlumaFoam® or **F,** traditional Stax; **G,** Protective taping is another option for return to play with a chronic injury.

and flexion of the DIP joint. It can result from failed treatment of mallet finger injuries and is more common in athletes with a hyperextensible PIP joint. A trial of immobilizing the DIP in extension and the PIP in flexion for 4 to 6 weeks can be initiated. Adjustments to the orthosis are made as the deformity begins to correct itself.

The duration of wear may be switched to part-time or nighttime use for maintenance. If there is a persistent deformity after nonoperative treatment of chronic mallet deformities, tendon rebalancing with a central slip tenotomy or spiral oblique retinacular ligament (SORL) reconstruction can be considered (Chauhan et al., 2014).

Mallet Orthosis

EMMA HIRST, OT
New Zealand

Consider longer design with the DIP in extension/slight hyperextension and the PIP flexed to 15° to 20° when patient presents with PIP hyperextension along with mallet injury. Orthosis will restrict PIP hyperextension and ensure the orthosis stays in the correct position.

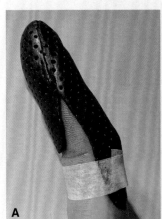

Anti-Swan Mallet Orthosis

ERFAN SHAFIEE, OT
Canada

Can be used in chronic and acute mallet finger patients who have developed swan-neck deformity. May be used for initial few weeks of immobilization and then modified to typical DIP orthosis. Orficast used here—easy to mold into desired position.

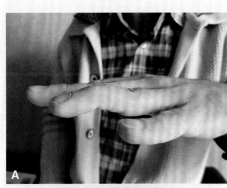

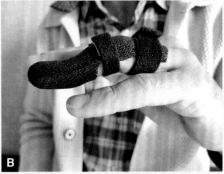

Other Soft Tissue Injuries

Overuse injuries in athletes can result from repetitive microtrauma that leads to inflammation of the involved muscle-tendon units and local tissue irritation and/or damage. These injuries are most likely to occur when an athlete changes the mode, intensity, or duration of training. Soft tissue injuries can occur from a single traumatic event or from repetitive stress due to overtraining. Soft tissue injuries can be managed not only with orthotic intervention, but consideration should be given to other materials such as taping and neoprene. These alternative materials can play a significant role in allowing healing while even returning to light activity.

Olecranon Bursitis

The olecranon bursa is a fluid-filled sac at the posterior elbow that may become inflamed from pressure or a direct blow to the olecranon process, with resultant olecranon bursitis. This is sometimes seen in golfers with repeated grounding of the club or during athletic competition from direct blows sustained to this region from a piece of playing equipment (hockey stick, baseball bat, tennis racket). Treatment options include aspiration, cortisone injection, edema control techniques, and the use of a soft compressive orthosis such as a soft elbow protective pad (Heelbo®) (Fig. 22–29). Return to sport is recommended when the athlete can use the piece of sporting equipment with adequate force and no pain. Weight bearing should be performed painlessly before returning to any sport requiring such maneuvers (e.g., gymnastics).

Wrist Ganglion

Dorsal wrist ganglia, although benign, can cause limitation in motion, endurance, and strength for athletes involved in impact sports. Because activity can cause the ganglion cyst to get larger, it may help to temporarily immobilize the area with a brace or orthosis (Fig. 22–24). As the cyst shrinks, it may release the pressure on nerves, relieving pain. Upon return to closed chain weight bearing or wrist deviation sporting tasks, a wrist tape support or neoprene support may be indicated (Fig. 22–30). Clinicians should be aware of other diagnoses that can replicate the presentation of a ganglion or occult ganglion cyst. The carpal boss is an osseous overgrowth that is occasionally mistaken for a ganglion cyst. The patients would be treated with rest and a wrist brace.

Hypothenar Hammer Syndrome

Athletes exposed to blunt trauma to the hands, for example, catchers in baseball, are at risk for injury to the ulnar artery called hypothenar hammer syndrome. This can result in ischemia to one or more digits depending on the athlete's palmar arch configuration. Use of custom padding (doughnut-shaped) in the glove to minimize trauma and vibration may be necessary to alleviate symptoms (Mueller, Mueller, Degreif, & Rommens, 2000) (Fig. 22–31). For the cyclist, handlebar and positional alterations may be necessary to complement the device dispensed.

Pisotriquetral Joint Synovitis

Pisotriquetral joint synovitis, or degeneration between the pisiform and triquetrum, can cause pain with activities that require gripping or pressure along the volar ulnar aspect of the palm, such as batting, gymnastics, and field sports. Arthritic changes in this joint can be an indication for pisiform excision. A gel-lined or cushioned orthosis may be helpful to protect this area from direct trauma during competition (Fig. 22–32).

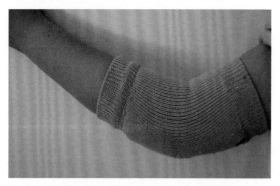

FIGURE 22–29 Soft elbow pad can be placed over posteriorly to prevent contact stress to the olecranon bursa.

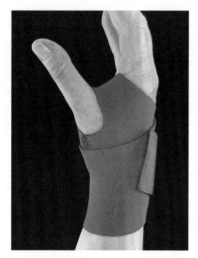

FIGURE 22–30 AliMed® Neoprene Wrist/Hand Wrap provides restriction of motion and light protection. (Photo courtesy of AliMed® (Dedham, MA).)

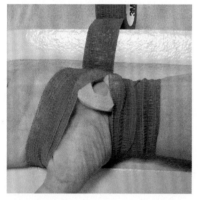

FIGURE 22–31 Padding to off-load pressure on hypothenar area applied with adhesive elasticized wrap; low profile to fit inside a glove. Custom fabricating an insert using neoprene and padding would provide a more permanent solution.

NERVE INJURIES

Sport-related nerve injuries are not as common as the bony and soft tissue injuries described previously. Many sports activities lead to compression and direct trauma to the nerves of the upper extremity. Refer Chapter 20 for more comprehensive information regarding orthotic management for nerve injuries.

Ulnar Nerve

Injury to the ulnar nerve in athletes most commonly occurs either at the elbow (cubital tunnel syndrome) or in the hand at Guyon canal (handlebar or cyclist palsy) (Kennedy, 2008; Wichmann & Martin,

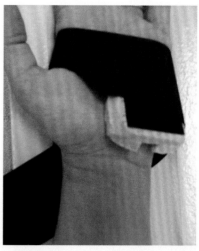

FIGURE 22–32 Soft padding secured to hand via hook and loop to protect the inflamed region and reduce pressure on the pisiform.

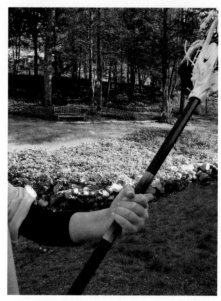

FIGURE 22–33 Custom restrictive elbow orthosis fabricated from neoprene for this lacrosse player to limit elbow extension and medial stress at elbow with cradling and throwing.

1996). Ulnar neuropathy at the elbow is often seen in throwing athletes secondary to the significant valgus stretch placed on the elbow and its surrounding soft tissue structures during the late cocking and acceleration phases of the pitch (Fig. 22–15A). In professional and collegiate athletes, ulnar nerve release or transposition surgery is often the treatment of choice. Orthosis use after surgery depends on the type of procedure and involvement of other structures (UCL reconstruction). Often, an elbow immobilization orthosis with the wrist included is fabricated for use during the early phases of rehabilitation. Transition to a soft elbow pad (Fig. 22–29), a neoprene restrictive orthosis, or taping can be used for return to competition in order to limit extension and valgus extremes (Fig. 22–33).

Compression of the ulnar nerve at Guyon canal is seen most commonly in cycling but can be seen in other sports in which the ulnar wrist is exposed to excessive pressure or sustained extreme wrist extension. Positioning and pressure of the hands on the handlebars in cycling is usually the biomechanical cause of injury. Clinical management consists of making adjustments to the type and position of the handlebars as well as use of padded cycling gloves or custom orthoses (Slane, Timmerman, & Ploeg, 2011) (Fig. 22–34A–C).

EXPERT PEARL 22–11

Padded Elbow Sleeve
LISA RAY, OTR/L, CHT
Virginia

Elasticized sleeve to provide for padding over prominent elbow hardware, olecranon, or ulnar nerve sensitivity at medial elbow. Use sleeves wider than needed to accommodate padding to prevent excessive pressure. Apply foam first after beveling edge (Temper Foam shown, Performance Health), then larger piece of thin liner piece to "seal" in. Position on arm overlying target area to relieve pressure.

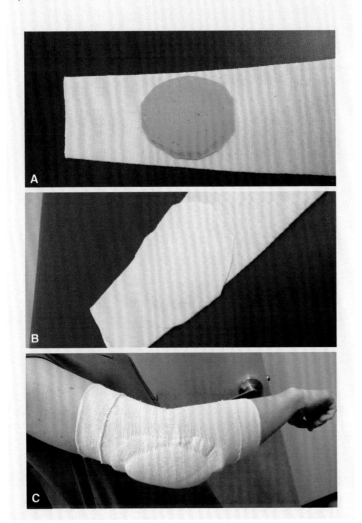

Median Nerve

Neuropathy of the median nerve at the wrist (CTS—carpal tunnel syndrome) can have a significant effect on the athlete's performance. Many sports run the risk of CTS including impact sports and those with tool use, custom gloves can be a great resolution with or without thermoplastic support. In horse racing, polo, and professional baseball, custom gloves by Dr. Harold Kleinert have shown dramatic improvement in the reports of symptoms (Fig. 22–35A,B). Nighttime use of a wrist immobilization orthoses, with the wrist positioned in neutral, is the initial conservative management for carpal tunnel syndrome (Fig. 22–24). Again, modification to the activity and equipment should be evaluated.

Pronator syndrome, or entrapment of the median nerve proximally, can occur at several sites, including the pronator teres, lacertus fibrosis, and proximal portion of the flexor digitorum superficialis (Servi, 1997). An arm- or forearm-based orthosis as well as activity modification may be helpful to place the structures at rest (Fig. 22–24). Techniques such as taping and soft orthoses offer an alternative to more restrictive orthoses and often can be used to transition back to play.

Radial Nerve

Acute trauma to the radial nerve can occur at multiple locations along its course, commonly at the spiral groove of the humerus or in the proximal forearm. Compression of the radial nerve, radial tunnel syndrome, can occur where the nerve enters the intermuscular septum or at the radial tunnel. These injuries are uncommon in sports but may be seen in athletes who perform repetitive pronation and supination (Jebsib & Engber, 1997; Long, 1995; Stanley, 2006) such as racquet sports, gymnastics, and field sports. An arm- or forearm-based orthosis that limits rotation may be helpful to place the structures at rest (Fig. 22–24).

Digital Nerves

One of the most common sites of neuropathy in the digital nerves is the thumb of bowlers (Sweet, Kroonen, & Weiss, 2011; Wright & Rettig, 1995). "Bowler's thumb" is a painful neuroma that can develop at the point where the thumb grips and releases the ball. Widening the size of the thumbhole in the bowling ball may be necessary to decrease pressure on the nerve. The use of padding, taping, or a gel sleeve at the base of the thumb may be useful for management of this condition (Fig. 22–36).

SPORT-SPECIFIC INFORMATION

BALL AND THROWING SPORTS

Ball sports are the leading cause of hand injuries in professional athletes (Netscher, Pham, & Goldie Staines, 2013). The use of the hand for ball control and contact with the opponent leaves the fingers exposed to injury. Multiple factors must be considered such as appropriate timing of treatment, long-term functional outcome, and often the most difficult issue—return to play. Most injuries in throwing athletes occur to the medial elbow, known generally as medial tension overload. This is seen in many throwing sports but not limited to baseball, softball, football, and cricket. The medial stress on the elbow during the late cocking phase of throwing cycle can create valgus stress on the stabilizers of the elbow.

CYCLE AND WHEELED SPORTS

The compressive forces incurred by the upper extremity in wheeled and cycling sports often result from repetitive gripping, shifting, excessive vibration, and repeated or sustained reaching. With the increased popularity of motorized or powered cycles, serious injuries are becoming more frequent. The ulnar nerve in Guyon canal is particularly vulnerable with handlebar sports. Often a result of sustained gripping and impact from intensive riding, carpal tunnel syndrome is thought to be the result of sustained positioning of the wrist in cycling activities as well as from vibration during long rides. The sustained wrist extension position during rides may induce tenosynovitis and increased pressure within the carpal tunnel.

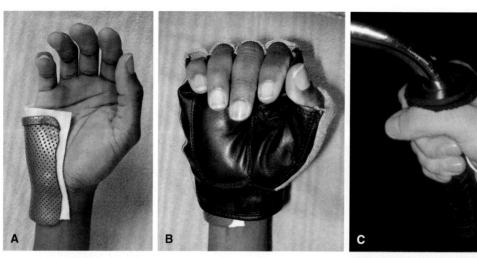

FIGURE 22–34 A and B, Custom thermoplastic insert for use under padded cycling gloves. **C,** Gel-lined options for thermoplastic material molded on the wrist of a weight lifter to reduce stress on the ulnar palm region.

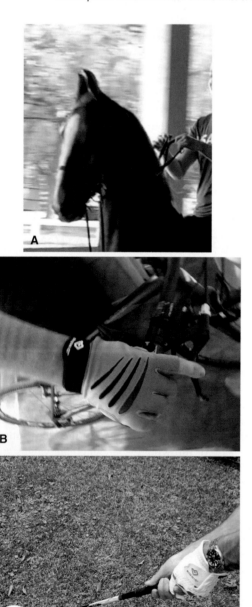

FIGURE 22–35 A, In equestrian events and other tooled sports, the sustained grasp and tension can exceed the capacity of many soft tissues in the hand. Adaptive gloves for nerve and joint protection. **B and C,** Bionic Gloves, as designed by Dr. Kleinert, have multiple specialty designs per sport (www.bionicgloves.com).

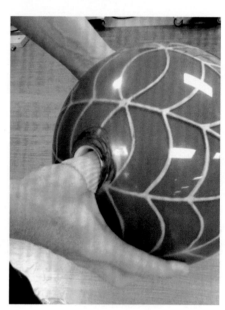

FIGURE 22–36 Note the lateral stress to the MP joint of the thumb while grasping the bowling ball. Gel-lined digit sleeves can pad the area and decrease pressure on the digital nerves.

IMPACT SPORTS

A FOOSH with the wrist in extension during the fall or with impact on another player or structure is a common cause of injury in football, rugby, gymnastics, and other sports. The resulting injuries are often fracture or dislocation. Carpal fractures and ligamentous injury can occur from sliding into bases or blocking other player momentum. Scaphoid fracture may not be easily recognized and is frequently diagnosed as a wrist sprain.

CLUB SPORTS

In baseball, hook of hamate fracture can occur from direct impact to the hypothenar eminence. The bat rests above the hamate on the butt of the hand, and the impact can cause a hook of hamate fracture. The repetitive motion of the golf swing or racquet swing and the stress of impact on the ball can lead to soft tissue injuries in the elbow, wrist, thumb, and fingers.

ADVENTURE AND GRAPPLING SPORTS

A wide variety of hand and upper extremities are reported annually in combat and grappling style sports. In 2012, a survey of martial arts participants demonstrated that 53% of upper extremity martial arts injuries occurred in the hand and wrist, followed by the shoulder and elbow at 27% and 19%, respectively (Diesselhorst et al., 2013). Combat sports can be classified into three main categories: striking sports, grappling sports, and a combination of these two types. Striking sports include boxing, kickboxing, karate, and taekwondo. Grappling sports include Brazilian jiu-jitsu and judo. Hybrids of these two styles include combinations of sticking, kicking, and grappling to achieve submission of the opponent (Drury et al., 2017). The hand and wrist injuries related to these categories are unique to the methods of combat. Diesselhorst and colleagues, in a survey of martial arts participants, found that the use of hand protection significantly reduced the likelihood of injury to the hand during participation. However, they did note slightly higher rate of injury to the elbow, forearm, and shoulder which was attributed to possible force dissipation more proximal in the limb as a result of hand and wrist protection. Other adventure activities such as rock climbing, hiking, roping, and riding sports have become increasingly popular in recent years. Hand and wrist injuries remain to highest reported among competitive climbers recognizing their susceptibility to certain injuries due to the unique biomechanical demands of grip positions for these sports (King & Lien, 2017). The predominant injury is to the finger flexor tendons or pulleys which account for 33% of all climbing injuries reported (Logan & Makwana, 2004). While these injuries are less common among the general population, they can occur with a sudden force against a flexed digit in any sport. Finally, the popularity of rugby across multiple countries has demonstrated further upper extremity injuries related to impact, throwing and grappling.

WATER SPORTS

Competitive water sports require great strength and flexibility as well as proprioception and kinesthetic sense to execute complex maneuver throughout the course of the sport (Haase, 2017). Not unlike a gymnast, a diver must maintain a high level of skills. Contact with the water accounts for a large proportion of diving injuries: 32.0% of men's portion of diving injuries and 16.2% of women's injuries according to one report (Kerr et al.,2015). Special consideration for orthotic use and tolerance become paramount in water-based sports including tissue tolerance, impedance to drag, and translation of the

orthosis while in the water. All of these issues should be especially considered in all care planning. Many water athletes use taping and strapping to support the wrist, elbow, and shoulder, the adhesion of tape can be problematic with exposure to water (Berkoff, & Boggess, 2011; Doyle, Lastayo, & Damore, 2006).

CONCLUSION

All school-aged children participate in sports, whether in gym class or as a member of the school's football team. In addition to the recreational and professional athletes, this makes for a large population at risk for an upper extremity injury. There are numerous benefits of physical activity well documented that include improved cardiopulmonary function (Braith & Stewart, 2006), glycemic control (Limke, Erbs, & Hambreacht, 2006), and psychological well-being (Lawlor & Hopker, 2001). Weight bearing structures directly affect an athlete's ability to move, overshadowing injuries to the upper extremity. The athlete moves well but may not be able to perform his or her sports. If neglected, upper extremity injuries can cause permanent damage and hinder daily activities as well as athletic performance. As such, upper extremity injuries in athletes confront therapists with often challenging situations. Complex issues such as the Houston Mystery must also be considered: in February 2019, there was a public disclosure of a medical problem with a dozen member of the University of Houston women's soccer team. Apparently after a particularly strenuous training session, a dozen members of the team were diagnosed with rhabdomyolysis and one member was hospitalized (Wojtys, 2019). While rhabdomyolysis can be diagnosed with medical tests, it is often obvious with brownish colored urine, extreme muscle soreness, weakness, and loss of ROM in the involved extremities. While this is not a common situation, it does none the less occur. With greater access to therapists without physician referral, knowledge of these complex complications specific to athletics remains very important. Although therapists are not expected to be experts on every sport, knowledge of the demands of the sport and a thorough understanding of the athlete's injury guide the therapist to appropriate orthosis selection. This chapter reviewed some of the common injuries therapists see in clinical practice and provided general guidelines for orthotic intervention.

FIELD NOTE: COLLABORATION WITH ATHLETE

Mojca (MO) Herman, MA,OTR/L, CHT
California

Through activity analysis and use of an athlete's sports equipment, a hand therapist can collaborate with an athlete in creating a tailored orthosis that both protects the healing tissue while simultaneously providing the ability to resume sport-specific components safely.

This is an example of a professional track cyclist, who was training for the Olympic Trials, sustained an injury and underwent a left triangular fibrocartilage complex (TFCC) repair. The athlete was sent to hand therapy postoperatively for custom fabrication of a Muenster orthosis. The traditional custom orthosis was fabricated; however,

the surgery and orthosis precluded the athlete from participating in any type of sport-related activities until the tissue was healed, thus removing any chance of qualifying for the Olympic team.

During the therapy visit, the athlete questioned the possibility of using a specialized stationary bike trainer in order to stay conditioned and simulate training in preparation for the Olympic Trials. This request required clearance from the referring physician; furthermore, a custom orthosis design that would allow the ability to grip the handle bars in a normal pattern, yet restrict forearm rotation to ensure the surgery was not compromised.

(Continued)

With input from the athlete, a second custom orthosis was designed for use only while riding the specialized bike on a trainer. The strategic orthosis design was a modification of the traditional orthosis whereby at the hand/wrist, the thermoplastic material was whittled away volarly to allow full grip/feel of the handlebars, but dorsally the material was extended to the metacarpophalangeal (MP) joints in order to immobilize the wrist and ensure that forearm rotation was restricted. The orthosis was further secured at the hand/wrist with a 2-inch Coban derivative.

This simple orthosis modification allowed normal "feel" for the athlete, furthermore, did not compromise the healing tissue or timelines for motion imposed by the referring physician. The athlete was able to resume sport-specific training and competition on a faster timetable because of the custom orthosis intervention.

* Permission granted by athlete to share images/case information for education purposes only

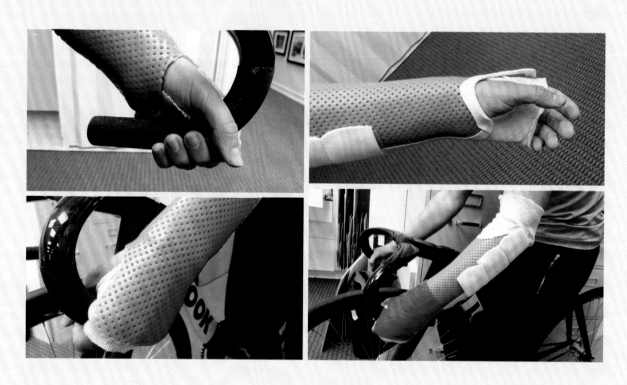

Case Study Section

The case studies presented here are meant as a teaching guideline only. Treatment and orthosis protocols vary greatly from surgeon to surgeon and from therapist to therapist. The therapist should check with the referring physicians and colleagues to define the preferred treatment and appropriate orthotic intervention.

Case Study 1: Fifth Metacarpal Fracture

RP is a 25-year-old right-handed professional hockey player. He sustained a fifth-metacarpal base fracture to his right SF during a fight. The fracture was managed by cast immobilization. The patient was referred to hand therapy at 3 weeks postinjury. RP presented with evidence of early fracture healing.

RP was placed in an ulnar wrist extension/RF-SF MCP flexion immobilization orthosis (wrist: 20° extension; MCP: 60° flexion; PIP/DIP: free) (Fig. 22–13A). He was instructed in orthosis removal for active ROM (AROM) exercises of the wrist and digits. At 4 weeks after injury, his orthosis was modified to include only the hand. The orthosis was small enough to fit into the hockey glove (Fig. 22–13D) and was used for protection during practice and, eventually, for safe return to competition.

Case Study 2: Mallet Finger

ML is a 28-year-old right hand–dominant professional baseball player. He sustained a mallet injury (rupture of the terminal extensor tendon) to his left MF while sliding into base during a game. He was immobilized for 8 weeks in a prefabricated dorsal DIP extension orthosis (Fig. 22–28F). After that time, he was referred to hand therapy for ROM and orthotic fabrication. He presented with limited DIP motion but was nontender over the dorsum of the DIP. A DIP immobilization cast orthosis that easily slid into ML's baseball glove was fabricated (Fig. 22–28C). This small orthosis allowed the patient to continue playing ball and provided him with the additional protection he needed to prevent reinjury of the newly healed terminal extensor tendon.

Case Study 3: Thumb Ulnar Collateral Ligament Injury

NA is a 34-year-old highly competitive lacrosse player who sustained a right thumb MP joint UCL avulsion injury during a game. Surgery was performed to repair the ligament using a suture anchor and percutaneous pinning. Postoperatively, he was placed in a wrist/thumb cast for 2 weeks (Fig. 22–12).

After cast removal, NA was placed in a wrist/thumb immobilization orthosis (wrist: extension; carpometacarpal [CMC]: midpalmar and radial abduction; MP: slight flexion and ulnar deviation; interphalangeal [IP] free (Fig. 22–4)) and was instructed in daily wrist and gentle thumb CMC, MP, and IP ROM exercises (avoiding MP radial deviation). The orthosis was fabricated from a 1/8-inch thermoplastic material.

At approximately 6 weeks, the orthosis was modified to allow unrestricted wrist motion. In order to return NA to play with minimal risk of reinjury, a thumb MP orthosis was fabricated out of 1/16″ thermoplastic material to be worn in a padded glove (Fig. 22–7). Both the glove and the lacrosse stick were brought to therapy for orthosis fabrication. This allowed the therapist to fabricate the orthosis to conform comfortably inside the patient's glove and to permit correct grip and control of the stick. The glove held the orthosis firmly in place so that straps were not required. Caution was used to make sure there were no jagged edges on the orthosis that would irritate the athlete's skin while playing. NA was able to return to competitive lacrosse and his job as a political cartoonist without functional deficit.

Case Study 4: Scaphoid Fracture

TB is a 30-year-old professional football player who sustained a right scaphoid fracture from a fall during practice. The patient underwent open reduction and internal fixation (ORIF) of the fracture; an interosseous compression screw was used. He was placed in a wrist/thumb cast after suture removal (Fig. 22–12).

At 4 weeks post surgery, TB was referred to therapy for a circumferential wrist/thumb immobilization orthosis with the IP joint included, along with a limited ROM program. The orthosis was made in two sections, a volar and a dorsal piece, and was fabricated out of a perforated 1/8-inch material (Fig. 22–11C). The dorsal component was added to the orthosis after the volar piece was molded and set. The therapist was careful to pad the ulnar styloid before applying the dorsal piece. This circumferential design further protected the wrist from moving dorsally out of the orthosis.

At 6 weeks, TB regained full wrist and thumb ROM. At that time, a playing cast was fabricated, which allowed the patient to return to practice and competition (Fig. 22–5A,B). He continued to use the thermoplastic orthosis for protection when not participating in football for an additional 3 weeks. The cast was used for the rest of the football season.

Case Study 5: Radial Styloid Fracture With Scapholunate Ligament Injury

Use of early controlled mobilization (ECM) approach that uses dart throwing motion (DTM) with a twist orthosis as an alternative to immobilization for conservative management of a minimally displaced and intra-articular distal radius styloid fracture with an associated scapholunate ligament injury in a 47-year-old female healthcare administrator (JP). Pain-free active DTM began at day 10 (5 times/d) with a dynamic DTM with a twist orthosis worn during the day from weeks 3 to 6 (Fig. 22–19A,B). At 6 weeks, JP had pain-free functional mobility and strength with minimal limitation in household and occupational activities, returning to her normal sporting activities by 3 months. ECM led to rapid return of normal functioning in the short term with no apparent impact on intermediate outcomes at 8 months.

CHAPTER REVIEW QUESTIONS

1. Describe the most appropriate material options for use with an athlete and explain how these options differ with other patient populations.
2. What is a playing orthosis? What must a therapist consider when fabricating one of these?
3. Describe a "jersey finger." Can the athlete return to sport after this injury? If so, when?
4. Name two common types of tendonitis in the hand and forearm. How would these diagnoses typically be managed in the athlete?
5. What is a mallet finger? What is one option to manage this so that the athlete may return to sport as quickly as possible?

ACKNOWLEDGMENT

Sincere thanks to Aida Galindo, OTR, CHT, Gerry Virtanen, OT, and Joshua Kluesner, OT, for their support in compiling this chapter.

23 Adult Neurologic Dysfunction[a]

Salvador Bondoc, OTD, OTR/L, BCPR, CHT, FAOTA

CHAPTER OBJECTIVES

After study of this chapter, the reader should be able to:
- Define terms that describe and influence the muscle and tissue response that a patient with neurological impairment may possess.
- Describe the clinical reasoning for selecting the most appropriate orthosis for a neurologically impaired patient.
- Explain the rationale for choice of orthotic materials in this patient population.
- Analyze the role orthoses can play in improving functional independence for the neurologically impaired.
- State the precautions for the use of casts, immobilization, or mobilization orthoses for this patient population.

KEY TERMS

Cerebrovascular accident
Decerebrate
Decorticate
Dependent distal edema
Dyssynergia
Elastic therapeutic tape
Flaccidity

Hyporeflexia
Hyperreflexia
Low-load prolonged stretch
Multiple sclerosis
Paresis
Postural control
Primitive reflexes
Spasticity

Spinal cord injury
Subluxed shoulder
Traumatic brain injury
Tremors
Weakness

MD NOTE

Dr. Alyse Sicklick
Connecticut

As a physiatrist working with patients with neurologically impaired upper extremities, I cannot overstate the importance of having a solid interdisciplinary/interprofessional collaboration with the rehabilitation team. One area where this collaboration is critically important is in spasticity management. In addition to medical/pharmacologic intervention, ongoing rehabilitation therapy is a key to ensure that the spasticity does not lead to pain, loss of range of motion, and disuse or nonuse of the arm and hand. A referral to an occupational therapist to provide functional training and provision of appropriate orthotic management in the upper extremity is often necessary.

FAQ

What is the recommended wearing schedule for patient with contractures due to spasticity?
There are three key factors to consider when prescribing a wearing schedule: (A) the severity of the spasticity and how it is being treated; (B) the characteristics of the contracture itself; and (C) the amount of functionality available to the contractured body part. Because of the dynamic nature of spasticity, the therapist has to factor into the schedule what makes the spasticity more pronounced (e.g., weather, emotional state, time of day, nature of activity, fatigue level, etc.) and identify periods of time when the muscle tone is more "relaxed."

---

[a]This chapter is based on the first-edition chapter written by Sue Ann Ordinetz, MS, CAS, OTR/L.

It is possible that the schedule will involve multiple shorter wearing periods versus a more prolonged single wearing period.

Secondly, determine if the contracture is musculotendinous or capsular. Shortening of the muscle creates a vicious cycle to the severity of spasticity. The more contractured a muscle is, the more sensitive the muscle is to stretch response. The goal of the wear schedule in this case is inhibition over time. Whereas in a capsular structure, the recommendation is to follow LLPS principles (refer Chapter 15 for more details). Finally, the orthotic wear should be balanced with concerns over learned nonuse or disuse. The single-most important aim for UE spasticity is restoration of function and the most effective approach is through volitional movement.

With so many conflicting literature on the risks versus benefits on the use of slings for the hemiplegic shoulder, how should I best approach this? Is it worth the time to train the patient with a sling?

In this chapter, an overview of different sling designs was presented. Table 23–1 should guide you on your decision-making based on the characteristics of your patient's upper extremity. With regards to evidence, more contemporary designs appear to fare better in terms of patient comfort, usability, functionality, and overall effectiveness to address shoulder subluxation and/or pain.

At what point it is best to discuss Botox injections (botulinum toxin A) as an option for patients with significant spasticity?

There is robust evidence that supports the use of BTA for patients that meet the inclusion criteria (i.e., where BTA is not a contraindication) throughout the stages of recovery, whether the onset is acute or chronic. Interprofessional collaboration naturally occurs in inpatient settings but should extend throughout the care continuum. In practical terms, it is good practice to include questions about medical spasticity management during the initial intake and clinically assess its effect not just on the upper extremity but in the overall function of the patient.

INTRODUCTION

This chapter addresses orthotic intervention for adults with central nervous system (CNS) disorders (Chapter 24 addresses the pediatric patient). This chapter discusses the common manifestations of neurologic dysfunction and offers the clinician guidance in clinical reasoning and problem solving when it comes to the application of an orthosis. Attempts have been made to ensure that the most current evidence is incorporated into this chapter. However, as literature on the use of orthotic devices for the neurologically impaired populations continues to emerge, the clinician is advised to keep current on this information and engage in critical reflection. Key to the success of integrating orthoses in practice is sound clinical reasoning based on evidence, theory, and assessment findings.

COMMON ADULT NEUROLOGIC CONDITIONS

Cerebrovascular accident (CVA), traumatic brain injury (TBI), spinal cord injury (SCI), and **multiple sclerosis (MS)** represent four common adult neurologic conditions seen in physical rehabilitation. Each condition has its own unique set of clinical considerations. Depending on the lesion site and the primary and secondary effects, an orthosis may be indicated. The orthosis can aid in addressing the presence of impairments in the upper extremity structures and functions. *Primary* effects or signs following an insult to the CNS are the direct manifestations of a neurologic lesion such as those that affect muscle tone (i.e., **flaccidity, spasticity**), stretch/deep tendon reflex (i.e., **hyporeflexia, hyperreflexia**), muscle strength and activation (i.e., **paresis** or **weakness**), and coordination (i.e., **tremors, dyssynergia**). On the other hand, *secondary* effects are manifestations that emerge because of the primary effects. Spasticity or flaccidity and weakness contribute to lack of mobility and functional use, which lead to complications including soft-tissue contractures, atrophy, edema, and pain. Furthermore, disuse along with the lack of normal muscle activation patterns around a joint and the loss of soft tissue support may lead to joint deformation or instability over time.

In developing an intervention plan that involves orthoses for the upper extremity, it is crucial for the therapist to take into consideration the onset of the condition, the current neurofunctional status of the upper extremity, and its progression. For instance, in the early stages of recovery where tone is likely to change, the need for an orthosis may also change. There is no one single most effective orthosis for each diagnostic condition. Therefore, the therapist must apply clinical reasoning based on knowledge of the condition, upper extremity biomechanics, evidence, and patient/client contexts and preferences during the design, fabrication, and training process.

CONSIDERATIONS FOR ORTHOTIC INTERVENTION

Depending on the goals of orthotic intervention, there may be instances when a specific orthosis may be applicable across conditions. For instance, the management of contracture by the use of a mobilization orthosis (such as serial static and static progressive designs) may follow the same treatment principle of low-load prolonged stretch (LLPS) (Glasgow, Tooth, & Fleming, 2010).

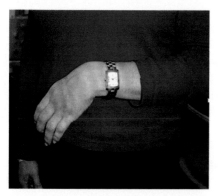

FIGURE 23–1 Patient presenting with wrist drop during the flaccid period following a cerebrovascular accident.

However, there are also typical patterns of impairment that may be specific to the condition and thus warrant special consideration when it comes to the use of orthoses. These will be described in the following text.

CEREBROVASCULAR ACCIDENT

Following an insult caused by ischemia or hemorrhage, the brain of a stroke survivor undergoes a series of physiologic events, which are considered as a part of spontaneous recovery. According to Teasell and Hussein (2016a), this period of recovery, which occurs around 4 to 6 weeks postinsult, constitutes resolution of cerebral edema and a return of circulation around the area of the ischemia. Although the spontaneous recovery period may continue for more weeks, another period of recovery marked by CNS reorganization ensues, lasting for several months (Teasell & Hussein, 2018). These two periods of recovery are apparent in the patient's clinical presentation.

During the acute recovery period, cortical functions immediately surrounding the area of ischemia are depressed. Consequently, muscle tone is marked by flaccidity, stretch reflexes are absent or decreased, and muscle activation is also absent or decreased. As the brain continues recovery, muscle tone and stretch reflexes increase, and voluntary muscle activation may then be possible. The extent of voluntary motor control and the evolution of spasticity and its severity vary from patient to patient. This makes early prediction, and thereby early intervention, of severely disabling spasticity challenging for clinicians (Wissel et al., 2010).

During the flaccid period, the hand and arm may rest in a dependent position. With the emergence of proximal control without return of extensor activity of the hand and wrist, the resulting posture may be a wrist drop configuration (Fig. 23–1). When the hand is unsupported, the finger extensors are placed in passive tension, causing the metacarpophalangeal (MCP) joint to be pulled into extension or hyperextension. From a flaccid state, spasticity may emerge in the upper extremity (Brunnstrom, 1970; Gowland, 1982; Wissel et al., 2010). The onset of spasticity varies in severity, timing, and location. However, there are muscle groups where spasticity becomes more pronounced and may lead to stereotypical posturing of the upper extremity. This posture includes the humeral adductors, humeral internal rotators and elbow flexors proximally, and digit/wrist flexors distally (Teasell & Hussein, 2016b) (Fig. 23–2). Such a stereotypical pattern is implicated

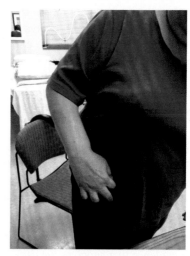

FIGURE 23–2 Spasticity becomes more pronounced, leading to a stereotypical posturing of the upper extremity.

in abnormality of reach, grasp, and manipulation, and, with disuse or nonuse of the arm and hand, the formation of contracture deformity becomes an inevitable sequel (Shumway-Cook & Wollacott, 2017).

During the flaccid stage, the glenohumeral joint is at risk for subluxation because of loss of contractile tension from the deltoid and supraspinatus muscles (Fig. 23–3A–C). In addition, with the humeral head slipping in inferior-lateral or inferior-anterior directions, the superior capsular structures become overstretched. During the spastic stage, shoulder subluxation may remain. The deformation is further complicated by the onset of increased spasticity in the subscapularis and pectoralis major muscles (Teasell & Hussein, 2016b). Hecht (1995) noted that spasticity in these muscles is the primary contributory factor in causing shoulder pain because of its tendency to restrict external rotation during humeral elevation. During humeral elevation (e.g., abduction), external rotation clears the greater tubercle of the humerus from coming in close contact with the acromion and thus preventing impingement.

Sling and Shoulder Support

Various sling and shoulder support designs have been commercially fabricated and studied to address shoulder subluxation. A simple *biomechanical design* comparison table is provided in Table 23–1. Regardless of the design, sling use has its own share of controversies in large part because of some of the risks associated with its use. The therapist must carefully monitor patients who are using slings to ensure that they are removing the sling, monitoring joint and soft tissue integrity, and providing exercise as recommended to prevent complications of stiffness and **dependent distal edema**. In a Cochrane systematic review, Ada, Foongchomcheay, and Canning (2005) found insufficient evidence that slings and positioning devices (i.e., shoulder supports) prevent or reduce shoulder subluxation. In addition, sling use has been criticized for its impact on a patient's **postural control** and body image. However, slings and shoulder supports are still clinically useful to the **subluxed shoulder** and the **flaccid upper extremity**. They can assist in prevention of further injury especially during transfers and ambulation by keeping the arm secure against the

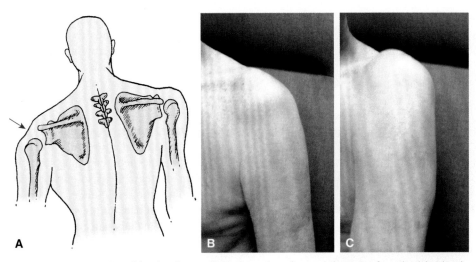

FIGURE 23–3 A, Subluxation of the glenohumeral joint due to loss of contractile tension from the deltoid and supraspinatus muscles with indentation just proximal to the humeral head. **B and C,** Note the flaccid right shoulder with atrophy of the deltoid muscle and the inferior displacement of the humeral head relative to the acromion. during attempt to elevate shoulder using the pectoralis major as substitution.

TABLE 23–1	**Comparison of Shoulder Slings**			
Characteristic	**Standard Sling**	**Arm Cuff**	**Holster Design**	**Saddle Design**
Commercial examples	North Coast Hemi Sling (North Coast Medical, Morgan Hill, CA)	AliMed® Hemi Sling (AliMed, Dedham, MA)	GivMohr® Sling (GivMohr® Corporation, Albuquerque, NM)	Omo Neurexa Plus (Ottobock USA, Minneapolis, MN)
Mechanism of support	Sling support is applied at the elbow, forearm, and wrist; a strap is attached to the sling and loops around the upper back to produce a superiorly directed pull on the arm and forearm.	Cuff support is applied at the mid-proximal arm; two to three straps are attached to the cuff and are anchored over the opposite shoulder. The straps are intended to apply a superior-posterior pull on the humerus.	The hand and forearm are supported by a wide semielastic figure-8 strap that loops around the hand through a plastic cylinder and crosses at the dorsal wrist. The straps continue proximally to the shoulder anteriorly and posteriorly that cross on the upper back and continue as a loop on the opposite shoulder. The flaccid extremity is supported from the palmar surface of the hand, providing compressive force through bones and joints of the arm, resulting in reduction of shoulder subluxation.	The forearm is supported by a cuff, i.e., attached to a neoprene-based shoulder saddle with two adjustable nylon straps. Proximal approximation of the upper limb to the shoulder girdle is achieved through two diagonally oriented nylon straps (one anterior, one posterior) across the glenohumeral joint. The anterior-posterior straps on the neoprene saddle also prevent anterior-posterior displacement of the humeral head. The saddle is further secured by a cross-body strap.
Effect on shoulder mobility	Immobilizes the glenohumeral joint in internal rotation and adduction but shoulder flexion is possible.	Affords shoulder abduction but restricts some movement in the sagittal (flexion-extension) and transverse planes (internal-external rotation).	Affords maximal shoulder abduction and extension and moderate flexion and external rotation.	Restricts the glenohumeral joint in the sagittal and frontal planes while keeping it in neutral rotation.
Effect on elbow, wrist, and hand	Elbow is immobilized in flexion; wrist may rest in flexion. Hand may not be used.	Affords full movement of the elbow and distal joints. Hand may be used.	Affords movement in the elbow; hand/wrist is saddled on a semiflexible plastic tube. Hand use is limited.	Affords near full forearm and elbow range of motion. The wrist and hand are free.
Effect on postural control and mobility	Shifts the center of gravity superiorly and anteriorly.	Allows arm swing during gait.	Facilitates thoracic extension; affords/facilitates arm swing during gait.	Facilitates stabilization of the scapula; affords arm swing during gait.
Potential sensory effects	Forearm and hand are not exposed.	Forearm and hand are fully exposed.	Moderate hand and forearm exposure to external environment; strapping configuration provides gentle joint compression; provides sensory input through dynamic compression.	Optimal hand and wrist exposure.

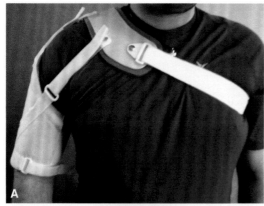

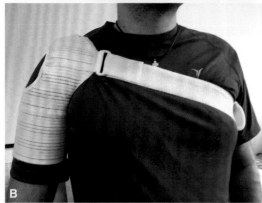

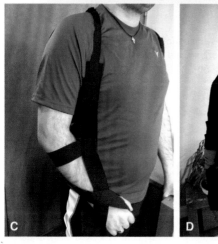

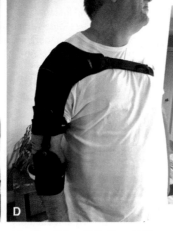

FIGURE 23–4 A, The AliMed˙ Hemi Shoulder Sling (Alimed˙, Dedham MA). **B,** The Rolyan˙ MFC Unilateral Shoulder Orthosis (Performance Health, Warrenville IL). **C,** The GivMohr˙ Sling (GivMohr˙ Corporation, Albuquerque, NM). **D,** The Ottobock˙ Omo Neurexa Plus shoulder orthosis (Ottobock USA, Minneapolis, MN).

patient's torso and lessening its tendency to flail around (Fig. 23–4A,B). As neuromuscular function improves, therapists may exercise judgment on the need for these devices. Several versions of slings that are used to support a subluxed shoulder are commercially available. In addition, there are alternative "sling" designs that have been shown to provide greater support. These include the GivMohr® Sling (GivMohr® Corporation, Albuquerque, NM) (Fig. 23–4C) and the Omo Neurexa Plus (Ottobock USA, Minneapolis, MN) (Fig. 23–4D). In two separate studies, both the GivMohr® (Dieruf, Poole, Gregory, Rodriguez, & Spizman, 2005) and the Omo Neurexa Plus (Hesse et al., 2013) have shown a reduction in the vertical displacement of the glenohumeral joint through x-ray studies.

The GivMohr® Sling applies an upward force through a thick elastic strap that extends to the hand and then loops in a figure-8 through a plastic cylinder. The hand rests on this plastic cylinder, and the wrist is stabilized where the straps intersect into a figure-8. The forearm is supported with a horizontal strap that also serves to stabilize the proximal part of the figure-8 loop.

The Omo Neurexa Plus consists of two major components: a shoulder saddle and a forearm cuff. The shoulder saddle is made of a high-grade neoprene material with silicone lining that is placed in strategic areas to ensure grip. A wide neoprene strap loops around the torso, under the opposite axilla, and the clips to the front and back of the shoulder saddle. The saddle also has nylon straps that diagonally cross the glenohumeral joint to ensure upward and medial compression of the humeral head against the glenoid. The cuff component is attached to two adjustable and detachable nylon straps—posteromedial and anterolateral that allows for forearm positioning. The wrist and the hand are free and unobstructed. A similar design to Omo Neurexa Plus is the Neuro-Lux II® (Sporlastic GmbH, Nurtingen, Germany) marketed only in Europe. In a randomized controlled experiment, the Neuro-Lux® not only facilitated improvements in the vertical alignment of the glenohumeral joint but also helped reduce signs and symptoms of shoulder hand syndrome (Hartwig, Gelbrich, & Griewing, 2012).

As a rule of thumb, sling use and shoulder supports should be diminished as the therapist notes evidence of muscle contraction of shoulder stabilizers. Persistent use of a sling may only encourage disuse, pain, and contracture. It must be noted that many traditional or universal sling designs place the upper extremity in humeral adduction and internal rotation with elbow flexion (Fig. 23–5). These positions may reinforce the synergy pattern described earlier and can be deleterious to upper extremity recovery. Instead, therapists should consider the use of more evidence-based shoulder orthoses previously described along with other evidence-based interventions for shoulder subluxation such as **neuromuscular electrical stimulation (NMES)**, task-oriented practice, and exercise. Information about these evidence-based interventions is beyond the scope of this text.

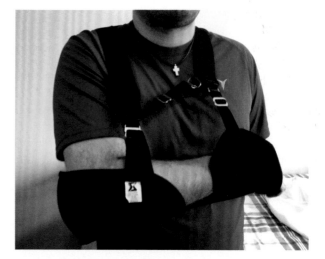

FIGURE 23–5 A Rolyan˙ Universal Sling promotes a pattern of shoulder adduction and internal rotation as well as elbow flexion (Performance Health).

EXPERT PEARL 23–1

Management of Hyperspasticity
CAROLYN BROWN, OTR/L, CLT, OTD CANDIDATE
Connecticut

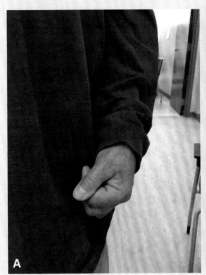 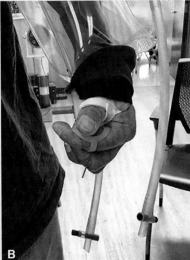 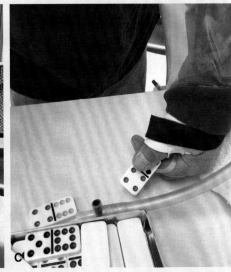

Orthoses can be used to address hyperspasticity in the finger flexors and thumb opponens in order to promote functional lateral pinch and release in patients with hemiparesis. This patient exhibits LUE hemiparesis and moderate hyperspasticity of the elbow, wrist, and finger flexors as well as the thumb opponens. His stage of motor recovery is Brunnstrom Stage III, mass grasp but no release. The patient's goal is to improve lateral pinch and release in order to use his hand as a moderate active assist. A: Patient exhibits lateral pinch, but no release. Patient also exhibits synergistic elbow flexion when he attempts to reach to table. B: An oval-8 orthosis placed on the IF proximal interphalangeal (PIP) prevents interphalangeal (IP) flexion. A rigid custom hand-based thumb abduction orthosis immobilizes the thumb MCP and prevents thumb opposition. An Aircast on the elbow reduces synergistic elbow flexion. C: The patient is now able to use his hand as a moderate active assist using compensatory release.

Taping

Another alternative to sling use is strategically applied tape. Tape application affords the clinician to directly influence at least partial alignment of the joint by constraining the joint and the movement of supportive bony structures. The application of tape to treat shoulder subluxation has its own share of controversies. Several approaches to taping or strapping have been proposed (Ancliffe, 1992; Hanger et al., 2000; Morin & Bravo, 1997). However, recent studies (Appel, Mayston, & Perry, 2011; Griffin & Bernhardt, 2006) point to the benefits of taping or strapping to manage pain, but evidence remains limited whether taping or strapping improves shoulder subluxation.

Two common taping options for shoulder subluxation are the **rigid taping** and **elastic therapeutic taping** (see Chapter 13 for more detail).

Rigid Taping

A commonly used approach combines a semi-elastic compliant adhesive layer that interfaces with the skin (i.e., undertape), and a rigid, less-compliant adhesive layer that is applied on top (Fig. 23–6). The undertape is extremely important because it protects the skin from shearing forces from the strong holding adhesive of the brown (overtape) tape. In general, rigid taping is employed to reduce pain and improve muscle function and biomechanics. Proper analysis of the underlying pathology is essential to maximize the effectiveness of the method, which focuses on reestablishing a proper length/tension relationship and motor control.

Rigid taping for the shoulder may occasionally cause skin irritation, depending on the condition of the muscle carrying the weight of the arm. The vertical strip serves to support the weight of the arm and provide upward lift of the humerus, and the transverse strip supports the humeral head in the glenoid, serving as a reinforcement of the anterior ligaments. When taping a patient who has suffered a CVA or who has weakened deltoids, the use of two vertical, parallel, and overlapping strips may assist in reducing the load on the skin. This taping may stay in place for 3 to 4 days depending on the patient's age, overall medical condition, diagnosis, and skin condition. Rigid taping for shoulder subluxation also works well for anterior instability because the tape strips create a perpendicular capsular support. In this case, a shorter vertical strip may be used to avoid upward compressive forces that may result in subacromial impingement.

Elastic Therapeutic Tape

Elastic therapeutic tapes are tapes made from cotton, which have varying degrees of stretch depending on the tape chosen (e.g., Kinesio® Tape, Balance Tex™ Tape, SpiderTech™ Tape; Patterson Medical, Warrenville, IL; Rocktape®, Durham, NC). Elastic therapeutic tape has become a popular option in part because of the ease of application and friendliness of wear. The elastic recoil of the tape combined with proper application affects the superficial fascia, creating a light skin "lift" on the tissue it rests on. Not only do these reactions cause a reduction in subcutaneous interstitial pressure and

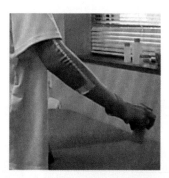

FIGURE 23-6 With this rigid taping technique, the tape applied posterior to the elbow provided stabilization of the arm during a functional reaching task.

improve lymphatic drainage, but also as movement occurs, there is constant tactile stimulus to the low-threshold cutaneous mechano-receptors of the skin. This stimulates muscle, decreases pain, and enhances proprioception for neuromuscular reeducation. The high elastic recoil of the tape also provides support to weak muscles, reducing fatigue and overstretching (Fig. 23-7A–C). The thickness and weight of the tape is approximately the same as skin so the patient does not normally perceive the tape.

Both the rigid and elastic therapeutic taping should be combined with a comprehensive strengthening program for the muscles affecting the joint to provide extrinsic stability and prevent further damage or stretching of supporting ligaments and joint structures. Whether the choice is taping or a sling/shoulder supportive device, the clinician must also consider preventive positioning. Typical positioning recommendations for the affected upper extremity are elbow/wrist extension and shoulder abduction and external rotation. Positioning options that may be used to prevent contractures and promote proper alignment include adjustable tables, lap trays, and arm troughs.

TRAUMATIC BRAIN INJURY

TBI is a form of acquired brain injury because of a sudden traumatic event that results in damage to the brain. There are different types of TBI based on the mechanism of injury—from a simple concussion to one that involves fracture or penetration into the skull. In addition to the initial trauma, damage to the brain is worsened by the shearing forces that the brain undergoes, heavy bleeding, development of hematoma, and a decrease or absence of oxygen supply (National Institute of Neurological Disorders and Stroke [NINDS], 2019a).

Patients with TBI may be seen for individualized rehabilitation from the early stages of recovery in the intensive care unit. The path of recovery may be progressive, starting from low levels of arousal, consciousness, and limited neuromotor activity to emerging levels of consciousness and the onset of spasticity and **primitive reflexes**. Early in the recovery process, the use of orthoses may be indicated to assist with appropriate positioning and prevention of contractures. More involved patients may exhibit exaggerated whole body stereotypical responses known as **decorticate** and **decerebrate** posturing or rigidity. In the upper extremity, decorticate rigidity consists of shoulder extension and internal rotation, elbow flexion and forearm pronation, and finger and wrist flexion. In contrast, decerebrate rigidity presents itself as shoulder adduction and internal rotation with elbow flexed, forearm pronated, and fingers and wrist flexed. When muscle tone is rigid, the resistance to passive movement is strong and constant throughout the range. Such condition places the patient at risk for contractures. Thus, the aim of therapy and the provision of an orthosis is to maintain and/or increase available range of motion (ROM) (Fig. 23-8).

To reduce contracture, prolonged stretch over an extended period of time may be favored. As detailed in Chapter 10, the use of serial casting is a preferred treatment option for this issue. One study suggested that in severe tone-induced contractures, the preferred approach is to apply a cast for short durations of 1 to 4 days to maximize ROM and minimize complications (Pohl et al., 2002) (Fig. 23-9). Complications such as pain, swelling, tissue breakdown, and contractures may arise. Therefore, the therapist must exercise extra caution when applying and removing a cast on a patient with severe tone. The advantages of serial casting are in the evenness of circumferential pressure or force application and its neutral warm inhibitory effect on muscle tone (Colditz, 2000, 2002, 2011). In a randomized controlled trial for the treatment of elbow contractures in adults with TBI (Moseley et al., 2008), serial casting was superior over positioning in increasing ROM. However, the effect was transient and/or not maintained after 4 weeks. This can be explained by the fact that elbow contractures in TBI are spasticity-induced. To mitigate this issue, the author recommends the intermittent application of a removable elbow orthosis during rest periods and referring the patient to determine whether the patient is a candidate for botulinum toxin A (BTA) injection. The use of BTA to manage spasticity has been shown promise in not only promoting reduction in tone but also in reducing pain, improving strength, and increased overall

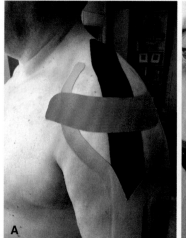
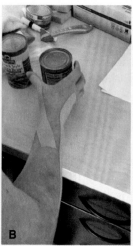
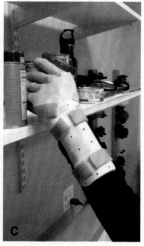

FIGURE 23-7 **A,** Elastic therapeutic taping to the shoulder using Kinesio® Tape. **B,** Elastic therapeutic taping applied to the dorsal wrist and thumb to facilitate stabilization of the wrist and increased hand aperture during a grasping task. **C,** Tape can be applied beneath an orthosis for additional facilitation of movement and digit/thumb alignment.

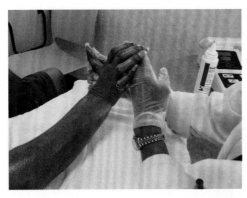

FIGURE 23–8 Passive stretching of the digital flexors being performed prior to reapplication of an orthosis.

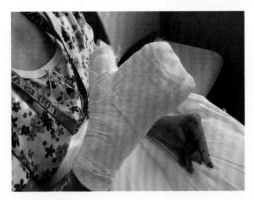

FIGURE 23–9 Initial cast application for dense digital flexion contractures. The cast provides a prolonged duration of gentle continual stress to these tight tissues. Note the posturing of the left hand.

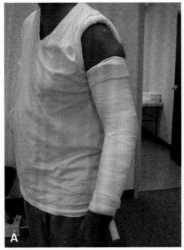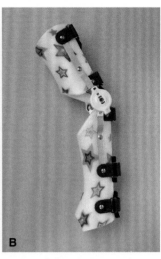

FIGURE 23–10 A, Serial static elbow extension mobilization cast using plaster of paris to obtain the serial static force. **B,** The Ultraflex™ EWHO (elbow-wrist-hand) Orthosis used to conservatively manage flexor/pronator length issues. (Photo courtesy of Ultraflex, Pottstown, PA).

function (Shaw et al.,2010). Furthermore, as a patient's level of consciousness improves, serial casting may continue with lesser risk for complications (Pohl, Mehrholz, & Rückriem, 2003) (Fig. 23-10A) or be substituted with hinged orthoses such as Ultraflex elbow-wrist-hand orthosis with or without rotation (Ultraflex™, Pottstown, PA) (Fig. 23–10B). For more sophisticated designs requiring minimal adjustments, rehabilitation therapists should collaborate with and seek the expertise of certified orthotists/prosthetists.

Many patients with acquired brain injury may continue to have functional return in their arm and hand function. However, compensatory patterns that combine flexor and extensor synergies or decorticate and decerebrate posturing are likely to persist (Fig. 23–11A–E).

SPINAL CORD INJURY

Some neuromotor signs such as spasticity and hyperreflexia found in SCI may share similarities with brain-based lesions (i.e., CVA, TBI), but the pattern of clinical manifestations and the course of recovery are unique. In SCI, the functional prognosis is directly linked to the level of injury. This is clearly illustrated by a series of practice guidelines published by the Consortium for Spinal Cord Medicine (2000). The goal of rehabilitation is to optimize the patient's function that corresponds to neurologic level. There is potential for improvement in the presence of partial innervation below the neurologic lesion known as the zone of partial preservation (McKinley, Jennings, & Pai, 2011). For instance, a patient with a neurologic level of C6 may have fair power in the long finger flexors, which corresponds with C8 functional level. Therefore, the therapist must regularly examine the patient's neuromuscular functions for any indication of functional return that exceeds the expected prognosis (Fig. 23–12). Depending on available motor

function and expected functional prognosis, orthoses may be used as adjunct to functional training by providing support to joints and substituting for denervated muscles. The following provides examples of orthotic intervention for the various levels:

- C5 tetraplegia without the functional ability to use the hand for manipulation—a wrist immobilization orthosis could be used with an attachment for a universal cuff (Fig. 23–13). This adaptation provides support to the wrist in the absence of wrist extension and would enable the patient to self-feed through the universal cuff because shoulder elevation and elbow flexion power may be adequate.
- C6 and C7 tetraplegia—the presence of innervated radial wrist extensors would enable them to use tenodesis action to achieve grasp (Fig. 23–14A,B). Harvey (1996) advocated for the use of progressive orthotic intervention to promote the development of tenodesis grasp. Wrist-driven wrist-hand orthoses based on the original design of the Rehabilitation Institute of Chicago (RIC) tenodesis orthosis (Michela, Sabine, & Sammons, 1959) may also be provided, especially when prehension is desired (Fig. 23–15A,B).
- C8 tetraplegia present with hand function based on the availability of innervated extrinsic finger and thumb flexors and extensors. Intrinsic function may be absent, and therefore, hand dexterity is limited. Without intrinsic power during grasp, the hand is subject to muscle forces that position the MCP joints in hyperextension and the IP joints in flexion. This claw hand or intrinsic-minus configuration is not functional especially when the task requires a cylindrical prehension pattern (e.g., grasping a cup). An MCP flexion immobilization orthosis with an opponens component may be one orthotic consideration used to augment the lack of muscle innervation of the intrinsics (Fig. 23–16A,B).

MULTIPLE SCLEROSIS

MS is an unpredictable CNS condition that is believed to be an autoimmune disease specifically attaching the myelin in the brain and the spinal cord (NINDS, 2019b). Most patients initially diagnosed with MS experience visual/visual motor symptoms and/or movement dysfunction that affects their balance and coordination. Other manifestations include cognitive, somatosensory, and psychosocial impairments. In the upper extremity, two of the more well-documented impairments associated with MS are a loss

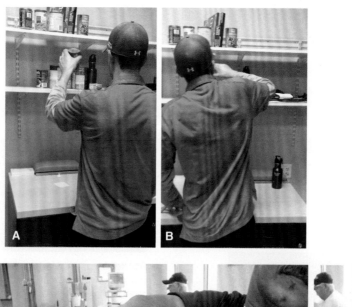

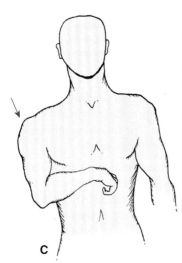

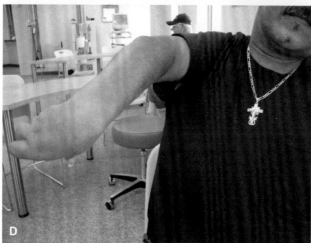

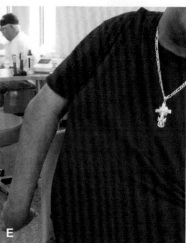

FIGURE 23–11 **A and B,** Note the comparison between the right (impaired) and left (intact) upper extremity during forward reach. The right arm demonstrates lasting patterns of a combined synergy including shoulder abduction with internal rotation, elbow flexion with pronation, and increased flexor tone in the hand (not visible). **C–E,** Decerebrate posturing including shoulder adduction and internal rotation, elbow flexion, and pronation with fingers and wrist flexed.

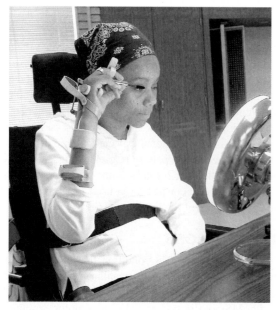

FIGURE 23–12 C6 complete tetraplegia using a wrist-driven, wrist-hand orthosis. (Reprinted with permission from Radomski, M. V., & Trombley Latham, C. A. (2008). *Occupational therapy for physical dysfunction* (6th ed.). Baltimore, MD: Lippincott Williams & Wilkins.)

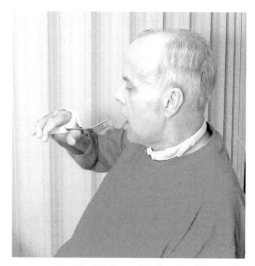

FIGURE 23–13 C5 tetraplegia using a universal cuff as part of a wrist immobilization orthosis. (Reprinted with permission from Radomski, M. V., & Trombley Latham, C. A. (2008). *Occupational therapy for physical dysfunction* (6th ed.). Baltimore, MD: Lippincott Williams & Wilkins.)

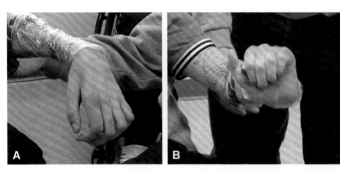

FIGURE 23-14 **Tenodesis. A,** Note the posturing of the wrist when flexed: MCP joints in extension and the IPs flexed. **B,** When the wrist is extended, the MCP joints posture in flexion as do the IPs.

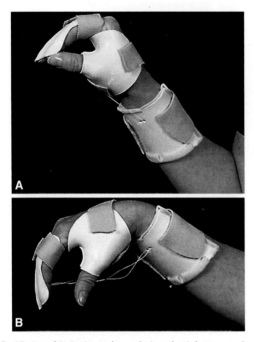

FIGURE 23-15 **A and B,** Reciprocal tenodesis orthosis harnesses the power from the radial nerve for light functional pinch/use. Wrist extension provides digit flexion and wrist flexion allows digit extension.

of coordination and joint position sense, especially in the shoulder girdle (Ünlüer, Ozkan, Yasa, Ates, & Anlar, 2019). Because of the unpredictable nature of MS, the functional presentation of the hand and upper extremity will vary from patient to patient. In a small study involving six participants with MS, a commercial wrist orthosis was used as one of the many strategies to limit tremors and enhance hand function (Hawes, Billups, & Forwell, 2010). Both the participants and the investigators of the study had a mixed reaction to the intervention effects.

The presence of contractures or functional hand deformities varies and may sometimes mimic a peripheral nerve injury. To date, there is no single "most effective" orthosis that may circumvent hand impairments. It is the therapist's clinical reasoning based on knowledge of hand biomechanics, motor control, and task analysis that are most critical in determining the most effective intervention tool (orthosis) for that patient. For instance, one common issue in patients with MS is lost of grip strength caused by weakness in extrinsic flexors and wrist extensors that minimize their ability to engage in self-care activities such as holding on a toothbrush or utensils; a therapist may try using a wrist

immobilization orthosis that positions the wrist in 20° of extension to optimize grip control (Fig. 23-17A). Another common issue is wasting of the intrinsic muscles of the hand resulting in flattening of the hand and loss of thumb opposition. Consequently, a patient with such problem may have difficulty with fine motor prehension (e.g., tripod or tip pinch). A simple solution is to provide a patient with a hand-based carpometacarpal immobilization orthosis that enables the approximation of the distal segments of the thumb and the index finger while maintaining the first web space for correct hand aperture (Fig. 23-17B).

Writing Strap
DEBBIE FISHER, MS, OTR, CHT
Texas

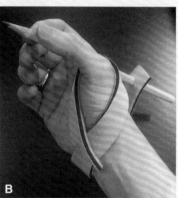
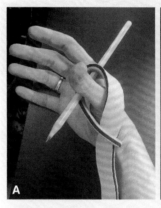

This adaptive device is ideal for a patient with limited ability to maintain a 3 point pinch. Simply measure a piece of 1/8″ neoprene around the wrist and double that before slitting one end and punching a small hole on the other end. Insert the pencil or pen in first, then wrap the strap around the thumb and wrist as pictured.

Adaptive Strap
DEBBIE FISHER, MS, OTR, CHT
Texas

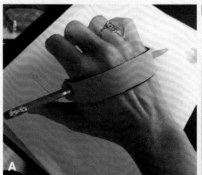

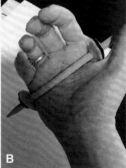

This strap is for a patient who needs assistance for gross grasp. In addition to modified writing, this can be used with silverware, toothbrush, and other items typically used with a universal cuff. Simply cut a piece of neoprene and punch small hole on each end to firmly hold the desired device.

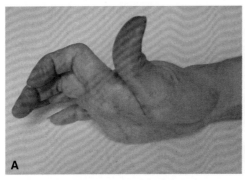
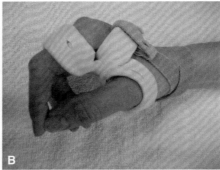

FIGURE 23–16 **A,** Severe claw hand deformity caused by longstanding brachioplexopathy. **B,** Metacarpophalangeal and thumb MP extension restriction orthosis. Note how the orthosis places the digits in a better position for attempts at functional use.

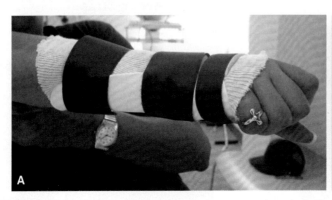
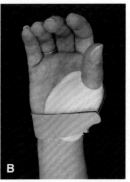

FIGURE 23–17 **A,** Wrist immobilization orthosis prevents excessive wrist flexion, allowing for functional grasp. **B,** Thumb carpometacarpal immobilization orthosis to maintain first web space and position thumb optimally for function.

CLINICAL REASONING ON THE USE OF ORTHOSES IN ADULT NEUROLOGIC CONDITIONS

There are three general purposes for the use of orthoses in adult neurologic conditions:

1. To prevent or manage an existing contracture/deformity
2. To provide joint support because of muscle weakness
3. To assist with neuromuscular reeducation

These purposes are not mutually exclusive. One type of orthosis may be used to satisfy more than one purpose. Furthermore, a patient may require the use of multiple orthoses to achieve various goals/objectives such as

- Support for the wrist while retraining manipulation (Fig. 23–17A)
- Protect and support postoperative procedures while providing some functional use (Fig. 23–18A,B)
- Prevent spasticity-induced contractures through separate orthoses on the elbow and the wrist and hand (Figs. 23–9 and 23–10)

MANAGING CONTRACTURES CAUSED BY SPASTICITY

Contractures may be defined as loss of extensibility of tissues leading to a loss of tissue and joint mobility. In patients with upper motor neuron lesions, contractures are proposed to be caused by degenerative changes in the elastic and contractile properties of muscle (Wissel et al., 2010). Because spasticity significantly limits

the coordinated control of movement, the onset of contractures or deformities in patients with neurologic conditions is largely caused by spasticity-induced movement restrictions. This is not to suggest that the presence of spasticity determines the onset of contractures; contractures are preventable depending on their nature. Contracture may occur in either or both the contractile (e.g., sarcomeres) or/and the connective tissue elements of a muscle. When muscle is immobilized and unused, the contractile elements atrophy because of the reduction of sarcomeres in either length or cross section (Farmer & James, 2001). Meanwhile, the connective tissue that lies within immobilized and disused muscles is lost at a slower rate and

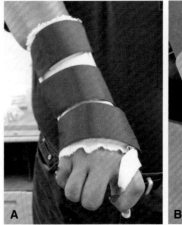
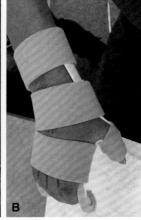

FIGURE 23–18 **A,** Custom-fabricated postoperative orthosis to support wrist. Additional index finger/middle finger web space thermoplastic "strut" was added to align index finger in opposition for pinch in order to assist with light functional use. **B,** Postoperative wrist/hand/thumb orthosis for optimal positioning during rest periods.

tends to thicken because of abnormal cross-linking between fibers (MacDougall, 1986). Spasticity leads to a loss of productive motion and joint/tissue contracture if muscle is not stretched and activated.

The loss of motion is confounded by the presence of spasticity because it may limit muscle excursion during active movement. In the absence of active movement or relative immobility, spasticity may further lead to muscle imbalance, which then leads to stereotypical positioning of the limb, causing further muscle disuse and shortening over time. Typically in antagonistic muscle groups, the degree of spasticity is greater or more pronounced in one of the muscle groups. For example, although spasticity and hyperreflexia may be clinically assessed in both elbow flexors and extensors, elbow flexor spasticity may be more pronounced than in the elbow extensors, resulting in a stereotypical elbow flexion posture.

A widely accepted clinical definition of spasticity is that it is a motor disorder characterized by a velocity-dependent increase in tonic stretch reflexes (muscle tone), resulting from hyperexcitability of the stretch reflex (Lance, 1980). Resistance may be felt or observed when a muscle is stretched passively or when joint movement accelerates, causing the antagonistic (spastic) muscle to trigger the stretch reflex. For instance, in patients with active elbow extension, rapid reaching will cause the hyperactive stretch reflex in the elbow flexors to limit elbow extension toward the end range. Thus, spasticity is also velocity-dependent. There are several theories proposed on the nature of spasticity; however, there remains a lack of consensus on a clinical definition that encompasses its complexity (Thibaut et al., 2013).

The use of orthoses to inhibit tone or address contracture formation in the neurologic population is wrought with controversy and confusion over proper nomenclature regarding these devices (Fig. 23–19A,B). A systematic review consisting of 21 studies of varying quantitative methodologies and study quality indicates a mixture of positive and insignificant outcomes (Lannin, Horsley, Herbert, McCluskey, & Cusick, 2003). The heterogeneity of the orthosis design, the intervention regimen, and the study population limits the generalizability of this systematic review's recommendations. From an evidence-based practice perspective, the ability of the clinician to *critically appraise* the literature without bias is of crucial importance in judging the usability of evidence in everyday practice.

DESIGNS OF ORTHOSES

The decision-making to fabricate an orthosis on a spastic upper extremity may fall under two general frames of reference:

1. Neurophysiologic tradition of tone inhibition
2. Biomechanical tradition of tissue lengthening or contracture prevention

Tone Reduction

Designs that aim to reduce tone include the following (Jamison & Dayoff, 1980; Langlois, Pederson, & Mackinnon, 1991; Mathiowetz, Bolding, & Trombly, 1983):

- Cone orthoses (Fig. 23–20A,B)
- Resting/immobilization orthoses (Fig. 23–21A–E)
- Finger/forearm abduction orthoses (Figs. 23–19A,B and 23–22A,B)

Most often, the resting hand position is characterized by positioning the wrist between 10° and 30° extension, MCP joints in 40° to 45° flexion, IP joints in neutral extension to 20° flexion, and the thumb in mid-palmar and radial abduction in order to maintain the first web space. Several variations of these orthotic designs exist through commercial and scientific literature.

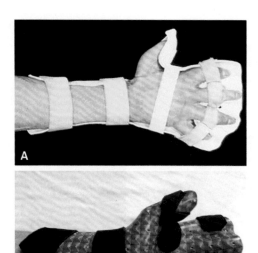

FIGURE 23–19 A and B, Several names have been used to describe these types of orthoses: finger spreader, hand abduction orthosis, or antispasticity orthosis.

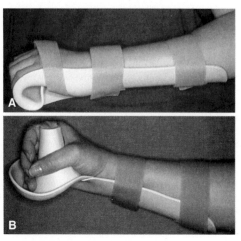

FIGURE 23–20 Rolling the finger platform on a wrist/hand immobilization orthosis **(A)** or forming a cone **(B)** in the hand portion of the orthosis may provide a low-load prolonged stretch to spastic digital flexors without overstretching them. Shown in B is a Preformed Spasticity Splint by DeRoyal, Powell, TN.

The mechanisms for how these orthoses exactly inhibit tone are theoretically based. The original work of pioneers in neuromuscular rehabilitation including Rood (1954), (1956) and Brunnstrom (1961) (1970) should be consulted for further details. The practice theories that emerged from these pioneers have spurned various designs over the years. To illustrate, Rood (1954) believes that pressure on tendon insertion has inhibitory effect. This theoretical influence may be seen in the volar orthosis or cone orthosis designs in which the purported pressure application on the tendon insertions of spastic flexors may trigger an inhibitory response (Fig. 23–20). The Bobaths, on the other hand, believed that maintaining abducted fingers and thumb has a "reflex inhibitory" effect; a resting hand orthotic design with the thumb positioned in abduction and/or a volar-based finger abduction orthosis design is aimed to meet the intention of their approach (Figs. 23–19A,B and 23–22A–C). Both cone and finger abduction orthotic designs and their modifications remain popular as indicated by their commercial presence in vendor catalogs.

The debate on the use of resting orthoses is further complicated by clinician preferences between volar and dorsal application of the

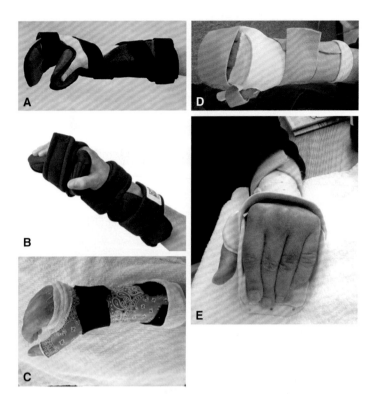

FIGURE 23–21 **A,** A soft immobilization orthosis can be often more comfortable than its hard thermoplastic counterpart. This Rolyan⁺ Kwik-Form⁺ Functional Resting Orthosis allows the therapist to adjust the joint positions. (Photo courtesy of Performance Health; Warrenville, IL, Rolyan is a registered Trademark of Performance Health.) **B,** This Comfy⁺ Hand/Thumb Orthosis is washable and easily modified to obtain a custom fit. Many options are available, including the thumb- and dorsal-based designs. (Photo courtesy of Comfy Splints, Gardena, CA.) **C,** A custom approach is sometimes warranted with this patient population. Post surgery, 3/32″ material is used to fabricate a custom wrist/thumb orthosis (dorsal approach) for a patient that underwent a wrist fusion and tendon transfer due to ongoing tone. This immobilization orthosis places the fused wrist and thumb transfer in a safe resting position encouraging gentle functional use of the thumb interphalangeal and uninvolved digits. **D,** Note that the dorsum of the hand is partially uncovered. This orthosis design allows for easy don/doffing. **E,** In this orthosis, the digits are positioned in maximal extension at metacarpophalangeal joints; any further extension would induce an increase in flexor tone distally.

resting hand orthosis. The rationalization for the choice of volar and/or dorsal application requires further study. Research studies are dated and do not indicate a clear advantage of one approach over the other (McPherson, Kreimeyer, Aalderks, & Gallagher, 1982; Rose & Shah, 1987; Takami, Fukui, Saitou, Sugiyama, & Terayama, 1992; Woodson, 1988). Design modifications that have emerged involve a volar hand support with a dorsal forearm base (Fig. 23–23A,B). One practical advantage of this design is class I

leverage at the wrist. The deforming forces that originate from the flexors are balanced by an opposing lever applied on the forearm while maintaining a highly stable wrist. In purely volar or purely dorsal orthosis, the counterforces are based on how secure the straps are. In cases of severe spasticity, despite the best fit, the wrist has a tendency to buckle into flexion in the volar design; whereas in the dorsal design, the fingers tend to buckle into flexion, causing a distal migration of the orthosis (Fig. 23–24).

In the biomechanical tradition, the purpose of orthotic management is to preserve as much as possible the relative muscle balance between flexors and extensors and the intrinsic and extrinsic muscles of the hand (Bondoc, 2005). An uneven return of motor control to antagonistic muscles results in muscle imbalance; however, the onset of contractures caused by muscle shortening on one muscle group and the passive elongation of its opposing muscle group can become a vicious cycle and thus requires immediate intervention. Clinicians should constantly evaluate the muscle length to determine the onset of contracture and use diagnostic reasoning to differentiate contracture from tone. It is best to compare the more involved with the uninvolved or less involved side to further determine the presence of impairment.

- *Tone* is sensitive to rapid passive stretch; therefore, resistance may be felt at any point within the joint ROM.
- *Contractures* are usually felt as resistance to passive stretch at end range. If one is dealing with contractures of the ligamentous structures, the clinician must also consider when joints are in loose- and close-packed positions. When joints are in loose-packed positions, there is greater accessory motion (e.g., mediolateral gliding) that may be produced. Joints with contractures will have a decrease in the accessory motions.

The clinician should also apply conditional reasoning by attending to the typical recovery pattern or progression of the upper extremity following a CNS lesion. For instance, a patient with a CVA who may begin with flaccid tone may progress into a spastic flexor tone along with stereotypical posturing of the limbs. In such case, the anticipation of arm and hand posturing should guide the choice for an orthotic design. During the flaccid stage, the recommended orthosis position is wrist extension of 20° to 30° with composite extension of the fingers and the thumb (Fig. 23–25A,B). This position will prevent overstretching of the wrist and finger extensors, which could lead to a decrease in their mechanical advantage when the patient begins to regain more motor control of the hand. As the person continues to experience recovery, the clinician must provide ongoing monitoring and, if necessary, make adaptations to the orthosis design and intervention plan.

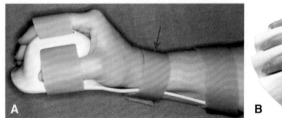
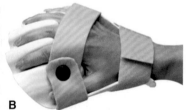
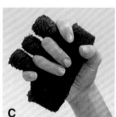

FIGURE 23–22 **A,** A Dorsal wrist strap placed just proximal to the thumb carpometacarpal joint can help prevent orthosis migration. Shown here is a Preformed Neutral Position Hand orthosis by DeRoyal. **B,** Hand-based Anti-spasticity Ball Orthosis by DeRoyal. **C,** The Rolyan⁺ Cone with Finger Separator prevents fingertips from digging into the palm and can prevent maceration in the palm and between the digits. (Photo courtesy of Performance Health; Rolyan is a registered Trademark of Performance Health, Warrenville, IL.)

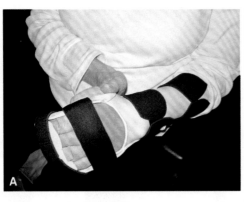
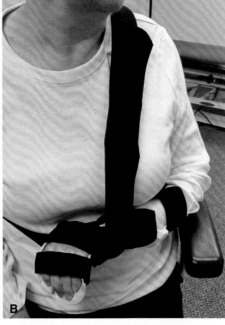

FIGURE 23–23 A, Dorsal/volar design using soft neoprene straps for closure. **B,** A custom neoprene shoulder support was made to assist the patient in holding up the weight of the orthosis/upper extremity because she had minimal active control of the extremity.

EXPERT PEARL 23–4

Web Spacers
KIMBERLY GOLDIE STAINES, OTR, CHT
Texas

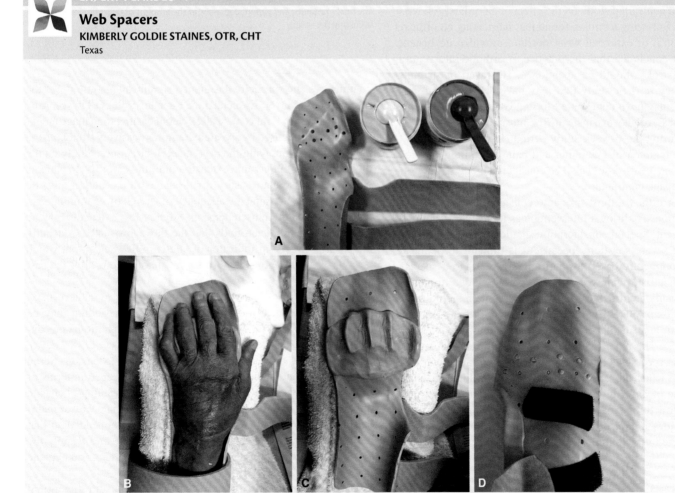

An alternative way to position fingers in a resting hand orthosis is to use elastomer putty to make a mold for web spacers. The putty will push through holes punched in the thermoplastic and that will secure it in place.

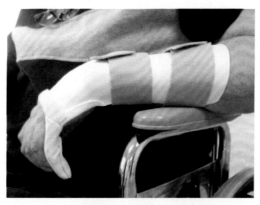

FIGURE 23-24 Dorsal/volar design. Note the counterforce generated through the orthosis and flexion posturing of digits because of tight flexor tendons. Over time, the orthosis can be serially positioned into more extension to lengthen the tendons.

Contracture Prevention

Using an orthosis to treat or prevent contractures is based on the concept of **LLPS**. Although the original basis for LLPS came from animal studies, Tardieu, Lespargot, Tabary, and Bret (1988) demonstrated in human spastic muscle that a minimum of 6 hours of sustained stretch is needed to preserve its normal physiologic length. However, the treatment or prevention of contracture caused by spasticity cannot be simply addressed using orthoses. Lannin, Cusick, McCluskey, and Herbert (2007), who conducted a randomized controlled study on the effect of an orthosis on wrist extensibility following a stroke, found that fabricating an orthosis in either neutral or extended wrist position provided no benefit. They further concluded that the practice of orthotic intervention following a stroke should be abandoned. However, one significant deficiency in their study that may have deviated from best practice and may have contributed to unfavorable outcomes was that "stretches" of the extrinsic flexor muscle groups were not performed during the 6-week study period (Lannin et al., 2007). Therefore, a regimen of stretching and pain-controlling physical modalities (e.g., heat) should also be considered along with orthosis use to manage contracture.

The use of orthoses must take into consideration the severity of the limitation. Traditional intervention as indicated earlier may not be sufficient. Special consideration should also be given when dealing with severe spasticity because it is difficult to delineate tone from contracture-based limitations. A referral to a specialist (e.g., physiatrist, neurologist) is appropriate to determine if a patient is a candidate for pharmacologic intervention including on a botulinum toxin A or BTA (Botox) injection or oral medications such as dantrolene and baclofen that target spasticity (Kheder & Nair, 2012). The reader is advised to consult reliable sources and physician specialists before discussing these matters with the patient. Even when the patient receives pharmacologic management, the use of an orthosis may continue to achieve maximum effect on contracture management. In some cases, the use of serial casting provides a complement or alternative to orthotic and/or pharmacologic intervention.

Serial Casting

The use of casts is commonplace to manage fractures and dislocations and is based on sound biomechanical principles to restrict movement and afford healing. The use of casts to manage

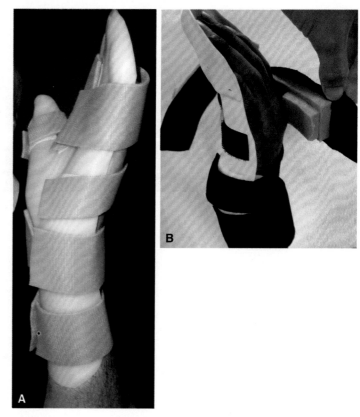

FIGURE 23-25 A, A Wrist/hand extension immobilization orthosis used to preserve muscle tendon length shortly after neurologic insult. **B,** Wide widths of foam can be placed over the dorsum of the digits to impart a gentle stretch to the flexor tendons. The patient can assist in the amount of tension delivered by adjusting the straps.

contractures and spasticity has gained significant attention over the past decades (Mayer, Esquenazi, & Keenan, 1996; O'Dwyer, Ada, & Neilson, 1996; Pohl et al., 2002). Serial casting to manage a flexion contracture caused by spasticity requires passively stretching the flexed joint and applying the cast material circumferentially on the limb at maximum tolerable extension until the cast sets. In patients with impaired somatosensory functions, extra precaution must be undertaken to determine the adequacy of stretch by examining skin color and palpating muscle tension. Slightly less extension may be indicated if the clinician finds that the flexor resistance is steadily increasing. This is an indicator of stretch reflex activation, which may further continue and cause some complications after the cast application.

It is recommended to apply minimal padding to achieve maximum surface contact and minimize shear. Gel padding may be strategically applied on bony prominences as an additional precautionary measure. The cast is left on for several days (e.g., 4–7 days), removed, and then reapplied with greater joint extension. Serial casting is discontinued when the patient has plateaued in terms of ROM gains or when there is no more clinically meaningful change that can be derived. A cast may still be an appropriate way to maintain gains. A bivalved cast configuration is recommended so that the patient or a caregiver may be able to remove and reapply the cast for skin inspection, ROM exercises if appropriate, and hygiene purposes (Fig. 23–26A,B).

Between cast applications, ROM exercises and functional training (whenever appropriate) are recommended. The cast should also be monitored during and after cast application and

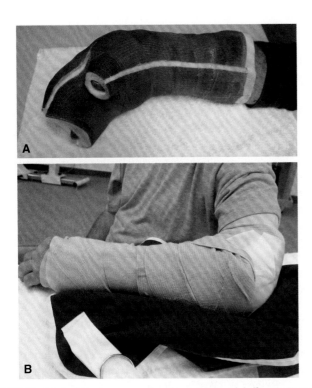

FIGURE 23-26 A, A Bivalve cast to allow for donning and doffing. **B,** Note the use of an elasticized wrap to allow for removal of this bivalve elbow cast.

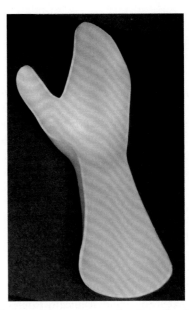

FIGURE 23-27 Preformed orthosis that can be reheated and *custom fit* to the patient.

before reapplication for presence of pain, swelling, pressure ulcers, or skin breakdown caused by stretch. The presence of these complications may require cast repositioning and/or an adjustment of the duration of wear (or even discontinuation of the cast). In one study (Pohl et al., 2003), complication rates ranged from 8% to 25% of the cases reviewed. The clinician should exercise judgment and caution with the use of casts as an intervention modality for contractures. The patient and/or appropriate parties should be well informed on the aforementioned complications in order to participate accurately in monitoring tissue responses to cast wear (see Chapter 10 for detailed information on fabrication of casts).

PROVIDING JOINT SUPPORT

A loss of motor control, especially when associated with weakness and hypotonia or flaccidity, renders the joint unstable. The goal for orthosis use is to provide support and achieve joint stability. When motor return is anticipated, such as in mild CVA or TBI, the clinician should consider the least restrictive orthosis to immobilize the targeted segment. For example, when a patient has poor control of the wrist but has the ability to partially grasp and release, a wrist immobilization orthosis may be sufficient (Fig. 23–17). But when motor return is not anticipated, the goal may be both protective and preventive. The hand and arm should be placed in a resting position that maintains musculotendinous balance and/or promotes optimal musculoskeletal function (Fig. 23–23).

Prefabricated or preformed immobilization orthoses are occasionally issued as a cost-saving measure and used for those patients who are too challenging to fabricate a custom orthosis. Chapter 9 reviews many of these orthoses in greater detail.

- *Preformed* (thermoplastic) orthoses with memory characteristics are preferable because the overall orthosis shape remains intact, and through heating, the clinician can then adjust the fit directly onto the patient (Figs. 23–20B, 23–22A,B, and 23–27).
- *Prefabricated* orthoses are generally soft and comfortable with a more forgiving and adjustable fit. Some have removable pieces or wire foam inserts that allow adjustment (Fig. 23–21A,B). Others contain air bladders that can be inflated to provide gentle stretch to the wrist and/or fingers. Prefabricated orthoses may be appropriate for patients with sensitive or fragile skin, such as the geriatric population. Softer orthoses, however, may be unable to provide adequate support for a large or heavy patient.

Whether a preformed or prefabricated orthosis is chosen for a patient, careful attention needs to be paid when evaluating for proper fit. Proper fit ensures against orthosis migration/slippage during wear. The importance of proper placement of the wrist strap cannot be overstated. This strap, when strategically placed, plays an important role in the orthosis's overall effectiveness that helps prevent migration (Fig. 23–22A).

CONSTRAINING EXTRANEOUS MOVEMENT JOINT SUPPORT

The lack of coordinated control of distal joints is a major barrier in achieving hand function for patients with spasticity and weakness. The delicate balance between the extrinsic flexors and extensors and between extrinsics and intrinsic muscles of the hand is often disrupted by excessive muscle tone and/or lack of muscle power. As a result, patients manifest with a functional form of mallet finger, boutonniere, or swan-neck deformation of the fingers. To address these tendencies, the therapist may custom-fabricate or use commercial preformed/prefabricated finger orthoses such as buddy straps, figure-8 type orthoses to constrain specific motions needed to facilitate grasp.

PROMOTING NEUROMUSCULAR REEDUCATION

Orthoses for the neurological population were historically designed to influence muscle tone, prevent contractures, and provide joint support. With more recent evidence from clinical neuroscience and neurorehabilitation, attention is steadily increasing toward the design and use of orthoses that may promote *active* use of the hand and arm and thus facilitate neuroplasticity with potentially long-lasting changes in motor behaviors (Hoffman & Blakey, 2011). Examples of such devices include the Saebo family of products (SaeboFlex®, SaeboReach®, SaeboStretch® and SaeboGlove®, Saebo, Inc, Charlotte, NC) and the Bioness H200 Hand Rehabilitation System (Bioness Inc, Valencia, CA).

SAEBOFLEX® (SAEBO, INC)

The SaeboFlex® is a dynamic orthosis that statically positions the wrist in optimal extension and dynamically extends the digits with spring-loaded traction in preparation for functional activities (Fig. 23–28A–C). The user is able to grasp an object by voluntarily flexing his or her fingers. The extension spring system assists in reopening the hand to release the object. The amount of tension may be adjustable to accommodate varying degrees of flexor spasticity.

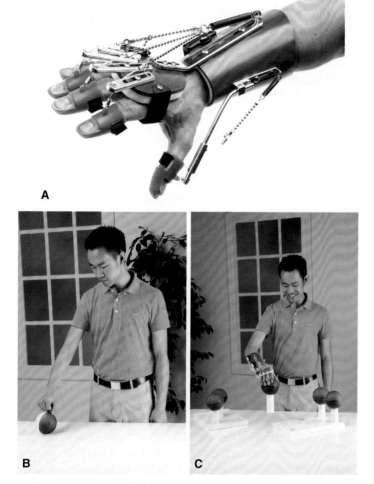

FIGURE 23–28 A, SaeboFlex˚. **B,** Grasping without and **(C)** with SaeboFlex˚, which dynamically extends the fingers, allowing for grasp and release activities. For a patient who has synergistic mass grasp ability but poor or no ability to release, this device affords hand use by providing assistance to release. (Photos courtesy of Saebo, Inc., Charlotte NC.)

This orthosis allows patients suffering from neurologic impairments such as stroke and the ability to incorporate their hand functionally in therapy and at home by supporting the weakened wrist, hand, and fingers.

SAEBOREACH® (SAEBO, INC)

If a patient has a strong flexor synergy influenced during reach and requires an extension assist to the elbow, the clinician can fabricate a custom elbow extension orthosis or consider the SaeboReach®, which may provide an alternative option (Fig. 23–29). The SaeboReach® is a SaeboFlex® device fitted with a dynamic elbow extension component. It must be noted, however, that either the SaeboFlex® or SaeboReach® orthosis is not designed as a device to substitute for a loss of function but rather as a training device to *prepare* a patient to perform functional tasks without or with minimal support. The training program for the patient involves highly repetitive practice of arm and hand tasks using the orthosis (Hoffman & Blakey, 2011). When a patient has gained substantial flexor tone inhibition from active use and some semblance of release, the patient is encouraged to use the arm and hand without the device. Pilot demonstration studies have shown promising results for stroke patients (Butler, Blanton, Rowe, & Wolfe, 2006; Farrell, Hoffman, Snyder, Giuliani, & Bohannon, 2007).

SAEBOSTRETCH® (SAEBO, INC)

The SaeboStretch® uses a "stretch technology," which allows the fingers to flex within the device when tone in the hand increases protecting the finger joints from excessive force (Fig. 23–30A,B). It uses a low-load, long duration of stretch to return the fingers into extension. The SaeboStretch® addresses issues such as deformity, joint damage, hypermobility, and contractures. This orthosis includes three hand pieces with various resistances to allow the therapist the ability to customize orthosis fit.

SAEBOGLOVE® (SAEBO, INC)

The SaeboGlove is a lightweight and low-profile dynamic orthosis that shares similar features as the SaeboFlex but provides lesser resistance and allows for greater excursion of joint movement at the fingers. Instead of spring-loaded traction, the SaeboGlove silicone-based elastic is proximally attached to a firm plastic base and distally attached to hooks embedded on a neoprene glove (Fig. 23–31A–C). The SaeboGlove is best used for patients with milder spasticity. It

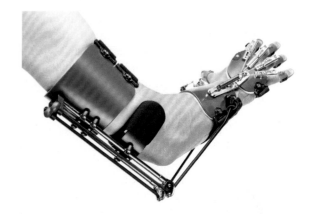

FIGURE 23–29 SaeboReach˚ addresses both elbow and hand involvement. Training in this device is part of both the clinic and home program; training includes repetitive task-oriented activities. (Photo courtesy of Saebo, Inc.)

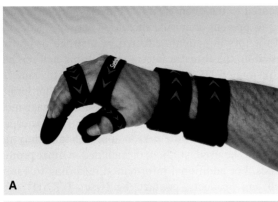

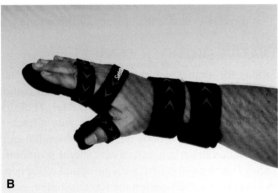

FIGURE 23-30 **A and B,** The SaeboStretch® liner is easily removable for routine cleaning. The straps are made of a nonskid material, which assists in preventing migration. (Photos courtesy of Saebo, Inc.)

can also be used by patients with posterior interosseous/radial nerve palsy, C7-pattern spinal cord/spinal root injury, or patients with decreased extensor power but have the capacity for controlled grip.

H200 HAND REHABILITATION SYSTEM® (BIONESS, INC.)

The H200 is primarily a functional electrical stimulation (FES) system that is built in a customizable orthotic base. The orthosis embeds the electric pads which can be repositioned for optimum stimulation. With a wireless control, the H200 can be used as a functional hand training device while optimally positioning the hand, wrist, and forearm. The H200 has been evaluated for use in patients with acquired brain injury (Alon, Sunnerhagen, Geurts, & Ohry, 2003; Ring & Rosenthal, 2005) but it can also be used for patients with SCI or other neurological conditions where FES is indicated (Fig. 23–32).

NEURO-INTEGRATIVE FUNCTIONAL REHABILITATION AND HABILITATION (NEURO-IFRAH®)

(Approach by Waleed Al-Oboudi, MOT, OTR/L)

Another family of commercially available orthoses and therapy equipment is known as Neuro-IFRAH® Products (San Diego, CA). The Neuro-IFRAH® orthoses and therapy equipment are designed to serve as adjuncts to the Neuro-IFRAH® Approach. These devices purport to aid motor recovery by integrating its own unique Neuro-IFRAH® Approach concepts and applications with self-evident rehabilitation principles. These products include, but are not limited to, custom and prefabricated orthoses designed to prevent and address secondary effects of abnormal muscle activity in patients affected by lesions at the level of the brain stem and above. For example, the Prefabricated EWHO (elbow-wrist-hand hinged orthosis) and WHO (wrist-hand orthosis) may be adjusted to provide composite wrist-hand (digits) and elbow-wrist-hand extension and counteract abnormal involuntary activity in the flexors (Fig. 23–33A). The unique flat hand paddle designs are alternated with curved designs following specific protocols and strategies. The company also offers shoulder orthoses such as the Shoulder Support and the Humeral External Rotator. The Shoulder Support consists of a forearm cuff that may be clipped or hooked to a belt worn by the patient. The forearm support can be adjusted at various angles providing many options for alignment and support. The target effect is to support the weight of the arm to protect the patient's shoulder. Meanwhile, the Humeral External Rotator consists of a forearm trough supported by an L-bar that extends to a semicylindrical

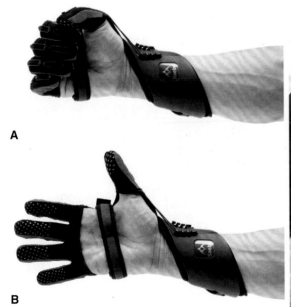

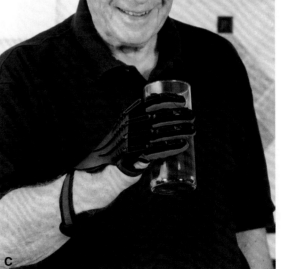

FIGURE 23-31 **A-C,** The SaeboGlove® helps clients suffering from neurological and orthopedic injuries incorporate their hand functionally in therapy and at home. (Photos courtesy of Saebo, Inc.)

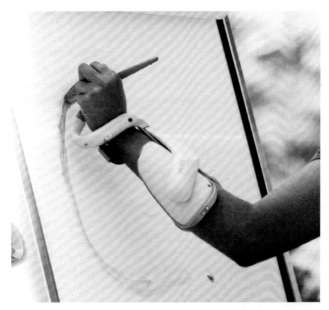

FIGURE 23–32 The H200 Wireless Hand Rehabilitation System (Bioness®) supports the wrist in a functioning position, allowing the fingers and thumb to move efficiently while reaching, grasping, and pinching. This can facilitate regaining hand function and complement a therapy program. The H200 Wireless Hand Rehabilitation System has two main parts that communicate wirelessly with each other: (1) the functional stimulation support (orthosis) and (2) the control unit (microprocessor). (Photo courtesy of Bioness, Valencia, CA.)

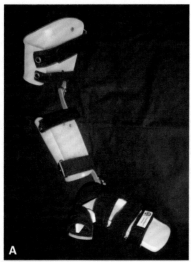

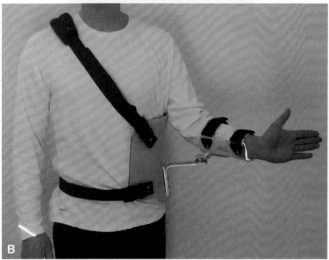

FIGURE 23–33 **A,** The Prefabricated EWHO (elbow-wrist-hand hinged orthosis) designed to decrease hypertonicity in flexors and increase passive mobility into extension. **B,** The Humeral External Rotator allows for adjusting of height, angle, and waist circumference. (Photos courtesy of Neuro-IFRAH® Organization, La Jolla, CA.)

plate secured to the client's waist (Fig. 23–33B). This device is intended to prevent abnormal increased activity in the humeral internal rotators in patients affected by a stroke or brain injury by positioning the forearm lateral to the trunk and the humerus externally rotated lateral to the humeral sagittal plane. All the devices found on their website are said to be proprietary in nature. The originator of the Neuro-IFRAH® Approach maintains that all Neuro-IFRAH® Products are adjuncts and are part of a highly individualized whole person approach, and thus all products are not to be used, studied, or included in other protocols or approaches. For additional information regarding this treatment approach and products, contact the Neuro-IFRAH® organization at www.neuro-ifrah.org. At this time, there are no published studies that directly evaluate the efficacy of these products.

ALTERNATIVE ORTHOTIC DEVICES

Other options for similar devices found both commercially and in research studies are those made from materials or combination of materials such as neoprene, Lycra, and elastic. These types of garments are most often made from heavy-duty stretch materials that contour well on the body and offer substantial *support* to joints or *restriction* to certain movements and/or positioning (Fig. 23–34). They can be hand-based, with the option of supporting the thumb in abduction and extension, or forearm-based, including a spiral wrap that provides a dynamic assist into thumb abduction and extension and forearm supination or pronation (Fig. 23–35). Wilton (1997) also describes the use of Lycra orthoses to achieve more normalized active movement patterns of the upper extremity, including a sleeve-length (axilla to wrist) dynamic assist (elbow extension forearm supination or elbow flexion forearm pronation) model, a gauntlet style with a thumb abduction sleeve, and a full glove style. Recent studies on the use of Lycra or neoprene-based orthoses for increased tone/spasticity have been geared toward children with cerebral palsy (Elliott, Reid, Alderson, & Elliott, 2011). Commercially available resting orthoses are also available and can provide an LLPS to the fingers. The stretch can be adjusted by the progressive inflation of an air bladder placed in a palmar roll (Fig. 23–36).

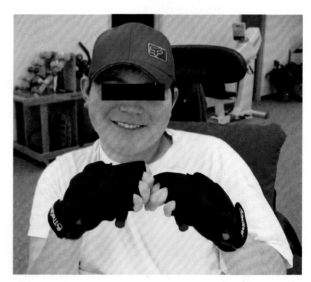

FIGURE 23–34 Thick neoprene and Lycra gloves support the metacarpophalangeal joints and position the thumb in this 16-year-old spinal cord injury patient.

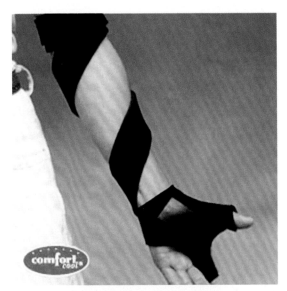

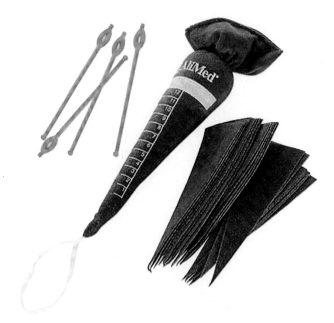

FIGURE 23–35 The Comfort Cool° Pronation-Supination Splint is made of neoprene and applied in either supination or pronation to patients of all age groups. The neoprene strap can be used with the included glove component or with a custom-fabricated thermoplastic wrist support. Neoprene's flexibility allows voluntary movement, whereas its elastic properties facilitate movement away from a spastic pattern. (Photo courtesy of North Coast Medical, Morgan Hill, CA.)

FIGURE 23–36 The Alimed° Hand Contracture Orthosis and Hygiene Kit is recommended for a quick solution or when a more conventional orthosis is not indicated. (Photo courtesy of Alimed, Dedham, MA.)

EXPERT PEARL 23–5

Tips for Keeping the Hand-Mind Connection
HandLab: Clinical Pearls
KAROL YOUNG, OTD, OTR/L, CHT
North Carolina

Have you ever had patients who will not use their finger although they have functional motion? They can move the finger while performing specific exercises in therapy, but as they leave the clinic, they resort to compensatory techniques and avoid using the finger to pick up car keys or an appointment card.

In addition to immobilization of the hand having negative effects on muscles, soft tissues, and joints, we must also consider how this immobilization has an adverse impact on the brain. A large portion of the brain is dedicated to the hand for both sensory and motor function. See image 1. When the hand is not used, these areas of the brain begin to change. Just 24 hours of disuse or immobilization decreases motor cortex excitability and reduces activation in the somatosensory cortex. Over time, this is likely to lead to difficulty with motor planning, altered sensibility, and pain (Burianová et al., 2016; Lissek et al., 2009).

The good news is when we engage the patient's brain, we decrease their pain, improve their sensibility, and increase their motor recovery. Here are some suggestions for engaging the brain to reverse the negative effects of immobilization.

Start Early and Positively

Early active motion is not only helpful to maintain the glide of soft tissues, muscles, and tendons, it is also good for the brain. Patients who require a period of immobilization for adequate healing can still start early by using guided imagery with imagined motions, working on laterality training by identifying images of their right and left extremities, and training with mirror therapy to keep the brain engaged (Bassolino, Campanella, Bove, Pozzo, & Fadiga, 2014; Gandolaa et al., 2019).

Include tactile stimulation early by exposing the extremity to a variety of textures with the eyes open and then closed. Keep an encouraging emphasis on therapy by using the term "discomfort" instead of pain and positively focus on even the smallest gains made in therapy (Fredrickson, 2009).

Make It Functional

As soon as possible, use functional task training. Performing meaningful activities that include both sensory and motor components improves functional outcomes (Che Daud et al., 2016; Lissek et al., 2009). Be sure to break tasks down into simple steps.

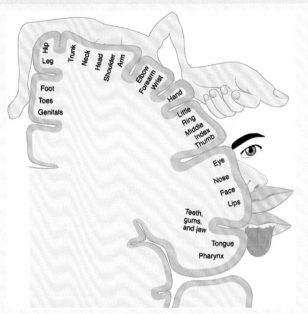

1. Homunculus of the human brain. (wikipedia.org)

Studies show that exercising the contralateral side of the brain will also stimulate the sensorimotor cortex of the involved extremity (Lee, Gandevia, & Carroll, 2009). Therefore, it is important to encourage use of both extremities while performing routine activities of daily living such as folding laundry and reading a magazine.

Include Proprioception

Activities that provide significant proprioceptive input stimulate both the peripheral nervous system and the central nervous system (the brain). Examples of activities that challenge awareness of joint position and joint motion are closed chain exercises, weight-bearing, scapular stabilization, perturbations (a small change in the regular movement), and isometrics (Karagiannopoulos & Michlovitz, 2016). See images 2 and 3.

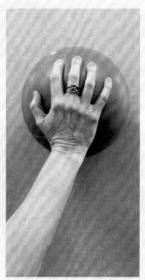

2. Closed chain exercise using a ball.

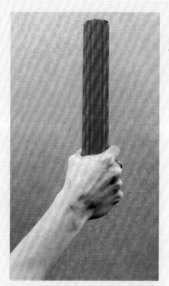

3. This semiflexible roll, when moved quickly, creates perturbations that provide proprioceptive input to the wrist.

References

Bassolino, M., Campanella, M., Bove, M., Pozzo, T., & Fadiga, L. (2014). Training the motor cortex by observing the actions of others during immobilization. *Cerebral Cortex, 24*(12), 3268–3276.

Burianová, H., Sowman, P. F., Marstaller, L., Rich, A. N., Williams, M. A., Savage, G., … Johnson, B. W. (2016). Adaptive motor imagery: A multimodal study of immobilization-induced brain plasticity. *Cerebral Cortex, 26*, 1072–1080.

Che Daud, A. Z., Yau, M. K., Barnett, F., Judd, J., Jones, R. E., & Muhammad Nawawi, R. F. (2016). Integration of occupation based intervention in hand injury rehabilitation: A randomized controlled trial. *Journal of Hand Therapy, 29*(1), 30–40.

Fredrickson, B. (2009). *Positivity.* New York, NY: Crown.

Gandolaa, M., Zapparolib, L., Saettac, G., De Santisb, A., Zerbib, A., Banfib, G., … Paulesub, E. (2019). Thumbs up: Imagined hand movements counteract the adverse effects of post-surgical hand immobilization. Clinical, behavioral, and fMRI longitudinal observations. *NeuroImage: Clinical, 23*, 101838. doi: 10.1016/j.nicl.2019.101838.

Karagiannopoulos, C., & Michlovitz, S. (2016). Rehabilitation strategies for wrist sensorimotor control impairment: From theory to practice. *Journal of Hand Therapy, 29*, 154–165.

Lee, M., Gandevia, S. C., & Carroll, T. J. (2009). Unilateral strength training increases voluntary activation of the opposite untrained limb. *Clinical Neurophysiology, 120*, 802–808.

Lissek, S., Wilimzig, C., Stude, P., Pleger, B., Kalisch, T., Maier, C., … Dinse, H. (2009). Immobilization impairs tactile perception and shrinks somatosensory cortical maps. *Current Biology, 19*, 837–842. doi 10.1016/j.cub.2009.03.065.

CONCLUSION

The decision to use orthoses for the neurologically impaired adult is complex. The clinician must consider various factors including the patient's diagnosis and course of recovery, current and anticipated functional abilities, patient's goals and motivation, the purpose of the orthosis, and the patient's or caregiver's ability to follow through with the intervention. The clinician must also exercise judgment based on the available updated theoretical body of knowledge and current evidence.

The lack of convincing evidence to support or refute the use of orthoses for addressing neurologic dysfunction continues to be a source of controversy among clinicians and researchers alike. Many large studies and systematic reviews have cast scientific doubt on the use of orthoses for the neurologic population. However, it may be argued that neurorehabilitation is a highly individualized practice, and that one regimen of intervention may not always work for two similar patients. The therapeutic efficacy of orthotic intervention is no exemption. Like many other adjunctive treatment methods, orthoses should not be used as a stand-alone treatment. The clinician is encouraged to use sound reasoning that translates into skillful documentation that justifies and clearly elucidates the rationale for orthosis use. As evidence for the rehabilitation of upper extremity motor control continues to emerge, clinicians are advised to keep abreast of scientific developments in order to provide the best service for their patients.

 FIELD NOTE: JOINT DEFORMITIES OF THE SPASTIC HEMIPARETIC WRIST AND HAND

Carolyn Brown, OTR/L, CLT, OTD Candidate
Connecticut

Upper limb spasticity impairs function by limiting active and passive ROM, resulting in a cascade of secondary impairments, including pain and joint deformity. Muscles that cross two joints tend to be disproportionately affected by spasticity (Black & Gaebler-Spira, 2018). The joints of the hemiparetic wrist and hand are subject to deformity due to muscle imbalances that place stress on the joint. Joint deformities can also result from improperly fitting orthoses. Common joint deformities seen in this population include carpal instability (A), swan-neck deformity (B), mallet finger (C), and ulnar deviation of the digits.

(continued)

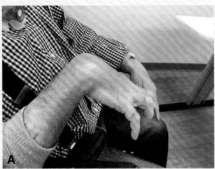

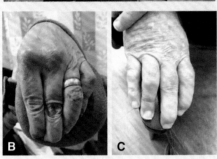

It is essential for the therapist to address joint deformities when fabricating custom orthoses or choosing prefabricated orthoses. Therapists may need to apply creative orthotic fabrication strategies to promote joint stability and prevent further deformity. Examples include padded strapping in an X-pattern across the dorsal wrist, buddy straps or finger separators to prevent ulnar deviation of digits, ring orthoses to reduce swan-neck deformity and mallet finger, and dense foam padding attached to orthoses to promote joint alignment and to avoid skin breakdown.

Reference

Black, L., & Gaebler-Spira, D. (2018). Nonsurgical treatment options for upper limb spasticity. *Hand Clinics*, 34(4), 455–464.

FIELD NOTE: ORTHOTIC CONSIDERATIONS FOR THE NEUROLOGICALLY AFFECTED HAND

Debbie Fisher, MS, OTR, CHT
Texas

Treating a patient with a neurological injury can be challenging on many levels. Common clinical concerns that may limit hand function include but are not limited to soft-tissue shortening, pain, joint contractures, weakness, spasticity, tone, and lack of volitional control.

When selecting an orthosis for a neurological condition such as a CVA, comfort and safety are critical to consider. Especially in light of involuntary tone that may occur, it is important to protect the joints from materials that are too rigid. Think about a patient that coughs, sneezes, or even laughs and his or her hand involuntary flexes into a hard, rigid resting hand orthosis. The opposing forces from the fingers flexing into the nongiving material can be painful and even harmful over time with the potential of causing joint deformities. One example of a customizable orthosis designed to limit soft tissue shortening is the Saebo Stretch. It is intended for someone with mild to moderate tone and comes with three variable hand plates that have different levels of flexibility. This allows for movement from the fingers when needed and springs back into extension when the patient relaxes. Another option is to fabricate a custom orthosis from a material with a thickness that provides some give in the material when the fingers involuntary flex. A thinner more springy material can be used to support the fingers, allowing some give if and when tone is active. A slightly more rigid material can be used proximally to stabilize the wrist and forearm.

When considering an orthosis to help facilitate repetitive functional grasp and release, a dynamic orthosis like the one pictured can be a very effective tool. This custom orthosis was inspired by both the traditional radial nerve palsy orthosis and the Saebo Flex (A–C). It is intended for the neurological patient that has slight to no soft-tissue shortening, active finger flexion, and functional ROM of the elbow and shoulder. Similar to a radial nerve palsy orthosis, it provides passive finger extension while allowing active finger flexion. In contrast, notice how the line of pull is coming from the distal interphalangeal (DIP) joints and that MCP and DIP flexion is restricted. This design limits the tendency of the entire hand from going into a full fist which could make it difficult for the hand to reset into extension. Because of this, it is not typically used as an adaptive orthosis or for fine motor tasks, but used as a tool for repetitive gross grasp and release activities. By minimizing composite finger flexion, the speed and number of repetitions are typically higher in a set amount of time. This is desirable for a number of reasons including the importance of mass repetition with the neurological impairment and how that can impact cortical plasticity. With appropriate training and cuing from the therapist, this orthosis can also aid with teaching the patient to relax and inhibit finger flexion which is required in the release phase essentially turning off the tendency to flex. The process for retraining a hand to do this independent of the orthosis should be attempted frequently after fatiguing the flexors. Complete progression from the brace may vary greatly from person to person depending on many factors.

Components that make up this device include Digitech outrigger kit (Performance Health), dynamic strapping—neoprene—for the thumb, static strapping for the fingers, variable tension rubber bands with separate attachment sites for each. Orficast (Orfit) can be utilized to fabricate the digit DIP component (D).

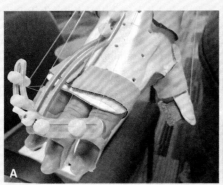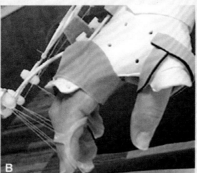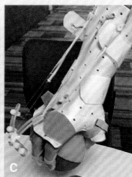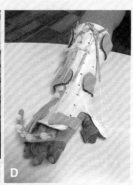

Case Study Section

The case studies presented here are meant as a teaching guideline only. Treatment and orthosis protocols vary greatly from surgeon to surgeon and from therapist to therapist. The therapist should check with the referring physicians and colleagues to define the preferred treatment and appropriate orthotic intervention.

Case Study 1

Part 1: Acute Cerebrovascular Accident—Inpatient Rehabilitation

Thomas is a 63-year-old male who sustained a left middle cerebral artery (MCA) infarct resulting in right hemiparesis and expressive aphasia. Past medical history is remarkable for hypertension. He worked for the fire department and was quite physically active prior to the stroke. After days of acute hospitalization, he was discharged to an inpatient rehabilitation facility for intensive occupational, physical, and speech therapy. At initial evaluation, Thomas presented with maximal assistance in self-care and functional mobility. He is capable of sitting on the edge of the bed/mat with supervision, transitioning from sit to stand, and maintaining standing for at most 90 seconds given moderate assistance on the right side.

In terms of his upper extremity, Thomas has scapular elevation and emerging flexor activity to the elbow and hand. Extensor activity of the wrist and the hand is absent. The hand and wrist rest in partial flexion while seated or standing because of emerging spasticity. Mild clonus is felt upon quick stretch of the wrist flexors. Because of lack of movement, the hand has dependent edema. Thomas reports dull pain with passive composite extension of the wrist and fingers past the neutral position. When constrained to perform active use of the right arm and hand, the upper extremity goes in stereotypical flexor synergy pattern of scapular and humeral elevation, elbow flexion and forearm supination, and finger/wrist flexion.

As part of the occupational therapy intervention plan, a program of flexor stretching and inhibitory weight bearing on the palm while seated is initiated as a preparatory intervention for repetitive task training with massed push–pull movements of the right upper extremity. NMES of the elbow, wrist, finger, and thumb extensors was also added into the treatment as a complement to task-oriented training. After 1 week of NMES, trace muscle contraction was possible along with emerging stretch reflex response to the extensors. However, flexor spasticity of the wrist and fingers increased significantly. To sustain gains in extensor activity, the occupational therapist added orthotic intervention into the therapy plan of care. To maintain a balance of flexors and extensors of the wrist and hand, a dorsal

forearm and hand-based immobilization orthosis was fabricated for use when Thomas was not active and for sleep (Fig. 23–37A).

Initially, Thomas needed minimal assistance to apply the orthosis. The occupational therapist collaborated with the nursing staff to ensure carryover of wearing schedule and to provide initial assistance to Thomas. Eventually, Thomas was able to independently wear the orthosis and report consistent compliance with wear and stretching schedule.

At the end of 4 weeks of intensive rehabilitation, Thomas was discharged to home with a plan for outpatient therapy services. At discharge, Thomas was able to dress and toilet with modified independence. He continued to need minimal assistance with heavy clothing and bathing. He ambulated at least 300 ft with a quad cane and contact guard assistance for safety. He formulated two to three word statements. He had greater upper extremity voluntary control as demonstrated by ~25% active shoulder elevation, ~75% active flexion of the elbow, massed flexion of the hand, and <25% extension during partial release.

During the last week of inpatient rehabilitation stay, Thomas was trained to use his massed flexion with greater functionality, such as grasping on a small ball or cylinder and carrying a small bag or weight using a hook grasp. But because of poor wrist extensor power, a dorsal wrist extension orthosis was fabricated to prevent passive wrist flexor posturing and to provide stability for active grip during task practice by maintaining functional wrist extension (Fig. 23–37B). Thomas continued the use of the immobilization orthosis for nighttime to prevent flexor

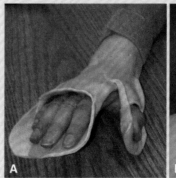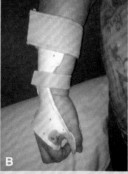

FIGURE 23–37 A, Note the additional finger-restraining straps added to prevent the tendency of the proximal interphalangeal joints to buckle into flexion that could eventually result in boutonniere positioning. **B,** Dorsal-based wrist immobilization orthosis including thumb positioning.

contracture development. As tone increased in the digital flexors, modifications were made by gradually increasing the wrist extension and thumb abduction angle.

Part 2: Acute Cerebrovascular Accident—Outpatient Rehabilitation

Thomas was a highly motivated individual continuing his recovery through the course of his outpatient therapy. Outpatient occupational therapy was geared toward restoring Thomas's upper extremity function through intensive task training. After his initial evaluation, he met the minimum criteria for the SaeboFlex® training program (Fig. 23–28). In addition to having substantial arm elevation and elbow flexion and extension, he also demonstrated mass grasp and emerging active release. He displayed tolerance of the immobilization orthosis that maintained his wrist and fingers in composite extension. Most importantly, Thomas demonstrated the motivation and capacity to carry out his home program.

Thomas had no known cardiac history prior to the stroke. But upon the occupational therapist's recommendation and with concurrence from his primary care provider, he underwent a stress test. The results of the stress test were highly favorable for him to begin a physical fitness program after 4 weeks of outpatient physical therapy. Upon discharge from physical therapy, he was walking with a small base quad cane and ankle-foot orthosis on even surfaces and close supervision on curbs and uneven surfaces. He was able to tolerate 30 minutes of cardio exercise using a combination of recumbent cycle and an ergometer with a hand strap attachment.

Thomas received authorization for a total of 20 outpatient occupational therapy visits by his insurance. The plan of care was established so that Thomas would receive treatment twice a week for 10 weeks. He began the SaeboFlex® program 2½ weeks into the course. The main objective of participating into the program was for Thomas to complete most of the requisite number of repetitions doing reach-to-grasp and transport-and-release drills at home. The role of the therapist was to facilitate transfer of training. At the clinic, the SaeboFlex® exercises were also used as a precursor to active practice with the hand without extensor assistance. The repetitive grasp against resistance and release mimicked the proprioceptive neuromuscular facilitation inhibitory technique of contract-hold-relax. With the SaeboFlex® orthosis off, Thomas was able to grasp and release tennis balls with the ulnar side of the hand. He developed improved control of mass grasp and release and was able to reach and transport objects away from the body with lesser compensatory movement. The biggest gain that Thomas made was his ability to move his arm in ipsilateral sideward, forward, and backward reach.

Thomas's next biggest barrier was the ability to use the radial side of the hand more functionally. Because most of the training with the SaeboFlex® orthosis was on gross grasp and release functions, the individual function of the fingers and thumb needed further training. In most MCA strokes, thumb adduction and flexion tone along with index finger flexor tone remain to be the most significant barriers to increased functional hand repertoire—especially one that involves precision grip and cylindrical grasp. The aperture of the hand required for pregrasp and the ability to assume precision finger patterns are grossly affected by the thumb-index hypertonic phenomenon. The flexor and adductor tone of the thumb and the index finger may be restrained using functional orthoses to directly address the fine motor control functions of the hand. Hence, the occupational therapist fabricated two orthoses: (1) PIP restriction orthoses and (2) first web space midpalmar/radial abduction orthosis (Fig. 23–38). These custom orthoses serve as adjunct

to forced use interventions such as modified constraint-induced therapy or repetitive task training. More specifically, these orthoses allowed Thomas to expand on the repertoire of tasks that he could perform.

Thomas would transition to only wearing the thumb abduction orthosis to practice more precision grasp activities beginning with cubes and then progressing to smaller objects. At the end of the 10-week period, Thomas had achieved a more advanced lateral grasp that mimics a basic tip and tripod pinch. With ongoing practice, Thomas will make more functional gains.

Additional case studies can be found on the companion website on thePoint.

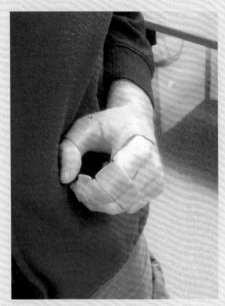

FIGURE 23–38 Functional orthoses used to promote improved use of left hand in completing daily tasks.

Case Study 2: Chronic Cerebrovascular Accident

Lillian is a 72-year-old female with history of multi-infarct vascular dementia. She lives in a residential care facility where she gets close supervision for mobility and self-care. Lillian ambulates with a cane and with minimal assistance for balance over short distances within her living suite. She requires setup for dressing and eating, supervision for toileting, and moderate assistance for bathing.

Three years ago, Lillian had a stroke, resulting in right hemiparesis. Prior to the therapy referral, caregivers and relatives reported that she used to function with the right arm and hand. However, since the stroke, her upper extremity was used less and less until it developed significant spasticity-induced flexor tightness and deformity. Learned nonuse, muscle weakness, and the biomechanical barrier imposed by the spasticity were contributing factors to her upper limb dysfunction.

At initial evaluation, Lillian presented with a stereotypical upper limb posture of shoulder adduction and internal rotation, elbow flexion and forearm supination, and wrist and fingers in composite flexion (Fig. 23–39A). Although Lillian had some mass voluntary movements in her proximal joints, her shoulders and elbow could be ranged with minimal discomfort, enough to assist her with bathing and dressing. Her wrist and fingers were severely contracted, so much so that the palm was macerated. The fingernails were untrimmed and curled inward as they dug into the palm. The hand had poor hygiene and emitted a foul odor. At Lillian's residential care facility, nursing care for the skin is not a required service unless requested by the client or client's family and there must be medical necessity established by a

(Continued)

physician provider. Lillian had been instructed by the nursing staff to apply a rolled washcloth in her palm; the carryover was poor because of decreasing memory retention. The therapy goal for Lillian was to increase hand opening to permit efficient and pain-free hygiene (including hand washing and nail trimming).

Lillian was conversant but had word-finding difficulties. She was alert, oriented to place and familiar persons, but needed occasional cues for time of day. Further into the evaluation, it was assessed that with the elbow flexed and the wrist in at least 50° of passive flexion, the MCP and DIP joints could be placed in neutral extension, whereas the PIP joints could be passively extended as follows: index, −45°; middle, −55°; ring, −60°; and small, −30°. The wrist was passively extended to −20° with the fingers compositely flexed. The occupational therapist collaborated with the nursing staff and Lillian's personal care assistant on how to best position the hand to provide proper hand hygiene. Because of hypertonicity, a small cylinder rolled in a washcloth was applied and became a temporary regimen. Lillian was referred to a specialist who could provide Botox injections. Meanwhile, the focus of treatment was to promote skin healing of the palm, increase the joint play of the PIP joints, and gradually increase Lillian's tolerance to sustained stretch of the finger and wrist flexors. To achieve this, a dorsal wrist immobilization orthosis was fabricated that restricted flexion to 30° to 40° along with the rolled washcloth in her palm.

Through therapist-physician collaboration, Lillian received her first round of Botox injections to the wrist and finger flexors as well as to the deep intrinsics of the hand. Within a week of the injection, the occupational therapist began to provide serial casting for each individual finger using three to four layers of plaster of paris (Fig. 23–39B,C). Because peak efficacy of the injection is normally not reached until a month, the casting progression began slowly, that is, casting the fingers approximately 15° to 20° greater than resting extension. The occupational therapist changed the cast every 5 to 7 days. By week 4 postinjection, the cast change was done twice weekly as needed.

Eight weeks from the initial evaluation, Lillian's PIP joints could be passively extended pain free with the wrist at −10° extension and the MCP joints in neutral as follows: index, −10°; middle, −20°; ring, −15°; and small, 0°. The caregivers and Lillian herself were able to efficiently cleanse the hand. Lillian can now have a simple manicure with ease. The occupational therapist discharged the wrist immobilization orthosis and replaced it with a soft prefabricated immobilization orthosis with rigid wrist and forearm support but semirigid hand support to accommodate tone fluctuations when Lillian ambulates. The strapping material used was flexible yet offered enough rigidity to effectively secure the joint segments.

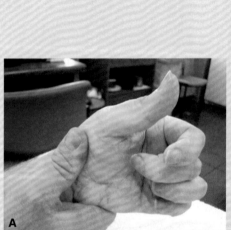 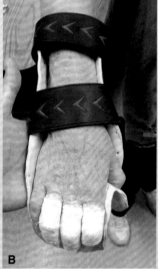 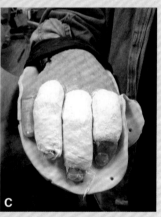

FIGURE 23–39 **A,** Flexion deformity of digits. **B,** Initial digit casting combined with volar wrist and hand immobilization orthosis to stretch tight flexors. **C,** Progression with more proximal interphalangeal extension in casts. Notice how the tone in the index finger is greater than the ulnar digits.

CHAPTER REVIEW QUESTIONS

1. What are common purposes for the use of orthoses in the adult with neurologic dysfunction?
2. What role can taping play in treating this population?
3. What is the theory behind the use of the Saebo products?
4. List a few prefabricated orthoses that may be indicated for use in joint contracture management.
5. What precautions must a therapist be mindful of when dispensing these devices?

ACKNOWLEDGMENT FROM SECOND EDITION

Sincere thanks to the following for providing input regarding their products/approaches included in this chapter: Paul Mohr, PT (GivMohr® Corporation), and Waleed Al-Oboudi, MOT, OTR/L (Neuro-IFRAH® Organization).

24 The Pediatric Patient[a]

Jill Peck-Murray, MOTR/L, CHT

CHAPTER OBJECTIVES

After study of this chapter, the reader should be able to:
• Appreciate the special developmental and environmental considerations in fabricating an orthosis for a pediatric patient.
• Describe the rationale for orthotic intervention in the pediatric population.
• List several common diagnoses and appropriate orthotic intervention for the pediatric patient.
• Give examples of design considerations for custom and prefabricated orthoses for children of various ages.
• List several ideas for gaining compliance with orthotic use from families and children.

KEY TERMS

Hand skill development

Neonate orthoses

Orthosis alignment

Orthosis compliance

Pediatric orthoses

Pediatric upper extremity conditions

MD NOTE

C. Douglas Wallace, MD
California

The role of the pediatric hand therapists in care of our patient population cannot be overstated in quality upper extremity care for children. Their skill and knowledge of the various pediatric upper extremity conditions, as well as, their ability to make therapy and home programs fun for our patients is critical to success. Pediatric patients have a myriad of needs, changes, and challenges based on age and maturity, both emotional and skeletal. Managing these patient-specific needs while striving for cooperation and adhering to sound biomechanical therapeutic principles is an engaging task with great rewards.

A well-made orthosis is one that fits the child comfortably and provides proper support as well as function. As a surgeon and a craftsman, I am always looking at ways to make something better. Consulting with my therapists about our shared goals for the orthosis and the design options yields optimal results for fit and function. I often brainstorm with my therapists on how to modify shape, composition, and unique design ideas. With my consult, they started using a Dremel tool to make slits in the orthosis, allowing the straps to hold the digits in the best positions. My favorite design for an orthosis is one that uses the lever principle to lift the body part (wrist or digit). Unfortunately, when I order it, I can never remember the name of the dorsal wrist orthosis, but I do remember that it looks like an old fashioned "cheese slicer," hence my nickname for this orthosis. Durability of the orthoses is another key characteristic, but most importantly, the child must want to wear it, so making it "kid friendly" is vital.

Creativity to gain cooperation with orthotic use, therapy, and home program are skills that are inherent to a successful pediatric hand therapist. I appreciate all their efforts and feel their role has been critical to the care of my patients.

FAQ

What advice would you give a therapist new to treating the pediatric patient?
a. Accept the challenges and rise to them without hesitation.
b. The infant is going to wiggle and squirm. The young child is probably not going to sit still in a chair for long periods. There may be some crying and tears, but this is the way an infant or young child communicates their frustrations.
c. Be prepared prior to the session with fun activities to keep the child busy while you are fabricating the orthosis.
d. Recognize that the child and family may be apprehensive about the process so take time to explain things completely with sample orthosis.
e. Read the sections of the chapter on ideas for compliance and acceptance of the orthosis.

---

[a]This chapter is based on the first edition chapter written by Elaine Charest, MA, MBA, OTR/L and the 2nd edition revised by this author.

f. Thoroughly, describe the application and use of the orthosis to the caregivers.

g. Praise the child for participation in the session and wearing the orthosis at home.

What is an easy method for preventing a child from removing their orthosis?

a. "Put a sock on it."

What do you do when a patient refuses to wear their orthosis?

a. Find out what is the issue underlying the refusal and try to solve it.

- Is it uncomfortable? Adjust it for comfort as needed.
- Does it make them sweat? Place a thin stockinette under the orthosis
- Are they self-conscience when wearing it? Can it be covered or decorated?
- Is it interfering with function? Can it be used at night only?
- Do they have trouble sleeping with it? Try using it during the day.

b. Remember an orthosis is not always the key to meeting the therapy goals.

INTRODUCTION

The pediatric patient is not just a "small adult." They are active, growing, and constantly changing in size and acquiring new developmental skills. Therapy and orthosis provision need to be tailored for each child with special consideration for factors that are unique to children. The purpose and types of orthoses are similar to adult orthoses, but there are often differences in design, material selection, strapping, and padding application. This chapter explains how an orthosis can be a part of the therapeutic intervention for children to address specific pediatric conditions, to enhance functional and developmental skills, and to provide comfort and protection. It offers suggestions to prevent self-removal and improve orthosis compliance. Also, this chapter describes a typical session for making an orthosis with suggestions for dealing with the challenges of fabrication and application of an orthosis on an infant or young child. The final part of this chapter presents case studies of common pediatric conditions and diagnoses with recommendations for possible options for orthoses. The author hopes to impart some knowledge and provide tools to assist with the assessment of pediatric hands to formulate an appropriate orthotic intervention for each child, but it is beyond the scope of this chapter to describe all the possible orthoses with the supporting literature to treat the hands of children.

PURPOSES OF ORTHOSES FOR THE PEDIATRIC PATIENT

The primary purposes of pediatric orthoses are to provide support and protection, to improve/maintain motion, and to enhance function and development (Hogan & Uditsky, 1998). After a child has undergone surgery or sustained an injury, the physician may request an orthosis to protect the healing tissue, skin, tendons, nerves, joints, and muscles. An immobilization type orthosis (see Chapter 1 of the Fabrication Manual) is commonly used with children to provide the proper support and positioning (Fig. 24–1A–C). There are custom or prefabricated orthotic options for children.

In certain congenital conditions, there is a need to maintain passive motion until surgical intervention. For example, an infant with type IV radial ray deficiency exhibits significant wrist radial deviation (Fig. 24–2A). To optimize joint flexibility, the parents are advised to perform a stretching program with every diaper change and use a wrist orthosis at all other times (Fig. 24–2B) (Moran & Tomhave, 2011).

Orthoses are often part of the therapeutic intervention plan to gain passive motion. A child with persistent stiffness after prolonged

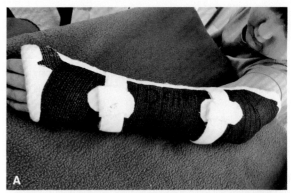
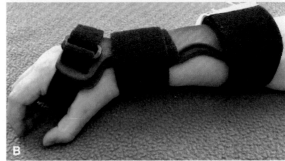
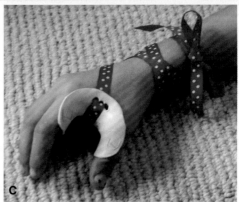

FIGURE 24–1 A, Circumferential orthosis made of casting tape provides support and protection after a forearm fracture. **B,** Dorsal-based prefabricated orthosis stabilizes the wrist but allows for functional freedom of fingers and thumb. **C,** Thermoplastic material of this orthosis conforms into the web space as well as supports the thumb and index finger.

immobilization in a cast will benefit from a static progressive mobilization orthosis (Fig. 24–3A,B). A child with congenital stiffness from conditions, such as camptodactyly or arthrogryposis, will benefit from the use of an orthosis with a serial static (Fig. 24–4A,B) or serial casting approach (Fig. 24–4C). By providing

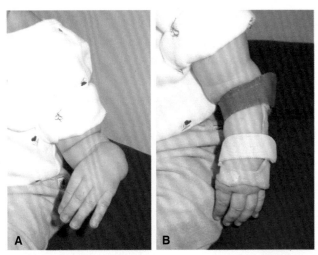

FIGURE 24–2 A, Child with radial ray deficiency exhibits significant radial deviation due to lack of structures on the radial side of the arm. **B,** The ulnar-based orthosis provides the leverage needed to position the wrist in neutral to maintain the available passive motion. Small vertical snips have been added to the proximal strap to improve comfort.

a low-load, prolonged stretch (LLPS), these types of mobilization orthoses maximize tissue length to improve passive motion (Duff & Charles, 2004; Yasukawa & Cassar, 2009; Schwartz, 2016; Grenier & Shankland, 2018).

Muscle imbalances caused by spasticity, abnormal tone, or peripheral nerve injury may result in the development of secondary joint contracture (Yasukawa & Cassar, 2009). The maintenance of normal anatomical relationships will help to maintain the tissue length. By providing proper positioning to align joints, the orthosis will help prevent the shortening of soft tissues (Fig. 24–5A,B) (Box 24–1). (Schoen & Anderson, 1999).

Also, muscle imbalances will affect the position of an arm, ultimately, interfering with functional use and normal developmental

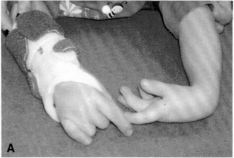
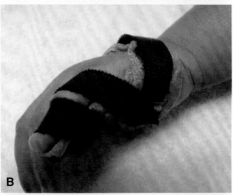
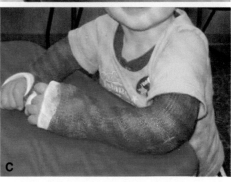

FIGURE 24–4 A, Child with arthrogryposis was unable to actively extend her wrist. If the wrist orthosis is used in a serial static manner, it can improve motion. **B,** Hand-based mobilization orthosis made of Orficast® will improve proximal interphalangeal (PIP) joint extension by weekly changes in a serial static manner (Orfit). **C,** A circumferential cast changed weekly should improve flexion in a child with congenital elbow extension contracture from arthrogryposis.

skills (Yasukawa & Cassar, 2009). An orthosis made of a stretchy material can provide a dynamic component to assist a weak muscle group. Fig. 24–6A shows a mobilization orthosis made of Fabrifoam® to encourage supination to orient the hand and arm in the position for improved hand use and finger dexterity (Azzam, 2012). Fig 24–6B exhibits how an orthosis will position the arm appropriately for weight-bearing and crawling. Crawling is a critical skill that promotes many areas of brain development and hand use (Clearfield, 2004; Visser & Franzsen, 2010). If the child's hand tends to fist, an alternative style orthosis will facilitate an open hand weight-bearing position (Fig. 24–6C).

The child born with a condition or who sustains an injury to the ligaments, tendons, joints, or neurovascular structures may have issues with joint stability. An unstable joint significantly alters the biomechanics of the hand or arm and thus affects function. For example, thumb hypoplasia or cerebral palsy can cause a thumb to be unstable at the metacarpal (MP) joint, so the child may not be able to hold objects or finger foods adequately. An orthosis can provide the biomechanical alignment to place the thumb tip in opposition to the fingers to optimize function (Keklicek, Uygur, & Yakut, 2015). This may be accomplished with the use of soft materials, such as therapeutic tape, neoprene (Fig. 24–7A,B), or thermoplastic material formed in the web space and around the thumb (Fig. 24–7C) (Box 24–2).

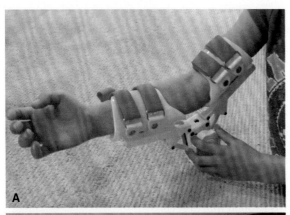
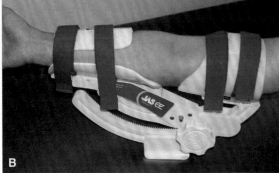

FIGURE 24–3 A, Elbow mobilization orthosis (JAS®) provides a static progressive stretch that is controlled by the patient to increase the tension with a turn of the knob. **B,** Gains made into full elbow extension within 1 month use of this orthosis. Joint Active Systems® (Effingham, IL).

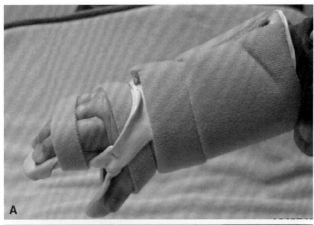

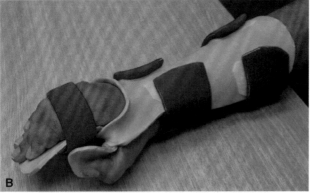

FIGURE 24–5 Volar/dorsal wrist and hand immobilization orthoses. **A,** Infant-sized custom orthosis with a dorsal forearm and volar hand piece. **B,** This immobilization orthosis with a dorsal forearm and volar hand piece can provide proper positioning to align joints and help prevent contractures.

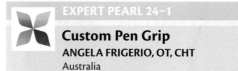

EXPERT PEARL 24–1

Custom Pen Grip
ANGELA FRIGERIO, OT, CHT
Australia

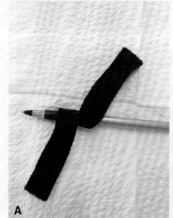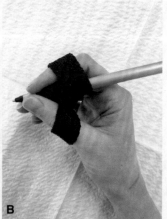

Orficast More thermoplastic tape cut into 3-cm strip. Wrap tape around pen and then apply to middle phalanx of index finger and proximal phalanx of thumb in a "figure-of-8" pattern. Experiment with tape placement, depending on patient's pencil grip or comfort.

BOX 24–1   VOLAR/DORSAL WRIST AND HAND IMMOBILIZATION ORTHOSIS

1. First heat the smaller hand segment.
2. Position child's hand by extending fingers with wrist in flexion.
3. Place material onto hand with base conforming into palmar arch.
4. While holding the thumb in abduction and extension, form thumb piece with gentle pressure, molding a trough for the thumb to rest.
5. Position the fingers into extension at IP joints and slight flexion at MCP joints while allowing the wrist to remain slightly flexed (except with significant extrinsic tightness, wrist should be moved into extension and fingers allowed to flex as needed).
6. Remove hand segment and prepare to heat and mold larger dorsal forearm-based segment.
7. Position child's arm by placing wrist into extension and allowing fingers to flex.
8. Place material onto dorsal forearm, gently smoothing down the sides. Distal edge should end at midmetacarpal region.
9. Allow the distal lateral pieces (wings), positioned ulnarly at the base of small finger and radially over web space, to "hang" while material sets.

10. Remove forearm segment.
11. Place hand segment on child and position wrist in maximal extension.
12. Reheat the "wings" on the forearm segment only in water to soften slightly.
13. Place dorsal forearm segment on child and gently mold "wings" around the ulnar and radial sides of the volar hand segment to attach in palm. Mark points where pieces overlap.
14. Remove both segments and permanently attach together. (Either use solvent or scratch off coating, followed by heating areas to bond with heat gun.)
15. Apply hook-and-loop straps as shown in **Figure 24–5A,B**.
16. Please note to wrist strap tension is key to help prevent slippage.
17. Be sure to choose a material with a protective coating to prevent inadvertent adherence during the molding process.

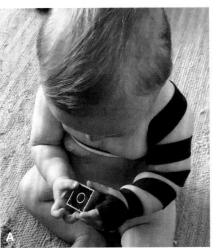
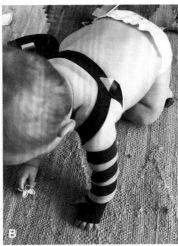
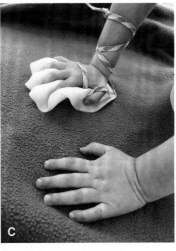

FIGURE 24–6 **A,** This mobilization orthosis made of Fabrifoam® (North Coast Medical, Morgan Hill CA) assists forearm supination and shoulder external rotation to position the hand for use. **B,** A long strip of Fabrifoam® can be used to position the entire arm for crawling or weight-bearing. **C,** Thermoplastic material molded between the web spaces on the volar surface of the hand can help position the hand for weight-bearing. A colorful shoelace tied over the fingers and thumb and then around the wrist in a figure-of-8 fashion secures the orthosis for crawling.

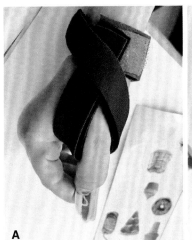
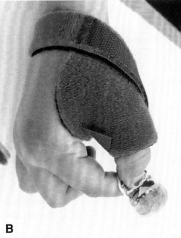
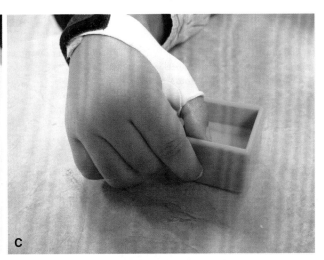

FIGURE 24–7 **A,** The original Joe Cool Thumb Splint is a prefabricated thumb abduction orthosis (The Joe Cool Company, South Jordan, UT) providing a subtle support and positioning of the thumb to allow for use. **B,** The McKie Thumb Splint is a neoprene thumb abduction orthosis (McKie, Duluth, MN) providing more support needed to mobilize the thumb for grasp. **C,** An orthosis made of thin thermoplastic provides a more rigid support to control the thumb metacarpal (MP) joint.

BOX 24–2   WEIGHT-BEARING ORTHOSIS

1. Use a piece of 3/32″ thermoplastic material 2″ wider and longer than the child's hand.
2. Place a ball of Theraputty onto a nonadherent surface.
3. Heat thermoplastic and mold onto supinated palm to form the palmar piece.
4. While abducting the fingers and thumb, allow material to drape between web spaces to form finger separators.
5. As material is partially set, carefully pronate hand into a weight-bearing position and press into the ball of Theraputty.
6. As material sets, direct attention to the ulnar and radial edges forming borders to improve fit.

7. After removal, use hole punch to make the following four slits in orthosis:
   a. First web space
   b. Index finger MCP joint
   c. Base of thumb carpometacarpal (CMC)
   d. Small finger MCP joint
8. Use a length of material (such as a ribbon or felt) and weave it through the slits and tie in a figure-of-8 around the wrist as shown in **Figure 24–6C, 24–12D**.
9. Another option includes using traditional hook-and-loop closure.

PLANNING ORTHOTIC INTERVENTION FOR THE CHILD

Understanding the issues that are unique to pediatric is critical to the success of the orthotic intervention. Their anatomy is often smaller than adults. Children go through stages of rapid growth and development and lead active lifestyles. There are some diagnoses and conditions that are specific to pediatrics, such as congenital anomalies, cerebral palsy, and juvenile arthritis. It is beyond the scope of this chapter to discuss the conditions in detail with the evidence-based rationale behind the therapeutic intervention and the use of specific orthoses. Table 24–1 provides a brief description of common pediatric upper extremity conditions, possible therapeutic approaches, and some suggested orthoses (custom or prefabricated) that are based on the available supporting literature.

In addition to a good understanding of the various diagnoses that are specific to the pediatric population, the therapist should select the most appropriate type of orthoses based on a complete evaluation of the affected structures and systems (tendons, muscles, nerves, ligaments, and bones). For instance, during the

TABLE 24–1	Orthotic Intervention for Common Pediatric Conditions	
Conditions	**Therapeutic Intervention**	**Suggested Orthoses**
Arthrogryposis Congenital condition characterized by joint contractures and weakness	Prolonged stretching to gain motion in involved joints Provide proper wrist position for hand use	**Custom:** Serial casting (Fig. 24–4C); serial static (Fig. 24–4A); static progressive mobilization orthoses **Prefabs:** JAS˙ Elbow (Effingham, IL) (Fig. 24–4A); Comfy™ Pediatric Goniometer Elbow Orthosis; Comfy™ Pediatric Finger Extender Orthosis (Lenjoy Med. Eng. Inc, Gardena, CA) **Custom:** Dorsal wrist orthosis (Fig. 24–6A) **Prefabs:** RCAI˙ Carpal Tunnel Orthosis (Restorative Care of America, St Petersburg, FL)
Brachial plexus palsy Stretch injury to the brachial plexus resulting in varying degrees of weakness in the involved arm	Provide proper positioning for the forearm and shoulder Correct elbow flexion contracture	**Custom:** Sup-ER Orthosis (see article Durlacher, Bellows, & Verchere, 2014); dynamic supination/ER strap (Figs. 24–6 A,B) **Custom:** Serial static elbow extension orthosis (Fig. 24–13B); serial casting (Fig. 24–4A) **Prefabs:** JAS˙ Elbow (Fig. 24–3A); Comfy™ Pediatric Goniometer Elbow Orthosis
Camptodactyly Congenital proximal interphalangeal (PIP) contracture, often of small finger	Reduce PIP flexion contracture	**Custom:** Finger extension mobilization serial static orthosis (Fig. 24–4B); serial casting; metacarpal (MP) blocking (Fig. 24–13); relative motion orthosis **Prefabs:** For older child only: OrthoFoam™ PIP Extension Orthosis (North Coast Medical)
Cerebral palsy Nonprogressive motor impairment caused by injury to the developing brain that causes irreversible upper motor neuron disorder characterized by abnormal tone, weakness, and progressive joint contractures	Maintain maximum length in elbow Provide proper position to hand, wrist, and forearm to help prevent contractures Supinate hand/forearm to enhance distal function Provide proper position to wrist to enhance distal function Provide proper position to thumb to enhance distal function	**Prefabs:** Posey˙ Pediatric Secure Sleeve˙ (Posey, Arcadia CA); Comfy™ Pediatric Goniometer Elbow Orthosis; Progress™ Pediatric Elbow Orthosis (North Coast Med.) **Custom:** Volar or volar/dorsal hand/wrist (Fig. 24–5B) **Prefabs:** Comfy™ Pediatric Hand Thumb Orthosis; Progress™ Pediatric Functional Orthosis (North Coast Medical) Orthosis; RMI˙ Neuroflex™ Restorative Pediatric Flex Hand (Restorative Medical) (Fig. 24–10C); Benik Volar Pan Extension (Silverdale, WA) (Fig. 24–10A) **Custom:** Serpentine style forearm strap made of neoprene or Fabrifoam˙ (Fig. 24–6A,B) **Prefabs:** Pediatric Comfort Cool˙ Supination Orthosis (North Coast) **Custom:** Dorsal wrist orthosis (Figs. 24–9A, and 24–12A) **Prefabs:** RCAI˙ Carpal Tunnel Orthosis (Fig. 24–8); North Coast Liberty™ Wrist Brace (Fig. 24–9B); Benik Neoprene Wrist Orthoses; RCAI Pediatric Wrist Forearm Orthosis **Custom:** Web space or thumb orthosis (Fig. 24–1C, and 24–7C) **Prefabs:** Joe Cool Thumb Orthoses (South Jordan, UT) (Fig. 24–7A); McKie Thumb Orthoses (Duluth, MN) (Fig. 24–7A); Benik Thumb Orthoses; RCAI˙ Thumb Abduction Support Strap; RCAI Neoprene Elastic Thumb Brace

TABLE 24–1	Orthotic Intervention for Common Pediatric Conditions (Continued)	
Conditions	**Therapeutic Intervention**	**Suggested Orthoses**
Charcot-Marie-Tooth Disease Hereditary sensorimotor polyneuropathy with progressive weakness primarily in intrinsic hand muscles	Provide finger positioning to enhance function Position thumb or fingers for use	**Custom:** Figure-of-8 orthosis; relative motion orthosis; MP-blocking orthosis (Fig. 24–13C) **Prefab:** Oval-8˚ Pediatric Finger Orthosis (3-Point Products, Stevensville, MD) **Custom:** Web space orthosis (Fig. 24–1C); neoprene thumb abduction orthosis **Prefabs:** Joe Cool Thumb Orthoses (Fig. 24–7A); McKie Web Stay Thumb Orthosis (Fig. 24–7B); RCAI˚ Thumb Abduction Support
Duchenne muscular dystrophy Slowly progressive proximal to distal muscle weakness finally including respiratory muscles	Provide positioning to prevent elbow contracture Provide positioning to prevent contractures of wrist and hand Provide positioning of wrists for use	**Custom:** Elbow extension orthosis (Fig. 24–13B) **Prefabs:** Posey˚ Soft-bead Elbow Orthosis; Comfy™ Pediatric Goniometer Elbow Orthosis; Progress™ Pediatric Elbow Orthosis **Custom:** Volar or volar/dorsal immobilization orthoses (Figs. 24–5B, and 24–14A) **Prefabs:** Comfy™ Pediatric Hand Thumb Orthosis; Progress™ Pediatric Functional Orthosis; RMI˚ Neuroflex™ Restorative Pediatric Flex Hand **Custom:** Dorsal wrist immobilization orthosis (Fig. 24–9A) **Prefabs:** North Coast Liberty™ Wrist Brace (Fig. 24–9B); Benik Neoprene Wrist Orthoses; Carpal Tunnel Brace from RCAI˚ (Fig. 24–8)
Fractures: Most common pediatric fracture site: Elbow	Reduce postsurgical or cast removal stiffness	**Custom:** Serial static (Fig. 24–13B); static progressive (turnbuckle) mobilization orthoses **Prefabs:** Ultraflex (Pottstown, PA); or JAS˚ Elbow; Comfy™ Pediatric Goniometer Elbow Orthosis; Progress™ Pediatric Elbow Orthosis
Hemiplegia due to stroke or TBI Weakness and tonal changes of upper and lower extremity on same side	Assist weak muscles in shoulder, forearm Provide proper wrist/thumb position for hand use Provide proper thumb positioning for use	**Custom:** Serpentine style strap which is made of neoprene or Fabrifoam˚ (Fig. 24–7B) **Prefabs:** Pediatric Comfort Cool˚ Supination Orthoses **Custom:** Static dorsal wrist immobilization orthosis (Fig. 24–9A); weight-bearing orthosis (Fig. 24–6C) **Prefabs:** Carpal Tunnel Brace from RCAI˚; North Coast Liberty™ Wrist Brace (Fig. 24–8); Benik Neoprene Wrist **Custom:** Web space or thumb orthosis (Figs. 24–1C, and 24–7C) **Prefabs:** Joe Cool Thumb Orthoses (Fig. 24–7A); McKie Thumb Orthosis (Fig. 24–7B); Benik Thumb Orthoses
Juvenile arthritis Persistent swelling of joints with onset before age 16 years	Provide proper night positioning Position wrist in extension to prevent loss of motion	**Custom:** Wrist/hand immobilization orthoses (Fig. 24–12B) **Custom:** Wrist immobilization orthoses (Fig. 24–9A) **Prefabs:** North Coast Liberty™ Wrist Brace (Fig. 24–9B); Benik Volar Pan Extension (Fig. 24–10A); Carpal Tunnel Brace from RCAI˚ (Fig. 24–1B)
Nerve injuries Radial nerve injuries Ulnar nerve injuries	Positioning to prevent contractures	**Custom:** Wrist immobilization orthoses (Fig. 24–9A) **Prefabs:** Benik Radial Nerve Tunnel˚ Orthoses; Liberty™ Wrist Orthosis (Fig. 24–9B); Carpal Tunnel Brace from RCAI˚ (Fig. 24–1B) **Custom:** Metacarpophalangeal (MCP)-blocking orthoses (Fig. 24–13C), relative motion orthoses
Osteogenesis imperfecta Hereditary connective tissue disorder resulting in bone fragility	Fracture management, Protection, and support	**Custom:** Immobilization orthoses supporting fracture sites or protecting vulnerable sites **Prefabs:** RCAI˚ Humeral Fracture Brace; RCAI˚ Wrist Fracture Orthosis

(Continued)

TABLE 24-1	**Orthotic Intervention for Common Pediatric Conditions** **(Continued)**	
Conditions	**Therapeutic Intervention**	**Suggested Orthoses**
Radial ray deficiency Congenital malformation of radial side of arm	Minimize soft tissue tightness due to radial wrist deviation posturing	**Custom:** Circumferential soft wrap (Fig. 24–17A); ulnar-based wrist immobilization orthosis (Fig. 24–2B) **Prefabs:** Benik Radial Dysplasia Orthosis; Comfy™ Wrist Deviation Hand Orthosis
Rett syndrome Progressive encephalopathy with loss of purposeful hand use with characteristic hand wringing and ataxia	Provide positioning to prevent excessive hand wringing or hand-to-mouth behavior	**Custom:** Elbow static orthosis **Prefabs:** Posey® Pediatric SecureSleeve®; Benik Neoprene Elbow Sleeve; Comfy™ Pediatric Elbow Orthosis; Progress™ Pediatric Elbow Orthosis; RCAI Pediatric Elbow Stabilizer, Benik Pediatric Hinged Elbow Orthosis
Syndactyly Lack of differentiation of fingers, skin, and/or bones	Postoperative scar extension management and maintain extension of fingers	**Custom:** Finger extension orthosis lined with moldable silicone putty
Sports injuries and tendonitis Overuse issues with pain, swelling, and limited use	Support to decrease pain and swelling	**Custom or Prefabs:** Immobilization orthoses as indicated by injury
Thumb hypoplasia Underdeveloped thumb with mild weakness to absent thumb	Maintain web and support thumb for use Postsurgical protection after surgery	**Custom:** Thumb orthosis (Fig. 24–7C) **Prefabs:** Joe Cool Thumb Orthoses (Fig. 24–7A); McKie Thumb Orthosis (Fig. 24–7B); Benik Thumb Orthoses **Custom:** Thumb spica static-type immobilization orthosis **Prefabs:** Joe Cool Thumb Orthoses (Fig. 24–7A); McKie Thumb Orthoses (Fig. 24–7B); Benik Thumb Orthoses
Thumb-in-palm deformities Flexion posturing of thumb due to lack of thumb extension musculature	Position in full extension at night Support thumb to allow for use	**Custom:** Thumb extension immobilization orthosis (Fig. 24–7C) **Custom:** Opponens thumb orthosis; web space orthosis (Fig. 24–1C); custom neoprene orthosis **Prefabs:** Benik Thumb Abduction Orthosis; Joe Cool Thumb Orthoses (Fig. 24–7A); McKie Thumb Orthoses (Fig. 24–7B)

Modified from Charest, E. (2003). The pediatric patient. In Austin N. & Jacobs M. (Eds.), Splinting the hand and upper extremity: Principles and process. Baltimore, MD: Lippincott Williams & Wilkins; Ho, E., Roy, T., Stephens, D., & Clarke, H. M. (2010). Serial casting and splinting of elbow contractures in children with obstetric brachial plexus palsy. Journal of Hand Surgery, 35A, 84–91; Fuller, M. (1999). Treatment of congenital differences of the upper extremity: Therapist's commentary. Journal of Hand Therapy, 12(2), 174–177; Moran, S. L., & Tomhave, W. (2011). Management of congenital hand anomalies. In Skiven T., Osterman L., Fedorczyk J., & Amadio P. (Eds.), Rehabilitation of the hand and upper extremity (6th ed., pp. 1631–1646). Philadelphia, PA: Mosby.

assessment of a teenager with a painful wrist, the therapist notes that weight bearing onto the gymnast's wrist is painful which may indicate a ligament strain (Trevithick, Mellifont, & Sayer, 2019). The therapist may then decide to promote healing by resting the wrist in a static style wrist orthosis for several weeks prior to beginning an isometric exercise program. Assessing the child from a developmental perspective as well as from an anatomical perspective will allow the therapist to determine the most appropriate intervention that may include an orthosis (Ho, 2010). Table 24–2 is a brief summary of normal grasp and hand skill development for the first 6 years of life. By doing an assessment of the child's current level of grasp and development, the therapist can plan an intervention to encourage the next stage of development. As the table describes, normal physiologic flexion and primitive reflexes predominate in the first few months of life. Parents may be concerned their infant is maintaining a thumb-in-palm posturing; however, the therapist can explain this is normal for babies until the age of 4 months. If there are major delays beyond that age, the child may not use the thumb or use the back of the thumb for prehension against the fingertips. A soft neoprene thumb orthosis will position the thumb to allow for more normal use (Fig. 24–7A–C). It is critical to position the thumb for use to provide sensory and motor feedback to facilitate normal functional brain mapping before the age of 3 years (Cheney, 2002).

To determine if an orthosis may be indicated to enhance function for the older child, an assessment of the child's functional abilities and desires for improved function should be completed using an appropriate functional outcome measure. A functional orthosis may support a proximal body part (i.e., weak wrist) to allow for distal hand function (Figs. 24–4A and 24–8). The orthosis may not always be the solution to enhance function, because it may interfere with a learned position of use (Ten Berge et al., 2012). The therapist needs to give the child the opportunity to practice with and without the orthosis to determine if it will help the child reach their functional goals (Jackman, Novak, Lannin, & Galea, 2019). Lastly, a determination of the child and family commitment to the use of the orthosis will complete the holistic approach to orthotic intervention.

PROPER SELECTION/DESIGN FOR PEDIATRIC PATIENTS

Proper design should always be based on good problem-solving that is grounded in proper biomechanical principles (see Chapter 4). Appropriate decisions about location, width, and length are critical in design plans, especially for children. Adapting an adult orthotic pattern to a smaller size does not allow for customization that is needed for a growing child. The design principles such as the use

TABLE 24–2	**Grasp and Hand Skill Development**
Age	**Developmental Level**
0–2 mo	**Reflexive Grasp** • Hand closes on objects placed in palm • Normal physiologic flexion (hands fisted), except with startle or stretching
2–3 mo	**Ulnar Palmar Grasp** • Holds toy or block placed in hand on ulnar side of hand • In supine, moves arms overhead and brings hands together on chest
4 mo	**Crude Palmar Grasp** • Contacts toy with palmar surface of hand • In prone, bears weight on ulnar side of forearms with good head control • Grasp reflex diminishing so thumb is no longer flexed in palm
5 mo	**Palmar Grasp** • Holds toy in palm enclosed by fingers with thumb adducted • In prone, pushes up on extended arms • In supine, can hold bottle with partial forearm supination
6 mo	**Raking Grasp** • Uses all fingers to rake small objects into palm • In prone, weight shifts on extended arms • In independent sitting, hands are now free for use • Grasp and release in purposeful manner
7 mo	**Radial Palmar Grasp** • Holds toy or block in radial side of hand • In prone, pivots and combat crawls • In sitting, transfers objects from one hand to another
8 mo	**Developmental Scissors Grasp** • Holds small object with thumb and radial side of index • Crawling with weight-bearing through shoulder, elbow, and wrist
9 mo	**Inferior Pincer Grasp** • Holds small object with thumb along distal radial side of extended index • Active forearm supination when reaching • Grasps toy or block using thumb and fingertips
10 mo	**Pincer Grasp** • Holds small object held with pads of index and thumb • Stands and cruises • Pokes with index finger • Beginning tool use (spoon)
12 mo	**Neat Pincer Grasp** • Holds small object with tip of index and thumb tip flexed • Walking independently, so more hand use • Uses hands in a coordinated manner (one hand stabilizes and other manipulates)
15 mo	**Forearm Neutral Palmar Grasp** • Holds marker in palm with forearm neutral • Releases object with wrist extension into container • Stacks two blocks • Holds ball in two hands
2–3 y	**Digital Pronated Grasp** • Holds marker with fingers and thumb with forearm pronated • Places small object into a hole with precision • Stacks 3–6 blocks into a tower

TABLE 24–2	**Grasp and Hand Skill Development (Continued)**
Age	**Developmental Level**
3.1–4 y	**Static Tripod Grasp** • Holds marker static with thumb, index, and long fingers • Stacks 7–9 blocks into a tower • Able to draw shapes • Beginning to cut with scissors
4.5–6 y	**Dynamic Tripod Grasp** • Holds marker with moving tips of thumb, index, and long fingers • Stacks 10–12 blocks into a tower • Able to write letters

Modified from Charest, E. (2003). The pediatric patient. In Austin N. & Jacobs M. (Eds.), Splinting the hand and upper extremity: Principles and process. Baltimore, MD: Lippincott Williams & Wilkins; Ho, E. S. (2010). Measuring hand function in the young child. Journal of Hand Therapy, 23(3), 323–328; Erhardt, R., & Lindley, S. (2000). Functional development of the hand. In Gupta A., Kay S., & Scheker L. (Eds.), The growing hand: Diagnosis and management of the upper extremity in children. London, United Kingdom: Mosby and McCoy-Powlen, J., Buckland Gallen, D., Edwards, S. (2017). Hand Development. In Wagenfeld A., Kaldenberg J., Honaker D. (Eds.) Foundations of pediatric practice for the occupational therapy assistant, 2nd ed. pp. 263–279), Thorofare, NJ, SLACK Inc.

of three points of pressure (one at each end in one direction and one in the middle in the other direction) and the use of first-class lever principle will be useful for a pediatric orthosis. By providing lift to the body part, rather than the straps forcing the body part into place, will make it easier for the patient or family to apply (Figs. 24–1B, 24–2B, and 24–4A). Because the body parts are often smaller in children than adults, the therapist needs to measure for the width and length of the orthosis. The width of the orthosis should be at least half the circumference of the body part, whether it is the upper arm, forearm, wrist, digit, or thumb (Fig. 24–9A). This will allow for maximal control from the straps when applied. The length should be as long as necessary to distribute the pressure appropriately, using joint creases as a guide to provide maximal length of levers. If the orthosis is a forearm based, then it should be fabricated to two-thirds of the length of the arm (Fig. 24–9A). The orthosis should be designed to support all necessary joints while allowing freedom of unaffected joints (Fig. 24–9B).

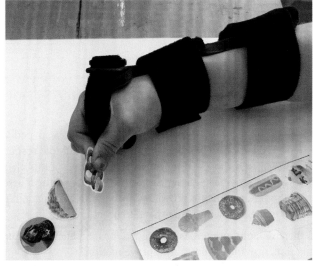

FIGURE 24–8 The Dorsal Carpal Tunnel Splint is a prefabricated wrist orthosis (Restorative Care of America, St Petersburg, FL) providing wrist support but allowing for distal function.

Pediatric Fabrication Tips
GINNY GIBSON OTD, OTR/L, CHT
California

Fabricating a thermoplastic orthosis for a young and awake child can be daunting, and more so if one attempts to fabricate the entire orthosis in one application. To ease the process, increase precision, and optimize aesthetics, consider fabricating the orthosis in phases. A series of steps for fabricating an orthosis for a child with ring and small finger camptodactyly is shown:

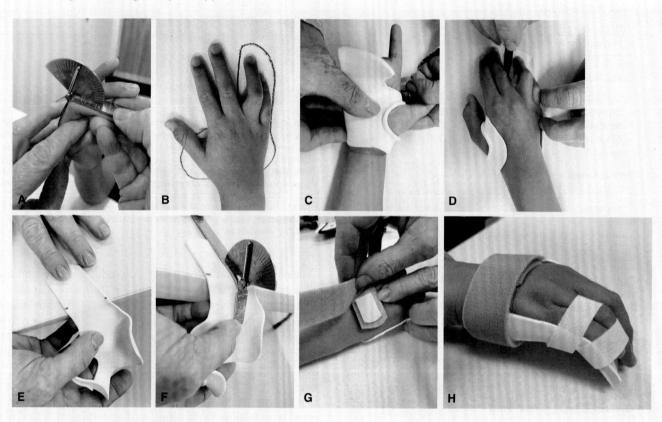

A. measure the flexion deformity and record the degree of limitation;

B. draw a pattern and cut out thermoplastic;

C. apply warm thermoplastic around thumb and on palm (the portion of thermoplastic that will rest against the volar digits is not shaped at this time); remove cooled thermoplastic; reheat the portion of thermoplastic that will rest against the volar digits and flatten;

D. apply cooled thermoplastic to the hand and mark edges of the digital pan at the level of the proximal interphalangeal (PIP) joint;

E. reheat the digital pan by dipping material in hot water to a depth that corresponds with the two pen marks; using a near straight edge of a flat surface;

F. bend the thermoplastic to an angle 5° or 10° less than the flexion deformity.

G. fold the most proximal strap around the dorsal aspect of the thumb hole and attach the two surfaces of the strap with Velcro (for older children) or sew (for infants and toddlers) to optimize a secure fit of the strap;

H. final fit of orthosis.

SELECTION OF PREFABRICATED ORTHOSES FOR THE PEDIATRIC PATIENT

Fortunately, more options for prefabricated orthoses in pediatric sizes have recently become available. There are multiple resources for prefabricated orthoses (refer to listing at the end of this chapter including web sites). The therapist needs to make a critical assessment of the orthosis before provision or ordering for a patient (see Chapter 9). The following issues need to be addressed:

- Is there an appropriate design needed for the patient to enhance function, provide support, or improve motion?
- Can the orthosis be ordered in the proper size? Having some sample sizes to try on the patient will help to determine if it provides proper positioning to aid function.
- Is it easy to apply for the family or patient? An orthosis that has multiple components may require complete understanding for proper application.
- Do the straps allow for proper positioning? A close examination of the strap placement is necessary to ensure that the appropriate forces are applied in the needed direction with necessary distribution of the pressure.
- Can the orthosis be adjusted for growth or change in position? Some of the newer styles are adjustable because they are embedded with a thin thermoplastic (Fig. 24–10A), malleable metal (Fig. 24–10B), or plastic (Fig. 24–10C).
- Can it be cleaned adequately? The materials should be washable and durable, especially if it is for long-term use.

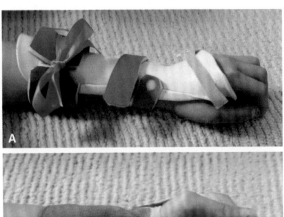

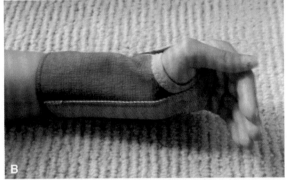

FIGURE 24–9 A, Wrist orthosis fabricated to two-thirds the length and one-half the width of the arm to help distribute the pressure from the orthosis or the straps on the arm. **B,** Child with radial nerve laceration was unable to actively extend his wrist. This prefabricated Liberty™ Wrist Brace (North Coast Medical) provided wrist support. The metacarpophalangeal (MCP) joints are free for motion, because this orthosis does not cross the distal palmar crease.

FABRICATION OF CUSTOM ORTHOSES FOR THE PEDIATRIC PATIENT

Material Selection

There are many material options to use for orthoses as described in Chapter 5. With children, it is important to start with the softest, thinnest, and lightest material possible and choose firmer options as needed. Examples of soft materials are neoprene, Velfoam®, Fabrifoam®, Plastazote®, and silicone-based putty. Foam cylinders (a pool noodle or cylindrical tubing) can be used for a soft hand orthosis or the hand piece in a forearm-based orthosis.

The hardest materials include casting materials, such as plaster, or polyester casting tapes, or thermoplastic tape (Orficast®). Casting materials are rigid, durable, conforming, and circumferential (Fig. 24–1A). They are often used for serially improving passive motion especially for patients with arthrogryposis (Fig. 24–4C) or camptodactyly (Fig. 24–4B). Some materials have the advantage of allowing the child to get them wet to swim or bathing. See Chapter 10 for more details on casting techniques and Chapter 11 for details on Orficast.

Thermoplastic materials are commonly used for pediatric orthoses, because they offer durability and can be adjusted easily. They come in various types, colors and thicknesses (Figs. 24–1C, 24–5A,B, 25–7C, and 24–9A). The selection of these depends on the requirements of the orthosis as part of the therapeutic intervention plan. Most materials come in various thicknesses: 1/16″, 3/32″, and 1/8″. A 1/16″ thickness material will make a lightweight orthosis which may be appropriate for a neonate or child with muscle weakness. This same thickness can be used to make a circumferential wrist orthosis that is supportive yet easy to apply for an older child. A circumferential design allows for the use of a thinner material because of how rigid an orthosis is when the final device has a curved shape. Most pediatric orthoses are made of the thinner (1/16″ or 3/32″) materials. Chapter 5 delves into greater detail on material and strapping selections.

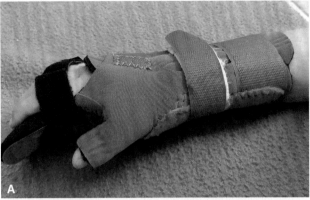

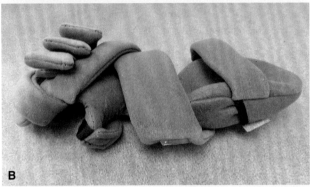

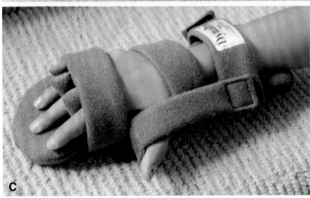

FIGURE 24–10 A, The Benik Wrist Support with Volar Pan Extension (Benik Corporation Silverdale, WA) has a thin thermoplastic embedded inside the neoprene which can be molded to the proper position. **B,** The HANZ WFHO™ (Performance Health, North Coast Medical) has a malleable metal with padding that is inside a fabric casing. It is easily bent into correct position for fingers, thumb, and wrist. **C,** The DynaPro Finger Flex Orthosis (Alimed Dedham, MA) is a prefabricated orthosis providing positioning to help maintain soft tissue length and adjust for changes with spasticity using a thin plastic insert.

Each type of thermoplastic material has different properties, and selection should be based on what is necessary to correctly form the orthosis. Armstrong (2005) explains the four major types of thermoplastics and how each can be used with children. The plastic-based thermoplastics (Polyform, Mulitform) have a great deal of conformability but can be easily overstretched, so they are best suited for small orthoses on the thumb or web space. Elastic-based thermoplastics (Orfit®, Aquaplast®) have good conformability with a high degree of memory (Figs. 24–2B, 24–4A, and 24–6C). This memory allows the entire orthosis to be remolded, but can make it difficult to reform sections and smooth edges. When utilizing a material with a protective coating, the temporary bonding ability in an antigravity position is helpful when fabricating orthoses; but the longer setup time may make this type of material difficult on young children. The rubber-based thermoplastics (Ezeform, Omega Plus) have a high resistance to stretch and minimal conformability making it a good choice for a rigid orthosis (Fig. 24–5A,B). The combined rubber-/plastic-based thermoplastics (Tailorsplint, NCM Preferred) are durable with balanced control and conformability. These have mild to moderate resistance to stretch and are easy to remold and edge. There is a relatively short working and setup time that makes them a good choice for pediatric patients (Figs. 24–1C, 24–7C, and 24–9A).

The color of the material for the orthosis may contribute to maximizing wear compliance. The young child may be more motivated to wear an orthosis made of colorful or patterned material, especially if they were allowed to choose it from a selection of materials. The teenager is often more compliant with a black orthosis or a neutral color with black straps. It should be noted that some of the thermoplastic materials that are embedded with a color or pattern may, on occasion, respond differently during the fabrication process leading to potential changes in the way it conforms to the body part.

Padding Selection

Some therapists feel a need to use moleskin or soft padding material to line an orthosis for the infant or child. Unfortunately, the bacteria, dirt, and moisture are absorbed by open-cell padding. If the orthosis is formed correctly, the material should be left unpadded. This will allow the orthosis to be wiped clean daily. If a softer internal feel is desired, a sleeve of stockinette or a thin sock of an appropriate length may be applied to the body segment under the orthosis. If there is a need to absorb perspiration, the use of a thin panty liner on the inside of orthosis can be beneficial since it can be easily removed and replaced (Fig. 24–11A).

Padding may be necessary for finger spreaders or over bony prominences to provide some pressure relief such as, the ulnar styloid in a patient with a radial ray deficiency. Closed-cell padding is easy to clean and comfortable and therefore a good option for children. An inexpensive and colorful padding can be made of adhesive-backed craft foam (Fig. 24–11B).

Strapping Selection and Placement

Strapping is critical especially with children because it holds the orthosis in the proper position. The therapist should consider the width, strength, durability, elasticity, and texture of the strap (Gabriel, 2008). If selected correctly, the strap should not cause irritation or excess pressure. If the edges of any strap cause issues, vertical snips can help to soften and flare the edge (Fig. 24–12A). Pediatric patients will benefit from straps that are soft as possible, yet, durable (Neoloop, Fabrifoam®, Soft Strap). Because the straps are often the third point of control that will exert a force, the width of the straps should be appropriate to the size of the body part to help maximally distribute the pressure. Orthoses for fingers or infants are often secured with 1/2″ straps (R-Thin® strap) (Fig. 24–4B). Straps across wrists are often secured with 1″ straps and forearms/upper arms can be secured 2″ or wider to distribute the pressure adequately for children (Fig. 24–12A). Maintaining the proper alignment of the orthosis is critical for an active child. On the volar surface, the strap should be placed just distal to the wrist crease, secured proximal to prevent distal migration of the orthosis (Fig. 24–12A). Providing the correct force from the strap can be a challenge. Placement of the strap in a slight diagonal may be helpful, and often two overlapping diagonals in an "X" pattern can facilitate a good hold on the dorsal surface (Fig. 24–12B,C). When attempting to gain finger positioning, it may be advisable to consider a finger strap in a spiral wrap which is placed just proximal to the joints (Fig. 24–4B).

The use of D-ring style straps to provide a "cinch" effect to hold the orthosis in place is often beneficial, especially for circumferential orthoses (Figs. 24–3A, and 24–8). The same effect can be accomplished by making a hole or slit into the material for the strap to run through (Fig. 24–12D). This may position the strap closer to the body part needing control (Fig. 24–6C).

Colorful straps may help increase the willingness of the child to accept the orthosis. Standard loop material comes in various colors (Figs. 24–4B, 24–5B). In addition, various types of soft strapping materials are now available, which can enhance comfort, compliance, and reduce issues of skin sensitivity (Figs. 24–12B,C). Ribbon or shoelaces can also be used in place of, or in addition to, the strapping materials (Figs. 24–1C, and 24–6C).

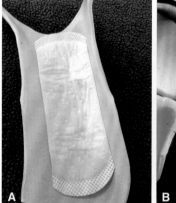
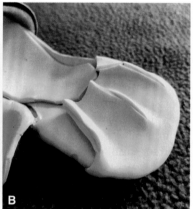

FIGURE 24–11 A, Generally, it is advisable not to pad the inside of an orthosis. If there is a need to absorb perspiration, the use of thin panty liner inside of the orthosis can be beneficial, because it can be easily removed and replaced.
B, When padding is needed, the use of closed-cell padding is recommended. Colorful adhesive back craft foam can be used as padding or formed to make comfortable finger spreaders. The edges can be heated with a heat gun to help form and adhere it to the orthosis. It is very inexpensive, comfortable, and easy to remove and replace.

Securing Thumb Orthosis
KIMBERLY GOLDIE STAINES, OTR, CHT
Texas

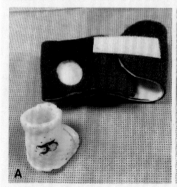
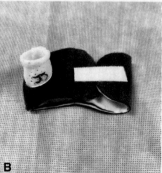

In tiny hands, it is sometime challenging to secure an orthosis on with traditional hook and loop. Using neoprene, cut a hole and push the thumb orthosis through—in addition to holding the orthosis on the extremity, the neoprene adds light compression.

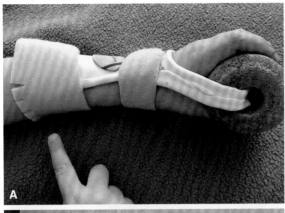
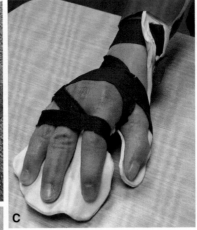
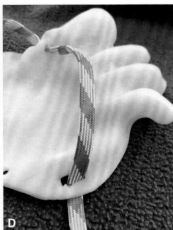
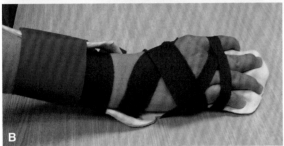

FIGURE 24–12 Strapping placement. A, The two-inch-wide soft strap is providing correct pressure on the forearm to hold the orthosis in place. This demonstrates how the edge can be flared by adding some small snips. Also, note that the one-inch strap around the wrist has been placed just proximal to the wrist crease to prevent distal migration of the orthosis. **B and C,** The third point of control is often the straps, and this one shows the use of crossed straps to secure the wrist into the orthosis. **D,** The use of a slit or hole for the strap to pass through can help position the strap closer to the body part and provides "cinch" effect to maintain the body part into the orthosis.

Enhancing Orthosis Use and Compliance

Therapists must take a multifaceted approach to **encouraging compliance with the orthosis for children**. A clear understanding and "buy in" is needed from the child and family to gain compliance with the orthosis use including the reason for use, wearing schedule, and application. To ensure proper application of the orthosis, it is often helpful to label the location of the orthosis (i.e., back of right wrist). A permanent marker can be used to label/number the corresponding hook-and-loop locations to aid in the ease of application (Fig. 24–13A). Providing the caregivers with a photo of the orthosis on the child or requesting that they take a photo or video with their mobile phone camera is advisable. Storing the orthosis in an obvious place, such as the nightstand or inside the patient's pillowcase may facilitate nightly use. Using a home program compliance grid to keep track of the wearing time allows the therapist to reward or praise the child for participation in the home program, including the use of the orthosis.

Making the orthosis unique is essential to improve compliance and acceptance of the orthosis. For example, the therapist can offer a choice of colors for the thermoplastic, strapping, and decorating options. The thermoplastic material can be decorated with an adhesive-backed foam shapes, stickers, permanent marker, fabric paints, jewels, beads, etc. (Fig. 24–13A–C). All decorations should be securely attached, especially for any child who may try to place the orthosis in his or her mouth. Decorative accents can be added using ribbons, bows, buttons, and lace that are sewn directly onto the straps (Fig. 24–14A–C). Naming the orthosis with appropriate child-friendly names may also help with compliance. For instance, an elbow orthosis decorated with an astronaut inside his "rocket ship" may help motivate the child to wear his orthosis (Fig. 24–13B).

Pediatric Orthoses
LAURA CARTER, OT
Australia

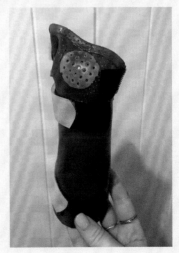

Where resources allow, creativity with pediatric orthoses can really help increase acceptance of and adherence to regimes. This "Ironman"-inspired orthosis came equipped with a blue "laser light" the patient could shoot beams from!

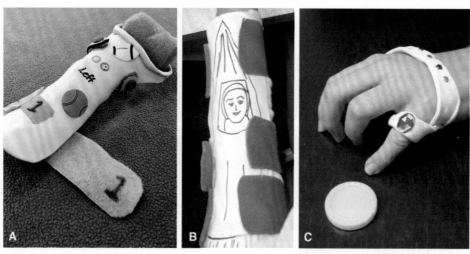

FIGURE 24–13 **Ideas to help with compliance and acceptance of the orthosis. A,** Labeling the orthosis with numbers or dots for corresponding hook and loop placement will aid in ease of application. Also, note the decorative additions using paper stickers and foam shapes, as well as, the buttons sewn on the straps. **B,** Drawing with a permanent marker can personalize the orthosis. The astronaut and his "rocket ship" motivated a young boy to wear his orthosis. **C,** Orthosis prevents hyperextension of the metacarpal (MP) joint while encouraging proximal interphalangeal (PIP) joint extension during exercise (pushing disc across table). Jewels were added with superglue and colors selected by patient.

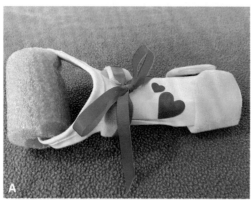

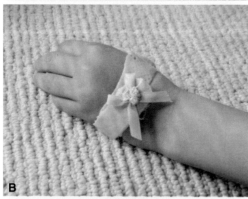

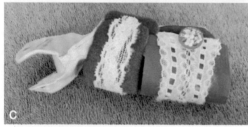

FIGURE 24–14 **A,** Dorsal-based orthosis provides a comfortable positioning with hand piece made from a pool noodle. The bow has been attached to the strap for decoration and prevention of self-removal. **B,** Pink bow was sewn onto the strap to help motivate a young girl to wear her orthosis. **C,** Lace and buttons were used to decorate this orthosis to maximize wearing compliance.

CHALLENGES OF ORTHOSIS PROVISION FOR A PEDIATRIC PATIENT

PREVENTING SELF-REMOVAL

There are various techniques to help secure an orthosis on a child. The first is the strapping. Unfortunately, simple hook and loop straps can easily be undone by a child of any age. Because of the small size of some straps, this can pose a choking hazard for the infant or young child. It is advisable to secure one end of the strap onto the thermoplastic material with a rivet (Fig. 24–15A) which is inserted into hole in the loop strap and then the end heated to press into an underlying piece of self-adhesive hook strap on the orthosis (Fig.24–15C). These options reduce the chance that the strap will be misplaced. To help **prevent self-removal of the orthosis**, the other end of the strap can be attached using the "double locking" method (Peck-Murray, 2016) (Fig. 24–15A–D). Placement of self-adhesive bandaging around the entire orthosis is another idea, but it should be applied without tight compression to avoid any circulatory compromise (Fig. 24–16A). Placing a sock or fingerless glove over the entire orthosis may deter the persistent child (Fig. 24–16B,C). Changing the strapping material or adding a shoestring or ribbon can allow for a more secure closure by tying a knot and bow (Figs. 24–1C, 24–6C, 24–9A, and 24–14A). Sewing a friendship bracelet with a plastic clasp onto the strap is another suggestion (Armstrong, 2005) for the older child (Fig. 24–16D).

ADDRESSING PRIMITIVE REFLEXES AND ABNORMAL TONE

The presence of primitive reflexes can influence the application of the orthosis. For instance, the asymmetrical tonic neck reflex (ATNR) can be used to help extend the elbow and open the hand as the head is moved toward that arm. Tonal issues (hypotonicity or hypertonicity) may be present in conditions such as cerebral palsy or hemiplegia. The orthoses will not treat the source of the abnormal tone but should help prevent contractures (Fig. 24–5B) or positioning the proximal body part to enhance distal function

(Fig. 24–8). The dynamic and inconsistent nature of spasticity will present a challenge even for the most experienced therapist (Fess, Gettle, Philips, & Janson, 2005). Relaxation techniques prior to the fabrication or application of the orthosis may allow for best positioning. A custom orthosis for a child with fluctuating spasticity may require rigid material with extra reinforcement and proper fabrication to allow for the optimal positioning without stress to the joints (Fig. 24–5B). Certain types of prefabricated orthoses (Fig. 24–10C) have an insert that is flexible, providing a spring-back effect delivering gentle stretch.

EXPERT PEARL 24–5

Orthosis for Constraint-Induced Movement Therapy (CIMT)
LAURA CARTER, OT
Australia

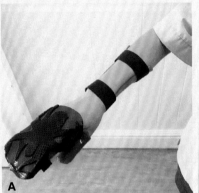
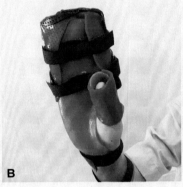

Young patient with cerebral palsy (CP) presenting with moderate spasticity in his "good" side and needed to restrain the arm in something sturdier than a mitt. The volar portion orthosis was fabricated first, and then the dorsal segment was molded. The dorsal piece was removable to allow for easy don/doffing, and the "Spiderman" color theme helped increase engagement with and acceptance of use.

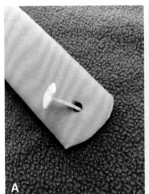
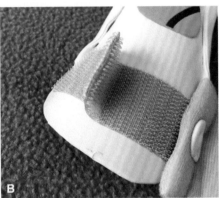
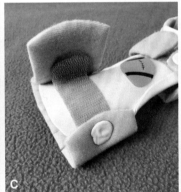
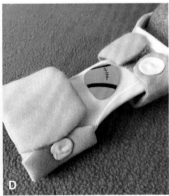

FIGURE 24–15 **Securing the straps to the orthosis. A,** A rivet made of strap thermoplastic is placed through a hole in the loop strap. **B,** A long piece of self-adhesive hook strap is placed onto the orthosis overlapping onto itself to make a tab. The end of rivet held in the loop strap is then heated and placed into one edge of the hook piece. **C and D,** The loop strap is placed around the arm over the tab and onto the remaining hook on the orthosis. As it will be difficult to remove with one hand, it deters self-removal of the orthosis.

SPECIAL CONSIDERATIONS FOR THE FRAGILE INFANT

The therapist who works in the neonatal intensive care unit (NICU) needs to decide on design, material, and strapping with consideration for fragile state of the infant, environmental issues, and nursing constraints (Tecklin, 2007). In addition, the therapist needs to use special care in fabrication and application. The infant may not tolerate handling or traction on nerves/joints/skin, and there is a greater risk of fracture, dislocation, and skin breakdown (Anderson & Anderson, 1988). Other concerns that affect the treating therapists include time constraints, fear of harming the child, lack of family participation, and nursing compliance issues.

The material used for the orthosis should be soft and supportive. Fig. 24–17A shows a soft elbow/wrist support made of 3″-wide Velfoam® wrapped circumferentially which was used to position the flexed arm of the neonate with radial ray dysplasia. **Soft hand supports for neonates** can be made of a tube of cylindrical foam with 1/2″ soft strapping in a figure-of-8 pattern to hold around the wrist (Fig. 28–17B) or constructed from a malleable foam IV board such as Accuboard (Fig. 24–17C). If needed, more rigid support can be made from 1/16″ thermoplastic materials which may be lined with closed-cell padding to protect the fragile skin. Simple instructions for orthosis application should be part of the care plan and posted at bedside with a photo. Coordinating the wearing schedule with feeding times may make it easier for nurses to comply with the wearing schedule.

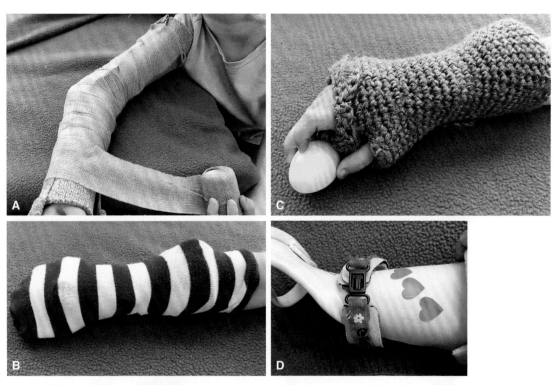

FIGURE 24–16 More ideas to deter self-removal of orthosis. A, Placement of self-adhesive bandaging around the entire orthosis which is applied without tight tension to avoid circulation compromise. **B,** Cover entire orthosis with a sock. **C,** Fingerless glove or cut sock over the orthosis will to allow use of the hand. **D,** Friendship bracelet with plastic locking closure sewn onto the strap.

EXPERT PEARL 24–5

Fabrication Tips

JILL PECK-MURRAY, MOTR/L, CHT
California

#1 A strap can be attached to an orthosis by placing it through a hole or slit.

Make a hole in the orthosis. Cut a hole into the end of the strap, insert it in orthosis and loop it through itself pulling tightly.

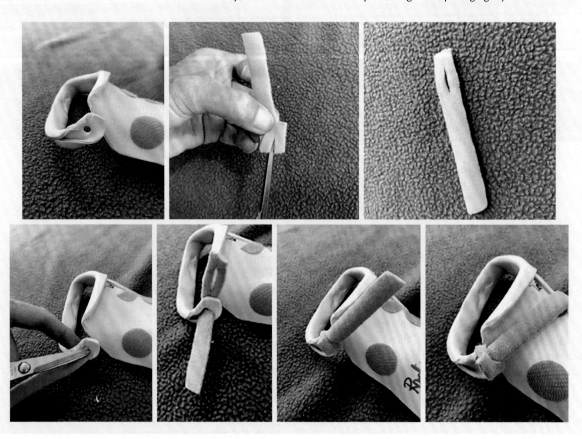

#2 A strap can be attached to an orthosis using a rivet made of thermoplastic.

Step 1. Use a long thin scrap of material. Hold it by the end with scissors over the heat gun to heat the end. Roll the heated end into a ball and flatten it with your fingers to make a "tack."

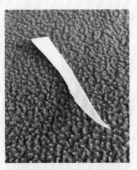

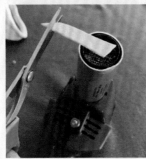

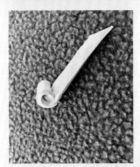

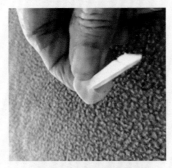

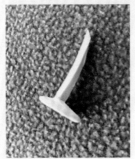

Step 2. Place the tack into a hole cut in the strap. Heat the end of it carefully without burning the strap. Press the heated end firmly into a piece of adhesive hook that is already attached to the orthosis.

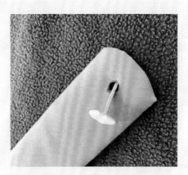

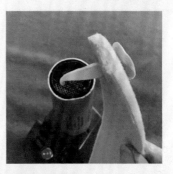

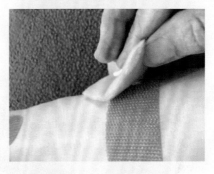

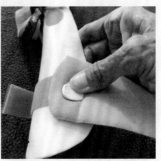

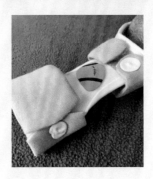

(Continued)

#3 To keep the strap in place or make it harder to self-remove, use the "double-locking" method.

Place a long piece of adhesive hook onto the orthosis making a tab by applying it onto itself. This tab should be two-thirds across the orthosis from the anchor of the loop strap (see above) which will wrap around to attach to it and then place the strap onto the remaining piece of hook on the orthosis.

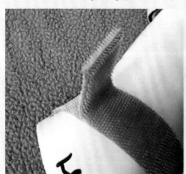 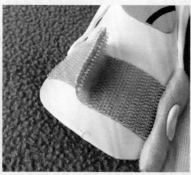 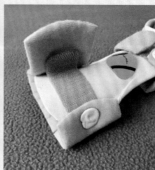 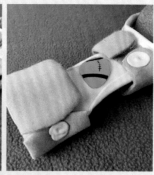

#4 Stretchy strapping materials can be used to provide a dynamic force to assist weak muscles and help position the body part for use.

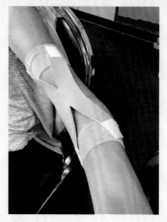

Assisting elbow flexion.

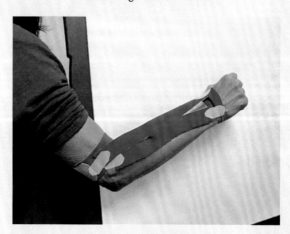

Assisting wrist extension.

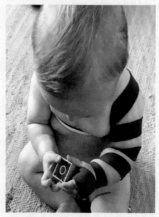

Assisting forearm supination and shoulder ER.

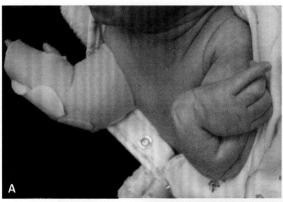
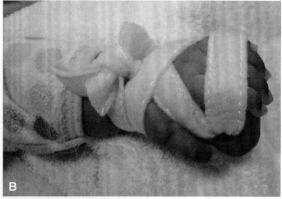
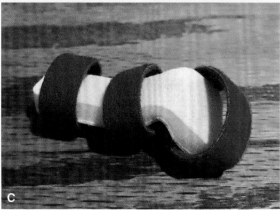

FIGURE 24-17 **A,** Neonate with bilateral radial ray deficiency was positioned on the right with a soft circumferential wrap of wide Velfoam® to hold the elbow, wrist, and hand extended. **B,** An orthosis made of cylindrical foam placed in the hand can be attached with soft ribbon and can provide a soft supportive position for the neonate. **C,** The orthosis can be made from IV board made of malleable metal with foam padding: Accuboard® (Kentec Medical, Irvine, CA).

TYPICAL SESSION OF ORTHOTIC FABRICATION FOR A PEDIATRIC PATIENT

The fabrication process can pose multiple challenges, especially if the child is an infant or young child. Changes to the environment and fabrication process make the process easier. The use of comfort positioning and distractions are recommended for medical procedures which can include orthotic intervention (Dastgheyb, Fishlock, Daskalakis, Kessel, & Rosen, 2018). Giving the infant a pacifier or bottle may be a good distraction for an infant (Fig. 24–18A). Holding the infant or toddler in a "bear hug" position provides comfort in the parent's lap while positioning the extremity out of view behind the parent (Fig. 24–18B). The older child, may feel less threatened if the area is free from sharp objects and imposing equipment. Offering a few toys or a puzzle will make the room more friendly and inviting. Having a sample orthosis available allows the child and parent to anticipate the final results (Fig. 24–18C). Allowing the child some opportunity to play with the softened material prior to fabrication may make the child less apprehensive when the warm material is later pulled out of the water to be placed on his or her arm (Schwartz, McKie, & Gabriel, 2015).

If possible, place the child's hand onto a piece of paper towel or a more durable shop towel to draw the pattern. Cut out the pattern on the towel and then place it on the child checking for proper fit prior to cutting out the material. Modify this paper pattern as needed to minimize the number of times that the warm material is placed onto the child for readjustments.

The therapist should then select a material for the orthosis with the correct thickness and properties for the child. If possible, allow the child to pick the color. The material should be placed into water of the correct temperature (150° for most plastic/rubber-based materials and 160° for elastic-based material). After the material is soft, it can be removed from the water and placed on a towel to cool. A piece of 1″ or 2″ stockinette can be placed onto the child's arm prior to provide a layer of protection.

When forming the orthosis, the therapist should place the material onto the arm or hand using gravity to assist, if possible (Fig. 24–18D). Working quickly, the orthosis needs to be allowed to harden enough to maintain the form. The elastic-based materials will need to be left on longer to allow them to completely cool to prevent shrinkage. It may be advisable to quicken the process by applying something cold, such as a washcloth that has been soaking in ice water or applying a baggie of ice. After it has hardened, the edges can be smoothed with a heat gun. Finally, the straps should be added with special attention to strap placement to make sure there is proper control of the position. If possible, let the child pick the color of the straps or shoe strings.

After the final adjustments, the therapist should allow time to make the orthosis fun to wear by decorating it, as well as adding labels to denote the location of the straps. The family or caregiver should be instructed in the application and strap orientation. They should be observed donning/doffing the orthosis and have any questions clarified. The therapist should provide a wearing schedule, request the caregivers to note any pressure problems from the orthosis, and remind them to bring the orthosis back at each visit for adjustments.

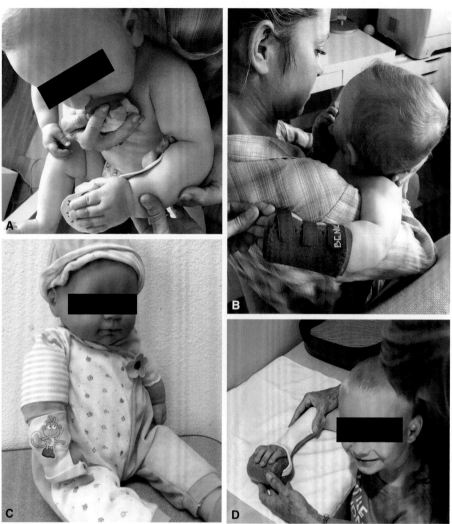

FIGURE 24-18 A, Providing a distraction such as a pacifier or bottle may allow the infant to tolerate the orthotic fabrication process. **B,** Holding the child in a "bear hug" position should comfort the child while positioning the extremity behind the parent and out of the child's view. **C,** Having a sample of the completed orthosis on a doll can help the child and family understand the final result. **D,** The cooperative child can be part of the process. Placing the arm on the table allows the therapist to use gravity to assist with the fabrication.

PEDIATRIC PREFABRICATED ORTHOSES SUPPLIERS

Accuboard (moldable IV board) www.KentecMedical.com.
3-Point Products (888) 378-7763 www.3pointproducts.com.
Benik Corporation (800) 442-8910 www.benik.com.
Bird & Cronin, Inc (800) 328-1095 www.birdcronin.com.
Comfy Splints (800) 582-5332 www.comfysplints.com.
Joe Cool Company (800) 399-2495 www.joecoolco.com.
Joint Active Systems (800) 879-0117 www.jointactivesystems.com.
McKie Splints (888) 477-5468 www.mckiesplints.com.
North Coast Medical (800) 821-9319 www.ncmedical.com.
Performance Health (800) 323-5547 www.performancehealth.com.
Restorative Care of America, Inc (800) 354-9321 www.rcai.com.
Restorative Medical (800) 793-5544 www.restorativemedical.com.

CONCLUSION

Orthosis provision for the pediatric patient can pose multiple hurdles. The therapist can rise to these challenges by using problem-solving ability that is grounded in good biomechanical principles to help design the most appropriate custom or prefabricated orthosis for each child. Additionally, there should be special consideration for factors that are unique to pediatrics, including methods to enhance orthosis use and compliance, prevent self-removal, address primitive reflexes or abnormal tone, and protect the fragile infant. The therapist should have a basic understanding of the various pediatric conditions to design the proper therapeutic intervention. This therapy program may involve the use of orthoses to enhance functional use, provide proper positioning, or provide protection before or after necessary surgical intervention.

FIELD NOTE: ORTHOSES FOR CHILDREN WITH ANOMALY OF THE THUMB

Ginny Gibson OTD, OTR/L, CHT
California

Three pathological conditions that may look similar upon first noting a flexion deformity of the thumb include trigger thumb due to an enlarged flexor pollicis longus tendon (FPL), clasped thumb due to hypoplasia of the thumb extrinsic extensors, and thumb-in-palm deformity due to muscle hypertonia. Orthotic management of children with these three conditions differ; therefore, careful observation to discern the nature the thumb deformity is essential. Trigger thumb is distinguished from other flexion deformities of the thumb because the interphalangeal (IP) joint is flexed[1]; whereas, excessive metacarpophalangeal (MCP) joint flexion with carpometacarpophalangeal joint adduction is characteristic of clasped thumb due to hypoplasia of the extensor pollicis longus (EPL) or extensor pollicis brevis (EPB),[2,3] or thumb-in-palm deformity due to cerebral palsy (CP) with hypertonia.[4]

Trigger thumb occurs due to thickening of the FPL tendon or tendon sheath at the level of the A1 pulley,[5] or a ganglion on the FPL,[6] and often presents with compensatory excessive hyperextension of the MCP joint.[7] Younger children with clasped-thumb due to hypoplasia of the EPL or EPB often have an extension lag at the IP or MCP joint, respectively[3,8]; that is, active range of motion (ROM) is incomplete, but passive ROM is full or near full. Children with thumb-in-palm deformity due to CP exhibit a range of contraction patterns but present with increased muscle tone.[4]

Despite the differing etiologies of the aforementioned thumb pathologies, an orthosis to reduce or prevent pain or contracture related to trigger thumb or clasped thumb due to hypoplasia may look quite similar (see Figure FN24–1), with greater variability seen among orthoses for indwelling thumb due to hypertonicity (see Figure FN24–2). Additionally, orthosis use for children with trigger thumb or thumb hypoplasia is likely to be time-limited; whereas, the chronicity of thumb-in-palm deformity due to CP with hypertonia may require long-term use of an orthosis—if the orthosis is found effective for reducing onset of soft-tissue shortening or increasing function.

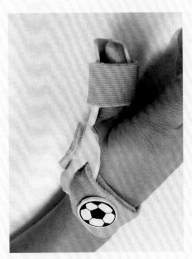

FIGURE FN24–1 Thermoplastic splint for trigger thumb or hypoplastic thumb.

Orthoses for Trigger Thumb

Applying an orthosis to the triggering thumb is done for comfort, to reduce triggering, and to preserve or increase ROM during growth. Because the IP joint is typically stuck in flexion, both the MCP and IP joints are crossed along the volar surface of the thumb. Outcomes of two similar studies provide weak evidence to suggest use of an orthoses may bring about more rapid resolution of triggering than observation alone. Koh reviewed medical records of children with a locked IP joint and compared use of a coil orthosis to hold the IP joint in extension at night to observation alone[9]. More children who were treated with an orthosis experienced complete resolution in a shorter period of time than children who were only observed; however, all but four patients (two in each group) ultimately had complete resolution. Lee also compared orthosis use to observation alone, but offered more than nighttime wear; the treatment group wore an orthosis all day for 6 to 12 weeks until active extension was achieved and then wore the orthosis at night.[10] Children receiving an orthosis achieved significantly improved extension without snapping. For both studies, researchers applied an orthosis that served to extend the IP joint of the thumb. Opting not to embark on an orthotic program should be considered in light of two studies that showed spontaneous resolution in 63% and 75.9% of the thumbs followed over 2 years.[1,11]

Orthoses for Clasped Thumb Due to Hypoplasia

Applying an extension orthosis to the thumb with EPL and EPB hypoplasia is done to increase function and preserve, or increase, ROM. If both the EPL and EPB appear to be hypoplastic, a therapist may decide to cross both the IP and MCP joints during sleep and at times the child is sedentary, but cross only the MCP joint when the child is more active.

Two older studies suggest children with passively correctable thumb hypoplasia may benefit from an orthosis.[12,13] After applying a short opponens orthosis to 17 thumbs with an extension lag at the thumb IP joint, MCP joint, or both joints due to hypoplasia of the extrinsic extensor muscles of the thumb, Lin et al.[12] observed 15 thumbs achieved "good" results when assessed with a standard measure. Tsuyuguchi et al.[13] examined three groups of children who had (1) no fixed contracture but had a flexion deformity, (2) had contracture, or (3) were deemed to have arthrogryposis multiplex congenital, and found children who benefitted most from use of an orthosis were those without a fixed contracture. In a more recent study by Ghani et al.,[6] researchers found eight hands of infants, 1 year of age or younger, with passively correctable thumbs (type I) received benefit from application of an orthosis. These infants achieved full active extension with full-time use of an orthosis for 6 months, followed by application of the orthosis at night for 6 more months. The same benefit was not observed for two hands categorized as having type II clasped thumb (presence of contracture).[6]

Orthoses for Thumb-in-Palm Deformity Due to Hypertonia

Greater variability of splint design, both for prefabricated and custom-made orthoses, may be considered for children with thumb-in-palm deformity due to CP; however, for the purpose of

(Continued)

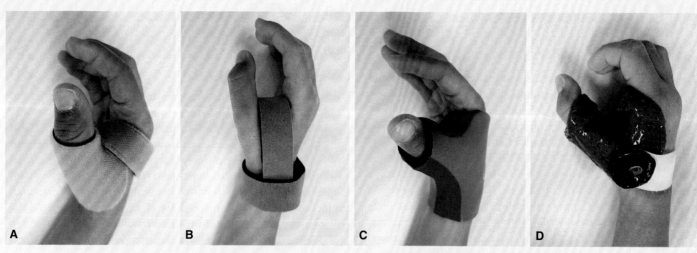

FIGURE FN24–2 Four orthoses used for thumb-in-palm deformity: **(A)** Mckie splints, McKie Splints, LLC, PO Box 242, Duluth, MN 55801 to 0242, **(B)** Joe Cool splints. The Joe Cool Company, 9448 Lady Dove Lane, South Jordan, UT 84095; **(C)** Benik splint. Benik Corporation, 11,871 Silverdale Way NW #107, Silverdale, WA 98383 USA; **(D)** thermosplastic short opponens splint.

this discussion, only thumb orthoses will be considered. Three small studies in which researchers evaluated a thumb-only orthosis for children with CP were located.[14-16] Currie and Mendiola[16] applied a thermoplastic orthosis to the thumb of five children, aged 20 to 26 months, with spastic hemiplegia due to CP to optimize thumb position and improve thumb function. At baseline, all children demonstrated a thumb-in-palm deformity at rest and during reach, and grasped objects with the ulnar side of the hand. Following application of the orthosis, all children showed emerging use of the radial side of the hand to grasp, such that they could hold objects between the thumb and fingers, and also began to explore toys bimanually.[16] Using an AB single-subject design, Goodman and Bazyk[15] evaluated the effectiveness of using a thermoplastic short thumb opponens orthosis for 6 hours per day in a child with unilateral CP. Researchers found clinically significant improvement for the Box and Blocks Test; grip, lateral pinch, and tip pinch strength; and active motion of the thumb in opposition, radial abduction, and palmer abduction.[15] Ten Berg et al.,[14] employed a multiple baseline design to investigate use of a neoprene thumb opponens orthosis on hand function for seven children, aged 2 to 7 years, with unilateral spastic CP presenting with thumb-in-palm deformity. Using goal attainment scaling as an outcome measure, after 2 months of daily wear for 4 hours, four children made functional gains with the orthosis on or off; whereas, two children made gains only with the orthosis on.[14]

References

1. Baek, G. H., Kim, J. H., Chung, M. S., Kang, S. B., Lee, Y. H., & Gong, H. S. (2008). The natural history of pediatric trigger thumb. *Journal of Bone and Joint Surgery*, 90(5), 980–985.
2. Ghani, H. A., El-Naggar, A., Hegazy, M., Hanna, A., Tarraf, Y., & Temtamy, S. (2007). Characteristics of patients with congenital clasped thumb: A prospective study of 40 patients with the results of treatment. *Journal of Children's Orthopedics*, 1, 313–322.
3. Tonkin, M. A. (2013). On the classification of congenital thumb hypoplasia. *Journal of Hand Surgery European*, 39E(9), 948–955.
4. Sakellarides, H. T., Mital, M. A., Matza, R. A., & Dimakopoulos, P. (1995). Classification and surgical treatment of the thumb-in-palm deformity in cerebral palsy and spastic paralysis. *Journal of Hand Surgery*, 20(3), 428–431.
5. Khoshhal, K. I., Jarvis, J. G., & Uhthoff, H. K. (2012). Congenital trigger thumb in children: Electron microscopy and immunohistochemical analysis of the first annular pulley. *Journal of Pediatric Orthopedics*, 21(4), 295e–299e.
6. Murgai, R. R. & Lightdale-Miric, N. (2020). Pediatric trigger thumb caused by a flexor tendon sheath ganglion. *Journal of Pediatric Orthopedics B*, 29, 203–205.
7. Li, Z., Wiesler, E. R., Smith, B. P., & Koman, L. A. (2009). Surgical treatment of pediatric trigger thumb with metacarpophalangeal hyperextension laxity. *Hand*, 4(4):,380–384.
8. Goldfarb, C. A., Wustrack, R., Pratt, J. A., Mender, A., & Manske, P. R. (2007). Thumb function and appearance in thrombocytopenia: Absent radius syndrome. *Journal of Hand Surgery*, 32(2), 157–161.
9. Koh, S., Horii, E., Hattori, T., et al. (2012). Pediatric trigger thumb with locked interphalangeal joint: Can observation or splinting be a treatment option? *Journal of Pediatric Orthopedics*, 32(7), 724–726.
10. Lee, Z., Chang, C., Yang, W., Hung, S., & Shih, C. (2006). Extension splint for trigger thumb in children. *Journal of Pediatric Orthopedics*, 26(6),785–787.
11. Baek, G. H. & Lee, H. J. (2011). The natural history of pediatric trigger thumb: A study with a minimum of 5 years follow-up. *Clinics in Orthopedic Surgery*, 3, 157–160.
12. Lin, S. C., Huang, T. H., Hsu, H. Y., Lin, C. J., & Chiu, H. Y. (1999). A simple splinting method for correction of supple congenital clasped thumbs in infants. *Journal of Hand Surgery British*, 24(5),612–614.
13. Tsuyuguchi, Y., Masada, K., Kawabata, H., Kawai, H., & Ono, K. (1985). Congenital clasped thumb: A review of forty-three cases. *Journal of Hand Surgery American*, 10(5), 613–618.
14. Ten BergeBoonstra, S. R. A. M., Dijkstra, P. U., Hadders-Algra, M., Haga, N., Maathuis, C. G. (2012). A systematic evaluation of the effect of thumb opponens splints on hand function in children with unilateral spastic cerebral palsy. *Clinical Rehabilitation*, 26(4), 362–371.
15. Goodman, G. & Bazyk, S. (1991). The effects of a short thumb opponens splint on hand function in cerebral palsy: A single-subject study. *American Journal of Occupational Therapy*, 45(8), 726–731.
16. Currie, D. M., & Mendiola, A. (1987). Cortical thumb orthosis for children with spastic hemiplegic cerebral palsy. *Archives of Physical Medicine and Rehabilitation*, 68(4), 214–216.

Case Study Section

The case studies presented here are meant as a teaching guideline only. Treatment and orthosis protocols vary greatly from surgeon to surgeon and from therapist to therapist. The therapist should check with the referring physicians and colleagues to define the preferred treatment and appropriate orthotic intervention.

Case Study 1: Camptodactyly

Jamie is an 11-year-old who noticed increasing flexion contractures of her small fingers on both hands in the last several years. She had no previous injuries that would have caused these PIP contractures. She was recently seen by the orthopedist who felt that these are contractures are due to an adolescent form of camptodactyly. He explained that the etiology is unknown, but may have to do with anomalous insertion of the lumbricals or shortening of the flexor tendon. He does not plan surgical release because there is risk of complications, such as the loss of flexion. He would like her to be managed more conservatively.

She presented for the first visit with both her small fingers held in flexion at rest. She admitted some concern about the appearance of her hands and frequently hides them under the sleeves of her sweatshirt. Her evaluation revealed that her ROM in both hands were within normal limits except in her bilateral small fingers, which lacked full PIP joint extension by 45° actively and 28° passively. Her grip strength was 20 pounds right and 18 pounds left. Manual muscle testing to lumbricals of both small fingers showed she exhibited a grade 3 strength. She denied any difficulty with use of hands in normal daily tasks, except she reported difficulty putting her hands in her pockets and placing her hands completely flat onto a table. She plays basketball and feels her ability to palm the ball has been diminished in the last few years.

Because her PIP joints could be reduced to less than 30° passively, she was a candidate for a serial static type mobilization orthosis (Fig. 24–4B). She wore them nightly for at least 10 hours. She also participated in a home program, which involved heated stretching, active extension exercises, and activities such as playing "penny soccer" while wearing an MCP joint–blocking orthosis (Fig. 24–13C). She received weekly therapy that included paraffin, fluidotherapy, intrinsic strengthening activities, and finger extension strengthening with putty. Her orthosis was adjusted for more extension at each visit. After 3 months, her motion had improved to 8° from full extension. She was discharged from weekly therapy but advised to continue her home program. Because it is advisable to wear her orthosis until she reaches skeletal maturity, she returned every several months for modification to accommodate for growth.

Additional case studies can be found on the companion web site on thePoint.

Case Study 2: Right Hemiplegia

Lilly is 14 months old with a diagnosis of right hemiplegia due to a stroke in utero. Her neurologist referred her for evaluation and treatment by an occupational therapist (OT).

At the first visit, her parents reported that she was noted to have limited use of her right arm as an infant. She does not crawl, and they noted she walked early. She has no cognitive or speech limitations. She tended to maintain her right arm in slight internal rotation of shoulder, mild elbow flexion, forearm in pronation, and thumb adducted and flexed into the palm. Her right arm evaluation revealed that the ROM was normal passively, except her elbow lacked full extension by 15°. Actively, she could flex her shoulder to 100°, move her elbow 30° to 120°, supinate to 10°, and extend her wrist to 30°. When asked to open her hand, she flexed her fingers when extending her wrist past neutral (composite finger and wrist extension at 0°). The thumb only extended at MP joint when the wrist was flexed. She preferred the left upper extremity for all tasks and used it age appropriately. She avoided use of the right upper extremity in spontaneous use. With verbal encouragement or when left was restrained, she attempted use of the right upper extremity. She could grasp objects, but her thumb was flexed so object rested on dorsum of the hand. She needed to flex her wrist to release. She could lift her arm to swipe at object at shoulder height with her forearm in pronation and her wrist in neutral. She would briefly weight bear on right arm when placed in side-sitting or in quadruped position. When given a ball, she could hold with both hands, but ball was held against the radial dorsal side of her hand.

Although her passive range was fairly good, she was at risk for developing further flexor tightness and contractures. A two-piece dorsal/volar immobilization orthosis was fabricated for night use (Fig. 24–14A). To enhance functional use, various alternatives were considered. A long strip of Fabrifoam° (Fig. 24–6A) could place the hand and forearm in a better position for use. The use of a weight-bearing orthosis held the hand open to encourage proximal strengthening (Fig. 24–6C). A dorsal wrist orthosis was provided to hold the wrist extended to use hand with wrist in more extended position (Fig. 24–8). Several options were tried to position the thumb for grasping objects on the volar surface (Fig. 24–7A,B).

Case Study 3: Elbow Fracture

Phillip is a 14-year-old who fell while skateboarding and fractured the medial epicondyle of his left humerus. He underwent open reduction and internal fixation (ORIF) and was casted for 4 weeks. At his follow-up orthopedic clinic visit, he was noted to have limited elbow and forearm motion with an ulnar nerve neuropraxia. He was referred for therapy at that time.

When he came for his first visit, he reported that he was a freshman in high school, an active teen who enjoyed skateboarding, surfing, and soccer. He was anxious to return to these activities as soon as possible. He denied any pain except with stretching to level 4 out of 10 on visual analog scale. He had numbness in his small finger and ulnar side of his ring finger. It was noted that he postures these fingers in hyperextension at the MCP joints with PIP joint flexion.

He had mild swelling around the elbow with a well-healed surgical incision area. He showed significant limitation in elbow motion (50°–90°) and forearm supination (20°). Because he was right hand dominant, he denied any difficulty with functional use, but the left arm had limited use for any reaching and carrying heavy objects. He had been told by his physician to avoid any contact sports, and he could not return to gym class for 2 months.

He was started on a therapy program focusing on gentle stretching and graded strengthening. Because his ulnar fingers were at risk for developing contractures, a soft loop style ulnar nerve orthosis was provided for day use. In addition, an MCP joint–blocking orthosis was fabricated for use during exercises (similar to Fig. 24–13C). He was given a home program to do several times per day.

By the second week of therapy, he made excellent progress in elbow and forearm motion but reported that he sleeps with his elbow in a flexed position. He was provided a custom, elbow extension mobilization orthosis (serial static) to wear at night that readjusted for more elbow extension at each therapy visit (similar to Fig. 24–13B).

After a month of therapy, he continued to have a lack of full elbow flexion and extension so the use of a Joint Active Systems (JAS°) brace was recommended (Fig. 24–3A). He was compliant with using it for 30 minutes three times per day in each direction. At the end of 3 months, he had gained all of his motion and was able to return to all of his sports, but he agreed to be more cautious when skateboarding (Fig. 24–3B).

Case Study 4: Radial Ray Deficiency

Abigail was born 5 weeks premature and noted to have severe abnormalities of her arms, hip dysplasia, and low platelet count. She was transferred to the NICU at the local children's hospital and diagnosed with thrombocytopenia-absent radius (TAR). Her first prescription for therapy was at 2 weeks of age while in the NICU. The OT focused on feeding and handling issues. She asked for a consultation with the pediatric hand therapist for orthosis recommendations. Brief assessment revealed that both upper extremity were held in tight shoulder adduction, elbows fully flexed, wrists fully flexed and radially deviated, fingers flexed at MCP and extended at IP joints, and thumbs were absent. When passively stretched, her arms lacked full motion: elbows, 100° from full extension; wrists, 50° from neutral; and the fingers lacked MCP extension by 25°.

Because surgical intervention is not indicated until the infant is about a year old, there was a need to maintain length of the soft tissue until that time. Because of her greater risk of fracture, dislocation, and the breakdown of fragile skin, the pediatric hand therapist fabricated a soft circumferential wrap (Fig. 24–17A). At the age of 6 months, this was changed to an ulnar-based orthosis (Fig. 24–2B).

CHAPTER REVIEW QUESTIONS

1. Describe three materials that were reviewed in this chapter that are appropriate for the pediatric patient. Provide rationale for these material choices.
2. Name three of the special developmental and environmental considerations when applying an orthosis on a pediatric patient.
3. Give two examples of creative, difficult to remove strapping applications for the pediatric orthosis.
4. Provide an example of an orthosis that enhances function for a pediatric patient.
5. Give two examples on how a clinician may encourage (patient and family) compliance and use of an orthosis to be worn on a pediatric patient.

25 Burns[a]

Courtney Condon, MEd, OTR/L
Katherine Hartigan Norris, MS, OTR/L

CHAPTER OBJECTIVES

After study of this chapter, the reader should be able to:

- Gain an understanding for burn injuries: severity, surface area, depth of wound, phases of healing, and long-term sequelae.
- Describe the considerations unique to orthotic intervention with the patient with burn injury.
- Identify the most common contractures seen in burn extremities.
- Understand the importance of material selection when addressing burn injuries and positioning.

KEY TERMS

Antideformity orthoses
Cutaneous functional units
Contracture
Compression garments
Depth of injury

Epidermal depth
Full thickness
Heterotopic ossification
Inflammatory stage
Neuropathies
Partial thickness

Position of function orthoses
Skin graft
Subdermal
Superficial thickness
Total body surface area (TBSA)

MD NOTE

Robert L. Sheridan, MD
Massachusetts

Deep hand burns have major adverse effects on function and quality of life. A perfect operation will not deliver a great result. A great result is only possible when a good operation is combined with skillful orthotic and therapy intervention. This critical component of care is particularly difficult to deliver for children who are unable to take the long view of their care. Tolerating immediate inconvenience and discomfort to enhance late function and appearance is difficult for young children. Providing humane and effective therapy to help children optimize their long-term outcome is extremely challenging but rewarding. Therapists who can do this are rare and valuable. These authors are among that small group and share in this chapter some of their unique skills and techniques.

FAQ

Our unit protocol does not allow for any ROM until 7 days post grafting, what should I as the therapist be doing during that time?
Some surgeons have very strict protocols after grafting to ensure graft adherence but OTs and PTs can still play a vital role. If orthoses are indicted, they should be doffed, cleaned, and donned daily to ensure no areas of pressure are caused and orthoses are fitting well to ensure functional positioning. If no orthoses are indicated, therapists can ensure joints at risk for contracture are supported and comfortably positioned including the neck, wrists, knees, and ankles.

Is it better to use a prefabricated orthoses to save time?
While prefabricated orthotics such as airplane orthoses can save time and material, they can often be very expensive and are difficult to modify with changing dressing size and to maximize therapy goals. If the therapist has the ability, the patient is better served with a conforming fabricated orthosis.

What material should I choose to fabricate a burn unit orthosis?
There are many differing opinions on material but ideally a low temperature, high memory perforated material seems to best serve this population. A high memory material allows for frequent modifications rather than prefabrication and the perforation allows for better exudate drainage.

---

[a]This chapter is based on the second-edition chapter written by Reg Richard, MS, PT, and Jonathan Niszczak, MS, OTR/L.

INTRODUCTION

Burn care is an ever evolving field that bases best practice on experiential interventions and consensus within practitioners in the community. The use of specialized orthoses to treat patients with burn injuries is one approach that may be used in the rehabilitation of these patients (Richard et al., 2008). Practitioners as a whole believe that the need for orthotic intervention in the acute and reconstructive burn populations positively impact long-term range of motion (ROM) and functional mobility. Fabrication of burn orthoses employs the basic orthotic principles described in Section I, and the focus of this chapter will address the uniqueness of burn injuries by highlighting principles that can contribute to successful patient outcomes. The most significant characteristic of orthoses fabricated for patients with burn injuries is that the orthosis is individualized to the specific needs of each patient. After detailed assessments, the ultimate goals of these orthoses are antideformity positioning and **contracture** prevention. The information in the following chapter pulls from different facets of rehabilitation research and relies heavily on the work of our colleagues to determine best orthotic practice for the burn population.

BURN INJURY CONSIDERATIONS

When fabricating a burn orthosis, the main considerations should be to

- Provide functional positioning of the limb to prevent burn scar contracture deformities.
- Preserve ROM either from baseline injury or after surgical intervention.
- Increase ROM after therapeutic interventions—correct a scar contracture.
- Protect delicate or exposed tendons, vessels, nerves, **skin grafts**, and flaps.
- Decrease pain (Richard & Ward, 2005).

A skilled therapist will consider several factors in selecting the optimal orthosis for a patient based on the patient profile. The joint(s) involved in the burn, for example, neck, shoulder, and hand, have a greater functional impact than a burn across the chest only. Fabricating an orthosis for a patient with a burn injury is based primarily on aspects related directly to the burn itself, including the following:

- Age of the patient and their perceived tolerance for wearing an orthosis.
- Depth and severity of the burn, including the expected time of wound healing.
- Patient's expected time of wound healing and prevention of surgical interventions.
- Patient's overall medical complexity, taking into account the total body surface area (TBSA) of the burn and burn distribution.
- Patient's mobility status while undergoing treatment.
- Patient's responsibilities and level of independence while undergoing burn treatment (i.e., will the patient be involved in self-care activities?).
- Comorbidities that might affect orthosis use, especially those involving impaired sensation.
- Patient's pain and anxiety burden and the team's ability to manage these.
- Patient and family's level of understanding.

Per national statistics, there has been a significant decline in the number of severe burns in the United States in the past 20 years

(American Burn Association). The ability of the burn therapist to accurately and precisely identify the correct plan for an orthosis is critical, especially for injuries involving the hand and upper extremity. A timely and clinically reasonable intervention has the ability to directly impact the patient's expected functional outcome and overall burn satisfaction as well as improved quality of life (Richard et al., 2009). Various burn care resources are available and may be helpful to gain a better understanding of this unique patient population (Box 25-1).

BURN WOUND SEVERITY

The severity of a burn wound is typically determined using **TBSA** calculations that take into account the distribution, **depth of injury**, and location of the burn (Fig. 25-1A,B). There is a direct correlation that exists between the TBSA and the expected number of scar contractures (Parry et al., 2019). Burn depth is also important in this assessment of potential functional loss in the face of scar contractures and is categorized into one of the four ways described below (Richard, 2000). From a rehabilitation perspective, the location of the burn injury is of concern when it involves skin creases overlying or adjacent to joint areas (Richard et al., 2009; Whitehead & Serghiou, 2009). In particular, skin recruitment (identified as **cutaneous functional units [CFUs]**) contributes to the motion of specific joints prone to burn scar contracture formation. A CFU involves a field of skin that extends well beyond the near proximity of the joint itself and uses up to 80% on average of available skin to produce specific ROM (Richard et al., 2009).

Burn injuries are classified based on the depth and levels of skin involved (**epidermal depth**); epidermal (**superficial**), **partial thickness, full thickness,** and **subdermal**. The depth of burn is classified as first-, second-, third-, and fourth-degree burns. As it pertains to wound healing, partial thickness wounds can be subdivided into superficial and deep by the amount of dermis involved (Rutan, 1998). The depth of injury is important from a wound healing perspective because it relates to the formation of scar tissue and the potential for subsequent contracture development.

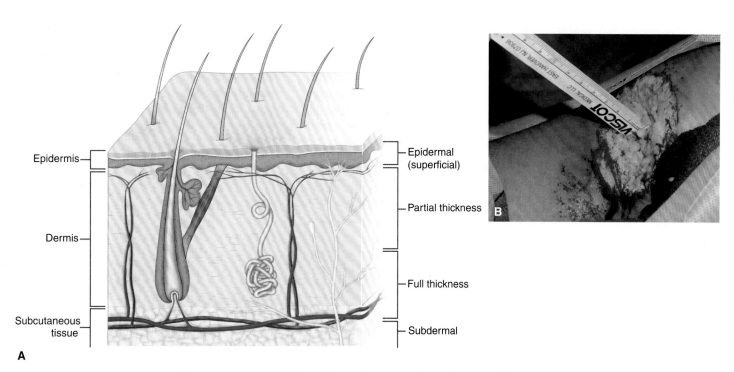

FIGURE 25-1 A, Layers of the skin and depth of tissue damage from the burn injury. **B,** Ruler utilized to measure depth. (Modified from Timby, B. K., Smith, N. E. (2018). *Introductory medical-surgical nursing* (12th ed.). Philadelphia, PA: Wolters Kluwer.)

Epidermal (superficial) burns are of little significance when considering functional positioning and healing (Fig. 25-2A–C). Most first- and second-degree burns heal within 14 days of injury and have minimal risk for scar contractures. Superficial partial thickness burns in the palms of the pediatric population can pose a risk to function when not properly positioned during healing (Greenhalgh & Stanley, 1994) (Fig. 25-3A–C). While this burn depth would not suggest scar formation, palmar creases that are allowed to heal together can lead to delayed wound healing and potentially impact hand function and growth over the life span of the child (Fig. 25-4A–C).

Deep partial thickness burns that heal primarily without surgical intervention do so through the formation of scar tissue that can potentially inhibit motion (Richard & Staley 1994b). Second- and third-degree burns that heal by secondary intention (i.e., from the base upward without surgical closure) do so by production of dense scar tissue. Deep partial thickness as well as full thickness burns that require skin grafting for wound closure pose a significant risk for scar contracture formation (Goverman et al., 2017) (Fig. 25-5A–C).

Subdermal burns, in particular those that are extensive in the damage to the underlying tissue, can also pose significant risk for contracture

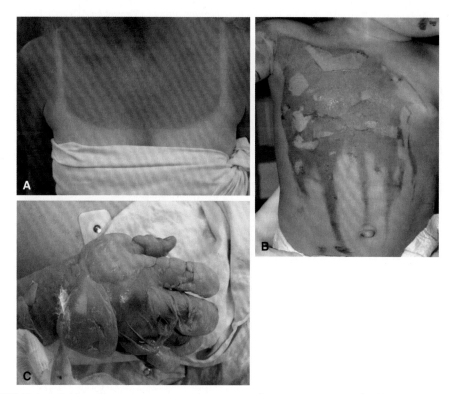

FIGURE 25-2 A, Epidermal burn, commonly seen in extreme sunburn exposure. **B,** Superficial scald injury distribution, commonly seen in pediatrics. **C,** Superficial partial thickness burn; note the erythema, blisters, and moist appearance of hand.

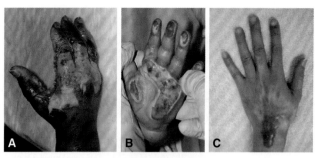

FIGURE 25-3 A, Deep partial thickness burn; note the pale appearance of skin and less erythema—scarring is likely to be visible as wounds will take greater than 14 days for closure. **B,** Superficial partial thickness burn in the palm will require a palmar extension orthosis. **C,** Deep partial thickness injury that healed by secondary intention; the thick scar with tension in surrounding dorsal skin impacts wrist flexion.

formation that would require the fabrication of an orthosis (Leblebici et al. 2006). Subdermal burns, commonly caused by electrical injury, exhibit extensive tissue damage underlying the skin, likewise can cause functional deficits that require an orthosis (Fig. 25-5D).

An important principle of orthotic fabrication in burns is the early application of an antideformity orthosis to ensure functional positioning during the healing phase. The timing of orthosis application must be skillfully judged as there is a likelihood of swelling or ongoing fluid shifts resulting in decreased blood flow. A second- or third-degree burn injury may present with significant changes in edema in the first 48 to 72 hours after injury (Fig. 25-6A,B). An already compromised blood flow has the potential to be negatively impacted by the application of an orthosis too early in the burn process resulting in possible tissue damage. Therefore, with the exception of positioning aids for immobility, an orthosis application should be withheld until the wound has declared itself and the extent of the burn is clearly demarcated (Holavanahalli, Helm, Parry, Dolezal, & Greenhalgh, 2011; Richard et al., 2009).

In the presence of a deeper burn, there is an increased risk for the involvement of underlying structures including the tendons, joint capsules, and ligaments as well as neurovascular structures. It is important, unless there is a direct medical contraindication, to position the structures in the position of least stress to prevent structural disruption and maintain functional positioning (Puri et al., 2013). In general, the orthosis should be positioned to prevent any excess stress that may disrupt the integrity of the wound and maintain a functional position.

Orthoses are applied on the surface of a burn to oppose the direction of the anticipated deformity. For example, a burn to the elbow antecubital surface requires an elbow extension immobilization

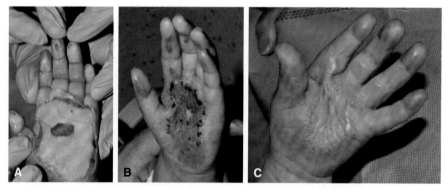

FIGURE 25-4 A–C, A full thickness injury that healed by STSG (split thickness skin graft). Note the tension in the thenar eminence and contracted 5th digit due to noncompliance with orthotic intervention.

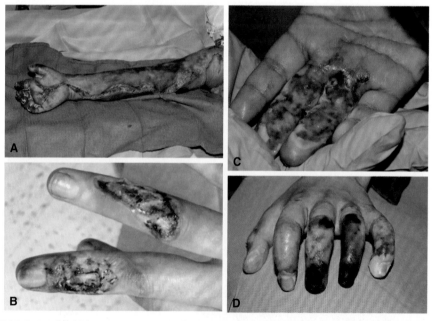

FIGURE 25-5 A, A full thickness upper extremity flame injury. A fasciotomy was performed, a procedure used to treat full thickness (third-degree) circumferential burns in order to prevent and treat compartment syndrome. **B,** Friction (treadmill injuries are common in pediatrics) requiring immobilization of the digits for prevention of burn scar contracture. Treadmill and friction injuries typically have exposed tendon and ligaments. **C,** Full thickness burn; note the depth on volar aspect contributing to the likelihood of significant contracture and loss of function. **D,** Post burn day 2 electrical injury; note the necrotic digits at the distal interphalangeal joints.

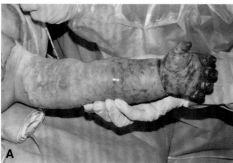

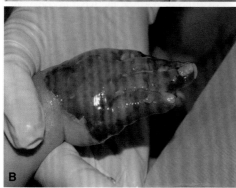

FIGURE 25-6 A, Significant edema in the hand and arm prior to removal of eschar. **B,** Increased edema as a result of a scald injury places the hand in a position that predisposes the development of claw hand deformity (metacarpophalangeal extension, interphalangeal flexion).

orthosis that is placed on the anterior surface of the extremity to prevent an elbow flexion **contracture** from occurring (Fig. 25-7A).

In circumferential or dorsal hand burns, the structures should be positioned to prevent any excess stress that may disrupt their integrity and maintain a functional position if the structures have already been disrupted. For a dorsal burn with questionable extensor tendon integrity, there are many issues to consider. Ideally, the wrist and metacarpophalangeal (MCP) joints should be positioned to place the tendons in a slack position (wrist and MCP extension); however, this position encourages functional complications of wrist and MCP extension contractures (Fig. 25-7B). Daily assessment of optimal ROM, functional movement, and orthosis positioning can ensure all goals are being met allowing for optimal patient recovery (Richard et al., 2009). Therapists must use their clinical judgment and constantly reevaluate their patient's needs, which change as tissue healing evolves. Ideally skilled therapeutic passive/active ROM

will coincide with dressing changes, wound care, and donning of orthosis. Therapists should consider clustering care in order to take advantage of patient medication usage required for manipulation.

Another aspect to consider with orthosis use on patients with burns is the development of **neuropathies**. A frequent site for development of an upper extremity neuropathy as a result of an orthosis is at the brachial plexus. Positioning a patient shoulder in horizontal abduction immobilization or in an airplane orthosis can cause increased risk of neuropathy (Fig. 25-8A). A brachial plexus injury may result from the patient being positioned in pure shoulder abduction over an extended period of time. Therapists typically recommend position of the shoulder at 90° abduction; however, pressure on the brachial plexus can be relieved by horizontally adducting the upper extremity 10° to 15°. However, in the pediatric setting, children have been positioned higher than 90° abduction without any reported effects (Fig. 25-8B).

Orthoses designed after a burn injury are customized for the patient with distinctive designs, configurations, and unique donning schedule depending on burn distribution. Troublesome contractures can be prevented by early orthotic intervention and antideformity positioning. Table 25-1 outlines orthosis designs that have been suggested for use with upper extremity burns.

The most common contractures associated with upper extremity burns are the following:

- Shoulder adduction/extension
- Shoulder internal rotation
- Elbow flexion
- Forearm pronation
- Wrist flexion

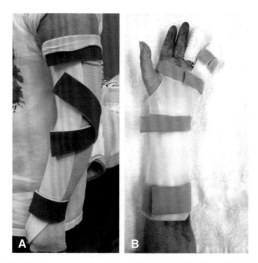

FIGURE 25-7 A, Elbow extension immobilization orthosis applied directly over healing skin grafts. **B,** Orthosis positioning wrist and small finger in extension to prevent undue stress on dorsal burn involving small digit extensors.

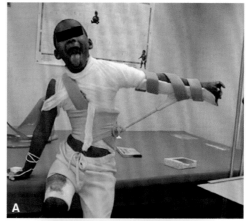

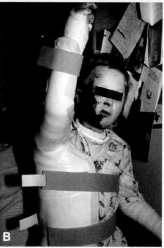

FIGURE 25-8 A, Pediatric axillary or airplane orthosis (shoulder abduction/elbow extension immobilization orthosis) fabricated at 90° (note donor site on the right thigh). **B,** Axilla orthosis fabricated greater than 90° of shoulder flexion and abduction used in the pediatric population.

- MCP joint extension
- Digit interphalangeal (IP) flexion
- Thumb adduction

If extremities are left immobile for many days, even in young children, capsular contractions and shortening of tendon and muscle groups crossing major joints will occur. When this happens, a predictable set of contractures will result. Some authorities believe that overly aggressive passive ROM can lead to **heterotopic ossification (HO)**, so this should be done with care, particularly at the elbow.

Burn contractures can be very difficult to counteract, but a working assumption of therapists in the burn unit is that restoring extension (once lost) is much more difficult than to regain flexion. The rationale for this is that the neurovascular bundle, once shortened, can only be lengthened with intensive and painful intervention, whereas activities like mobilization, functional use, and weight bearing naturally restore flexion (Puri et al. 2013).

The exception to this is with the suspicion of HO in the elbows. Clinically it can be difficult to diagnose HO in the presence of a large and deep burn injury. However, if the clinician suspects HO in the elbow joint either by increased pain with ROM or with a hard end range feel during ROM, it is prudent to immediately initiate an alternating elbow flexion/extension orthosis protocol with orthoses being switched at a minimum every 12 hours.

BASIC BURN ORTHOSES

While there remains a lack of researched consensus on the "correct" burn orthosis, the burn therapist community has two goals in mind when fabricating and implementing interventions: ensuring the position of function and positioning to decrease risk of deformity (Whitehead & Serghiou, 2009). The position of function considerations varies greatly between the pediatric and adult populations in particular due to the hypermobility of pediatric joints (Cooney, 1984). Therefore, in the adult population, it is important for the burn therapist to consider adult biomechanical principles of underlying structures when fabricating orthosis, in particular for the hand and wrist (Daugherty & Carr-Collins, 1994).

Selecting, implementing, and designing the appropriate burn hand orthosis are of critical importance to the burn therapist providing therapy (Richard et al., 2009). Orthoses in this category are referred to by various names, but they essentially sort out into two groups: **position of function orthoses** and **antideformity orthoses** (Fig. 25-9).

Both types of orthoses position the wrist in some degree of extension. In general, position of function orthoses allows for some degree of flexion at the proximal interphalangeal (PIP) and distal interphalangeal (DIP) joints, whereas antideformity orthoses hold those joints in extension. The discriminating factor between the orthoses is the amount of flexion allowed at the MCP joints. Position of function orthoses places the joints at 60° or less of flexion, whereas antideformity orthoses position the MCP joints in greater than 60° of flexion. Individualized fabrication is directly guided by the burn severity and location on the fingers as well as the risk to the underlying structures. When considering antideformity positioning, it is vital that the therapist takes into account the patient's level of activity and arousal to determine the position of function. Especially in the ankles and wrists, even if unaffected, antideformity orthoses should be considered to decrease the risk of foot or wrist drop once the acute stage has passed (Richard & Ward, 2005). Several suggested positions for the thumb were noted, which probably coincided with burn location based on clinical experience.

A further consideration related to burn location is when the injury involves skin creases over multiple consecutive joints. Previous work has shown that the position of an adjacent joint has an influence on skin excursion at the next joint in the series (Richard et al., 1994). Therapists need to consider designs that incorporate all areas of involvement to ensure maximal benefit of an orthotic intervention by the placement of an elongation stress over multiple

TABLE 25-1	**Common Upper Extremity Burn Orthoses**	
Burn Wound Location	**Common Orthosis Name**	**References**
Axilla or shoulder	• Airplane • Conformer/figure of 8 • Abduction wedge • Clavicular strap	• Malick and Carr (1982), Richard and Stanley (1994b), Walters (1987), Richard et al. (2005), Manigandan et al. (2005), and Chow (2006) • Malick and Carr (1982), Richard and Stanley (1994b), Walters (1987), Obaidullah et al. (2005), and Richard et al. (2005) • Malick and Carr (1982), Richard & Stanley (1994b), and Richard et al. (2005)
Elbow	• Dynamic • Gutter or trough • Conformer • Three point • Spiral	• Malick and Carr (1982), Richard and Stanley (1994b), Walters (1987), and Richard et al. (2005) • Richard et al. (1995) and Richard et al. (2005) • Richard et al. (1994) and Richard et al. (2005) • Richard et al. (1994), Malick and Carr (1982), Walters (1987), and Richard et al. (2005)
Wrist and hand	• Palmar pan • Position of function • Antideformity • Thumb spica • C-bar thumb web spacer • Palmar or dorsal extension • Traction or banjo • Halo • Flexion glove • Sandwich • Bivalve • Gutter	• Richard et al. (1994), Malick and Carr (1982), Richard et al. (2005), and Wallace et al. (2009) • Richard et al. (1994) and Richard et al. (2005) • Richard et al. (1994), Malick and Carr (1982), Walters (1987), Richard et al. (2005), and Agrawal and Bhattacharya (2011) • Richard and Staley. (1994a), (1994b), Van Straten and Sagi (2000), Richard et al. (2005), and Kaine et al. (2008) • Richard and Staley. (1994a), (1994b), Van Straten and Sagi (2000), Richard et al. (2005), and Kaine et al. (2008) • Daugherty and Carr-Collins (1994), Richard et al. (1994), and Richard et al. (2005) • Richard et al. (1994), Walters (1987), and Richard et al. (2005) • Malick and Carr (1982), Richard et al. (1994), Schwanholt et al. (1992), Yotsuyanagi, Yokoi, and Omizo (1994), and Richard et al. (2005) • Malick and Carr (1982), Richard and Stanley (1994b), and Richard et al. (2005) • Richard et al. (1994), Walters (1987), and Richard et al. (2005) • Richard et al. (1994), and Richard et al. (2005) • Gilliam et al. (1993), Richard et al. (1994), Walters (1987), and Richard et al. (2005) • Richard et al. (1994), and Richard et al. (2005) • Rivers, Collin, Fisher, Solem, and Ahrenholz (1984), and Richard et al. (2005)

consecutive joint skin crease surface areas (discussed in the following text) (Cooney, 1984).

In particular to the total hand burn, special consideration must be paid to both the first and fifth digits because the dynamic pulling forces of developing scar tissue and the multiple planes of motion within each of these digits can create significant long-term complications if not continuously monitored with precise management of orthoses and carefully guided rehabilitation.

WOUND HEALING PHASES

Wound healing can be divided into three phases that have some amount of overlap (see Chapter 3 for more specific details) (Greenhalgh & Staley, 1994). During the **inflammatory stage** or the initial stage, wound repair lasts 3 to 5 days under normal circumstances. Depending on the burn distribution, orthoses should be avoided primarily for two reasons, unless needed to stabilize a joint. First, an orthosis fabricated and applied too early can cause vascular compromise when edema increases, making the orthosis too small. Therapists should consider wrapping orthoses using gauze rolls versus traditional loop strapping (Fig. 25-10A). For the same reason, straps used to hold the orthosis in place can become constrictive, potentially impeding circulation. When orthoses are used during the acute phase of injury, they should be nonconforming to accommodate for fluctuations in edema (Fig. 25-10B).

EXPERT PEARL 25-1

Dressing Changes With Surgitube
BOB PHILLIPS OTR/L, CHT
Georgia

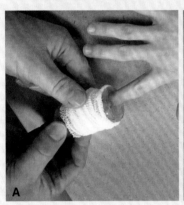 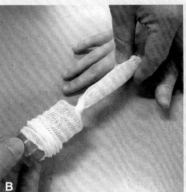 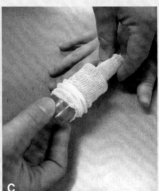 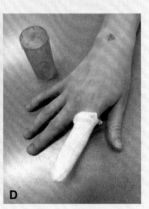

Easy hack great for applying surgitube or a similar tubular product. Use a pill bottle without the label to allow for easy donning.

EXPERT PEARL 25-2

Fabrication Over Bandages
THERESA BELL-NAGLE, OTR/L, CHT
Massachusetts

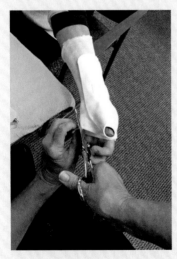

Cover wound dressing with extra layer of stockinette so that the warm material doesn't stick, then cut the stockinette and remove the orthosis easily without disturbing the dressing.

The use of orthoses for patients who have moved beyond the emergent phase of treatment and into the **proliferative** and **wound maturation phases** depends on several factors (Richard, Staley, Miller, & Warden, 1996, 1997; Richard et al., 2009). In burns that have a high risk on contracture development, the practice is that an orthosis is fabricated early in the admission or treatment phase and used at all times until the skin grafts have healed with a focus on daily active and passive ROM as indicated by the location of skin grafts.

In general, immobilization orthoses are commonly used to prevent scar contractures, whereas mobilization orthoses are used to correct any existing scar contracture (Richard et al., 2009; Richard, Shanesy, & Miller, 1995). Part of the reasoning for this difference is based on the biomechanical principles that underlie each type of orthosis.

Bacteria-Controlled Nursing Unit

A system of patient protection from bacterial cross infection called the bacteria-controlled nursing unit (BCNU) is utilized at a variety of different facilities. The BCNU allows for the patient's bed to be in strict environmental control of 6 × 10 feet area rather than the patient's entire room being controlled (Fig. 25-11A). BCNU allows the ability to deliver all medical care without entering the protective environment and maintaining all monitoring, life support, and intravenous equipment outside the

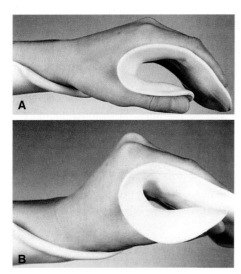

FIGURE 25-9 **A,** Position of function orthosis. **B,** Antideformity orthosis. Note difference in degree of metacarpophalangeal and interphalangeal joint flexion.

controlled environment. The clinical effectiveness of this system in the treatment of burn patients has been studied and compared with the effectiveness of single room isolation on a burn isolation ward and conventional isolation techniques on an open burn ward. The studies show that the BCNU is significantly more effective in preventing bacterial cross-contamination than conventional precautions (3.8% vs. 13.1%, $P < .001$; and 8% vs. 22.8%, $P < .001$) over a 2- and 4-week period (Glenn, Burke) (Fig. 25-11B).

BIOMECHANICAL PRINCIPLES

Immobilization orthoses, which statically place a joint in a specific position, use the principle of stress relaxation on scar tissue (Richard & Staley, 1994a). Based on this principle, the amount of force required to maintain a given position of angularity decreases over time (Fig. 25-12). Essentially, tissues adapt to the stress placed on them. Due to the high contractibility of burn wounds, it is important to start the use of therapist fabricated orthosis as soon as the wound has declared itself. Burn wounds that remain open during the healing process are painful. Forceful stress on the tender tissues may increase the amount of pain experienced by the patient. When an immobilization orthosis is initially applied to a patient, there should

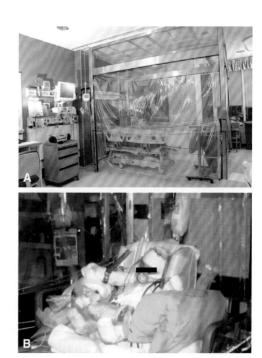

FIGURE 25-11 **A,** BCNU (bacteria-controlled nursing unit) is a strict environmental unit for patients who require isolation. **B,** Early mobilization and positioning while restricted in the BCNU walls.

be only slight discomfort, which lessens in a short period of time, owing to accommodation of the tissues. To avoid generating too much stress on delicate tissue, there is a tendency to use immobilization orthoses more than mobilization orthoses during this time.

After burn wound closure, as scar tissue continues to mature and contract, the ongoing biologic force needs to be counteracted by an equal or greater force. Once a burn wound is covered with new tissue, the primary source of pain is essentially removed and a greater demand can be placed on the tissue with less discomfort. If the patient has developed a scar tissue contracture during this phase of scar maturation, mobilization orthoses that operate under the principle of tissue creep are suggested. Tissue creep is the process whereby the length of biologic tissue continues to elongate if tension is kept constant and maintained over a prolonged period of time (Richard & Staley, 1994b). The key to this principle is the constant application of force, which provides a stimulus for the tissue to lengthen by production and growth of additional tissue (refer to Chapter 15).

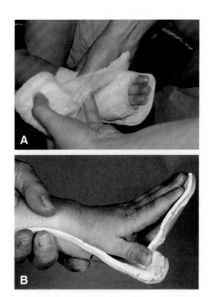

FIGURE 25-10 **A,** Pediatric palmar extension orthosis donned with gauze roll (Kerlix). **B,** Volar orthosis; note the wrist extension and thumb abduction.

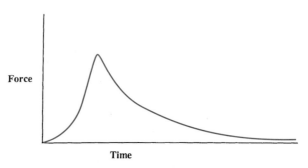

FIGURE 25-12 Soft-tissue stress relaxation. After the peak stress is reached from the application of an immobilization orthosis, the amount of stress experienced by the tissue decreases. (Reprinted with permission from Richard, R. L., & Staley, M. J. (1994). Biophysical aspects of normal skin and burn scar. In Richard R. L. & Staley M. J. (Eds.), *Burn care and rehabilitation – Principles and practice* (pp. 65). Philadelphia, PA: Davis.)

IMPLICATIONS FOR ORTHOTIC INTERVENTION

GENERAL CONSIDERATIONS

Therapists on the burn unit have many options in selecting the best orthoses for their patients. Orthotic literature commonly makes distinctions between a conforming and nonconforming orthosis, with conforming orthosis fabricated directly on the patient and nonconforming generally being off the shelf and prefabricated with general sizes (Parry et al. 2019). Caution should be used when applying nonconforming orthoses over wound dressings because their more generalized fit may lead to excessive pressure along the orthotic borders. Nonconforming or off-the-shelf orthoses are commercially available for several joints and are typically sized using one measurement. A positive aspect of using prefabricated nonconforming orthoses is they can be made readily available to clinicians during emergencies and may be useful at other times when therapists are not available, such as nights, weekends, and holidays. Conforming orthoses are fabricated by a therapist directly on the patient or with several measurements taken from the patient. They typically have improved distribution of pressure and a lesser tendency to migrate or shift once applied correctly. A well-made conforming orthosis can provide more effective antideformity positioning as it can be customized to the patient. Special attention also should be afforded when fabricating an orthosis over bony prominences to prevent skin breakdown. These orthoses can be applied relatively safely over bulky dressings by nursing personnel. Fabricating safe and effective conforming orthoses requires experience and skill in patient positioning, manipulation of the orthotic material, and correct application with strapping or bandages. Staff should be instructed in proper application, fit, and precautions with fabricated orthosis. Frequent reeducation in the application and use should be provided and monitored closely to ensure no detriment to the patient (Manigandan et al, 2005).

In some settings, there is a concern that any orthosis applied over a new skin graft might affect graft take and wound closure. While the vascularity of a new skin graft is a concern, there should be no limitation to the use of positioning orthosis (Richard et al., 1997) (Fig. 25-13). The therapist must ensure that donning and doffing the orthosis does not increase shear or pressure over the grafted areas. Whenever possible, a post-surgical orthosis should be used for optimal positioning and immobilization of fresh hand graft. The use of overly bulky post-surgical dressings should be limited whenever possible to ensure functional and/or antideformity positioning is maintained (Schwanholt, Daugherty, Gaboury, & Warden, 1992).

At this time, there continues to be no general consensus for postoperative orthosis wear schedule and many protocols are facility-specific. Therapists should consider multiple indicators including the age of the patient, pre-existing conditions such as arthritis, and physician specifications (Daugherty & Carr-Collins, 1994). For example, young children typically possess flexible joints within these cases, positions of hyperextension of the MCP joints can be made for palmar burns with minimal potential for causing MCP joint extension contractures (Schwanholt et al., 1992) (Fig. 25-10B).

After burn wound closure, the body continues to heal itself by producing scar tissue, which typically has a detrimental effect on motion. As scar tissue continues to mature and contract, the main focus is on scar management, increasing mobility and preserving function. If the patient has developed a scar tissue contracture during this phase of scar maturation, mobilization or dynamic orthoses that operate under the principle of tissue creep are suggested. Tissue creep is the process whereby the length of biologic tissue continues to elongate if tension is kept constant and maintained over a prolonged period of time (Richard & Staley, 1994b). The key to this principle is the constant application of force, which provides a stimulus for the tissue to lengthen by production and growth of additional tissue. Mobilization or dynamic orthoses may be progressed by the therapist or patient as the joint's ROM improves.

The optimal amount of time that an orthosis should be worn has yet to be determined (Richard et al., 2009). Each patient presents differently and should be approached individually. Initially, adults and children should wear orthoses at all times with breaks only for functional activities or active and passive ROM. A scar contracture problem that is unique to patients with hand burns is a web space syndactyly. This condition can occur on the dorsum of the hand between any two fingers, but it is functionally most problematic at the first web space. A burn in this area may cause the thumb to contract into adduction or hyperextension. When applying an orthosis to the thumb, caution is needed to avoid damage to the collateral ligaments and subsequent instability of the thumb and also with the goal to maximize the space in the first web space to prevent creep (Fig. 25-14).

Unconscious patients may or may not need burn orthoses (Fig. 25-15A,B). However, unconscious patients always require protection of the ankle to prevent foot drop. Foot drop can be a functionally devastating outcome of prolonged bed rest even if the feet are unburned (refer to Field Note). These patients are at high risk for developing contractures and demand a therapist's attention regarding proper positioning, orthosis use, and exercise. A key burn therapist axiom is "the position of comfort is the position of contracture"; continuous and vigilant monitoring of the burn treatment intervention will help to achieve long-lasting functional recovery and outcomes.

A deep burn of the anterior or lateral neck, if left untreated, can cause significant functional deficits as this skin contracts to heal. At times, therapeutic intervention in the Intensive Care Unit (ICU) is limited by the medical complexity of the patient, but long-term functional outcomes can be improved by deliberate antideformity

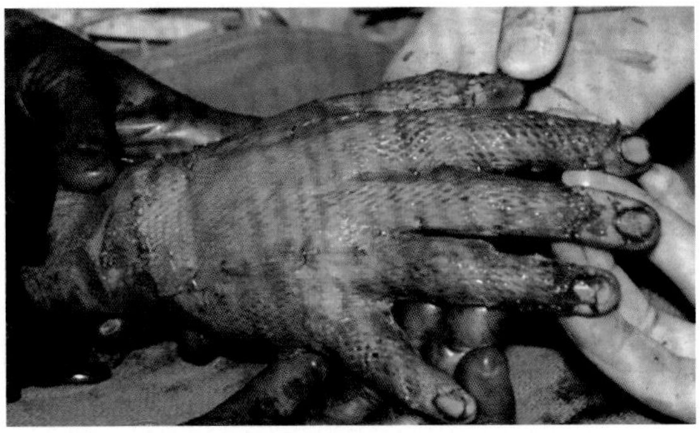

FIGURE 25-13 A meshed, split thickness skin graft that will require immediate postoperative immobilization in a volar orthosis to prevent graft loss.

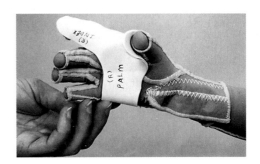

FIGURE 25-14 A pediatric carpometacarpophalangeal abduction immobilization orthosis (c-bar orthosis) for treating burns to the first web space.

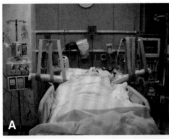
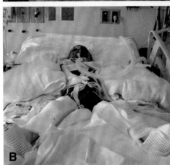
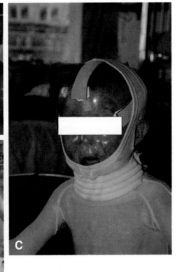

FIGURE 25-15 **A,** Modified bilateral shoulder abduction orthoses suspended with intravenous (IV) poles. These devices can be moved more easily than airplane orthoses with sedated patient and allow for easier positioning with a ventilator, multiple IV pumps, and nursing care. **B,** Positioning a patient using a variety of materials: pillows for the upper extremities and knees. Ankle orthoses are used for foot and ankle positioning and note no pillows behind the head in order to keep the head in a neutral position. **C,** Watusi collar assists in the management of neck contractures and positioning.

positioning, regular ROM activities, and appropriate orthoses that do not interfere with the patient's medical treatment.

Cervical neck contracture can be common with medically complex patients due to the frequent patient repositioning from nursing staff. The therapist must take responsibility to provide adequate education regarding positioning and orthotic wearing routines to nursing staff in order to prevent a cervical contracture. One fabricated orthosis that has proven to help prevent scar contracture formation is a Watusi collar (Fig. 25-15C). This orthosis is inexpensive and can be easily made in-house using cloth, loop strapping, and commercial plastic tubing. Generally, this orthosis is comfortable for the patient to wear and allows for cervical rotation ensuring safety during community mobility. A Watusi collar can be progressed by the therapist by adding additional rungs of tubing and can also be used in adjunctive pressure device with conformers and silicone sheeting.

Orthoses should be checked frequently for proper fit and adjustments made accordingly. During the day, mobility of alert patients should be encouraged as appropriate. However, orthosis wear should be continuous except for dressing changes when exposed joints are present or in the presence of already existing contractures. Clinically, a patient's ROM guides the wearing schedule of an orthosis. If the patient's ROM is decreasing, the time spent in orthoses should be increased with all other treatment interventions and activity program considerations (Fig. 25-16). Disinfectant cleaning of orthoses was found more beneficial than air drying for burn orthoses (Richard & Staley, 1994a; Staley, Richard, Daugherty, & Warden, 1991).

Scarring usually develops within the first few weeks after wound closure but it can be difficult to predict who will develop scarring. Scars can appear poorest at 6 months until they mature between 12 and 18 months. As scars mature, they will fade in color, increase in pliability, and become less sensitive. Hypertrophic scars stay in the area of original burn and appear textured, raised, and red/purple in color. Hypertrophic burn scars develop when the collagen fibers are laid down in a very disorganized manner. Patients often experience intense itching after their burn injury due to oil glands damage.

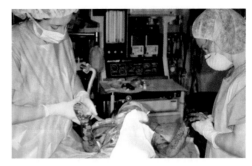

FIGURE 25-16 Patients who are unable to move should have PROM completed in order to maintain range of motion (ROM) and prevent stiffness from developing.

Patients are recommended to apply a moisturizer with high water content frequently throughout the day. As burn scars mature, moisturizers should be applied by massaging with adequate pressure to help in softening and loosening scars.

When pressure garments are incorporated into the patient's scar management routine, pieces of loop strapping can be sewn to the garment material to secure the orthosis. Oftentimes, when burns affect several areas, it is helpful to incorporate multiple orthoses into one design pattern or fabricate each orthosis to fit precisely with the others. The more orthoses there are, the greater the chance of losing one. Furthermore, an all-inclusive orthosis design makes donning the orthosis easier for caregivers. For example, with small children particularly, a shoulder abduction and elbow extension immobilization orthosis can be combined (Fig. 25-8A) (Richard, Schall, Staley, & Miller, 1994). As another example, the hand, wrist, and elbow can be incorporated into one orthosis (Richard et al., 1994). A novel orthosis for treating bilateral axillary burns simultaneously is the T-shirt orthosis (Fig. 25-17) (Daugherty & Carr-Collins, 1994; Manigandan, Gupta, Venugopal, Ninan, & Cherian, 2003). The orthosis is worn on the anterior torso and secured with straps that cross over the back.

Pressure therapy for scar management, also known as compression therapy, is extremely important for modulating formation of scar tissue after wound closure. Pressure garments are utilized to minimize the development of scar by interfering with the production of collagen and development of scar tissue. Pressure garments may also be used to protect fragile skin, reduce the risk of hypertrophic scarring (thick, hard scar), and decrease itching. Pressure garments are initiated once the skin is durable enough to tolerate donning and doffing without blistering. Close monitoring of the affected area is indicated, particularly over the first few days, to ensure patient tolerance with mobility tasks and ongoing fluid shifts. Burn therapists typically initiate pressure therapy using an intervention with the least risk for causing shearing or blistering, such as Ace bandages. With successful tolerance for this, they may progress the patient to

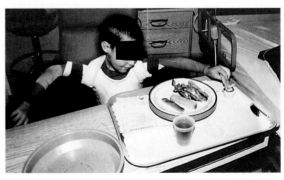

FIGURE 25-17 T-shirt orthosis (bilateral abduction immobilization orthosis) used to position both extremities after injury.

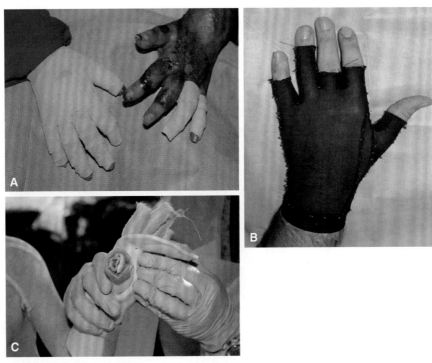

FIGURE 25-18 Pressure garments are worn after a burn to control scarring, help the scar mature, and improve overall cosmetic appearance. **A,** Least restrictive interim garment (Coban) that is applied by wrapping, allowing for minimal shearing. **B,** Custom compression garments are designed to patient's measurements and burn distribution. **C,** Custom compression garments with hand orthosis during the scar remodeling phase of rehabilitation.

more aggressive interventions, including rolled elastic gauze such as Conform, self-adherent wraps (Coban, CoWrap), elastic tubular bandages (Tubigrip, Spandagrip), interim pressure garments, and custom-made garments (Fig. 25-18A). Interim garments are available off-the-shelf and are used as a transition until custom fitting garments are available. Custom-made pressure garments (nylon spandex) garments are made to the patient's measurements and burn distribution (Fig. 25-18B). Some custom garment companies allow patients to select a color choice, which can help with patient compliance.

For maximum effectiveness, pressure garments should be worn as much as possible, ideally 7 days a week, 23 hours daily. Patients will remove pressure garments in order to complete their scar management routine of bathing, moisturizing, and scar massage (Fig. 25-18C). Garments are worn until the scar is mature as deemed by their physician. A mature scar typically presents as soft, pliable, and flat, with normal vascularity. A typical course of pressure therapy will last between 8 months and 1 to 2 years following wound closure. Silicone sheeting, foam, elastomer, or other materials may be placed under the **compression garments** to improve conformity and to provide additional pressure to hypertrophic areas. It is important that the patient's scar management routine is frequently evaluated and progressed as their scar tissue matures over time.

EXPERT PEARL 25-3

Scar Management
ANNA OVSYANNIKOVA, MD, HAND THERAPY
Russia

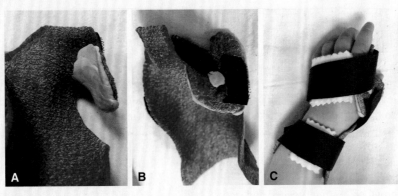

To fixate scar mold with orthosis: Make a little hole or two in the orthosis with hole punch/scissors. Prepare the silicone and while it is setting push it into the hole and mold the internal surface.

Custom Pressure Glove
TRISH GRIFFITHS, OT
South Africa

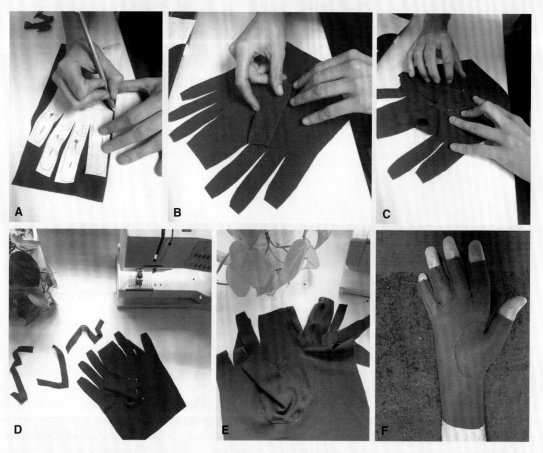

Steps to fabricate a pressure garment glove:

- Elasticized material is used which has a unidirectional stretch (Elastonet used here).
- Pattern taken of patient's hand and circumference measured at wrist, distal palmar crease, and proximal phalanges.
- Material folded with fold running along the border of the index finger.
- Glove is fabricated at 85% of the circumference of the wrist and distal palmar crease and therefore 15% of the circumference is subtracted from wrist and distal palmar crease before transferring the pattern on to the material.
- Thumb piece sewn on first, 1 cm toward to volar aspect of the hand to allow for a slightly opposed resting position in the glove.
- Finger gussets of 1.5 cm are sewn on to the material on the dorsal aspect to maintain a good web space. Pressure around the fingers is measured using the following formula to take the gussets into account.
  - Index and little finger: (Circumference of finger—1.5 cm gusset)/2
  - Middle and ring finger: (Circumference of finger—[1.5 cm × 2])/2
- Gussets attached to volar part of material and ulna border of glove sewn together.

MATERIAL SELECTION

When fabricating an orthosis for an acute burn patient, it is important to take into account the size of the dressings needed to protect underlying tissue as well as consider the potential change in dressing bulk. The girth of a dressed extremity may change regularly throughout an inpatient stay secondary to edema, muscle atrophy, bleeding, or even provider preference. Therapists will observe the dressing size depending on the provider, healing process, and status of the patient (Richard & Staley, 1994). It is therefore important to choose a material with good memory to allow for frequent orthotic modification in order to improve conformity to the affected areas. Burn units and therapists have orthosis materials of preference, but in general terms, therapists will utilize materials for specific body parts and rationale for orthotic intervention (Staley et al, 1991). Considerations in selecting orthosis materials include strength, rigidity, durability, memory, conformity, and ease of fabrication (Canelon, 1995). Orthoses that do not fit correctly can place body segments in positions that encourage development of scar tissue

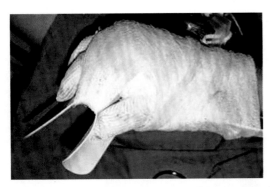

FIGURE 25-19 Poorly applied orthoses can further influence undesired positioning and contractures. Look closely at the position of the metacarpophalangeal and proximal interphalangeal joints relative to the orthosis platform; this position is supporting an intrinsic minus (claw hand) and not an intrinsic plus (antideformity) position.

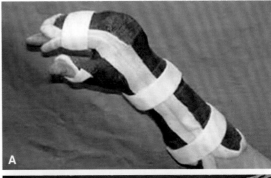

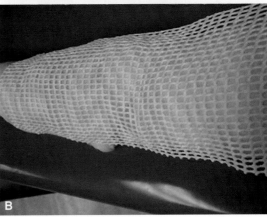

FIGURE 25-20 **A,** Bivalve Delta-Cast immobilization orthosis for burn hand (Essity, Charlotte NC). **B,** This elbow extension orthosis is made of Hexalite; note the open weave allows for breathability and passage of heavy exudates.

contractures. Therefore, the adage "no orthosis is better than a poorly fitted orthosis" is one to heed in burn care (Fig. 25-19). For best practice, all orthoses should be labeled with the patient's name and hospital-approved method of identification.

Owing to the small anatomical structures of patients younger than 1 year of age, fabrication of orthoses on this patient population is difficult and requires some experience to achieve a successful outcome. Depending on the child's size, it may be easier to position the extremities with the use of bulky dressing or inserted material, such as Elastomer or foam, in lieu of an orthosis.

Body orthosis in adults and older pediatrics patients needs to be able to sustain large loads from heavy appendages, be easily remoldable as the size and shape of an appendage changes, and be perforated to allow for soaking medicine and wound exudate to pass through. Most therapists choose a 1/8″ perforated thermoplastic material with medium to high memory and medium conformity (Richard & Staley 1994a, 1994b). For best practice, all orthoses should be labeled with the patient's name and hospital-approved method of identification as well as orientation of orthosis for any staff helping with orthotic donning outside of scheduled therapy sessions. As most orthotic material tends to be the same color as dressing supplies, it is prudent to use color or have the patients, where able, personalize their orthoses.

If therapists fabricate custom orthoses early during a patient's hospitalization, then a material that can be frequently remolded is recommended because of the number of modifications that may be needed to accommodate fluctuations in edema and bandage thickness. In 1969, the first use of a thermoplastic material to customize a burn orthosis was described (Willis, 1969). Since that time, a host of materials for orthoses have been advocated and used (Cox, Taddonio, & Thompson, 1991; Richard & Staley, 1994a; Willis, 1970). Generally, 1/16″ material can be used with the pediatric population and in areas that do not bear much weight, such as the fingers. Thicker materials, 1/8″, should be used for pediatric orthoses crossing larger joints such as the elbows, knees, and axillas as well as for adult orthoses to ensure a rigid orthosis with adequate positioning. The material of choice for the burn therapist is largely dependent on the current stage of the wound healing process. Ideally, thermoplastics with moderate memory that have perforations but still maintain the rigidity to counteract positional forces are essential to support the modifications required from dressing and bandaging adaptations during the initial phases of healing and/or skin grafting. Fabrication of orthoses for the burned upper extremity can incorporate various types of materials (including aluminum,

wood, high-temperature polycarbonates, and thermoformable foams), and the optimal selection is only limited to the imagination and resourcefulness of the treating clinician and the presenting wound/scar presentation (Agrawal & Bhattacharya, 2011; Forbes-Duchart & Niszczak, 2010).

Perforated or open-weave material is best used for patients who have a large amount of wound exudate or transudate and when topical antibiotic solutions are in use; the perforations allow the exudate to escape and the medicine to penetrate through the dressings. Also, these plain thermoplastics (without combinations of foam, padding, or antibiotic properties) are more commonly used for ease of application and to create a well-fitting orthosis with bandaging or with pressure garments. Perforated material also allows for some air to reach the dressings, drying them and preventing wounds from becoming macerated.

Traditional plaster cast material provides a cost-effective alternative to thermoplastics in some cases. Other casting type materials have been used (including 3M™ Scotchcast™ Plus fiberglass, Hexalite®, and Delta-Cast® Conformable polyester tape) in similar fashion to traditional casting to support optimal prolonged position and provide lightweight stability (Fig. 25-20A,B). These techniques and materials may not be the best choice during the acute phase of wound healing because frequent cast changes would be required. Cast material tends to absorb the wound exudate, which necessitates removal and application of a new device. However, when patient compliance is an issue, serial casting can be a more effective medium than thermoplastic orthosis use. Also, consider thermoplastics when orthosis hygiene is an issue. These materials can be easily wiped clean, disinfected, and reapplied to the extremity. Casting may help in the later stages of wound healing to position joint(s) for a mobilization orthosis using serial static stress to improve and facilitate long-term ROM improvements (Daugherty & Carr-Collins, 1994).

Web Space Tightness
SHERI B. FELDSCHER, OTR/L, CHT
Pennsylvania

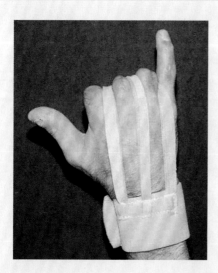

Velfoam was used for this quick, easy-to-fabricate digit web space stretcher (courtesy of Evelyn Mackin) to apply a low-load long duration stress to the web spaces. Used to increase the surface area of the digit and allow for prosthetic use in digits not having enough length for a prosthesis to be applied.

STRAPPING SELECTION

The strapping methods used in adult and pediatric populations may differ; however, in the acute phase, rolled gauze offers an effective means of securing an orthosis. Strapping is not financially feasible for the acute patient who is undergoing frequent dressing changes or has damp dressings due to soaking medicine or wound exudate. The use of bandage material without stretch or elastic to secure and increase conformity of orthosis is preferred with the acute population. The use of bandage material allows for easy and cost-effective orthotic management and also has the added benefit of familiarity with the use of the product for all members of the burn team (Fig. 25-21A). This method of securing the orthosis in the pediatric population allows for correct positioning without excess pressure points. This method ensures the orthosis is difficult for a child to remove and can improve compliance for the intervention (Serghiou & Niszczak, 2011).

Once a patient has transitioned out of the acute stage or if the patient requires frequent doffing/donning of the orthosis for exercises or functional use, strapping of the orthosis may be warranted (Fig. 25-21B). For compliant adults, a rolled gauze bandage, elastic wrap (e.g., Ace or Coban), or foam straps (e.g., Velfoam) offer an effective means to secure an orthoses (Fig. 25-21C). One method is to use a sandwich orthosis (Gilliam, Hatler, Adams, & Helm, 1993; Ward, Schnebly, Kravitz, Warden, & Saffle, 1989). With this type of orthosis, recommended for use with the hand, a dorsal and volar piece is made that encases the hand. As an alternative, a bivalve hand cast can act as a type of sandwich orthosis. It is always important to consider that the pediatric population is not always good at accurately describing pain or tingling as a result of compromised blood flow due to orthosis position, so the therapist needs to closely monitor any of these orthoses. An abundance of caution must be used when utilizing elastic wraps to secure an orthosis in the pediatric

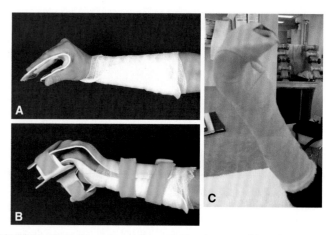

FIGURE 25-21 **A,** Circumferentially applied bandage material used to secure orthosis. **B,** Hook and loop straps make it easier for the patient and care providers when donning and doffing this "clamshell" orthosis used post contracture release. **C,** Circumferential elasticized bandage used to secure a volar wrist/hand immobilization orthosis.

and noncompliant patient due to increased compression. When choosing a strapping material, it is important that the material be easy to clean to reduce the risk of infection, secure, and provide good conformity with the orthosis (Wright, Taddonio, Prasad, & Thompson, 1989).

Another technique for holding an orthosis in place and preventing distal slippage is to line the orthosis with Dycem or a similar nonskid material. This tacky material acts as a good interface between the orthosis and material in which it comes into contact, especially slick pressure garments commonly employed for burn management. Finally, simply increasing the angle of wrist extension in a hand orthosis, if appropriate, can prevent distal migration of the hand beyond the end of the orthosis. With all of these methods, it is important to teach the caregiver what the orthosis looks like when correctly positioned and when appropriate provide caregiver training to reposition the orthosis.

CONCLUSION

A skilled burn therapist can be an invaluable member of the interdisciplinary team on a burn unit, providing insight on positioning and orthosis selection in the acute stages of burn care. Early intervention in the ICU can help patients maximize their long-term functional outcomes and ease the transition to outpatient treatment. The use of orthoses in the rehabilitation of patients with burn injuries is an integral part of a comprehensive treatment program. It takes experience and clinical expertise to decide when, how, and which orthoses to fabricate to ensure that all functional and surgical goals are met. A therapist must carefully consider the burn location, depth, and mechanism as well as the patient's age and any other confounding factors as all of these can significantly impact the outcome. Biomechanical principles should be taken into account based on the treatment objectives and special considerations should be extended to pediatric and geriatric patients.

Successful strategies demand a decision on whether to custom fabricate an orthosis or to use a prefabricated or commercially available orthosis. If an orthosis is custom made, attention should be paid to design and the type of material selected. There still remains room for much research into time of application, duration of use, and the benefits of prefabricated versus custom orthoses, but this chapter is an attempt to provide a snapshot of the philosophy of orthosis use on a working burn unit.

FIELD NOTE: LOWER EXTREMITY BURN INJURY

Aimee Chiasson, PT, DPT
Massachusetts

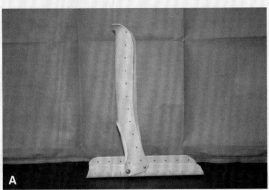

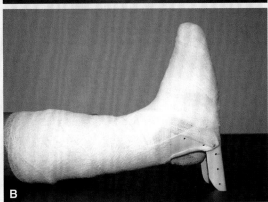

Patients with burn injuries can often have involvement of multiple areas of their body, so it is not uncommon for their lower extremities to be affected. In the acute setting, lower extremity orthoses should not only support positioning to counteract potential scar contractures but also facilitate appropriate joint kinematics once weight bearing is indicated (Figures A,B). For example, when treating a patient with an anterior ankle burn, a therapist should consider both positioning to counteract the contracture (plantarflexion) and positioning that supports weight bearing (neutral ankle position). Orthoses are applied to the limb from distal joint to proximal joint to maintain proper alignment and positioning of all joints involved in the burn injury. Lower extremity orthoses may be used in conjunction with inserts and pressure therapy to prevent and treat lower extremity contractures, especially those in the metatarsophalangeal joints. Upon wound closure, semirigid casting may also be used for static progressive correction of knee and ankle contractures. It is important to note that a patient may need a lower extremity orthosis in an area that is not affected by their burn injury as a precaution against

the effects of prolonged immobility. In these scenarios, the orthosis is often used to prevent muscle tightness (e.g., plantarflexion contracture) or to relieve pressure and prevent pressure ulcer. Below is a description of common lower extremity orthoses used in the burn population with a focus on the purpose of positioning as well as special considerations for this patient population.

Orthosis	Purpose	Special Considerations
Two piece foot	• A hinged orthosis used to maintain the ankle in a functional position and prevent plantarflexion contracture/deformity. • Design also off weights the heel, eliminating pressure and decreasing likelihood of skin breakdown.	• May be customized for patients with ongoing plantarflexion contractures. • Patient cannot stand/weight bear when wearing this orthosis. • Improved durability over Multi Podus boots when patient is being treated with soaks or has significant wound drainage.
Knee extension	• To maintain knee in extended position to prevent knee flexion contracture and/or immobilize joint for graft protection. • Can also assist in maintaining proper hip alignment by reducing hip flexion momentum.	• May be customized for patients with ongoing knee flexion contractures. • Improved durability over knee immobilizer while the patient is being treated with soaking medication or has significant wound drainage.
Hip abduction wedge	• To maintain hips in an abducted position to prevent skin contracture, muscle tightness, and/or for graft protection.	• Limits hip adduction but does not limit hip flexion. • Most commonly be used for protection of grafts in the groin area. • Needs to be removed for toileting and mobility.
Hip spica	• To maintain the hips in a neutral position and/or abduction. • Mainly used to prevent hip flexion/adduction contracture and/or for graft protection.	• Limits hip flexion and can be fabricated to place the patient in variable degrees of hip abduction. • Needs to be removed for toileting and mobility.

Case Study Section

The case studies presented here are meant as a teaching guideline only. Treatment and orthosis protocols vary greatly from surgeon to surgeon and from therapist to therapist. The therapist should check with the referring physicians and colleagues to define the preferred treatment and appropriate orthotic intervention.

Case Study 1: Upper Extremity Burn Injury With Skin Grafting

MJS, a 41-year-old left-dominant female, was preparing supper and used an accelerant on smoldering briquettes in her outdoor barbecue grill when the charcoal suddenly erupted into flames.

The previously healthy patient was estimated to have experienced a 7% surface area burn of her dominant upper extremity. The palm of her hand was spared along with an area of skin on the medial aspect of her upper arm. She was diagnosed as having mixed deep partial and full thickness burns throughout (Fig. 25-22). When the therapist first evaluated the patient the morning after the injury, the patient's hand and upper extremity were markedly edematous, and the hand and fingers were in a slightly flexed position. Joint motion was moderately restricted throughout, secondary to edema and pain. Surgery to apply skin grafts to the areas of full thickness injury was scheduled for 2 days after injury. Owing to the swelling and impending surgery, the therapist placed the upper extremity in an elevated position and instructed MJS to perform active ROM to tolerance to aid in edema reduction and maintenance of ROM.

By the time of surgery, the edema had subsided remarkably, and the areas of full thickness burn had demarked themselves and were confined to the volar aspect of the arm and forearm, which involved the antecubital space. These areas were excised and covered with split thickness sheet skin grafts harvested from a superior posterior thigh donor site. The surgeon requested the therapist's attendance in the operating room, where a position of function hand orthosis was fabricated to immobilize the deep partial thickness burns and an elbow extension immobilization orthosis was formed and applied over the bulky dressings. MJS's elbow area was kept immobilized for 5 days to allow for adherence of the skin graft.

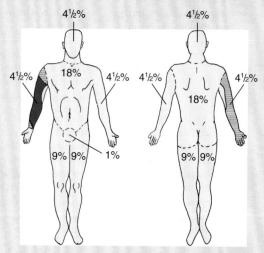

FIGURE 25-22 Distribution and depth of burns. The hatched areas represent partial thickness burns, and the solid areas represent full thickness burns.

After surgery and throughout the remainder of MJS's hospitalization, the hand orthosis was modified into more of an antideformity position (Fig. 25-23). The patient's finger ROM increased through a program of progressive exercise. At 2 weeks after surgery, the patient demonstrated ROM and strength within normal limits, so she was transitioned to the orthosis at night; the schedule progressed to an as-needed basis after the patient was discharged from the hospital.

When the elbow area was undressed for the first time after surgery and ROM was reinitiated, the patient lacked 25° of elbow extension with noticeable blanching of the skin graft when stress was applied. Apparently, her elbow had been slightly flexed when the bulky outer bandages were applied in the operating room, which was not apparent by visual inspection. MJS's existing postoperative

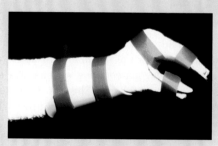

FIGURE 25-23 Antideformity position orthosis.

elbow orthosis was remolded to form an elbow extension mobilization orthosis (Fig. 25-7A).

The patient received twice-daily therapy treatments. She showed minimal improvements in ROM, and the orthosis was modified as necessary. The nurses began having difficulty applying the orthosis at night owing to increasing elbow flexion tightness. A decision was made to change the intervention to MJS wearing the orthosis at all times with breaks only for therapies. The rationale was that MJS could receive gentle stress applied consistently throughout the day and night while being able to participate in strengthening and ROM activities during therapy. Once she demonstrated full elbow ROM, the orthosis schedule was changed to at night only.

Case Study 2: Bilateral Upper Extremity Burns, Inhalation Injury, and Skin Grafting

CS is a 40-year-old, left hand–dominant female who sustained a 20% total body surface area (TBSA) burn to her bilateral upper extremities, anterior chest, neck, face, and hands as a result of a house fire. CS also suffered significant smoke inhalation and survived the fire only by jumping out of a second-story window to escape the flames. On initial presentation to the Burn Intensive Care Unit (BICU), she was intubated and placed on a ventilator. Initial x-rays and MRIs were negative for any other fractures or trauma, but she was noted to have deep dermal injuries to her hands and upper arms that would require skin grafting. The remainder of her burns appeared as more superficial partial thickness and therefore would not require grafting. On the third day after admission, CS received split thickness skin grafting to the affected areas and was immediately placed in upper extremity orthoses as well as hand orthoses to support graft take, minimize edema, and maintain functional position (Fig. 25-24A). The surgeon requested the therapist's attendance in the operating room, where position of function hand orthoses was fabricated to immobilize the deep partial thickness burns to her hand grafts. While CS was weaning from the ventilator, therapy was focused on

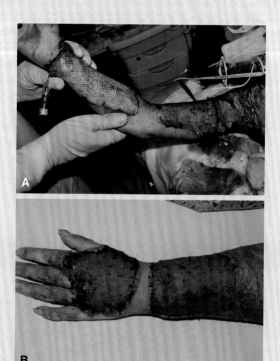

FIGURE 25-24 Healed meshed split thickness skin grafts performed on post burn day 3 **(A)** and on dorsal forearm/hand **(B)**.

use of the orthoses for positioning upper extremities after grafting and to maintain available ROM while in bed. Once CS weaned from the ventilator on postburn day 7, therapy focused on active ROM (AROM) and participation in activities of daily living (ADLs) skills. Rehabilitation also addressed cardiovascular conditioning to support good pulmonary function to regain normal cardiac endurance. Wound demarcation throughout the remainder of her chest and bilateral axillas, proximal upper extremities, neck, and face demonstrated signs of good intrinsic healing with limited scar formation. Both of her dorsal-based skin grafts to the hands and distal forearms demonstrated good healing; however, the left hand was noted to still be having small areas of wounds (mostly dorsal hand) that did not support optimal graft take (Fig. 25-24B). On postburn day 9, CS was able to demonstrate full AROM of her upper extremities (except for her left hand), good functional use with ADLs, and mobility; therefore, shoulder positioning was discontinued. Active self-positioning and AROM was employed. Orthosis at night was still used for the left hand, secondary to wounds and decreased AROM. CS favored the use of the right hand because the left had slightly delayed healing and was often more painful to move than the right, especially with full digit flexion.

CS was discharged from the BICU directly to home at 3 weeks and was immediately started on outpatient therapy to address wounds and healing skin grafts. During her first outpatient visit, CS was fitted for a right hand pressure garment. Unfortunately, her left hand still had many open areas and was unable to tolerate a garment but was able to be started with pressure therapy in the form of a disposable self-adherent elastic bandage. Night positioning with the orthosis was continued, secondary to the potential for contracture development and loss of ROM.

CS continued to attend therapy as an outpatient, but her left hand continued to be limited by wound healing and pain. CS refused to wear an orthosis for her left hand and did not want to consider another skin graft to promote wound closure. Wound healing continued to be a problem especially for the dorsal PIP joints, resulting in joint contracture (MCP joint extension and PIP joint flexion) along with significant loss of hand function. The patient underwent an excision of the scar tissue, dorsal digit skin grafting with pinning of all PIP joints in extension. An antideformity orthosis was made intraoperatively to maintain MCP flexion and PIP extension to support the graft and maintain extension position of the PIP joints. The orthosis was changed daily to assess for areas of pressure or potential for skin breakdown and gentle ROM was performed prior to reapplication. The skin grafts healed well, and at 10 days, the pins

were removed to allow for gradual mobilization of the PIP joints. Coban™ wrapping was used because the skin was too fragile for a pressure garment.

A dorsal-based orthosis was chosen to position the MCP joints in flexion while maintaining pressure over the dorsal grafted area. This functional orthosis was used all day except for specific ADL and bathing. By blocking extension, this orthosis prevented the scars from pulling the MCP joints into extension and PIP joints back into flexion. CS became a diligent participant in her therapy and was compliant with her orthosis schedule. She continued therapy focusing on bilateral hand use, increasing left hand mobility, pressure garment monitoring, and scar management.

At 18 months after the initial injury and grafting procedures, CS was successfully discharged from therapy with full functional use of her hands, minimal scar formation, full wound closure, and functional ROM. CS's left hand still lacked her preinjury level of digit extensibility, but she had regained the use of her dominant hand successfully and returned to her life independently.

Case Study 3: Pediatric Case

KN is a 2-year-old male who was in the care of his grandparents when he pulled a hot pot of coffee down on himself sustaining a 21% TBSA second- and third-degree scald to his face, neck, right axilla, R arm circumferentially, and his right dorsal hand. Prior to this injury, he was typically developing. Upon admission to the pediatric Inpatient Burn Unit, he was brought to the operating room for wound evaluation and debridement with allograft placement, at that time the therapist evaluated and determined KN had full ROM but due to the burn locations was at risk for axillary and elbow flexion contractures. In the operating room after allografting, the therapist fabricated an axillary orthosis placing KN's shoulder in 90° of abduction, external rotation, and neutral horizontal abduction. Due to KN's age and size, the therapist was able to fabricate the axillary orthosis to include the elbow placing it in full extension and also fabricated a wrist cock-up orthosis to protect the wrist from wrist drop while positioned away from the body. KN was immobilized for 5 days and then the therapist initiated gentle passive ROM until stent down when the patient was cleared for active ROM.

Two weeks post, KN was demonstrating limited AROM of the shoulder and elbow but all wounds were grafted and closed. The therapist initiated an interim pressure vest and sleeve and provided education to the parents that both garments should be worn at all times and the orthoses should be off for time in the morning and evening for play only.

CHAPTER REVIEW QUESTIONS

1. What important facts should the therapist consider when asked to apply an orthosis to a patient with burn injury? Discuss tissue considerations as well as material selections.
2. Describe the depths of burn injury and how this relates to orthotic intervention.
3. What is important about burn injuries that are over skin creases and what should the management involve in these situations?
4. How should a total hand burn be managed? Explain positions of each joint and list the precautions to look for.
5. What is web space syndactyly? Why is this significant and how can this condition be managed?

26 The Musician[a]

Aviva Wolff, EdD, OT/L, CHT

CHAPTER OBJECTIVES

After study of this chapter, the reader should be able to:
- Understand the unique evaluation and treatment approaches for the injured musician.
- Recognize the indications for use of orthoses and taping techniques for this patient population.
- Appreciate the diverse treatment approaches for the two main categories of injuries to the musician: traumatic injuries and performance-related musculoskeletal injuries.
- Explain the fabrication of an orthosis for injuries related to handling instruments and playing orthoses for age-related problems.

KEY TERMS

Functional movement analysis   Playing orthoses   Traumatic injuries
Performance-related musculoskeletal injuries Training orthosis

MD NOTE

Alfred Gelhorn, MD
New York

As a physiatrist board certified in sports medicine, I treat many performing artists with various acute and chronic injuries. Many of these injuries are a result of poor musculoskeletal practice patterns including poor posture, focal weakness, or tightness in joints that are involved in playing the instrument. It is a research and clinical priority for me not only to treat these performing artists once injury occurs but also to work toward a goal of injury prevention, which has historically been a low priority in musician training curricula. A multidisciplinary approach is most effective in treating and preventing these injuries, and I rely heavily on the assessments and recommendations of the physical and occupational (hand) therapists that I work closely with. I depend on the specific skill and expertise of hand therapists in functional task analysis, musculoskeletal assessment, and orthotic fabrication to provide comprehensive care for my patients and to lead them on the path to recovery. The creative fabrication of customized orthoses by hand therapists whether designed to provide feedback to correct a faulty position, to provide additional support to an injured structure, or to protect a healing structure allows my musician patients to honor their professional commitment and return to safe playing early. The information shared with me by the therapists from a comprehensive video analysis of playing posture and performance provides invaluable information that allows us as a team to jointly solve problem and address the root cause of the injury. Without this information, we are treating symptoms without cause. When we address the faulty playing postures and musculoskeletal imbalance, we are providing musicians with lifelong healthy practice habits to optimize their musculoskeletal health and performance longevity.

FAQ

How do you determine what level of immobilization/support to provide in cases of nonspecific musculoskeletal pain and overuse?
I utilize a multifaceted approach that includes education in warm-up, pacing, return to play schedule, smart practice habits, and often proximal stabilization exercises. For physical support while playing, I prefer to assess the pain level from least to most restrictive. I first assess the playing of a soft, slow, brief segment with either an elastic stockinette or elastic taping. If that is not enough to alleviate the pain, I will add a flexible prefabricated neoprene type wrap or an orthosis made of hybrid fabric type material. From there, I may add nonelastic tape and then progress to a thin thermoplastic material.

---

[a]This chapter is based on previous editions written by Caryl Johnson, OTR/L, CHT, and Coleen Lowe, MPH, OTR/L, CHT.

How do you approach an acute tendinitis where a musician has an injury that would benefit from rest but insists on playing for an important commitment?

When the musician will play at all costs, I instruct in playing the minimal amount required with as much support as the musician is willing to use. I always preface by stating: "My clinical recommendation is that you rest and not play." Sometimes this is not an option, and in those cases I will advise to practice repertoire using mental imagery, the contralateral hand, and "shadow playing" or "ghosting" where the user is not actually applying any pressure on the keys or strings. For the actual performance, I recommend heating the injured area prior to playing, applying elastic tape to match the skin color.

INTRODUCTION

Injured musicians present with unique challenges for orthotic fabrication because of the complexity and range of musical instruments, the musculoskeletal demands of playing an instrument, and the high stakes involved. Performance commitments and fear of career jeopardy often result in musicians continuing to perform while in pain or while injured. Orthoses may be fabricated for a range of injuries with multiple purposes: to protect, correct, and/or assist (Boyette, 2005). **Performance-related musculoskeletal disorders (PRMDs)** are the most common injuries affecting the hands and arms of musicians and include overuse and misuse injuries. In fact, the reported lifetime prevalence of PRMD affecting all musicians is 93% (Ackermann, 2012). Other injury categories and conditions observed in the musician population include hypermobility, acute injuries, and musician dystonia. The type of injury and condition will dictate how to approach the assessment, intervention, and choice of appropriate orthosis. Depending on the type and stage of injury, the purpose and material choice will vary. In the presence of an acute or PRMD injury, an orthosis is used to protect injured structures while allowing for playing in a protected range in situations where performance is required and allowed. In these cases, the fabrication of the orthosis must account for the instrument features and the playing position. Similarly, a different type of orthosis is selected for a case of a misuse injury to correct an awkward or excessive joint position. Orthoses that address dystonic movements are designed to constrain or control sensorimotor input.

This chapter will review the range of available orthoses and how to choose the correct orthosis for an injured musician by providing a step-by-step approach to the assessment and treatment approach for each injury category. The first part of the chapter will provide a thorough review of the musician's assessment: the musician's medical and performance history, the musculoskeletal examination, and an analysis of the playing position and posture. The second part will cover common musician injuries and relevant orthoses including how to select the appropriate design and material to achieve the treatment goal without interfering with musical production when possible. Regardless of the injury or purpose of the orthoses, there are special considerations in fabrication that are unique to instrumental musicians. These will be discussed in context below.

EVALUATION AND TREATMENT APPROACH

Injuries vary by type of injury and by instrument played in frequency, location, and type. The highest level of PRMDs is reported to occur in string players and the most frequently affected areas include the neck, jaw, shoulders, arms, and back. A wide range of risk factors have been implicated in the development of PRMD, including repetitive movements over extended periods of time. These are often further exacerbated by sudden changes to practice schedules, repertoire, and technique (Brandfonbrener, 2003). Awkward postures are demanded by the shape and weight of the instrument and often prolonged asymmetrical postures. For example, the asymmetrical playing demands required of bowing instrumentalists often contribute to neck and shoulder pain (Rensing, Schemmann, & Zalpour, 2018). To treat musicians' injuries effectively, the therapist must have a thorough understanding of anatomy and kinesiology and a keen ability to observe and analyze dysfunctional movement patterns and muscle imbalances.

ASSESSMENT

The evaluation and assessment consist of the following components: the medical and performance history, the musculoskeletal and functional assessment, and an analysis of playing posture and performance. In addition to the standard medical history, a performance history provides valuable information when assessing this population. The performance history is designed to gather information on the musician's practice history and habits and includes questions that relate to practice schedules, warm-ups, and length of practice. Any recent changes in playing time, technique, teacher, style, or repertoire should be noted. Additional questions concerning changes in the musician's artistry, work, leisure, and personal life are also important as they may contribute to the musician's physical well-being and recovery.

When treating musicians' injuries, a thorough examination of posture, with and without the instrument, is essential (Fig. 26–1A–D). The therapist uses clinical problem-solving and standard provocative tests to screen the upper quadrant and cervical spine for impingement and nerve compression as well as instability and tendon/ligament injuries. The musculoskeletal and functional examination should be thorough with a focus on observation and testing for any proximal muscle imbalance as well as neural tension tests. Testing for muscle tightness and weakness will identify the specific muscles to target in treatment with stretching and strengthening exercises.

Resting posture is assessed in sitting and standing to note any asymmetries at the shoulder, scapula, and neck position. Abnormal postures such as forward head, lateral tilt, shoulder anterior rotation, scapular winging, or protraction should be noted. Resting playing posture is observed next and any abnormalities and asymmetries are noted.

Observation of the playing posture and position is unique to this population and critical for both proper evaluation and effective treatment. This must be done with the instrument preferably

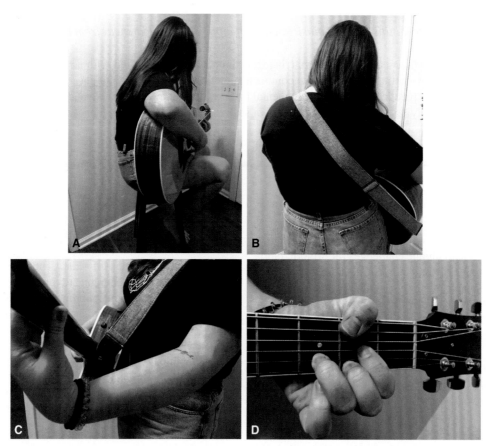

FIGURE 26–1 A, Assessment of guitarist's posture in sitting where decreased lumbar lordosis, rounded shoulders, and protracted scapulae are evident. **B,** Potential areas of concern on the guitarist's left side include the deviated cervical spine along with the compressive strap across the clavicle. **C,** Sustained wrist flexed position visualized from lateral view. **D,** Soft tissue impact at the fingertips on the strings noted as well.

in the natural playing environment to determine proper setup, position, and placement of music sheet and music stand. Playing posture is assessed first during a slow easy segment followed by a fast and technically more challenging segment. The assessment should be performed in both seated and standing positions for musicians who play in both positions. Likewise, if a musician plays multiple instruments, each instrument should be assessed separately. During the playing assessment, each joint is observed for abnormal or awkward posture or excessive mobility. Hypermobility and excessive joint angulation while playing is recorded preferably via video when possible. A 360-degree video of playing performance allows for observation of each joint as it interfaces with the instrument from multiple angles. This can be accomplished easily using a cellular phone camera by walking around the player while recording. A video recording allows for review in detail and slow motion and is helpful in identifying abnormal postures that may be contributing factors. Knowledge of the characteristics and position requirements of each instrument is important to understand the unique playing demands required by the interface between musician and instrument.

TREATMENT

Once the cause of the pain or injury has been identified, a treatment plan is developed to address the immediate symptoms and cause of the problem. The initial treatment of any acute symptoms involves pain and edema control and possibly immobilization followed by gradual mobilization and a graded return to play schedule. Once the acute stage has subsided, the therapist educates the musician in balanced and efficient body mechanics when performing and practicing and works with the musician to begin a realistic long-term strengthening and conditioning program to prevent further injury or reinjury. General musician health education is also addressed and includes information about a physical warm-up prior to playing, stretches, pacing, and measures to increase circulation to the arms and avoid musculoskeletal fatigue.

Certain helpful parallels may be drawn between the treatment of musicians and the treatment of athletes. The fine motor control and elaborate coordination necessary to play an instrument requires regular physical conditioning and training, such as that required to achieve an elite skill in a sport. Musicians and athletes spend many hours each day training to improve their specific physical skills and enhance their innate talent-activating, efficient muscle synergies that are unique to the person and use-dependent (Safavynia, Torres-Oviedo, & Ting, 2011; Ting & McKay, 2007). For both of these groups, external and internal demands for performance success may drive the person beyond his or her conditioning tolerance and/or abilities, resulting in injury. Gathering information about the correct playing position for the patient's instrument, the patient's level of skill, the demands of the repertoire, and the role music plays in his or her life assists the therapist in developing a plan of care. Treatment of the injury alone is not enough to enable the musician to resume performance; a total

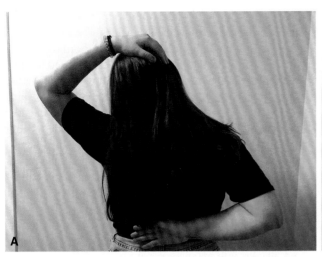 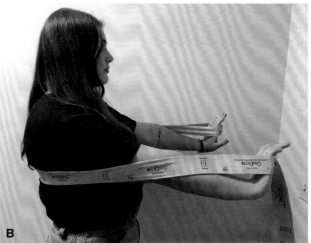

FIGURE 26–2 A, Stretching of lateral cervical spine and associated musculature and **(B)** serratus anterior strengthening exercise to address proximal weakness in upper extremity.

body conditioning program should be implemented to improve overall strength and endurance along with thorough patient education about posture, body mechanics, and flexibility, and a balance of work and leisure is important to help the musician understand how to avoid reinjury (Fig. 26–2A,B).

Another important aspect for a successful recovery is a graded plan and schedule for return to the instrument. It is not simply enough to tell the musician to resume playing slowly. The amount of playing he or she can do should be progressive, based on the injury, stage of tissue healing, preinjury practicing habits, and general physical status. From the student to the amateur to the professional performer, musicians frequently have strong emotional drives to play their instruments, which add intensity and anxiety to their responses to their injury, including fears about losing the ability to play and losing their artistic expression. Frequent reassurance, education about tissue healing and timing, guidance on how to resume full performance on their instrument, and support during the course of rehabilitation are important to the recovery of musicians.

INDICATIONS FOR ORTHOTIC INTERVENTION

Regardless of injury type, musicians of all levels (unlike the general population, but similar to athletes) face enormous pressure to continue or return to play as soon as possible (Norris, 2002; Wilson, 1998). Limits on playing time can result in profound financial and psychological losses. Therefore, the approach and decision-making process to use an orthosis that allows early return to play is multifaceted and must account for expectations, rules, guidelines, performance commitments, and the specific demands of the instrument. The first priority is protection of the injury and healing structures. The decision to immobilize and protect is based on the evaluation of the health status and is a synthesis of the information collected from the medical and performance history, the physical examination, laboratory and imaging results, and communication with the referring physician. The next step is to evaluate the playing/participation risk. Creighton, Schrier, Shultz, Meeuwisse, and Matheson (2010) propose a decision-making return to play algorithm for sports injuries that can be adapted for musicians. In their model the participation risk is assessed by the type of sport/instrument,

position played, limb dominance, competitive level, and ability to protect while playing (Creighton et al., 2010). Additional factors that affect the decision-making include the timing, season (performance demands), pressure from the player, external pressure, masking of the injury, and legal concerns.

Orthoses that can be worn by the instrumentalist during recovery have been used successfully. This chapter describes the possibilities and practical considerations of creating **playing orthoses** for musicians, which are orthoses made to be worn and used while playing an instrument. Playing orthoses maximize extremity function by

- Immobilizing and protecting healing structures
- Stabilizing joints
- Rebalancing deforming forces
- Improving joint alignment
- Assisting and training muscle action
- Correcting abnormal positions or excessive joint motion
- Correcting abnormal movement

Playing orthoses are immobilizing, supportive, restricting, or assistive devices that serve a dynamic function. They can be constructed for the elbow, wrist, hand, fingers, or thumb. The upper extremity movements needed for playing the instrument together with the clinical purpose for the orthosis determine its design (Johnson, 1992a). The playing orthosis is designed to do the following:

- Limit or assist the joint motion needed.
- Conform closely to the body.
- Minimally interfere with the body motions of playing (Van Lede & Van Veldhoven, 1998).
- Not chafe the skin or rub against bony prominences.
- Be as lightweight as possible.
- Be used with minimal or no strapping.
- Not touch the instrument or interfere with its moving parts.

A differentiation should be made between PRACTICE versus PLAYING orthoses. Practice orthoses are used privately during practice and can therefore be a bit bulkier to allow for added protection. Practice orthoses often are the first orthosis the player uses while attempting to play the instrument and may include the joint above and below for additional protection. PLAYING orthoses are used publicly during performance, so thin, unobtrusive material is essential as well as tape in place of straps to minimize bulk and add stability.

Orthotic Fabrication for Performance-Related Musculoskeletal Injuries

Musicians frequently present with conditions resulting from playing their instruments, such as inflammation of muscle and tendon (usually related to insufficient conditioning or increased use or force), compression neuropathies (related to repetitive motion at extreme joint angles), and soft-tissue injuries (related to repetitive impact to palm or finger and related to sustained static stretch of a muscle, e.g., scapular adductors, rotator cuff) when an instrument must be held or supported for long periods of time (Fig. 26–1A–D). The most common performance-related injuries present as tendinitis, synovitis, nerve compression, or vague nonspecific pain and are usually the result of misuse of the upper extremity or of insufficient conditioning for the physical demands placed on the player (e.g., increased playing time and intensity before an audition or performance, overusing distal muscles, and underusing proximal muscles). The challenging muscular coordination and specialized repetitive use of the musician's body and upper extremity require good posture and muscular balance at the instrument originating from a strong supportive framework, comprising strong trunk musculature, a stable pelvis and shoulder girdle, a flexible and relaxed forearm and hand, and overall strength and endurance to prevent injury.

Repetitive stress injuries, including tendonitis, synovitis, myositis, and compression neuropathies, are frequent presenting diagnoses for musicians (Johnson, 1992a; 1992b). A broad spectrum of therapeutic interventions can be used to treat these conditions, including heat/ice, soft tissue and joint mobilization, therapeutic exercise, and orthoses. Complete immobilization is sometimes indicated as an early intervention to rest inflamed tissues and inhibit provocative movements. After the acute phase, when pain and swelling have diminished, a playing orthosis in conjunction with a graded return to play schedule can be used to block extreme or symptom-producing motions and allow the patient to gradually return to his or her instrument. There are times that playing commitments will prevent musicians from being able to adhere to a strict "no playing" window. In these cases, the orthotic recommendation for a playing orthosis will be like those described below for acute injuries. Playing orthoses and support for nonacute repetitive stress injuries such as medial and lateral epicondylitis and ulnar wrist pain are fabricated to provide the amount of support required while allowing for maximum mobility while playing. The material should be as thin and flexible as possible and applied with thin straps or tape to minimize bulk and add stability.

A player with extensor carpi ulnaris (ECU) tendonitis may be fitted with a playing orthosis to immobilize the wrist. The wrist is positioned in 20° of extension and the orthosis molded generously around the hypothenar eminence to restrict ulnar deviation. This orthosis supports the wrist in extension and prevents repetitive ulnar deviation placing the ECU on slack. The orthosis helps to educate the musician to avoid ulnar deviation when playing by providing tactile biofeedback (Fig. 26–3A). When indicated, elastic tape can also be used to support the ECU and restrict some wrist flexion and ulnar deviation while providing tactile biofeedback during use to educate the instrumentalist to play in safe positions (Fig. 26–3B). With the violinist, elastic tape can be used to support the painful ulnar side of his right wrist during bowing and to prevent excessive left wrist flexion and ulnar deviation while fingering (Fig. 26–4A,B). For the percussionist, elastic tape can support the ulnar wrist and prevent excessive ulnar deviation (Fig. 26–4C). Some instrumentalists will prefer a neutral color tape or orthosis to avoid attention to the injury.

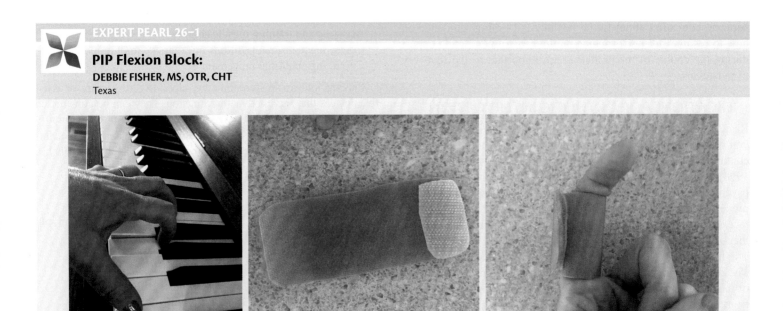

EXPERT PEARL 26–1

PIP Flexion Block:
DEBBIE FISHER, MS, OTR, CHT
Texas

Fabricated from loop strapping material and a small strip of adhesive hook secured on the back for closure. Alternative to use at night for a patient with trigger finger aggravated by repetitive piano playing—adjustable for comfort and swelling.

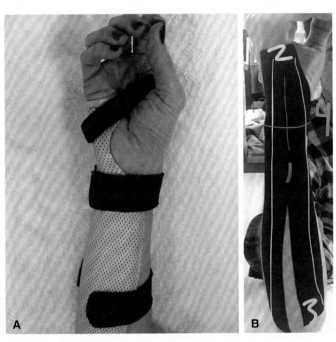

FIGURE 26-3 A, Because it is lightweight and has some flexibility, 1/16″ perforated material with memory was used to support the wrist in slight ulnar deviation in this wrist immobilization orthosis. Note full clearance of the metacarpophalangeal joints and thenar muscles. Neoprene material utilized to allow muscle movement beneath strapping. **B,** Elastic therapeutic tape applied to the ulnar wrist to support the extensor carpi ulnaris and provide feedback to avoid excessive ulnar deviation. Note the smartphone markup application can be used to number the tape strips for instruction in self-taping.

Progressive ligament injuries may result from prolonged stress to the joints of the fingers and thumb from extended playing and awkward postures. Thumb metacarpophalangeal (MP) ligament injuries and joint pain are often seen in guitarists and low string players when too much tension is generated by the thumb against the guitar, cello or bass neck, and in woodwinds (Fig. 26–5). Woodwind and brass players who support the instrument on their right thumb may develop a chronic ulnar collateral ligament injury from either the weight of the instrument resting on the thumb or repetitive stretching of the thumb at the MP joint (Fig. 26–6A,B). A digital gel cap can be used both preventively to provide feedback and alert the player to reduce tension and lessen the instrument weight and for early stage injury and pain (Fig. 26–6C,D). For more advanced injury, where immobilization and protection are indicated, a low-profile thumb MP immobilization playing orthosis provides static alignment and additional support to the thumb MP joint (Fig. 26–7A–D). The interphalangeal (IP) joint can be included as well when indicated. This orthosis functions to decrease inflammation and decrease the external deforming force at the thumb MP joint as seen in the cellist.

There are many variations of thumb MP immobilization playing orthosis that can be used. Playing orthoses can be constructed to stabilize any of the thumb joints laterally or longitudinally. The carpometacarpal (CMC) joint can be blocked from excess adduction and/or dorsal subluxation, and the MP and IP joints can be stabilized laterally to prevent stress on the collateral ligaments (Bean, Tencer, & Trumble, 1999; Brandsma, Oudenaarde, & Oostendorp, 1996; Glickel, Malerich, Pearce, & Littler, 1993; Haelterman, 1996; Heyman, Gelberman, Duncan, & Hip, 1993).

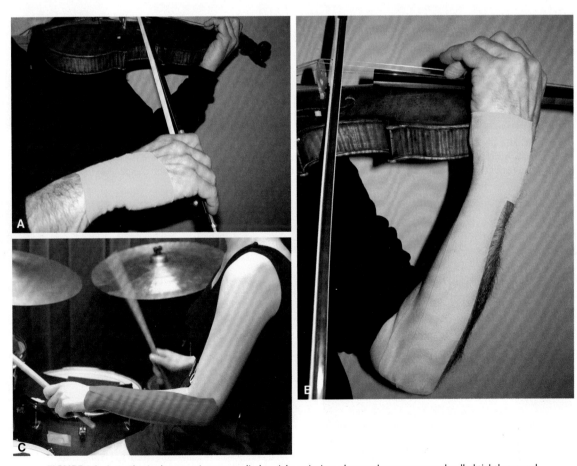

FIGURE 26-4 A, Elastic therapeutic tape applied to right wrist just ulnar to thenar crease and pulled tightly around dorsum of hand, supporting ulnar carpus and distal radioulnar joint. **B,** Elastic tape applied to left wrist and ulnar forearm to support extensor carpi ulnaris and ulnar side of wrist and forearm to provide tactile feedback to help musician recognize when he is flexing and ulnarly deviating his wrist too much. **C,** Elastic tape is applied along the wrist extensor muscles to provide external support in this percussionist with lateral elbow pain.

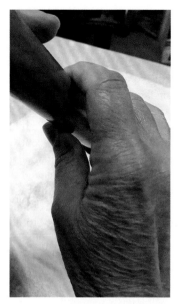

FIGURE 26-5 Tension generated by the thumb grip against the recorder creates a lateral stress across the thumb interphalangeal and metacarpophalangeal joint.

The finger IP joints may also sustain ligamentous injuries from repetitive playing, particularly in percussive instrumentalists. Figure 26-8 illustrates the case of a pianist who injured her right index finger (IF) and middle finger (MF) following prolonged excessive practice of a percussive repertoire. In order to generate a specific sound, she was attempting a forceful technique of downward movement creating a stress across the proximal interphalangeal (PIP) joints into extension. The constant pain at the PIP joints of right left IF and MF worsened with this movement into PIP extension. She was able to play without pain using PIP extension restriction orthoses that positioned the inflamed joints into slight flexion and restricted hyperextension (Fig. 26-8).

Soft tissue impact injuries are also seen in musicians. The palmar skin, fingertips, and sides of the fingers are areas that receive repetitive mechanical stresses from some instruments. They are subject to reactive injury, painful and inflamed soft tissues, digital nerve irritation, or development of small masses. Reactive soft tissue problems on the finger or fingertips of players may be successfully protected with soft materials, such as elastic tape (Fig. 26-9A,B). Low string players (bass and cello) are particularly

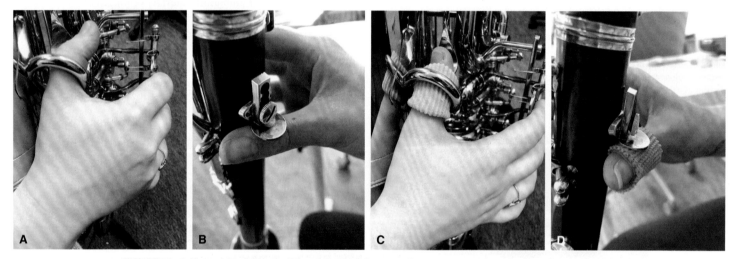

FIGURE 26-6 The weight of the tuba **(A)** and clarinet **(B)** creates ulnar stress across the right thumb metacarpophalangeal joint. A digital gel cap provides feedback and alerts to player to lessen the weight of the instrument in a tuba player **(C)** and a clarinetist **(D)**. This can also be used to provide relief for early pain and digital nerve irritation.

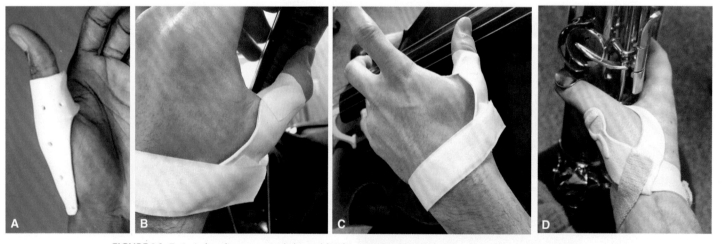

FIGURE 26-7 **A,** A thumb metacarpophalangeal (MP) immobilization orthosis for ulnar collateral ligament injury to prevent lateral stress on healing tissue fabricated out of rigid thermoplastic to allow early return to playing. Note the minimal amount of material used to provide stability while not interfering with playing. **B and C,** A thermoplastic playing orthosis to provide rigid support to the thumb MP joint to decrease the external deforming force in a cellist. Note tape utilized distally versus traditional loop for securing orthosis. **D,** This playing orthosis supports both the thumb CMC and MP joints by restricting excessive radial deviation and hyperextension via the distal radial portion of the orthosis. In the way the orthosis is fabricated, it also provides a dorsal volar stabilization of the first CMC joint.

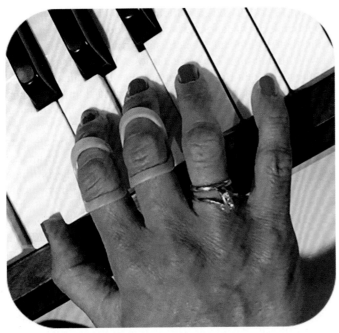

FIGURE 26–8 Oval-8® Finger Splints on pianist's left middle finger and ring finger proximal interphalangeal joints to prevent hyperextension and reduce pain while playing (3-Point Products®).

add an additional layer of complexity and challenge to treatment. Protection of injured and repaired structures is always prioritized over early return to play, and a joint decision is made between the musician, hand therapist, physician, and music teacher that accounts for all factors. First and foremost, return to play is dependent on the safety and stability of the injury. Other factors include upcoming commitments, contractual obligations, and the season of injury. Fear of delayed return to play and anxiety over recovery is common among instrumentalists.

Patients who have suffered **traumatic injuries**, including nondisplaced and/or stable upper extremity fractures, can be fitted with playing orthoses that brace the fracture against deforming forces. The orthosis can support and immobilize the healing bone to allow safe use when playing the instrument. Gutter playing orthoses (three-sided, U-shaped orthoses) can be used on long bones (distal radius and ulna), metacarpals, and on the phalanges. Evidence shows that longitudinal stress can hasten the formation of callus if alignment is not disturbed (Schenk, 1992). The nonarticular orthosis allows playing and provides additional longitudinal support to the fracture. An immobilization orthosis is worn when the patient is not playing to provide support and protection.

For example, a guitar player with a nondisplaced distal radius fracture may be immobilized in a volar forearm-based orthosis that is removed only for exercise. In the later stages of healing, the patient may be able to safely return to the instrument by being fitted with a prefabricated wrist orthosis to support the fractured area (Fig. 26–10A,B).

Many traumatic ligament injuries are amenable to the fabrication of an orthosis in a way that allows the performer to continue playing. The degree or nature of instability, alignment, and amount of swelling determine the choice of design of the orthosis (Fess, 2002; Mayer & McCue, 1990; Sadler & Koepfer, 1992). Acute and chronic triangular fibrocartilage complex injuries can be immobilized in an ulnar gutter type orthosis that can be removed and replaced with a supportive wrist strap for playing (Fig. 26–11).

Orthoses used for acute injuries must be adjusted as swelling and contours change to ensure an appropriate fit. Although musicians who are able to make an earlier return to music will be more able to cope with the psychological feelings of loss caused by the injury,

susceptible to painful fingertip subcallus blisters, neuromas, or small glomus tumors on the finger pads of the left hand from the repeated pressure against thick metal strings. Callus injuries tend to resolve over a period of months if they are not irritated further. Although the use of any material on the fingertip can be unacceptable to some players, in a concert, some musicians can often tolerate the use of a digital gel cap (Fig. 26–9C) or a very thin material such as Orficast® (Fig. 26–9D).

Orthotic Fabrication for Traumatic Injuries

Musicians are susceptible to the same range of acute hand injuries as the general population, and these include fractures, sprains, lacerations, crush injuries, and contusions. Although the initial phases of treatment are the same as those for a similar injury in any patient, the return to play demands and contractual and financial obligations

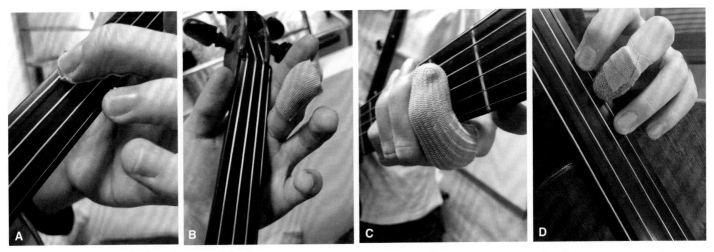

FIGURE 26–9 A and B, Use of elastic tape on the fingertip of a cellist with digital nerve irritation resulting from excessive forceful pressing on string. **C,** A digital gel cap used to protect a guitarist who has an index finger neuroma. The sleeve can be trimmed to the distal interphalangeal or proximal interphalangeal crease to allow greater freedom of movement. **D,** Orficast® used on the middle finger of a cellist with fingertip pain who was unable to play with the elastic tape (Orfit Industries).

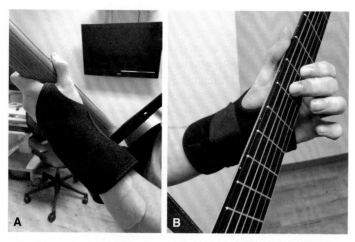

FIGURE 26–10 A and B, A prefabricated wrist immobilization orthosis for the left wrist of a guitar player with a stable distal radius fracture in the late stages of healing.

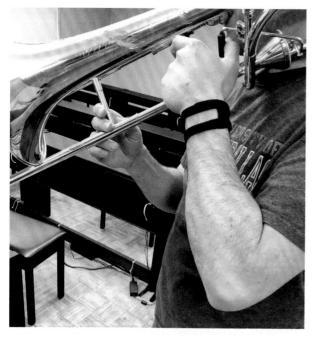

FIGURE 26–11 A prefabricated wrist strap to support and protect the ulnar wrist from the ulnar directed force and weight of the trombone. WristWidget® shown here.

the use of playing orthoses should create no disruption to alignment, bony reduction, or healing, nor should playing orthoses create compensatory or substitution movements proximal or distal to the injury in the kinetic chain of the functional movement pattern. Lacerations or other skin lesions may need orthoses fabricated to provide wound protection from contact, pressure, or percussion to avoid irritating the healing tissues.

Orthotic Fabrication for Injuries Related to Handling Instruments

Many instruments must be held to the mouth or lifted in some way for playing, resulting in injuries related to lifting and positioning the instrument. Woodwind instruments are good examples; all must be supported and held near the body and mouth for playing. Lifting the weight of these instruments places stress on the upper extremity, especially the joints of the thumb. Playing orthoses can support the instrument by transferring part of the instrument weight to a more proximal joint and muscle group

(Johnson, 1992a). Two types of custom-molded playing orthoses for the thumb can be fabricated to assist woodwind players in supporting their instrument. A more supportive orthosis is a variant of a wrist/thumb immobilization orthosis that transfers part of the instrument's weight from the thumb to the dorsal ulnar wrist (Fig. 26–12A). The other orthosis is a hand-based thumb MP immobilization orthosis wrapped from ulnar to radial and around the thumb (Fig. 26–12B–D). When constructing supportive orthoses, care must be taken to never mold material directly on the instrument to avoid damage to the finish of an expensive instrument. Any orthoses that come into direct contact with the instrument must be constructed with care to not damage the instrument or interfere with sound production (Boyette, 2005).

Prefabricated orthoses can be challenging to fit perfectly for instrument support compared to the intimate fit achieved from a well-molded, custom-fabricated orthosis. In the absence of a custom option, a form-fitting, prefabricated wrist or thumb orthosis may give partial support to the wrist, MP, and/or IP joints (Fig. 26–10A,B). When choosing a prefabricated orthosis, it is helpful to consider the same factors as when designing a custom-molded orthosis: Avoid any obstruction to the instrument or its moving parts and respect the player's customary hand and wrist position. Custom-fabricated neoprene orthoses are an additional option.

Other commercially available adaptive devices used for instrument support include neck straps (Fig. 26–13A), oboe or English horn support (rests on the chair and supports the instrument on a rigid stem), and the post (holds the instrument out from the body braced against the player's abdomen). There are multiple websites that also offer various straps, stands, supports for musical instruments, and other accessories that might be helpful for the musician to prevent injury. Adjustable thumb rests move the instrument's weight more proximal to eliminate pressure on the thumb IP joint and distal phalanx (Fig. 26–13B).

Playing Orthoses for Age-Related Problems

Age-related changes such as development of osteoarthritis (OA) can have a profound effect on the music and sound quality, playing speed, and the ability to reach certain notes. OA of the IP joints often results in radial and ulnar deviation. These small joint displacements cause difficulty in the fine and precise finger coordination required for playing most instruments. Finger gutter orthoses that are applied dorsally can allow for better alignment of the joints and placement of the digits on the fingerboard and keyboard. Elastic taping is also effective particularly for strumming and picking. Figure 26–14A demonstrates the use of a dorsal-based orthosis for the left MF distal interphalangeal (DIP) joint in a cellist. She has OA in the left MF DIP joint with ulnar deviation and her PIP joint rotates radially, preventing her from placing her digit down on the string correctly, affecting the sound of the note. Also, she cannot maintain the space between her fingers, which affects her ability to reach the correct note. She was fitted with a dorsal PIP and DIP joint orthosis that was molded as she positioned her fingers on the cello strings (Fig. 26–14A). The orthosis prevents her DIP joint from deviating and allows her fingers to maintain the correct spacing on the strings because of the improved alignment of her PIP and DIP joints. Figure 26–14B demonstrates the use of elastic tape to provide a radial pull and correct ulnar deviation at the PIP joint in a guitarist with a similar presentation (Fig. 26–14B). A volar gutter orthosis was worn at night to provide better alignment while not playing and the elastic taping was worn for playing.

EXPERT PEARL 26–2

Functional Orthosis

ANNE WAJON, PT
Australia

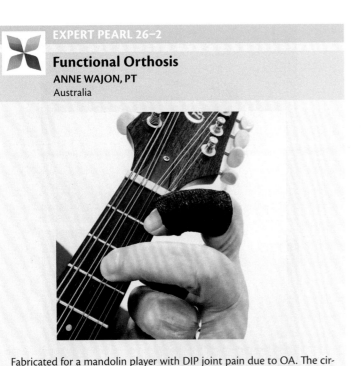

Fabricated for a mandolin player with DIP joint pain due to OA. The circumferential orthosis is made from Orficast thermoplastic tape and positions the DIP in slight flexion to allow for playing.

OA with pain at the CMC joint is common in musicians. A custom-molded thumb CMC joint immobilization orthosis that does not include the MP joint (Colditz, 2000) has helped some musicians during practice sessions but was noted to be too restrictive during performance (Fig. 26–15A,B). The Push CMC orthosis allows for more flexibility while providing stability at the thumb CMC joint (Colditz & Koekebakker, 2010). Some musicians may be able to practice with using this orthosis, although most report that the speed and flexibility required for performance is inhibited by its use. Additionally, many musicians will opt to play without anything to avoid any attention to injury.

Constructing a Playing Orthosis

As noted above in the assessment section, a thorough physical and musical history and evaluation (with and without the instrument) precede construction of a playing orthosis. If the patient has an acute or traumatic injury, they will need two or three orthoses: a resting or protective orthosis and, when the injury allows, a practice and playing orthosis to assist the return to the instrument. If the patient has an inflammatory or chronic problem, observation of the musician playing his or her instrument must be included as part of the assessment. This observation method is often referred to as a **functional movement analysis**. During this functional movement

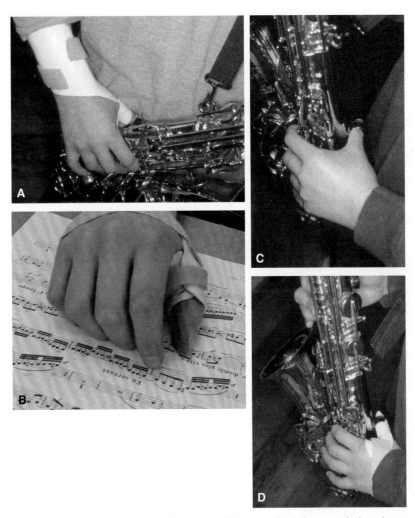

FIGURE 26–12 **A,** This spiral design of a wrist/thumb immobilization orthosis decreases the lateral stress on the thumb for this saxophonist. **B,** Thumb metacarpophalangeal (MP) immobilization orthosis for ulnar collateral ligament injury to prevent lateral stress on healing tissue. **C and D,** Note lateral stress on thumb MP joints from holding saxophone and hand-based immobilization orthosis that includes the interphalangeal joint to help support the weight of the instrument.

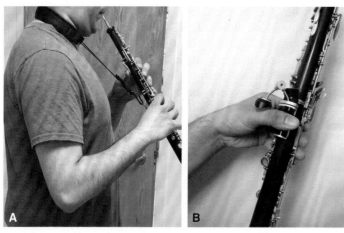

FIGURE 26–13 A, A neck strap to support the weight of the Oboe. **B,** An adjustable thumb rest to direct the oboe weight more proximally and distribute pressure away from the thumb interphalangeal joint and distal phalanx.

analysis with his or her instrument, the following information is collected:

- Musician's posture
- Head position
- Upper extremity balance and imbalances
- Joint positions during playing

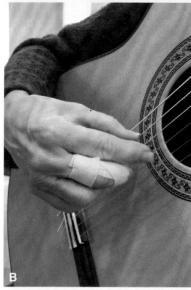

FIGURE 26–14 A, Lateral view of proximal interphalangeal (PIP) and distal interphalangeal orthosis to align joints with osteoarthritis (OA) into a better playing position. **B,** Elastic tape provides a radial directed force to counteract the ulnar deviation in this guitarist with OA at the PIP joint of the middle finger.

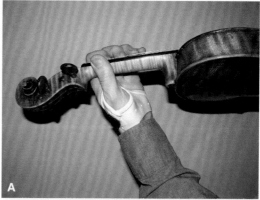

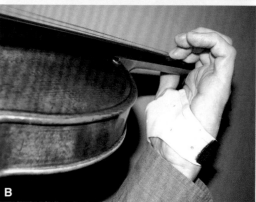

FIGURE 26–15 A and B, A thumb CMC joint immobilization orthosis to lessen CMC joint pain. Notice how this design does not restrict movement at the thumb metacarpophalangeal joint.

- Body mechanics
- Excessive tension in muscle groups
- Increases in body or facial tension
- Playing endurance
- Correctness of functional movement
- Note any substitutions and/or compensatory movements (especially with repetitive use injuries; be sure to educate musician)

The therapist analyzes these observations and then develops the multifaceted treatment plan. A comprehensive treatment plan will include education in general musical health habits: warm-up, pacing, practice habits, stretches for tight muscles, strengthening exercises for weak muscles, and ergonomic and biomechanic modifications to position and posture as well as the use of a playing orthosis as soon as clinically possible. If a playing orthosis is appropriate, consulting with the physician about any restrictions or contraindications is important (Norris, 2002; Stephens & Leilich, 1998; Stotko, 1998). The patient should bring the instrument to the fabrication appointment, and the therapist should schedule a generous amount of time if possible. Table 26–1 outlines a step-by-step procedure for evaluation and fabrication of a playing orthosis.

ORTHOTIC FABRICATION

Material Selection

Thermoplastic materials with a longer working time and less memory are usually preferred for playing orthoses. A high degree of conformability is necessary to ensure comfort and optimal fit. A longer working time allows for adjustments before the position of the orthosis is finalized. Thicker thermoplastic materials (1/8″), with

TABLE 26–1	**Evaluation and Fabrication of a Playing Orthosis**

1. When possible, observe the patient as he or she plays the instrument. Note the synergistic movement patterns of the bones, joints, and soft tissues in relation to the instrument.
2. Determine an appropriate orthosis pattern by taking into account the goals for the playing orthosis based on the diagnosis, stage of healing or symptoms, and the treatment plan.
3. Choose a suitable material based on the function and fit needed.
4. Measure to fabricate an orthosis pattern from a paper towel.
5. Again, observe the patient playing the instrument and review the rationale for the design. Try the pattern on the patient, and test for interference with instrument parts.
6. Cut and prepare the material. The patient should be ready to play the instrument for the fitting.
7. Mold the material on the extremity while the patient maintains a playing position with the instrument; take great care when conforming the material to avoid the moving parts of the hand and instrument.
8. Apply straps or tape if needed, making sure they do not interfere with the hand or instrument; the material used should be the patient's choice.
9. Test the orthosis. Ask the patient to try playing with the orthosis firmly in place. Encourage him or her to identify any parts that are uncomfortable or hinder playing. Take time with this step; if the patient is unable to play with the orthosis, they are likely not to use it and may slow down or hinder the healing process.
10. Test the orthosis while the patient plays in several musical contexts: a slow passage, a fast passage, and a technically demanding section. Note: Some players have to change instruments or dress in the course of a performance; check the patient's ability to remove and apply the orthosis.
11. Once the orthosis is comfortable, fits well, does not interfere with playing ability, and has been determined that the design achieves the goals of support, assist, and/or restriction of movement, check the general effect of wearing the orthosis on the movement of the upper extremity. Does the orthosis cause abnormal movements, compensations, and/or substitutions that may lead to other musculoskeletal problems? If noted, the cause of the movement problem should be identified and addressed.
12. Plan a follow-up visit for the patient with his or her instrument to make any necessary alterations. Be sure the patient is able to play at his or her level of ability in the orthosis.

some degree of conformability, are best used for instrument weight bearing orthoses and orthoses that cross the wrist. Thicker materials are also more suited for larger hands. Thinner thermoplastic materials, such as 1/16″ and 3/32″, are best used for orthoses of the digits and thumb and for **training orthoses**—not to provide rigidity but to serve as a gentle reminder (tactile biofeedback) of proper joint position.

The choice of perforated or nonperforated thermoplastics depends on the purpose and function of the orthosis and the amount of adjustment time needed for construction. Perforated materials are desirable to allow for breathing yet tend to set up more quickly and may not allow for the multiple adjustments needed when making a playing orthosis comfortable. The choice of coated versus uncoated material will depend on the design and whether any part of the orthosis requires bonding (Austin, 2003; Breger-Lee & Buford, 1992; Moberg, 1984). Another consideration when choosing a material is that musicians who will be performing in public with their orthosis may prefer a material that blends in with their skin color to minimize visibility. The newer hybrid materials that combine textile-like thermoplastic properties (Orficast® Orfit Industries, Belgium) are thin, lightweight, flexible, and nonbulky—an ideal choice for musicians when appropriate (Fig. 26–9D).

Strapping Selection

Straps are best made of traditional hook and loop when firm stabilization is required for protection. Taping and elastic wraps are always preferred for playing orthoses to minimize bulk (Fig. 26–7B,C). When soft tissues must move beneath the straps, softer materials, such as elastic, neoprene, or foam, are a more appropriate choice (Fig. 26–3A). Finger orthoses that require stabilization can be applied with an elasticized wrap or elastic tape (Fig. 26–9D). Care must be taken to wrap these materials without applying too much tension to avoid compression of the neurovascular structures.

Taping techniques such as elastic tape or static tape can be used in lieu of a playing orthosis when light support or gentle feedback to guide movement is required. Taping provides the player with the opportunity to play with minimal restriction while providing support. Taping may also be appropriate as a short-term emergency solution when a player must perform with an injury. Useful taping patterns for musicians include figure of 8 taping to allow a joint to move while being supported. Figure 26–16A demonstrates the use of a figure of 8 technique for the thumb CMC joint for the left hand of an acoustic guitarist with mild CMC OA joint pain. Figure 26–16B–H demonstrates a taping technique for a pianist with ulnar wrist pain resulting from excessive wrist ulnar deviation while playing the center of the keyboard. The technique gently guides the movement out of ulnar deviation by providing resistance in the opposite direction. The smartphone draw feature can be used to label and order the tape strips as a patient education guide for self-taping. Taping is not recommended as long-term solution for musicians because it requires frequent and sometimes expert application. Prolonged use may also irritate the skin (Reese, Burruss, & Patten, 1990).

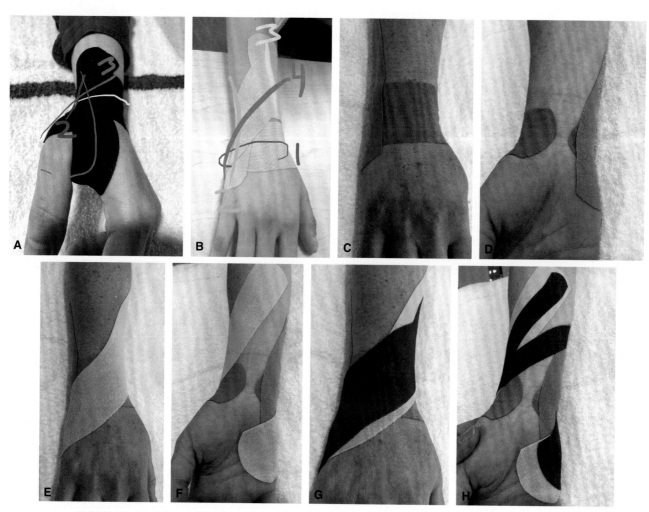

FIGURE 26–16 A, Figure of 8 taping technique for the thumb CMC joint of an acoustic guitarist. **B,** Elastic taping technique in a pianist to correct excessive ulnar deviation (consider labeling images for self-taping guidance). **C and D,** Taping for ulnar wrist pain and to prevent excessive ulnar deviation: volar wrist and ulnar longitudinal strips; **E and F,** deep oblique strip; and **G and H,** final superficial oblique strip.

CONCLUSION

Orthotic fabrication for the musician with an injury requires a complex synthesis of knowledge, skill, expertise, and creativity. A good understanding of the anatomy and mechanics of the hand and upper extremity must be combined with an appreciation of the instrument design and demands along with the unique characteristics of the player. Additionally, the performance commitments and psychological ramifications of the injury must also be considered and addressed. Proper orthotic design and fabrication is predicated on these factors in order to ensure that the musical performance and physical structures are not adversely affected. A thorough assessment with appropriate design, proper selection of materials, and a thoughtful delivery and approach will ensure the best outcome and compliance without jeopardizing healing structures and music quality.

 FIELD NOTE: ESTABLISHING RAPPORT

Aviva Wolff, EdD, OT/L, CHT
New York

Establishing a trusting clinician-patient rapport is the key to success with the musician population. In order to build a successful rapport, it is important to be familiar with the musician psyche. Musicians by nature are accustomed to pushing the limits of ability from a physiological, emotional, and performance perspective. They are, as a group, highly disciplined and intense. A hand injury, no matter how minor, creates an understandable source of anxiety and distress over perceived and real short-term and long-term ramifications. Performances may be canceled, livelihood may be affected, and the potential of career jeopardy is terrifying. There is also a stigma associated with the perception of injury, and many musicians will try to hide their injury from colleagues and the public at all costs. The hand therapist is thus in an important position of setting expectations and deescalating the fear. Empathy is critical in making the musician feel validated and understood. A musician who that the clinician understands the demands of their vocation and schedule will trust you with their care and likely comply with the treatment program. During the initial visit, clinicians can expect to spend a fair amount of time discussing concerns and explaining the trajectory of the injury and rehabilitation/protective/return to play process. Providing a concrete timeline with the appropriate caveats is helpful to provide perspective, set expectations, and deliver much needed reassurance and hope for recovery and full return to play when possible.

Once the trusting relationship is established, the problem-solving process of fabricating a protective or playing orthosis for musicians is analogous to the provision of protective gear for a competitive athlete on the field. The goals are similar to prevent further injury, to protect repaired/injured structures, and to promote comfort. The approach is similar as well. While the priority is always to protect repaired and injured structures, individual factors and contractual/financial obligations are also heavily considered when determining the protection method and timing of orthotic use.

Case Study Section

The case studies presented here are meant as a teaching guideline only. Treatment and orthosis protocols vary greatly from surgeon to surgeon and from therapist to therapist. The therapist should check with the referring physicians and colleagues to define the preferred treatment and appropriate orthotic intervention.

Case Study 1: Guitarist With Wrist Tendonitis

A 19-year-old jazz guitar conservatory student presented with complaints of pain in the left volar wrist and forearm. The onset of his symptoms developed over the past few months, during which time his playing schedule had increased dramatically as new conservatory student. During the playing posture analysis, he demonstrated excessive left thumb IP hyperextension and excessive left wrist flexion that were causing excess tension in the wrist and thumb flexor tendons and muscle belly (Fig. 26–17A,B). Further physical examination revealed hypermobility at the thumb joint as the cause of the thumb joint hyperextension. An oval 8 playing orthosis for the thumb was helpful in

repositioning the thumb IP joint in a more neutral position to avoid hyperextension and reduce tension (Fig. 26–17C). Dorsal elastic taping provided feedback to avoid excessive wrist angulation while playing (Fig. 26–17D).

Case Study 2: Trumpet Player With Proximal Phalanx Fracture

A 49-year-old professional trumpet player fell while playing softball and fractured the proximal phalanx of his left thumb. He was treated surgically with an open reduction internal fixation and fit with a volar forearm-based thumb spica orthosis postoperatively. He was cleared to begin a gradual return to play schedule 5 weeks postoperatively. Initially, a short opponens orthosis was fabricated as a playing orthosis to support the thumb, but it did not allow for enough flexibility to hold the instrument and play. To provide support during the return to play schedule, elastic taping was applied in a figure of 8 pattern to the thumb MP and CMC joints with an additional lateral piece across the radial wrist (Fig. 26–18).

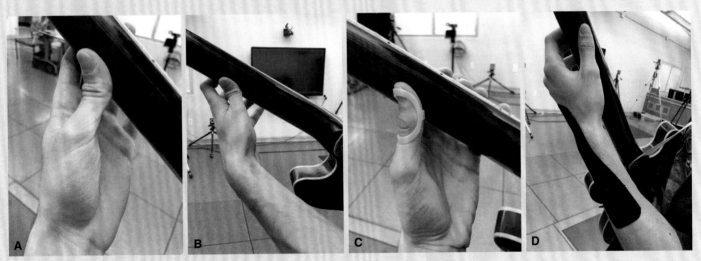

FIGURE 26–17 **A,** Excessive thumb interphalangeal (IP) hyperextension in an acoustic guitarist with left volar wrist pain and **(B)** excessive wrist flexion. **C,** Correction of thumb IP hyperextension with an Oval-8 orthosis and **(D)** correction of wrist hyperflexion with elastic tape placed dorsally.

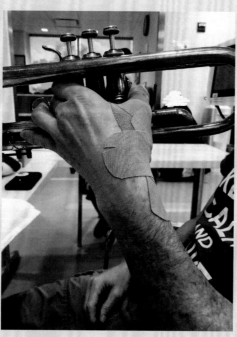

FIGURE 26–18 Figure 8 taping to the thumb metacarpophalangeal and CMC of a trumpet player recovering from a right thumb proximal phalanx fracture.

CHAPTER REVIEW QUESTIONS

1. What are the main objectives of a playing orthosis in a musician?
2. Describe the considerations and orthotic intervention for a musician that has sustained a forearm repetitive trauma. Include what orthosis or taping techniques can be applied throughout the course of healing.
3. What injury to the thumb does the woodwind player often acquire? Why does this happen and how can this injury be managed?
4. What musicians may have soft tissue injuries? What are two examples of these injuries and what are the appropriate orthotic intervention choices for each?
5. During a functional movement analysis with the musician's instrument, what information should be collected in order to develop the most appropriate treatment plan that includes the orthosis?

27 Hand and Upper Extremity Transplantation

Gayle Severance, MS, OT/L, CHT
Amy Vissing, MHS, OTR/L, CHT

CHAPTER OBJECTIVES

After study of this chapter, the reader should be able to:

- Describe the preoperative and postoperative role of the hand therapist in the care of the hand transplant patient.
- Understand anatomical and functional recovery differences between proximal and distal level transplants.
- Recognize the importance of orthotic intervention in both protection and functional recovery for the hand transplant patient.
- Identify concepts for postoperative therapeutic intervention and functional recovery.
- Identify potential postoperative complications to graft survival and functional recovery after hand transplantation.

KEY TERMS

Acute rejection
Allograft
Body wholeness
Cortical plasticity
Cortical reorganization
Distal level forearm transplants
Doppler readings

Graft rejection
Hand transplant candidate selection
Hand transplantation
Hand transplantation team
Joint position sense
Motor imagery
Motor re-education
Muscle activation

Neuromuscular electrical stimulation
Osteosynthesis
Peripheral nerve regeneration
Quality of life
Regenerative Peripheral Nerve Interface
Sensory re-education
Target Muscle Reinnervation
Vascular composite tissue allotransplantation

MD NOTE

L. Scott Levin, MD, FACS
Pennsylvania
Benjamin Chang, MD, FACS
Pennsylvania

It has been two decades since the first successful hand transplant in the United States. Since that time there have been approximately 150 upper extremity (UE) transplantations performed in over 100 patients worldwide (Mendenhall, Brown, Ben-Amotz, Neumeister, & Levin, 2018; Shores et al., 2017; Tasigiorgos et al., 2017). Hand transplantation is also referred to as vascular composite tissue allotransplantation because it includes the diverse composition of heterogenic tissues that make up a human limb including skin, fat, nerves, arteries, veins, lymphatic vessels, bone, cartilage, tendons, and ligaments. Together, these anatomical structures are needed to restore a structural, functional, and aesthetically pleasing limb (Siemionow, Kulahci, & Bozkurt, 2009). There are challenges related to graft acceptance, immunological tolerance, nerve regeneration, and restoration of function. In addition to the technical complexity of hand transplantation, it is critical to address the psychological well-being of the patient undergoing this life changing procedure. For the emerging field of hand transplantation to be a successful option in amputee care, it is essential to assemble a cohesive and knowledgeable multidisciplinary team. The hand transplant team consists of some 20 different specialties in the fields of medicine, surgery, nursing, pharmacy, social work, psychiatry, finance/hospital administration, and therapy (Amirlak et al., 2007; Gordon & Siemionow, 2009; Severance & Walsh, 2013). Among this team, there is a shared responsibility for effective communication and collaboration that lends to an integrated treatment plan.

As hand surgeons and leaders of the transplant team, we recognize the vital role of our hand therapy colleagues. The hand therapist's presurgical functional assessment and patient education supports the candidate selection process. Postoperatively, we rely on their rehabilitative expertise to construct orthoses to protect the newly grafted limb, to initiate a progressive exercise program to facilitate musculoskeletal integrity and minimize adverse scarring and edema, to engage the patient in cortical retraining and support neuromuscular recovery, to educate and train the patient and caregiver, and to offer the ongoing emotional and psychological support required after this life altering procedure. The hand therapists are intimately involved with the patients care from day one and spend lengthy amounts of time with the patient and caregivers providing rehabilitative expertise, physical support, and emotional encouragement.

The close relationship between hand surgeon and hand therapist has long been an essential component to successful patient outcomes. It is through a culture of mutual respect and teamwork that we deliver quality care to the hand transplant patient.

FAQ

What are the precautions/special considerations in orthotic fitting for patients with hand transplantation?

In the early weeks of rehabilitation, frequent adjustments may be required. Special considerations include preventing shearing, protecting bony prominence, and designing the orthosis to allow frequent vital checks and monitoring for skin breakdown due to lack of sensation of the transplanted hand and use of the orthosis for long periods. Pictures and labeling of straps and components help to ensure proper application by multiple team members and the caregiver. Later on, modifications are necessary to ensure fit and patient adherence as most patients will require orthoses for about 1 year following surgery to address muscle imbalance.

When inspecting the patient skin for signs of rejection, should we inspect the entire limb or just the donor skin?

During a rejection period, one of the early, visible signs will be maculopapular lesions or small red bumps resembling a rash. This will occur only on the donated skin and not on the patient's native skin. It has not been the experience of these authors for patients to report the bumps or rashes as itchy or painful. Topical medications are one of the methods for treating rejection episodes, and patients may continue to use their orthoses. Patients and caregivers are advised to wash their orthoses with each medication application and then apply new, clean stockinette as a useful barrier between the medicated limb and the orthosis. Therapy intervention may continue during this time, unless there are other patient factors or medical guidance to hold therapy.

"In a proximal level transplant, I have seen anterior and posterior long arm orthosis used to support the arm/forearm. Why did you choose the posterior approach?"

These authors choose the posterior approach for the long arm orthosis because it is felt that this approach would offer greater pressure distribution, comfort, and edema control. The posterior approach would also be easier to don and doff for various staff members (MD's, nursing, caregivers, etc.). Moreover, the patient has a better view of their new limb which may promote acceptance of the new body part.

How do anti-claw orthoses for hand transplantation differ from those used in nerve palsies?

MCP extension restriction orthoses (anti-claw orthoses) for hand transplantation provide the same mechanical support as those used in patients with combined median and ulnar nerve palsies in which the intrinsic muscle function is absent. One difference and consideration in orthotic fabrication and design is to ensure that the dorsal aspect of the orthosis covers the greatest surface area possible in order to truly dissipate pressure. The fabricating clinician must appreciate the complete asensate nature of this body part.

Recovery of different intrinsic muscle groups may be incomplete following hand transplantation and warrants adaptations of the MCP extension restriction orthosis to support motor recovery and augment function. Due to the long-term effects of amputation on cortical reorganization, patients with hand transplantation may require the use of these orthoses in conjunction with cortical and sensorimotor retraining to improve motor planning and execution throughout the extremity.

INTRODUCTION

With significant limb loss due to traumatic injury or serious illness, options to restore a functional limb are limited to primary reconstruction/replantation, prosthetic devices, or transplantation (Pace & Zeske-McGuire, 2013). Hand transplantation and hand replantation are very different. Hand replantation surgically reattaches the patient's own limb after a traumatic injury severed it from the body, and this must occur within a very limited time frame. Hand transplantation is a reconstructive option for a person who has been living, often for years, with hand or UE amputation(s). Hand transplantation attaches the limb(s) from a recently deceased organ donor to the healthy residual limb of living person. Similar to solid donor transplant (i.e., heart, lung), patients are required to take lifelong immunosuppressive medications to prevent rejecting the donor limb (Ravindra et al., 2008).

Both procedures are surgically complex, but the challenges differ. A replantation usually occurs in the setting of tissue loss with or without mutilation and contamination of limb components (Kvernmo, Gorantla, Gonzalez, & Breidenbach, 2005), which can make postoperative rehabilitation complicated. Conversely, hand transplantation is strategically planned by an extensive healthcare team, and surgery is rehearsed in advance. Candidates go through a thorough selection process, and hand therapists evaluate and educate the patient before surgery.

HAND TRANSPLANTATION

GENERAL CONSIDERATIONS

The objective of amputee care, whether through transplantation or prosthetics using Targeting Muscle Reinnervation (TMR) or Regenerative Peripheral Nerve Interface (RPNI), is to improve the quality of life (QOL). But QOL is highly subjective and a hand, or the loss of a hand, may mean different things to different people (M. Nassimizadeh, A.K. Nassimizadeh, & Power, 2014). Every patient possesses their own reasons and goals for hand transplantation but there are common themes including a desire to restore body wholeness; regain the experience of sensation; and improve strength, functionality, and appearance. In broad terms, these goals may be similar among patients but the depth and meaning are as unique as the individual. As such, each individual patient and their unique experiences and expectations need to be thoroughly considered before and after the hand transplantation.

PATIENT SELECTION

The importance of the patient candidate selection process cannot be understated and should be understood in more detail than is pertinent to this chapter. Suffice it to say, persons interested in hand transplantation must participate in a comprehensive selection process involving a medical evaluation, psychological assessment, financial counseling, rehabilitative functional evaluation, and extensive patient and caregiver education. Hand therapists meet with the candidate to assess their current functional status, review their experience with prosthetics and rehabilitation, and discuss their goals and expectations. A patient's beliefs and attitudes about their condition, expected treatment, and ability to influence the outcome are all important factors to adherence in chronic hand injuries (O'Brien, 2010). Therefore, therapists should allow ample time for candidate interview and provide detailed education about the lengthy rehabilitation and recovery period. Studies show that the use of pictures along with written and spoken language can increase a patient's attention, comprehension, recall, and adherence (Houts, Doak, Doak, & Loscalzo, 2006) and should be utilized along with videos of orthoses, therapy interventions, and previous hand transplant patients' functional outcomes during the education process for hand transplantation.

LEVELS OF TRANSPLANTATION

The level of attachment of transplanted limb to the recipient limb is the single most influencing factor in designing a post-op rehabilitation program (Severance & Walsh, 2013; Pace & Zeske-McGuire, 2013) (Fig. 27–1A,B).

DISTAL FOREARM TRANSPLANTATIONS

In distal forearm level transplants (distal transplants), a patient maintains their native extrinsic muscles and the intrinsics come from the donor. Early hand movement is possible in a matter of days through the patient's native long flexors and extensors. In time, recovery of some intrinsic function and discriminative sensory function is expected because of the shorter distance for nerve regeneration (Shores et al., 2017).

PROXIMAL AND MID-FOREARM TRANSPLANTATIONS

With proximal and mid-forearm level transplants (proximal transplants), the extrinsic and intrinsic muscles that power the hand are from the donor limb. Nerve regeneration must occur before sensory and motor recovery is possible and this may take several months. Significant functional improvement is noted in both distal and proximal level transplantations, but proximal level transplants may result in weaker grip, more limited sensory recovery, and limited or no intrinsic function compared with distal transplants (Shores et al., 2017). Regardless of transplant level, early post-op precautions and limited sensory and motor activity produce an initial phase of functional decline for all patients. It is important that patients and caregivers are made aware of this before surgery so that they are prepared for this sudden change.

GENERAL THERAPY TIMELINE

Providing a specific and accurate timeline for each stage of rehabilitation and functional recovery would be misleading and arbitrary given the variability in each hand transplant case (Severance & Walsh, 2013). Yet, it is essential for patient and caregiver to have a general outline of the time commitment that is required. After transplantation, the patient will stay in the acute care hospital for 1 to 4 weeks in order to establish medical stability and functional safety. After hospital discharge, the patient remains in the area for another 1 to 3 months for medical, psychological, and rehabilitative

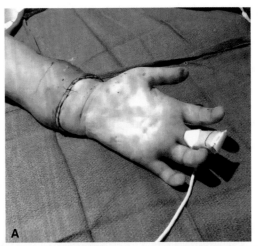
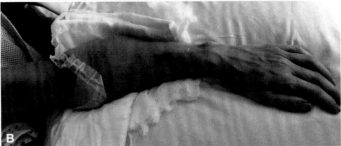

FIGURE 27–1 Distal **(A)** and proximal **(B)** level transplantation.

management, during which time, the patient attends outpatient therapy 5 days a week, 2 to 6 hours a day (Severance & Walsh, 2013; Pace & Zeske-McGuire, 2013; Bueno et al., 2014; Wessenbacher et al., 2014). When patients return to their hometown, the therapy schedule may taper down depending on level of transplant and therapeutic need. A reduced schedule also allows the patient to integrate back into their lives, family roles, and community.

ORTHOTIC CONSIDERATIONS

The initial purpose of the orthosis after hand transplantation is to protect the newly transplanted limb including the osteosynthesis, muscle-tendon balance, nerve(s), vascular, and integumentary integrity (Table 27–1). In the first few weeks, frequent orthotic adjustments are needed as wounds heal and edema subsides. The first year following surgery will involve multiple design changes as precautions retire and motor function returns to the new limb. It is important that any changes to the orthotic design and schedule are based on neuromotor recovery, functional utility, clinical reasoning, and patient safety. Patients may grow weary of using orthoses and are eager to use their new limbs free of external devices. To improve the patient's acceptance and adherence, patient should understand the purpose and wear schedule. The therapist should help the patient understand the orthoses are not permanent fixtures to their new limbs, rather temporary rehabilitative tool(s) to maximizing their functional outcome. Additionally, all members of the team should comply and support the orthosis regimen.

MONITORING REJECTION

Acute rejection (AR) occurs in 85% of hand transplant recipients in the first year (Schneeberger, Khalifian, & Brandacher, 2013). The skin is the principal target for the body's immune response. So careful and frequent inspection of the skin allows for earlier detection

TABLE 27–1	Orthosis Table: Mid–Proximal Level Transplant	
Mid–Proximal Level Transplant		
Phase/Time	**Orthosis**	**Comments**
Early 0–2 mo	Two-piece orthosis (Fig. 27–3). 1. Proximally: dorsal long arm orthosis (discharge 6–8 wk) 2. Distally: forearm resting hand	Protect osteosynthesis, coaptation of tissues, and nerve and vascular systems. Balance extensors and flexors
Intermediate 2 mo to 1.5–2 y	1. Continue forearm immobilization orthosis (night/rest) (Fig. 27–6) 2. Helmet orthosis (day) (Fig. 27–9)	Once patient can control/stabilize their wrists movement
Late	Corrective or assistive orthoses as needed	To aid in motor recovery, function, and/or address any contracture
Distal Level Transplant		
Early 0–3 wk	1. Forearm immobilization (Fig. 27–6) 2. Forearm-based "Crane Outrigger" mobilization orthosis (Fig. 27–10) or Helmet orthosis with therapy only (Fig. 27–17)	Allows for early protective motion
Intermediate 3 wk to 1 y	1. Forearm or hand-based immobilization (night/rest) 2. Helmet orthosis (day) (Fig. 27–11)	After edema resolved and improve tissue equilibrium
Late	Same as mid-proximal	Same as mid-proximal

and treatment with steroids and tacrolimus, an immunosuppressant drug (Siemionow et al., 2009; Schneeberger et al., 2013; Murphy, Zuker, & Borschel, 2013). The hand therapist should be attuned to early clinical manifestations of AR, which may include diffuse or focal pattern of erythematous maculopapular lesion or rash. Typical patterns will present over the dorsal aspects of the forearm and hands (Schneeberger et al., 2013; Sarhane et al., 2013; Fisher, Lian, & Kueckelhaus, 2014). Palmar presentations have been associated with mechanical stress (Wessenbacher et al., 2014). Not all skin changes implicate rejection. Pressure areas from orthoses should be distinguished from acute rejection.

PSYCHOLOGICAL CONSIDERATIONS

The outcome of hand transplantation is not only defined by physical and functional status but also the psychological well-being of the patient. Due to the visible nature of the allograft, postoperatively the patient must adapt to seeing and wearing someone else's hand(s) and adjust to a new body image. While the majority of patients have reported positive changes in QOL and body image, there are reports of rejection and graft loss linked to nonadherence to post-op regimens as the result of psychological complications (Kumnig et al., 2012).

PSYCHOLOGICAL REGRESSION

Psychological regression is most prevalent in the early days after surgery due to initial loss of function, lack of social/family support, feelings of isolation, intensive therapy schedule, and side effects of medication (Kumnig, Jowsey, & DiMartini, 2014; Salminger et al., 2016). Self-consciousness about the physical difference between the allograft and a normal hand may trigger a range of concealing behaviors and social avoidance (Kumnig et al., 2012). Body image adjustment also depends on the patient's perception of the family's level of acceptance of the allograft (Jowsey-Gregoire et al., 2016). When left unchecked, negative emotions including stress, anxiety, loneliness, and helplessness further diminish the patient's coping mechanism, resulting in decreased motivation and adherence to medication and therapy regimens which in turn leads to rejection (Kumnig et al., 2012; Piza-Katzer & Estermann, 2007). Therefore, managing patient

expectations and fostering a sense of ownership of the new hands facilitate a positive body image and better adjustment following hand transplantation (Kumnig et al., 2012; Jowsey-Gregoire et al., 2016).

The therapy team can play an important role in recognizing psychosocial and adjustment issues. In spending extensive one-on-one time together, the therapist may be more attuned to changes in mood, affect, and behavioral pattern of the patient and often becomes the person to whom the patient confides his/her negative emotions. The therapist can support the patient during the adjustment period by collaborating with the transplant team for psychological intervention.

CORTICAL REORGANIZATION

Following an amputation, maladaptive changes occur locally on the cortical map and throughout the sensorimotor network due to sensory deprivation. Studies on cortical plasticity show that those changes are reversible through cortical remapping after hand transplantation once the transplanted hand is integrated (Vargas et al., 2009). Muscle and sensory re-education help to integrate the transplanted hand at the cortical level (Hsu et al., 2019; Huchon et al., 2016; Rosen et al., 2015).

MOTOR RE-EDUCATION

Motor re-education aims at improving the activation and coordination of the available muscle groups. The patient engages the innervated extrinsic muscles in gross motor tasks and progresses to prehension and object manipulation as intrinsic muscle function returns. The program should incorporate objects of different sizes and shapes and utilize different contact surfaces to improve carryover to ADLs (Huchon et al., 2016) (Fig. 27–2A–C). While immediate activation is possible in some muscle groups after hand transplantation, motor planning and performance depend on the recovery of tactile sensation and proprioception (Salles et al., 2017). Because recovering tactile sensation in the hand can take many months, motor retraining should include neurocognitive strategies such as motor imagery and joint position sense training (Hsu

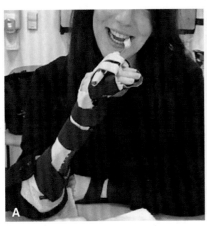
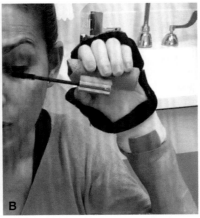
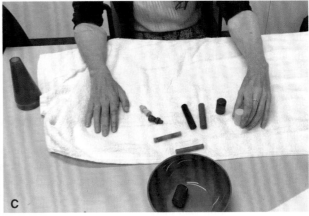

FIGURE 27–2 A–C, Through different stages of neuromotor recovery, patients engage in ADL activities using tools and objects of different shape for motor re-education.

et al., 2019; Rosen et al., 2015; Salles et al., 2017). The patient practices motor imagery by constructing a mental image of performing different movements and activities with the transplanted hand. For patients who have difficulty with imagining hand movements, guided observation of another person performing an activity is an alternative technique to activate the motor centers of the brain (Hsu et al., 2019). Joint position sense training is performed with and without vision of the patient to improve awareness of which joint is being moved, the direction of movement, and joint positions in different segments of the extremity (Salles et al., 2017).

SENSORY RE-EDUCATION

A sensory re-education program is divided into cortical stimulation and sensory discrimination training following peripheral nerve repairs (Rosen et al., 2015). In the early days after nerve repair, a visual-perceptual technique is used for cortical stimulation and has been shown to enhance sensorimotor function (Hsu et al., 2019; Rosen et al., 2015). Hence, the authors have adopted this technique for patients with hand transplantation. First, the patient observes the insensate hand being touched with a familiar texture or object and perceives what the sensation should be. The sensation is then verified by touching the native skin with the same texture/object. Given the close proximity of the face and hand on the homunculus, the face was often used as the native skin surface. Once protective sensation is available, the patient continues with traditional sensory re-education including localization of touch, tactile discrimination, and stereognosis (Rosen et al., 2015).

REHABILITATION: PROXIMAL AND MID-FOREARM LEVEL TRANSPLANTATION

EARLY PHASE

Hand therapy may be initiated 5 to 7 days postoperatively, while occupational therapy (OT) and physical therapy (PT) may be consulted earlier to initiate edge of bed and out of bed mobility.

Orthosis

For the patient with proximal level transplants, the orthosis incorporates multiple joints from elbow to fingers and can be challenging and time-consuming to fabricate. The patient is required to wear these initial orthoses continuously, and because they cover so much of the arm, they can be cumbersome and uncomfortable. Additionally, they can migrate and, if applied incorrectly, cause a change in position and

a risk to tissue integrity. A two-piece orthosis can be fabricated to help mitigate these concerns (Fig. 27–3A,B). The proximal component is a long arm orthosis for the purpose of supporting the boney anastomosis around the elbow. This piece starts at the proximal humerus and extends to the distal forearm. With grafting close to the elbow, the joint elbow is positioned at 30° to 40° of extension to prevent compression of vascular and nerve structures and protect musculoskeletal integrity, but the exact position should be reviewed with the surgeons. The distal orthosis is essentially a forearm-based wrist-hand immobilization orthosis designed to balance the extensor and flexor systems with the wrist in slight extension. The metacarpophalangeal (MCP) joints are positioned at 30° to 45° of flexion, the interphalangeal (IP) joints are positioned in extension, and the thumb is resting between radial and palmar extension. This two-piece design allows the clinician and caregiver to remove one piece for range of motion (ROM) while protecting the adjacent area. Moreover, breaking it down to smaller components makes it easier to mold, adjust, and contour each area appropriately, lessening the risk for improper fit. A cutout hole at the wrist level provides direct access for frequent pulse checks and

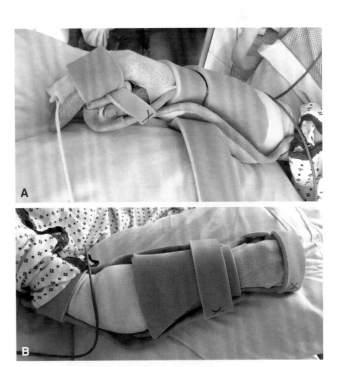

FIGURE 27–3 A and B, Two-piece orthosis to support a proximal level hand transplant. The distal hand immobilization orthosis may lie over or under (as in this photo) to the proximal long arm orthosis, depending on the level of the graft, limb presentation, and patient comfort. Velfoam® straps seen here provided comfort but are not as durable as neoprene straps used in later cases.

Doppler readings by the medical team without disturbing the orthosis position (Fig. 27–4). During fabrication, there should be special attention to protecting the surgical incisions with adequate soft dressing and closed cell padding. The orthosis should allocate additional space about the elbow where post-op edema is likely to accumulate. Surgical incisions are dressed with Xeroform® (or nonadherent sterile wound dressings), high absorbency pads for fluid collection, and loose gauze bandage wraps. All is then covered with noncompressive cotton stockinette.

Compressive garments are not recommended during in this early phase so to protect vascular structures and to allow easy accessibility to the skin for Doppler readings and to monitor for signs of rejections. Postoperative edema is managed with the light dressings, ROM program, and modest elevation of the limbs during rest periods (Fig. 27–5). Once bone stability is established, the proximal long arm support is discharged while still maintaining the distal piece to support the hand and forearm. The distal piece may need to be adjusted to ensure adequate forearm support.

Fabrication Process and Considerations

It is advisable to have two fabricators: one to hold and protect the new limb and manage medical lines while the second does the molding. Clinicians should use materials that work best with their fabrication skills. For the proximal orthosis, a material with good memory and rigidity supports the larger joint and is easier to mold over bandages and the distal orthosis. Materials with some drapability are helpful in conforming around the wrist and hand. Contours in the distal component reduce the risk for migration. All materials should be durable enough to withstand the consistent use and frequent remolding but not so heavy as to add undue weight and stress on the patient's UE during activities such as transfers.

Perforated materials may improve airflow and reduce the heaviness of the orthosis on the patient's limb. For strapping, the therapist should consider a soft loop material (i.e., such as Velfoam®, neoprene) because these types of traps are lightweight and conform easily to the orthosis and involved body part. These soft strapping systems afford satisfactory distribution of pressure. They also come in a variety of widths and/or can be cut to fit a particular design (Fig. 27–3A,B). However, strapping materials made of foam may become less durable and fray over time with frequent donning and doffing. Neoprene material can be equally accommodating; it can

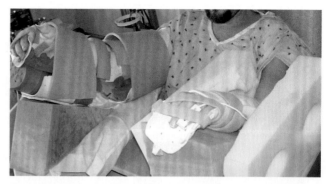

FIGURE 27–5 Positioning for vascular flow and edema control in this patient with bilateral transplantations. Notice the Carter˜ pillow elevating his left upper extremity.

also be cut to various widths and lengths and is extremely durable as well as aesthetically pleasing (Fig. 27–6). Another consideration is the use of closed cell padding which tends to resist odors, perspiration, and bacteria and can be wiped clean (Coppard, 1996). As always, the limbs should be inspected frequently for any pressure areas, friction locations, or other "fit" problems. This is especially important when there is insensate skin, surgical incisions, and changes in limb size due to edema.

Exercises

Maintaining activity within the muscle with active range of motion (AROM) and passive range of motion (PROM) may increase trophic factor release on regenerating motor neurons (Udina, Puigdemasa, & Navarro, 2011). ROM exercises are based on tissue and boney stability following surgery and at this level typically begins within the postoperative day (POD) five to seven. The patient maintains their native muscles to control of the shoulder and elbow, so active assisted range of motion (AAROM) may be performed here. Assistance is required by the therapy and trained caregivers to support the heavy distal limb during proximal AAROM.

Elbow ROM may be restricted to midrange to prevent vascular and nerve compromise by compression with elbow flexion and attenuation with extension. Forearm ROM may be guarded to protect osteosynthesis and thus is moved according to the surgical team. PROM is performed to the wrist and hands because the newly transplanted deinnervated muscles move these joints. PROM is in a tenodesis pattern to maintain balance between the extensor and flexor system.

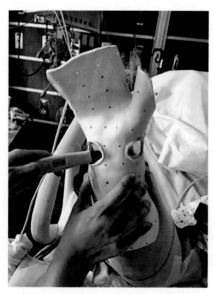

FIGURE 27–4 Cutouts on the volar aspect allow the medical staff to perform Doppler reading and monitor vascular flow to the hand.

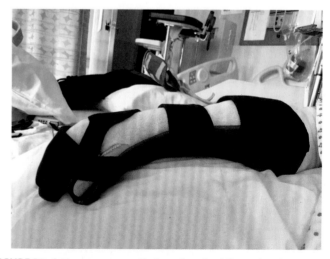

FIGURE 27–6 Neoprene straps afford comfort, durability, and aesthetics. Forearm-based resting wrist-hand orthosis is used for support and to maintain equilibrium between flexors and extensors until patient has sufficient motor control of wrist and digits.

ADL and Functional Mobility

OT and PT may be consulted within the first few PODs to assist the patient with edge of bed and out-of-bed mobilization and transfers. This is particularly important for patients with lower extremity (LE) amputations. Out of bed activity helps the patient get used to the weight and altered body habitus with their new limbs. Initially, a platform walker is used to support the new limbs. As standing balance improves and elbow ROM is cleared and tolerated, the patient uses adapted arm slings to protect transplanted limbs and orthoses (Fig. 27–7). What may come as some surprise to the patient is the amount of people and effort it takes to do a simple out of bed transfer to the chair or to the commode.

Assistance is needed for donning of LE prosthetics and clothing, managing medical lines, maneuvering around hospital room, and maintaining dynamic balance. Custom fabricated cuffs and tools can be attached to the orthosis to allow for some independence with eating and grooming (Fig. 27–2A). Stylus tools can be adapted to operate touchscreen phones and tablets so the patient can communicate with friends and family back home (Fig. 27–8A,B). However, these should be designed to allow visualization of the screen with proper stylus placement in order to safely position the limb during movement without stressing the coaptation site.

INTERMEDIATE PHASE

Orthosis

Several months after surgery, the patient should have enough strength to stabilize their wrists and progress to a less bulky, more functional dorsal hand-based MCP extension blocking orthosis with a component that also holds the thumb in a functionally abducted position (Fig. 27–9A,B). This orthosis is more commonly referred to as the Helmet orthosis and is akin to a lumbrical plus, anti-claw orthosis or formally described (ASHT nomenclature) as an extension restriction orthosis. For the purpose of this chapter, we will refer to it as a Helmet orthosis. Due to the distance between

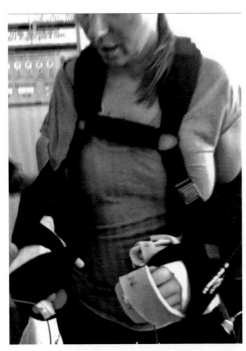

FIGURE 27–7 Modifying the strap placement on shoulder slings helps carry and protect the newly grafted limbs during ambulation. Left and right straps cross posteriorly and connect to the contralateral anterior wrist level D-ring. The straps can stay hooked in place and the patient don the sling like a jacket. A sternal level strap connects the two straps in front and prevents sliding off the shoulder.

peripheral nerve coaptation and the muscle motor end plate, innervation of intrinsic muscles is slow and not assured. A Helmet orthosis serves to balance out absent or weak intrinsics against more powerful extrinsic muscles. Maintaining an intrinsic plus position while waiting for intrinsic return can help create some intrinsic and capsular tightness that may prevent a longstanding claw deformity (Scheker & Hodges, 2001). The reader is referred to Chapter 20 for more detailed information on peripheral nerve injuries and orthosis intervention. The Helmet orthosis can enhance grasp and release for improved engagement of the limb in functional tasks further integrating cortical reorganization and patient satisfaction (Fig. 27–9C,D). Patients may need to wear this orthosis consistently for up to a year or longer, but the MCP position can be adjusted over time to a more extended position if the patient is able to simultaneously engage IP extension. Consider using a lightweight durable material (1/16th inch thermoplastic) that is conformable and aesthetically pleasing to garner patient acceptance and functionality. Due to impaired sensation, unremitting patient education around skin inspection and sensory protection is paramount.

Exercises

Nerve regeneration will dictate exercise and activity selection, with attention toward newly innervated muscles, balancing extensors and flexors, and engaging in bilateral activity and cortical reorganization. With regard to neuromuscular electrical stimulation (NMES), Novak and von der Heyde (2015) cite a lack of literature supporting its use to maintain viability for reinnervation following long duration deinnervation. However, the use of alternating current electrical stimulation may be used once muscle reinnervation has occurred (Novak & von der Heyde, 2015), and electrodes should be placed on skin where there is protective sensation. NMES should augment muscle rehabilitation and not take precedence over sensory motor re-education techniques such as biofeedback, repetition, and engaging in familiar, functional tasks. Still, newly reinnervated muscles are quick to fatigue, and therefore, short low intensity exercise is preferred over high-intensity exercise for axonal regeneration (Novak & von der Heyde, 2015; Sabatier, Redmon, Schwartz, & English, 2008; Kahn & Moore, 2016.)

With early muscle return, patients should perform isometric contractions in midrange with gravity eliminated or assisted planes progressing the arc of motion and gravitational challenge as motor movement improves. These authors advise targeting muscle groups that recruit specific motor nerve groups (i.e., all median) or those groups that move synergistically.

As the patient begins to use their new hands, care is taken to avoid injury due to diminished sensation. Placing a mirror in front of the patient during attempted exercise offers the patient an expanded view to monitor their hands for both sensory protection and self-assessment of their performance.

LATE PHASE

Between 1 and 2 years post-op, there is increase in extrinsic strength and signs of intrinsic recovery are expected. The Helmet orthosis should be continued until there is adequate IP extension and no appearance of claw deformity. Continued use of a forearm-based resting wrist-hand immobilization orthosis (or can be hand-based if appropriate) at night maintains anatomical balance (Fig. 27–6). If there is intrinsic return, the return will be spotty and considerably weaker than the extrinsic muscles. By this time, sensation in the hand is likely improved, so NMES to the intrinsics may be beneficial. Higher-level neuromotor rehabilitation and sensory retraining techniques previously discussed, along with occupational based skill acquisition, predominate this phase.

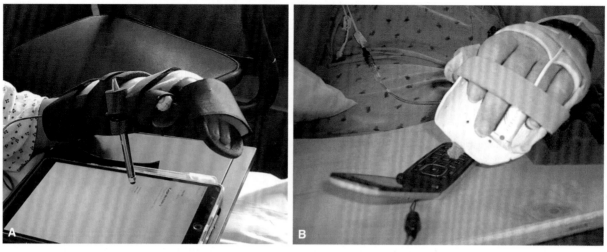

FIGURE 27–8 **A and B,** During early stages of both proximal and distal level transplants, patients may not have enough finger strength or sensory awareness to maneuver a touchscreen or home button, so fabricating removable stylus cuffs allows patient to use devices to stay in touch with friends and family.

DISTAL FOREARM TRANSPLANTATION

EARLY PHASE

As in proximal transplantation, the early phase of rehabilitation for distal forearm transplantation emphasizes graft protection, protected ROM, edema and pain management, and education of the patient and caregiver. However, because distal forearm transplants maintain native extrinsic muscles of the hand and wrist, hand therapy begins within 1 to 3 days after surgery for orthotic fabrication and ROM of the hand. Early AAROM and controlled AROM maintain tendon gliding and promote motor function that is not achieved by PROM alone.

The absence of low ulnar and median nerve function perpetuates the intrinsic minus hand position in the presence of the native extrinsic flexor and extensor muscle function in a distal level transplant. Patients are educated on the risk of hand contractures and the importance of wearing resting and functional orthoses until intrinsic muscle function returns. Skin protection and monitoring of skin integrity is emphasized to prevent injury during ADLs due to the initial absence of protective sensation in the transplanted hand.

Orthosis

Hand mobilization begins in a forearm-based mobilization orthosis which substitutes for intrinsic muscle function and offers biomechanical balance to the extrinsic and intrinsic muscle-tendon

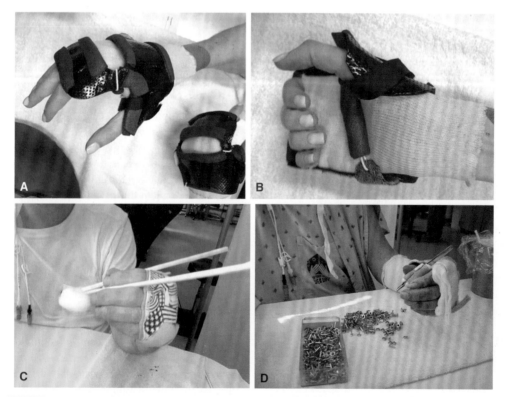

FIGURE 27–9 **A,** Dorsal-based Helmet orthosis with thumb in radial-palmar abduction. **B,** A padded elasticize strap across the palm ensures comfort, secures fit, and helps prevent clawing by applying light palmar pressure to offset extension forces. **C and D,** Functional use is to enhance with the positioning the Helmet orthosis provides (metacarpophalangeal flexion and thumb opposition).

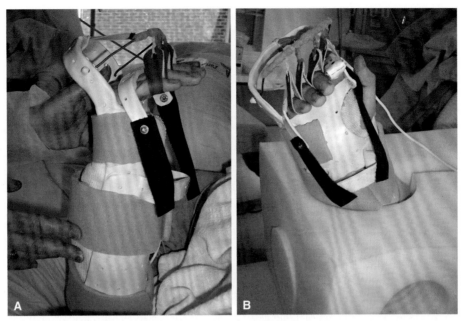

FIGURE 27–10 A and B, The Crane Outrigger connects to the static tower component and to the finger slings via rubber bands. Moving in an arc over the digits, this outrigger dissipates tension during active composite flexion. During extension, the outrigger recoils up toward the tower base and assists with interphalangeal extension.

groups and is known commonly as the "Crane Outrigger" (Scheker & Hodges, 2001) (Fig. 27–10A,B).

The Crane Outrigger was first described by Chesher et al. (1988) for use in hand replantation and later utilized for the very first hand transplantation in Louisville, Kentucky, in 1999 (Chesher et al,. 1988). It is composed of a forearm-based orthosis with the wrist in neutral, a custom bent wire outrigger, a static tower base, and an extension restriction bar that work together to facilitate active digit flexion and active assisted IP extension. Due to the absence of the thenar muscle function, the thumb is placed midway between radial extension and palmar abduction with a separate outrigger to maintain functional positioning for pinch. The patient uses a forearm-based wrist and hand immobilization orthosis at night similar to the one shown in Figure 27–6.

The patient may initially require passive assistance to mobilize the orthosis if they present with muscle weakness and limited motor control. Chesher advises the axis for the wire outrigger to be placed precisely at 2 cm dorsal and 1.25 cm distal to the MCP joints of the digits. Soft and gently conforming IP slings are placed on each digit and connected to the wire outrigger with No. 12 rubber bands. A removable extension restriction bar maintains MCP flexion and is adjusted progressively to achieve a maximum of 60° to 75° of flexion as edema subsides. It is beneficial for the therapist to become familiar with the tools and specifications for configuring this specialized orthosis by practicing fabrication preoperatively. To improve efficiency, a template can be made to provide a reference point for setting the axis of the outrigger.

The Crane Outrigger should be worn during therapy and for as much time as possible to encourage frequent mobilization of the digits (Scheker & Hodges, 2001). Due to the complexity of the Crane Outrigger, caregivers and nursing staff should practice applying it with the hand therapist's supervision before orthosis wear is extended outside of therapy hours. This orthosis may require frequent adjustments due to tissue changes, dressing needs, and overall gains in mobility. A wrist and hand immobilization orthosis is worn at night and during rest periods to maintain muscle balance (Fig. 27–6). These authors will note that although the Crane Outrigger is commonly used for distal level transplants,

an alternative design may be appropriate for mobilization in the early phase and will be discussed further in the case study at the end of this chapter.

Early Phase Exercises

Active, active-assisted, or passive digit motion is performed only in the Crane Outrigger until 3 weeks post-op. Shoulder AROM, elbow and forearm AAROM are performed with the distal joints supported. Nursing and caregivers are instructed to assist with exercise programs several times a day.

INTERMEDIATE PHASE

Orthosis

Weaning of the Crane Outrigger begins at 3 weeks post-op. The patient is then transitioned to the Helmet orthosis during therapy and light activity. As previously mentioned, the Helmet maintains MCP flexion and shortening of the intrinsics for muscle balance to minimize the tendency toward clawing. A Bouvier maneuver (a test for ulnar nerve function) is performed to determine the MCP flexion position that optimizes digit IP extension in the Helmet. In the first 12 weeks, full MCP extension is avoided during hand hygiene, changing between orthoses and during exercises. This will minimize the tendency for clawing of the digits (Scheker & Hodges, 2001). Perforated materials promote airflow and each therapy session should include an orthotic check to ensure fit and the monitoring of patient adherence to its use during light daily activities.

Similar to proximal transplants, as ROM and sensation improve, the Helmet orthosis can be streamlined to allow for more skin contact for better function and to ensure patient adherence during functional activities (Fig. 27–11 A,B). Daily use of the Helmet continues until the patient regains intrinsic motor function and is no longer at risk for clawing. At night, the wrist-hand immobilization orthosis helps prevent deformity (Fig. 27–6) and muscle tightness and is worn until the patient has adequate wrist control and is cleared for weight bearing. After this clearance, the forearm-based wrist and hand orthosis can be modified to hand-based and continued at night until intrinsic muscle function returns.

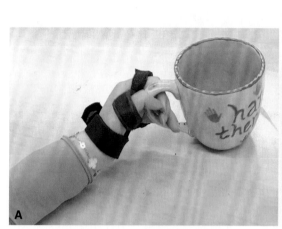
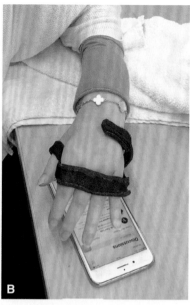

FIGURE 27–11 **A and B,** A streamlined Helmet design allows more skin contact for better function. Metacarpophalangeal joints can move into more extension as motor recovery progresses.

Intermediate Phase Exercises

In the Helmet orthosis, the patient begins with active or active assistive tenodesis exercises. When the osteosynthesis is determined to be stable, the patient engages in gross motor tasks, light ADLs using adapted tools, and sensorimotor retraining. The orthosis should accommodate a variety of adapted tools such as grooming devices and feeding utensils to maximize independence in the home and community setting (Fig. 27–12A,B). Stretching of the forearm and the wrist is performed in a tenodesis pattern for any joint stiffness. The therapist should monitor extensor digitorum communis function and differential gliding of flexor digitorum superficialis and flexor digitorum profundus periodically,

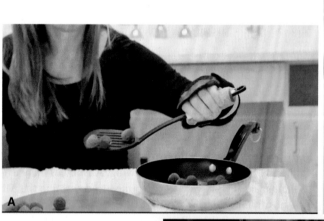
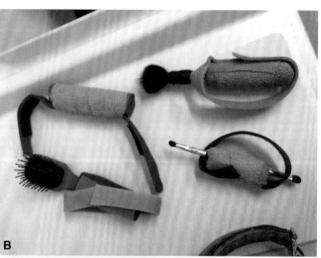
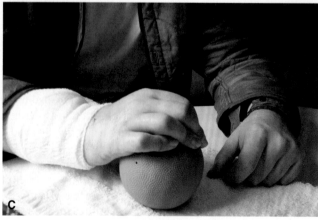

FIGURE 27–12 **A,** Engaging the transplanted hand with familiar household tools can maximize therapy carryover to the home setting. Orthosis should be worn for ADL retraining to maintain muscle-tendon balance until intrinsic muscles are innervated. (Photo courtesy of PENN Medicine.) **B,** Common grooming tools can be modified and attached to the orthosis to engage the patient in cortical reorganization and functional independence. Coban˚, loop strapping, and tubing help to prevent tool migration. **C,** Gentle wrist motion performed over a therapy ball.

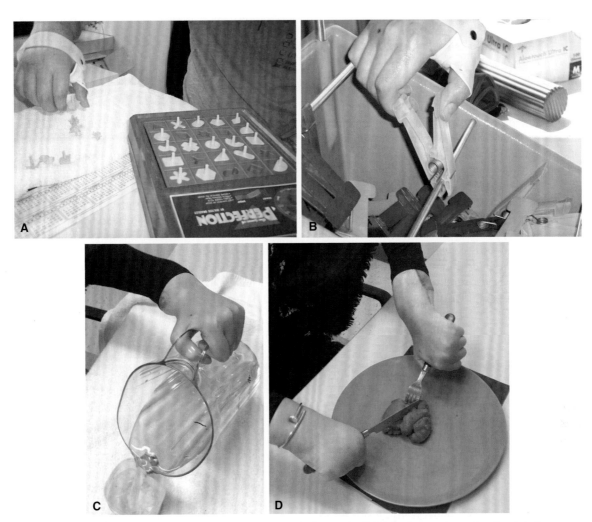

FIGURE 27–13 **A and B,** The thumb is positioned in mid palmar and radial abduction to enhance functional pinch. **C and D,** Improving motor strength and sensation allow more activity out of the constraints of orthoses.

in a safe range to prevent MCP extension lag and intertendinous adhesions (Fig. 27–12C).

At 8 to 10 weeks and with radiological evidence of bone healing, the patient may begin progressive strengthening exercises from a proximal to distal manner to promote functional stability. The exercise program should continue to integrate motor skill and kinesthesia in all segments of the extremity and provide sensory challenges for the hand (i.e., performed with and without visual cueing) to maximize sensorimotor control.

LATE PHASE

Orthosis

Orthosis design in the late phase continues to address muscle imbalance between extrinsic and intrinsic muscles. The Helmet orthosis is progressively weaned as the patient regains functional digit extension without clawing. A hand-based thumb orthosis may be needed for pinching and grasping until thenar muscles return (Fig. 27–13A,B). The hand-based night orthosis is continued for 1 year or until patient has sufficient ulnar and median intrinsic muscle function and is no longer at risk for hand deformities.

Late Phase Exercises

Exercises in the late phase improve balance between extrinsic and intrinsic muscles, coordination of movement, and integration of sensory and motor functions into higher-level ADL skills (Fig. 27–13C,D). Manual muscle testing of intrinsic muscle groups continues to monitor nerve regeneration and strength. Neuromuscular retraining incorporates place and hold exercise, AROM, prehension tasks, and fine motor activities to engage the intrinsics. The patient is instructed to avoid co-contraction from extrinsic muscles or stronger proximal muscles during activities using verbal and tactile cues. NMES and biofeedback aid intrinsic functional and neuromotor recovery. As the patient becomes more independent in ADLs and demonstrates adherence to home exercise program, therapy visits are reduced to as needed basis.

CONCLUSION

Hand transplantation offers the potential for restoration of appearance, sensation, function, and participation, and by extension a physical and mental confidence that can be lost along with the loss of a limb. Hand transplantation candidates should be carefully screened for their medical stability, rehabilitative commitment, and psychological resilience. Hand therapists working with transplantation patients should possess a solid foundation in musculoskeletal and peripheral nerve rehabilitation, be skillful and creative in orthotic fabrication and therapeutic interventions, and adept at counseling patients during a recovery period that can be emotionally and psychologically challenging.

Orthotic devices are essential for protection during the initial post-op phase and facilitate structural balance during the extended period of nerve regeneration. Hand therapists should be familiar with the fabrication and purpose of the orthoses used for this unique patient population and should accommodate the individual needs of each patient into the design. Patients need to understand the utility of each device and adhere to the orthotic routine to maximize optimal functional recovery after hand transplantation.

FIELD NOTE: THE TRANSPLANTED HAND VERSUS THE REPLANTED HAND

Marie Pace, OTR/L, CHT
Kimberly Zeske-Maquire, MS, OTR/L, CHT
Pennsylvania

Treating the transplanted UE is unique from replantation for several reasons. After an injury that requires replantation, there is often a significant amount of tissue trauma that must be overcome in order to eventually have functional outcomes. Surgeons have to make use of the viable tissue that remains in order to create a working hand or limb. For example, if a patient has an amputation transcarpally and the surgeons are able to replant the hand, the carpus must be fused due to bone loss and ligament damage. Permanent loss of wrist motion would result, but it is likely that sensation and motor function to the fingers would be spared. The post-surgical orthosis would be the same as with a transplant except wrist support would continue longer to ensure proper fusion. The goals for restoring tendon glide, functional use, and intrinsic muscle function would be the same. Compensatory strategies for loss of wrist motion would be addressed in therapy.

In the case of a hand transplant, the donated hand is chosen in part because it is not damaged. The optimal level of transplantation is carefully planned to closely restore normal anatomy. There is time to plan and enlist the cooperation of a full team of skilled surgeons to harvest the donor tissue and prepare the recipient's residual arm(s). The team carefully and securely attaches the allograft in order to maximize the eventual function of the reconstruction.

Case Study Section

The case studies presented here are meant as a teaching guideline only. Treatment and orthosis protocols vary greatly from surgeon to surgeon and from therapist to therapist. The therapist should check with the referring physicians and colleagues to define the preferred treatment and appropriate orthotic intervention.

Case Study 1: Proximal Forearm Bilateral Transplantation Case

At the age of 19, Patient X lost all four limbs to sepsis; bilateral upper extremities just proximal to the elbow joint and bilateral lower extremities just below the knee. Patient X participated in therapy and was trained on LE prosthetics and UE myoelectric prosthetics. While she valued and used her prosthetics for some basic ADLs, they did not offer a path to complete independence. Cosmetically, the UE prosthetics offered some satisfaction, but they were "clunky," had no sensation, often appeared dirty, and were difficult to clean. At times she felt like a "robot." Patient X sought out hand transplantation to increase her functional independence, feel better in an intimate relationship, safely care for children, perform her own self-care/grooming, "to feel," and to avoid the stares of others.

Nearly 2 years after her transplant candidate assessment, Patient X received her bilateral hand transplants.

After surgery, the patient's upper extremities were immobilized in postoperative bandages. On POD 3, acute care PT and OT met with the patient at bedside to begin out-of-bed mobilization. Hand therapy started at POD 6 for fabrication of a two-piece long arm orthoses as previously described (Fig. 27–3A,B). Surgical precautions restricted the elbow to 0° to 40° of passive motion for the first 2 weeks and slowly progressed to more flexion over the next 2 weeks. While she maintained her native biceps and triceps muscles, AROM of the elbow was restricted to prevent undue tension on her boney anastomoses. Exercises also included AAROM of shoulders, short arc forearm ROM, and passive tenodesis of the wrist and hand. Treatment included cortical reorganization, activities to accept the new limb, and family training. When the patient experienced her first rejection episode, therapy continued and much time was spent addressing anxiety and adjustment strategies related to some early medical complications and her postoperative functional limitations. The only postoperative pain the patient reported was in the first few postoperative weeks, and this was localized to the shoulder and elbow on the limb that required a surgical seroma evacuation.

Transcutaneous electrical stimulation was utilized to address shoulder pain with electrodes placed on her native skin, but due to the insensate skin NMES was not used on the transplanted portion of the limb. Postoperative edema was addressed with elevation and ROM. Compression garments were not used in order to protect the vascular structures from needless pressure and to allow for easy inspection of the skin for rejection monitoring.

By 4 weeks, she was cleared for AROM of her elbows, which permitted discharge of the proximal orthoses and training with adaptive devices for eating, grooming, and using an iPhone/iPad to communicate with family and friends back home. She was able to mobilize without a walker using UE slings to support her upper extremities. These functional gains along with medical stability enhanced with her psychological well-being and ensured her readiness for hospital discharge.

Patient X participated in outpatient therapy at the transplant facility 5 days a week, 2 hours a day for approximately 1 month until she was discharged home. Awaiting sensory motor return in the transplanted limb, therapy engaged the patient with ADL adaptive devices and limb safety education (Fig. 27–14). There was an eagerness for independence in toileting and personal care, and while attempts should be made to accommodate the patient's short-term goals, these high-level skills may not yet be physically possible in the early stages, so support and guidance is needed to help the patient redirect attention to more timely activities.

Patient X participated in exercises for balance, endurance and core strengthening, continuation of cortical reorganization activities, and monitoring of sensorimotor recovery. In preparation for discharge to her home site, we communicated with her home therapist to provide a thorough medical history and therapy treatment plan. She was fitted with bilateral Helmet orthoses to be used once she transitioned out of her forearm-based orthoses (Fig. 27–9A–D). At two and a half months post-op, she had palpable recovery of pronator teres and deep touch sensation to all the sensory nerves distal to grafting. Signs of extrinsic wrist and finger recovery began around three and a half months postoperative. By this time the patient had returned to her hometown where she attended outpatient therapy 3 days a week. At 7 months she returned for her medical and therapy assessment and was noted with 2/5 to 3/5 strength in the extrinsic wrist and digit muscles, but no intrinsic function. While she was ready to transition to the Helmet orthoses, she was apprehensive and required training and encouragement to feel comfortable with reduced external support. After 1 to 2 days of training, she successfully transitioned, practicing light grasp and release tasks, but adapted tools for tasks like writing and eating were still needed to compensate for the lack of intrinsic function (Fig. 27–15). Fortunately, Patient X was committed to her therapy program and using her orthoses.

By 1 year, she had protective sensation in her right hand in all three peripheral nerves and tactile sensation in the right median nerve. Her Helmet orthoses were working well as noted by no hyperextension at the MCP joints. She reported no pain including and no neuroregenerative discomfort. She had returned to important aspects of her life including travel and was able to drive which facilitated her return to work. At 17 months, thenar motor regeneration was noted.

Two years after surgery, Patient X returned to the transplant facility for reassessment and recommendations to take home to her local therapist. There was significant neuromotor and sensory innervation and she no longer required her orthoses. However, while she had extrinsic and intrinsic innervation and protective sensation, there were imbalances between her right and left hand

skills, intrinsic and extrinsic strength, and gross and fine motor control. Since resuming work and engaging more in her own self-care, the demands of daily life had resulted in compensatory movement patterns that were starting to hinder progression of sensorimotor control of coordinated grasp and release, development of thenar muscles, and recognition of sensory stimuli. Her therapists worked with her to develop a home program that focused on these skills and included fine motor ADL activities without the use of adaptive aides. She began to show remarkable improvement with typing, buttoning, tying her shoes, opening containers, and making a ponytail (Fig. 27–16A,B). These multifaceted movements required problem-solving, observational and physical practice, and mindful execution. The patient was encouraged to attend to the external task rather than her internal motor challenges that can lead to self-critique and frustration. Choice of treatment activities should consider both the physical and psychological stressors in honing new skills and grade steps to facilitate successful experiences.

Psychologically, Patient X expressed a healthy resilience and dedication to her postoperative regimen. She was an active listener, asked timely questions related to her care, managed external distractions, and was motivated to manage her care if not physically, then verbally by engaging family and nursing as needed. As in many cases where one is recovering from an injury or illness and moving from acuity to wellness, it is hard to stay attentive and motivated to a rehabilitative regimen. At this 2-year point, Patient X recognized this critical juncture and requested a weekly activity and exercise task list to keep her attentive to her functional recovery as she integrated back into her busy daily routine. A tracking log was provided coupling specific therapeutic exercises (i.e., electrical simulation of intrinsic muscles, sensory retraining) with practical, daily activities (i.e., week 1: tie shoes 1 × a day every day, use left hand to apply lipstick and blush). The therapists also utilized the "Handwriting for Heroes" (Yancosek, Gulick, & Sammons, 2015) program bilaterally to improve fine motor coordination, intrinsic strength, and hand-eye coordination. The therapists continue to stay in touch with Patient X via frequent video chats and annual therapy visits and reassessments. At this writing, Patient X is 3.5 years post-op and continues to make progress in her functional recovery.

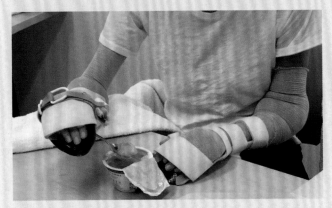

FIGURE 27–14 Early phase of proximal level transplant. Adaptive tools attached to FAB resting wrist-hand orthosis give the patient self-control over basic skills while waiting for extrinsic motor recovery.

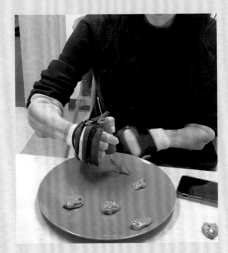

FIGURE 27–15 Intermediate phase proximal transplant. Patients have extrinsic motor activity and some sensory recovery which allows them good basic function in the Helmet orthotic.

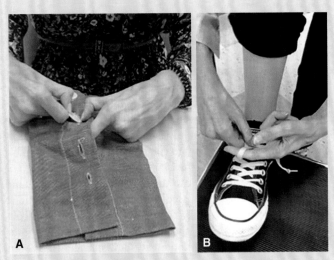

FIGURE 27–16 A and B, Late phase proximal transplant. Patients are particularly eager to gain independence in self-care. Nerve regeneration affords opportunity to train the patient on functional skill acquisition. Efforts should be made to engage intrinsic muscles and limit compensatory movement through the more powerful extrinsics.

(Continued)

Case Study 2: Distal Forearm Transplantation Case

Patient Y is a 44-year-old shopkeeper and mother of three who required amputations after contracting septicemia subsequent to a surgical procedure. She underwent bilateral below knee, right proximal forearm, and left trans-metacarpal amputations. The left thumb was partially intact which enabled a functional pinch. She used cosmetic UE prostheses but reported better function with the residual limbs. During her preoperative evaluation, Patient Y stated that the loss of her limbs took away her life and feminine features. Although she wanted to preserve the left residual thumb, a partial hand approach was inferior to a distal forearm transplant due to anatomic, cosmetic, and functional concerns (Shubinets et al., 2018). Eight years following amputations, Patient Y received left distal forearm and right proximal forearm transplantations.

The hand therapy began on POD 3 to fabricate orthoses and begin mobilization of the left distal forearm transplant. Right proximal forearm transplant proceeded as described in the previous case on POD 6. The initial plan to use a Crane Outrigger (Fig. 27–10A,B) was revised in consultation with the surgeons. During surgery, extra tension of the wrist extensors was applied to facilitate tenodesis grasp. After surgery, Patient Y demonstrated effective mechanism for tenodesis and could actively extend the IP joints to neutral with passive MCP flexion. Due to strong osteosynthesis and tensile strength, it was deemed safe to initiate early short arc tenodesis mobilization with therapy supervision in a Helmet orthosis instead of using the Crane Orthosis (Fig. 27–17A,B), thereby accelerating through the early phases of rehabilitation and into the intermediate phase as previously described earlier in this chapter. At all other times she was in a forearm-based wrist-hand immobilization orthosis (Fig. 27–6). Adaptive tools were provided on POD 9 for light ADL and iPad® use. Lightweight materials and training with therapy minimized muscle fatigue and co-contraction from the stronger, more proximal structures.

Around this time Patient Y reported nerve regeneration discomfort and hypersensitivity on the left dorsal radial and ulnar sensory nerves distributions. The orthoses were adjusted and therapy reinforced gentle handling of the limb.

Since the left UE was more active, cortical reorganization training included using the left hand to reach for targets and crossing midline to engage with the right UE (Fig. 27–18). Patient Y utilized a graded motor imagery app for laterality training to improve awareness of her transplanted hands at the cortical level.

During her hospital stay, Patient Y had two caregivers. Extra time and therapy support were needed for both caregivers to feel comfortable with handling the grafts and assisting with therapy regimens. Games such as Connect-4 and playing cards promoted visual-motor control and increased mutual comfort between the patient and her significant others around the new limbs (Fig. 27–19). Patient Y also played an important role in educating the caregivers by showing them videos of exercises and cuing them during ROM exercises, transfers, and for managing the LE prostheses.

Psychological adjustment to the new hands was a gradual process. Initially, Patient Y expressed apprehension to the appearance of her new limbs, specifically the nails, limb size, and skin color. To alleviate her concerns, she was shown pictures of another hand transplant case to demonstrate how changes in size and color of the graft can evolve over time. The medical team referred Patient Y to dermatology for education on nail care while on immunosuppression.

At 4 weeks following transplantation, Patient Y was cleared for weight bearing as tolerated in the distal level transplant. She

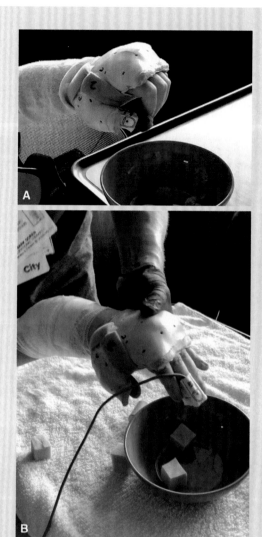

FIGURE 27–17 A and B, Distal level transplant. Patients can start engaging extrinsic muscle activity with active-assisted tenodesis motion and activities. In the early days post-op, this patient required facilitation of wrist flexion to activate synergistic digit extension due to surgical tensioning of the wrist extensors.

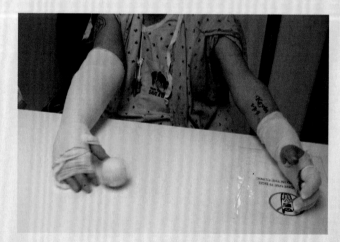

FIGURE 27–18 Active range of motion in the gravity eliminated plane—using cortical reorganization training techniques.

required setup and occasional standby assistance for feeding, applying makeup, and operating her iPhone® and iPad®. She continued to require moderate to maximum assistance to drink from a cup, dressing, bathing, and managing prostheses. She demonstrated safety in bathroom transfers and was deemed ready for hospital discharge.

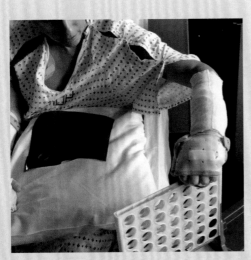

FIGURE 27–19 Distal level transplant. Engaging the patient and family in fun games is an effective way to improve acceptance of the new limbs and working on therapeutic activities.

Patient Y participated in outpatient therapy with the same hand therapists for 2 weeks. As she progressed, the caregivers were updated on her exercise regimen. After several revisions to accommodate the changes in her limbs, her orthoses were showing some wear and tear. Now that she was in more public settings, the appearance of her orthoses was more important to her. New orthoses were made to address the physical and psychological well-being of the patient and ensure user adherence.

At 6 weeks post-op, Patient Y returned home to continue therapy with a local hand therapist. The authors have continued to follow her regularly through video conferencing. At 2 months she reported not using the Helmet orthoses during daily activities since she had more hand movement. She was re-educated to the purpose of the orthosis, and additional assistance by local therapists was recruited to reinforcing orthosis use for at least 1 year. Patient Y was receptive and agreed to continue orthosis regime.

At 3 months post-op, Patient Y demonstrated motor recovery in the right proximal transplant including reinnervation of pronator teres and had active wrist flexion and extension. She also regained active digit flexion in the same limb.

At four and a half months, Patient Y was able to perform oral hygiene, drive, and apply LE prostheses with her left hand and stabilizing with the right forearm. Immature sensory recovery to the left hand resulted in a blister to her small finger after handling hot food. She acknowledged the need for skin protection and consistent self-inspection and has not had further injury since.

At 6 months, Patient Y remained committed to her recovery and attended therapy 3 to 5 days per week. She is pleased with the ability to gesture with both hands and actively engage in self-care and raising her children. At 9 months, Patient Y demonstrated emerging intrinsic muscle function in the distal forearm transplant and protective sensation in some areas of the hand. Her day and night orthoses were modified to reduce MCP extension restriction to address flexor tightness and included a pull loop for each strap to enable donning and doffing by the patient.

By 1 year, she demonstrated ability to open jars with her distal transplant and was able to turn a key using lateral pinch in both hands. She had 2/5 thumb abduction strength on the left, but hand extrinsic co-contraction affected thenar control during functional tasks. Orthotic modifications, exercises, and NMES activities were recommended to her home site therapist. She continues to attend therapy 1 to 2 times per week to improve independence in household chores, hair care, and writing skills.

CHAPTER REVIEW QUESTIONS

1. What is allotransplantation? Who are the candidates?
2. Explain the preoperative and postoperative role of the hand therapist in this patient population.
3. Explain the difference between the transplanted hand and the replanted hand.
4. How important is the level of attachment, how does this influence the postoperative protocol, and what are some of the postoperative complications that a therapist should be keenly aware of?

ACKNOWLEDGMENT

We would like to acknowledge our 2nd edition authors of this chapter: Marie Pace, OTR/L, CHT and Kimberly Zeske-Maguire, MS, OTR/L, CHT and their contribution to the knowledge related to treating this special patient population.

Index

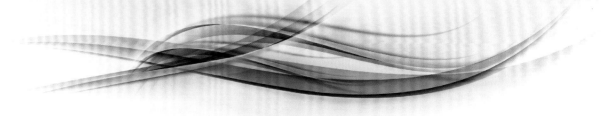

Note: Page numbers followed by 'f' indicate figures, 't' indicate tables and 'b' indicate boxes.